Textbook of CLINICAL CHIROPRACTIC

A SPECIFIC BIOMECHANICAL APPROACH

Textbook of CLINICAL CHIROPRACTIC

A SPECIFIC BIOMECHANICAL APPROACH

Editor
GREGORY PLAUGHER, D.C.
Assistant Professor, Palmer College of Chiropractic West, Sunnyvale, California
Director of Research, Gonstead Clinical Studies Society, Mt. Horeb, Wisconsin

Associate Editor
MARK A. LOPES, D.C.
Private Practice
Fremont, California
Research Associate
Gonstead Clinical Studies Society
Mt. Horeb, Wisconsin

Editorial Advisors
DARALD E. BOLIN, D.C.
Salem, Oregon

DAVID L. CICHY, D.C.
Providence, Rhode Island

T. RAYMOND CLINTON, D.C.
Mt. Horeb, Wisconsin

DOUGLAS B. COX, D.C.
Mt. Horeb, Wisconsin

W. ALEX COX, D.C.
Mt. Horeb, Wisconsin

DANIEL T. HANSEN, D.C.
Olympia, Washington

STEPHEN G. RAY, D.C.
Kihei, Maui, Hawaii

JAMES T. STOENNER, D.C.
Mt. Horeb, Wisconsin

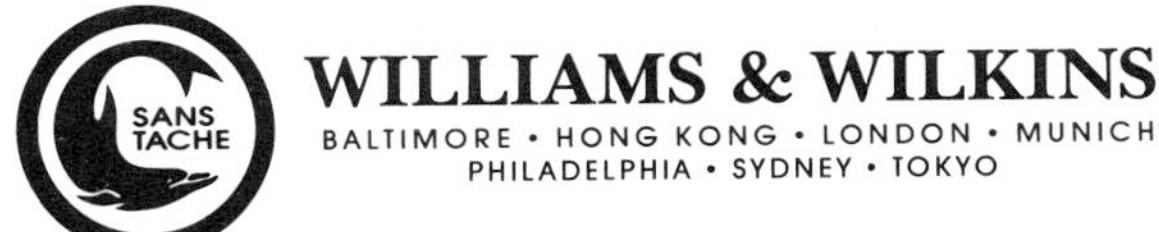

WILLIAMS & WILKINS
BALTIMORE • HONG KONG • LONDON • MUNICH
PHILADELPHIA • SYDNEY • TOKYO

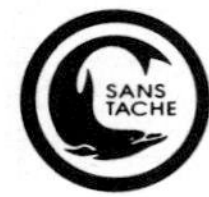

Editor: John P. Butler
Managing Editor: Linda Napora
Copy Editor: Mary Woodman
Designer: Dan Pfisterer
Illustration Planner: Wayne Hubbel
Production Coordinator: Charles E. Zeller

Williams & Wilkins
428 East Preston Street
Baltimore, Maryland 21202, USA

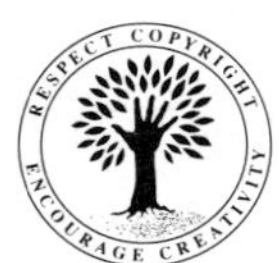

Printed in the United States of America

Library of Congress Cataloging in Publication Data

Textbook of clinical chiropractic : a specific biomechanical approach
/ editor, Gregory Plaugher ;
associate editor, Mark A. Lopes.
p. cm.
Includes index.
ISBN 0-683-06897-0
1. Chiropractic. 2. Manipulation (Therapeutics) I. Plaugher, Gregory. II. Lopes, Mark A.
[DNLM: 1. Chiropractic—methods.]
RZ255.T48 1993
615.5′34—dc20
DNLM/DLC
for Library of Congress 92-5613
CIP

92 93 94 95 96
1 2 3 4 5 6 7 8 9 10

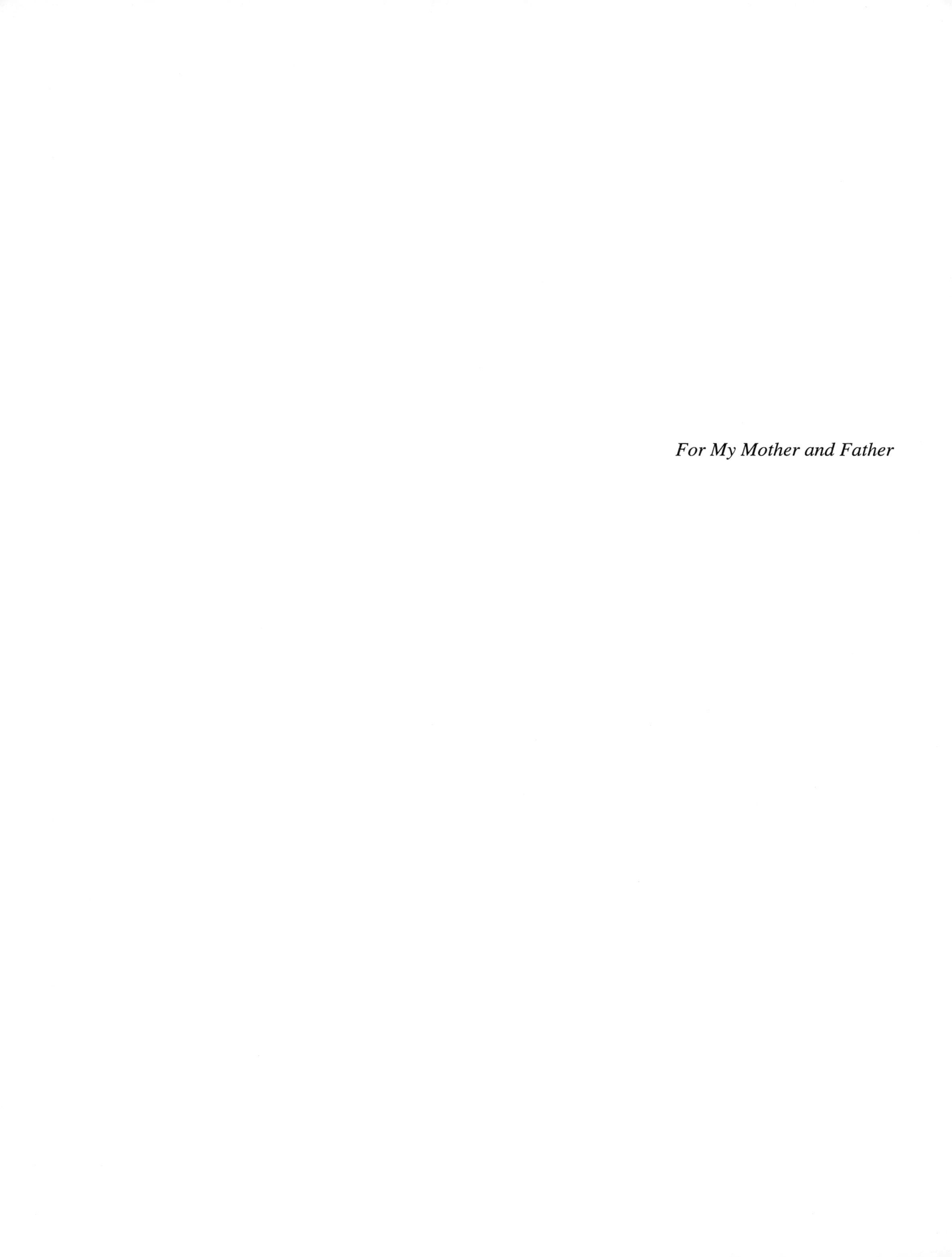

For My Mother and Father

Preface

Clinicians often find it difficult to communicate the techniques that they practice. Due to the isolation of clinical practice, there has been a paucity of literature available for the practicing chiropractor or student, since few clinicians have taken on the task of documenting what they do. This text focuses in a specific manner on the clinical applications that chiropractors provide on a day-to-day basis. The list of contributors, practicing chiropractors as well as academicians, demonstrates that the clinical practice of chiropractic serves as the basis for the book.

Textbook of Clinical Chiropractic provides a very specific approach to the art of spinal adjusting; the adjustive maneuvers presented facilitate normal biomechanics. Too often, manipulative procedures have been applied with blatant disregard for normal physiology and anatomy. Care in applying the adjustive art is stressed throughout the text. The flexible pediatric spine, which is resilient to seemingly innocuous forces, deserves the same carefully applied adjustment that an adult's spine would require. If the clinician carefully applies the adjustment in all instances, regardless of the age or state of the patient, then he or she should be more able to accommodate the patient suffering from severe spinal trauma, such as a disc herniation, spinal fracture, or dislocation.

In Chapter 1 we present a brief discussion of some philosophical principles integral to the practice of chiropractic. We have attempted to show the integration and mutual dependency of the philosophy, science, and art in chiropractic. Often, an ambiguous notion of any of the above aspects hinders the intellectual progress of the practicing clinician. A refreshing perspective is presented, free from dogma and pseudophilosophical constructs. We close the chapter with a look at how the adjustive art is applied and how one can most effectively learn this skill. Ease of learning was never a parameter in the development of the adjustive strategies presented throughout the text. Perhaps an insight into the psychomotor aspects of learning the adjustive art will facilitate competence in this area.

It is not enough to know in a general way how the spine moves, to have an ability to motion palpate to determine a fixation, and then follow up with a manipulation. Just as the neurosurgeon must have an intense understanding of the anatomy of the brain prior to operation, so the chiropractor should be an expert in the anatomy and biomechanics of the region in question. In Chapter 2 we provide a valuable reference source on the biomechanics of the spinal column. The reader will appreciate the clinical extrapolations that are derived from the biomechanics literature.

The vertebral subluxation complex and its component signs and symptoms are presented in Chapter 3. It has not been sufficient for us to describe the functional lesion in an abstract manner. Instead, we have integrated the pathological information into two case studies to demonstrate how the nature of the pathology can provide useful information toward the ultimate application of an adjustment.

Chapters 4 and 5 cover the spinal examination procedures from a clinical and radiologic standpoint. Aspects of general orthopaedics and neurology are not presented in detail, since much of this information is readily available elsewhere. The palpatory aspects of the examination and how to recognize normal and abnormal spinal function from a radiologic perspective are described. The numerous radiologic illustrations and roentgenometric analyses should facilitate a practical understanding of the role of plain film radiology in chiropractic.

Chapters 6 and 7 are devoted to the low back. The reader will appreciate how each adjustive maneuver is described in a comprehensive manner with a focus on the interactive biomechanics. A three-dimensional coordinate system superimposed over each illustrated adjustment is found throughout. Only through visualizing the three-dimensionality of the pattern of thrust can the clinician hope to deliver the most comfortable and effective adjustment.

The subject of scoliosis, especially the adolescent idiopathic variety, is presented in Chapter 9. We believe that chiropractors can make a substantial contribution in this area. With a thorough knowledge of the relevant subject matter, the importance of early screening and appropriate management can be appreciated.

Chapters 8, 10, and 11 cover the diagnosis and management of mechanical disorders of the thoracic and cervical spine. Where applicable, specific disorders are discussed in detail and appropriate adjustive maneuvers are presented. The subjects of interscapular pain, acceleration-deceleration injuries, and torticollis are presented with specific clinical management strategies.

Dr. Rowe has done an excellent job of explaining the role of chiropractic care in the management of patients who have suffered spinal fractures or dislocations. Chapter 12 reviews the concept of spinal stability in relation to these severe injuries. The radiologic and clinical findings of numerous case studies are presented. Broad generalizations are difficult for any patient suffering from severe spinal trauma, but a case-specific approach should provide the doctor with a basic understanding of how these patients, when appropriate, can be carefully managed.

The need for information regarding appropriate spinal management in patients with a visceral concomitant disorder has long been overdue. Despite a lengthy history of chiropractic therapy for these manifestations, only recently have case studies and clinical trials begun to appear in the literature. Of course, many individuals may require combined allopathic and chiropractic care. However, should the patient have a spinal lesion, it is imprudent to withhold treatment, provided such therapy does not hinder other management approaches.

Pediatric care is presented in Chapter 14. It is becoming increasingly apparent that a preventive approach is especially relevant to spinal pathology and the subsequent neurologic manifestations that can result. The numerous illustrations will provide the doctor with a foundation for applying the adjustment in the newborn or toddler patient. Applications of chiropractic care during pregnancy are also presented.

Extravertebral disorders such as temporomandibular joint dysfunction and extremity afflictions are presented in Chapters 15 and 16. Each specific disorder is followed by ample illustrations, enabling the doctor to immediately implement the adjustive maneuvers into his or her practice.

Perhaps the practicing clinician will comprehend the tremendous need for participation in research. Research by practitioners is critical for the growth and scientific development of our profession. This text should serve as an agenda for future clinical research rather than as a final statement of facts. For the student, it is hoped that this book will facilitate the sometimes difficult process of learning the art of being a doctor.

The patients, whom we all will ultimately provide our services for, have provided the necessary impetus for the completion of this work. Their needs can best be served through the development of standards of practice based on clinical methods that have been subjected to scientific scrutiny. It is now time for all of us to accelerate our efforts toward this end.

Gregory Plaugher, D.C.
Sunnyvale, California

Acknowledgments

Many individuals have been involved in the completion of this textbook. One particular individual deserves special mention. Bong Mo Yeun illustrated the book in rapid fashion despite his tremendous personal loss during the process. His wife, Bo, succumbed to a long struggle with cancer while the final line drawings were being completed. The suffering of humanity has inspired this writing, and if the book helps the patients we have dedicated our lives to serving, then our efforts will not have been in vain.

My associate editor, Dr. Mark Lopes, has been a mentor of mine for several years. When I was overwhelmed by the magnitude and pace of the project, he provided the necessary push for completion. Two other mentors, Dr. Richard Gohl and Dr. Edward Cremata, provided many case materials and generally served as sources of inspiration in the clinical realm. All of the contributors deserve much appreciation. The majority of these individuals took time away from their private practices or academic duties to finish their assignments in a timely manner. The tone set by each chapter should provide the reader with a refreshingly clinical perspective.

The Editorial Advisors perused the drafts of the manuscripts for grammatical errors and content. Several members also provided case materials. Drs. Alex and Douglas Cox served as willing models for the majority of the photographs of the adjustment set-ups. Several patient models also helped: Beth Sneidar, Twyla Sederstrom, Wendi Marks, Julie Lumley, Melissa Cox, and Victoria Jette. Sue Adler provided library assistance, and Laura Tucker and Joy Rasmussen helped with typing. Dr. Bill Ruch provided the cadaveric illustrations.

Many individuals participated in the editing, commentary, and retrieval of literature and other case materials: Jane Ho, John Culp, Dr. Serge Froment, Dr. Roger Heschong, Dr. Mark Werking, Dr. Karen O'Brien, Dr. Janet Roh, Dr. Loretta O'Brien, Joe Saccoman, Dr. Eileen Cremata, Dr. Jack Peterson, Dr. Vince Hoffart, Dr. Bob Swiryn, Dr. Thomas Sherman, Dr. Peter Thibodeau, Dr. Charles Martin, Dr. Martin Rowe, Betty Rowe, Dr. John Sipple, Dr. Robert Katona, Dr. Peter O'Hara, Carol Mann, Dr. Eugene Allison, Vince Giovannoni, Michael Putnam, Dr. Craig Ripley, Dr. Daryll Curl, Debbie Pinney, Dr. Joe Martin, Dr. Tim Shabazian, Dr. Jeffrey Wong, Deborah Emory, Dr. Louis Cofrancesco, Dr. Meridel Gatterman, Dr. David Philipson, Dr. Max Joseph, and Dr. Cherie Goble. They all have my deepest gratitude.

The National Institute for Chiropractic Research provided assistance for Dr. Keating's contribution. The ultimate completion of *Textbook of Clinical Chiropractic* could not have occurred without the foresight of the Board of Directors of the Gonstead Clinical Studies Society.

For those I have neglected to mention due to the harried nature of my existence for the past two years, I extend my appreciation.

Most importantly, this book is dedicated to the memory of C. S. Gonstead (1898-1978), who provided the foundation upon which this text is based.

G.P.

Contributors

CLAUDIA ANRIG HOWE, D.C.
Private Practice, Fresno, California

H. JASON ARAGHI, D.C.
Private Practice, Los Gatos, California, Clinical Sciences Instructor, Life Chiropractic College West, San Lorenzo, California, Research Associate, Gonstead Clinical Studies Society, Mt. Horeb, Wisconsin

TRENT R. BACHMAN, D.C.
Private Practice, Fremont, California, Clinical Sciences Instructor, Life Chiropractic College West, San Lorenzo, California, Research Associate, Gonstead Clinical Studies Society, Mt. Horeb, Wisconsin

STEPHEN L. COLLINS, D.C., C.C.S.P.
Private Practice, Fremont, California, Clinical Sciences Instructor, Post Graduate Faculty, Life Chiropractic College West, San Lorenzo, California

EDWARD E. CREMATA, D.C.
Private Practice, Fremont, California, Clinical Sciences Instructor, Life Chiropractic College West, San Lorenzo, California, Research Associate, Gonstead Clinical Studies Society, Mt. Horeb, Wisconsin

RICHARD W. DOBLE, JR., D.C.
Research Associate, Gonstead Clinical Studies Society, Mt. Horeb, Wisconsin

DAVID A. GINSBERG, D.C.
Private Practice, Fremont, California

ANTONI M. JAKUBOWSKI, D.C.
Private Practice, London, England

JOSEPH C. KEATING, JR., Ph.D.
Professor, Palmer College of Chiropractic West, Sunnyvale, California, Member, Board of Directors, Association for the History of Chiropractic

JAMES E. KONLANDE, Ph.D.
Professor and Co-Chairman, Department of Anatomy and Chemistry, Life Chiropractic College West, San Lorenzo, California

MARK A. LOPES, D.C.
Private Practice, Fremont, California, Research Associate, Gonstead Clinical Studies Society, Mt. Horeb, Wisconsin

RONALD J. PICARDI, D.C.
Private Practice, Bardonia, New York, Post Graduate Faculty, Life Chiropractic College West, San Lorenzo, California

GREGORY PLAUGHER, D.C.
Assistant Professor, Palmer College of Chiropractic West, Sunnyvale, California, Director of Research, Gonstead Clinical Studies Society, Mt. Horeb, Wisconsin

STEPHEN G. RAY, D.C.
Private Practice, Kihei, Maui, Hawaii

DAVID J. ROWE, D.C.
Private Practice, New York, New York

STEPHEN H. ROWE, D.C.
Private Practice, New York, New York, Post Graduate Faculty, Life Chiropractic College West, San Lorenzo, California

MITCHELL S. SILL, D.C., C.C.S.P.
Private Practice, Castro Valley, California

STEVEN S. TANAKA, D.C.
Private Practice, Watsonville, California

PETER J. WALTERS, M.Sc., D.C.
Private Practice, Parramatta, New South Wales, Australia, Member, Advisory Board and Education Committee, Centre for Chiropractic, Macquarie University, Sydney, New South Wales, Australia

Contents

1 Introduction to Clinical Chiropractic

JOSEPH C. KEATING, JR., GREGORY PLAUGHER, MARK A. LOPES, and EDWARD E. CREMATA

ROLE OF PHILOSOPHY AND SCIENCE IN CHIROPRACTIC

More substantive scientific investigation in chiropractic has occurred in the past decade than in all the previous history of the profession. This long overdue revolution has been welcomed by some, feared by others, and ignored by many. It may be premature to expect otherwise, for the accumulating volume of scientific data has not yet had a significant impact on the ways in which chiropractic is actually practiced. The sorts of decisive clinical experiments that could determine the disadvantages and relative merits of various chiropractic methods of helping back pain patients, for example, are only now beginning to appear in the literature (1). Studies to determine the effectiveness and relative effectiveness of chiropractic interventions for patients with visceral and behavioral health problems, however, are not yet on the drawing board.

Necessarily, therefore, chiropractic has been and will continue to be practiced based on less-than-ideal information. The same can also be said for all other health disciplines, and were we to return in a millennium we would still be confronted with the uncertainty of the individual, for science will never be so complete as to offer precise answers for all the idiosyncratic problems that patients bring to us. The problem of inadequate information is especially severe in chiropractic, however, because of our long survival struggle with organized medicine. Chiropractors have insisted, based on a century of clinical experience, that there is value to the art and that patients have a right to receive the alternative, complementary, primary care, and specialty services that doctors of chiropractic provide. Although successful to a point in the legislative halls of various states and provinces (e.g., in obtaining licensing laws and independent boards of chiropractic examiners), the claims and political strategies that have helped to win legal relief have also served to warp attitudes toward the nature of science and its role in health care (2,3).

Consequently, an extraordinary diversity of (frequently contradictory) misconceptions about clinical science can be identified (4,5) (Table 1.1), ranging from the error of equating science with medicine to the untenable notion that science is "truth." Along the way, we have likewise become confused about the relationships among science, philosophy, and technique. These uncertainties provide barriers to developing the science and art of chiropractic to its full potential.

This is a book about technique in the clinical science of chiropractic. Although the authors repeatedly and most appropriately caution the reader about the tentative and largely untested nature of patient care, it may be well to review the characteristics of a genuine philosophy of the science of chiropractic. An appreciation of the appropriate philosophical and scientific context within which clinical methods are offered herein, can provide several benefits (such as guidance, inspiration, and comfort) to those who value and wish to understand better and apply the wisdom gained through practical experience. For those for whom this work serves as an introduction to chiropractic, a consideration of the character of philosophy in health science may encourage the sort of open-mindedness and tolerance for uncertainty that are so essential to both research and clinical practice.

Philosophical Principles in the Science of Chiropractic

All scientific activity is based on assumptions, some of which are shared by all sciences and some of which are unique to particular disciplines. Medical scientists, for example, have long adhered to the concept of disease. From this prescientific assumption, many testable hypotheses have been explored, some of which have been abandoned, some of which are generally accepted, and others which are still too poorly studied to permit firm conclusions. The discipline of physics has no use for medicine's disease construct but shares with medicine and astronomy an *a priori* (untestable) belief in the orderliness of causes and effects, and in the potential discoverability of cause-effect sequences.

Table 1.1.
Common Misconceptions About Research in Chiropractic

1. Chiropractic is a proven, complete science
2. Research is unnecessary, since chiropractic is a "deductive science"
3. The purpose of research is to prove that chiropractic works
4. The primary goal of chiropractic research is to prove the neurological basis of the subluxation
5. Research is someone else's responsibility
6. Research is too expensive for chiropractic
7. Chiropractors cannot do research because they have not been trained

No one can prove or disprove the existence of disease, nor can we objectively test whether causation is "true" or "false." The *a priori* assumptions (principles) of science are not subject to the scientific method of hypothesis-testing. Although the surgeon may mistakenly believe that in identifying a lesion he or she has discovered the disease, in fact only a sign of disease has actually been observed. The disease construct (which includes homogeneous clustering of signs and symptoms, knowledge of prognosis, knowledge of etiology, and derivative implications for patient care) cannot be located in space. Disease has no physical location, except in the minds of those who find it a more or less useful means of thinking about the health problems that patients bring to doctors. The concept of disease can no more be verified or falsified than can the idea of a supreme being. Such matters of faith (assumptions) may be more or less useful but cannot be scientifically proven or disproven; they are prescientific. These assumptions provide a part of the philosophical base of science. Exemplary of the prescientific principles and metaphors of chiropractic are the "supremacy of the nervous system," the "healing power of nature," and the concept of reciprocal influence between the structure and the function of the body.

The testable propositions offered by the members of a scientific discipline are known as hypotheses and theories. A theory may be thought of as one or more hypotheses; a hypothesis is a tentatively offered assertion about some aspect of the natural world that can potentially be verified or refuted by examining the natural world. For example, if we believe that a particular method of adjustive intervention will produce change in spinal motion at a particular segmental level, we might design an experiment to test the validity of this proposition. A well-designed experiment would include methods of controlling for or eliminating rival hypotheses, such as spontaneous change, natural oscillation, or instrument error. Publication of the results of such an experiment will lend credibility (or cast doubt) on our hypothesis, and may prompt other investigators to attempt to replicate or extend our research. If positive (confirmatory) evidence accumulates in the scientific literature, our hypothesis may eventually become widely accepted, not as truth, but as the best available approximation to truth.

It is important to note the tentativeness of hypotheses and theories, whether they have been tested, inadequately tested, or not yet tested at all. There is no absolute threshold of confidence in science, no plateau beyond which all doubt is forever abandoned. To doubt the tentative nature of all scientific knowledge is to forget the many lessons of the history of science. Consider, for example, the confidence with which physicists adhered to the relatively simple mechanical concepts of Newton for several centuries. Yet, in the face of the wisdom offered by Einstein's theory, Newtonian "truths" were abandoned (or absorbed) in favor of the more comprehensive theory of relativity. Although we ordinarily have more confidence in hypotheses that have repeatedly survived rigorous experimental tests than in those that are yet untested, we must be prepared to alter our theories in the face of better explanations (i.e., more comprehensive, better evidence). Science and scientists have much to be humble about.

Chiropractic is not merely science but is also a profession with a social purpose: to improve the health and welfare of human beings. Like other applied or clinical sciences, therefore, chiropractic has adopted a number of principles that guide the acquisition and implementation of scientific knowledge. For instance, chiropractors (like other health professionals) adhere to the Hippocratic maxim to "do no harm." Such ethical precepts are not scientifically testable, are neither true nor false, and do not ordinarily give rise to testable propositions. These sorts of principles, unlike the concepts of disease or causation, are not prescientific; they might be thought of as extrascientific, or as part of the professional principles of the discipline rather than as part of the philosophy of science. All health professions and applied sciences, however, seem to agree on the appropriateness of such principles. These professional principles can also supersede scientific principles and motivations. For instance, the surgeon might wish to know the efficacy of a particular operation, yet be unable to conduct the required placebo-controlled clinical experiment because of ethical barriers. In such instances the needs of the patients (as protected by professional principles) outweigh the clinician-investigator's desire to know.

Chiropractic encompasses all three of these sorts of ideas: prescientific assumptions, testable hypotheses, and professional principles (Table 1.2). During our century of clinical practice and political struggle, however, we have sometimes failed to distinguish among these categories. *A priori* assumptions have been offered as incontrovertible philosophical truths; scientifically untested hypotheses have been proclaimed as proven facts; professional principles have been misconstrued as scientific explanations. Although a historical analysis of how political and legal machinations have produced this confusion is beyond the scope of this chapter, it is important to recognize the confusion to plan for a legitimate philosophy of the science of

Table 1.2.
Principles and Metaphors of a Philosophy of the Science of Chiropractic

- *Clinical conservatism (first, do no harm)
- *Disease (reliable clusterings of signs and symptoms)
- *Epistemology of science (scientific method)
- *Holism
- *Homeostasis and the self-healing capacity ("Innate Intelligence")
- *Professional autonomy
- *Structure-function reciprocity
- *Supremacy of the nervous system (strategic role of the nervous system)

chiropractic. If we can distinguish among assumptions, hypotheses, and ethical and professional imperatives, we can then also take pride in developing a first-class science and art of chiropractic, and thereby improve our technique and increase patient benefits.

Let us consider a few of the constructs that have traditionally been offered by chiropractors.

Innate Intelligence

Since its introduction by D.D. Palmer in 1906 the concept of "Innate Intelligence" has been a source of derision (6), not infrequently from critics who themselves acknowledge the "healing power of nature." The source of this criticism is not the idea that humans are self-repairing and self-maintaining biological entities (which is a legitimate prescientific assumption). Neither have chiropractors been criticized because their recognition of an intrinsic healing capacity has encouraged a conservative orientation to health care by chiropractors, nor because the Innate metaphor encourages (or should encourage) a humility about the great limits to our understanding of human biology. Indeed, these are very positive aspects of Palmer's theory of Innate Intelligence. These aspects are mirrored in other sciences and professions by other names. The famous physiologist Walter Cannon poetically termed his heuristic notion of homeostasis the "Wisdom of the Body," and chiropractors share their respect for the *vis medicatrix naturae* and conservative health care with biofeedback psychologists, naturopaths, osteopaths, and others.

Why has an idea with so many positive and useful connotations brought such scorn on chiropractic and divisiveness within the chiropractic ranks? There are at least two reasons. Firstly, D.D. Palmer and many of his successors have defined the intrinsic healing capacity of patients as a fraction of Universal Intelligence (God), and in so doing have offered a religious construct as part of a scientific explanation (theory). In so doing, Palmer rendered his theories untestable, because spirits and deities are outside the realm of the observable and testable. Innate Intelligence cannot "explain" physiological functions but is instead another label for them. The development of scientific explanations for biological processes is the work of biologists, who are not content to offer names in place of testable cause-effect sequences. In this context, Innate serves as a substitute for biological curiosity and scientific investigation; better to acknowledge our infinite ignorance of the complexities of human physiology than to mask such ignorance by attributing physical processes to spiritual entities. Moreover, the spiritual intricacies of the Innate concept, such as the triune of Innate, Educated and Universal Intelligence, or the distinctions Palmer made between the "spirit" and the "soul," are viewed as superfluous from the perspective of science. Fortunately, the founder of chiropractic allowed that chiropractic could be competently practiced without adherence to his ideas about Innate/God.

Secondly, D.D. Palmer offered Innate Intelligence as a source of his knowledge of the correctness of his hypotheses; he tells us (7) that his 1910 volume, *The Chiropractor's Adjuster,* was written "under spiritual promptings." Spiritual insight has no role in science, however, and is contrary to the epistemology of science. *Epistemology is that branch of philosophy which concerns itself with the nature of knowledge* (See below). As noted earlier, science proceeds to construct knowledge of the natural world by posing and testing hypotheses, by discarding those which fail to stand up to scientific tests, and by pursuing those which seem to best explain the facts determined in objective investigations. This epistemology, also known as the *scientific method,* is certainly not the only way in which we may come to know "reality." It is the method used in science, however, and knowledge systems that offer spiritual insights to support their beliefs are inherently at odds with the philosophy of science.

Despite these criticisms, Palmer's notion of Innate includes a number of connotations that are quite legitimate and appropriate for a science of chiropractic. Palmer originally devised chiropractic in reaction to the horrendous abuses suffered by patients at the hands of the trial-and-error empiricism of turn-of-the-century heroic medicine in the Midwest. Recognition of the organism's ability to repair itself and to maintain health under appropriate conditions encouraged Palmer (and has prompted chiropractors ever since) to maintain a conservative, relatively noninvasive orientation to assisting patients. This is not to say that chiropractic is risk-free (8) but rather to acknowledge that chiropractic methods are probably less risky overall than the rapid advance of high-technology medicine and surgery in this century (9). Recognition and respect for biological self-regulation by chiropractors may be seen to perpetuate the ancient Hippocratic maxim "first do no harm." In this sense, then, the construct of Innate may be considered to promote caution in clinical practice, and hopefully also a thirst among doctors for ever better information about how the body works. As a practical matter, the practitioner of any chiropractic system must decide, in each and every case, what would be the best way to facilitate the patient's inherent recuperative powers: to do nothing, to apply a particular chiropractic method, or to seek additional or alternative health services.

Epistemology of Science

As suggested above, the branch of classical philosophy that concerns itself with the nature of knowledge is known as *epistemology.* In addition to the unfortunate offering of spiritual insight as a way of knowing the value of chiropractic, D.D. Palmer also offered several other epistemologies for his theories and methods (5,10). These epistemologies include founding authority, rationalism and private, uncritical empiricism; none of these methods of knowing the value of chiropractic are consistent with the philosophy of science, although two of these (rationalism and private empiricism) are legitimate sources of chiropractic hypotheses. Regrettably, Palmer did not offer his theories with the tentativeness that characterizes a clinical experimenter:

> Chiropractic is a proven fact—it is a science demonstrated by the art of adjusting. As we become acquainted with its principles, founded upon laws as old as the vertebra, we make less failures. The science can only be developed along the lines laid down by the Founder (11).

A genuine science of the art of chiropractic cannot be shackled to the theories and methods of its seminal thinker. Rather, science requires the flexibility to pose and test new hypotheses and techniques and the ability to discard those procedures and ideas that do not stand up to the rigorous reality testing of the scientific method. Similarly, the idea that a hypothesis or procedure is valid or effective merely because it is consistent with or can be deduced from the knowledge of the basic sciences must be rejected: just because a procedure makes sense is no guarantee that "it works." Nor can the private, unsystematic or uncritically published observations of doctors substitute for the rigors of controlled trials of chiropractic methods. Although clinical observations and deductions from basic science do have valuable roles to play in the clinical discipline of chiropractic (as sources of hunches, hypotheses, and theories), these are necessary but not sufficient (12) to establish the scientific validity and effectiveness of the theories and methods that comprise the chiropractic art.

The alternative is an epistemology in which hypotheses are offered tentatively, tested carefully, and conclusions are published in scientific periodicals where everyone has the opportunity to criticize investigators' assumptions, research methods, and interpretations of results. This process is central to science: a system of gradual public accumulation and refinement of the knowledge base. Moreover, this is a process for and to which the chiropractor is especially well situated to contribute; who better to observe, record, and publish the phenomena of chiropractic science than the Doctor of Chiropractic? The tangible product of this activity is the chiropractic scientific literature, as represented by the outstanding periodicals noted in Table 1.3. The goal is not to "prove that chiropractic works" (which is little more than an advertising slogan) but rather to develop and demonstrate improved quality of care for patients.

These comments (and perhaps the epistemology of science) may not sit well with many doctors; a century of struggle with political medicine has taught the profession that adamant, albeit unsubstantiated, assertions and claims have great political value (3). Nevertheless, as we now commence the era of chiropractic science, the very same bold claims, anti-scientific epistemologies and philosophical strategies that have earned the profession some measure of legal security impede chiropractic's development.

Most of the technique knowledge offered throughout the rest of this volume is based on a sound knowledge of the basic sciences and accumulated clinical chiropractic experiences. Shall we be embarrassed at how little of this information has undergone rigorous scientific testing, or should we be excited about the possibilities to be explored? An appreciation of the epistemology of science leads us to the latter. The attitude of the chiropractic clinician-investigator ought to be a balance between caution and humility (in drawing conclusion and making claims) and creativity and enthusiasm for the possibilities inherent in the chiropractic art (13).

Supremacy of the Nervous System

Since the time of D.D. Palmer's second theory (11,14) and those theories of Solon M. Langworthy, D.C. (15), chiropractors have adhered to the prescientific construct of neural supremacy (16). Although originally offered as a scientific truism (17), this construct is more appropriately and usefully construed as an *a priori* assumption. For instance, biopsychologists and others have explored the possibilities of training the nervous system (e.g., through biofeedback procedures) to alter and improve disturbed physiological processes. Similarly, chiropractors also use a variety of methods that may be derived from the notion that the nervous system exerts a profound and pervasive influence in health and illness. For example, hypotheses about the meaningfulness of subluxation and the usefulness of adjusting are testable propositions that are consistent and derivable from the metaphor of neural supremacy. Interestingly, the legal mandate of the chiropractor in California is to maintain the "structural and functional integrity of the nervous system." We should note that no one can prove or disprove that the nervous system is supreme, any more than we could prove that the kidney or the liver is the "master organ." Nevertheless, the metaphor of neural supremacy can and has given rise to many testable hypotheses and methods, and in this capacity is quite appropriate.

A philosophical challenge for chiropractic practitioners is to formulate testable propositions about the nature and potential consequences of neural dysfunction as a consequence of structural abnormality and about the role of adjusting in resolving such lesions. Of course, these philosophical imperatives lead directly to the even more daunting task of designing, conducting and reporting (in scholarly journals) the results of such trials of chiropractic theories and methods. Although such tests will not prove or disprove the metaphor of neural supremacy, they can demonstrate the usefulness of this *a priori* principle for a genuine science of chiropractic.

Table 1.3.
Recommended Scholarly, Professional and Scientific Periodicals for the Chiropractor

Journal Title	Editor and Editorial Address	Annual Subscription Cost (1990–1991)	Comprehensive Indexing	Topics
Chiropractic History	Russell W. Gibbons; 207 Grandview Drive South, Pittsburgh, PA 15215 U.S.A.	$35 (included in dues of the Association for the History of Chiropractic)	Bibliography of the History of Medicine of the National Library of Medicine (USA), CLIBCON Index[a]	History
Chiropractic Journal of Australia	Rolf E. Peters, D.C. and Mary Ann Chance, D.C.; P.O. Box 748 Wagga Wagga, NSW 2650 Australia	$50 (Australian) within Australia, $65 overseas	Australasian Medical Index, British Library Complementary Medicine Index, CLIBCON Index[a]	Science, history, professional and educational issues
Chiropractic Sports Medicine	Robert Hazel, Jr., D.C.; 220 Vroom Avenue, Spring Lake NJ 07762 U.S.A.	$50; students: $35	Biosciences Info Services, CLIBCON Index[a] Excerpta Medica, Phys Ed Index	Science, professional issues
European Journal of Chiropractic	Simon Leyson, D.C.; Gwendwr, 16 Uplands Crescent, Uplands, Swansea SA2 OPB Great Britain	$76.50 (U.S.)	CLIBCON Index,[a] Current Awareness Topics Service (British Library)	Science, history, professional and educational issues
Journal of the Canadian Chiropractic Association	Alan Gotlib, D.C.; 1396 Eglinton Avenue West, Toronto, Ontario, Canada, M6C 2E4	$57 (Canadian)	CLIBCON Index[a]	Science, history, professional and educational issues
Journal of Chiropractic Education	Grace E. Jacobs, D.A.; 590 N. Vermont Ave., Los Angeles, CA 90004 U.S.A.	$25	CLIBCON Index[a]	Educational issues, scholarly research in education, science, history
Journal of Chiropractic Technique	Thomas F. Bergmann, D.C.; 735 Keokuk Lane, Mendota Heights MN 55120 U.S.A.	$48; students: $25	CLIBCON Index[a]	Science, history, professional and educational issues
Journal of Manipulative & Physiological Therapeutics	Dana J. Lawrence, D.C.; 200 E. Roosevelt Road, Lombard, IL 60148 U.S.A.	$68; students: $40	BIOSIS, CLIBCON Index,[a] Current Contents Excerpta Medica, Index Medicus, USSR Academy of Sciences	Science, some history, professional and educational issues
Journal of Manual Medicine	J. Dvorak, M.D.; Dept. of Neurology Wilhelm Schulthess Hospital Neumunsterallee 3 CH-8008 Zurich Switzerland	$119 (U.S.); DM 158.00		Science, professional issues

[a]CLIBCON (Chiropractic Library Consortium) Index to the Chiropractic Literature

Clinical Conservatism

The chiropractor's use of relatively less risky health-care procedures has already been noted. This self-imposed limitation does not, however, absolve the doctor of responsibility for wrestling with the thorny ethical dilemmas that practice presents. Respect for patient welfare and the inherent recuperative powers of the body demands that chiropractors question their use of all methods, because the risks of all health-care procedures are always relative. The doctor ought to weigh how much better or worse off a patient would be if nothing is done, or if referral were made to another kind of doctor.

Clinical conservatism also implies a concern for the ethical dilemmas involved in chiropractic research. For instance, when are posttreatment x-rays justified? Does the doctor's desire to know whether structural changes have resulted from adjusting justify further radiation exposure, or must potential patient benefit outweigh such risks? Can the chiropractor assume that "chiropractic works" so as to justify any form of assessment or intervention? What ethical conflicts would be presented in a comparative trial of chiropractic versus medical/surgical methods for patients with scoliosis? A commitment to clinical conservatism implies a willingness to think such issues through and to be guided firstly by the patient's best interests.

Subluxation

Is the chiropractic notion of subluxation a philosophical principle (i.e., an *a priori* assumption or metaphor) or is it a scientific proposition? Could it be both? Is subluxation a scientifically proven fact? Is the existence of a chirolesion essential to the profession (18)?

Most chiropractors are able to agree at a conceptual level on a definition of the classic chiropractic lesion.

Likely to be included in that definition is some combination of structural abnormality and consequential alteration of function. Agreement ends here. To the authors' knowledge, no operational definition of subluxation has ever been scientifically substantiated, although a great many different theories and methods of subluxation-detection have been offered. What little consistency and agreement there are on the definition of the chiropractic lesion revolve around the reality and meaningfulness of subluxation, whatever the ubiquitous critter may be. We rarely question whether subluxations are "real." Are subluxations more or less real than the concept of disease?

The idea of subluxation is so overburdened by connotations and political implications (10) that the use of the term "subluxation" as a catchall label for the "manipulable lesion" sometimes hinders rather than promotes good clinical science. Worthy first steps in resolving the confusion over "subluxation" involve: 1) differentiating among its philosophical (metaphoric) versus scientific/hypothetical/operational versus dogmatic definitions, 2) loosening our rigid grip on the subluxation concept as the *sine qua non* of chiropractic, 3) increasing research efforts to establish an objectively reproducible and clinically relevant subluxation definition, and 4) lessening reliance on the subluxation in the political arena. Chiropractic as a profession has the right and the ability to sustain itself whether or not subluxation is a meaningful concept.

Professional Autonomy

The overwhelming majority of chiropractors agree that the chiropractic art and science is the privilege and responsibility of doctors of chiropractic and that chiropractors have a right to organize and self-regulate. The organization of the profession ought to proceed in a manner consistent with DCs' self-professed mission to improve the health of patients. Like the concepts of neural supremacy and clinical conservatism, the principle of professional autonomy is a matter of choice and is neither true nor false.

The principle has its limits, however. To the extent that chiropractic-the-profession aspires also to be chiropractic-the-science, it necessarily assumes the responsibilities of a science. Prominent among these is the obligation to share its knowledge and wisdom freely with all interested parties (19). As we noted earlier, science is a public process of information refinement through publication and critical debate. There can be no private science of chiropractic, and contributions from nonchiropractors ought to be judged according to their content rather than their profession of origin.

Professional autonomy and self-regulation also require that individual doctors participate in the collective activities of the whole, and abide by the ethical standards of the profession. If chiropractic-the-profession aspires to be a scientific discipline, then it must assume responsibility for policing itself. We might also expect the profession to pool its knowledge and resources so as to further knowledge development and implementation. The recent initiatives to develop standards of quality of care through publication (20) and standard-setting conferences (21) are encouraging.

ART IN CHIROPRACTIC

Clinical Art

The interactive process between patient and physician is complex. Coulehan (22) has discussed the clinical art of chiropractic, offering suggestions on how to optimize the patient encounter. The physical skill of the spinal adjustment has often been referred to as the art of chiropractic. Coulehan considers the adjustment the manual art, and the interactive process between doctor and patient, the clinical art. Qualities of the clinical art include: a) empathy, the ability to sense a patient's experience and feeling accurately and to communicate this understanding to the patient; b) genuineness, the ability to be oneself without hiding behind a role or facade; c) unconditional positive regard, the ability to accept and validate patients just as they are. The patient will respond to these qualities by developing trust, thus reducing anxiety. Relieving tension in the mind is at least as important as in the spinal column. The strategic role of the nervous system in maintaining homeostasis and the chiropractor's role in facilitating it does not stop at the foramen magnum.

Doctors are trained to identify and treat lesions, diseases, maladies, infirmities, etc. Patients, on the other hand, suffer illnesses that are experiences of disparagement in states of being and in social function—the human experience of sickness (23). The identifiable lesion is not always directly related to the patient's state of being. It is important for the doctor to recognize this potentially dichotomous relationship between lesion and illness in facilitating patient recovery. Whether the doctor wills it or not, all doctor/patient encounters are sets of social and interpersonal transactions (24). The patient is inevitably going to be affected in important ways by the relationship with the doctor. To render quality patient care, it is imperative that the doctor increase the knowledge and the skill he or she brings to bear on that relationship. We must abandon the notion that we need to "subtract" the patient to get to the disease; rather we must learn to observe the body **and** to hear the patient (23,25).

Manual Art

In keeping with the clinically practical focus of this text, we have chosen to present some of the nuances of the chiropractic manual art. A discussion of how the student can optimize the learning environment and the rationale behind the specific techniques presented follows.

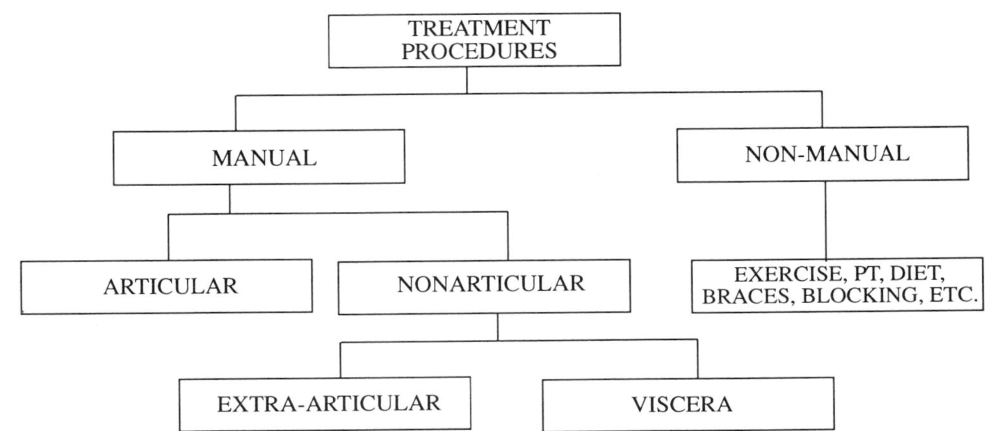

Figure 1.1. Chiropractic treatment procedures. Modified from Bartol KM. A model for the categorization of chiropractic treatment procedures. J Chiropractic Technique 1991;3:79.

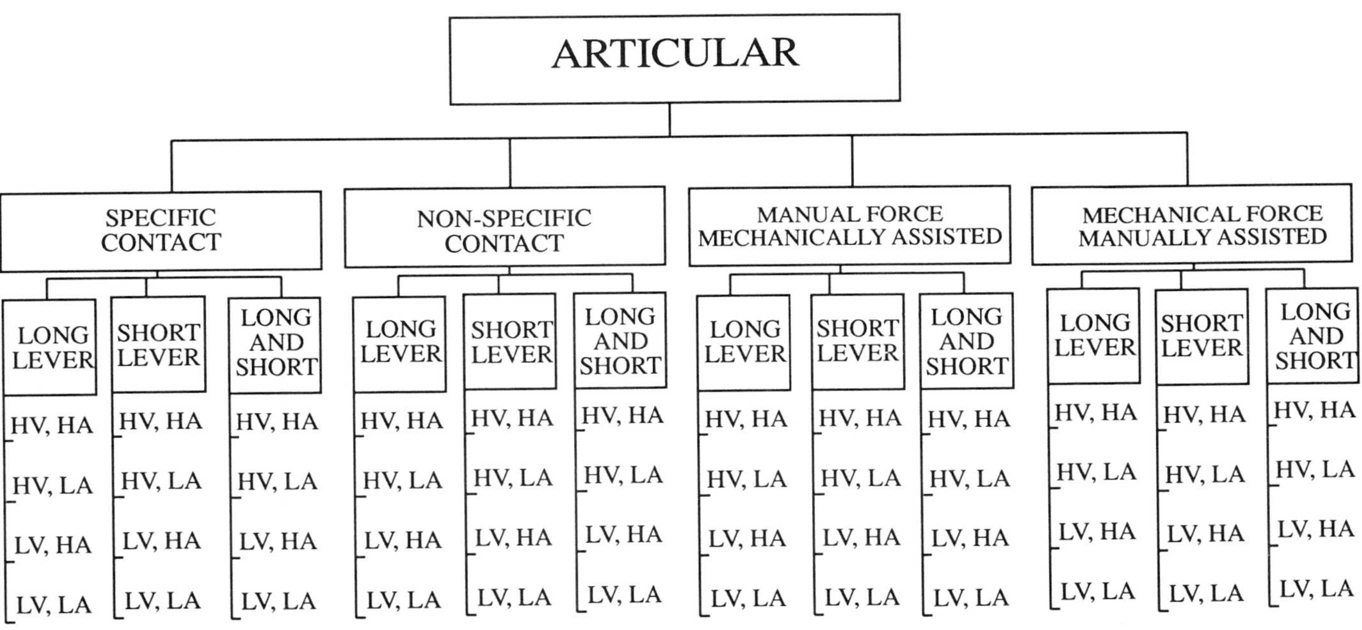

Figure 1.2. Articular procedure descriptions. H = High, L = Low, V = Velocity, A = Amplitude. Modified from Bartol KM. A model for the categorization of chiropractic treatment procedures. J Chiropractic Technique 1991;3:79.

SHORT LEVER SPECIFIC CONTACT PROCEDURES

A model for the categorization of chiropractic treatment procedures has been presented by Bartol (26). The ACA Council on Technique has developed this flow chart based on the "method of delivery" as a means for categorizing the different technique procedures (Figs. 1.1-1.2). An emphasis on specific, short lever arm adjustments will be found throughout this text. There are several reasons why we have adopted this approach.

Primum Non Nocere. "Above all, do no harm," is a principle that all health care providers must consider first before performing any examination or treatment procedure. A listing system is used to determine the relative position (positional dyskinesia) of the subluxated segment in need of an adjustment. The articulation will assume a position that is reflective of the ligamentous damage that is present. The use of a specific adjustment, three-dimensionally directed away from the direction of misalignment, is to avoid additional harm to the supporting ligamentous elements.

The specific adjustment also protects normal, nonsubluxated segments. By using mechanically advantageous pretensioning (preload), end-range positions, the practitioner can protect the normal segments from any trauma caused by the adjustive thrust.

Patient Management. Specificity during the adjustive thrust combined with limiting the number of spinal segments adjusted at any one time, assists the practitioner in the clinical management of the patient. A more direct or causal relationship may be inferred, when fewer spinal segments are adjusted at one time or in a series. These adjustments are then compared with both subjective and objective factors of the patient's response to treatment. The clinical importance of this approach is quite obvious when comparison is made to the rigors of a clinical trial (i.e. controlled clinical trials), where the limiting of variables is necessary to determine the effects of interventions.

Compensation. Gonstead, Gillet, Jirout, and others have taught that the spine compensates for subluxated/fixated motion segments. These compensatory segments or spinal regions are often hypermobile, edematous, and tender. Specificity during adjustive thrusts may protect these irritated areas from manipulative thrusts. A comprehensive examination will assist the practitioner in differentiating primary subluxations from secondary compensations.

LEARNING THE ADJUSTIVE ART

Learning the psychomotor skills of adjusting within the confines of a college curriculum, has been problematic. Because highly complex, coordinated movements require considerable time to master, the student is usually faced with insufficient skills when beginning patient care. There are many ways in which to optimize the learning environment. Perhaps a look at how technique is typically taught with an analogy from baseball can provide a useful perspective:

> The novice pitcher is being instructed on how to throw baseballs across home plate in the strike zone. Instead of allowing the pitcher to see the strike zone, it is covered with a shadow.
>
> The first pitch is thrown into the abyss. It does not result in a strike (or joint movement for that matter). The instructor moves the elbows, shoulders, arms, and legs of the pupil, to a position which, on release of the throw (or thrust), will theoretically result in a strike. The throw is repeated, with a similar outcome.

The key to someone throwing strikes, or making a successful adjustment, is to know, to see, or to imagine the result of each pitch or thrust. Alterations can then be made (some subconsciously) in the motor system to change the throw or release of the ball or thrust. If chiropractic students could see the effect (i.e., joint displacement) of the thrust both during and after, then their bodies could conform to the new requirements more easily.

Videotaping the student's movements can sometimes provide useful information. It is more important for the student to study the movements of a successful adjust-

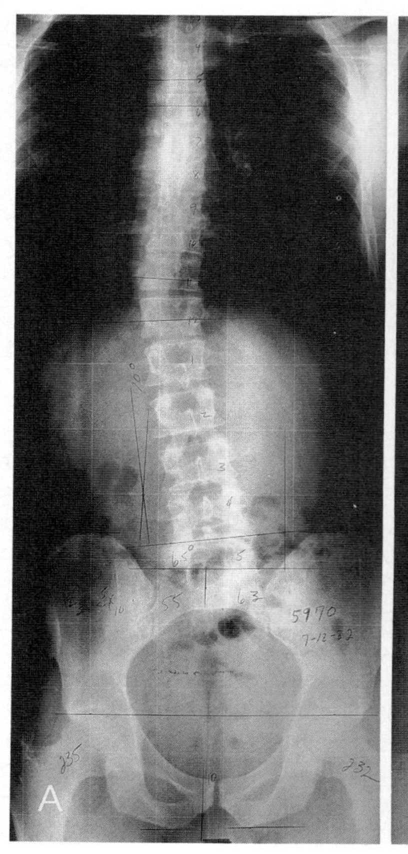

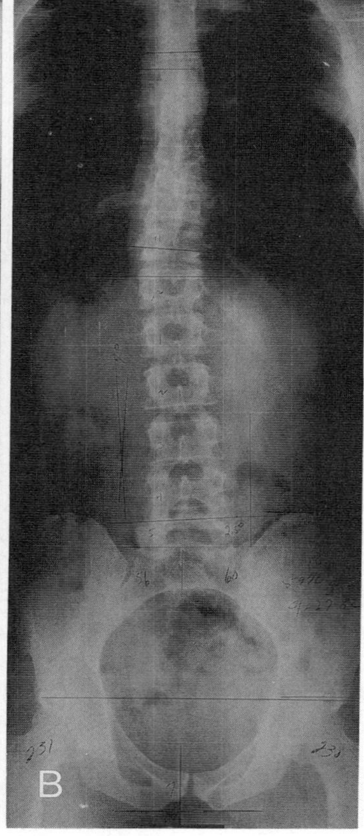

Figure 1.3A, Pretreatment radiograph demonstrating a left convex scoliosis, a lateral flexion malposition at L5, and positional dyskinesias of the sacrum and innominates. **B,** Post-treatment radiograph showing improvement in scoliosis and intersegmental displacement of the lower back. Patient was not antalgic and comparative examination was made after 6 weeks of care.

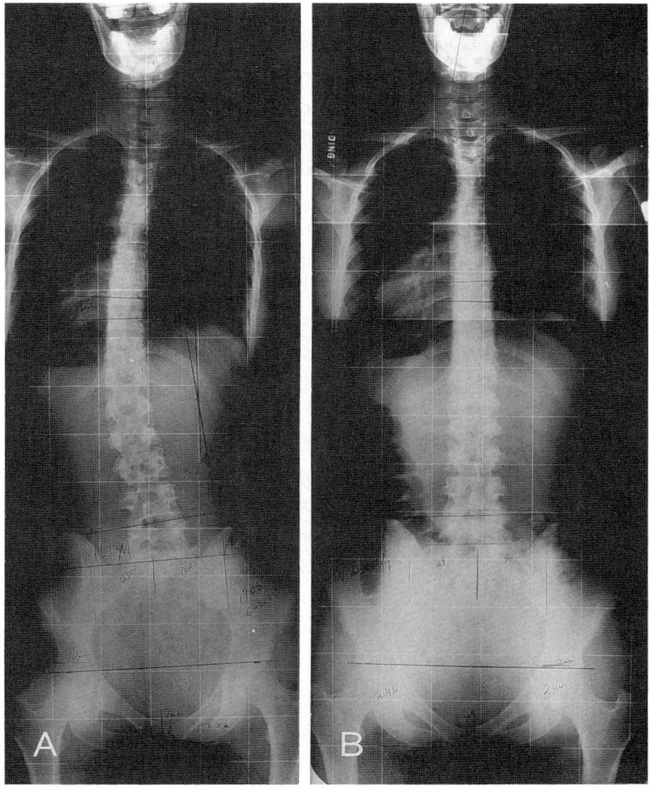

Figure 1.4A, Pretreatment radiograph. Patient is not antalgic. **B,** Posttreatment radiograph shows dramatic improvement in the intersegmental and postural displacements. Unfortunately, it is not always so easy.

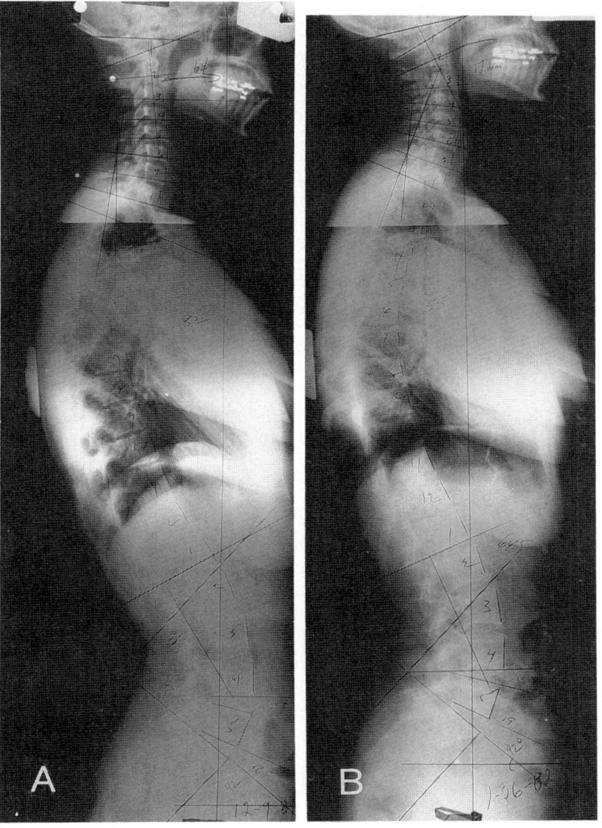

Figure 1.5A, Pretreatment radiograph. Notice the failure of the cervical lordosis to be balanced over the lumbar lordosis. **B,** Posttreatment radiograph after approximately 6 weeks of care. Notice the return of the cervical lordosis and the overall improvement in the postural configuration of the full spine.

ment either through video or direct observation. The attempt is then to duplicate the instructor's actions.

There are many ways to image the spinal column, but at present, only those methods using ionizing radiation have widespread availability. How then can the radiograph be used as a strike zone to maximize the effectiveness of a thrust? First, the positions of the various segments and their global postural configurations can be readily determined. For many adjustments the primary objective will be to move the segment forward (i.e. posterior to anterior). If the force is not directed through the center of mass of the segment this will cause forces to be dispersed more at adjacent levels (27). Second, pre- and postradiographs after successful and unsuccessful adjustments can provide the student with a visual picture of the effects from differently directed forces. If the radiograph demonstrates improvement in position or movement, then this can be used as a conceptual "goal," as it were, similar to how a baseball pitcher will conceptualize a strike before the throw (Figs. 1.3–1.6). If the force is directed inappropriately, then this too will be evident (Fig. 1.7). These mental pictures cannot be emphasized enough. When the novice positions for a set-up, at best, they will be thinking about line of drive in relation to the spinous process being contacted. The doctor, however, will have a mental picture of the three-dimensionality of the listing and the pattern of thrust that will be directed through the center of mass of the segment.

The cerebellum is chiefly concerned with coordinated movements. The cerebrum can interfere with these activities. Let us say, for example, that one hundred red bricks were placed end on end on a flat terrain. Most people would have no trouble at all walking along the narrow row of bricks, placing one foot in front of the other. If an individual was intoxicated in the above scenario, impaired cerebellar activity would hinder the walk. To show how the cerebrum can interfere with the task the row is now raised 50 feet above the ground. Most people would now have tremendous difficulty in negotiating the task. This is because they would be thinking (i.e., a cerebral activity) about the possibility of falling. The same scenario applies to the adjustment. Although a visual picture of the pattern of thrust is necessary, thinking intensely about the event or other matters tends to incoordinate the activity (Fig. 1.8A). Many times, the reason for an unsuccessful adjustment is that the individual is concentrating on matters

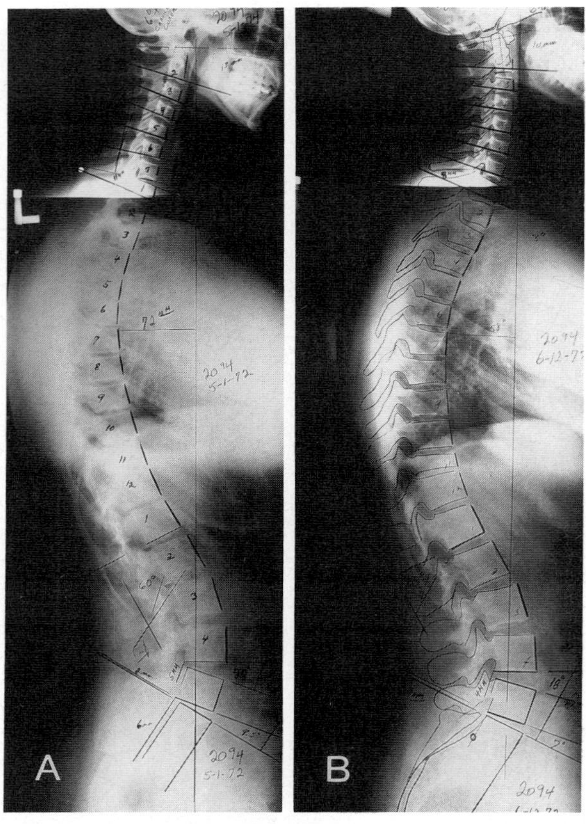

Figure 1.6A, Pretreatment radiograph showing retrolisthesis at L5 and L4 and a kyphotic cervical spine. **B,** Posttreatment radiograph after approximately 6 weeks of care. Notice the return of the cervical lordosis and reduction of the retrolisthesis at L5.

unrelated to the performance of the coordinated thrust. These distractions must be kept to a minimum, especially when one is beginning to learn the adjustive process (Fig. 1.8B). Cerebral activities are of course extremely important during the diagnostic work-up. The doctor must then "switch gears" when performing the psychomotor activity.

Scientific investigation into the role of imagery in facilitating the learning of adjustive skills has been provided by Josefowitz et al. (28). Two groups of students were evaluated for their ability in performing a spinous push adjustment for the lumbar spine. The first group mentally rehearsed performing the adjustment, and the second group imagined the spine and the positive outcome of the adjustment. The performance of the group who imagined the spine improved significantly more than the group who rehearsed the physical aspects of the adjustment. It is clear from this report that the continued practice of having students observe an instructor making an adjustment is suspect. Students are likely to benefit more from studying the intricacies of the biomechanics of the spine and pre- and comparative radiographs (both static and dynamic) and from imagining the positive outcome of the adjustment.

SUMMARY

This excursion into the philosophy, science, and art of chiropractic has been far from comprehensive. Nevertheless, it is hoped that the reader will have sensed the mutual

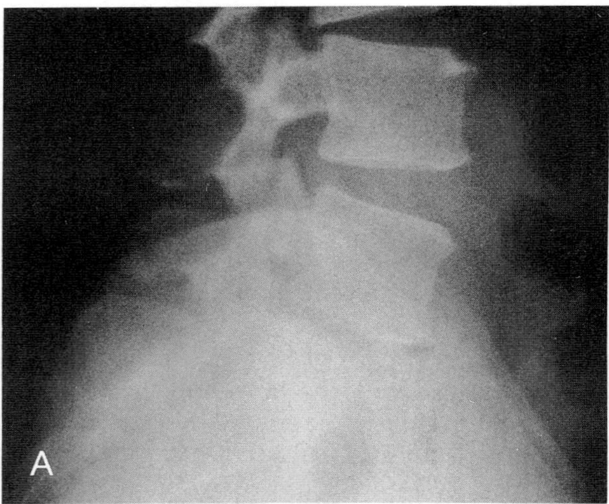

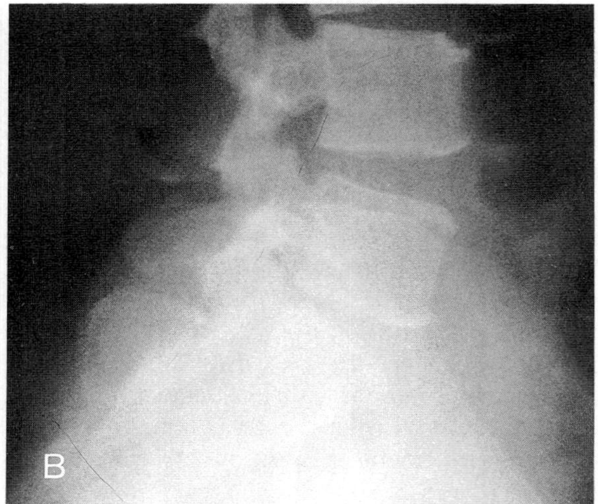

Figure 1.7A, Pretreatment radiograph demonstrating minimal retrolisthesis of L5 on sacrum. Motion palpation assessment revealed marked restriction in forward translation (+Z) of the sacrum. The patient was adjusted 10 times. Clinical findings suggested marked improvement in motion of the sacrum, a condition which was inconsistent with the radiologic picture. A comparative radiological examination was therefore performed. **B,** Posttreatment radiograph after (12 adjustments) demonstrating a clear retrolisthesis of L5, most likely caused by adjusting the sacral base forward. Even in the absence of clear contraindications to manipulation (e.g., lytic metastasis of the contact vertebra), chiropractic procedures are not entirely benign.

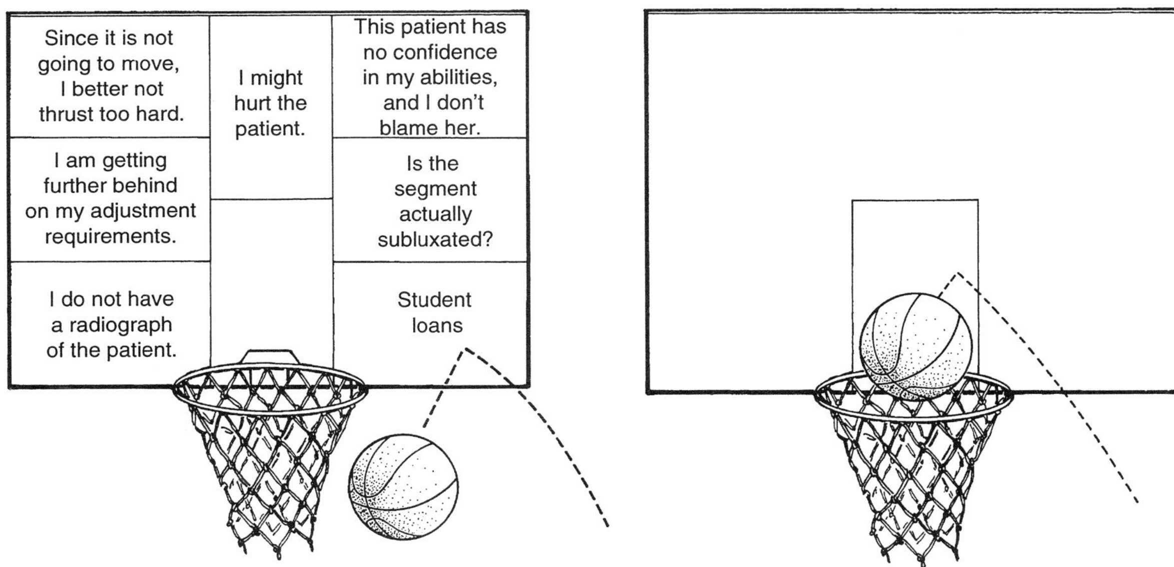

Figure 1.8 (**Left**) Thinking about matters disrupts cerebellar function and leads to a missed basket. (**Right**) A clear backboard results in two points.

dependence among philosophy, science, and technique (art) in chiropractic. The exchange among components of the discipline of chiropractic is necessary and desirable, and requires some mental exertion. Rather than serving as a defensive, political crutch for the profession, philosophy ought to be a source of guidance and inspiration for the development of a first-class science of chiropractic technique. Prepared by a familiarity with the legitimate roles of all three areas of chiropractic thought, the chiropractor can take pride in what we have learned so far and maintain enthusiasm for the task awaiting us.

REFERENCES

1. Meade TW, Dyer S, Browne W, Townsend J, Frank AO. Low back pain of mechanical origin: randomized comparison of chiropractic and hospital outpatient treatment. Br Med J 1990;300:1431–1437.
2. Keating JC, Mootz RD. Five contributions to a philosophy of the science of chiropractic. J Manipulative Physiol Ther 1987;10:25–29.
3. Keating JC, Mootz RD. The influence of political medicine on chiropractic dogma: implications for scientific development. J Manipulative Physiol Ther 1989;12:393–398.
4. Keating JC. Common misconceptions about research in chiropractic. J Minnesota Chiro Assoc 1986;(November):14–15.
5. Keating JC. Rationalism, empiricism and the philosophy of science in chiropractic. Chiropractic History 1990;10(2):23–30.
6. Donahue JH. D.D. Palmer and innate intelligence: development, division, and derision. Chiropractic History 1986;6:30–36.
7. Palmer DD. The chiropractor. Los Angeles: Beacon Light Printing, 1914.
8. Terret AGJ. It is more important to know when not to adjust. Chiropractic Technique 1990;2:1–9.
9. Robbins ER. Matters of life and death: the risks vs. benefits of medical care. New York: WH Freeman, 1984.
10. Keating JC. Philosophical barriers to technique research in chiropractic. Chiropractic Technique 1989;1:23–29.
11. Palmer DD. The chiropractor's adjuster: the science, art and philosophy of chiropractic. Portland, OR: Portland Printing House, 1910.
12. Kaminski M, Boal R, Gillette RG, Peterson DH, Villnave TJ. A model for the evaluation of chiropractic methods. J Manipulative Physiol Ther 1987;10:61–64.
13. Keating JC. The chiropractic practitioner-scientist: an old idea revisited. Am J Chiro Med 1988;1:17–23.
14. Palmer DD. Who discovered that the body is heated by nerves during health and disease. The Chiropractor. 1904 (Dec);1(1):12.
15. Smith OG, Paxson MC, Langworthy SM. A textbook of modernized chiropractic. Cedar Rapids, IA: Laurance Press, 1906.
16. Keating JC. The embryology of chiropractic thought. Europ J Chiropractic 1991;39:75–89.
17. Rehm WS. Legally defensible: chiropractic in the courtroom and after, 1907. Chiropractic History 1986;6:50–55.
18. Keating JC. Science and politics and the subluxation. Am J Chiro Med 1988;1:107–110.
19. Keating JC, Bergmann TF. Editorial: public domain. Chiropractic Technique 1989;1:111–112.
20. Vear HJ, ed. Chiropractic standards of practice and quality of care. Gaithersburg, MD: Aspen Publishers, 1992.
21. Chiropractic Technique 1990 (August). A special issue devoted to the proceedings of the Consensus Conference on Validation of Chiropractic Methods in Seattle, WA.
22. Coulehan JL. The treatment act: an analysis of the clinical art in chiropractic. J Manipulative Physiol Ther 1991;14:5–13.
23. Kleinman A, Eisenberg L, Good B. Culture, illness, and care. Clinical lessons from anthropologic and cross-cultural research. Ann Intern Med 1978;88:251–258.
24. Eisenberg L. What makes persons "patients" and patients "well?" Am J Med 1980;69:277–285.
25. Cassel EJ. The nature of suffering and the goals of medicine. N Engl J Med 1982;306:639–645.
26. Bartol KM. A model for the categorization of chiropractic treatment procedures. J Chiropractic Technique 1991;3:78–80.
27. Lee M. Mechanics of spinal joint manipulation in the thoracic and lumbar spine: a theoretical study of posteroanterior force techniques. Clin Biomech 1989;4:249–251.
28. Josefowitz N, Stermac L, Grice A, et al. Cognitive processes in learning chiropractic skills: the role of imagery. J Can Chiro Assoc 1986;30:195–199.

2 Clinical Anatomy and Biomechanics of the Spine

GREGORY PLAUGHER with the assistance of MARK A. LOPES

Biomechanics of the spine has historically been presented as an abstract subject, somehow separate from clinical applications. This chapter has been written to bring each anatomical and biomechanical premise or fact directly into the clinical situation, thus providing a central focus. The chiropractor must be an expert in spinal biomechanics and have the ability to apply the information in the clinical situation.

The spinal column is a complex structure. This complexity can often confuse the student clinician. Fortunately, some areas of the spine are well studied, such as the lumbar spine. There are insufficient basic science data or clinical research for other regions of the spine. Furthermore, the organization of such a complex topic is difficult because of the multiple interactions between the separate anatomical parts and physiological components.

The spinal column has the primary function of protecting the delicate spinal cord and nerve roots from injury. Protection of the nervous system is provided primarily by the articular structures (e.g., bone, ligament), but mechanisms do exist in the nervous system itself (e.g., spinal cord) that protect it from injury.

The function of protection takes place in a very hostile environment, one in which large loads and bending moments are encountered and transmitted, during which demands of normal physiologic movement must necessarily be preserved. In this awkward environment, things often go awry and injury results.

The presentation of clinical anatomy and biomechanics of the spine can take a number of directions. This discussion proceeds from the inside out, highlighting the major focus of the chiropractic physician, the nervous system.

SPINAL CORD

Biomechanics

Much more is to be learned about the physical properties and the functional mechanics of the spinal cord. When removed of circumferential attachments, nerves, and dentate ligaments, the spinal cord will lengthen by 10% under its own weight in the vertical position. This very flexible behavior changes to stiff resistance when an attempt is made to deform it further (1). The load-displacement curve for the spinal cord, therefore, has two distinct phases (Fig. 2.1):

1. The first is characterized by a large displacement with minimal applied forces.
2. The next phase shows little deformation under larger forces.

Forces in the initial phase are up to 0.01 N (0.04 oz.). The second phase can support 20–30 N (4.5–6.7 lb/f) before the tissues begin to rupture.

The spinal cord must adapt to the changes in length of the spinal canal during physiological motion. Flexion and lateral bending will effectively lengthen the spinal canal, necessitating accommodation by the cord and nerve roots (Fig. 2.2). Most of the change in length occurs at the posterior portion of the spinal cord (Fig. 2.3A-B). Two mechanisms are responsible for the change in length. The first is characterized by a folding/unfolding accordion-like action of the posterior cord. The second, which is only responsible for approximately 25 to 30% of the length change, is due to the elastic stretch/compression of the spinal cord tissue itself. In the cervical spine, the neutral, lordotic cervical region shows the posterior cord folded like an accordion (Fig. 2.3A). During flexion, the cord first

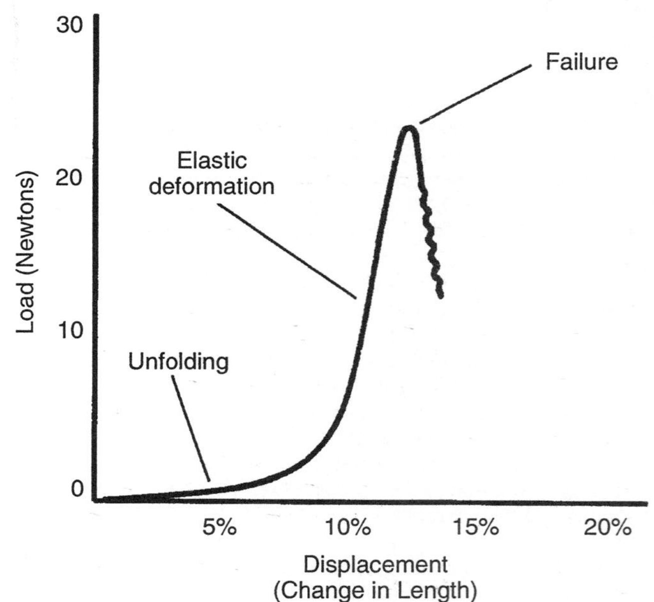

Figure 2.1. The load displacement curve for the spinal cord. Based on data from Brieg A. Adverse mechanical tension in the central nervous system. Stockholm: Almqvist & Wiksell International, 1978.

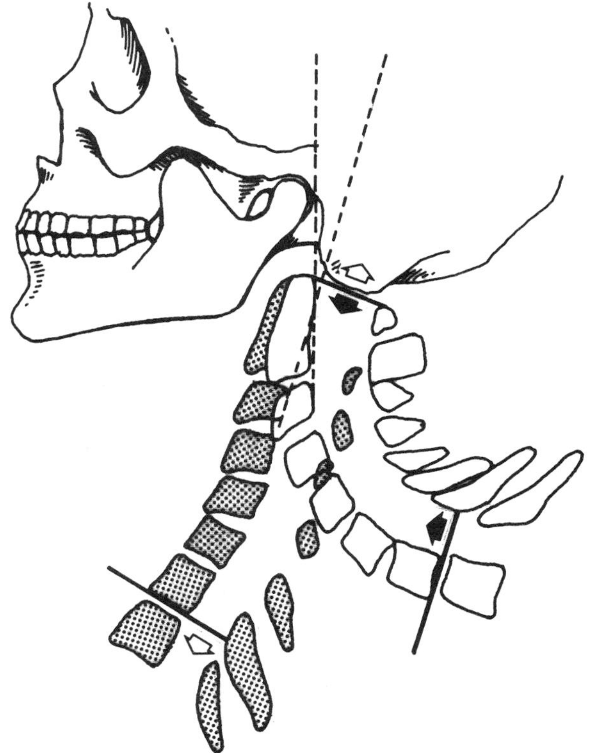

Figure 2.2. The spinal canal shortens during extension and lengthens during flexion.

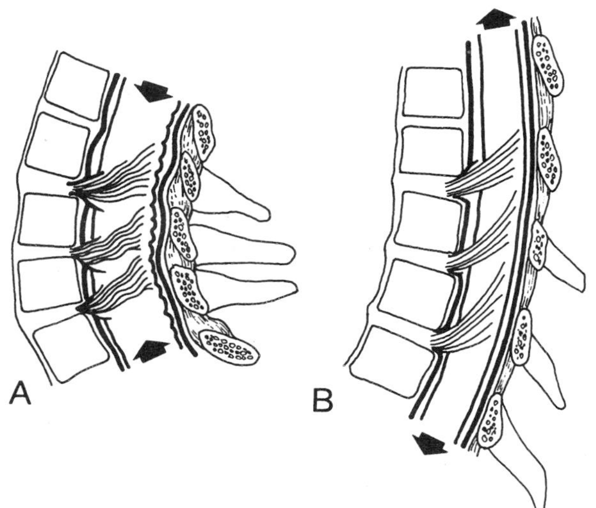

Figure 2.3. Mechanism by which the spinal cord changes length (See text). **A,** Neutral Position. **B,** Flexion.

unfolds with a minimal increase in its tension, followed by some elastic deformation near full flexion (Fig. 2.3B). When moving into extension, the spinal cord first folds, then elastically compresses. With hyperflexion of the neck or static postures of marked kyphotic angulation, the potential for spinal cord stretch is increased. Central nervous system disorders, such as tic douloureux or cervical migraine, can often be provoked with cervical flexion (1).

FUNCTIONAL SPINAL UNIT

The term functional spinal unit (FSU) or motion segment refers to two adjacent vertebrae and the ligamentous and soft tissue elements that connect them. In the thoracic spine the posterior rib articulations are also included in the description. The motion segment has the same functional characteristics as the region of the spine of which it is a part (2,3). The articulations from occiput to C2, and the sacroiliac region, are described in detail in Chapters 6 and 11. The anatomical parts of the FSU or motion segment from C2 to S1 are as follows (Fig. 2.4):

1. The central joint: vertebral bodies, intervertebral disc (annulus and nucleus), anterior and posterior longitudinal ligaments;
2. The posterior joints and articular capsule; and
3. The ligaments between the neural arches: supraspinous, interspinous, intertransverse, and the ligamentum flavum.

The effect of annular and nuclear injury at a single FSU on movement has been demonstrated by Panjabi et al. (4). A lumbar motion segment was tested before and after annulus removal, and later, with a combination of annulus and nucleus removal. The mechanical properties were determined by imposing a predetermined torque around each of the cardinal axes (X,Y, Z) (Fig. 2.5). Vertebral movement after each application of torque was then measured in degrees. As can be seen in Figure 2.6, although both injuries had effects, nucleus removal (with annulus injury) caused the most increase in motion. This occurred in all directions, excluding compression (−Y)

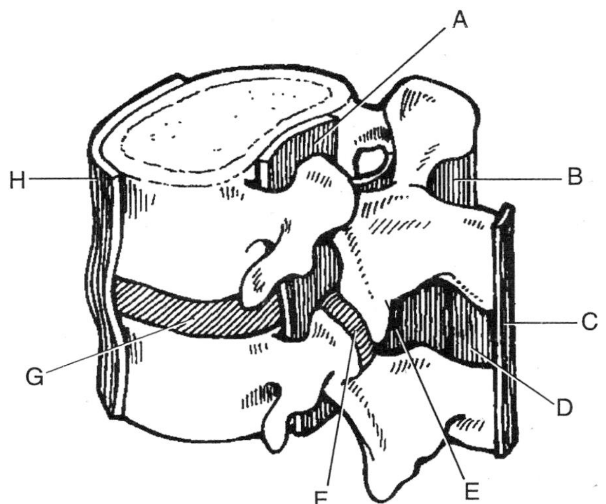

Figure 2.4. The functional spinal unit or motion segment. A) posterior longitudinal lig., B) intertransverse lig., C) supraspinous lig., D) interspinous lig., E) ligamentum flavum, F) articular capsule, G) intervertebral disc, H) anterior longitudinal lig.

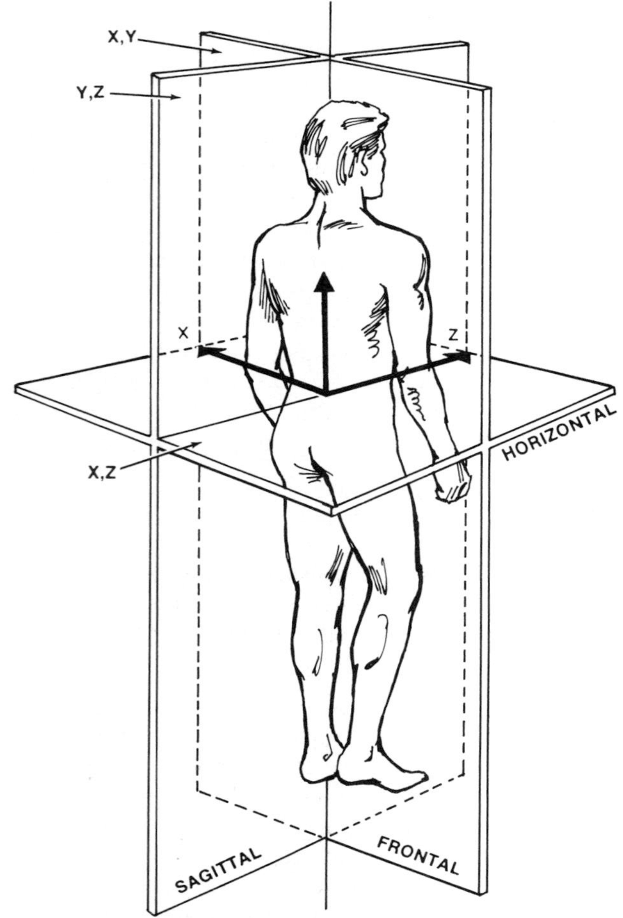

Figure 2.5. The cardinal planes of the human. Each plane is formed by two axes. The sagittal plane is formed by the Y and Z axes, the coronal plane by the Y and X axes, and the transverse plane by the X and Z axes.

or bending towards the side of injury ($+\theta Z$). The lack of significant biomechanical change after experimental injury at the disc of the motion segment when loaded under compression has been termed the "self sealing phenomenon" (5).

With the effects of specific disc injuries in mind, the implications for exercise or ergonomic prescription, are as follows:

1. The patient should not laterally flex away from the side of injury as this will cause the greatest increase in motion.
2. Movements that cause compression at the site of the injury, such as extension for a posterior, central annular bulge, or right lateral bending in the case of right sided disc injury, should be encouraged. If these movements increase pain or dysfunction, then they should be discontinued.

Panjabi et al. (4) have postulated the process whereby the effects from injury at a single FSU spread to the surrounding motion segments, thus influencing entire spinal regions (Fig. 2.7). Unequal movement of the FSU caused by central injury will then spread to the posterior articulations (Fig. 2.8).

Three-Joint Complex

Function and dysfunction at the motion segment should be analyzed from a three-joint perspective (6). The disc and the two facet joints make up a tripod of complex joint interactions. The center of axial rotation (θY) for the disc and the facets is close to the center of the disc (7). This center, about which the vertebra rotates, will change position when there is motion restriction (fixation dysfunction). This is usually due to trauma and adhesions in portions of the disc or facet joints. The center or axis of rotation can also change position because of ligamentous laxity or rupture. The changed axis will load the joints of the FSU in an asymmetrical manner. This asymmetrical loading renders the individual susceptible to continued reinjury when the spine is loaded symmetrically, because the dysfunctional motion segment will cause loads to be focused at particular sites. The abnormal movement of the FSU, from damage to the disc alone, will gradually lead to subsequent injury and degeneration at the posterior joints. Lumbar facet degeneration rarely occurs before disc degeneration (8).

Intervertebral Disc

Annulus Fibrosis. The annulus fibrosis consists of a narrow outer zone of collagenous fibers and a wider inner zone of fibrocartilage which surrounds the nucleus pulposus (9). The annulus consists of approximately 15 to 25 distinct layers—depending on the circumferential location, the spine level and the age of the individual (10). The architectural pattern of the annulus is a fabric of lamellae with all the fibers in each lamina running in the same direction. The adjacent laminae have a similar structure, but these collagen fibers run in the opposite direction. The fiber angle, with respect to the horizontal, varies within the lamellae. Gallante (11) has determined that the fiber angle is approximately 28 degrees for the outer layers and 22 degrees for the inner lamellae (Fig. 2.9).

This angle to the horizontal increases when the posterior annulus is distracted, such as during forward bending. Collagen fibers are strongest when loaded along their longitudinal axis. Gallante (11) has further shown that the annular fibers tensed at 30 degrees to the horizontal are approximately three times stronger than those fibers that are loaded horizontally.

The tensile strength of the lumbar annulus is greatest at the posterior and anterior periphery (12). These areas are loaded most during flexion and extension motion. Although there is added strength for resisting flexion this is not true for axial rotation (Y axis). During axial rotation, the torque is applied perpendicular to the fiber orientation (Fig. 2.10) of the annulus. The annulus is

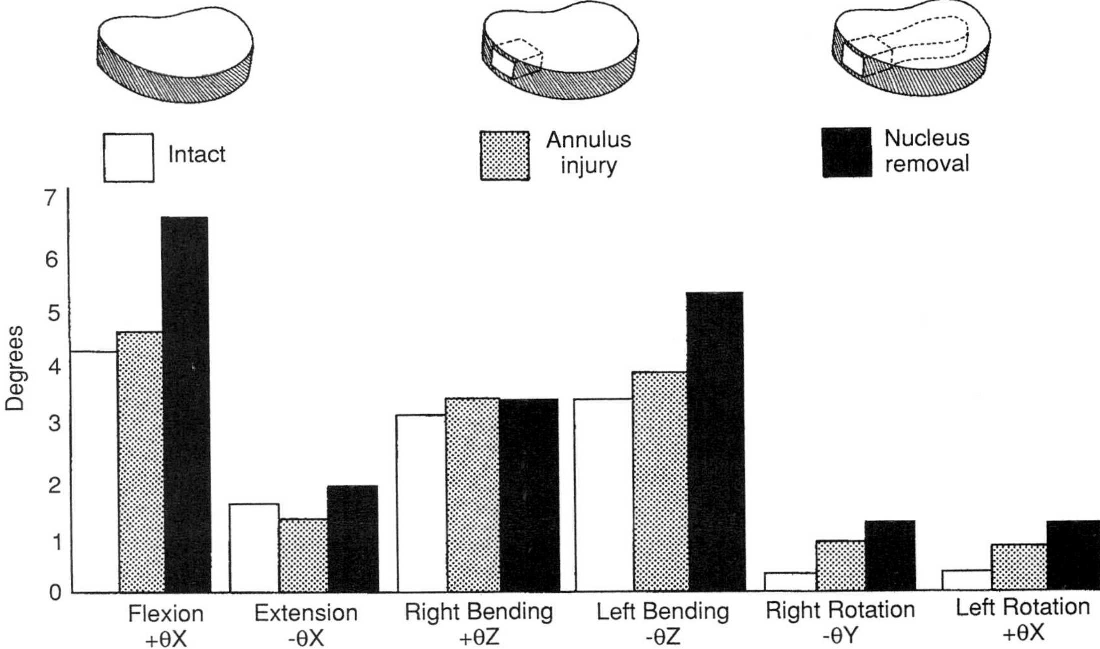

Figure 2.6. Six instability tests for a lumbar motion segment after experimental partial annular injury and, partial annular and nuclear removal. Modified from White AA, Panjabi MM. Clinical biomechanics of the spine. 2nd Ed. Philadelphia: J.B. Lippincott, 1990:13.

STRUCTURAL INJURY RESULTS IN ASYMMETRIC MOVEMENT OF ONE VERTEBRA WITH RESPECT TO THE SUBJACENT VERTEBRA

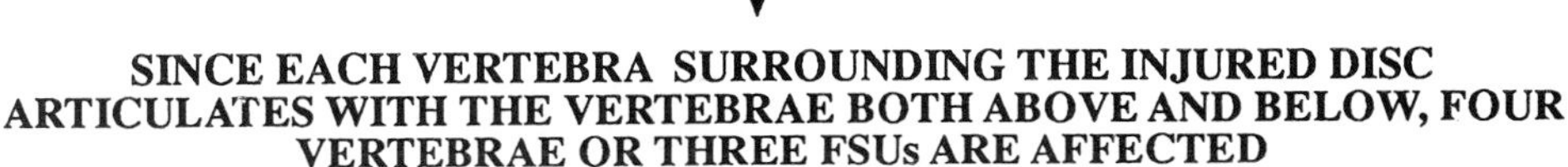
SINCE EACH VERTEBRA SURROUNDING THE INJURED DISC ARTICULATES WITH THE VERTEBRAE BOTH ABOVE AND BELOW, FOUR VERTEBRAE OR THREE FSUs ARE AFFECTED

Figure 2.7. Single joint injury leads to multiple levels of involvement.

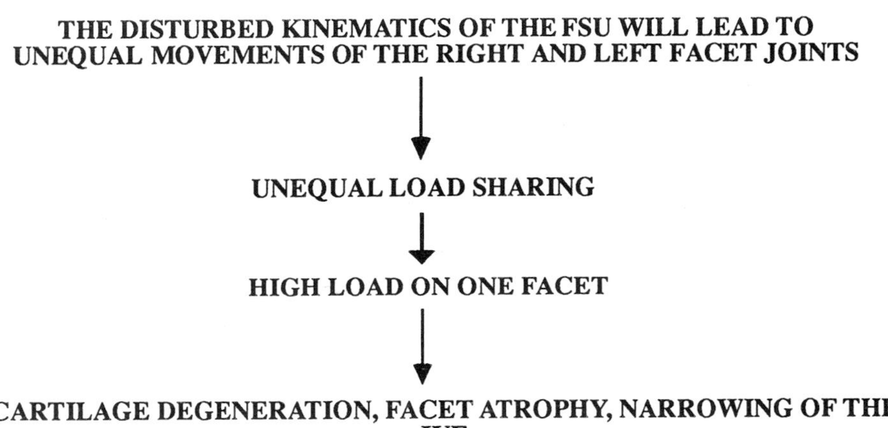

Figure 2.8. The pathogenesis of spinal degeneration.

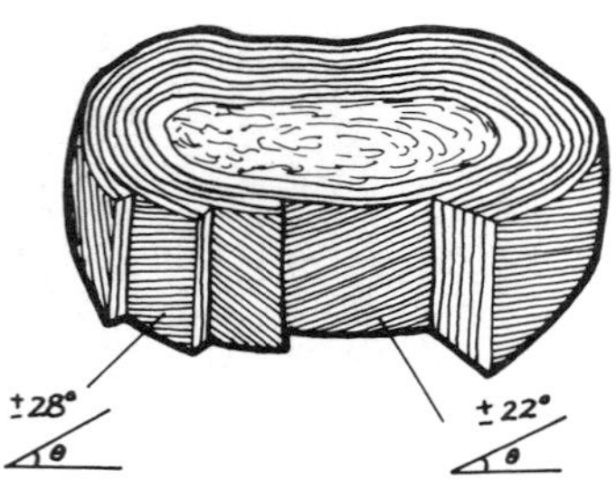

Figure 2.9. The fiber orientation of the annulus fibrosis. The orientation is nearly 30 degrees from the horizontal at the periphery when the motion segment is not flexed or extended. The fiber angle approaches 20 degrees near the nucleus. Based on data from Galante JO. Tensile properties of the human lumbar annulus fibrosis. Acta Orthopaedica Scand 1967; Suppl. 100.

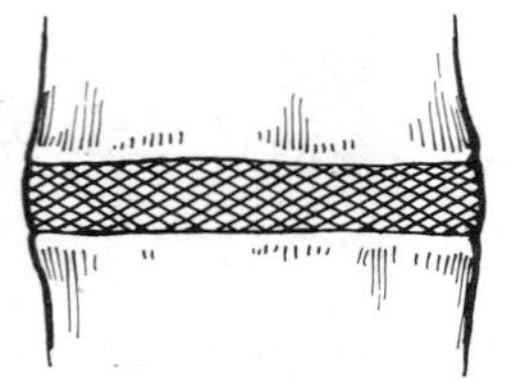

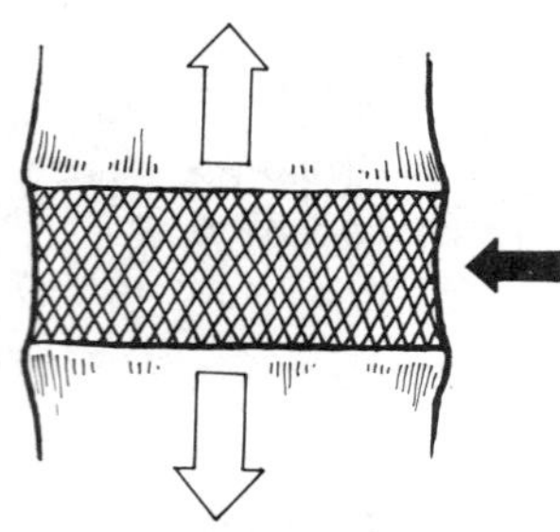

Figure 2.10. During flexion, the posterior annulus is distracted. Under this type of loading (white arrows) the annulus is quite capable of resisting the external force. In the distracted position the annulus is less able to resist axial torsion (dark arrow).

extremely vulnerable under this type of load (13). The disc is a highly specialized structure but by virtue of its specialization it cannot resist all loads in an equal manner. This is the anisotropic[a] character of the annulus.

The annulus is extensively connected to the vertebrae it separates. In the adult, the outer laminations attach to the cortex of the vertebral body via Sharpey's fibers thus creating a strong junction. The intermediate fibers pass from one end-plate to the other, whereas the innermost fibers attach to the periphery of the cartilaginous portion of the end-plate (3). The proximity of the entire posterior annular border and the posterior longitudinal ligament to the anterior aspect of the spinal canal and lateral recesses is clinically important if a space occupying lesion is present (e.g., disc protrusion). Because of the attachment of the disc to the vertebral body, adjustments can be delivered to the vertebra in an attempt to influence the position of displaced annular or nuclear material.

Nucleus Pulposus. The nucleus pulposus, a gel-like mucopolysaccharide structure, resides in the posterior central axis of the disc (Fig. 2.11). It has a dry weight of only 15% of its wet weight. This percentage of water varies considerably with age as well as with the state of health of the disc and the surrounding osseous structures (3). Fluids are passed in and out of the annulus and nucleus primarily by diffusion (15). The adult nucleus contains no blood or nerve supply. Nutrients are delivered to the tissues and cells through diffusion. The diurnal variation in water content, and joint movement, are necessary for optimal disc function.

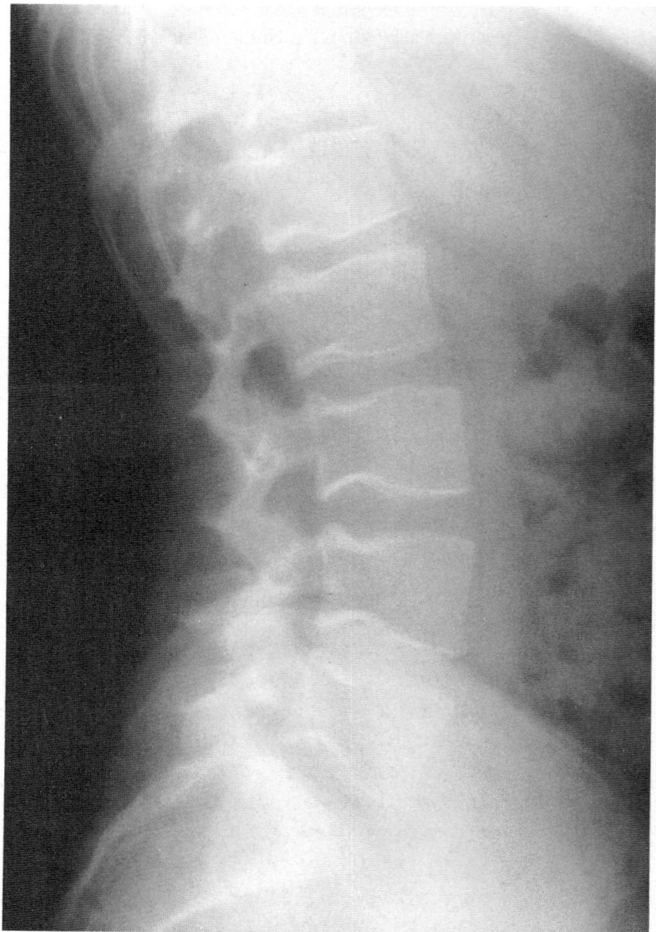

Figure 2.11. The nucleus pulposus lies in the posterior center portion of the disc, as evidenced in this individual with multiple nuclear invaginations into the vertebral bodies.

[a] *Anisotropy:* Having different mechanical properties with unlike directions or spatial orientations (2,14). For example, the intervertebral disc is much stiffer when loaded in compression than when tensile forces are applied, due to the increase in hydrostatic pressure of the nucleus during compression. This is an example of disc anisotropy. Movements of the spine also have anisotropic patterns. The lumbar spine for example, is more flexible (less stiff) during flexion and extension than axial rotation (Y axis). This behavior is due, in part, to the configuration of the posterior joints.

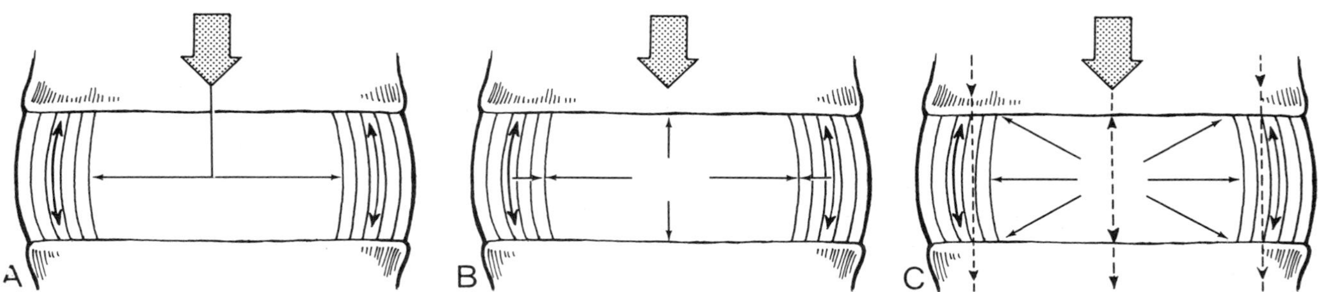

Figure 2.12. **A,** Axial compressive loads are transmitted from the end-plate of the superior vertebra to the nucleus pulposus, thus raising internal pressures. The rise in nucleus pressure exerts forces radially onto the annulus. **B,** The tension developed in the annulus prevents the nucleus from expanding. **C,** The increased nuclear pressure then exerts forces on the vertebral end-plates. Modified from Bogduk N, Twomey LT. Clinical anatomy of the lumbar spine. Melbourne: Churchill-Livingstone, 1987:20.

The lumbar nucleus occupies approximately 30 to 50% of the total disc cross sectional area (2). The spherical shape of the nucleus is readily recognizable in the young or normal spine (3,7,16). With degeneration from trauma, the nucleus begins a gradual process of dehydration that renders it less distinct from the annulus fibrosis. The spherical shape can be markedly distorted in the degenerated spine (12). It has been stated that the normal nucleus is dumbbell shaped (17). This is based on the preliminary work of Brown et al. (12), in which two aged specimens displayed this appearance. A dumbbell-shaped nucleus is most likely related to degeneration of the motion segment.

The annulus and nucleus constitute a functional unit, the effectiveness of which depends on the integrity of each component. Any major dysfunction of the motion segment must be accompanied by, if not chiefly caused by, a breakdown in normal nucleus-annulus structural and functional relationships.

Compression loads applied to the central articulation involve the redistribution of axial compressive forces from the nucleus horizontally outward, to the annulus (18) (Fig. 2.12). The nucleus is tightly bound peripherally and held under pressure by the annulus. A nucleus pulposus dehydrated from degeneration is less able to sustain fluid pressure. This decreases the central load on the end-plates during compression and distributes the axial load more peripherally.

The danger of compressive overload at the central joint is an argument for limiting certain sport activities for the young. Activities such as powerlifting and gymnastics can cause severe axial (Y axis) compression. End-plate invagination and Schmorl's nodes are more likely in the compressed young or nondegenerated disc, because of the prominent, highly pressurized nucleus (19,20).

A study by Horne et al. (21) found that competitive water ski jumping leads to a higher incidence of vertebral trauma, including the abnormalities associated with Scheuermann's disease. Sward et al. (22) showed that elite male gymnasts had a higher incidence of disc degeneration (evaluated by magnetic resonance imaging, MRI), thoracolumbar abnormalities (e.g., Schmorl's nodes), and back pain. Jackson et al. (23) found a history of low-back pain significant enough to disrupt training in 25% of female gymnasts. The mean age of this group was 14 years.

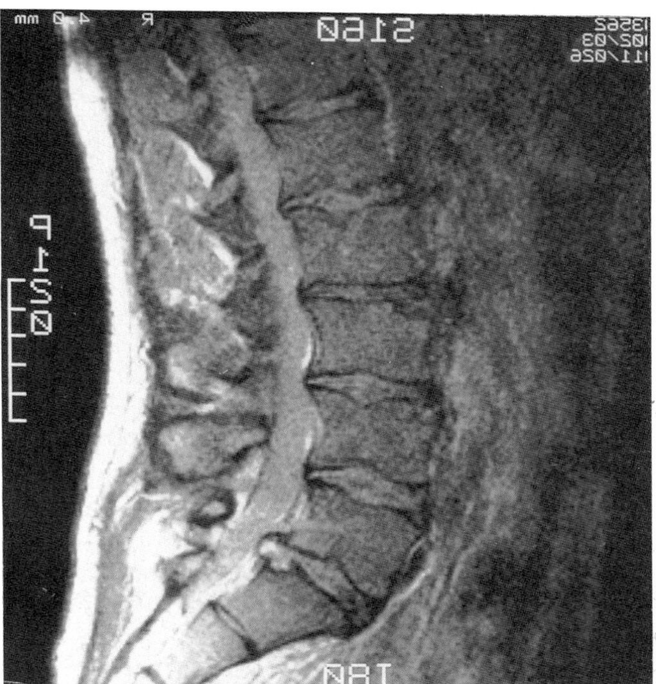

Figure 2.13. The MRI shows evidence of disc degeneration and Schmorl's nodes at multiple levels, and a herniation at L5-S1 in this former weightlifter. Courtesy Michael J. Cuneo.

Wrestlers (24), football players (25), heavy weight lifters (26), gymnasts (22,24) and other athletes who subject their spines to extreme axial loads seem to be at risk (Figs. 2.13–2.18). The radiological findings of the study by Sward et al. (24) suggests both traumatic changes to the motion segments as well as disturbed vertebral growth.

Both the age of onset of athletic activity and the degree of mechanical load on the axial skeleton are important factors in the development of these abnormalities. Sward

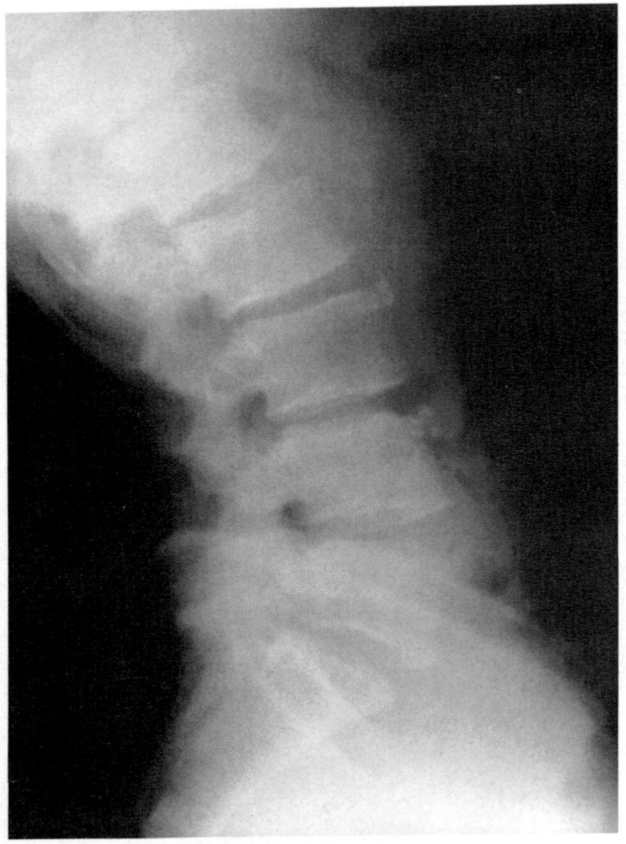

Figure 2.14. The lateral lumbar radiograph of the patient in Figure 2.13. demonstrating multiple Schmorl's nodes, disc space narrowing, and a spondylolisthesis at L5.

et al. (24) raise a number of important questions regarding these findings: At what age should vigorous athletic training begin and what loads are acceptable to avoid damage to the back? Who takes the responsibility to prevent and detect injuries in young athletes—the athletes themselves, the trainer, the club, the sport federation, the physicians or the parents? What can be done in terms of age limits or modification of rules? All these issues must be faced, especially as the intensity of training seems to increase while the age at onset seems to decrease.

The movement of the nucleus during certain postures has been somewhat controversial (2,15,16). In the most definitive study to date (27), it was determined that the nucleus bulges posteriorly during forward flexion of the lumbar and thoracic spine (Fig. 2.19). The annulus, in contrast, bulges anteriorward during forward bending.

Inflammation and its concomitant edema can occur at virtually any spinal level when there is trauma to the disc. Damaging forces disrupt the collagen fibers. This disruption interferes with the protein-polysaccharide synthesis-depolymerization equilibrium, in favor of an increased or unbalanced depolymerization. The increased proteoglycan degradation is associated with an increased fluid uptake, thus raising intradiscal tension and pressure (28) (Fig. 2.20). Although the nucleus has no nerve endings, the outer layers of the annulus are innervated by pain fibers from the recurrent meningeal nerve which are stimulated when there is injury in the area (18). It may take up to three days after a trauma for the disc to swell to its maximum. It is important to relate this information to the patient if they are examined immediately after a trauma because the pain may increase substantially over the ensuing few days. The cervical and lumbar discs have the greatest ability to imbibe fluid (2). This can occur during recumbency or antigravity, and after trauma.

Diurnal changes in the straight leg raising test have been investigated by Porter and Trailescu (29). They found that patients with lower lumbar disc protrusion had a decrease in straight leg raising after two hours of recumbency. Diurnal change in straight leg raising is probably related to the disc's proteoglycan content, its hydration, and other factors. Clinical observations have shown that a patient with an inflamed lumbar disc is more difficult to adjust immediately after a night's sleep. It is therefore preferable to treat these patients later in the day, or after they have spent several hours upright or moving about. The degenerated disc, in contrast, is more easily adjusted when more fluid is present in the disc, because this will usually facilitate movement.

The increase in fluid in the nucleus after recumbency was analyzed in vivo by Adams et al. (30). The results showed that the range of movement of the lumbar spine increased about 5° during the day. In a separate analysis of cadaver lumbar segments they determined that creep loading of the joint increases the range of lumbar flexion by about 12.5°. Their conclusions were that forward bending movements subject the spine to higher bending stresses in the morning compared with later in the day. The increase is about 80% for the ligaments of the neural arch and 300% for the intervertebral disc. Lumbar discs and ligaments are therefore at greater risk of injury in the early morning.

End-plate

The hyaline cartilage vertebral end-plates have an important role in transporting nutrients to the avascular disc. Brown and Tsaltas (31) found that there is a decrease in diffusion of substances in aging end-plates. Fractures of these structures are the most common pathology detected during lumbar spine dissection (3). Bernick and Cailliet (32) studied lumbar vertebrae varying in age from birth to 73 years. Their findings indicated that there is a gradual calcification of the end-plate with age. Abnormalities were commonly detected in the microvasculature and nutrient spaces or canals that would then retard the passage of substances from the blood into the bone, cartilage and disc. Roberts et al. (33) have determined that when

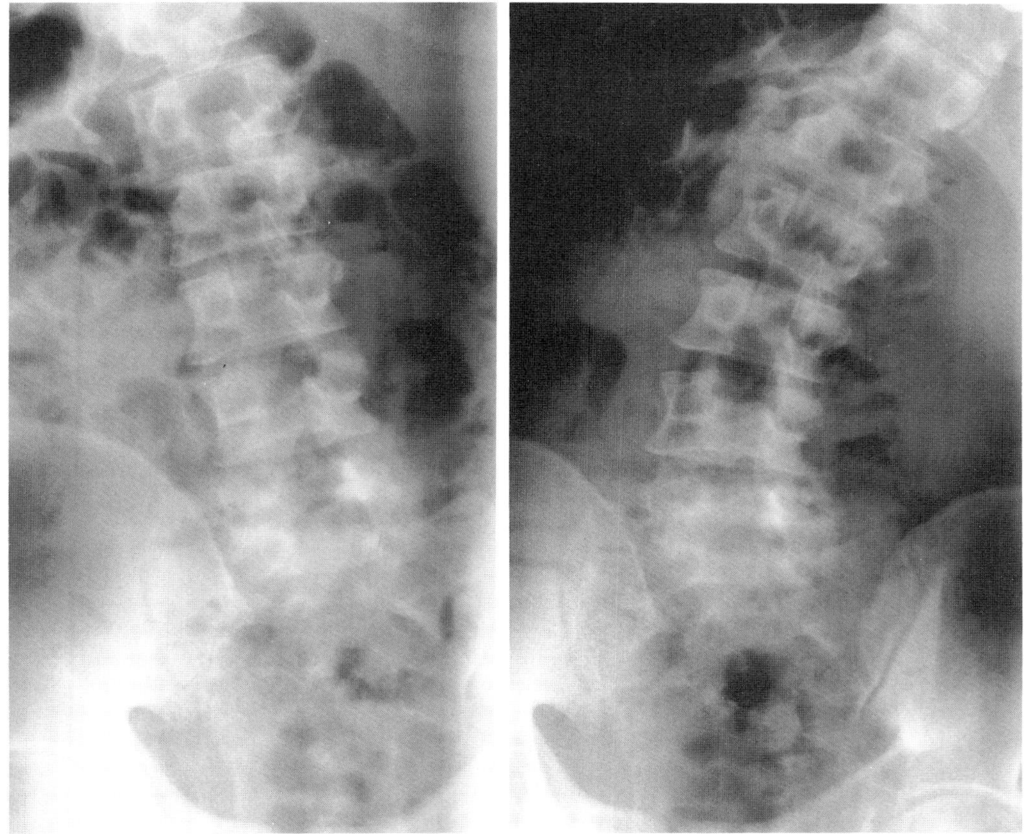

Figure 2.15. Right and left lateral bending radiographs of the patient in Figure 2.13 demonstrating abnormal coupling patterns and fixation dysfunction.

Schmorl's nodes are present, the disc and end-plate at the location of the node show loss of proteoglycan compared with the surrounding tissues.

Disc Shape

The normal disc shape is slightly thicker anteriorly in the lordotic cervical and lumbar spine, and thus helps to form the secondary curves. The kyphosis of the thoracic spine is formed by the wedge shape of the thoracic vertebral bodies; the discs are relatively equal in anterior and posterior thickness (9).

The disc space can best be observed on the lateral spinal radiograph. Its appearance provides important information for the practitioner in locating and evaluating the VSC (See Radiographic Disc Evaluation and Chapters 4 and 5).

Biomechanics of the Disc

The crossed arrangement of the annulus allows and resists axial torsion (θY), flexion/extension (θX), lateral bending (θZ), and shear ($\pm$Z, $\pm$X). The disc is an extremely stiff structure when subjected to mechanical loading. For example, during compression of the spine, the disc is much stiffer than the vertebral body. The latter will fracture when the FSU is overloaded.

Compression. The disc is more stiff under compression than when under tension. This is due to the increase in hydrostatic pressure of the nucleus pulposus (2,34). Compression overload causes the vertebral body or end-plate to fail rather than the disc. Experiments by Virgin (5) failed to herniate the lumbar discs under compression overload, even in the presence of an open communication to the nucleus through annular removal. End-plate invaginations and sclerosis, Schmorl's nodes, and compression or burst fractures, are all radiographic signs of trauma from compression overload.

Compression of the disc causes increased internal pressures, which have been measured experimentally by Nachemson (35). As can be seen in Figure 2.21, the load on the L3–4 disc varies considerably with different body positions (See Chapter 7).

Modeling of human mechanics using only data from disc pressure measurements is inadequate. In most cases the different body positions represent quasistatic condi-

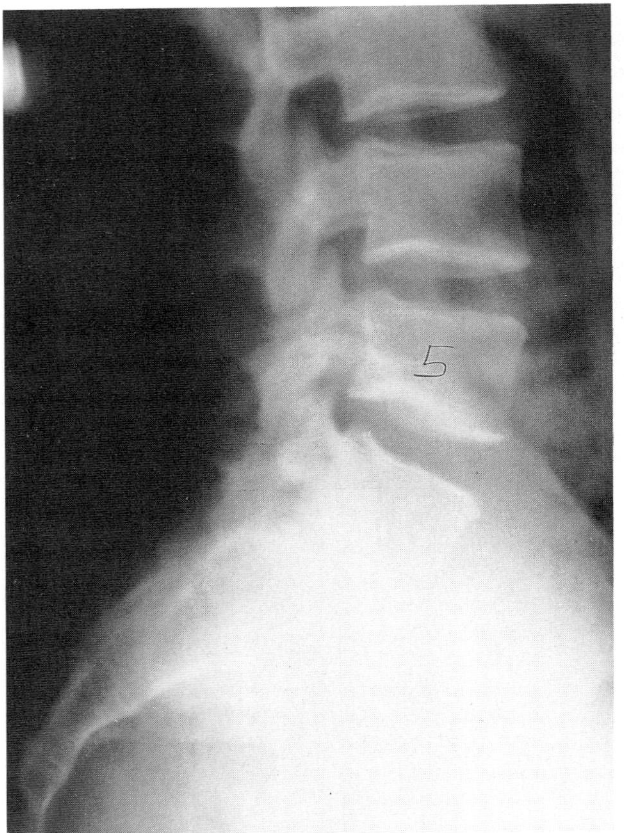

Figure 2.16. The lateral lumbar radiograph demonstrates a Schmorl's node at L5. This individual began powerlifting at the age of twelve. At age thirteen he was lifting 425 lbs in the dead lift event. Courtesy Dr. Robert Katona.

tions that are generally not reflective of how the individual would execute a task (e.g., lifting) (36). For example, as the various measurements are taken in a static, forward flexed position, the ligamentous stretch or creep of the lumbodorsal fascia and midline ligaments will cause progressive recruitment of the erector spinae muscles thus increasing internal disc pressures. The contribution of the ligamentous system to the execution of a dynamic lift is substantial (See Biomechanics of Lifting) (Fig. 2.22).

Torsion (Y axis). The intervertebral disc resists rotational displacement by developing tension in the annular fibers. Resistance is also offered by the posterior joints. Their contribution is substantial in the upper lumbar spine where their sagittal orientation causes impaction of the joint on forced rotation. In the lower lumbar spine, however, where the facets are more oblique, they play less of a role in limiting rotation (See Chapter 7). Here, the zygapophyseal joints are designed to resist anterior shear, which is greatest in the lower lumbars, especially L5-S1. To counter axial rotation of the L5-S1 motion segment, the iliolumbar ligaments provide added resistance (37). Torsion is restricted at the thoracolumbar junction by the mortice-like configuration of the posterior joints (38).

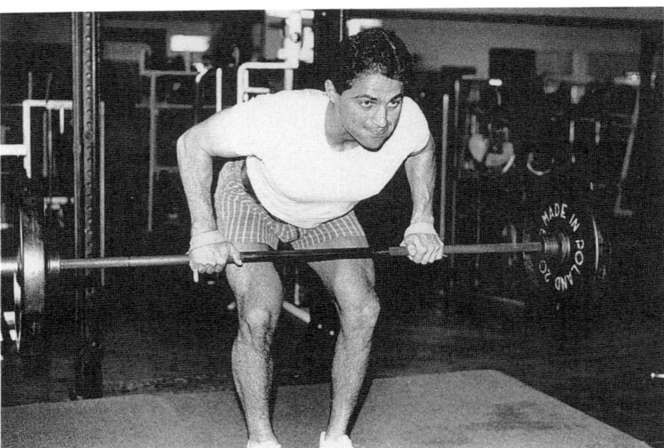

Figure 2.17. Rowing exercise with a barbell (135 lbs). Although this maneuver helps to strengthen the back muscles, it does so at the price of extreme axial compressive loads applied to the intervertebral joints.

More cephalad, the rib cage has a primary role in limiting axial rotation.

Farfan et al. (39) rotated lower lumbar disc specimens to failure in an attempt to determine their torque strength. The average failure torque was 25% less in degenerated discs indicating a decreased ability to resist this motion. Degeneration consisted of dehydration of the nucleus, and circumferential and radial fissures of the annulus. There tended to be greater torque strength for the more rounded discs. Under mechanical loading, Farfan (3) determined that the lumbar annulus begins to develop tension at approximately 2 degrees of rotation with microdamage occurring shortly thereafter in some cases (Fig. 2.23). Loud snapping sounds were often heard from some specimens because of annular tearing. These sounds were reminiscent of the "snap" often reported by patients during lumbar spine injury. Factors that decrease the torque strength of the motion segment include:

1. Little contribution from the posterior joints as in the lower lumbar spine;
2. Iliolumbar ligaments (present at L5 but not at L4);
3. Retrolisthesis of the segment causing a separation of the facet joints which decreases their effectiveness in resisting rotation;
4. Previous degeneration: circumferential tears, radial fissures, etc.;
5. Flexion of the motion segment. This orients the posterior fibers more vertically thus decreasing their ability to resist forces perpendicular to the longitudinal axis of the collagen fibers (13) (Fig. 2.10); and
6. An ovoid disc shape.

Shear. Horizontal translational displacements of the disc ($\pm Z$, $\pm X$) are markedly restricted by the annulus. A high force is required to cause an abnormal displacement in horizontal translation. Although stiffness of the spine is greatest during compression, large values are also seen during shear loading. It is greater, for example, during

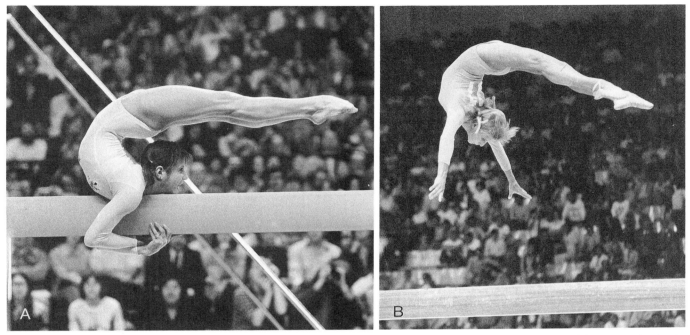

Figure 2.18. The incredible artistic and athletic expression of this Olympic gold medal winner does more than "chill" the spine of the observer. **A,** Various strains are placed on the ligamentous elements during the balance beam routine. **B,** High axial compressive loads are applied to the intervertebral joints during launch and landing. Courtesy AP/World Wide Photos.

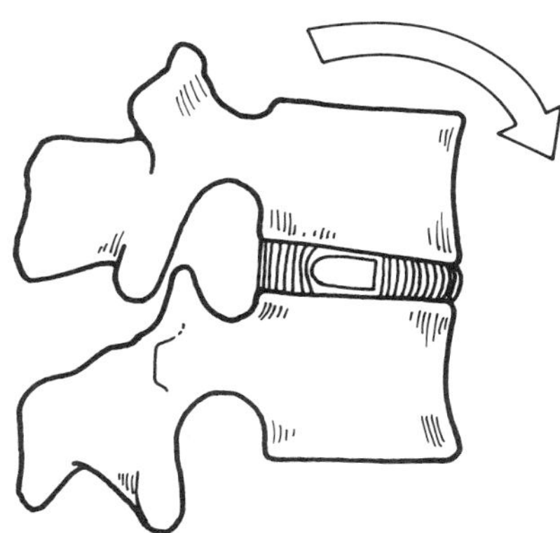

Figure 2.19. The nucleus bulges posteriorward during flexion and the annulus bulges anteriorward.

shear than during axial rotation or lateral bending (5,12,40–42). The presence of laterolisthesis or retrolisthesis is indicative of severe disruption of the restraining mechanisms of the annulus (11,43). This disruption often does not manifest itself radiologically until severe plastic deformation of the annulus has occurred, usually over the course of many years. For this reason, laterolisthesis is more common in the geriatric spine.

The lumbar posterior joints also have a role in limiting shear forces in the lumbar spine, especially during anterior (+Z) and lateral shear (±X). Depending upon the extent of the initial trauma to the disc, retrolisthesis can often be detected radiographically at an early age (Fig. 2.24). The zygapophyseal joints offer little resistance to posterior shear forces. The cervical and upper thoracic zygapophyseal joints tend to restrict anteroposterior (Z axis) shear and flexion extension (θX) much more than the central joint of that region, in contrast to the lumbar disc.

Vibration. Sullivan and McGill (44) examined the relation between whole-body vibration and decreases in spine length beyond normal diurnal changes. Their results indicated that there is a loss of height in the spine after 30 minutes of vibration. There appeared to be a recovery in height on the day the subject underwent vibration, such that these subjects were even taller than the controls at the end of the day. The authors speculated that this could be caused by an inflammatory response in the disc substance from vibrational injury.

Creep. Creep is defined as a deformation of a viscoelastic tissue (e.g., ligament) in response to a constant, suddenly applied load (2) (Fig. 2.25). Higher forces or loads tend to produce greater deformation of spinal ligaments as well as faster rates of creep. Kazarian (45) performed creep tests on lumbar discs during compression loading (Fig. 2.26). The discs were graded based on their level of degeneration. Non-degenerated discs creep slowly and reach their final deformation value after considerable time. In contrast, the more degenerated disc has a faster rate of creep.

Creep effects are noticeable for all ligaments that are under constant loads. Injury seems to increase creep,

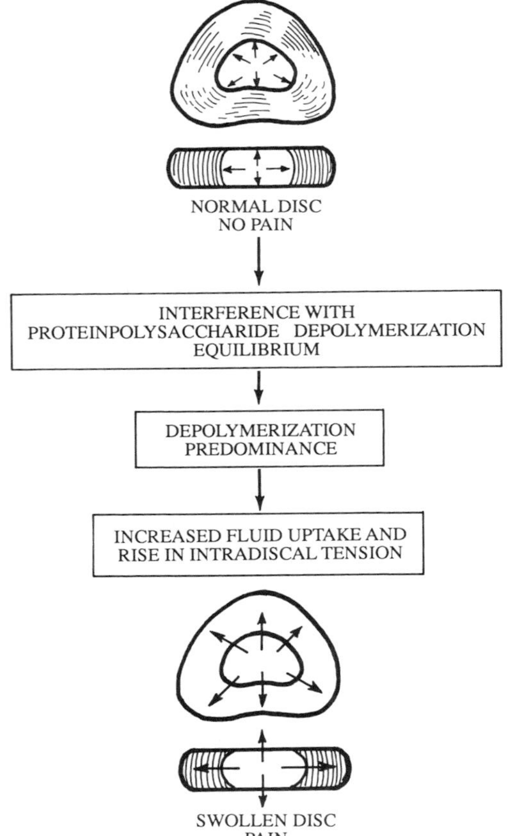

Figure 2.20. The mechanism of the swollen disc and production of pain. Modified from White AA, Panjabi MM. Clinical biomechanics of the spine. 2nd. ed. Philadelphia: J.B. Lippincott Co., 1990:397. Based on data from Naylor A. Intervertebral disc prolapse and degeneration; the biochemical and biophysical approach. Spine 1976;1:108–114.

which implies that adjusting the motion segment into the direction of ligamentous laxity would accelerate this effect.

Hysteresis. Hysteresis is defined as a failure of either one or two related phenomena to keep pace with the other (14). Loading produces a particular load-displacement curve for ligamentous structures (e.g., intervertebral disc), but gradual release of the load produces a different load-displacement curve (Fig. 2.27). This loss of energy (i.e. delay) is referred to as hysteresis and is a characteristic of all biological tissues when subjected to a load/unload cycle. Hysteresis in action occurs, for example, when a person jumps down from a height. The shock energy from impact is absorbed (i.e. a delayed return) all the way from the feet to the brain by the vertebrae, discs, and extremity joints (2). Virgin (5) found that the larger the load applied, the greater the hysteresis. He also determined that hysteresis decreased when the disc was loaded a second time. This loss of hysteresis after the second load implies that the disc may not be able to withstand repetitive loads effectively (See Fatigue Tolerance). Hysteresis is much

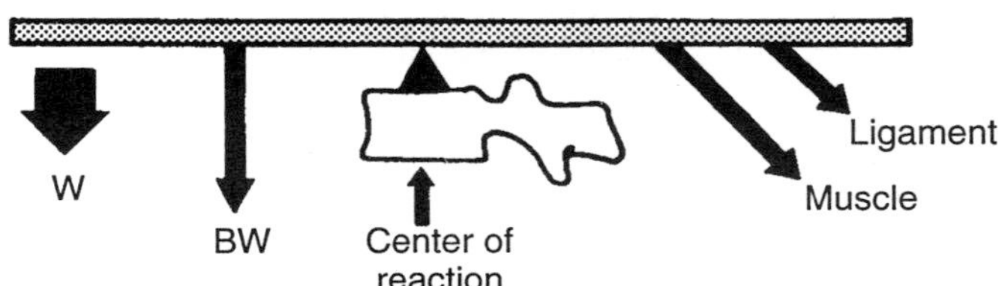

Figure 2.22. The role of the ligamentous and muscular elements in balancing the loads of body weight (BW) and a weight held in the hands (W). Modified from Gracovetsky S. Function of the spine. J Biomed Eng 1986;8:219.

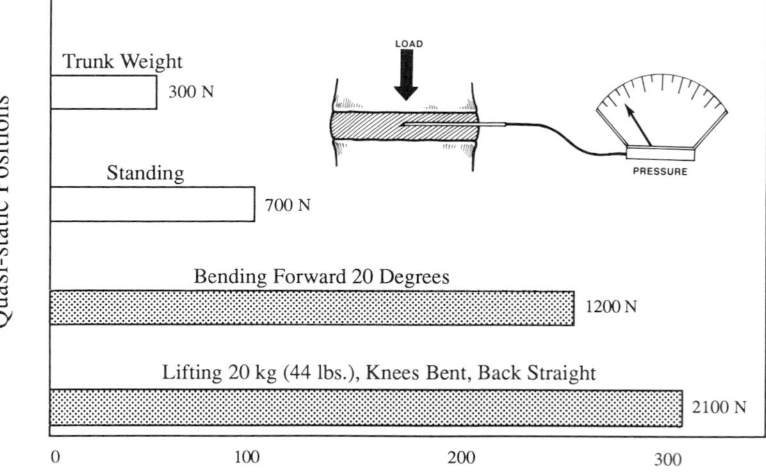

Figure 2.21. Intradiscal pressures under varying postures and lifts. Modified from White AA, Panjabi MM. Clinical biomechanics of the spine. 2nd Ed. Philadelphia: J.B. Lippincott Co., 1990:11. Based on data from Nachemson A. The load on lumbar discs in different positions of the body. Clin Orthop 1966;45:107–122.

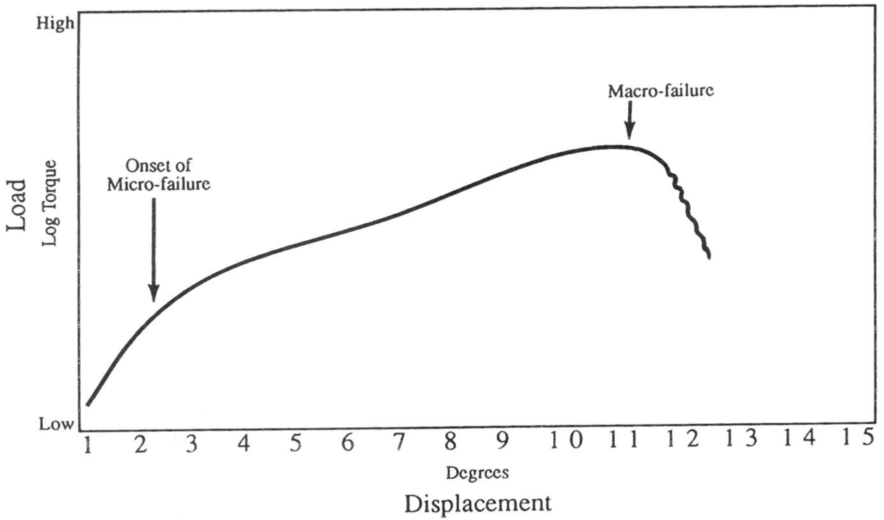

Figure 2.23. Load displacement curve for a lumbar intervertebral disc during axial rotation. Modified from Bogduk N, Twomey LT. Clinical anatomy of the lumbar spine. Melbourne: Churchill Livingstone, 1987:65.

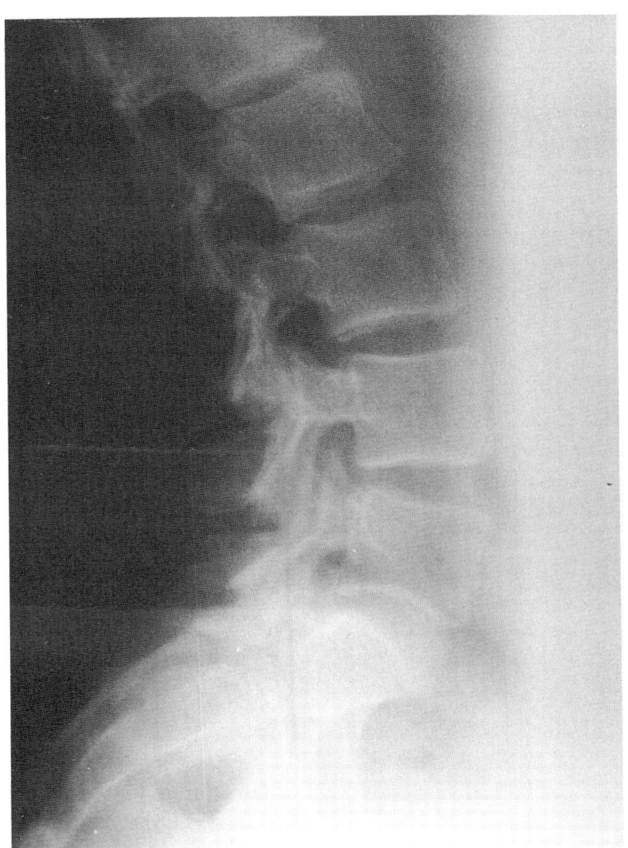

Figure. 2.24. The radiograph of this 13-yr-old illustrates retrolisthesis at L5, indicative of disc injury at that level.

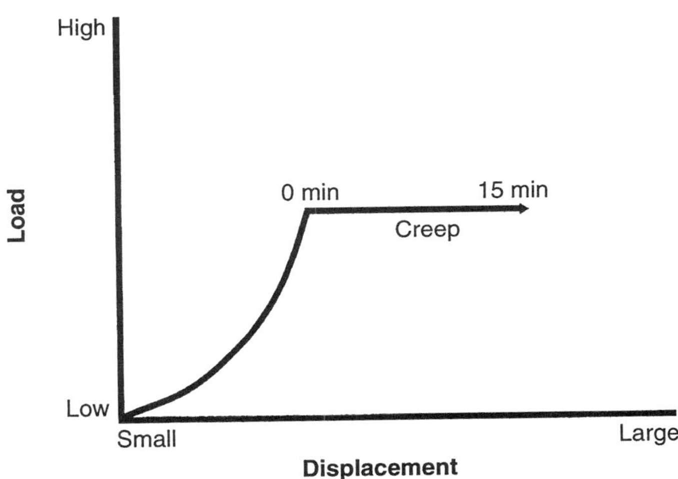

Figure 2.25. The load-displacement curve depicts the phenomenon of creep. Modified from Bogduk N, Twomey LT. Clinical anatomy of the lumbar spine. Melbourne: Churchill Livingstone, 1987:55.

less in the aged or degenerated disc, making the elderly more susceptible to trauma from external forces.

Fatigue Tolerance. The disc is not able to withstand repetitive cyclic loading and unloading for long periods of time. Fatigue induced failure leads to degeneration of the motion segment (46). Brown et al. (12) performed a fatigue tolerance test on a lumbar disc. A repetitive (1100 cycles/min.) forward bending motion of 5 degrees with axial compression of 15 lbs was induced on a lumbar motion segment. The disc began to show signs of failure after only 200 cycles and completely failed after 1000 cycles (less than one minute). The fatigue life of the disc is low in vitro and is difficult to determine in vivo. Individuals in occupations involving repetitive load/unload cycles, such as in the trucking industry, often have a higher incidence of low back pain and disc herniation (47). This may be due, in part, to hysteresis and fatigue tolerance characteristics of the motion segment.

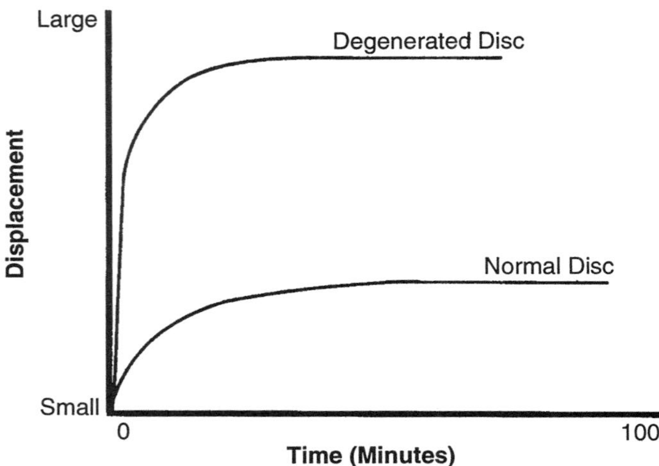

Figure 2.26. The creep curves for a degenerated and normal disc under a constant, suddenly applied compression load. Based on data from Kazarian LE. Creep characteristics of the human spinal column. Orthop Clin North Am 1975;6:3–19.

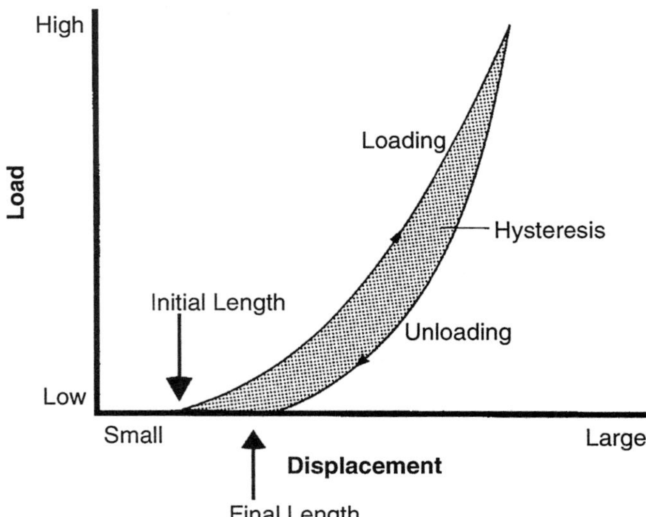

Figure 2.27. Hysteresis. Loading and unloading of a ligament produces two distinct load-displacement curves. Modified from Bogduk N, Twomey LT. Clinical anatomy of the lumbar spine. Melbourne: Churchill Livingstone, 1987:56

Goel et al. (48) found an increase in retrodisplacement of the motion segment after experimental pure cyclic flexion bending of a ligamentous lumbar spine for five hours. This displacement is due to a loosening of the disc substance, primarily the annulus.

Liu et al. (49) studied the effects of cyclic torsional loads on lumbar discs. They found that torsional fatigue loads had a number of undesirable effects: (*a*) leakage of synovial fluid at the apophyseal joints, (*b*) fibrillation of the facet cartilage surface, and (*c*) fracture of various elements of the vertebra. Their conclusions suggested that prolonged exposure to cyclic torsional loads producing more than 1.5 degrees of angular displacement per segment is detrimental to elements of the lumbar spine.

Degeneration

The onset of disc degeneration in the early stages corresponds with the onset of symptoms (3,50). Some individuals, however, experience no symptoms at all. In these cases, early signs of spinal degeneration can only be determined through objective analytical procedures, such as MRI.

There is some certainty that the first pathological changes occur in the annulus. These early changes take the form of small circumferential separations between the annular lamellae. Evidence of lamellar separation has been reported as early as eight years of age (3). In the vast majority of disc injuries, healing occurs in the form of granulation tissue and vascularization. The new blood supply comes from the outer annulus and the end-plate. If there is damage to either of these tissues, the rate of healing will be slowed. The repair mechanisms tend to hydrolyze the disc contents and remove loose fragments while stabilizing the remainder of the disc (3). The neutralizing of the loose material within the disc secures the joint and provides less material for possible extrusion or entrapment.

The usual progressive nature of the degeneration of the intervertebral disc includes increasing involvement of the annular lamellae as more concentric cracks appear. These fissures do not communicate at first with the nucleus. The location of the lamellar separations varies with the particular disc. At the L4 and L5 levels they occur most commonly in the posterior and posterolateral annulus (3).

Degenerative changes of the disc occur peripherally before involving the nucleus. No nucleus change occurs without advanced structural changes in the annulus (3). Radial fissures in the annulus appear much later and coalesce with previously existing circumferential tears. These radial fissures begin in the innermost lamellae near the nucleus and progress outward. Interestingly, these radial fissures are most commonly found in the thoracic spine (51).

With injury and degeneration the disc becomes less resistant to torsional forces. After repeated postural stressing, the already compromised disc is the weak link in the closed kinematic chain and will be the first to be reinjured.

Zygapophyseal Joints

The zygapophyseal joints consist of cartilaginous facet surfaces, synovium, and capsular ligaments. Supporting the facet joints are the capsular ligaments that are relatively "baggy" to allow for a large range of motion, especially in the cervical spine. The anteromedial border of the capsule makes up the posterior portion of the inter-

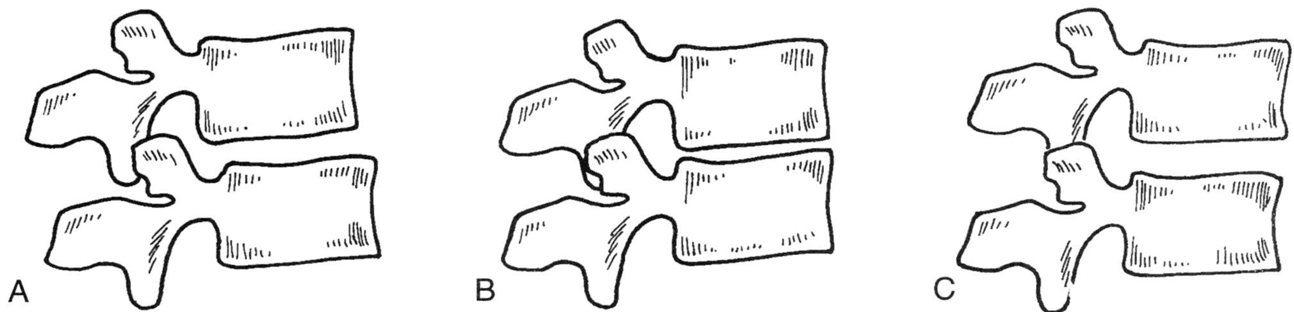

Figure 2.28. **A,** The effect of retrolisthesis (−Z) on the intervertebral foramen. Because of the elliptical shape of the foramen, this type of displacement has a more marked effect on the IVF contents than does height reduction (−Y) from disc degeneration (**B**). **C,** Normal disc.

vertebral foramen. This close relationship is of significance when telescoping of the facet joints occurs during retrolisthesis (Fig. 2.28). The proximity to the IVF is also of importance when hypertrophy of the capsule or surrounding bone occurs.

The shapes of the facet joints vary considerably from one level to the next, and with the state of health of the joint. Differences in shape from one side of the same motion segment to the other are relatively common. This anomaly alters the normal functional aspects of the joint accordingly. Facet anomaly developed after birth may well be associated with asymmetrical development of the disc and vertebral body in response to unequal torsional stresses in early life (3). Radiographically evaluating vertebral positions in stressed postures must be accompanied by the appropriate analysis of the facet planes in the neutral position. Functional changes caused by anomaly must not be confused with interarticular dysfunction from soft tissue disturbance.

The zygapophyseal joints function mainly to guide and limit movement of the motion segment (15). They are not designed for the support of a significant percentage of weight in axial compression in the lumbar spine (2). The mid cervical spine has facets that support a greater proportion of the axial compressive load. The compressive loads of the cervical region are normally not relatively high. Because of the minimal strength of the region, compression injury of the cervical spine can take the form of fracture, partial and full dislocations, and severe soft tissue disruptions.

When the intervertebral disc is normal, gross injuries of the neural arch and facet joints are not seen (3). Computerized tomographic evidence of lumbar facet pathology has not been detected in the absence of degenerative changes at the disc, as evaluated with MRI (8). Abnormalities of the disc will lead to increased free motion at the facet joints. Compression fractures of the lamina of these joints are commonplace (3).

Disruption of a zygapophyseal joint follows a progressive pattern common to any diarthrodial joint. Early changes include synovitis with possible synovial folding between the joint. Interarticular adhesions occur as the degenerative process continues. With repeated strains, capsular laxity and osteophyte formation occur.

Degeneration commonly leads to positional dyskinesia, especially retrolisthesis (52). A gradual reduction in disc height, enlargement of the facets, and posterior displacement result in stenosis of the spinal canal and lateral recesses.

Aging and Degeneration

It is the opinion of Farfan (6) that aging and degenerative processes are not synonymous. His conclusion is based on the fact that many elderly and young joints behave similarly with regards to their mechanical properties. Degenerated joints, however, behave stiffer than normal articulations. An increase in stiffness in the joint is characteristic of scar formation. Scar formation only occurs after injury. The accumulation of effects from various traumas throughout an individual's life is most likely responsible for the changes in mechanical properties seen in many aged specimens.

Scar formation alters the mechanical properties of the joint, rendering it less able to withstand external loads which heightens the possibility of reinjury. A downward spiral of degenerative processes usually affects the joint. The more often it is reinjured and scarred, the more likely it will be injured again. This is one of the reasons there cannot be a 100% structural and functional recovery after injury to the three-joint complex.

With these considerations in mind, an adjustive maneuver directed into a joint should not compromise the soft tissue structures. This precaution will avoid injury and inflammation with subsequent scar formation. As restricted mobility in the three-joint complex is diminished, close monitoring of the joint with reliable methods of movement assessment is essential. The results of follow-up examinations will determine the need and frequency of adjustive procedures. There is no indication for adjusting or manipulating a normally functioning or hypermobile articulation.

The aim of chiropractic care of the degenerated joint is slightly different from that of care for one less deranged. Symptoms play a more critical role in determining the frequency of adjustments, because normalization of the functional or structural aspects of a degenerated joint is unlikely. The clinician should be cautious in attempting to reverse years of joint pathology.

Spine Ligaments

Spinal ligaments (e.g., PLL, supraspinous, ligamentum flavum, etc.) are uniaxial structures and are most effective in resisting loads in the direction in which the collagen fibers run. The interspinous ligament, for example, resists flexion of the spine much more effectively than axial rotation or shear forces.

During physiologic ranges of motion, very little force is required to move the motion segment because of the relatively low resistance provided by the various ligaments. This force becomes great, however, as the FSU approaches the trauma range. For the ligamentum flavum, approximately seven times more energy is absorbed in the trauma range compared to the physiological range (53). Thus, ligaments perform two quite contrasting functions:

1. To allow and guide smooth motion in the physiological range with a minimum of resistance and expenditure of energy from the organism, and
2. To absorb large quantities of energy near the trauma range thereby protecting the spinal cord during potentially traumatic situations.

As the ligaments reach the end of their elastic range they influence the position of the instantaneous axis of rotation for the FSU. This is especially true if pathologies exist such as adhesion formation or ligamentous laxity. Ligamentous injury will manifest itself as abnormal positions of the FSU when the segment is put through a particular motion. Alar or transverse ligament disruptions can be detected radiographically (cine or plain film) by moving the upper cervical spine in axial rotation (Y axis), lateral bending (Z axis) or flexion ($+\theta X$) (See Chapter 11). If the ligament stays within its physiologic range of motion, it will stretch and elastically recover during various movements, termed elastic deformation. If the ligament is stretched beyond its range of motion, it will recover to some extent but portions of it will remain stretched. This is known as plastic deformation. The amount of plastic deformation that takes place during a trauma is dependent, in large part, on the magnitude of the forces involved. Ligamentous injury also results in scar formation which reduces the content of elastic fibers in the structure. Less elasticity will tend to make the joint function abnormally and make it more prone to reinjury.

After experimental injury, it takes at least six weeks for a tendon to regain 80% of its tensile strength (54). The recovery time for a ligamentous injury is probably close to this value, depending on the blood supply in the region. This fact is important to consider in the management of the patient who may obtain rapid symptomatic improvement but has not functionally recovered enough to participate in rigorous activity, hard labor, or rehabilitative exercises. These activities may put a strain on ligaments not yet fully healed. Bed rest, however, is not indicated except in extreme circumstances. Passive movements and walking should be encouraged as a form of therapy. Movement during repair diminishes collagen cross-linking and allows scar tissue to be laid down along the stress points of the motion segment. The antigravity effect of walking in a pool may enable a patient to actively move various articulations, even if normal ambulation is impossible.

The role of stretching in spinal rehabilitation deserves some discussion. In the athlete where joint flexibility is requisite to performing a particular activity, flexible ligamentous and muscle elements are important. Athletes usually have well-developed musculature and it is the muscles that provide an important role in stability for the motion segments. When these individuals cease to participate in their particular sporting activities, their muscles atrophy, and more of a burden is placed on the ligaments. If their occupation involves sedentary ergonomics, creep of the ligaments could increase symptomatology. After an extremely flexible athlete (e.g., gymnast) has retired from sporting activities, it would be wise to avoid sedentary occupations. In contrast, the inflexible person will do much better in a more sedentary occupation. If this individual is placed in a job where large demands are made on the flexibility of the spine, there may be increased risk for injury. Stretching activities must therefore be implemented with regard to the demands placed on the individual's spine throughout the day. Stretching of chronically shortened ligaments and tendons caused by scarring and fixation dysfunction of the motion segment will be beneficial for the individual. Caution must be taken to avoid further stretching of ligaments that have undergone plastic deformation.

The Vertebrae

Landmark Identification. It is important to be aware of the various shapes of the vertebrae in a particular spinal region to enhance accuracy in locating the appropriate dysfunctional motion segment. Accuracy of vertebral count is critical in ensuring specificity of contact and force when applying manual therapy. Static palpation for determining motion segment location must be compared with the radiograph, because anomalies in the number of vertebrae often occurs. For example, there can be thirteen thoracic vertebrae or six lumbars, which if unknown, could lead to the application of a force at the wrong motion segment. Also, the shapes of the various spinous processes can vary from their "common appearance."

Because it is often difficult to palpate the mid-cervical spine, landmarks of the lower cervical spine are often used to determine the location of the dysfunctional motion segment in this region. The vertebral prominence is such a landmark but is not always the seventh cervical vertebra. In the past, a method whereby the cervical spine was extended hypothetically aided the practitioner in determining the C7 vertebra. It was said that the sixth cervical "tucks" on extension. The cervical spine does not "tuck." In fact, the sixth and all cervical vertebrae tip inferiorward ($-\theta X$) and often posteriorward (if disc damage is present) during extension movement. The palpator detects a disappearance of the bone under the fingertips when extending the cervical spine. This has led to the assumption that the vertebra is moving away during this movement. The ligamentum nuchae is actually buckling and bulging over the spinous processes, increasing the distance between fingertip and spinous process. If T1 is actually vertebral prominence and C7 is relatively small, then C7 may feel as if it is "tucking." A better, but by no means foolproof, method to determine the spinal levels, is to flex the cervical spine and determine the most prominent vertebra(e). Generally during flexion, C7 and T1 should have the most protuberant spinous processes. If in doubt, a flexion radiograph can be made of the cervical spine with a small radiopaque object attached to the skin over a boney protuberance. The physical count can then be considered in light of the radiograph.

It is a good rule to palpate at least twice when locating a vertebral segment, unless the count is unambiguous. When moving the patient from the sitting to a prone position, a point marked on the skin may move away from the vertebral location it is intended to identify. Usually the mark moves cephalad in the cervical and thoracic spine, but to ensure specificity, the spinous process can be contacted while the patient changes positions. This becomes more critical when the patient is difficult to palpate, such as in obesity. The use of the inferior border of the scapulae to determine vertebral location should be avoided because of its inherent inaccuracy.

Caution is advised when asking the patient to identify the offending motion segment while the doctor palpates. The most symptomatic spinous process may be a hypermobile motion segment which is contraindicated for a manipulation. Palpable tenderness is an important finding in isolating the VSC (See Chapter 4) but does not substitute for a comprehensive examination.

Trabeculae. The trabeculae of the vertebral body are arranged both vertically (columns) and horizontally (ties), much like the frame of a skyscraper (Fig. 2.29 A and B). The horizontal trabeculae effectively increase the compressive strength of the vertebral body. This can be explained by the engineering principle or theory of Euler (2). There is a gradual loss in the horizontal trabeculae and progressive thickening of the vertical trabeculae with age (55) (Fig. 2.30 A and B). A fifty percent reduction of the horizontal trabeculae will reduce the compressive strength of the bone to ¼ of its original value (56). Reduction in the cross sectional area of the vertical trabeculae will reduce the compressive strength as well. Trabecular loss and thinning occur in osteoporosis, making the bone susceptible to fracture.

It seems that the rate of bone loss with age is similar for both males and females. Women, however, seem to start this gradual loss with less bone than their male counterparts. Bone mineral content of lumbar vertebrae also correlates with the height and weight of the individual (57). This correlation is in agreement with the findings of Nilsson (58), who showed that the majority of femoral neck fractures occurred in slender women. Compressive strength of the vertebral body decreases considerably beyond the age of forty.

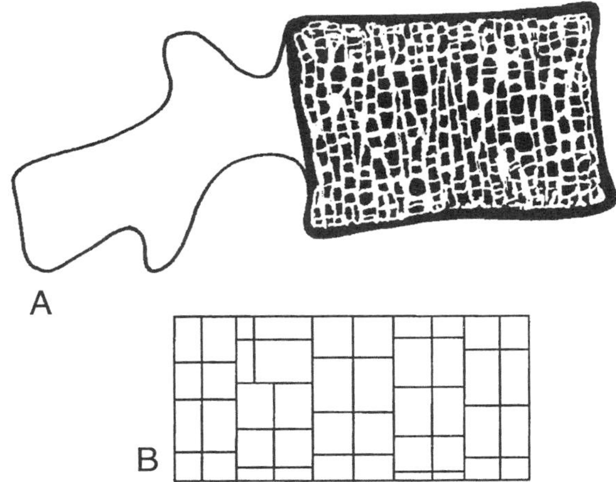

Figure 2.29A,B. The trabeculae of the vertebral body are arranged both vertically and horizontally.

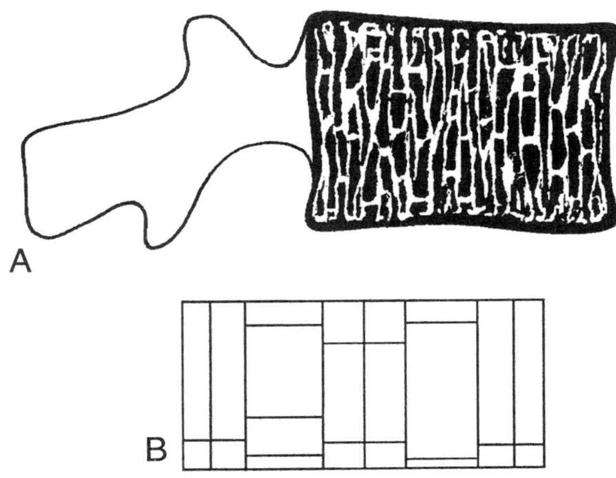

Figure 2.30A,B. With age and various disorders (e.g., osteoporosis), there is a gradual loss of both horizontal and vertical trabeculae thus weakening the structure.

Biomechanics. The intervertebral disc is *not* the shock absorber for the spine. Spinal shock absorption is provided to some extent by the sagittal curves (59) and primarily by a hydraulic mechanism of the vertebral body (6). During loading there is a collapse of the intertrabecular spaces. This collapse constrains the movement of the bone marrow thus providing a hydraulic cushion. The cancellous core of the vertebral body deforms approximately 9.5% before failing, compared with only 2% for the cortical shell (2). The disc, much stiffer than the vertebral body, will cause the end-plate/cortex to fail during compression overload.

The compression strength of the vertebral body increases caudally, in proportion to the progressive increase in axial compression loads (2). The center portion of the end-plate has the greatest compressive strength (60). This strength counters the increased pressure in the area by the nucleus pulposus. If compression overload occurs, however, the central portion will be the first to fail because of the concentrated amount of stress placed there. In degenerated discs, where the nucleus has dehydrated, compression loads are distributed more peripherally. In these patients, peripheral fractures of the end-plate or vertebral body are more common (2). The young are at more risk for developing nuclear invaginations of the end-plate or Schmorl's nodes, due to compressive overload. A well-hydrated nucleus pulposus will burst through the end-plate during loading. If a fracture is characteristic of an injury that occurred when the nucleus was well hydrated (e.g., central end-plate depression), it is often the case that the injury occurred when the individual was younger. A fracture of the periphery of the vertebral body usually means that more load was transferred through the annulus which often occurs when there is dehydration of the nucleus. There is a tendency towards dehydration of the nucleus as one ages.

Because bone is a dynamic tissue, it will readily adapt to a changing environment. Bone remodeling from mechanical stress (Wolff's Law) is an example of adaptation. The effects of gravitational stress on the posture of the spine is an important argument for attempting to maintain the sagittal curves of the spinal column. In the cervical spine, for example, a kyphotic cervical curve will place more compressive stress on the anterior vertebral bodies. The increased load will cause their normal box-like shape to become deformed, creating a protuberance at the anterior (Fig. 2.31).

Bone compensation caused by alterations in the mobility of the FSU can be detected radiographically. The appearance of a traction osteophyte (Fig. 2.32) at the ante-

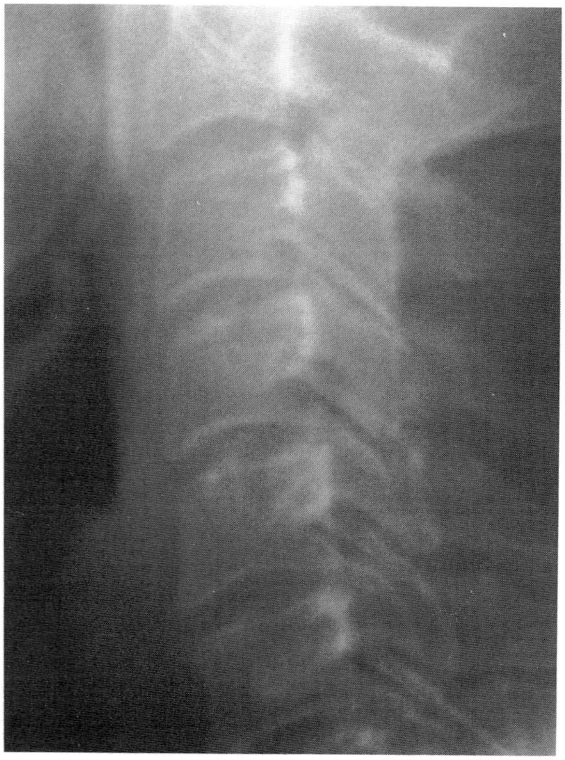

Figure 2.31. The lateral cervical radiograph demonstrates bone remodeling of the anterior portion of the vertebral bodies due to abnormal stresses in this individual with a hypolordotic cervical spine.

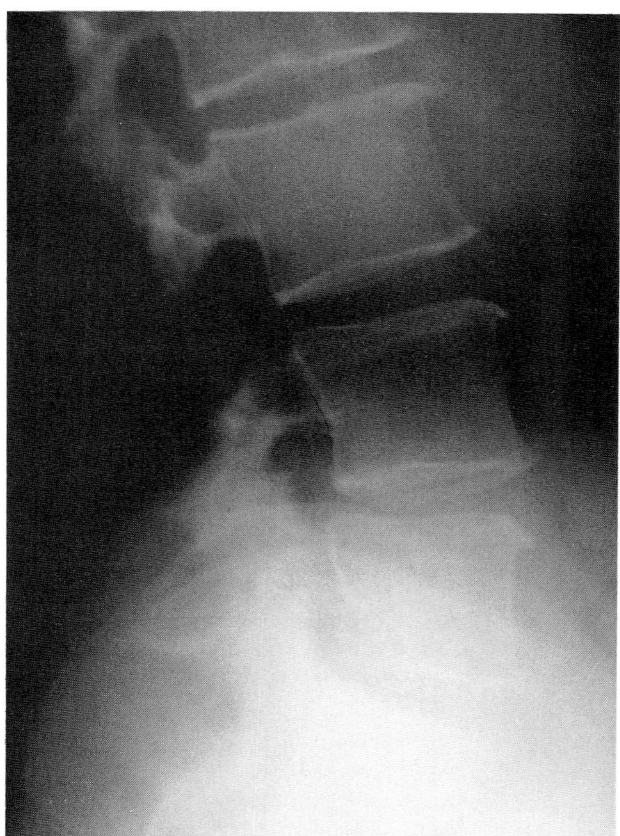

Figure 2.32. Anterior traction osteophytes caused by hypermobility at the motion segment. There is a degenerative spondylolisthesis at L4.

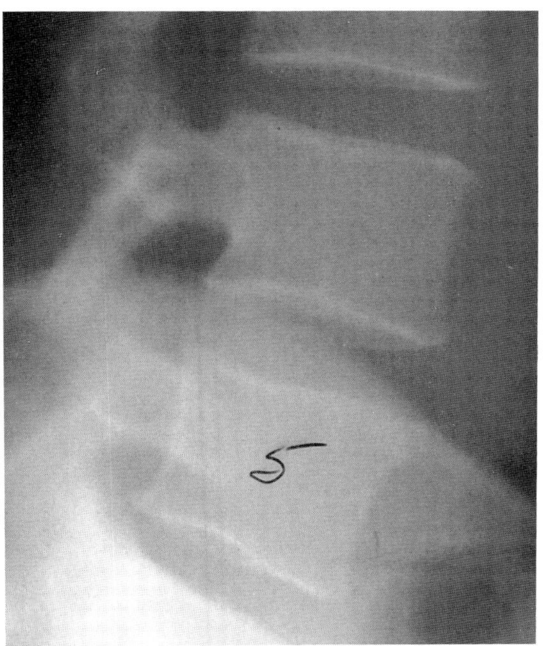

Figure 2.33. The radiograph shows the effect of an acutely swollen disc (D1) on the L4-L5 intervertebral joint space.

rior or posterior portion of the vertebral body may imply increased tractional forces at the annulus and longitudinal ligaments because of hypermobility or instability.

Radiographic Disc Evaluation

An evaluation of the disc space height on the lateral radiograph has led to a numerical classification system of the stages of disc swelling through degeneration (61). A widened disc space appearance on the lateral film, correlated with the clinical picture, may be due to an increased fluid uptake within the disc and is designated as a D1 disc (Fig. 2.33). The remainder of the classification scheme is reserved for progressive stages of the degenerative process.

When the disc space height begins to decrease, most of the diminishment in size occurs posterior to the nucleus because of previous injury at the annulus. This is true primarily of the cervical and lumbar regions. Degeneration of the thoracic motion segments is presented in Chapter 8. In lumbar spine injury, 90% of the damage is posterior to the nucleus. The first stage of disc degeneration is called a D2 disc and shows a small decrease in the posterior aspect of the disc space with a concomitant slight posteriority (retrolisthesis) of the vertebral body (Fig. 2.34). Because of the angulation of the facet joints and the diminishment of the posterior disc, the vertebral body shows a slight inferiorward tipping ($-\theta X$).

As the creep properties of the deranged joint continue, the disc height diminishes and the positional dyskinesia increases. There is a tendency towards greater malalignment of the FSU in the geriatric, due entirely to the degenerative process. The D3 disc is very thin at the posterior

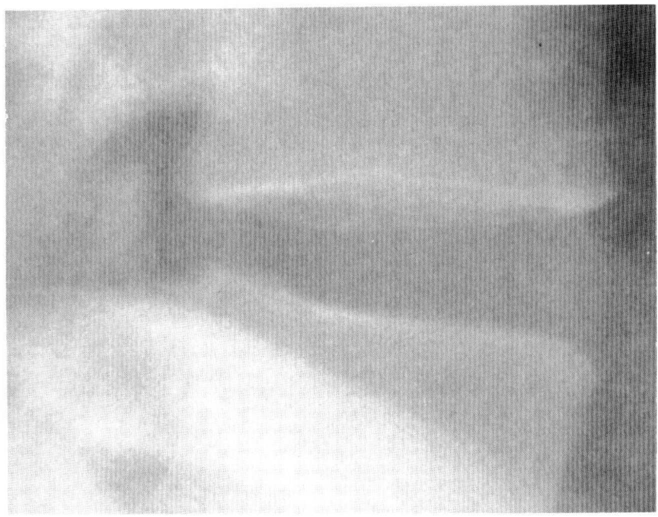

Figure 2.34. The radiographic appearance of a D2 disc.

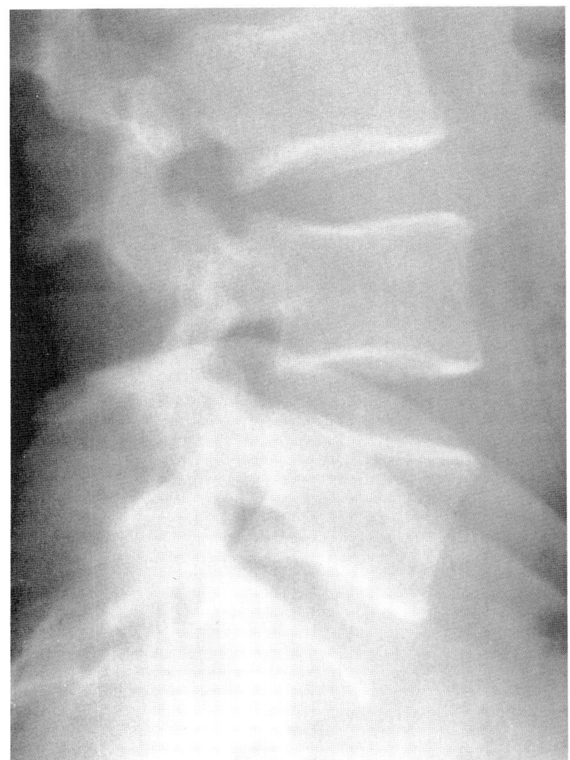

Figure 2.35. The radiographic appearance of a D3 disc at L5-S1.

with very little change occurring at the anterior portion of the disc (Fig. 2.35).

As the destructive processes in the disc continue, the anterior portion becomes progressively more involved. The early stage of total disc thinning is classified as a D4. Here, the dimensions of the disc have been reduced to approximately two-thirds of the original height (Fig. 2.36). Disc narrowing can cause the zygapophyseal joints to carry up to 70% of the intervertebral load. This will

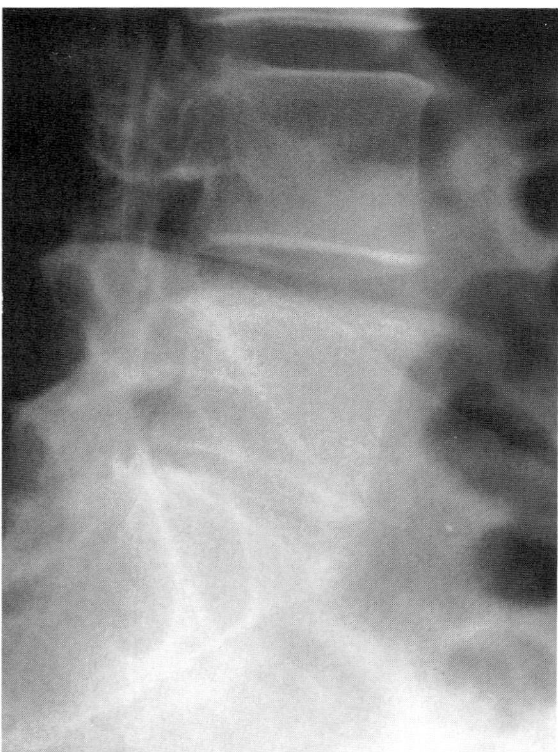

Figure 2.36. The radiographic appearance of a D4 disc at L5-S1.

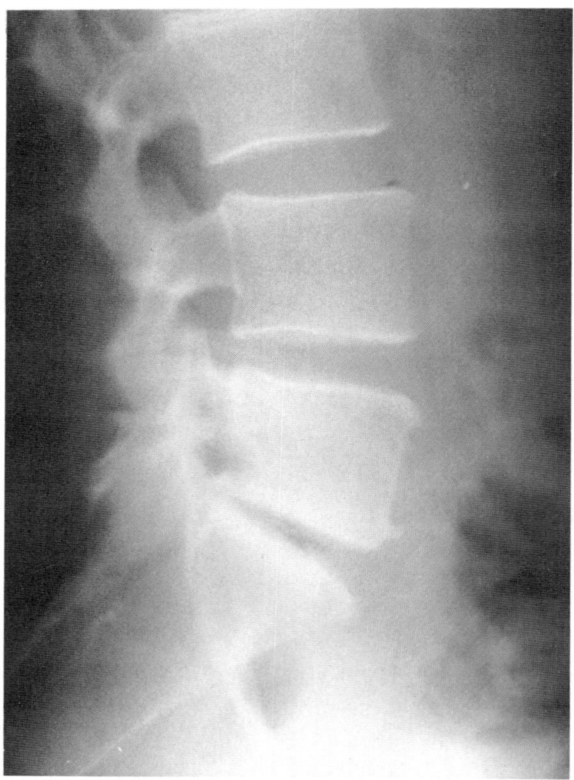

Figure 2.37. The radiographic appearance of a D5 disc at L5-S1. Notice the presence of the vacuum phenomenon, indicative of severe internal disc disruption.

then lead to secondary osteoarthritic changes occurring within the hyaline articular cartilage (62).

A D5 disc shows the space reduced to ⅛ of its original height (Fig. 2.37). Depending on the extent of injury and reinjury, a D5 disc shows up from 5 to 20 years after the initial trauma. The development of a D5 disc within five years of injury would signify enormous trauma to the motion segment or disc surgery such as chemonucleolysis (chymopapain injection).

When the disc is nearly gone and the vertebral bodies are about to undergo natural fusion, this is termed a D6 disc (Fig. 2.38). The greater the extent of degeneration, the more prolonged the care and the worse the prognosis for alleviation of objective findings. At some stage, however, symptomatology will gradually diminish. This is likely caused by the lessened amount of tissue able to become inflamed, provided the individual is relatively sedentary. Individuals with degenerative joint disease usually have reduced functional capacities. For example, range of motion can be markedly reduced, depending on the extent of degeneration. The D6 disc holds the worse prognosis and the D2 or D1 disc, the more favorable. Knowledge of the classification scheme is helpful when conferring with another doctor about a patient.

Coordinate System

The right-handed orthogonal coordinate system (RHOCS) is used for communication of the kinematic aspects of the spinal column (63,64). Vertebral position and movement can be accurately and unambiguously described with this listing system for all six degrees of freedom of the motion segment. Because the RHOCS has been proposed as an international standard for defining body parts, it will be referred to as the "international system" (65). This system should be the primary method of communication for the various configurations and movements of the motion segment and should be adopted by the chiropractic profession (65–67). Continuation of multiple, sometimes arbitrary listing systems leads to confusion in the student and among practitioners, especially when referral of a patient is required.

By convention, the listing of movement or position of the motion segment is with respect to the vertebra below (2). This is an important point to consider, especially when we present the kinematics and subluxation complexes of the upper cervical region. This is in contrast to many "upper cervical" listing schemes that list the atlas with respect to the occiput.

The X axis runs from the center of the motion segment straight left (+X) or right (−X). The Z axis runs from the posterior (−Z), to the anterior (+Z) through the X axis, whereas the Y axis, which is also referred to as the longitudinal axis, runs in a caudal (−Y) cephalad (+Y) direction. Rotation clockwise ($+\theta$), or counterclockwise

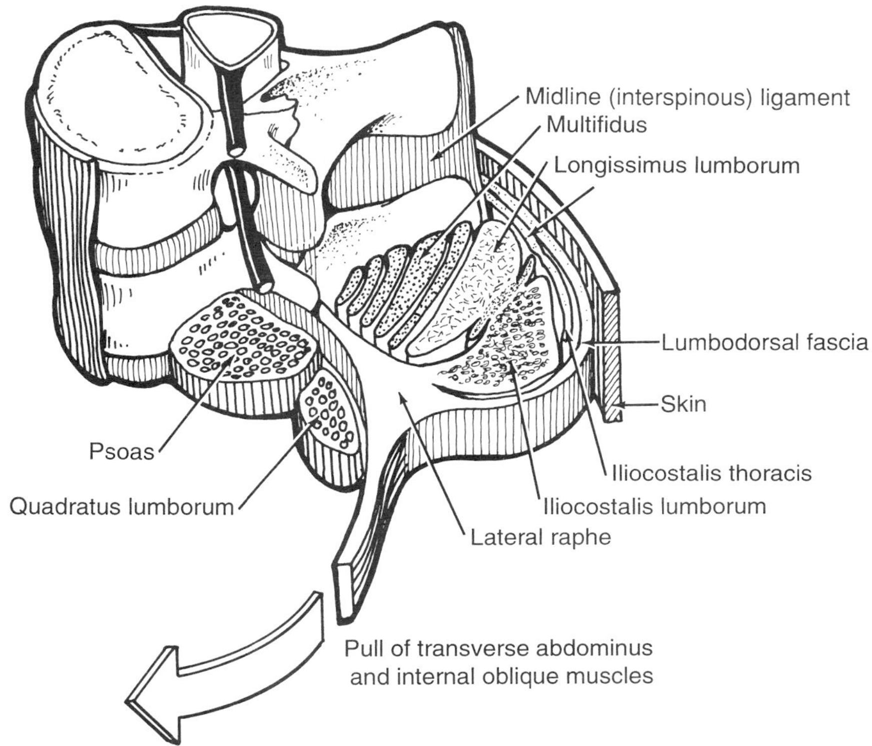

Figure 2.59. The anatomy of the lumbar spine and pull of the lumdodorsal fascia by the transverse abdominus and internal oblique muscles. Modified from Gracovetsky S. The spinal engine. Wien: Springer-Verlag, 1988:98.

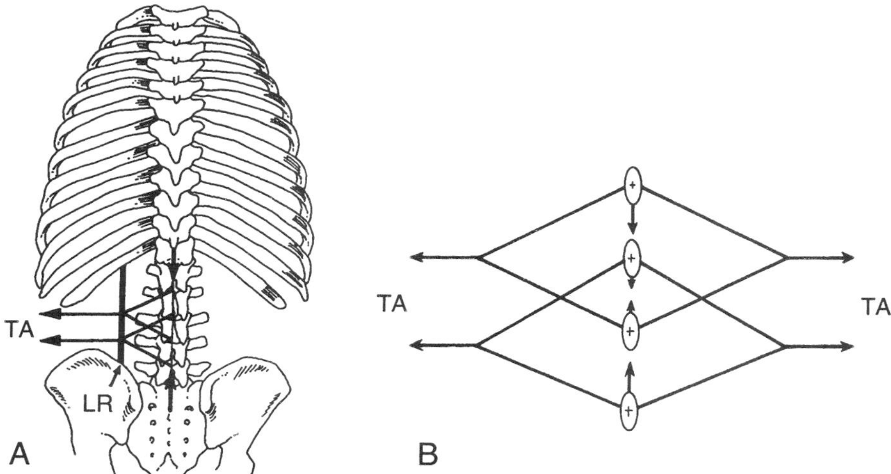

Figure 2.60. Contraction of the transverse abdominus and internal oblique muscles provides a lateralward pull on the lumbodorsal fascia (**A**), thus exerting an extensor moment on the lumbar spine (**B**). Modified from Gracovetsky S. Function of the spine. J Biomed Eng 1986;6:217–223.

during forward flexion because of this effect. This occurs only in the presence of disc injury, where the restraining elements of the annulus to posterior shear are weakened. The posteriorward pull of the fascia will counteract the increased anterior shear force that occurs as the sacral base angle increases during forward bending. If a large spinous process is present (Fig. 2.63B), the pull will change to an anterior shear force during forward bending. Interestingly, individuals with spondylolisthesis of L5 usually have a large spinous process at that level. The ineffectiveness of the fascia in creating a posterior shear force to counter the anterior shear could be one of the mechanisms in the development of a fatigue fracture of the pars interarticularis in these individuals.

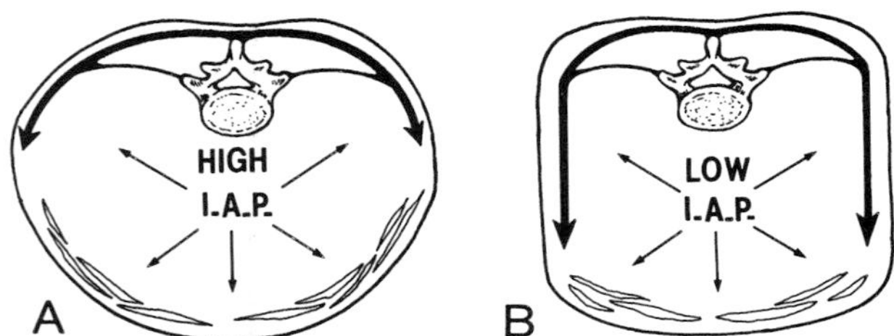

Figure 2.61. Pressurization of the abdominal cavity facilitates the lift by optimizing the pull of the LDF. Modified from Gracovetsky S. The spinal engine. Wien: Springer-Verlag, 1988:114.

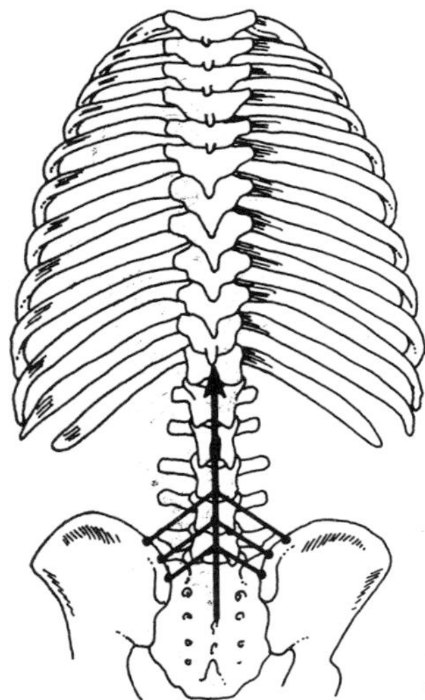

Figure 2.62. Attachment sites of the lumbodorsal fascia at the iliac crests enables it to passively raise the spinal column during contraction of the powerful hip extensors. Modified from Gracovetsky S. The spinal engine. Wien: Springer-Verlag, 1988:95.

Midline Ligaments

The midline ligaments consist of the supraspinous, interspinous, facet capsules, ligamentum flavum and the posterior annulus. These ligaments exert an extension bending moment when the lumbar spine is flexed. Because the amount of resistance increases with progressive forward flexion they are termed posture dependent, and are passive in their contribution to the lift. They also have time dependent characteristics such as creep. The ligaments' contribution is minimized if the subject lifts too slowly because creep of the ligaments will reduce the amount of force that is generated by these structures.

Muscles

Muscles provide stability for the spinal column in three ways:

1. The powerful hip extensors such as gluteus maximus are used primarily in duties requiring heavy exertion;

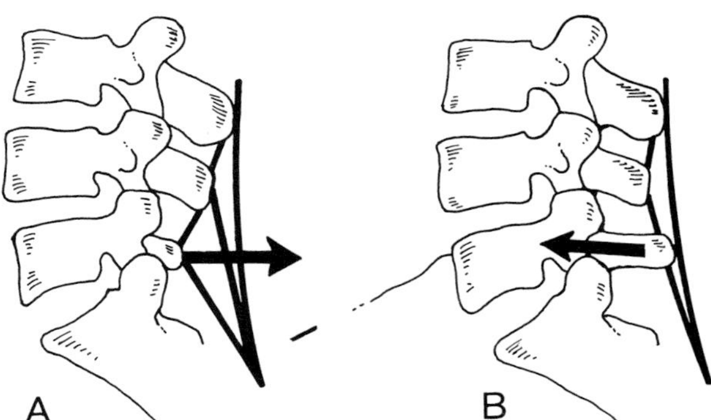

Figure 2.63. **A,** Posterior pull of the lumbodorsal fascia (small spinous process). **B,** Anterior pull of the lumbodorsal fascia (large spinous process). Modified from Gracovetsky S. The spinal engine. Wien: Springer-Verlag, 1988:108.

2. The paraspinal musculature is used for lighter tasks; and
3. The abdominal muscles are used for integrating the ligamentous system with the muscular system and adjusting the entire complex to the particular task at hand (76).

Figures 2.64 and 2.65 illustrate the integration of the ligamentous and muscular systems during the lift and free fall. As can be seen, the erector spinae are relatively inactive during the lower position of the lift, in contrast to the hip extensors that are very active (93).

The "danger point" is defined as the crossover point where the individual is going from a predominantly muscular to a ligamentous strategy or visa versa. This portion of the lift must be executed with great care.

The uneven distribution of stress that occurs when an individual uses a muscle strategy during a lift results in the highest stresses at the L3-L4 intervertebral joint (76). This corresponds to the finding that Schmorl's nodes occur with the highest frequency in the L3 vertebral body endplates (3). Figure 2.66 demonstrates integration of the muscular and ligamentous systems during backpacking.

Creep

It is important to execute a substantial lift at speed due to the creep properties of the LDF and midline ligaments. Their contribution to the lift is minimized if the subject remains in a flexed posture before initiating the lift. Rapid acceleration during the lift should be avoided, however, because this would increase the overall force required (F = MA).

Pathomechanics

The relaxation phenomenon is observed when the lumbar spine and pelvis are forwardly flexed to horizontal. In this position, the paraspinal muscles become inactive as evaluated by EMG. Freefall is prevented because of the tension in the midline ligaments and the lumbodorsal fascia.

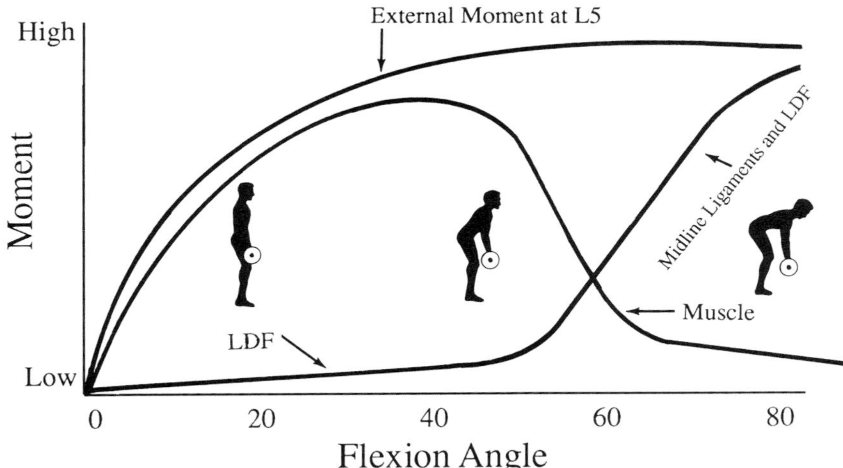

Figure 2.64. The distribution of forces developed in the ligamentous and muscular systems for a lift with a small external load. Activity of the hip extensors is not depicted. Their contribution would be relatively great during the early portion of the lift. Modified from Gracovetsky S. Function of the spine. J Biomed Eng 1986;8:220.

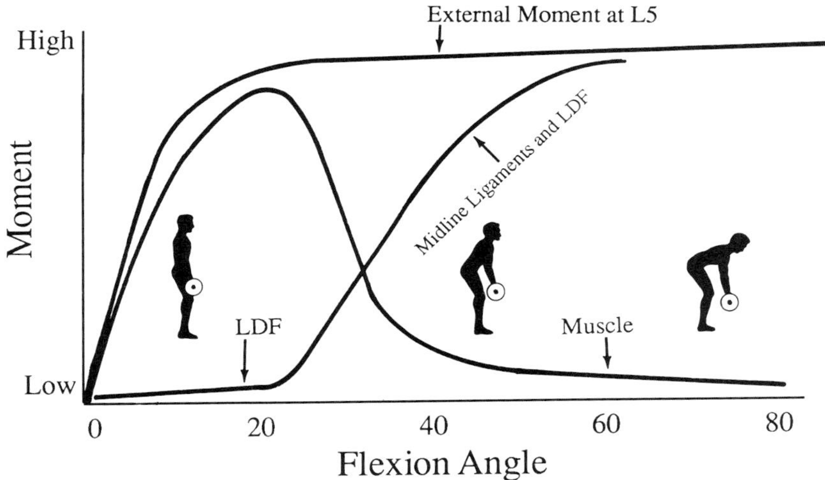

Figure 2.65 The distribution of forces developed in the muscular and ligamentous systems during a substantial lift. Notice the engagement of the ligamentous elements earlier in the lift. Activity of the hip extensors is not depicted. Modified from Gracovetsky S. Function of the spine. J Biomed Eng 1986;8:220.

The relaxation phenomenon also exists on maximal lateral bend (94). It is easy to see why many lumbar spine injuries occur with the spine flexed forward and laterally bent. In this posture, the ligaments take the majority of any load applied; this usually leads to failure of the system. The combined movement of flexion with axial rotation poses the greatest threat to the integrity of collagen fibers in the annulus fibrosis (3,13).

The individual should always avoid asymmetrically loading the spine because this seems to be a common injury mechanism (Fig. 2.67). Even if the lift is executed with good posture, overload situations do occur. Often, previous injury or asymmetrical motion at the FSU will precipitate injury in an otherwise benign environment. Lifting too much weight or executing the lift at too great a speed can lead to injury. The central nervous system seems to have an innate mechanism that minimizes many potential overload situations.

Fail-Safe Mechanism

Mathematical modeling of the spine has determined that the maximal lift a person should be able to accomplish is roughly one-third greater than the maximal recorded effort in vivo. It is interesting to note that the relative strengths of muscle, ligament and bone are stressed equally as they approach their ultimate strength. Apparently, the organism senses impending injury and shuts

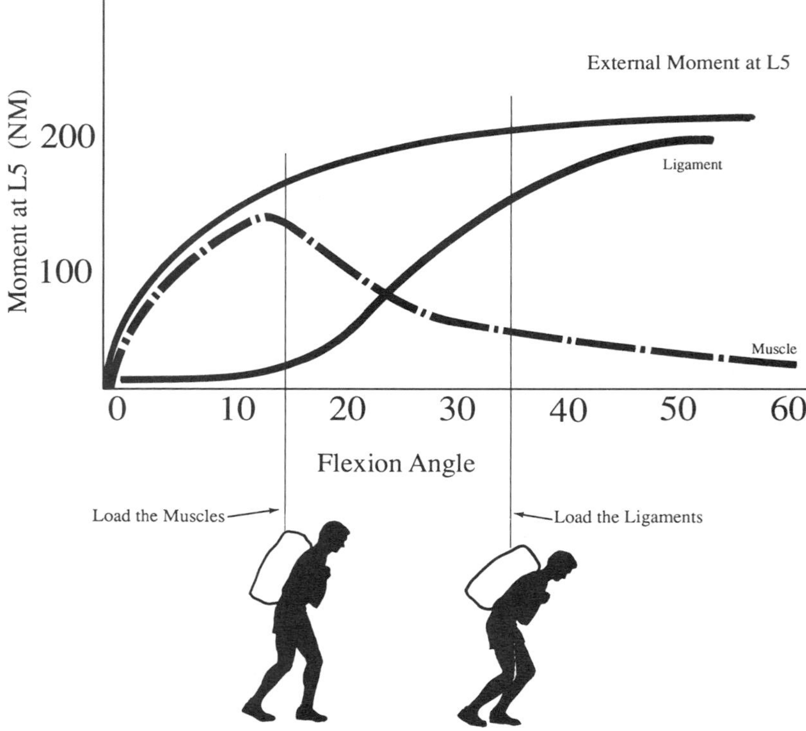

Figure 2.66. During backpacking or other activities, the individual can alternately increase and decrease the lordosis, switching from a muscle-predominant to a ligament-predominant strategy. By performing this alternating pattern it is possible to avoid loading either structure continuously, thus reducing the likelihood of fatigue. Modified from Gracovetsky S. The spinal engine. Wien: Springer-Verlag, 1988:155.

down, by refusing or aborting the task. Gracovetsky has termed this the "fail-safe mechanism" (36).

BIOMECHANICS OF THE SPINAL ADJUSTMENT

If one were to drop an object of one kilogram from a height of one meter it would exert less force on impact than if it were dropped from a height of two meters. Although both objects accelerate equally during freefall caused by gravity, and the masses of both objects are equal, the forces they exert on impact are not. The second object accelerates for a longer period of time, therefore increasing its instantaneous velocity when impact finally occurs. A greater impact velocity requires a greater rate of deceleration, assuming equal deceleration times for both objects. The force of impact is equal to the acceleration, in actuality a deceleration, multiplied by the mass of the object ($F = ma$).

The force received by a patient during an adjustment represents the mass of the doctor while decelerating after impact with the patient. Haas (95) states that the adjustment can be broken up into a two phase acceleration-deceleration process. In the acceleration or thrust phase, the product of the doctor's mass and acceleration of the adjustive thrust yields the force employed by the doctor to reach the desired impact velocity. In the deceleration or impact phase, the doctor's mass multiplied by the deceleration quantifies the actual adjustive force produced by the doctor-patient collision.

Several other factors are at work in determining how much force the patient receives. The tissue overlying the doctor's contact point (e.g., pisiform) as well as over the contact point of the patient (e.g., mamillary process), will contribute to the overall equation. The more soft tissue, the greater the dissipation of force and a slower transference of energy from the doctor to the patient (96,97). The doctor attempting a specific adjustment should use doctor and patient contact points that minimize this force dampening effect, while allowing adequate comfort for the patient. For specificity, the pisiform contact is often preferred to the thenar eminence, and adjustments using the spinous process of the lumbar spine, are preferred to transverse (L5 only) process and mamillary process contacts. In patients where much tissue lies between the skin contact point and the actual segment (as in the obese, where a mamillary contact is needed), a greater amount of force is generally required, all other factors being equal. This may come at a sacrifice of specificity and patient comfort in some cases.

The patient-doctor contact point area is also important in the determination of the amount of force the patient receives. A broader contact on the vertebra will

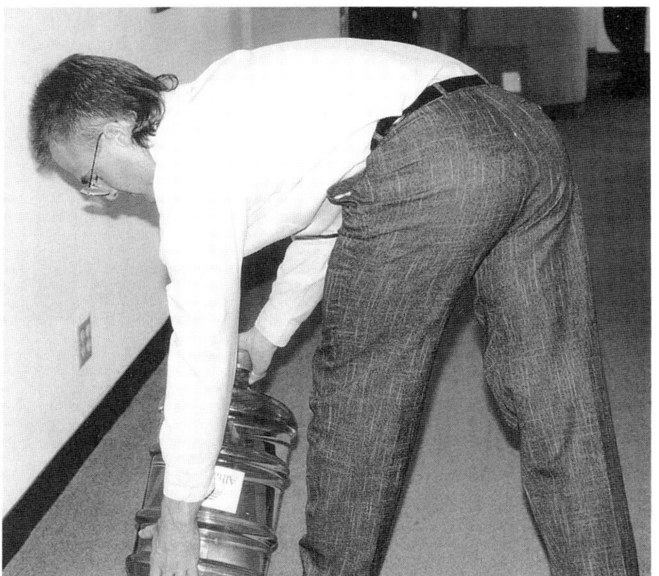

Figure 2.67. The pathomechanics of lumbar spine injury.

dissipate the force over a larger area, some of which will not be acting to produce the desired bone or joint movement. It is critical for the doctor to have as specific a contact as possible and direct that force through a combination of the center of mass of the vertebra and the plane lines of the three-joint complex. The use of broader and less specific contacts (such as in long lever manipulations) will often more easily cavitate a joint. Joint cavitation is not the ultimate goal, although it does occur with a successful adjustment. Inexperienced practitioners, without proper instruction, will assume that when a "crack" is elicited, a successful adjustment has taken place. When a thrust is attempted and no movement occurs, this is rationalized as "it didn't need to go." There are more rational means for determining where and how to thrust into a patient's spine.

The specificity of the adjustment, and applying it to a motion segment that needs it, is one key to limiting variables and predicting outcomes for the patient, and should not be lightly discarded as unimportant. The art of specific adjusting can be frustrating to learn at times. Understanding the biomechanics of the spine and the various pathological entities that affect it will facilitate the learning process.

Force Measurements

Peak force for low back adjustments is generally greater for experienced doctors than inexperienced adjusters (98). Greater grip strength, height, and weight were generally correlated with increased peak force for low back simulator adjustments (99). Wood and Adams (100) reported average force values of approximately 255 Newtons (57 lbs) for simulator posterior ilium adjustments in the prone position which is similar to values obtained on actual patients by Hessell et al. (101) using the Thompson technique.

Herzog (102) found there was a wide variation between chiropractors, and for the same chiropractor, for the peak forces used for sacroiliac adjustments. The point of application of the treatment force was applied as much as five centimeters away from the desired contact point; pretension forces and peak treatment forces were found to be positively related. Wood and Adams (100) detected slightly lower forces using the Thompson technique for simulator adjustments of the lumbar spine when compared to sacroiliac adjustments.

Herzog et al. (103) determined the forces used during a thoracic adjustment. A hypothenar contact on the transverse process of T4 was followed by a posterior to anterior thrust and the forces developed were then recorded. The preload force was approximately 150 N (34 lbs). The preload was then followed by a rapid thrust that reached a peak value of approximately 380 N (85 lbs) at 113 msec. Greater preload and greater peak force were seen with the thoracic adjustment when compared to the ilium adjustment using the Thompson technique.

Manual adjustments of the cervical spine seem to have much less force than for either the thoracic spine or the sacroiliac joint (104). There is also some evidence that cervical adjustments are applied twice as fast as those applied to the T4 area or to the sacroiliac joints (103).

Manual vs. Instrument Procedures

Advocates of instrument adjusting cite the relative safety of a reproducible, very controlled, predetermined force (105). Indeed, many of these advocates (106) see no situation where a manual contact procedure would be superior to an instrument. One instrument, the Activator Adjusting Instrument (AAI), has undergone some rather rigorous experimental testing with a laboratory animal. Piezoelectric accelerometers were attached to the bone of an anesthetized dog. Small, relative 1-mm translations and 0.5-degree rotations occurred during the first 19 msec after percussive thrusts at the L2-L3 motion segment (107).

There are several parameters of the adjustive process that instruments do not address. The first involves the direction of thrust. Whereas instruments are confined to a predetermined line of drive, a manual contact procedure can actually change the vector of application during the process of bone movement. To move a C7 vertebrae from a fixated extended position to a neutral or flexed position, it is necessary to gradually change the direction of thrust to accommodate the pattern of motion of the vertebra. This can be termed the "pattern of thrust." As can be seen in Figure 2.68, the pattern of thrust for a C2 vertebra has a much flatter arc than that of C4 or C7. This is due primarily to the facet angles, which are more ver-

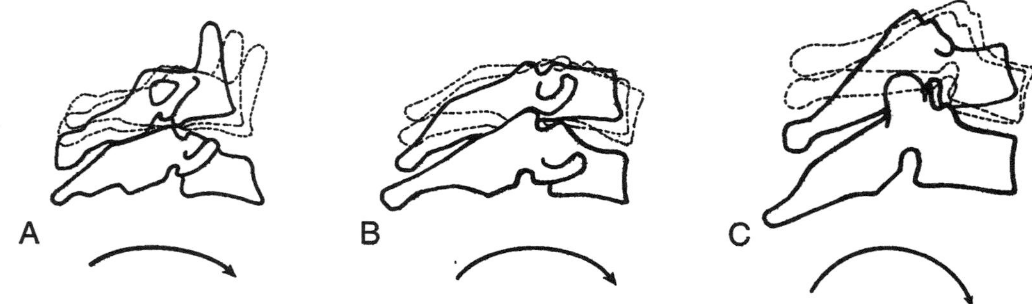

Figure 2.68A-C. Pattern of thrusts for upper cervical (C2), mid (C4) and lower cervical (C7) motion segments.

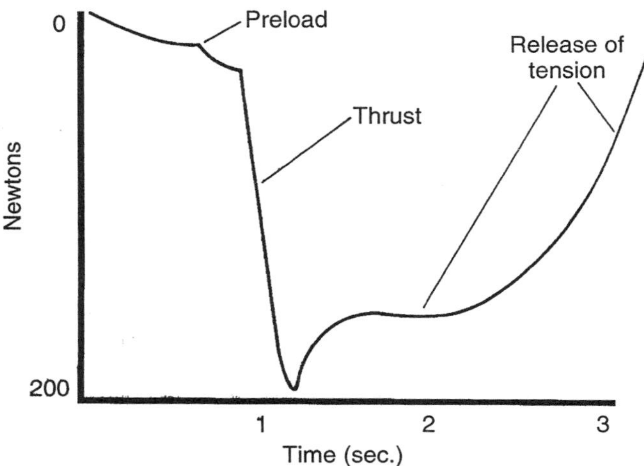

Figure 2.69. A qualitative analysis of a set-hold type of adjustment.

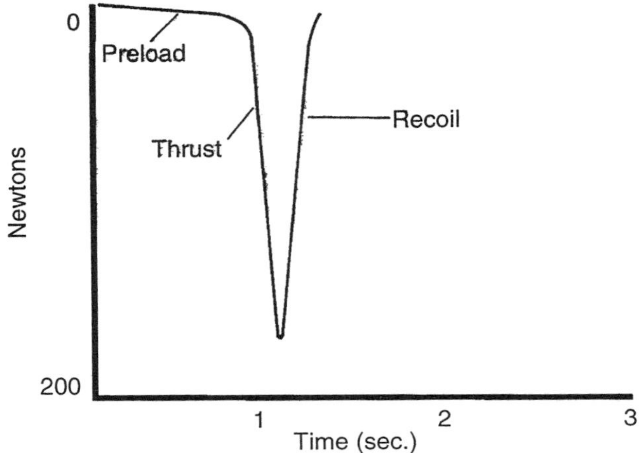

Figure 2.70. A qualitative analysis of a toggle-recoil adjustment.

tical in the lower cervical spine. The application of torque or screw motion towards the end of the thrust also cannot be performed with the typical adjusting instruments.

Another situation where manual adjusting procedures are preferred lies in the duration of thrust. The general approach advocated here for spinal adjustments, is to apply the force in the specified pattern of motion, and "hold" the segment contacted for 1–2 sec after the thrust. The force should then be gradually released after the thrust (Fig. 2.69) (66). In contrast, a toggle-recoil adjustment involves a rapid release of tension after the thrust (Fig. 2.70).

The "holding" after the thrust is an attempt to affect the viscoelastic tissues with a more lengthy time component, thereby increasing the effectiveness of the adjustment on these elements. It is known that viscoelastic tissues respond by lengthening to loads applied over long time durations. An adjusting instrument cannot affect the motion segment in this way.

All spines have somewhat different functional characteristics, which prohibit broad generalizations on the characteristics of an adjustment. The geriatric patient, or the patient with a severely degenerated motion segment, is adjusted much differently (i.e. generally with less amplitude) than a pediatric or young adult. Two people of similar morphological characteristics may require vastly different preloading, set-up time, relaxation, and force needed for a successful adjustment. Manual contacts help the doctor "feel" the patient's tolerances and adjustment needs. This feedback is then used to make the next adjustment even more comfortable than the last.

Another difference between manual and instrument adjusting lies in the fact that instrument adjusting almost never results in cavitation of the articulation. This cavitation appears to increase, at least temporarily, the range of motion of the articulation.

The foregoing theoretical arguments regarding the superiority of hand versus instrument adjusting await clinical trials using various outcome measures (e.g., patient function, spine function, neurological function, etc), to determine the most effective methods for reducing vertebral dysfunction.

REFERENCES

1. Brieg A. Adverse mechanical tension in the central nervous system. Stockholm: Almqvist & Wiksell International, 1978.
2. White AA, Panjabi MM. Clinical biomechanics of the spine. 2nd ed. Philadelphia: J.B. Lippincott Co., 1990.

3. Farfan HF. Mechanical disorders of the low back. Philadelphia: Lea & Febiger, 1973.
4. Panjabi MM, Krag MH, Chung TQ. Effects of disc injury on mechanical behavior of the human spine. Spine 1984; 9:707–713.
5. Virgin W. Experimental investigations into physical properties of intervertebral disc. J Bone Joint Surg 1951; 33B:607–611.
6. Farfan HF. Biomechanics of the lumbar spine. In: Kirkaldy-Willis WH, ed. Managing low back pain. New York: Churchill Livingstone, 1983:9–21.
7. Cossette JW, Farfan HF, Robertson GH, Wells RV. The instantaneous center of rotation of the third lumbar intervertebral joint. J Biomech 1971; 4:149–153.
8. Butler D, Trafimow JH, Andersson GBJ, McNeil TW, Hockman MS. Discs degenerate before facets. Spine 1990; 15:111–13.
9. Williams PL, Warwick R, eds. Gray's anatomy. 36th British ed. Philadelphia: W. B. Saunders, 1980.
10. Marchand F, Ahmed AM. Investigation of the laminate structure of lumbar disc anulus fibrosus. Spine 1990; 15:402–410.
11. Galante JO. Tensile properties of the human lumbar annulus fibrosis. Acta Orthopaedica Scand 1967; suppl. 100.
12. Brown T, Hanson R, Yorra A. Some mechanical tests on the lumbo-sacral spine with particular reference to the intervertebral discs: a preliminary report. J Bone Joint Surg 1957; 39A:1135–1164.
13. Pearcy MJ. Inferred strains in the intervertebral discs during physiological movements. J Manual Med 1990;5:68–71.
14. Stedman TL. Stedman's medical dictionary. 25th ed. Baltimore: Williams & Wilkins, 1990.
15. Kapandji I. The physiology of the joints. Vol. 3. New York: Churchill Livingstone, 1974.
16. Grieve GP. Common vertebral joint problems. New York: Churchill-Livingstone, 1981:504–505.
17. Greenstein GM, Summers DJ. Biomechanics. In: Lawrence DJ, ed. Fundamentals of chiropractic diagnosis and management. Baltimore: Williams & Wilkins, 1990:24.
18. Bogduk N, Twomey LT. Clinical anatomy of the lumbar spine. New York: Churchill-Livingstone, 1987.
19. Kurowski P, Kubo A. The relationship of degeneration of the intervertebral disc to mechanical loading conditions on lumbar vertebrae. Spine 1986;11:726–731.
20. Taylor JR. The development and adult structure of lumbar intervertebral discs. J Manual Med 1990;5:43–47.
21. Horne J, Cockshott WP, Shannon HS. Spinal column damage from water ski jumping. Skeletal Radiol 1987;16:612–16.
22. Sward L, Hellstrom M, Jacobsson B, Nyman R, Peterson L. Disc degeneration and associated abnormalities of the spine in elite gymnasts: a magnetic resonance imaging study. Spine 1991;16:437–443.
23. Jackson DW, Wiltse LL, Cirincione RJ. Spondylolysis in the female gymnast. Clin Orthop 1976;117:68–73.
24. Sward L, Hellstrom M, Jacobsson B, Peterson L. Back pain and radiologic changes in the thoraco-lumbar spine of athletes. Spine 1990;15:124–129.
25. Ferguson RJ, McMaster JH, Stanitski CL. Low back pain in college football linemen. J Sports Med 1974;2:63–69.
26. Granhed H, Morelli B. Low back pain among retired wrestlers and heavy-weight lifters. Am J Sports Med 1988;16:530–533.
27. Krag MH, Seroussi RE, Wilder DG, Pope MH. Internal displacement distribution from in vitro loading of human thoracic and lumbar spinal motion segments: experimental results and theoretical predictions. Spine 1987;12:1001–1007.
28. Naylor A. Intervertebral disc prolapse and degeneration; the biochemical and biophysical approach. Spine 1976;1:108–114.
29. Porter RW, Trailescu IF. Diurnal changes in straight leg raising. Spine 1990;15:103–106.
30. Adams MA, Dolan P, Hutton WC. Diurnal variations in the stresses on the lumbar spine. Spine 1987;12:130–37.
31. Brown MD, Tsaltas TT. Studies on the permeability of the intervertebral disc during skeletal maturation. Spine 1976;1:240–244.
32. Bernick S, Cailliet R. Vertebral end-plate changes with aging of human vertebrae. Spine 1982;7:97–102.
33. Roberts S, Menage J, Urban JPG. Biochemical and structural properties of the cartilage end-plate and its relation to the intervertebral disc. Spine 1989;14:166–173.
34. Kulak RF, Belytschko TB, Schultz AB, Galante JO. Nonlinear behavior of the human intervertebral disc under axial load. J Biomech 1976;9:377–386.
35. Nachemson A. The load on lumbar discs in different positions of the body. Clin Orthop 1966;45:107–122.
36. Gracovetsky S. The spinal engine. Wien: Springer-Verlag, 1988.
37. Chow DHK, Luk KDK, Leong JCY, Woo CW. Torsional stability of the lumbosacral junction: significance of the iliolumbar ligament. Spine 1989;14:611–615.
38. Singer KP, Giles LGF. Manual therapy considerations at the thoracolumbar junction: an anatomical and functional perspective. J Manipulative Physiol Ther 1990;13:83–88.
39. Farfan HF, Cossette JW, Robertson GH, Wells RV, Kraus H. The effects of torsion on the lumbar intervertebral joints: the role of torsion in the production of disc degeneration. J Bone Joint Surg 1970;52A:468–497.
40. Markolf KL, Morris JM. The structural components of the intervertebral disc. J Bone Joint Surg 1974;56A:675–87.
41. Moroney SP, Schultz AB, Miller JAA, Andersson GBJ. Load-displacement properties of lower cervical spine motion segments. J Biomech 1988;21:769–779.
42. Liu YK, Ray G, Hirsch C. The resistance of the lumbar spine to direct shear. Orthop Clin North Am 1975;6:33–48.
43. Henson J, McCall IW, O'Brien JP. Disc damage above a spondylolisthesis. Br J Radiol 1987;60:69–72.
44. Sullivan A, McGill SM. Changes in spine length during and after seated whole-body vibration. Spine 1990;15:1257–1260.
45. Kazarian LE. Creep characteristics of the human spinal column. Orthop Clin North Am 1975;6:3–19.
46. Sandover J. Dynamic loading as a possible source of low-back disorders. Spine 1983;8:652–658.
47. Kelsey JL, Hardy RJ. Driving of motor vehicles as a risk factor for acute herniated intervertebral disc. Am J Epidemiol 1975;102:63–73.
48. Goel VK, Voo L-M, Weinstein JN, et al. Response of the ligamentous lumbar spine to cyclic bending loads. Spine 1988;13:294–300.
49. Liu YK, Goel VK, Dejong A, et al. Torsional fatigue of the lumbar intervertebral joints. Spine 1985;10:894–900.
50. Ritchie JH, Fahrini WJ. Age changes in the lumbar intervertebral disc. Can J Surg 1970;13:65–71.
51. Eckert G, Decker A. Pathological studies of the intervertebral discs. J Bone Joint Surg 1947;29:447.
52. Hadley LA. Anatomico-roentgenographic studies of the spine. Springfield: Charles C Thomas, 1964.
53. Nachemson A, Evans J. Some mechanical properties of the third lumbar inter-laminar ligament (ligamentum flavum). J Biomech 1968;1:211–220
54. Farfan HF. Symptomatology in terms of the pathomechanics of low-back pain and sciatica. In: Haldeman S, ed. Modern developments in the principles and practice of chiropractic. New York: Appleton-Century-Crofts, 1980.
55. Atkinson PJ. Variation in trabecular structure of vertebrae with age. Calc Tiss Res 1967;1:24–32.
56. Bell GH, Dunbar O, Beck JS, Gibb A. Variation in strength of vertebrae with age and their relation to osteoporosis. Calc Tiss Res 1967;1:75–86.
57. Hansson T, Roos B. The influence of age, height, and weight, on the bone mineral content of lumbar vertebrae. Spine 1980;5:545–551.

58. Nilsson BE. Spinal osteoporosis and femoral neck fracture. Clin Orthop 1970;68:93–95.
59. Panjabi MM, White AA. Basic biomechanics of the spine. Neurosurgery 1980;7:76–93.
60. Keller TS, Hansson TH, Abram AC, Spengler DM, Panjabi MM. Regional variations in the compressive properties of lumbar vertebral trabeculae: effects of disc degeneration. Spine 1989; 14:1012–19.
61. Herbst RW. Gonstead chiropractic science and art. Mt Horeb, WI: Sci-Chi Publications, 1968.
62. Giles LGF, Kaveri MJP. Lumbosacral intervertebral disc degeneration revisited: a radiological and histological correlation. J Manual Med 1991;6:62–66.
63. Panjabi MM, White AA, Brand RA. A note on defining body parts configurations. J Biomech 1974;7:385–87.
64. White AA, Panjabi MM, Brand RA. A system for defining position and motion of the human body parts. Med Biol Eng 1975;13:261–65.
65. Gerow G. Osseous configurations of the axial skeleton: specific application to spatial relationships of vertebrae. J Manipulative Physiol Ther 1984;7:33–38.
66. Plaugher G, Lopes MA. The knee-chest table: indications and contraindications. Chiropractic Tech 1990;2:163–167.
67. Cremata EE, Plaugher G, Cox WA. Technique system application: the Gonstead approach. Chiropractic Tech 1991;3:19–25.
68. Macintosh JE, Bogduk N. Basic biomechanics pertinent to the study of the lumbar disc. J Manual Med 1990;5:52–57.
69. Seligman JV, Gertzbein SD, Tile M, Kapasouri A. Computer analysis of spinal segment motion in degenerative disc disease with and without axial loading. Spine 1984;9:566–573.
70. Gertzbein SD, Seligman J, Holtby R, et al. Centrode patterns and segmental instability in degenerative disc disease. Spine 1985;10:257–261.
71. Ogston NG, King GJ, Gertzbein SD, et al. Centrode patterns in the lumbar spine: baseline studies in normal subjects. Spine 1986;11:591–595.
72. Panjabi MM, Goel VK, Summers D. Effects of disc degeneration on the instability of a motion segment. Trans Orthop Res Soc 1983;8:212.
73. Panjabi M, Abumi K, Duranceau J, Oxland T. Spinal stability and intersegmental muscle forces: a biomechanical model. Spine 1989;14:194–199.
74. Arkin AM. The mechanism of rotation in combination with lateral deviation in the normal spine. J Bone Joint Surg 1950;32A:180–188.
75. Lysell E. Motion in the cervical spine. Acta Orthop Scand 1969:123(suppl).
76. Gracovetsky S, Farfan HF, Lamy C. The mechanism of the lumbar spine. Spine 1981;6:249–262.
77. Speiser RM, Aragona RJ, Heffernan JP. The application of therapeutic exercises based upon lateral flexion roentgenography to restore biomechanical function in the lumbar spine. Chiro Res J 1990;1(4):7–16.
78. Gjelsivick A. Bone remodeling and piezoelectricity. J Biomech 1973;6:69–77.
79. Brickley-Parsons D, Glimcher MJ. Is the chemistry of collagen in intervertebral discs an expression of Wolff's law? A study of the human lumbar spine. Spine 1984;9:148–159.
80. Gatterman MI. Chiropractic management of spine related disorders. Baltimore: Williams & Wilkins, 1990.
81. Bernhardt M, Bridwell KH. Segmental analysis of the sagittal plane alignment of the normal thoracic and lumbar spines and thoracolumbar junction. Spine 1989;14:717–721.
82. Mosner EA, Bryan JM, Stull MA, Shippee R. A comparison of actual and apparent lumbar lordosis in black and white adult females. Spine 1989;14:310–314.
83. Farfan HF, Huberdeau RM, Dubow HI. Lumbar intervertebral disc degeneration. J Bone Joint Surg 1972;54A:492–510.
84. Gonstead CS. Audiotape from the Gonstead Seminar of Chiropractic. Mount Horeb, WI, circa 1968.
85. Voutsinas SA, MacEwen GD. Sagittal profiles of the spine. Clin Orthop 1986;210:235–242.
86. Andriacchi TP, Schultz AB, Belytschko TB, Galante JO. A model for studies of mechanical interactions between the human spine and rib cage. J Biomech 1974;7:497–507.
87. Gracovetsky S. An hypothesis for the role of the spine in human locomotion: a challenge to current thinking. J Biomed Eng 1985;7:205–216.
88. Thurston AJ, Harris JD. Normal kinematics of the lumbar spine and pelvis. Spine 1983;8:199–205.
89. Gracovetsky S. Function of the spine. J Biomed Eng 1986;8:217–223.
90. Anderson CK, Chaffin DB, Herrin GD. A study of lumbosacral orientation under varied static loads. Spine 1986;11:456–461.
91. Floyd WF, Silver PHS. The function of the erector spinae muscles in certain movements and postures in man. J Physiol 1955;129:184–203.
92. Bogduk N, Macintosh JE. The applied anatomy of the thoracolumbar fascia. Spine 1984;9:164–170.
93. Hinz B, Seidel H. On time relation between erector spinae muscle activity and force development during initial isometric stage of back lifts. Clin Biomech 1989;4:5–10.
94. Raftopoulos DD, Rafko MC, Green M, Schultz AB. Relaxation phenomenon in lumbar trunk muscles during lateral bending. Clin Biomech 1988;3:166–172.
95. Haas M. The physics of spinal manipulation. Part I. The myth of F = ma. J Manipulative Physiol Ther 1990;13:204–206.
96. Haas M. The physics of spinal manipulation. Part II. A theoretical consideration of the adjustive force. J Manipulative Physiol Ther 1990;13:253–256.
97. Haas M. The physics of spinal manipulation. Part III. Some characteristics of adjusting that facilitate joint distraction. J Manipulative Physiol Ther 1990;13:305–308.
98. Wood J, Adams AA. Comparison of forces used in selected adjustments of the low back by experienced chiropractors and chiropractic students with no clinical experience: a preliminary study. Proceedings: 14th Annual Biomechanics Conference on the Spine. Boulder: University of Colorado, 1983:73–98.
99. Adams AA, Wood J. Changes in force parameters with practice experience for selected low back adjustments. Proceedings: 15th Annual Biomechanics on the Spine. Boulder: University of Colorado, 1984:143–167.
100. Adams AA, Wood J. Forces used in selected chiropractic adjustments of the low back: a preliminary study. Proceedings: 14th Annual Biomechanics Conference on the Spine. Boulder: University of Colorado, 1983:51–71.
101. Hessell BW, Herzog W, Conway PJW, McEwen MC. Experimental measurement of the force exerted during spinal manipulation using the Thompson technique. J Manipulative Physiol Ther 1990;13:448–453.
102. Herzog W. Clinical biomechanics of the sacroiliac joint (Abstract from Low Back '90). J Manipulative Physiol Ther 1991;14:277.
103. Herzog W, Conway PJ, Zhang EM, Hasler EM, Ladly K. Forces exerted during spinal manipulative treatments of the thoracic spine. Proceedings of the 1991 International Conference on Spinal Manipulation. Arlington, Virginia: Foundation for Chiropractic Education and Research, 1991:275–280.
104. Triano JJ, Schultz AB. Cervical spine manipulation: applied loads, motions and myoelectric responses. Proceedings: American Society of Biomechanics, 1990;14:187–188.
105. Fuhr AW, Smith DB. Accuracy of piezoelectric accelerometers

measuring displacement of a spinal adjusting instrument. J Manipulative Physiol Ther 1986;9:15–21.

106. Fuhr AW. Verbal response to a gallery question as to any situation where a manual contact procedure would be superior to that of an instrument. Sixth Annual Conference on Research and Education: Emphasis on Consensus. Monterey, CA, 1991.

107. Smith DB, Fuhr AW, Davis BP. Skin accelerometer displacement and relative bone movement of adjacent vertebrae in response to chiropractic percussion thrusts. J Manipulative Physiol Ther 1989;12:26–37.

3 Vertebral Subluxation Complex

MARK A. LOPES with the assistance of GREGORY PLAUGHER

This chapter explores the nature of the various aspects of the vertebral subluxation complex (VSC). It is beyond the scope of this writing to describe in detail all the possible entities included in the broad category of the VSC. The purpose of the material presented is to focus on selected aspects of the VSC relevant to chiropractic care.

Several distinct types of physical changes that occur in relation to the VSC have been described. These changes include those affecting kinesiologic, histologic, neurologic, myologic, biochemical, vascular, inflammatory, and connective tissue characteristics (1,2). This chapter will pay particular attention to the following clinical manifestations resulting from the physical changes listed above:

1. The relative positions of the vertebrae above and below an articulation involved in subluxation;
2. Interarticular motion abnormalities in any or all of the six degrees of freedom of the motion segment; and
3. Neurophysiologic involvement caused by interarticular abnormalities.

Clinical presentation of a complex disorder can lead to treatment approaches that vary considerably, even within the same health field. One of the reasons for this variation results from approaching these problems from an isolated perspective of assessment. A multiparameter approach is requisite to provide for a working system of analysis and correction appropriate for each individual case presentation. One of the most important fundamentals of systematic full spine treatment is the recognition of the multiparameter nature of the VSC. The chiropractor should use examination procedures that are both sensitive and specific to all of the parameters of the VSC. Analysis procedures for the VSC will be covered in Chapters 4 and 5.

A complete understanding of normal anatomy and physiology of the structures involved is necessary to fully appreciate the clinical approach to the VSC. The subluxation is essentially an interarticular phenomenon (3). The reader is encouraged to pursue an in-depth study of normal articular structure and function and the effects of injury on the motion segment. Literature on the subject of spinal related conditions is extensive. Most research on spinal injuries has been performed on the lumbar spine. Many references for this chapter are taken from lumbar studies and may be cautiously extrapolated to other spinal regions.

POSITIONAL DYSKINESIA

Chiropractors have considered the interarticular alignment of spinal structures an important aspect of the VSC ever since the first chiropractic adjustment was given (4). The understanding of positional dyskinesia (misalignment of one vertebra on another) has evolved considerably since the original chiropractic "bone out of place" theory was formed.

The importance of the identification of positional dyskinesia is easily illustrated by the development of radiographic analysis of spinal structures. Widely taught at chiropractic colleges are literally dozens of methods of radiographic analysis (3). Positional dyskinesia is a factor in the etiology of neurophysiologic disorders, especially in the cervical and lumbar areas (5–11).

Etiology

Causes of positional dyskinesia have been postulated to involve the most basic circumstances of life, such as posture, the influence of gravity and cerebral dominance. The apparently high incidence of spinal subluxation of our species, in relation to other animals may be associated with the evolutionary theory of development from the quadruped to the upright stance (3). The spine is also under constant influence of cerebral dominance. The upper thoracic spine, for example, has the tendency for a lateral deviation with the convexity towards the side of the dominant hand (12).

Clinical Considerations

Positional dyskinesia is an important aspect of the subluxation. Malalignment of contiguous vertebral structures that support weight and guide movement, alters the ability of the involved functional spinal unit (FSU) to continue normal function. It is questionable, however, that positional dyskinesia by itself can cause direct neurophysiologic dysfunction. The association of positional dyskinesia with the degeneration of soft tissues and disruption of normal mechanics has been reported (13–15).

Mechanisms of Injury

It is important to recognize that positional dyskinesia can occur in any direction along the planes of possible movement, and in any combination of directions, as are applicable to the articulation in question. The nature of positional dyskinesia varies with the shape and function of each articulation, and from region to region in the spine.

The mechanisms by which any given positional dyskinesia of the spine occurs is not always clear. The existence of positional abnormalities in the spine can best be explained by a discussion pertaining to interarticular soft tissue disruption.

Two probable mechanisms of positional dyskinesia of the spine will be presented. One mechanism involves a sudden application of a damaging force. The other is a mechanism occurring more gradually over a period of time. These mechanisms are put forth as probable but not as the only possible causes of positional dyskinesia.

MACROTRAUMA

Sudden forces that overcome the strength of the paraspinal soft tissue can cause immediate damage to the joint capsules, disc, and ligaments that support a vertebral articulation (16). The nature of the damaging force, whether torsional, compressive, tensile, shearing, or a combination thereof, is the principle factor determining exactly which soft or hard tissue elements will be affected most (Fig. 3.1).

Interarticular injuries can damage any or all of its components. The main effects of injury are to the intervertebral disc, the two zygapophyseal joints, as well as the interspinous area. The reactions that occur in the spine in response to the different injury vectors have all been well described by various authors (17–19).

MICROTRAUMA

The second suggested mechanism of injury involves the spine's reaction to long-term subthreshold (not causing irritant damage) forces. The forces of gravity on posture in combination with weakness or unbalanced contraction of postural muscles, inevitably take their toll on spinal structure (Fig. 3.2).

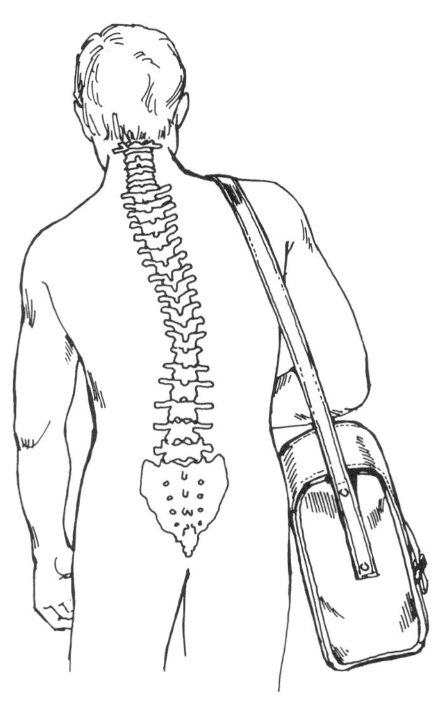

Figure 3.2. Chronic asymmetrical loading of the spine resulting in scoliosis in a mail carrier.

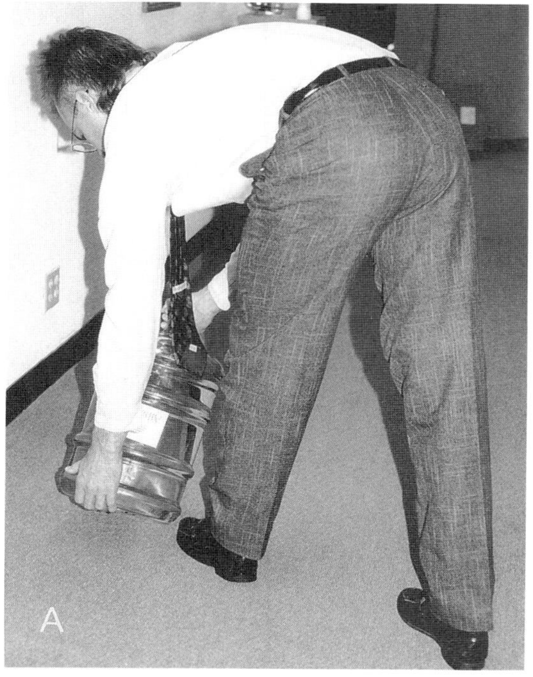

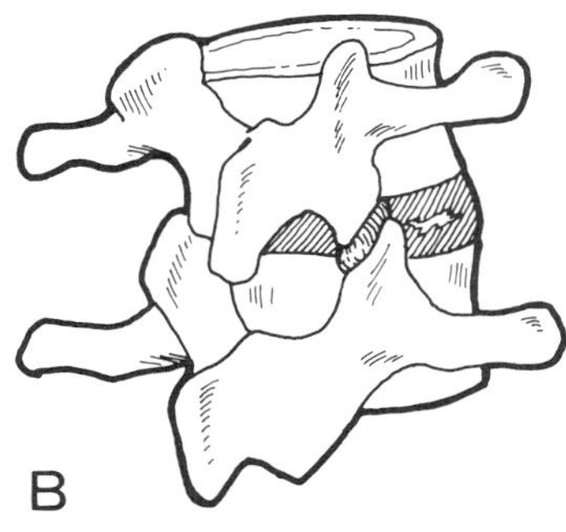

Figure 3.1. **A,** A common mechanism of sudden macrotrauma to the lumbar spine with resultant injury to the annulus and facet capsule depicted in (**B**).

The intervertebral joint loses stiffness after injury and the creep characteristics of the joint are changed. Creep is the gradual deformation of the intervertebral joint (ligamentous structures) under a constant load. Creep deformation occurs most in the direction of the injury, thus with a fractured end-plate the disc creeps to a reduced thickness. With torsional (Y axis) failure the joint tends to creep into the rotated position of injury (18).

Another example of the effects of long-term physical stress is seen as a compensation reaction. Anatomically normal FSUs are subjected to increasing amounts of stress during routine motions by compensating for other areas in the spine which are relatively restricted in their ability to move in one or more planes of normal motion (20). Intervertebral misalignment may well be the result of the injured spine's specific reaction to singular or accumulative traumatic forces.

Retrolisthesis

Retrolisthesis positional dyskinesia occurs most obviously in the normally lordotic cervical and lumbar areas and is best seen on the lateral spinal radiograph. Retrolisthesis is often accompanied by segmental hyperextension ($-\theta X$). This type of positional dyskinesia is capable of narrowing the spinal canal (21) and alters the weight bearing status of the FSU. This weight-bearing change sets the stage for compensatory weight bearing changes that can affect the entire spine, especially above the retrolisthesis. On the lateral spinal radiograph the shape of the disc space, the posterior edges of the vertebral bodies, as well as the interspinous spaces, can reveal the presence of $-Z$ and $-\theta X$ positional dyskinesia. Shifts in weight bearing with resultant changes in spinal curves as seen on x-ray can aid the clinician in determining which subluxated areas of the spine are affecting the overall structure. Subluxations that appear to significantly affect the functional, and postural status of entire regions of the spine are termed primary subluxations, and are of major clinical importance.

Retrolisthesis in the thoracic spine is usually less apparent and is commonly accompanied by flexion ($+\theta X$) misalignment. The theoretical importance of retrolisthesis in this area evolved from clinical observations of patient improvement after posterior to anterior adjustive techniques.

Evidence of abnormal weight bearing by the facets is often seen on the lateral spinal radiograph, accompanied by $-Z$ translation (retrolisthesis) of one vertebra on the segment below. This results in the degenerative changes (sclerosis) seen in the facet articular surfaces. Persistent $-Z$ translation, or any other type of displacement, stretches the facet capsular ligaments, and would not occur without significant failure and destruction of intervertebral disc substance (Fig. 3.3). The classic "facet syndrome," and/or instability, is likely secondary to disc abnormalities (13). The management of patients diagnosed with what some practitioners consider facet syndrome must, therefore, include attempts to restore normal intervertebral disc mechanics (as opposed to symptom relief only) if correction is to be attained. After clinical observations, Gonstead theorized that the most significant direction of positional dyskinesia of a vertebrae from C2 to L5 is retrolisthesis ($-Z$) (22).

Clinical Considerations

The structural integrity of the spinal canal and lateral recesses are altered by positional dyskinesia. Encroachment on the neural and other soft tissue structures within

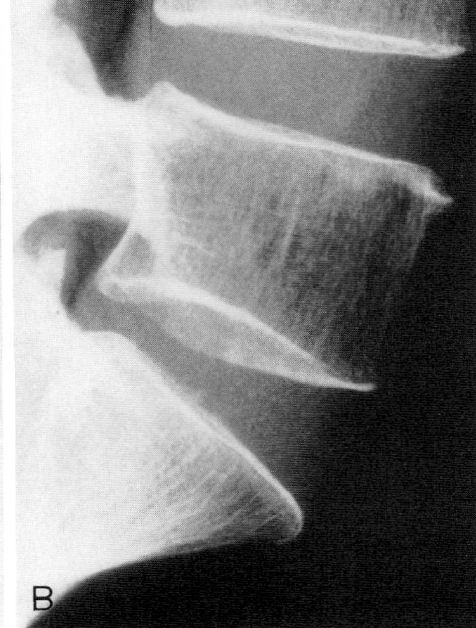

Figure 3.3A-B. Retrolisthesis of L5 vertebra on S1, secondary to annular disruption.

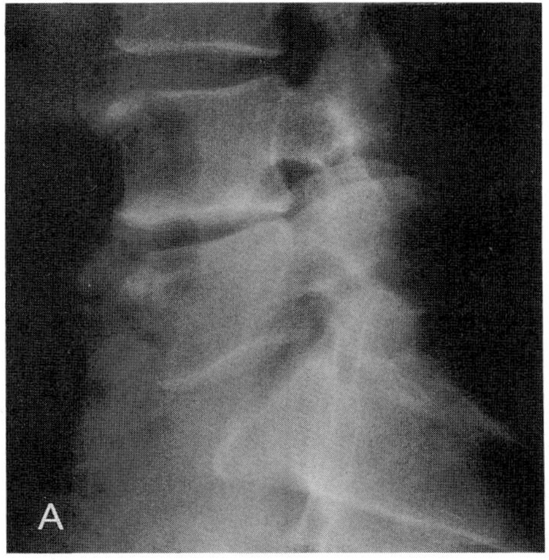

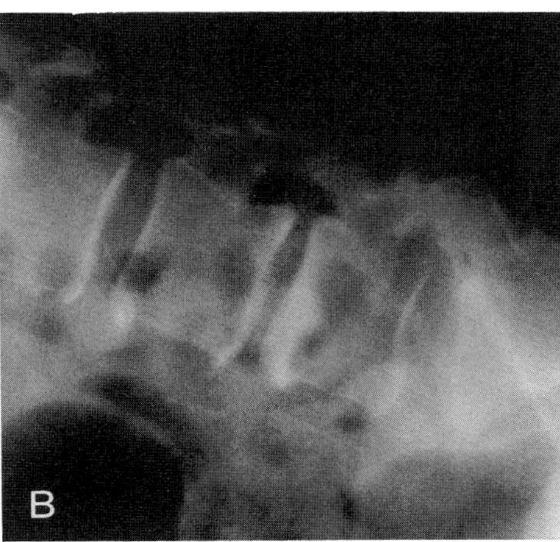

Figure 3.4. **A,** Standing neutral lateral lumbar radiograph showing retrolisthesis of L4. **B,** Flexion view of the patient in **A** revealing freedom of movement of the "misaligned" L4.

the canal may lead to adverse mechanical tension on these structures. Stenosis secondary to persistent malalignment has been reported (5).

It is interesting to note that many manipulative procedures employ primarily rotational (Y axis) forces as a major component of the maneuver. These forces not only have the most potential for harm to the annulus and the posterior joints but are also ineffective in reducing retrolisthesis or extension positional dyskinesia.

Primum Non Nocere

One of the foremost postulates of any health care practitioner, is to "above all do no harm." Knowledge of the relative positions of vertebrae is necessary, to avoid the potential for further distortion of the neural elements and articular ligaments, cartilage, and disc during adjustments.

For example, if the L4 vertebra is rotated $+\theta Y$ (spinous right) on L5 and an adjustment is performed at L4 in the $+\theta Y$ direction, further torsional injury may result. One of the most common malpractice actions against chiropractors is related to incidents involving excessive axial rotation to the lumbar spine in the side posture position. To lessen the likelihood of malpractice litigation, one should consider the alignment characteristics of the involved FSU and apply manual forces in the opposite direction of the positional dyskinesia.

Positional information is of little use if one has no knowledge of the dynamics of the articulation. *No adjustment (i.e., grade 5 mobilization*[a]*) should be administered to an apparent positional dyskinesia without concomitant evidence of a relative decrease in mobility at that articulation.* It is well known that misaligned vertebrae may be freely movable (Fig. 3.4). These freely movable misalignments must be distinguished from articulations that exhibit a relatively fixed position when x-rayed in different postures (23). Fixation dysfunction is a dynamic component of the structural and functional characteristics of spinal subluxations. The knowledge of the presence of fixation dysfunction in combination with that of the relative positions of vertebrae surrounding the subluxated articulation, is a prerequisite to the administration of the adjustment.

In summary, the chiropractor should evaluate positional dyskinesia by applying the same engineering principles that govern all structures under the effects of gravity. These principles must then be combined with the overall posture and the history of trauma of the patient, to properly establish the likely causes and clinical relevance of positional dyskinesia.

FIXATION DYSFUNCTION

Dysfunction, in strict definition, simply means ill operation of the described entity (24). Applied to the functional spinal unit, the term dysfunction implies that abnormal motion characteristics are present.

Abnormal structure, such as anomaly, positional dyskinesia, etc., can lead to dysfunction, and dysfunction can lead to abnormal structure, such as articular degeneration. The motion coupling of the lumbar spine, for example, is dependant on the lordotic posture of that area (See Chapter 7).

Fixation is a term describing a specific type of dysfunction that is applied to a FSU that is restricted in any or all of its six degrees of freedom.

Besides the limitation of the intersegmental range of motion, fixation dysfunction can be manifested by alterations in the instantaneous axis of rotation (25). A restriction in one direction of the articulation may be accompanied by an increased range of motion in the opposite direction.

[a]Grade I-IV mobilization descriptions:

Grade I: Small amplitude movements performed at the beginning of the range of motion of an articulation
Grade II: Large amplitude movements that do not reach the limit of the range
Grade III: Large amplitude movements performed up to the limit of the range
Grade IV: Small amplitude movements performed at the limit of the range
Grade V: Movement into the paraphysiologic range

Clinical Considerations

Fixation dysfunction is an important aspect of vertebral subluxation and it must be analyzed, corrected, and managed, along with the alignment and neurophysiologic aspects of the VSC. Prolonged fixation can cause abnormal somato-autonomic and somato-somatic reflexes (26), compensatory hypermobility at other spinal articulations (20), and spinal articular degeneration (27).

The importance of the intervertebral disc to spinal function has been discussed in an earlier section. One major mechanism involved in the maintenance of homeostasis of the disc is the process of imbibition. The physical properties of the intervertebral disc have been conceived as depending mainly on the water binding capacity of the nuclear pulp. The hydration of the nucleus is predominantly due to the imbibition pressure exerted by its mucopolysaccharide gel (17). The influx of nutrition, and the effusion of waste products from the disc, relies on imbibition due to the disc's inherent lack of blood supply (12). Prolonged fixation can be a cause of degenerative change of the disc by interfering with its ability to maintain itself through imbibition (Fig. 3.5) (19). The lack of motion impedes the flow of fluids through the intervertebral articulations.

Interarticular movement is necessary for the prevention of contracture and adhesion formation, as well as for the proper orientation of collagen fibers. Extracellular water loss, glycosaminoglycan depletion, and collagen cross linking accompany persistent immobility. The above response is uniform throughout ligaments, capsules, tendons, and fascia (27).

Compensatory Hypermobility and Instability

Hypermobility dysfunction is seen when any particular range of motion of the articulation(s) has increased beyond what is considered normal for articulations within the same region of the spine (28). It is not uncommon for hypermobile segments to be the cause of symptomatology in an individual (28).

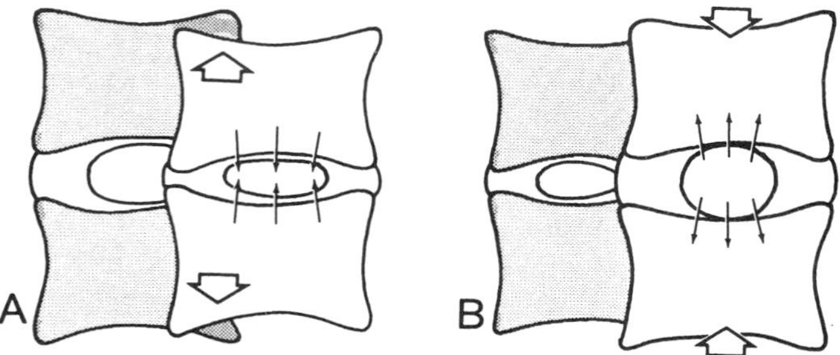

Figure 3.5. The imbibition of fluids into (**A**) and diffusion out of (**B**) the nucleus of the intervertebral disc. The hydrophilic nature of the healthy nucleus maintains the fluid pressure within.

It has been said that for every subluxation, there is compensation (22). Hypermobile articulations have been considered as a compensatory phenomenon, secondary to the presence of fixation dysfunction elsewhere in the spine (usually at adjacent or nearby segments) (20). Compensatory hypermobility above the level of surgical fusion is well known (29). The explanation given for the compensation has been that when an individual attempts to move the spinal region near the fixation dysfunction, other articulations nearby are forced to move through a greater range of motion. The total spine will attempt to maintain normal global or end-range of motion, sometimes sacrificing the integrity of an individual spinal unit.

It has been reasoned that the stress of compensatory hypermobility and abnormal weight bearing results in the breakdown of the interarticular soft tissues. This degeneration is commonly seen on the lateral radiograph of the cervical spine in the form of traction osteophytes at spinal levels above the area of subluxation, usually between the C4 and C6 FSUs.

Case studies have described adjustments applied to areas of hypomobility that have resulted in increased movement of previously restricted articulations (30–33). Jirout (30) describes compensatory hypermobility reduction from adjusting nearby levels involved in fixation dysfunction.

We saw earlier in the chapter that persistent positional dyskinesia in one area can result in compensatory alignment changes elsewhere. Here we have presented the compensation mechanisms involving motion characteristics. It can be seen that specific adjustments, applied to reduce positional dyskinesia and improve mobility, have biomechanical effects that extend to spinal regions beyond those directly treated.

Etiology

Much is to be learned about the factors involved in restricted vertebral mobility. A literature review by Rahlman (34) describes fixation dysfunction as, "acute joint fixation, locking, binding, blocking" which includes localized muscle spasm and can be ameliorated immediately after a manipulation.

Theories of fixation dysfunction must encompass not only those mechanisms involved in acute, but also chronic fixation. It is common for the VSC to occur and progress insidiously. Many acute presentations, therefore, are actually an acute stage of a chronic condition.

It is likely that most occurrences of articular fixation are multifactorial. Possible mechanisms of fixation include muscle spasm, meniscoid entrapment, articular adhesions, edema, and disc derangement. Contracture of the ligaments, muscles, and tendons may also resist intersegmental motion. Abnormalities in articular structure, especially in the facets, may affect joint function and be mistaken for fixation dysfunction (See Chapter 7).

MENISCOIDS

An entrapped meniscus-like body in the apophyseal joints called a meniscoid is an attractive theory behind vertebral fixation. A meniscoid is attached at its base to the articular capsule of the zygapophyseal joint with a free end that invaginates into the articulation (35). Meniscoids have been found in all regions of the spine. Meniscoid entrapment may not only lead to the restriction of motion, but also to pain and muscle spasm secondary to joint capsule traction.

Further investigation by Bogduk and Engel (36) into the structure and the arrangement of meniscoids reveals that they are a weak combination of fibrous connective and adipose tissue. The type of strong tissue necessary to cause joint locking and generate tension in the joint capsule was not observed in their own work or in the studies they cited. Several other investigators have studied meniscoids and their conclusions are variable as to the significance of meniscoid entrapment relating to joint lock.

Meniscoids may contribute to some part of joint derangement in specific cases, especially in the cervical spine where the facets are large relative to the three joint complex. Capsular proliferation secondary to degeneration of a large facet joint may result in a larger meniscoid. Derangement of a cervical facet may hypothetically have a greater influence on the function of the three joint complex than in the thoracic or lumbar spine.

Some cases may begin with a pinching pain that initiates a cycle of events and produces restricted intervertebral range of motion accompanied by painful and spasmed musculature. The degenerative changes associated with meniscoid entrapment may be similar to that of the detached cartilage of knee joint derangement. Although meriting further research, the meniscoid theory of joint fixation does not appear to be a mechanism that is a major contributor to fixation dysfunction found at primary sites of the VSC.

MUSCLE SPASM

Muscle spasm is known to reduce spinal mobility. The possible mechanisms eliciting muscle spasm are many and varied. Reflex mechanisms involving muscle are never unisegmental; that is to say that they are relayed to segments above and below the level of the direct initiation of the neurologic impulse (37). Muscle spasm often exists at multiple spinal levels. This phenomenon is often elucidated on stress radiography by the presence of restricted mobility of a section of the spine, which may consist of a few to many vertebral articulations. This type of grouped hypomobility is different from the unilevel intersegmental fixation that the chiropractor must look for in determining specifically which articulation is to be adjusted.

Muscle spasm is not likely the chief cause of most cases of intersegmental hypomobility (35). In one experiment, evidence of fixation dysfunction existed even after patients were completely under anesthesia, which included myorelaxants. Movement restriction was even more recognizable during narcosis, as the patients were totally relaxed (38).

Muscle spasm has been implicated as one possible reason for fixation dysfunction. The reflex mechanism involved in muscle spasm may be interrupted by the adjustment, leading to an instantaneous restoration of motion. We must look further, however, to uncover the mechanisms that are primarily responsible for intersegmental fixation dysfunction.

ADHESIONS

Disorganized fibrous cross-linking (scarring) between parallel collagen fibers is termed adhesion formation (27). Adhesions may form in ligaments, cartilage, muscles, tendons, or fascia. Articular adhesions are the by-product of the process of degeneration, and may result from trauma or immobilization (35). Ligamentous and cartilaginous tissue disruption involves healing mechanisms that replace normal tissue with fibrotic tissues of a lesser grade (17). Degeneration often begins at an early age and may result from persistent malalignment and fixation. The acute case presentation usually involves an acute stage of a chronic underlying condition. It is common that considerable disruption of supportive spinal soft tissue exists by the time most patients seek care for their condition.

Articular adhesions are likely to be part of the manifestation of intersegmental fixation dysfunction, especially as degenerative changes progress. The breaking up of adhesions from a spinal adjustment could account for some of the reason that an instantaneous change in intersegmental motion may occur after an adjustment is given. In cases of post adjustment pain, the cause may be inflammation in reaction to tissue damage from the tearing of adhesions.

The retraction of adhesions may progressively restrict interarticular movement. This process occurs over a relatively long period, thus necessitating recurrent adjustive interventions. Adhesion formation and gross soft tissue disorganization are the likely reasons that prolonged supportive chiropractic care may be necessary for patients with chronic VSC.

INFLAMMATION

The effects of inflammation on restricting mobility of an articulation is exemplified by the painful restriction of edematous joints. In the acute stage, intersegmental motion may be inhibited by the presence of inflammatory fluids in the joint space (Fig. 3.6).

Movement of fluids away from the articulation, when indicated during the acute stage of injury, can be accomplished by "pumping" the articulation in the direction of

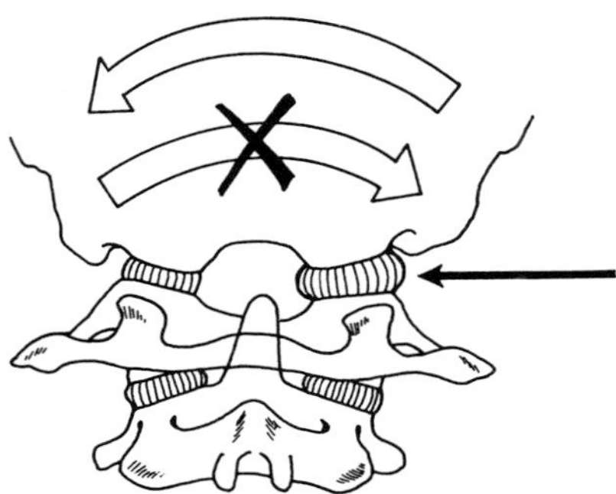

Figure 3.6. Intraarticular edema on the right at C0-C1 inhibiting movement which requires approximation of the articulating surfaces.

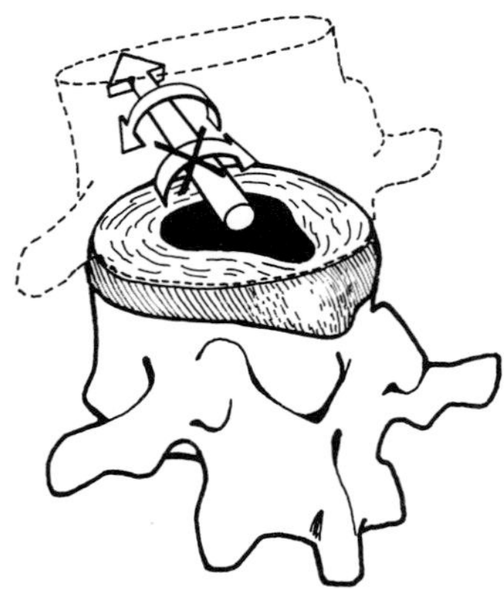

Figure 3.7. A displaced nucleus pulposus may act as a barrier to the approximation of the vertebral end-plates during motion.

correction. Pumping the joint involves intermittent manual grade 3 and 4 mobilization of the articulation. This mobilization can be combined with mild intermittent manual traction and cryotherapy to help disperse fluids and decrease pressure from inflammation, thereby reducing articular pressures.

DISC DERANGEMENT

Intervertebral disc derangement can easily disturb intersegmental function. An important aspect of intersegmental fixation is the disruption of the functional relationships of the nucleus pulposus to the annulus fibrosis. It is especially important to recognize nuclear-annular relationship disturbances in the management of patients with subluxation at levels where significant disc tissue still remains.

The sequestration of a part of the nucleus through a fissure in the annulus, causing the entrapment of nuclear material in an abnormal position, may lead to a mechanical barrier of motion between the vertebral body endplates (Fig. 3.7) (39–42).

Normal disc function exemplifies the extent to which intersegmental fixation of spinal levels from C2 to L5 can be influenced by nucleus/annulus disrelationships. The relatively large interarticular surface area occupied by the disc, as well as the fact that the disc supports most of the weight of axial compression forces, illustrates its potential to be a major factor in the manifestation of fixation dysfunction.

Both the insidious progression of major biomechanical disturbances of the spine, and the permanent effects of subluxation on spinal integrity, can be explained by disc related mechanisms. Instantaneous improvement in intersegmental mobility from spinal adjusting may be explained by the release of entrapped and sequestered disc material (39).

Hypermobility. Disc degeneration may lead to hypermobility. It is safe to say that hypermobility of the motion segment is impossible without significant disc dessication. Kirkaldy-Willis (28) describes a process of lumbar spine degeneration that involves a gradual progression of variable events which eventually leads from dysfunction to instability to stablization. The incidence of hypomobility versus hypermobility resulting from progressive disc degeneration is not clear.

It is not to be assumed that abnormal discs are the only factors necessary to be considered in subluxation. Intervertebral disc derangement, however, is of paramount importance to the biomechanical aspects of the VSC.

CONTRACTURE

Soft tissue adaptation in the form of contracture (shortening) of muscles, ligaments, and tendons may act to restrict intervertebral motion (17). Reduction of contractures is probably one of the mechanisms involved in the restoration of joint movement and improvement in spinal curvatures. Prolonged fixation dysfunction from other mechanisms, however, likely precedes gross contracture.

DISC PROTRUSIONS

Abnormal disc changes can and do affect any and all levels from C2 to L5 (5). The highest incidence of clinically significant protrusions occur in the lower lumbar discs. Any disruption in the disc must be accompanied by altered mechanics of the three-joint complex. Marked disc protrusion is seen as an advanced stage of the process of degeneration, which begins very insidiously from an early age (16).

Substantial controversy exists regarding the indications for chiropractic treatment for patients with disc protrusions. Before advanced imaging techniques (e.g., MRI, computerized tomography), many patients with protruded discs were adjusted without consideration for the extent of the underlying disc derangement. Some chiropractors appear to be shifting the emphasis in therapeutic approach away from manipulative procedures for these cases. Clinical experience, however, has been that most intervertebral disc displacements are manipulable lesions (39,43). The omission of the adjustment in treatment of many cases of disc protrusion likely results in unnecessary patient suffering.

Some feel flexion distraction techniques are preferable to manipulation for treatment of disc lesions. Others point out that the only studies showing efficacious manipulative treatment for disc protrusions used long lever rotational manipulations (44). The potential danger of worsening a disc protrusion by rotational maneuvers is related to axial torsion damage or failure. Flexion distraction's proposed effect is longitudinal traction of the posterior annulus and posterior longitudinal ligament (PLL) in an attempt to produce a negative pressure within the disc thereby creating a centripetal effect on the nucleus (45). The flexion distraction techniques apply tension to nerves and ligaments that may be disrupted. Most of the damage to the annulus occurs posterior to the nucleus pulposus; therefore, traction would have the effect of stretch on the sprained ligaments. It is likely, however, that substantially more people with pain from disc protrusions have been helped than hurt via both of the above approaches.

The specific adjustment can be used in attempts to directly push the displaced nucleus anteriorly. We advocate specific, short lever adjustments, primarily in the +Z (posterior to anterior) direction for posterior disc displacements whenever possible (Fig. 3.8). Tolerance by the patient is most important. Any increase in leg pain during set-up or thrust should be considered a contraindication for that position and an alternative position or contact should be attempted. Each patient must be matched with the correct table and position. The spinous contact (at least initially) is preferred, as this contact produces the least rotational lever while maximizing +Z force (See Chapter 7).

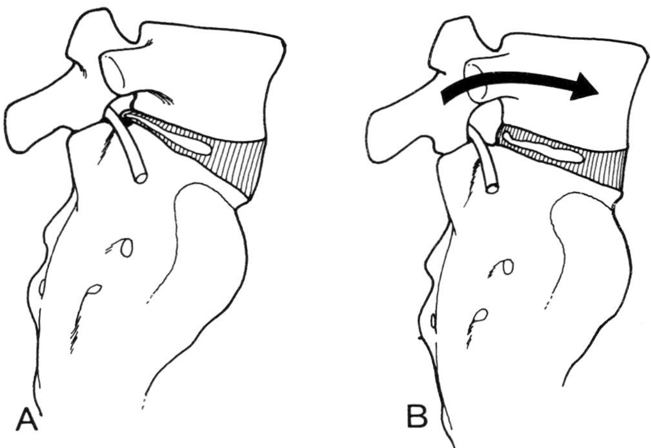

Figure 3.8. **A,** Displaced disc material with concomitant retrolisthesis of L5 vertebra. **B,** The +Z force applied during a specific adjustment attempts to influence the position of the displaced disc material.

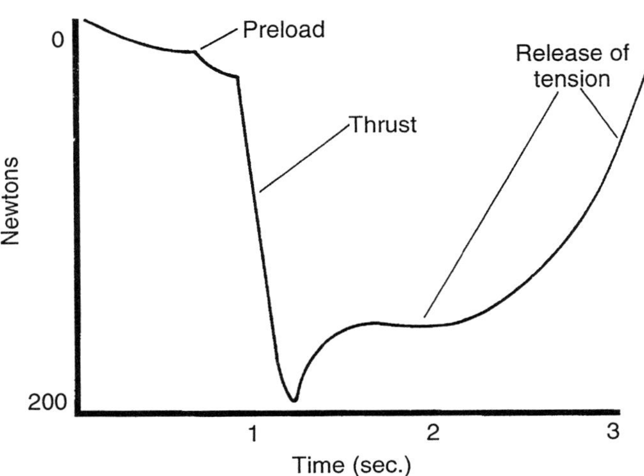

Figure 3.9. The graph demonstrates in a qualitative way, the set-hold feature of the specific adjustment.

Creep properties of ligaments are time dependent (46). A force applied for a long duration, as in flexion distraction or posterior to anterior (+Z) long amplitude maneuvers, is likely to create a greater effect on the intervertebral ligaments when compared to short duration loads. A combination of the direct adjustment along with long duration forces is most likely to maneuver the sequestered disc material. In administering an adjustment, the doctor is advised to set, then hold pressure forward for several seconds, followed by a gradual release (Fig. 3.9).

The reduction of a protrusion as viewed with MRI or CT is not necessary for a substantial resolution of the patient's signs and symptoms (47). Disc protrusions, though of great importance, do not always result in the direct production of symptoms (16,17). The disc can be the cause of pain without protrusion, as derangement may stimulate the recurrent meningeal nerve. Disc protrusion can reportedly account for lumbar pain anywhere from one to thirty percent of the time (48). Intervertebral dysfunction is also common with disc derangement in the absence of protrusion.

OPEN WEDGE

The original Gonstead subluxation theory revolved around the intervertebral disc and the changes it undergoes in response to trauma (22). The shape of the disc space on X-ray is used to infer the state of the disc. *Locating an "open wedge" on the antero-posterior (AP) radiograph or a degenerated disc on the lateral projection is not, however, pathognomonic of subluxation.* Many of the most misaligned FSUs are likely compensations for subluxations elsewhere in the spine (22).

It is incorrect to assume that the appearance of an open wedge on the AP radiograph indicates that the nucleus has moved towards the open side of the wedge. The direction of a nucleus shift or protruding annulus may well be on the side opposite the open wedge. MRI, CT, or obvious clinical findings indicative of protrusion are much more accurate in determining the location of displaced disc material.

Vertebral end-plate invaginations may reveal the location of the nucleus (49). A variant of this is the classic Schmorl's node (Fig. 3.10A-B) (5). Please refer to Chapter 7 for disc space findings in relation to spondylolisthesis and base posterior sacrum subluxations.

Examination

The potential cause of fixation-dysfunction must be determined if proper management of the VSC is to be achieved. To determine the cause of spinal joint fixation in a presenting patient, the chiropractor must first have an understanding of all the known causes of fixation as well as expertise in the analysis of spinal motion.

One of the greatest potential pitfalls in the differential diagnosis of the VSC relates to determining aberrant motion characteristics via palpation. Despite repeated attempts, investigations into joint end-feel motion palpation of the lumbar spine have yet to show good levels of interexaminer reliability (50). Intersegmental range-of-motion palpation (both passive and active) has not been researched adequately (51). Perceived results of an intersegmental range of motion assessment determined through palpation should not be weighed heavily relative to other means of assessment of vertebral motion (e.g., stress x-ray, videofluoroscopy). Radiography has been suggested as the most objective method of assessing intersegmental motion abnormalities (52). The risks associated with excessive x-ray exposure limits radiography as a means of frequent follow-up assessment. See Chapter 4 for a detailed description of the chiropractic examination.

NEUROPHYSIOLOGIC DYSFUNCTION

Any attempt at providing a complete, concise summary of the ramifications of a neurologic disorder is lacking, due to the inherent want for knowledge that exists with respect to the central nervous system. What is presented here is a working theoretical basis for the approach to the neurologic interference involved in the VSC.

Space Occupying Lesions

Neurologic ramifications from tumors, fractures, and other pathologies may be severe but are likely much less common than those occurring from degenerative changes of the intervertebral articulation. Neurologic interference can be seen as both a direct and an indirect result of subluxation. Lesions of a persistent space occupying nature predispose the nerve root complex to direct irritation (3). These conditions are exacerbated by the effects of tension placed on nervous tissue during movement and from pressure secondary to edema (10). A decrease in the cross sectional area of the spinal canal and intervertebral foramen has been shown to occur as a result of vertebral positional dyskinesia and disc displacement, as well as from changes accompanying the inflammatory and degenerative processes (28). The persistence of fixated positional dyskinesia at levels of subluxation ensures the longevity of the existence of the space occupying aspect of the lesion.

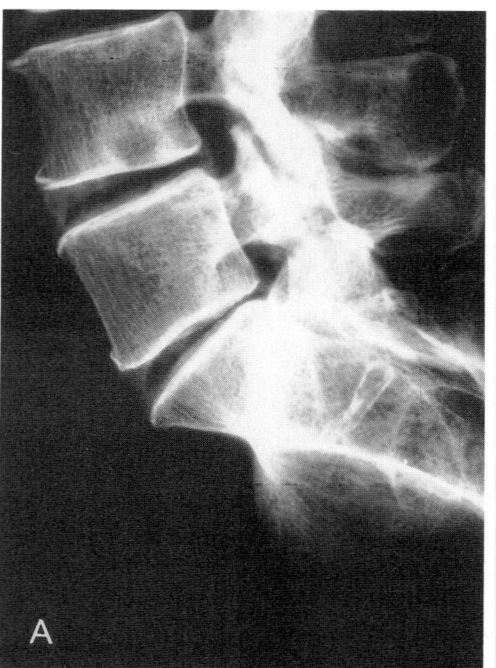

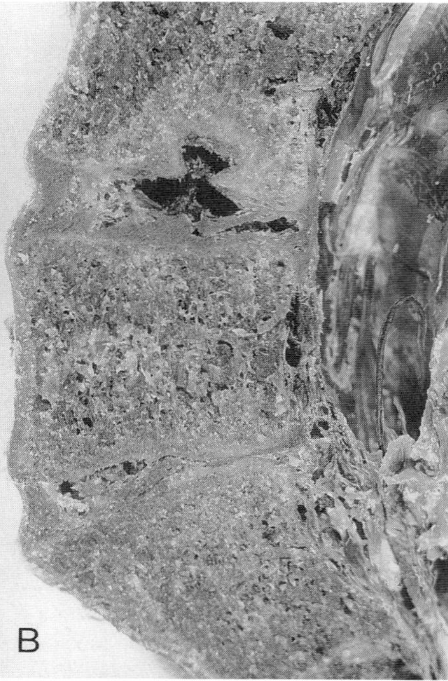

Figure 3.10. A, Lateral radiograph of a cadaveric specimen exhibiting a lucency of the inferior vertebral body of L4 indicative of an invagination of nuclear material through a fractured end-plate. Notice the subtle invagination in the L5 inferior vertebral body. **B,** A sagittal slice of the specimen in **A** exposing the gap in the L4 end-plate. The remains of the degenerated nucleus of the L5 disc are seen under the upward invagination of the L5 inferior end-plate.

Hadley (5) has suggested that abnormal constriction in the size of a normal intervertebral foramen, if not actually causing nerve root pressure, nevertheless decreases the reserve safety cushion space surrounding the nerve and may predispose it to pressure. The subsequent development of edema, hemorrhage, disc pressure, or movement of adjacent structures may be sufficient to produce radicular symptoms. He found evidence that cervical, thoracic, and lumbar articulations could produce intervertebral foramen encroachment when persistent malposition of one vertebra on another existed.

Kirkaldy-Willis (28) has suggested that nerve compression in the lumbar spine is most commonly associated with disc degeneration, either by itself, or in combination with degenerative and/or developmental stenosis of the spinal canal. Once stenosis occurs, the neurologic elements are more susceptible to insult from relatively small changes in disc displacement. This apparent predisposition to nerve involvement may explain why some individuals, with relatively minor physical exam findings present with more discomfort than others with apparently more objective evidence of dysfunction. The radiographic, CT, and MRI evaluations often illustrate this stenosis component.

Adverse Mechanical Tension

The effects of tension on the nerve elements must be considered when studying the neurologic ramifications of the VSC. The primary source of meningeal and neural tension is the lengthening of the spinal canal on forward bending and lateral flexion (53). Limb movements will also transmit tension to the nerve roots, causing piston-like movements of the root complex within the intervertebral foramen (17). Normally, the soft tissues adapt freely to these skeletal movements, but in the presence of space occupying lesions involving the spinal canal and intervertebral foramen, and when there are sclerotic or fibrotic lesions that restrict the mobility or extensibility of nervous and meningeal tissues, the tension may be greatly increased (17,53). Even when the lesion appears to be exerting an essentially compressive effect, the resulting deformation leads to a local increase in tension. An important cause of functional disturbances, both of the nerve access cylinders and the blood vessels, lies in the reduction of their cross-sectional areas, resulting from tension and/or compression (53).

Grieve (17) cites over fifty investigative reports of conduction block, ischemia, and post-ischemic paresthesia. "Severe and prolonged compression blocks the nerves' blood supply and produces other damage. It then loses its ability to conduct impulses. Prolonged inflammation appears to produce the same effect. Temporary compression will produce temporary loss of conduction, from minutes to days, depending on the degree and duration of the compression. Intermittent compression or mechanical irritation may lead to inflammatory changes with space occupying effects produced by edema, and thus some or all of the changes and clinical features after inflammation. Traction of sufficient force to disrupt the nerve, will cause irritation and consequent neuritis." Swelling of the nerve root elements may be associated with some cases of neuritis (54).

Persistent and prolonged fixation, positional dyskinesia, and ensuing degeneration can create a stenotic predisposition to nerve involvement. Disc displacement, inflammation, and movement of nerve elements through the stenotic spinal canal and foramenal areas are all significant factors contributing to the manifestation of neurologically related conditions of the VSC.

COMPRESSION EFFECTS

Let us pursue some basic information about the nature of abnormal nerve function under compression and how the restoration of function ensues when pressure is removed. The "all or none" law refers to the principle that nerve tissue will either respond to stimuli completely or not at all. This law is applicable to the individual nerve fibers only. Studies of nerve compression have demonstrated that blockage of only some nerve fibers in the nerve is possible. The remaining fibers in a nerve root complex under compression respond to stimulus normally (21). The importance of this phenomenon is that the manifestation of compressive effects depends on those parts of the nervous system that are being affected. Conscious awareness of nerve involvement by the patient would only be possible if nerve pathways under voluntary control were involved. When objective findings of subluxation exist in the absence of subjective complaints, the necessity for the correction of the subluxation still exists. This necessity is not only for biomechanical reasons but also for the underlying potential for neurologic involvement that may result without notice.

There are reversible and irreversible conduction blocks that result from compression. A completely reversible conduction block seems to leave the nerve undamaged. The usual explanation of the reversible block is anoxia. The nerve deprived of oxygen ceases to conduct in 16 to 35 minutes. If neither axons nor blood vessels are damaged during the constriction, conductibility returns soon after the compression is removed (17).

The irreversible conduction block is characterized by disturbances in nerve continuity and degenerative structural changes in nerve and or vascular tissues. A greater amount of constriction and/or compression over a longer time period is necessary to produce an irreversible conduction block (17).

Neurologic findings that are almost instantaneously improved after the administration of an adjustment, such as deep tendon reflexes, motor power as measured by grip strength, and dermatomal sensory loss (55), may be due to the removal of constriction in the area of a completely reversible conduction block.

Different types of nerve fibers appear to react differently to compression and its consequences. The number of fibers affected in the nerve varies with the degree of constriction (17). When a patient presents with seemingly irreversible signs of nerve damage, it should not be assumed that attempts at the correction of the subluxation will be of no neurologic value. Interruption of the constriction, although not likely resulting in the healing of tissues already lost to degeneration, may help to prevent further degenerative changes of nerve tissue by relieving compression and tension on elements not yet permanently affected.

CLINICAL CONSIDERATIONS

Compensatory hypermobility of the motion segment can be a potential cause of nerve irritation and degeneration. The major difference between compensatory and subluxated levels in their ability to produce direct nerve involvement is that compensatory areas are highly moveable and are not likely able to produce fixed stenotic lesions. Symptoms are often reported by patients in areas of compensation. These symptoms are usually temporary in nature and are generally easily abated by rest and/or applying corrective measures to areas of primary subluxation.

Denervation Supersensitivity

Injury or pathology may result in peripheral nerve or dorsal root ganglion (DRG) damage. Ensuing nerve fiber degeneration mainly takes the form of either axonal or segmental degeneration. Trauma induced axonal degeneration leading to secondary myelin sheath breakdown is termed Wallerian degeneration (56). Segmental demyelination occurs when Schwann cells and the myelin sheath are damaged without effect to the axon anatomically, yet the conduction of impulses may be impeded (57). After denervation, changes occur in the muscle and receptor sites that are characteristic of denervation supersensitivity (DS).

SIGNS

Denervation supersensitivity of peripheral nerves can be, at least to some degree, related to the VSC. Muscle and peripheral receptors become hypersensitive to circulating neurotransmitters and other stimuli after denervation of some neurons. Associated signs and symptoms of this phenomenon include cutaneous and myalgic hyperalgesia, autonomic dysfunction, trophic changes and increased muscle tone (57). These findings have been reported in "low back sprain" patients without otherwise obvious physical findings (58).

MUSCLE CHANGES

Denervation resulting from degeneration and inflammation local to the spine may lead to peripheral supersensitivity at the neuromuscular receptors. The area of response to acetylcholine spreads from that immediately adjacent to the receptor end-plate, along the surface membrane, and sometimes involves the entire nerve fiber (59). Normal muscle presents as relatively soft and undefined at rest (resting tonus is present). In the presence of DS, palpation reveals hypertonicity of resting muscle due to hyperexcitation of the muscle by the spindle. The muscle may become abnormally shortened because of this effect (57). Asymmetrical muscle shortening may eventually contribute to skeletal asymmetry.

MOTOR POINTS

The "motor point" is that skin region overlying the terminals of the neurovascular hilus at the point where the principle blood vessels enter the deep surface of the muscle. These motor points are not normally tender. Mild tenderness at motor points may be found in normal individuals after exercise. In patients with DS, the amount of tenderness at motor points is directly proportional to the severity of the radiculopathy (57).

TROPHIC CHANGES

The "boggy" or "doughy" characteristics of tissues overlying a subluxated FSU's paraspinal area, detected through palpation, may be due to a phenomenon termed trophedema. Partial interruption of a peripheral nerve causes gradual fibrosis of the subcutaneous tissue (60).

AUTONOMIC CHANGES

Vasomotor, sudomotor, and pilomotor dysfunction may be caused by DS. "Mottling" of the skin, palor and cyanosis, lower skin temperature, and rarely, pigmentation resembling erythema *ab igne* are vasomotor disturbances that have been related to DS (57).

Hyperhidrosis resulting from DS may be seen beyond the confines of the involved nerve's distribution. Extensive sweating areas may include the axillae, palms and soles (57).

"Goose pimples" may occur as a result of brisk cool air exposure (as the patient undresses) over the skin of an affected area. This reflex may only be observable for a brief moment and can be a pilomotor effect of DS in the dermotomes of the involved nerves (57). This phenomenon can only be detected in the absence of a generalized pilomotor response.

Autonomic nervous system dysfunction via neurologic involvement at the spinal cord, nerve root and inter-

doctors to assume a primary psychogenic etiology in patients with confusing clinical pictures involving muscle pain. It is doubtful that psychologic factors represent the primary etiology in most of these cases. Prolonged physical dysfunction, however, will almost assuredly involve some psychologic component and vice versa. Referral for concomitant psychologic counseling should be considered in the management of these patients.

Chiropractic intervention with regards to viscerosomatic dysfunction revolves around normalizing the primary visceral etiology (See Chapter 13). Psychologically induced somatic dysfunction may involve similar mechanisms as viscerosomatic conditions. Overall chiropractic spinal management may be indicated in these conditions, possibly reducing the likelihood of exacerbations of previously present subluxations during the acute phase, and contributing to the overall patient well-being (89). Future research is needed to clearly define the role of chiropractic care in aiding the patient in the acute and recovery stages of these disorders. It is possible that early mobilization of the concomitant spinal areas may minimize the exaggerated muscular responses and subsequent production of pain. Referral for medical care should be considered in all of these cases. A primary visceral etiology should be suspected in patients that do not otherwise respond to adjustments. It is the authors' opinion that primary visceral causes of the VSC are relatively rare; however, these mechanisms should be considered in light of the potentially devastating consequences from mismanagement.

INFLAMMATION

Interarticular inflammation from trauma causes edema that reduces joint movement. Immobilization can cause degenerative joint disease (DJD) (90). Arthritis or DJD is usually diagnosed radiologically by the presence of bony proliferation and decreased soft tissue at the joint space. Chronic or repeated episodes of inflammation may eventually result in ossification of paraspinal ligaments (91). The restoration of motion leads to a decrease in the degenerative process (2).

Inflammation results in hyperexcitable nerves and causes ganglia to continue firing long after stimulation has ceased (2). Inflammation is a potentially powerful enhancer of pain production and prolongation, as well as increased muscle tone (which also may restrict movement) through hyperexcitation of the nerves exposed to inflammatory byproducts.

VASCULAR CHANGES

Alterations in the arterial supply and venous drainage of the spinal column has been suggested as a contributing factor to interarticular degeneration after immobility (2). Experimental occlusion of the arterial supply and/or venous drainage can lead to joint stiffness (91). Lantz (2) suspects that when venous stasis occurs the reduced rate of removal of cellular toxins leads to inflammation and accelerates the degenerative process. Immobilization, disc herniation compressing on epidural veins (92), or SNS dysfunction creating arterial constriction may be involved in VSC progression. Blood flow restriction may heighten the effects of trauma and the interarticular dehydration that follows immobilization.

ARTICULAR NOISE

Evidence suggests that the cracking sound of the articulation that occurs in response to manipulation is due to coaptation of articular gases in synovial joints (93). When the separation of the joint surfaces is great enough to coaptate the articulation, an abrupt liberation of gas from the synovial fluid occurs (Fig. 3.13). Once this coaptation of gas has occurred, there is a refractory period during which the articulation experiences a greater degree of interarticular freedom of movement. Manipulation of the joint during the refractory period may not produce another audible crack. It takes approximately twenty minutes for the gas to slowly redissolve and end the refractory period (93).

Repeating a thrust into an articulation after fully coaptating the joint by a prior thrust may result in ligamentous strain more readily than would be expected to occur in an uncoaptated joint. The coaptation forces are thought to provide an elastic barrier of resistance to gapping of the articulation (94). It requires less force to overcome coaptative forces in an unrestricted joint than in an articulation restricted by previous interarticular changes (95). Specific adjustments aimed directly at restricted articulations are indicated in preference to long lever, regional manipulations for the above reason.

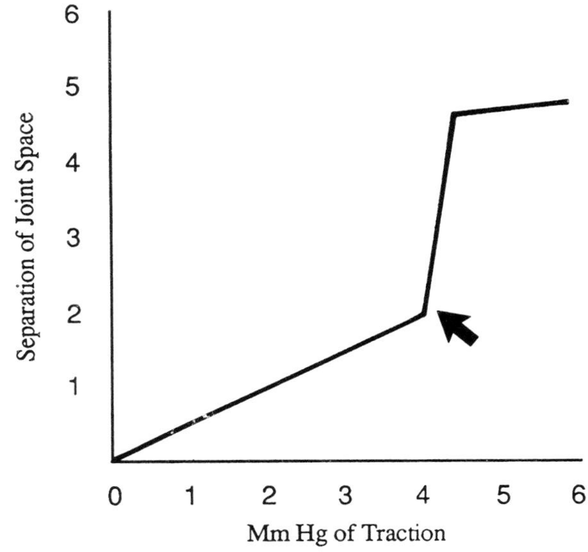

Figure 3.13. The graph depicts the progressive application of force to separate a synovial joint (*arrow* = the point of coaptation).

CORRECTION OF THE VSC

The clinical application of our understanding of specific full spine chiropractic management is illustrated in the following examples of the VSC.

Example One

Consider one common type of subluxation pattern encountered in the cervicothoracic spine. A patient is suffering from midline, lower neck pain, and objective signs of the VSC (as will be discussed in Chapter 4) are found on the patient at the C7-T1 motion segment. The static upright neutral A-P x-ray of the area involved reveals the presence of $-\theta Z$ (left lateral flexion) and a $+\theta Y$ (spinous process rotated to the right side) alignment of the C7 vertebra on T1. The lateral radiograph exhibits the presence of $-\theta X$ alignment (an extension malposition) of C7 on the T1 vertebra with concomitant C7 $-Z$ alignment. The translation into Gonstead nomenclature of the above positional dyskinesia is PRS-inf (22). The motion characteristics of the C7-T1 articulation are analyzed, and the C7 vertebra is found to be restricted in $+\theta Z/-\theta Y$ (coupled right lateral flexion and contralateral spinous rotation) and $+\theta X$ (forward flexion) motions.

The positional dyskinesia and the fixation dysfunction are considered secondary components to the disruption of the normal functional and structural characteristics of the FSU. The alignment of the joint will help to determine the mechanism of injury. The trauma in this example most likely involved forces of compression ($-Y$), left lateral bending ($-\theta Z$) and or axial rotation ($+\theta Y$) of the head and neck, and possibly flexion or extension ($\pm\theta X$). This then led to the motion segment assuming a position of $-Z$ (P), $+\theta Y$ (R), $-\theta Z$ (S), and $-\theta X$ (inf). The effects of weight bearing and posture help to further the accelerated plastic deformation of the damaged interarticular soft tissue. The vertebra(e) settles into the direction of the ligamentous weakness. Inflammation and scarring with fibrous adhesions add to the articular dysfunction.

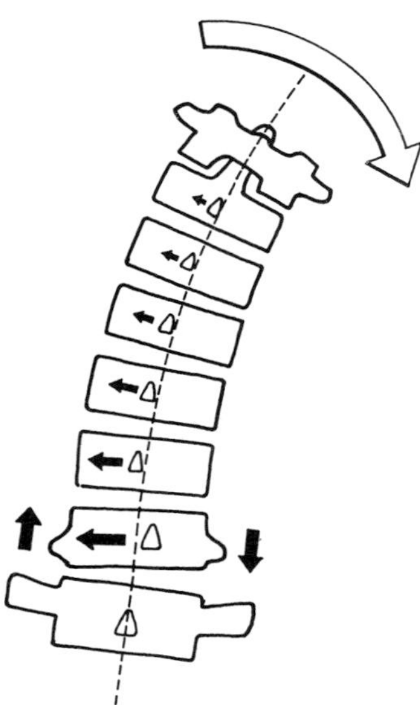

Figure 3.14. This line drawing illustrates the effects of prepositioning the spine for a specific adjustment designed to correct a C7 PRS subluxation.

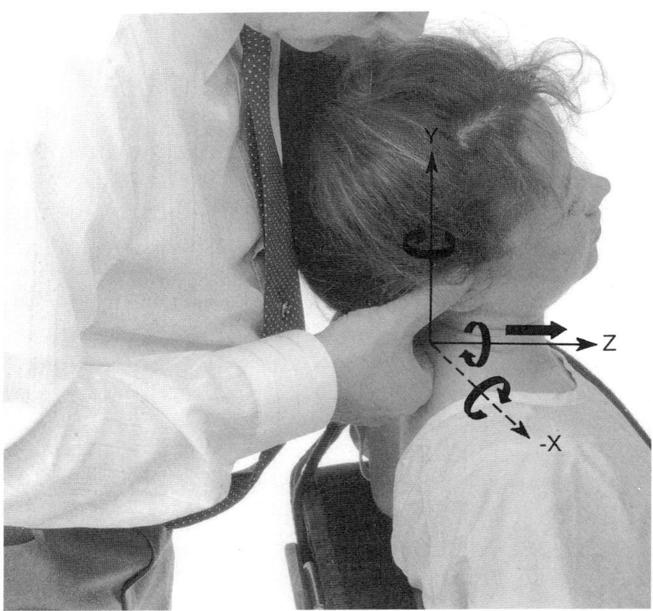

Figure 3.15. A photograph demonstrating the correct set-up and multiple directions of forces that combine to make-up the desired correction of a C7 PRS subluxation.

An adjustment chosen to correct such a subluxation would include pretensioning and applying a force in the opposite direction of the positional dyskinesia, usually with the patient's neck in $+\theta Z$ (right lateral flexion) (Fig. 3.14). The thrust would be from posterior to anterior, with inferior to superior lifting of C7 on T1, from the right side contacting the right posterior inferior portion of the spinous process (Fig. 3.15).

The goals of the application of force in this maneuver are to improve mobility in the direction the articulation was lacking (fixation dysfunction) and to normalize the interarticular alignment (positional dyskinesia). After the adjustment, the motion is reanalyzed to determine if improvement occurred. Alignment changes, if any, are seen on comparative radiographic examinations.

CLINICAL CONSIDERATIONS

As mentioned earlier, many cases are acute presentations of a chronic underlying condition. The fixation dysfunction in the above example likely represents the combination of nuclear-annular disrelationships, adhesions, maligned joint surfaces, edema and muscle spasm. In the presence of nuclear displacement it is important to first separate the vertebral end-plates before applying the force aimed at directing the nuclear material towards a more normal position. Because of the extensive connections of the annulus to the vertebral body, forced translation of one vertebra on another can potentially affect disc position. Rotary manipulation has undergone controlled clinical trials showing effectiveness in the management of patients with disc lesions (47). More research in this area is necessary. If function is to remain more normal after a correction is made, intradiscal healing must occur, sealing the fissures and preventing nuclear remigration. Repetitive adjustments, and possibly nutritional supplementation, may be necessary to aid the FSU in its return to normal function, because of the slow repair process of the tissues involved. Proper patient ergonomics are imperative to this healing process. Over time the disruption of function and persistent malalignment will lead to degeneration of all supportive soft tissues which further ensures the persistence of dysfunction.

Example Two

A common subluxation of the lumbosacral articulation involves a posterior nucleus shift through radial fissures in the annulus. This eccentric nuclear position creates blockage to extension movement at L5-S1. The lateral radiograph will show the discal abnormality, by exhibiting a more parallel or open posterior configuration of the usually anteriorly wedged appearance of the L5-S1 disc space (Fig. 3.16). Severe low back pain and concomitant sciatica or referred leg pain (at times bilaterally), can accompany the above lumbosacral subluxation.

Correction of this type of subluxation (termed a base posterior sacrum subluxation, See Chapter 7) is easily accomplished in the side posture position, but can also be achieved in the knee-chest or prone position. The doctor manually contacts the posterior-superior aspect of the sacrum at the S1 or S2 tubercle and applies a +Z (posterior to anterior) force, following through with an inferior to superior arcing motion of the contact hand. The anterior aspect of the L5-S1 disc space is separated and the base of the sacrum is pushed forward, allowing disc material to be moved forward away from the spinal canal. The inferior to superior motion at the end of the forward thrust is aimed to further force nuclear material out of the posterior aspect of the disc space. L5-S1 is then re-evaluated for the presence of extension movement. Clinical observations suggest that the positional dyskinesia of the base posterior sacrum appears reduced on x-rays taken after a series of corrections have been made, relatively more often when compared to other positional dyskinesias.

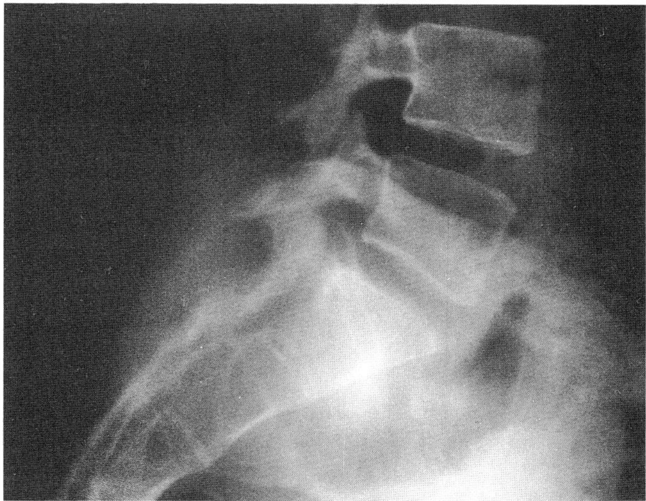

Figure 3.16. Base posterior sacral positional dyskinesia.

The above examples represent only a small sample of the potential subluxation configurations encountered on a daily basis in a chiropractic practice. Much of what is applied in chiropractic practice is based on the inductive reasoning from clinical observations in combination with known experimental results. The paradigm is far from complete however.

SELECTIVE ADJUSTING

Mixing Systems

A common question proposed by chiropractic students, that is not often clearly answered, pertains to when it is acceptable to "mix (autonomic) systems." The clinically relevant aspect of this question centers on the separation of adjustments applied to the lower cervical, thoracic, and lumbar vertebrae, from those delivered to the upper cervical or sacral regions. To address this question completely, one must consider more than just parasympathetic nervous system (PNS) and sympathetic nervous system (SNS) effects.

Gonstead advocated the separation of adjustments affecting both of the main divisions of the autonomic nervous system. Affecting either the PNS or the SNS is considered especially important in the management of patients with a visceral concomitant. When a specific visceral effect is desired (e.g., increasing intestinal motility), selective adjusting of subluxations influencing only one autonomic division at a time may be indicated (See Chapter 13).

Reducing Variables

During the initial phase of chiropractic care, reducing the number of VSCs adjusted will diminish the number of variables the doctor must consider in evaluating the response to treatment. By adjusting less motion segments each session, it is easier to determine the apparent cause and effect relationships between the patient's response and the treatment applied. This concept is also applicable to mixing types of treatments as with chiropractic and adjunctive therapies. If a patient responds favorably to a treatment administered then all is well. If, however, the doctor applied more than one type of treatment or adjusted more than one FSU (especially in close proximity) and the patient did not respond favorably, it may prove difficult to determine what steps to take next. *It is important to remember that treatment is partially diagnostic.* The "shotgun" approach of applying multiple therapeutic modalities together may prove to relieve initial symptoms more rapidly than spinal adjusting alone (96). In long-term corrective care, however, a step by step systematic approach to treatment will be more valuable. Through the limitation of variables, the chiropractor progressively learns about specific adjustments and their outcomes. Eventually, more levels can be adjusted at one time or additional care can be prescribed when adequate information has been obtained from the treatment trial.

Selectively separating lumbar adjustments from those directed to the sacroiliac joint may be useful not only for separating autonomic divisions but also for mechanical reasons. Lumbar subluxations can refer pain to one, or less commonly to both sacroiliac articulations. An example of reducing the number of variables in the initial treatment phase may occur when the patient presents with signs and symptoms of a VSC in both the lumbar and sacroiliac areas. By limiting treatment to one area or the other, the potential mechanical effects of the adjustment can be more clearly delineated.

In instances where the patient is seen on an infrequent basis, multilevel adjustments, when indicated, may be more effective since a lack of attention to some motion segments may result in a deterioration of the patient's condition. In some cases, normalizing the structural and neurologic balance in the body by correcting subluxations in multiple regions of the spine can be advantageous.

Proprioceptive Effects

The upper cervical area is richly endowed with proprioceptors. This abundant supply is responsible for head-to-body proprioceptive balance (97,98). The potential neurologic effects of upper cervical adjustments is evidenced by the fact that nerve dysfunction at this level may potentially affect any spinal cord pathway. To more accurately assess the effects of upper cervical adjustments, it is often necessary to adjust this region alone.

SUMMARY

The understanding of mechanisms involved in the VSC will evolve with further knowledge, which is a by-product of continued investigation. The practical application of chiropractic has developed empirically after millions of clinical observations. It is likely that many of these applications will withstand the test of time and clinical research; those that do not should be refined or discarded. This work is but a foundation open to the addition of any new developments related to the care and maintenance of spine related disorders.

REFERENCES

1. Lantz CA. The vertebral subluxation complex. Int Rev Chiro 1989 Sept/Oct:37–61.
2. Lantz CA. The vertebral subluxation complex part 2: the neuropathological and myopathological components. Chiro Res J 1990;1(4):19–38.
3. Leach RA. The chiropractic theories. 2nd Ed. Baltimore: Williams & Wilkins, 1986.
4. Palmer DD. The science, art, and philosophy of chiropractic. Portland: Portland Printing House Co, 1910:189.
5. Hadley L.A. Anatomico-roentgenographic studies of the spine. Springfield: Charles C Thomas, 1964.
6. Hadley LA. Intervertebral joint subluxation, bony impingement, and foramen encroachment. Am J Roentgenological Rad Ther 1951;65:377–402.
7. Epstein JA. Sciatica caused by nerve root entrapment in the lateral recess: the superior facet syndrome. J Neurosurg 1972;36:584–589.
8. Grogono BJS. Injuries of the atlas and axis. J Bone Joint Surg 1954;36B:397–410.
9. Sunderland S. Nerves and nerve injuries. 2nd. ed. Edinburgh: Churchill Livingstone, 1978.
10. Sunderland S. The anatomy of the intervertebral foramen and the mechanisms of compression and stretch of nerve roots. In: Haldeman S, ed. Modern developments in the principles and practice of chiropractic. New York: Appleton-Century Crofts, 1980:45–64.
11. Sunderland S. Meningeal-neural relations in the intervertebral foramen. J Neurosurg. 1974;40:756–763.
12. Warwick R, Williams PL eds. Gray's Anatomy. 35th British ed. Philadelphia: W.B. Saunders Co, 1973.
13. Yochum T. Essentials of skeletal radiology. Baltimore: Williams & Wilkins, 1987:192–193.
14. Panjabi MM, Yamamoto I, Oxland T, Crisco JJ. How does posture affect the coupling? Spine 1989;14:1002.
15. Knutsson F. The instability associated with disc degeneration in the lumbar spine. Acta Radiol 1944;24:593–609.
16. Farfan HF. Mechanical disorders of the low back. Philadelphia: Lea and Febiger, 1973.
17. Grieve GP. Common vertebral joint problems. New York: Churchill and Livingstone, 1981.
18. Farfan HF. Biomechanics of the lumbar spine. In: Kirkaldy-Willis WH, ed. Managing low back pain. New York: Churchill Livingstone, 1983:9–21.
19. Junghanns H. Clinical implications of normal biomechanical stresses. English language ed. Rockville: Aspen Publishers Inc, 1990.
20. Jirout J. The effect of mobilization of the segmental blockade on the sagittal component of the reaction on lateral flexion of the cervical spine. Neuroradiology 1972;3:210.
21. Sharpless S.K. Susceptibility of spinal nerve roots to compression block. In: Goldstein M, ed. The research status of spinal manipulative therapy. Washington D.C: Government Printing Office, 1975:155–161.
22. Herbst RW. Gonstead chiropractic science and art. Mt. Horeb, WI: Sci-Chi Publications, 1968.
23. Schalimtzek M. Roentgenological examination of the function of the lumbar spine. Universitetsforlaget I Aarhus: Denmark 1958:155–167.
24. Webster's New world dictionary, 2nd ed. Simon and Schuster: New York, 1982.
25. Van Buskirk RL. Nociceptive reflexes and the somatic dysfunction: a model. J Am Osteopath Assoc 1990;90:792–809.
26. Coote JH. Somatic sources of afferent input as factors in aberrant autonomic, sensory, and motor function. In: Korr I, ed. The neu-

robiologic mechanisms in manipulative therapy. New York: Plenum Press, 1978.
27. Dishman RW. Review of the literature supporting a scientific basis for the chiropractic subluxation complex. J Manipulative Physiol Ther 1985;8:163–174.
28. Kirkaldy-Willis WH. Managing low back pain. New York: Churchill and Livingstone, 1983:82.
29. Lehmann TR, Spratt KF, Tozzi JE, et al. Long-term follow-up of lower lumbar fusion patients. Spine 1987;12:97–104.
30. Carrick FR. Treatment of pathomechanics of the lumbar spine by manipulation. J Manipulative Physiol Ther 1981;4:173.
31. Grice AS. Radiographic, biomechanical and clinical factors in lumbar lateral flexion: part I. J Manipulative Physiol Ther 1979;2:26–39.
32. Hviid H. The influence of chiropractic treatment on the rotatory mobility of the cervical spine—a kinesiometric and statistical study. Ann Swiss Chir Assoc 1971;5:31.
33. Sandoz R. Technique and interpretation of functional radiography of the lumbar spine. Ann Swiss Chiro Assoc 1965;3:66.
34. Rahlman J. Mechanisms of intervertebral joint fixation. J Manipulative Physiol Ther 1987;10:177–187.
35. Gatterman MI. Chiropractic management of spine related disorders. Baltimore: Williams & Wilkins, 1990: 45.
36. Bogduk N, Engel R. The menisci of the lumbar zygapophyseal joints: a review of their anatomy and clinical significance. Spine 1984;5:454.
37. Wyke B. Workshop on the clinical neurology of joints. Audio cassette program. Dallas: Nov. 22–23, 1980.
38. Lewit K. The contribution of clinical observation to neurological mechanisms in manipulative therapy. In: Korr I, ed. The neurobiologic mechanisms in manipulative therapy. New York: Plenum, 1978: 43–52.
39. Cyriax J. Textbook of orthopedic medicine, 11th ed. Eastbourne: Bailliere and Tindall, 1984: 36–42.
40. Duncan W, Hoen T. A new approach to the diagnosis of herniation of the intervertebral disc. Surg Gynec Obstet 1942;75:257–267.
41. Maigne T. Orthopedic medicine: a new approach to vertebral manipulations. Springfield: Charles C Thomas, 1972.
42. Sandoz R. Newer trends in the pathogenesis of spinal disorders. Ann Swiss Chiro Assoc 1971;V:93.
43. Hubka MJ, Taylor JAM, Schultz GD, Traina AD. Lumbar intervertebral disc herniation: chiropractic management using flexion, extension, and rotational manipulative therapy. Chiropractic Technique 1991;3:5–12.
44. Cassidy JD, Quon JA, Kirkaldy-Willis WH. Letter to the editor. J Manipulative Physiol Ther 1990;13:40–41.
45. Cox JM. Low back pain mechanism, diagnosis and treatment. 4th ed. Baltimore: Williams & Wilkins, 1985.
46. White AA, Panjabi MM. Clinical biomechanics of the spine. 2nd. ed. Philadelphia: J.B. Lippincott, 1990.
47. Quon JA, Cassidy JD, O'Connor SM, Kirkaldy-Willis WH. Lumbar intervertebral disc herniation: treatment by rotational manipulation. J Manipulative Physiol Ther 1989;12:220–278.
48. Bogduk N. Pathology of lumbar disc pain. Manual Med 1990;5:72–79.
49. Twomey L, Taylor JR. Structural and mechanical disc changes with age. Manual Med 1990;5:58–61.
50. Keating JC. Inter-examiner reliability of motion palpation of the lumbar spine: a review of quantitative literature. Am J Chiro Med 1989;2:107–110.
51. Keating JC, Bergmann TF, Jacobs GE, Finer BA, Larson K. Interexaminer reliability of eight evaluative dimensions of lumbar segmental abnormality. J Manipulative Physiol Ther 1990;13:463–470.
52. Portek I, Pearcy NJ, Reader GP, Mowat AG. Correlation between radiographic and clinical measurement of lumbar spine movement. Br J Rheum 1983;22:197.
53. Brieg A. Adverse mechanical tension in the central nervous system. Stockholm: Almqvist & Wiksell International, 1978.
54. Takata K, Shun-Ichi I, Kazuhisa T, Yoshinori O. Swelling of the cauda equina in patients who have herniation of a lumbar disc. J Bone Joint Surg 1988;70:361–368.
55. Carrick F. Cervical radiculopathy: the diagnosis and treatment of pathomechanics in the cervical spine. J Manipulative Physiol Ther 1983;6:129–137.
56. Bradley WG. Disorders of peripheral nerves. Oxford: Blackwell Scientific Publications, 1974:129–145.
57. Gunn C, Milbrandt W. Early and subtle signs in low back sprain. Spine 1978;3:267–281.
58. Gunn CC, Milbrandt WE. Tenderness at motor points—a diagnostic and prognostic aid for low back injury. J Bone Joint Surg 1976;58A:815–825.
59. Axellson J, Theslett S. A study of supersensitivity in denervation mammalian skeletal muscles. J Physiol 1959;147:178–193.
60. Haymaker W, Woodhall B. Peripheral nerve injuries. Philadelphia: W.B. Saunders Co, 1953:145–151.
61. Korr I, ed. The neurobiologic mechanisms in manipulative therapy. New York: Plenum Press, 1978:229–268.
62. A dictionary of life sciences. London: Pam Brooks LTD, 1978.
63. Byrne JH. Cellular analysis of associative learning. Physiol Rev 1987;67:329–439.
64. Groves PM, Thompson RF. Habituation: a dual-process theory. Psychological Rev 1970;77:419–450.
65. Thompson RF, Spencer WA. Habituation: a model phenomenon for the study of neuronal substrates of behavior. Psychol Rev 1966;73:16–43.
66. Slosberg M. Spinal learning: central modulation of pain processing and long-term alteration of interneuronal excitability as a result of nociceptive peripheral input. J Manipulative Physiol Ther 1990;13:326–336.
67. Denslow JS, Hassett CC. The central excitatory state associated with postural abnormalities. J Neurophysiol 1942;5:393–401.
68. Patterson MM, Steinmetz JE. Long-lasting alterations of spinal reflexes: a potential basis for somatic dysfunction. Manual Med 1986;2:38–42.
69. Malliani A, Pagani M, Lombardi F. Visceral versus somatic mechanisms. In: Wall PD, Melzack R, eds. Textbook of Pain. New York: Churchill Livingstone, 1984:100–109.
70. Wyke B. The neurology of back pain. In: Jason MIV, ed. The lumbar spine and back pain. 3rd ed. Edinburgh: Churchill Livingstone, 1987.
71. Bogduk N. The innervation of intervertebral discs. In: Ghosh P, ed. The biology of the intervertebral disc. Vol 1. Boca Raton: CRC Press, 1988:135–149.
72. Ruch TC. Pathophysiology of pain. In: Ruch T, Patton HD, eds. Physiology and biophysics: the brain and neural function. 2nd ed. Philadelphia: WB Saunders Co, 1979:272–324.
73. Mountcastle VB, ed. Medical physiology. St Louis: CV Mosby Co, 1980:391–427.
74. Feindel WH, Weddell G, Sinclair DC. Pain sensibility in deep somatic structures. J Neurol Neurosurg Psychiatry 1948;11:113–117.
75. Stacey MJ. Free nerve endings in skeletal muscle of the cat. J Anat 1961;105:231–254.
76. Stilwell DL. Regional variations in the innervation of deep fascia and aponeuroses. Anat Rec 1957: 127:635–653.
77. Stilwell DL Jr. The innervation of tendons and aponeuroses. Am J Anat 1957;100:289–317.
78. Wall PD, Melzack R, eds. Textbook of Pain. London: Churchill Livingstone, 1985:2–15.
79. Mathews JA, Yates DAH. Reduction of lumbar disc prolapse by manipulation. Br Med J 1969;3:696–697.
80. Mathews JA. Dynamic discography: a study of lumbar traction. Ann Phys Med 1968 7:275.

81. Neumann HD. A concept of manual medicine. In: Buerger AA, Greenman PE, eds. Empirical approaches to the validation of spinal manipulation. Springfield: Charles C Thomas, 1985:267–272.
82. Tardieu C, Tabary JC, Tabar C, Tardieu G. Adaptation of connective tissue length to immobilization in the lengthened and shortened positions in cat soleus muscle. J Physiol (Paris) 1982;78:214–220.
83. Huet De La Tour E, Tardieu C, Tabary JC, Tabary C. Decrease of muscle extensibility and reduction of sarcomere number in soleus muscle following a local injection of tetanus toxin. J Neuro Sci 1979;40:123–131.
84. Maier A, Eldred E, Edgerton V. The effects of spindles on muscle atrophy and hypertrophy. Exper Neuro 1972;37:100–123.
85. Esaki K. Morphological study of muscle spindle in atrophic muscle induced by immobilization. Nagoya Med J 1966;12:185–201.
86. Shambaugh P. Changes in electrical activity in muscles resulting from chiropractic adjustment: a pilot study. J Manipulative Physiol Ther 1987;10:300–304.
87. Gracovetsky S, Farfan HF, Lamy C. The mechanism of the lumbar spine. Spine 1981;6:249.
88. Salter RB. Textbook of disorders and injuries of the musculoskeletal system. Baltimore: Williams & Wilkins, 1970:220.
89. Wiles MR. Visceral disorders related to the spine. In: Gatterman MI, ed. Chiropractic management of spine related disorders. Baltimore: Williams & Wilkins, 1990:379–280.
90. Videman T. Experimental osteoarthritis in the rabbit. ACTA Orthop Scand 1982;53:339–347.
91. Lussier A, Demedicus R. Correlation between ossification and inflammation using a rat experimental model. J Rheum 1983;11:114–117.
92. Theron J, Moret J. Spinal phlebography. New York: Springer-Verlag, 1978.
93. Roston JB, Haines RW. Cracking in the metacarpophalangeal joint. J Anat 1947;81:165–173.
94. Cassidy JD, Kirkaldy-Willis WH, McGregor M. Spinal manipulation for the treatment of chronic low-back and leg pain: an observational study. In: Buerger AA, Greenman PE, eds. Empirical approaches to the validation of spinal manipulation. Springfield: Charles C Thomas, 1985:119–48.
95. Meal GM, Scott RA. Analysis of the joint crack by simultaneous recording of sound and tension. J Manipulative Physiol Ther 1986: 9:189–195.
96. Coxhead CE, Inskip H, Meade TW, North WRS, Troup JDG. Multicentre trial of physiotherapy in the management of sciatic symptoms. Lancet 1981 May 16:1065–1068.
97. Cohen LA. Role of eye and neck proprioceptive mechanisms in body orientation and motor coordination. J Neurophysiol 1961;24:1–11.
98. De Jong PTYM, De Jong JMBV, Cohen B, Jonkees LBW. Ataxia and nystagmus induced by local anesthetics in the neck. Annals Neurol 1977;1:240–246.

4 Spinal Examination

MARK A. LOPES with the assistance of GREGORY PLAUGHER, PETER J. WALTERS, and EDWARD E. CREMATA

The goal of the spinal examination is to assess normal and abnormal spinal function accurately. Neuromechanical disorders such as the vertebral subluxation complex (VSC) will manifest characteristic signs and symptoms that are readily identifiable. The effects of intersegmental dysfunction on the global posture of the spine are also analyzed. The doctor must be able to evaluate the entire locomotor system and its related areas to obtain a comprehensive assessment of the patient. The spinal examination therefore, has a number of components.

A differential diagnosis of the major complaints should always be performed. The patient assessment includes a determination of spinal levels or thrusting actions that are contraindicated for treatment.

Chiropractors need to be aware of the multitude of conditions that subjectively and/or objectively mimic the signs and symptoms associated with a VSC. Viscerosomatic referred pain patterns are encountered in practice and can include such etiologies as kidney or bladder infection, myocardial infarction, and gall bladder disease.

Determining the treatment of choice in patient management requires reliable and valid multiparameter procedures (i.e., multitest regimen). Chiropractors should use analytical tools that are both sensitive and specific to the manifestations of a VSC. At this point, the usefulness of most of the examination strategies available to the chiropractor, including those presented here, is unknown. The information presented here is largely based on clinical observation from various sources and is corroborated with scientific information wherever possible.

In addition to clinical necessity, third-party payers and independent examiners will increasingly require documentation and rationale that support treatment regimes. Little uniformity exists regarding the desired approach to a given clinical situation. Some consensus exists, however, for manipulation as a treatment for low back pain (1). Unfortunately, the vast majority of legal precedence for the substantiation of the need for treatment of physical injuries are orthopaedic and neurologic tests aimed at detecting gross pathology, neuropathy, and dysfunction. The complete clinical picture of all the characteristics of the VSC may be subtle and easily missed with traditional orthopaedic or neurologic examinations. For example, it is common for an individual to have intersegmental dysfunction without symptomatic or apparent limitations (2). An orthopaedic test showing a full range of motion is not sensitive to abnormalities of individual motion segments. Another example of an inappropriate examination is the use of a neurologic test that can only detect gross motor weakness, when only minor changes may be present. Subtle, early signs may exist in individuals with partial involvement of the neural elements. Such subtle signs may take the form of trophic skin changes or vascular dysfunction from abnormalities in autonomic or sensory function (3).

Chiropractors are a primary portal of entry for public health care. When a patient enters a chiropractor's office, the doctor must first decide whether or not that patient is a candidate for chiropractic treatment. Without the proper skills of clinical evaluation, the doctor may not be able to determine if the presenting signs and symptoms originate from a VSC or from a condition beyond the scope of chiropractic practice. Appropriate treatment is possible only after using adequate examination procedures and arriving at an accurate assessment.

RELIABILITY AND VALIDITY OF DIAGNOSTIC TESTS

One of the major research activities in the profession focuses on determining the reliability and validity of various diagnostic instruments or tests (e.g., lumbar motion palpation). The reliability and validity of most of our common means for assessing the status of the patient with a VSC are largely unexplored. When adequate research is performed, some of our traditional examination procedures may prove to be unreliable for certain patient groups. Those procedures that have been researched, have been tested primarily for reliability and not for validity. The results of trials performed on end-feel motion palpation for example, have not, thus far, shown acceptable levels of reliability (4). Most of these experiments lack clinical extrapolation because a large portion of them were performed using relatively pain-free individuals as subjects. Other procedures, such as palpation for tenderness (5) and bilateral thermocouple skin temperature analysis (6), have shown reliability in some instances but have yet to be tested for validity.

Sensitivity is defined as the proportion of subjects with the disease who have a positive test. Sensitivity indicates how good a test is at identifying the diseased. *Specificity* is the proportion of subjects without the disease who have a negative test. Specificity indicates how good a test is at identifying normal individuals. The usefulness of a diagnostic test depends not only on its sensitivity and specificity, but also on the prevalence of the disease in the population. As the prevalence of a disease decreases, it becomes less likely that someone with a positive test actually has the disease and more likely that the test represents a false positive (7). The more rare a disease is, the more specific a test must be to be clinically useful. If the disease is relatively common, then the test must be very sensitive to be useful. Otherwise, a negative test is likely to represent a false negative (7).

CLINICAL RELEVANCE

Scientific studies do not always give us information that is clinically applicable. It is difficult to design experiments to duplicate the manner in which an examination tool is used in the clinical setting. Practitioners must use caution in extrapolating too much from one or a few studies, unless the design of the experiment is close to the clinical use of the procedure. For example, studies that are done on pain-free subjects testing procedures commonly used on patients with symptoms of back pain may not be applicable to the clinical setting. The preceding hypothetical experiment may be more appropriate in determining the ability of the test to identify normal individuals (i.e., specificity).

Perhaps one reason for the marginal reliability found when testing examination procedures relates to the researcher's inability to reproduce the actual clinical use of the instrument tested during the experiment. Often, the design of a research project dictates blinding or controlling parameters that demand a modified use of the examination tool, thus allowing uninterpretable data or data that cannot be interpreted as a direct measurement of clinical usefulness of the examination tool tested. In motion palpation studies, perhaps we have discovered several ways in which not to use motion palpation, but it is still premature to comment on the test's clinical usefulness in perhaps a slightly different application, particularly if this modified use more closely resembles the actual clinical use (7). Perhaps the use of diagnostic tests in pain-free subjects, sometimes not reproducing the test's usual clinical use, adversely influences the outcome and interpretability of some reliability testing. Caution is advised when attempting to apply the results of these investigations to modify clinical protocols. Until further research is completed, chiropractors and other health care practitioners must rely primarily on clinical experience and informed logical thought progression for decision making in regards to the diagnosis and treatment of choice.

CLINICAL DECISION MAKING

The potential for variability in spinal assessment is illustrated in the following example. Schalimtzek (8) reported that of a total of 420 lumbar segments analyzed with functional radiography, more than half (i.e., 220 segments) demonstrated signs of dysfunction.

A complex disorder such as the VSC requires different types of assessment procedures to obtain a comprehensive evaluation. The different parameters (i.e., signs and symptoms) of the VSC, such as the neurologic and biomechanical components, require their respective examination strategies. Although a multitest examination protocol is advocated here, occasionally the doctor must rely on one or a few important findings to decide on the treatment that is indicated or contraindicated. One factor may weigh more heavily than any other if it appears that this factor is pathognomonic of the presenting disorder. Consider the following example. A patient presents with localized, upper neck pain. Examination reveals equivocal x-ray and instrumentation findings, palpable muscle spasm and tenderness on the right between the C2 and C3 vertebrae. Let us assume that the doctor has ruled out the possibility that the muscular and tenderness findings are compensatory in nature. With an awareness of the possible underlying causes of these findings (e.g., meniscoid entrapment, reflex spasm, etc.), the doctor may speculate from these few findings and decide to apply a safe, short, manipulative trial.

Test Magnitude

In the interpretation of some diagnostic tests, a cut-off point needs to be determined to differentiate a negative from a positive test. Often the magnitude of the positive findings of a test helps in the determination of the amount of weight that the test deserves. A cholesterol test showing twice the normal amount expected for a particular patient should be given much more weight than a cholesterol test showing only marginal elevation above "normal" (normal values are usually a mean of a given population). Retrolisthesis of 3 millimeters on a lateral weight-bearing radiograph is much more likely to interfere with the neural contents of the foramina than a 1-millimeter displacement. This likelihood is due to the fact that the transverse diameter of the IVF, when diminished, will interfere with the neural contents contained within (9). In contrast, reduction of the vertical dimension, will have little effect.

A reproducible bilateral thermocouple difference of 15 points on the meter, will likely be more reliable, because it can be more easily differentiated from normal, than a three point difference. If only those patients with the magnitude of findings for either of the above examples were selected for interexaminer reliability studies of these parameters, reliability coefficients might be more encouraging. Reliance on high magnitude (clinically obvious) tests and the discarding of marginal tests, therefore, is one way that the clinician can increase the accuracy of the examination. The discarding of marginally positive tests (slight fixation, slight positional dyskinesia, suggestive but not definitively positive orthopaedic tests) will likely help the clinician in the reduction of error during the interpretation of the examination.

Diagnostic Treatment

The fact that chiropractic adjustments are partially diagnostic can assist in patient management. Even if two doctors do not agree on where to adjust a patient at the beginning of treatment, the step by step approach to the follow-up of a series of adjustments may eventually lead the two practitioners to the same "primary" area. Adjustments administered to areas of secondary involvement, or compensations, often result in symptomatic exacerbations of primary areas. Unsuccessful treatment in this situation will usually direct treatment to another level involved in VSC, given that more than one level exists in that patient. Adjusting one segment too high will often direct the force to a compensatory hypermobile articulation, causing irritation. Hypermobility and instability commonly occurs above the level of fixation dysfunction as in the case of surgical fusion for the lumbar spine (10). Adjustments applied below the level of subluxation commonly cause less irritation unless provided on an ongoing basis.

Outcome Measures

Clinical assessment tools are essentially outcome measures used to determine the effectiveness of health care. Outcome measures are categorized according to whether the information they reflect is physiologically or clinically relevant (11). The dependability of the assessment procedure is its most important attribute. Unfortunately, few outcome measures that are pertinent to chiropractic care have unambiguous literature support or consensus among clinicians. Electromyographic, thermographic, radiographic, and palpatory findings are used as outcome measures for a patient, but without strong data as to their reliability and validity it is sometimes difficult to determine their clinical usefulness. The absence of absolute certainty does not preclude their use in clinical practice for the time being, because most current applications are largely based on empirical evidence.

Valid outcome measures that have strong research support include assessments of regional mobility (e.g., goniometric) (12), pain reporting instruments (e.g., pain drawing, McGill Pain Questionnaire, Visual Analog Scale) (13), self-care activities, and limited performance measures (e.g., Sickness Impact Profile, Oswestry Disability Score) (14). Because many individuals can have spinal lesions that are relatively silent in terms of symptomatology or functional limitations, there is a preference for "hard data" (objective) over "soft data" (subjective) types of measures in the spinal evaluation, where an adjustment may be indicated.

One very interesting test is the Schema Assessment Instrument (SAI). In a study by Lacroix et al. (15), the SAI was the only measure that accurately predicted the return to work for patients with low back pain. Other measures investigated in that study were orthopaedic physical evaluations and other soft data measures. The SAI is an assessment of the accuracy of the patient's understanding of his or her own condition. The above findings strongly suggest that patient education is important in the recovery from low back pain conditions. Patient education and awareness has a significant effect on the percentage of those patients that successfully return to work after an episode of low back pain. White (16) believes that once a patient understands and takes responsibility for the condition, the ability to control the pain is enhanced.

DIAGNOSTIC USEFULNESS

Several criteria are used to determine the usefulness of an assessment procedure. Some of these factors include applicability, practicality, reliability, validity, sensitivity, and specificity (17). Vendors selling an instrument or procedure to practitioners often present data suggesting that their instrument has been adequately tested for some of the above criteria. Unless scientific evidence is presented, no firm conclusions should be made. Not being prepared to make a qualified decision, practitioners are often sold on the instrument based on income potential or technical appeal rather than diagnostic usefulness. It is easy to increase a doctor's income by artificially inflating the cost per visit average through the addition of unnecessary diagnostic testing. Sackett et al. (18) have developed the following guidelines for determining the clinical usefulness of a diagnostic test:

1. Has there been an independent, "blind" comparison with a "gold standard" of diagnosis?
2. Has the diagnostic test been evaluated in a patient sample that included an appropriate spectrum of mild and severe, treated and untreated disease, as well as individuals with different but commonly confused disorders?
3. Was the setting for this evaluation, as well as the filter through which the study patients passed, adequately described?
4. Have the reproducibility of the test result (precision) and its interpretation (observer variation) been determined?
5. Has the term "normal" been defined sensibly as it applies to this test?
6. If the test is advocated as part of a cluster or sequence of tests, has its individual contribution to the overall validity of the cluster or sequence been determined?
7. Have the tactics for carrying out the test been described in sufficient detail to permit their exact replication?
8. Has the utility of the test been determined? (Will the patient be better off for it?)

The above is a rigorous but necessary protocol for evaluating any assessment strategy. Most diagnostic tests, in any health field, will not satisfy many of the above guidelines. Often Guideline 1 cannot be met, simply because of the lack of a valid "gold standard" or reference test.

Diagnostic Strategies

Diagnostic approaches have been described as one or a combination of the following four types (18). The first is pattern recognition—often unconsciously used by the seasoned clinician. A second type is the multiple branching method, which is an algorithmic progression of logical steps toward the correct diagnosis. The third type of diagnostic approach is the exhaustion method, the "complete" history and physical exam used by the novice directly out of the classroom setting. Finally, the most widely used strategy is the hypothetico-deductive approach. The hypothetico-deductive strategy is the formulation of a short list of potential diagnoses or actions followed by clinical actions that will best reduce the length of the list. The initial short probabilities list is formulated on average within 28 seconds after exposure to the earliest clues (19).

If clinicians can ferret out the key observations, their effectiveness and efficiency will sharply increase. One must determine which data are useful and which should be ignored. One must also know how to obtain the relevant data in a reliable and accurate manner. The clinician is the most important factor in the advancement of the art and science of examination (20).

CLINICAL DISAGREEMENT

Patient Histories

Even experienced clinicians often disagree over patient histories. In one study (21), two senior British surgeons independently interviewed the same group of patients who had undergone operations for peptic ulcers. Using the same set of clinical criteria, the two surgeons agreed on whether or not the operation had been successful in less than two-thirds of the cases. Such clinical disagreement is of major concern, in light of the fact that the history is often the most important factor in clinical assessment.

Physical Findings

Because most clinical manifestations of the VSC do not lend themselves to simplistic evaluations, decisions regarding the treatment of choice (e.g., segment to be adjusted) may vary from doctor to doctor. This variation is true even when both providers share the same techniques and philosophies of approach. Neuroradiologists tested for agreement of interpretation of lumbar CT scans showed that total agreement was obtained in only 6 of the 52 asymptomatic subjects (22). Chiropractors tested for interexaminer reliability of lumbar radiographic analysis of 56 different measures showed statistically significant agreement for only 6 of the 56 marking procedures used (23). When clinicians examine the same patient twice, they are only slightly more likely to agree with themselves than with another clinician (24).

The interpretation of diagnostic tests is a common source of disagreement. Among the medical diagnostic tests interpreted inconsistently are mammograms, coronary angiograms, ECGs, and pathology specimens (18). Assessment of patient compliance may also be inaccurate. Clinicians in one study were no more accurate than random chance in assessing patient compliance (25). Patients were found to be accurate in assessing their own compliance in another study (26). These same patients tended to be biased, however, and overestimated their compliance by an average of 20%.

Keating et al. (5) tested the interexaminer reliability of a multitest regimen for lumbar segmental dysfunction. Of the eight assessment strategies tested, only the determination of palpatory pain over osseous or paraspinal tissues showed good agreement beyond that expected by chance alone. Weaker agreement levels were noted for skin temperature differences and for visual inspection of segmental abnormality. Little agreement was detected for passive or active lumbar motion palpation.

Diagnosis and Treatment Recommendations

The least agreement seems to exist with respect to diagnostic or management decisions. Researchers have tested clinicians on several occasions about agreement of diagnosis and management. A most glaring example of inaccuracy occurred in the following study (27). Three hundred eighty-nine children with intact tonsils were examined by a group of physicians; tonsillectomy was recommended for 45%. The remaining children not recommended for surgery were then reexamined by another group of clinicians for a second opinion. Of the second opinion group, 46% were then recommended for surgery. The rest of the children, twice passed over for surgical recommendations, were examined a third time. Remarkably, 44% of these children were recommended for tonsillectomy. More recent examples of the above type of inaccuracies suggest that the contemporary situation is relatively unchanged (18).

Suppose, for example, a study similar to the one above was designed to test whether or not a motion segment exhibited fixation dysfunction and needed an adjustment, using motion palpation findings as the inclusion/exclusion criteria. As the clinicians are asked to scrutinize segments that were previously determined to be normal, there is likely to be a tendency to try and identify a dysfunctional level. When a clinician is forced to make a decision, bias becomes a considerable confounding variable.

Sources of Clinical Disagreement

The difficulties in maintaining consistency in clinical decision making are evident. Clinical disagreement can arise from the examiner, the examined, and the examination. Factors influencing clinical consistency are the biologic variation in the senses, the tendency to record inference rather than evidence, getting overcome by diagnostic classification schemes, entrapment by prior expectation, and ignorance (18).

It is most important to reduce clinical disagreement in the crucial areas of the history, examination, and diagnosis to ensure proper patient management. One must pay particular attention to certain questions and answers in the history, skillfully use the most reliable examination procedures, eliminate the most variable methods, and approach the decision from an unbiased perspective.

When a specific element has a crucial effect on the management of the patient, the clinician must be certain to prevent or minimize the inaccuracy and inconsistency in determining its presence and significance. Table 4.1 is a list of strategies for maximizing accurate and consistent clinical assessment.

ACCURACY AND BIAS

Consistency between clinicians is essential, but consistency by itself is insufficient. Clinicians may agree but be inaccurate. To illustrate the difference between accuracy and consistency, we will consider an example involving motion palpation. Palpation of the range of motion of an articulation lacks acceptable gold standards for comparison and is therefore subject to variation and bias. Bias is a systematic distortion or a preconceived opinion about something (28). One may develop bias about the meaning or interpretation of a procedure such as motion palpation, as one is left to freely interpret the evidence obtained from clinical experience, because of the lack of a gold standard for comparison. If a biased clinician sets out to teach motion palpation, that bias will likely be systematically shared. The students of that clinician may skillfully and consistently agree with the findings of the instructor after enough practical experience. The accuracy of these consistent palpators may still be poor, if the initial instructor's interpretations are invalid.

The authors conclude that a pragmatic approach by knowledgeable clinicians, striving to eliminate bias, inconsistency, and inaccuracy, will provide the most useful information. Applying a judicious trial of chiropractic care after diligent evaluation may help reveal the effectiveness of the treatments and assessments used.

Table 4.1.
Strategies for Minimizing Inaccuracy and Inconsistency in Clinical Assessment[a]

1. Seek agreement of critical factors
   a. Repeat the evaluation
   b. Ask a blinded colleague to repeat the evaluation
   c. Confirm or refute findings using a gold standard when available
   d. Seek documentation or witnesses for corroboration of key findings
2. Differentiate between inference and evidence in case notations
3. Use appropriate tests and tools
4. Blind each assessment from other data
5. Continually seek to improve academic knowledge and the skill of assessment

[a]Modified from Sackett DL, Haynes RB, Tugwell P. Clinical epidemiology: a basic science for clinical medicine. Boston: Little, Brown & Co, 1985:14–49.

INTEGRATING ELEMENTS OF THE EXAMINATION

When attempting to determine whether or not the source of low back pain is stemming from a lower lumbar disc region or the sacroiliac area, the historical facts of the timing and location of the pain are crucial. Sacroiliac pain less often refers or radiates below the knee, is rarely severe and incapacitating, and is commonly relieved by sitting and worsened by walking or lying down. Pain generated from the lower lumbar areas is more commonly referred below the knee, can be excruciating in intensity, and is generally worsened by sitting and reduced by walking or lying recumbent.

Examination of the sacroiliac and lumbar spine may take various paths. In assessing the sacroiliac area for motion abnormalities, inspection, motion palpation, or lateral bending radiographs are readily available options. The most tested of the above procedures is the Gillet motion palpation test, with preliminary evidence that the intraexaminer reliability of the assessment is acceptable (29,30).

Radiographic findings are important differentiating factors in these patients. The lateral radiograph is often the most direct way to assess the structural position of the lower spine and may quickly point to one area or the other as being potentially involved. A lumbar retrolisthesis (31) indicates a likely disc injury, whereas a gross abnormality of the lumbar lordosis may imply a compensatory reaction from a lower level, such as the sacroiliac joint. A properly exposed, well-positioned lateral lumbar radiograph, and a Gillet motion palpation test of the sacroiliac articulations, in combination with a history of the timing and location of the pain are valuable components for this type of evaluation. The above protocol does not encompass a complete work-up. Particular attention should be paid to the carrying out of the above tasks if one expects to assess this type of condition in reliable fashion.

If the findings from the above assessment are equivocal, a logical progression should follow. Suppose there are two levels that show the presence of retrolisthesis (e.g., L4 and L5). A lumbar flexion radiograph may be helpful. If the joint is not fixated, the segment will move anteriorward on flexion due to the anterior shear that is increased during forward flexion. If L4 moves anteriorward (as is often the case) and L5 remains posterior, then a posterior to anterior (+Z) adjustment at L4 is contraindicated because of the instability that is present at that level (See Chapter 7). Lateral bending radiographs may detect dysfunction in another dimension of possible movement. Lateral bending radiography may be useful, especially if sagittal plane motion is relatively normal.

EXAMINATION

A comprehensive chiropractic examination hinges on the ability of the practitioner to combine the history taking, orthopaedic, neurologic, and chiropractic examinations into one smooth, flowing procedure under clinical conditions. The first visit to a doctor's office may leave a lasting impression. The confidence a patient has in the doctor can be greatly enhanced by a quality interaction during the initial encounter.

The physical confines of the clinical setting will provide certain limitations to the format of the initial visit. Streamlining procedures for the expedition of business practices may jeopardize the quality of the examination and treatment process.

Patient Interview

History taking is enhanced when the doctor waits until most of the communication is completed before writing down what was reported. One wants to project the image of a doctor that listens and cares, as well as one who understands the presenting complaints of the patient. Projecting this image is difficult when the doctor is looking down and writing while the patient is talking. The conversation flows and becomes more natural when it is not interrupted.

If certain questions are of a rhetorical nature or if the response the patient is going to give is likely to be false, then the question should not be asked. For example, a parent is unlikely to volunteer information that they have been abusing a child.

Meaningful history taking is a skillful art. If the doctor is going to be rushed during the process, then the examination should be postponed to a later time. It is often difficult to elicit a lengthy history from a patient in acute pain. If the patient is extremely uncomfortable, the doctor should be thorough enough to assess only those needs of the patient that are immediate.

Experienced clinicians manage clinical disorders ranging from the common to the obscure. Patterns of symptoms may allow the astute practitioner to develop initial impressions of the cause of the patient's condition before any examination. The doctor should use an eclectic approach during the history to determine whether or not the patient's condition is amenable to chiropractic treatment, as well as which levels of the spine may be involved in subluxation.

Notations

The initial history notations are essentially the same for all practitioners. The chiropractor, however, must use a slightly different note taking procedure than other health care disciplines. The follow-up visit notations are very specific and are modified from initial history and examination findings. S.O.A.P. notes are common to both medicine and chiropractic. The "S" stands for subjective complaints, "O" for objective findings, "A" for assessment, "P" for prognosis and prescription.

Vernon (32) advocates the use of S.O.R.E. notes for chiropractic practice. The "S" stands for subjective, "O" for objective, but the "R" stands for prescription (as in Rx or treatment; i.e., adjustment), and "E" represents exercises and ergonomics. The rationale for the use of S.O.R.E. rather than S.O.A.P. notes is due to the frequency of chiropractic visits. Assessment and prognostic indicators are not as useful on a routine visit to the chiropractor as they are to the medical doctor. The medical doctor usually sees the patient after considerable time has elapsed and may make an assessment that changes the prognosis or prescription. The chiropractor may see the patient more frequently and can use the "R" and the "E" to list treatment rendered and exercise or ergonomic instruction on an ongoing basis. The occasional use of S.O.A.P. notes with the frequent use of S.O.R.E. notes, provides a useful balance of information in monitoring the progress of the chiropractic patient.

Abbreviations that are universally understood are useful. Specific to a multiparameter approach are notations concerned with each of the parameters of the VSC. Each of these are then monitored at each visit.

Edema, hyperemia, motion characteristics, instrumentation findings, muscle characteristics, and tenderness are commonly checked each visit. These objective findings may be supplemented with traditional history taking as well as orthopaedic and neurologic test results. Follow-up instructions concerned with the "R" and "E" portions are continually reassessed. Abbreviated notations are acceptable if interpretable by others, such as independent examiners, because patient records are often subjected to outside review.

Abbreviations for decreased symptoms, an exacerbation, or no change may take the form of arrows pointing down, up, or sideways (e.g., → LBP stands for no change in low back pain). A positive instrumentation finding with a thermocouple skin temperature device could be: TD C7-T1. The "TD" represents a temperature differential (See Appendix 4A).

LISTINGS

The Palmer-Gonstead-Firth (PGF) listing system of vertebral misalignments are abbreviations for descriptions of interarticular alignment characteristics (33). Keeping current with the standards of practice necessitates the entry of more than these traditional listings into treatment records. For example, a data entry on a particular visit cannot consist solely of the segment contacted and how it was adjusted; progress is equally as important. Without careful documentation, especially in the busy practice, patient management can include a large proportion of guess work.

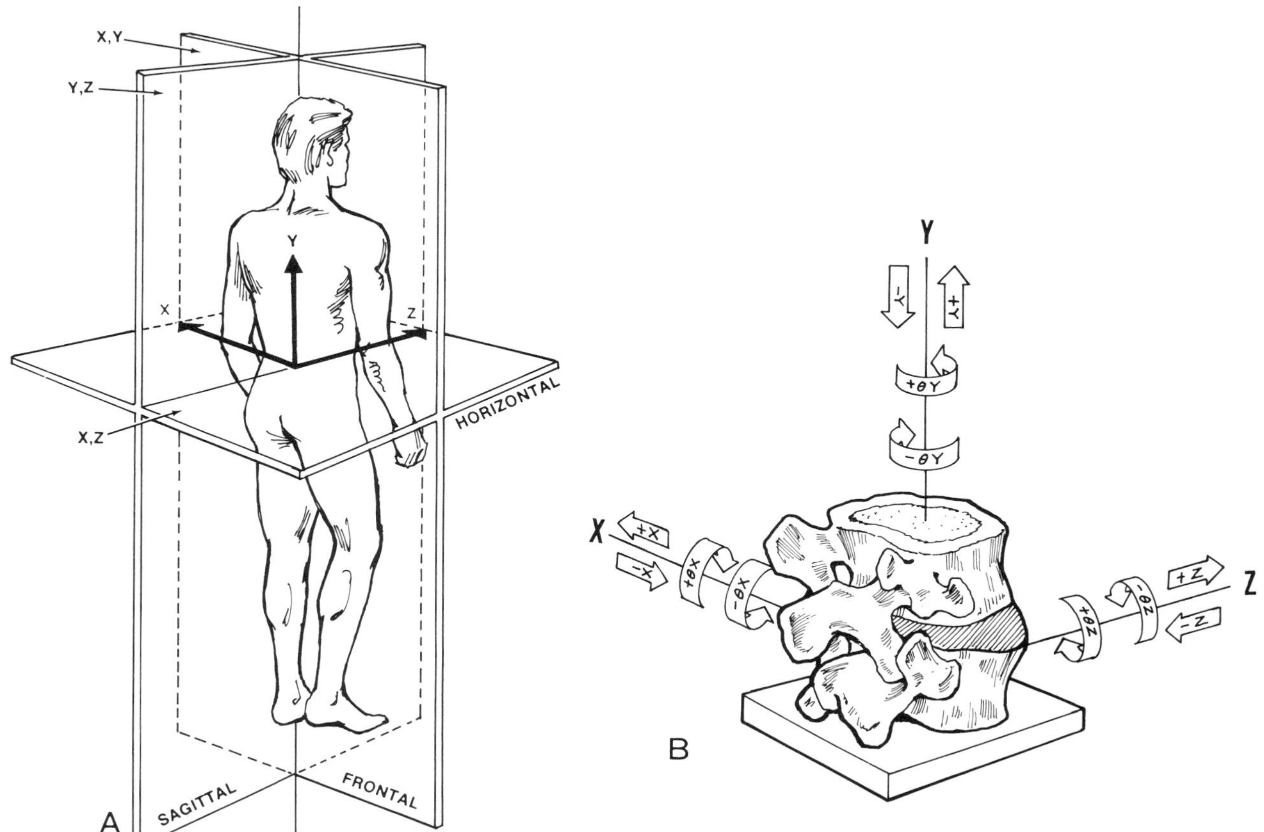

Figure 4.1. A, The cardinal planes of the human. Each plane is formed by two axes. The sagittal plane is formed by the Y and Z axes, the coronal plane by the Y and X axes, and the transverse plane by the X and Z axes. **B,** The international system for defining movements and positions of the functional spinal unit.

The listing describes the positional state of a vertebra relative to its subjacent foundation. We have included a table that shows what each letter of a listing represents. This has been combined with the right-handed orthogonal coordinate system (See Chapter 2) (Fig. 4.1A-B). Because this method has been proposed for international acceptance (34–36), it will be referred to here as the International System (33). The letters used in the PGF and International listing systems and their meaning are presented. Generally, the first letter of the listing denotes translation along the Z axis, the second letter is for rotation of the vertebrae around the Y axis. The third letter is for listing any lateral flexion positional dyskinesia.

Direction	PGF	International
Anterior	A	$+Z$
Posterior	P	$-Z$
Right (Spinous)	R	$+\theta Y$
Left (Spinous)	L	$-\theta Y$

If there is a lateral flexion malposition of the vertebra, this is listed with the PGF system in relation to the direction of spinous rotation (i.e., right or left). If the spinous has rotated towards the open or superior side of the wedge (opposite the direction of lateral flexion), this is noted as an "S." If the spinous has rotated towards the closed or inferior side of the wedge, this is listed with an "I." Two examples are presented that also have the component of posteriority listed with them.

PRS PLI

The International system lists lateral flexion positional dyskinesia as a rotation, around the Z axis (clockwise $(+\theta)$ or counterclockwise $(-\theta)$). The preceding examples would be listed as follows.

$-Z, +\theta Y, -\theta Z \qquad -Z, -\theta Y, -\theta Z$

Listings for the pelvic ring are somewhat more complex. Gonstead (37) is the originator for most of these listings. Some assumptions must be made regarding the axes of rotation for the pelvic bones to describe their positional states meaningfully.

Ilium. Internal or external rotation of the ilium with respect to the sacrum is essentially a rotation around the Y axis (See Chapter 6). The ilium is listed with respect to the sacrum. External ilium movement (Posterior superior iliac spine (PSIS) moving away from midline) is listed with an "Ex" and internal movement with an "In." The international system denotes internal and external ilium rotations relative to the sacrum as movements around the Y axis. An Ex ilium on the right would be a clockwise rotation around the Y axis and would be listed as $+\theta Y$. An In ilium on the left side would also be a clockwise rotation and would be listed as $+\theta Y$. It therefore becomes important to list the side of the sacroiliac involvement.

Antero-superior motion of the PSIS relative to the sacrum ipsilaterally is listed as "AS" and postero-inferior motion as "PI." This type of movement is essentially a rotation around the X axis. In the International System an AS would be listed as $+\theta X$ and a PI as $-\theta X$.

Sacrum. Rotation of the sacrum relative to the ilium at the sacroiliac joints in the Gonstead system is listed as a posterior rotation on either the right or left side (e.g., P-R or P-L). There is no listing for anterior sacrum rotation because the ilium would be adjusted from posterior to anterior in this instance. A P-R sacrum is essentially a counterclockwise rotation around the Y axis and would be listed as $-\theta Y$. A P-L sacrum would be listed as $+\theta Y$.

C2-L5. Hyperextension of the vertebral body is commonly listed as inferior or "inf." This movement is a rotation around the X axis and would be listed as $-\theta X$ in the international system. Contact points for adjusting the vertebrae are abbreviated and follow the main listing:

m = mamillary process, sp = spinous process,

t = transverse process, la = lamina

One would not apply a listing to a motion segment unless the articulation in question met the criteria of a VSC, a prerequisite of which is fixation dysfunction (See Chapter 3).

Movements of the motion segment are easily listed with the International system. Fixation dysfunction can be represented with a descending arrow just preceding the listing of the particular movement. If motion is increased in a particular direction, then the arrow preceding the listing can be oriented upward. If the movement of the joint is the same as when last examined a "no change" could be listed with a horizontal arrow or by "noΔ."

Flexion = $+\theta X$
Anterior Translation = $+Z$
Right Lateral bending = $+\theta Z$
Right Translation = $-X$
Body Right Rotation (Spinous Left) = $-\theta Y$
Body Left
Rotation (Spinous Right) = $+\theta Y$
Caudal Translation = $-Y$

Extension = $-\theta X$
Posterior Translation = $-Z$
Left Lateral Bending = $-\theta Z$
Left Translation = $+X$
Cephalad Translation = $+Y$

A complete list of chart abbreviations used frequently in chiropractic practice is presented in Appendix 4A (38).

S - MDLN LBP w/ Ⓡ Lat hip P, 2 wks drtn, wrs to sit, insdius onset

O - edema, HE, TNDR L2/3; T L2, L5;↓ $-\theta X$ L5

A - flare-up

P - L5 PL adj Ⓡ PB, ice, ergnmc cnslt; (W,F)

Figure 4.2. Notations from an office visit after a few weeks of inactive care. SOAP notes were used because an assessment was made regarding the patient's overall status. The patient presented with an insidious flare-up of two weeks duration. The patient had midline low back pain with right lateral hip pain that was worsened by sitting. Objective findings included edema, hyperemia, and tenderness at the L2 and L3 levels, skin temperature alterations at L2 and L5, and restricted extension of L5 vertebra on S1 detected with motion palpation. Treatment consisted of adjustment of the L5 vertebra on S1 in the right pelvic bench position, cryotherapy, and ergonomic consultation for prevention of further injury. The patient was rescheduled for Wednesday and Friday.

S - Nk Pn imp 50%, sl HA post adj, LBP no Δ

O - ↑ $+\theta X$ & dim edema C7-T1; TD C7, L5; HE L5-S1, ↓ $+\theta X$ L5

Rx - C7 PLS-inf, L5 P; watch UC; 3X/2wks

E - exs next wk, reduce sting

Figure 4.3. Notations from a routine follow-up visit during the initial phase of relief care. S.O.R.E. notes were used as they are more appropriate for routine visits with chiropractic care. The patient experienced a fifty percent improvement in neck symptoms since the last visit. A slight headache was reported after the last adjustment. There was no change in the low back symptoms. Limited examination revealed increased flexion range of motion and diminished edema of the C7-T1 articulation. Skin temperature alterations were noted at C7 and L5. Hyperemia and restricted flexion range of motion was evident at L5-S1. Treatment consisted of specific adjustment of C7 and L5 vertebrae with the listings noted. Concern for possible indications for treatment of the upper cervical region on future visits was noted. Further treatment is scheduled at three times per week for two weeks. Exercises will be implemented the following week and the patient was advised to decrease the amount of sitting for the ergonomic reduction in postural stress.

An example of typical chiropractic office visit notations is illustrated in Figure 4.2. The notations are exemplary of a patient seen for reevaluation or for treatment for an exacerbation. Figure 4.3 represents notations more commonly used for routine or multiple visits for chiropractic care. Large amounts of narrative information may be gleaned from the brief notations written in this format. The S.O.R.E. format is illustrated.

GENERAL GUIDELINES

Differential Spinal Pain Assessment. Guidelines for assessing cases of spinal pain have been provided by Hogan (39). These general guidelines are as follows:

1. Neuromuscular skeletal disorders will have their symptoms caused or aggravated by stressing the part involved with movement or activity.

2. Referred pain usually shows no local signs or stiffness, full range of motion, and no increase in pain when the part is stressed. The patient may, however, suggest that some positions are more comfortable than others.
3. Neoplasia should be considered when the symptoms of the patient are that of a constant or relentless pain unrelieved by rest and usually worse at night. Usually, the primary site of the neoplasia is overlooked or asymptomatic.
4. Infections should be suspected when the pain is increased by motion but not relieved by rest. Range of motion will be decreased and there will be local tenderness. The patient is usually afebrile. The white blood cell count is usually normal, but the erythrocyte sedimentation rate will be elevated. The condition is usually subacute or chronic.
5. When dealing with viscerosomatic pain radiating to the low back, consider the following: *a*) sacral pain usually indicates disease of pelvic organs; *b*) lumbar pain usually indicates disease of lower abdominal organs; and *c*) lower thoracic/upper lumbar pain usually relates to diseases of the upper abdominal organs.
6. Simple mechanical low back pain rarely extends below the knee.
7. Acute pain in the abdomen is usually not a common feature in patients with low back problems. It should be remembered that pain in the abdomen for longer than 12 hours may indicate appendicitis. If nausea and vomiting, constipation or diarrhea are present, one should strongly consider a visceral origin.
8. Women of child-bearing age who have missed their period by 10 days may be pregnant. When evaluating female patients with low back pain, it is important to determine the date of the last period and the expected date of the next period, and suggest a pregnancy test if the possibility of pregnancy exists.
9. No one is too ill to examine.
10. It is unlikely that someone electing to visit a physician for any reason is "healthy."

The doctor should work backwards from the history of any visceral symptoms (when present) to the possible area of spinal involvement. The reader is directed to the appropriate chapter for differential diagnosis of specific regional subluxation patterns, and management of the patient with a visceral concomitant.

Order of the Examination

It is helpful to organize the examination into postural categories, so that it can flow from the standing tests to those of sitting, supine, and prone. One may mingle orthopaedic and neurologic tests with the chiropractic analysis. Some choose to go from history taking directly into the comprehensive chiropractic analysis, then on to a complete orthopaedic and neurologic exam, before deciding which radiographic examination, if any, is indicated. It is generally best to work continuously and concisely, and avoid interruptions of exam procedures with manual recording of results after each test. Try to perform a group of tests, then record.

Patient with Acute Pain

Static evaluations are preferred over dynamic tests when examining the acute pain patient where movement is restricted by the severity of the pain. A complete history may be followed by static palpation, instrumentation, and radiographic examination. At times, a patient will be unable to bear weight long enough to be examined in the sitting or standing positions. A hi-lo table with hydraulic raising and lowering capabilities facilitates the changing of positions. Static evaluations may be done in the prone position. In rare cases, a radiograph taken non-weight bearing on the floor, or on a table top, may be the only radiographic exposure tolerated by the patient in severe pain. If only one exposure is possible in the above rare cases, the lateral radiograph is preferred. The lateral radiograph usually provides more useful information for determining the levels indicated and contraindicated for chiropractic adjustment.

IATROGENICS

It is important to remember that many tests function to isolate the problem at hand by reproducing the pain. It is not uncommon for the patient to suffer an exacerbation of pain due to rigorous examination. Care must be taken to adapt the examination to each patient. Streamlining examination procedures may be necessary to eliminate unnecessary patient discomfort. One must do what is required to make an accurate determination of the patient's status, yet avoid duplication of similar tests when possible.

FOLLOW-UP EXAMINATIONS

Chiropractic care requires more frequent and numerous patient visits than medical outpatient care for similar conditions during the early stages of care. The initial examination provides the "working diagnosis" that enables the doctor to prescribe necessary treatment for the first few visits. Follow-up visits provide additional information each time the patient is seen, allowing the doctor to modify the diagnosis and treatment plan as necessary. Commonly, several sessions are required to assess the initial success of the treatment plan.

Adequate examination must include at least a brief analysis of the spine on each follow-up visit, in addition to the initial comprehensive examination. It is unfortunate for patients that some chiropractors do not gown patients (i.e., female patients) on follow-up visits and continue to treat patients on an ongoing basis without direct exposure to the skin overlying the spine. One should never administer an indiscriminate adjustment. It is an act of malpractice to treat without adequate examination.

A description of the methods of each examination procedure follows. Procedures that are performed routinely on most patients such as visual analysis, palpation, instrumentation, and plain film radiography are described first. Additional procedures that supplement the differential diagnosis are discussed after the routine procedures. Analytical methods in this section are described primarily on the basis of their relevance to the VSC. Orthopaedic and neurologic tests complete the diagnostic work-up and are listed at the end of the chapter.

MECHANISMS OF INJURY

For a number of injuries, a description of the trauma by the patient or a third party can aid in isolating an area of joint dysfunction. For example, if the lumbar spine is unable to resist a flexion moment, the result will be injury of the posterior ligamentous structures. The ligaments furthest from the center of rotation, such as the supraspinous, will have to move through a large arc and will usually undergo plastic deformation before other ligamentous elements. This ligament is easily palpated for the presence of tenderness, edema, or scar tissue.

A rotational injury to the pelvis would displace the ilium if the ligaments have been stretched beyond their ability to resist the tension. A common example of such a mechanism would be a blow to the ASIS, as can occur in contact sports. The well-positioned antero-posterior radiograph of the pelvis would likely show evidence of a positional dyskinesia in the region (40–41).

A torticollis presentation may be due to an atlanto-axial rotatory fixation/subluxation (See Chapter 11). This condition can be caused by sleeping with an awkward, rotated, neck posture such as in the prone position. The radiograph will often show the displacement as will a movement assessment of the upper neck (e.g., Dvorak Test).

INSPECTION

The most important aspects of the visual inspection are gait and postural analysis, static and dynamic intersegmental visualization, and global movement visualization. The chiropractor attempts to discover the presence of the VSC by picking up visual clues of positional dyskinesia (intervertebral misalignment) and fixation dysfunction at the skin surface. Body symmetry or asymmetry of posture and motion is scrutinized. A complex approach is advocated here where elements of the history (e.g., mechanism of injury), examination findings, and potential treatment choices are continually integrated and compared. This process provides for a thorough and eclectic understanding of the patient's needs and allows for proper follow-up assessments.

Gait

In the absence of profound neurologic disorders, gait analysis may reveal subtle signs of VSC. Distress during ambulation, as well as functional manifestations of lumbo-pelvic and upper cervical subluxation may be observed while the patient is walking. A patient in noticeable pain will reveal guarded movement of the affected area with or without postural deviation. For example, in cases with severe neck pain, a distinct lack of head movement will be observable.

Sacrum and ilium subluxations may have noticeable effects on lower limb positions and movements. Fixation dysfunction of the sacro-iliac joint will often result in a decrease in the length of the stride ipsilaterally. Functional lower limb length inequalities are likely to occur if sufficient positional dyskinesia accompanies the fixation dysfunction. An internal or external foot flare with concomitant uneven heel or sole wear of the shoe may be caused by Ex or In ilium subluxations. Heel wear on the medial side of the shoe may indicate the side of a functional or anatomical long leg; laterally worn heels may indicate the short leg side.

A fixed, extended positional dyskinesia of the sacrum with respect to the L5 disc space ($-\theta X$ sacral base or "base posterior" sacrum), or a posterior first or second sacral segment (S1 or 2, $-Z$), may result in bilateral toe-in foot flare and/or a genu valgus waddling appearance to the gait. Because adaptive mechanisms often occur in a patient with a long-standing lesion, this particular gait pattern is often more noticeable in the pediatric patient, and warrants early intervention.

Gonstead recognized a relationship between persistent occiput/atlas disrelationships and gait (42). An AS occiput ($-\theta X$ restricted position of the occiput on the atlas) may be accompanied by bilateral outward toe flare. A PS occiput ($+\theta X$) and other upper cervical subluxations may cause toe walking.

Posture

An individual's posture reflects the disposition of the interrelationships of the structural architecture. Standing posture requires little muscular activity (43). The conformation of bone, as well as the articulations between the bones, most directly influence the postural attitude. The posture of the spine is extremely important to its biomechanical function (44).

Biomechanical adaptation is the biologically mediated change in the structures and material properties of the body. In the growing skeleton, these alterations in epiphyseal growth rates can be altered by asymmetrical loads. This phenomenon has been termed the Heuter-Volkmann (HV) Law. This law states that increased pressure across the epiphyseal growth plate inhibits vertical growth, and decreased pressure across the plate accelerates growth (36). The HV Law and Wolff's Law, as well as the phenomenon of creep (See Chapter 2), generally explain an individual's posture. Deviations from optimal intersegmental alignment will be reflected as abnormal

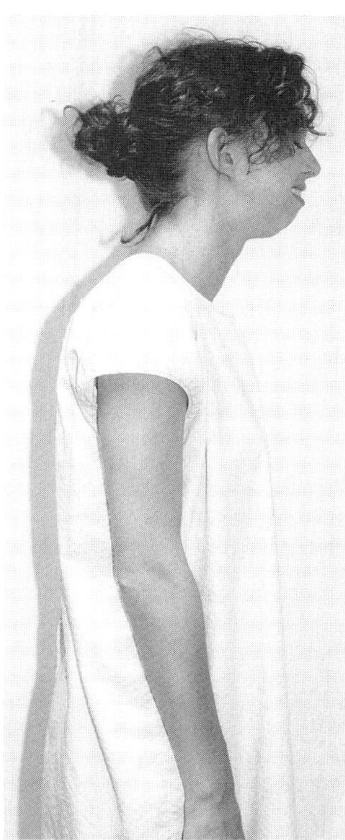

Figure 4.4. Posture in the sagittal plane showing regional adaptation resulting in forward carriage of the head. Flexion ($+\theta X$) malpositions of a few to several upper thoracic vertebra levels is the likely etiology. Tall people, those occupations involving forward bending and lazy posture, commonly show these findings.

posture, provided the changes are of sufficient magnitude to affect more than a few functional spinal units (FSUs) (Fig. 4.4). Constant asymmetric postural loads on the vertebral elements will eventually lead to dysfunction.

The posture of the spine during various movements should also be scrutinized. "Inflexion points" in the intersegmental alignment, present in either static or stressed postures, indicate probable local structural anomaly or intersegmental dysfunction. An inflexion point is an abrupt change in the contour of the spine. This change can be detected in the neutral posture or when the patient moves into a particular position, such as lateral bending (Fig. 4.5A-B). Hypertrophy, atrophy, or asymmetry of musculature, edema, hyperemia, and deviation from bilateral symmetry of any bony landmarks may indicate potential areas of subluxation.

Standing

PATIENT PREPARATION

The patient should be gowned and barefoot with the posterior spine exposed. Instruct the patient to stand upright and walk in place or backwards while looking directly forwards, and come to rest with the feet hip width apart, heels even, and the knees fully extended. Next, have the patient bend the neck, head, and upper body, forward, back, and side to the side, while maintaining the eyes closed. The patient should then come to rest in a position that feels as if the eyes are looking directly forward and the spine is straight.

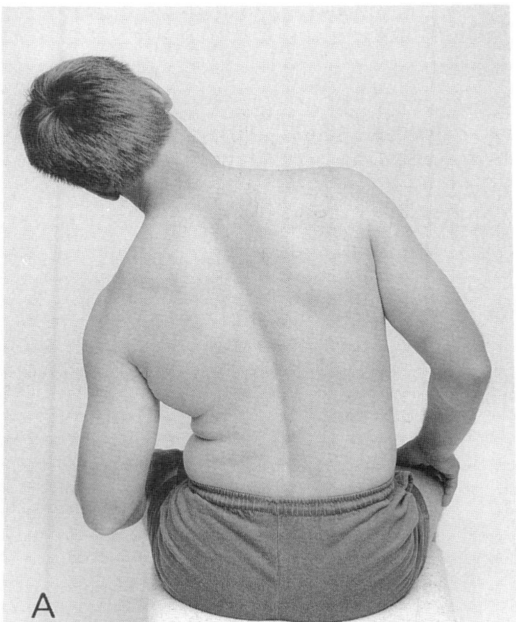

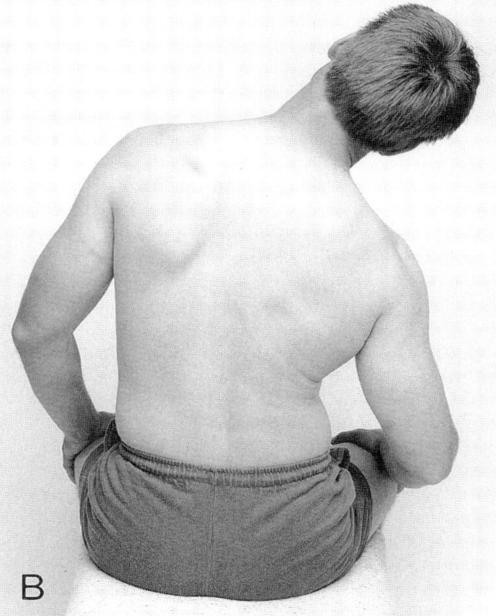

Figure 4.5. **A,** Left lateral bending shows a smooth arcing motion of the thoracolumbar spine with slight dysfunction noted from approximately T5 to T9. **B,** Posture during right lateral bending. Notice the overall restriction compared to **A**. An abrupt inflexion point is seen at T9.

Standing visual examination may be aided by the use of a plumb line for more precise analysis. Visualizing the patient from the back, the structural landmarks include: the feet, knees, gluteal folds, intergluteal line, hips, waist, spine, scapulae, shoulders, and ears. Visual inspection of the trunk should begin with gross visual inspection for scoliosis (See Chapter 9).

Sagittal Plane. From the side one should examine the balance of the three main centers of mass (head, thorax, and pelvis), and inclination of the lower limbs. The spinal curves should also be scrutinized from the side view. Relaxed or "lazy" posture is best observed in this view (See Fig. 4.4). Disorders of intersegmental and global ligamentous and muscular function will commonly be revealed as forward weight bearing of the head, hyperkyphosis of the thoracic spine, and/or hyperlordosis of the lumbar spine. Lateral postural assessment exposes the "poker spine," which is characterized by a decreased lumbar lordosis, flattened thoracic kyphosis, and a kyphotic cervical spine (Fig. 4.6). Genu recurvatum of the lower extremities may have effects on the lumbopelvic area. The altered inclination of the femur, as seen in the lateral view, may rock the pelvis in the $-\theta X$ direction, thus leading to a tendency for compensatory [lumbar] hyperlordosis.

Forward head carriage is common and may indicate flexion ($+\theta X$) positional dyskinesia of the middle to upper thoracic spine. Marked anterior weight bearing of the head may be accompanied by upper cervical hyperextension and lower cervical kyphosis, although each case should be considered individually. Patients with this forward head carriage have a tendency for symptoms related to increased mechanical tension in the spinal cord (e.g., headache, etc.), cervical muscle tension, and the mechanics of intervertebral strain in the compensatory middle cervical area. Decreased anterior height of the thoracic vertebral bodies also creates forward flexion of the area involved, with compensatory changes above.

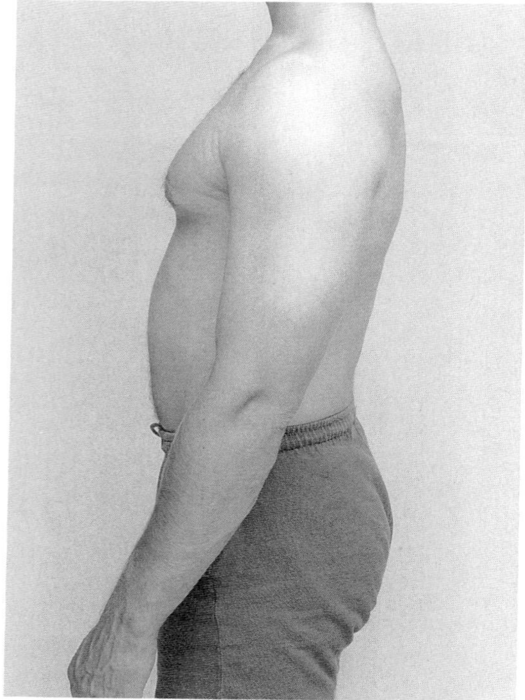

Figure 4.6. Sagittal profile. This patient has diminished sagittal curves. The thoracic curve is especially flattened. There is an associated AS ilium subluxation on the patient's AP radiograph (not shown). This is the same patient as in Figure 4.5.

Senile kyphosis is detected in older patients and appears as a prominent upper thoracic spine or hump. Upper to middle thoracic kyphosis is commonly associated with osteoporosis, especially in older women. Longstanding hyperkyphosis may increase when the patient grows old. With age, the female kyphosis tends to increase in magnitude at a greater rate than the male. Aside from obvious effects of compression fractures, this increase is due primarily to anterior degeneration of the intervertebral discs. Degeneration in this area, caused by increased pressure on the anterior annulus, appears to compound the effect of the hump (45).

In a controlled study investigating the relative effects of chiropractic adjustments and exercise in geriatric kyphosis, three groups were observed over a period of 4 months. The group that received chiropractic adjustments revealed a decreased kyphosis of 11.4 mm, the exercise group improved 7.1 mm, and no change was seen in the control (46).

The stance of the patient with a disc protrusion creating lumbar nerve root compression is characteristically hypolordotic. This flattened lumbar lordosis reduces the posterior bulge of the disc, whereas flexion of the hips and knees reduces the stretch on the sciatic nerve roots (36). Findings from the postural assessment can be correlated with a lateral full-spine radiograph (See Chapter 5).

Coronal Plane (viewed from the posterior). A scoliotic spine can be detected with postural analysis of the coronal plane. Abnormal curvature in this view appears as a lateral deviation of the normally erect spinal column, with raised musculature on the side of posterior rotation of the transverse processes. Noticeably raised musculature over the transverse processes will not occur without grouped rotation of several levels, such as in patients with scoliosis. Intersegmental rotation will likely not be visible in this manner.

Segmental inconsistencies of skin pigmentation, patches of hair, fatty or fluid cysts, increased subcutaneous tissue thickness, mottled skin, and singular moles near the spine may give clues to areas of trophic disturbances from chronic, subtle nerve dysfunction (3).

Visual assessment of leg length inequality (LLI) can be accomplished in the standing position. Several points of reference can be used, including the iliac crests, sacral base, gluteal folds, and the PSISs. The presence or absence of scoliosis should be noted. Asymmetry of structures when compared bilaterally or the presence of scoliosis is not pathognomonic of LLI. Leg length inequality is best evaluated with a standing antero-posterior radiograph of the pelvis. Postural evidence of possible LLI, necessitating orthotic correction, is erroneous unless corroborated by a radiograph.

Standing assessment may also be used to make a gross determination of the effectiveness of shoe lift implementation. Place the desired amount of lift under the short leg side while visually assessing the attitude and posture of the lower spine and pelvis using the above mentioned landmarks. This type of assessment should be used only in the interim or in cases for whom radiography is contraindicated. Follow-up radiographic assessment after approximately one month is indicated in most cases (See Chapter 6).

In the P to A view, the AS or PI ilium is easily visualized as asymmetric gluteal folds and iliac crest heights. Asymmetry in the dimples normally seen just below the PSIS may also reveal the AS or PI ilium. Notice any asymmetry in the posterolateral iliac crests, suggestive of an In or Ex ilium. In ($-\theta$Y) ilium movement on the right sacrum may cause a more flattened appearance of the soft tissue overlying the postero-lateral portion of the ilium. The Ex ilium will demonstrate a more protuberant gluteus.

Anterior to Posterior View. The important landmarks from the standing front view include: the feet, knees, hanging hand position, head, eyes, and ears. Hand position may reveal regional thoracolumbar rotation. A relative difference in the distance between the hands and the torso is indicative of rotational distortions. Foot flare and biomechanical alterations of the feet are easily viewed from the anterior. Inspection of the level of the eyes and ears may reveal head/torso deviations.

SITTING POSTURE

Static visual assessment in the sitting position can demonstrate many of the same findings as the standing assessment. When the patient assumes the sitting position, however, posture may appear vastly different. For example, in cases with "slouched" posture and hyperlordosis of the lumbar spine evident on standing analysis, sitting posture may reveal a lumbar kyphosis. This difference is likely due to compensatory laxity of the thoracolumbar ligaments or poor muscle tone. Slouched posture puts unnecessary stress on the ligaments because of inactivity of the paraspinal musculature (See Chapter 2 for muscle/ligament relationships).

The In or Ex ilium is sometimes more easily detected in the sitting versus the standing position. These asymmetries are seen as a flattened and wider gluteal appearance on the In side and a more rounded and narrower appearance on the Ex side. A fixed rotated (θY) positional dyskinesia of the sacrum may deviate the intergluteal cleft to one side. The distance between the cleft and the ilium will be wider on the posteriorly rotated side.

Stressed Posture Inspection

Motion characteristics can be visualized in the standing or sitting position. As the patient bends the neck and trunk in various directions, asymmetrical and atypical motion may be evident. Fixation dysfunction in one area may result in a compensatory increase in motion in a nearby region. Asymmetrical structure can lead to atypical motion patterns. The radiograph can be of help in determining whether or not motion patterns are the result of structural asymmetries.

The doctor should be very specific in directing the patient through motions to isolate the problem, as the patient may have adapted to a restriction by developing regional movement patterns that appear to be quite normal on gross inspection. During dynamic inspection, the examiner should be attentive to patient remarks referring to symptoms brought on by the movement being assessed. Pain or stiffness while stressing the structure is often of considerable diagnostic value. Pain from contractile elements would typically present itself on stretching the involved muscle during contralateral bending. Active movements will also provoke pain of muscle origin. Pain from noncontractile tissue (e.g., ligaments) is characteristically worsened by movements that stretch these elements. Flexion movement that worsens the compression of a pain sensitive structure such as cartilage or neural elements may elicit a pain response. Both passive and active motion can provoke symptomatology.

Sitting

All six degrees of freedom of each region may be visualized in the sitting position. Sitting assessment of the spine in chiropractic practice is common, as this position facilitates multiple phases of the evaluation (e.g., skin temperature analysis, motion and static palpation, etc). To visualize (or palpate) intersegmental motion, it is important to instruct the patient to assume postures that will aid the discovery of restrictions in each area. The following positions aid intersegmental motion analysis in lateral flexion:

1. Sacroiliac dysfunction is easily tested with the spine in lumbar lordosis, which locks the lumbar facets and isolates movement to the pelvis.
2. A neutral lumbar lordosis enables analysis of lumbar motion.
3. The thoracic spine is isolated for analysis when the lumbar region is in lordosis.
4. The cervical and upper thoracic spine is best viewed with the thoracic spine upright, and the cervical area very slightly flexed.

Intersegmental lateral flexion dysfunction is most easily seen in the thoracic and lumbar areas. A "blocking" of vertebrae on the side of restriction and an abrupt "kinking" of the spine on the side of hyperflexion expose dysfunction in lateral bending (See Fig. 4.5A-B).

The coupling motion of rotation on lateral bending should be examined also. Watch for the lumbar erector spinae muscles to depress on the side of lateral bending, and protrude on the opposite side. Erector spinae motion on lateral bending is usually not as pronounced in the thoracic spine as it is in the cervical and lumbar area. The cervical and thoracic areas should be checked for coupling. In this area the spinous processes will move to the convexity of bend.

Unilateral restriction of lateral flexion (θZ) motion in the lower cervical and upper thoracic spine may result in visible and palpable tension in the lateral superficial neck muscles on the opposite side of lateral flexion. The mid to upper cervical vertebrae yield to the lower restriction in lateral flexion and as a result may be pulling on the opposite lateral neck musculature, thus causing the band-like protruding muscles.

Lateral flexion dynamic visual analysis may help to differentiate a primary muscle etiology from that of primary nerve involvement causing pain. If the presenting pain is reproduced or worsened by lateral flexion ipsilaterally, nerve etiology is more likely, because entrapment of an irritated nerve caused by the compression of the movement is increased. Pain increased or reproduced by contralateral lateral flexion is more likely due to the stretching of a sore muscle or ligament.

Flexion/extension inspection is useful to determine the presence of dysfunction in the cervical, low thoracic, and lumbar regions, as this motion is relatively great in these areas compared with other movements (e.g., axial rotation). A smooth fanning out of the spinous processes in flexion, and even accentuation of the lordotic curvatures on extension should be observed during normal motion. Look for an abrupt inflexion in curvature or spinous process separation as evidence of possible intersegmental dysfunction (e.g., fixation dysfunction or hypermobility).

To view lower spine function, direct the patient to "arch and slouch" the low back. An obvious restriction at the end-range of lumbo-sacral extension ($-\theta X$) often reveals a "blocked" appearance in the lumbosacral area with a concomitant hyperlordotic curvature in the thoraco-lumbar area. A "base posterior" sacrum or retrolisthesis of L5 may produce the above scenario. Flexion/extension of the cervicothoracic junction is readily visible because of the protuberant spinous processes in the region.

Axial rotation visualization is particularly useful for the analysis of the cervical spine. Dvorak and Dvorak (47) propose functional examination of the cervical spine in rotation by isolating either the atlantoaxial or the lower cervical spine. Flexion of the head and neck permits primarily upper cervical rotation, whereas extension of the neck and straightening of the thoracic spine, isolates the lower cervical vertebrae for axial rotation analysis (Fig. 4.7A-B).

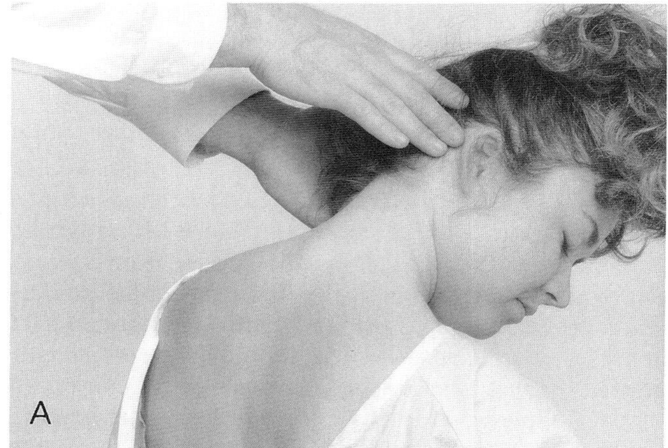

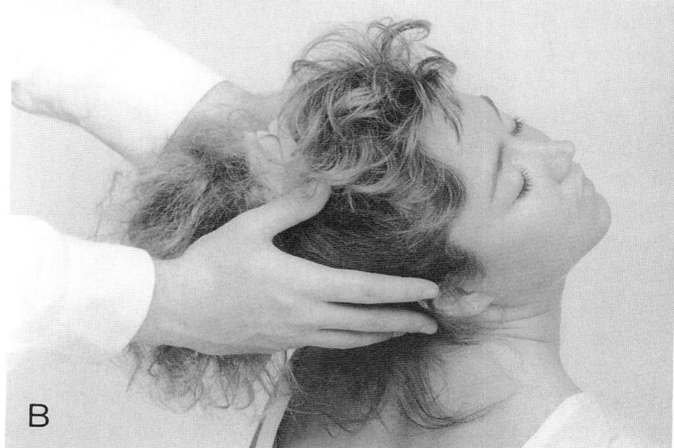

Figure 4.7. **A,** The Dvorak test is illustrated. Flexion of the head will isolate the upper cervical region, especially C1-C2 during axial rotation. The patient's head is rotated from side to side to determine the presence of upper cervical rotatory fixation dysfunction. **B,** Extension will isolate movement restriction due to lower cervical and upper thoracic involvement. This maneuver is contraindicated for the patient with vertebrobasilar artery insufficiency.

Palpation

STATIC

Digital palpation is one of the chiropractor's chief means of directly assessing the patient's condition. Palpation for tenderness is integral to the examination because it can indicate pathology of the superficial fascial and ligamentous elements or referral pain patterns. A firm pressure should be applied to the tip of the spinous process followed by a "rolling up" motion along the length of the spinous. The "laying on of hands" in itself is manual communication to the patient that the doctor understands and can locate the involved areas. Gonstead (42) thought it useful to identify tender spinal levels by pressing on the spinous process enough to elicit a pain response. He felt that the patient would be aware that the doctor knew where the problem was and that the severity of the tenderness would alert the patient to the gravity of the condition.

Soft Tissue Palpation. Palpation is a method used to search for signs of damage and inflammation in the paraspinal soft tissues. The paraspinal areas reveal injury of the interspinous/supraspinous ligaments (48). The paraspinal musculature may show evidence of abnormal anatomic and physiologic phenomena.

Superficial, localized edema is characterized by a detectable accumulation of excessive fluid in the subcutaneous tissues (49). Localized inflammatory edema (as opposed to other edematogenic conditions) may be found at traumatized spinal levels (48). Clinical experience has been that palpation close to the spinous processes most readily reveals VSC related edema. Edematous areas over the spinous may reflect damage to the supraspinous ligament. Moving the palmar aspect of finger caudocephalad and cephalocaudal, asymmetries in tissue texture can be determined which may be indicative of underlying edema, muscular hyper or hypotonicity or autonomic nervous system dysfunction (e.g., denervation supersensitivity).

Hyperemia or Red Response. A superficial vascular response of vasodilation may result from stimulation of the paraspinal soft tissue due to pressure from digital palpation or skin-contact instrumentation scanning. The red response can persist for several minutes and is most evident in the thoracic region (50). This response may be related to the local autonomic nervous system dysfunction secondary to VSC in that area.

Tenderness. The most tender segment is often associated with the etiology of the patient's pain. Spinous process tenderness is commonly used to locate the potential subluxation. Pressure should be applied to the spinous tip while moving cephalad. The lowest, most tender thoracic or cervical spinous have been reported by Gonstead as likely candidates for adjustment (42). Facet area tenderness in the cervical region can be indicative of a symptomatic facet articulation. Tenderness at the lower aspect of the sacroiliac joint may indicate an AS ilium subluxation, whereas tenderness at the upper sacroiliac may reflect a PI ilium. If the entire sacroiliac articulation is tender, the doctor should suspect a posteriorly rotated sacrum or an Ex ilium. Palpation of tenderness in the thoracic spine is more likely related to the level of involvement, due to the lack of intersegmental connections between the nerves supplying contiguous spinal segments (51). One must be careful not to assume that these findings of tenderness are in themselves indications for an adjustment to that articulation. Hypermobility can cause tenderness yet would be a contraindication for an adjustment.

Musculature. Normal muscle is soft and pliable. Hypertonicity of paraspinal musculature may relate segmentally to the area of nerve irritation or dysfunction. Inspect the paraspinal musculature for active trigger points as a possible cause of local symptomatology. Trigger points may or may not be segmentally related. An area of hypertonicity is often related to hypermobility, because the reflex neurologic mechanisms will attempt to splint or stabilize the area (i.e., arthrokinetic reflex; see Chapter 2). The area of subluxation may exhibit a very edematous and boggy texture of the affected tissues (Fig. 4.8A-B). Hypertonicity of paraspinal muscles can also occur in areas of fixation dysfunction secondary to reflexes initiated by increased mechanoreceptor activity (See Chapter 3).

Trophic Changes. A boggy or doughy consistency felt on palpation near the spinous process is a very common finding that may reveal the intersegmental level of subluxation. A combination of neurologic dysfunction and soft tissue reaction to injury of the supraspinous/interspinous ligaments and muscles may be responsible for these findings.

Lateral Flexion. Inflexion points in spinal symmetry can be accentuated by placing the spine in lateral flexion. Isolate the areas being assessed and laterally flex the area almost to its end range. Next, in this sidebent position, run your finger(s) along the concavity of the spinal curvature, then along its convexity (Fig. 4.8A). Note any deviation from a smooth curvature. Often, at a fixed inflexion point, one will detect an abrupt spinous deviation relative to the adjacent spinous process(es).

MOTION PALPATION

The two main types of chiropractic motion palpation are "end-feel" palpation and intersegmental range of motion palpation. Several studies have tested the reliability of end-feel palpation; whereas little has been done to test intersegmental range of motion palpation (4). There is no conclusive evidence that motion palpation is a reliable or valid procedure. The lack of evidence supporting motion palpation does not, however, indicate that it should be abandoned as a clinical procedure. Future research must incorporate larger sample sizes with symptomatic subjects.

One very interesting study illustrates the potential practicality of the procedure as an examiner was asked to determine the presence or absence of symptomatic cervical zygapophyseal joints (52). The examiner's accuracy was tested against radiologically controlled, diagnostic cervical nerve blocks. A positive motion palpation finding indicating a symptomatic joint was defined as meeting all of the following three criteria: abnormal end-feel, abnormal quality of resistance to motion, and reproduction of pain (either local or referred) when passive accessory movements (end-feel) were tested). Of the 20 subjects in the study, the examiner correctly identified all 15 patients with proven symptomatic zygapophyseal joints, and all

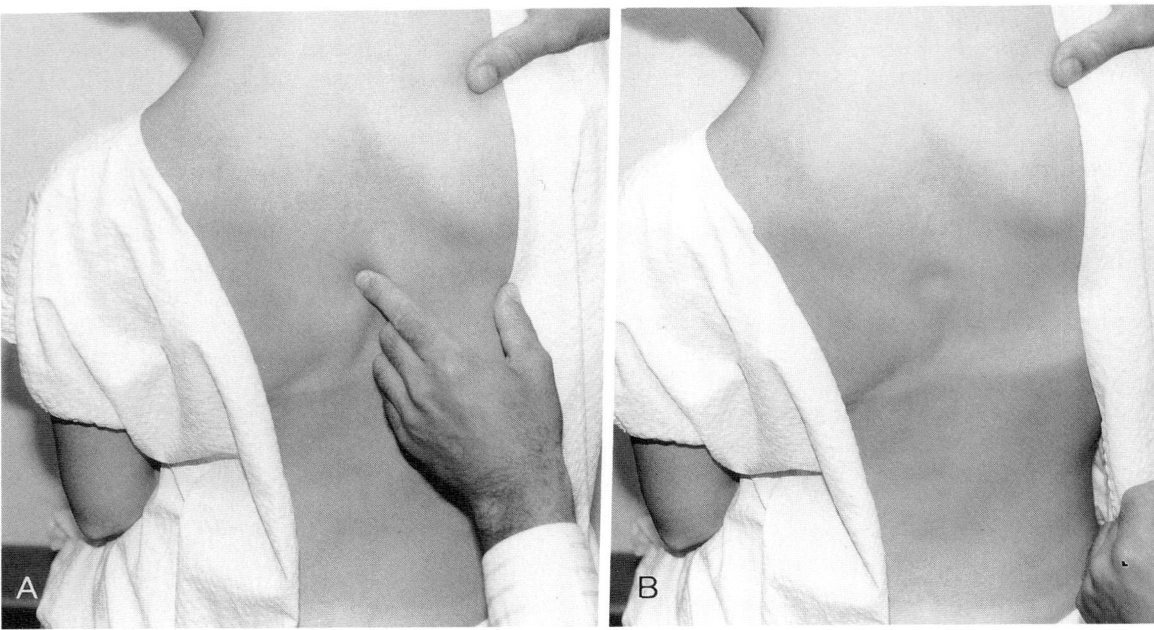

Figure 4.8. **A,** Static palpation for soft tissue texture changes, which can be performed in the neutral position or during stressed postures. Inflexion points during side bending may also be detected in this manner. **B,** Pitting edema is demonstrated in the midthoracic area.

five without. The examiner further singled out the correct segmental levels of symptomatic joints in all cases. The authors concluded that manual diagnosis can be as accurate as radiologically controlled, diagnostic nerve blocks in the diagnosis of cervical zygapophyseal joints.

INTERSEGMENTAL RANGE OF MOTION PALPATION

The authors advocate the use of intersegmental range of motion palpation (IRMP) as the primary method of motion palpation. IRMP is described here as the palpation of intervertebral movement assessed during passive and/or patient-assisted motion. Passive intersegmental motion assessment is conducted while the patient is directed by the examiner to allow the examiner to move the area through the desired range of motion. Clinical experience has been that if the patient assists the movement, it is more difficult to determine intersegmental range of motion because of the global movement tendencies of muscle action. Active intersegmental motion is assessed when passive motion assessment is not possible due to the size or position of the area. The lumbar and sacroiliac areas are commonly palpated during patient assisted motions, whereas the cervical and thoracic spinal areas are easily palpated during passive motions.

Often the patient will experience pain when a relatively restricted articulation is moved towards the restricted end-range of motion. The patient will commonly and sometimes unconsciously resist the movement in the above situation. This abnormal quality of resistance to motion can be sensed by the examiner. An abnormal resistance to motion may be noticeable during either or both types of intersegmental range of motion palpation. When present, this resistance may indicate a positive finding for a symptomatic articulation. It is commonly found in the cervical spine over a hard mass of soft tissue overlying the facet articulation.

Many manual practitioners will manipulate a cervical articulation on the basis of an apparent symptomatic articulation alone, especially when radiographic examination is not part of the assessment. The above application of manipulation may or may not provide rapid symptomatic relief. The doctor must take care to make certain that the manipulation is not only for pain relief. Chiropractors must be aware of the complex array of compensation mechanisms that can be responsible for such painful cervical facet articulations. Often, further examination will reveal subluxations in the mid to upper thoracic spine that are responsible for painful compensatory reactions above.

The contact point of the examiner's hand for intersegmental palpation is usually the tip of the finger(s). The segmental contact point of the bone depends on the level being palpated. Most commonly the spinous process is used. In the cervical spine from C1-C7 the interlaminar area of the articular pillars may be contacted. From C0-C2, the mastoid, articular condyle areas, and transverse processes may be used. Intersegmental range of motion palpation of the sacroiliac joint can be determined by contacting above and below the PSIS in the joint space between the sacrum and ilium.

OPTIMIZING THE MOTION PALPATION ASSESSMENT

Prepositioning the area to be assessed with motion palpation is the same as for visual inspection. A light touch is essential when motion palpating (37). If the patient's pain is exacerbated during the assessment, then the adjustment might be more difficult to perform. Too much pressure may also decrease the ability of the fingertips to detect subtle changes in movement. It is important that intersegmental movements are evaluated rather than the total global posture. The global motion may not be reflective of the intersegmental biomechanics of the joint in question.

The most accurate means for assessing the movement of the intervertebral joint is likely through stress radiography (See Chapter 5). Comparing the radiographic results to the palpation assessment will increase the examiner's ability to know what he/she is feeling. As the patient undergoes a course of treatment, the movement can be compared to previous findings. It is not prudent to repeat x-rays continually to determine the movement of the joint after each adjustment. Stress radiography may not be indicated for the initial examination in all cases.

Pelvic Motion Palpation. Fixation dysfunction may be revealed by palpating the relative motions of the sacrum and the ilium during different types of movements. Sacroiliac range of motion palpation has shown more interexaminer reliability than motion palpation of the lumbar spine. The Gillet motion palpation test exhibited moderate levels of intraexaminer reliability in one study (29). This test is performed in the standing position. The doctor contacts the PSIS on one side with the ipsilateral thumb and the S2 tubercle of the sacrum with the opposite thumb. The patient is directed to slowly raise the ipsilateral leg with the knee bent, until the knee is waist high. Motion between the PSIS and S2 are compared bilaterally for differences. The downward motion of the PSIS relative to S2 is diminished on the side of fixation dysfunction.

A variation of the above procedure is performed by contacting each PSIS with the examiner's thumbs (Fig. 4.9). As the patient raises the flexed knee, the PSIS on the side of the raised knee should lower. Relative movements of the PSISs are compared.

Another test is conducted in the sitting position. The doctor contacts the PSISs bilaterally with the thumbs and instructs the patient to bend forward at the waist. Symmetry of PSIS movement is monitored and compared bilaterally. The PSIS that raises more is likely the restricted articulation because as the lumbar spine flexes and pulls the sacrum forward (i.e., nutation), fixation at the SI joint will move the PSIS upward ipsilaterally (Fig. 4.10A-B).

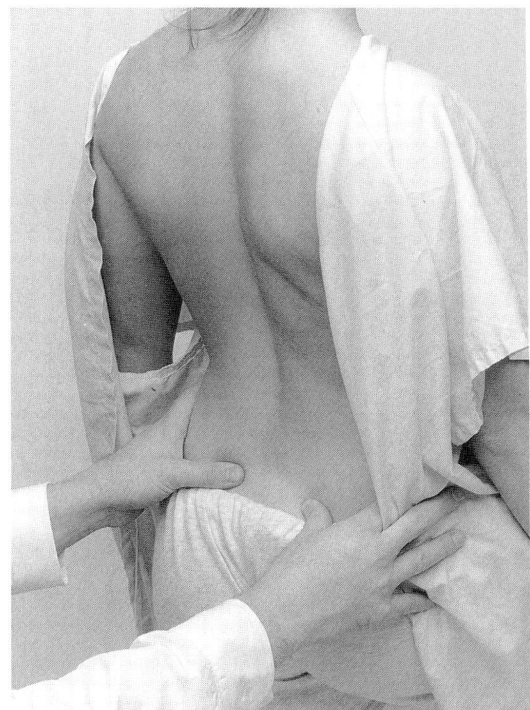

Figure 4.9. Motion palpation of the sacroiliac joints. The examiner is contacting both PSISs. As the patient raises each leg the examiner notes the inferiorward excursion of each PSIS. Failure of the PSIS to drop in comparison to the contralateral side may be indicative of SI joint fixation dysfunction. Because rotation of the fifth lumbar vertebra could cause unilateral tensioning of the iliolumbar ligament and thus failure of the ilium to move inferiorward, this type of positional dyskinesia should be ruled out before assuming a SI fixation is present.

Lateral flexion of the sacroiliac articulation is evaluated by placing the tips of two digits just medial to the PSIS. As the subject is laterally flexed ipsi- and contralaterally to the side of contact, the examiner detects movement at the SI joint. Palpation can be performed at both the superior and inferior margins of the joint (Fig. 4.11A-B). If a marked fixation is present, inspection may reveal that the contralateral buttock will raise when the spine is laterally flexed ipsilateral to the side of contact.

Lumbar Motion Palpation. Lumbar motion palpation is usually performed in the seated position but can be done standing. Here, the doctor will attempt to detect lateral flexion of the motion segment by placing the finger(s) just lateral and inferior to the spinous process of the segment in question. The spine is then laterally flexed. If lateral flexion motion is present, there will be a relaxation of the ipsilateral soft tissues lateral and inferior to the spinous process of the segment in question (Fig. 4.12). Normal coupled motion of the lumbar spine occurs when the spinous moves toward the concavity of lateral bend (See

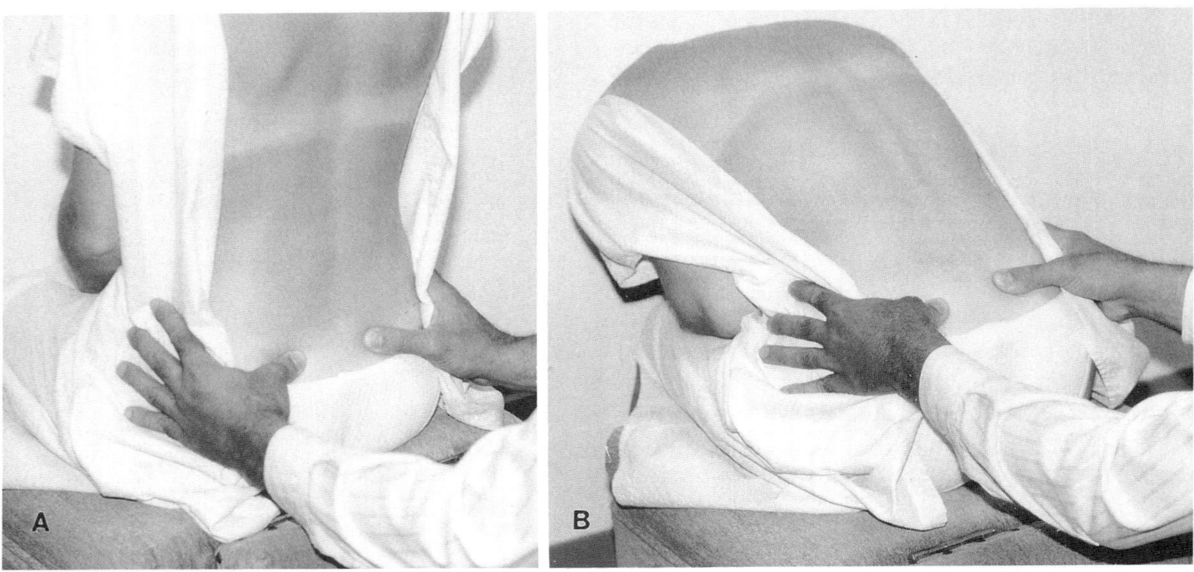

Figure 4.10. **A,** Motion palpation of the sacroiliac joints. The examiner is contacting each PSIS. **B,** During flexion, if a PSIS moves more superiorward, this may be indicative of SI joint fixation on the same side.

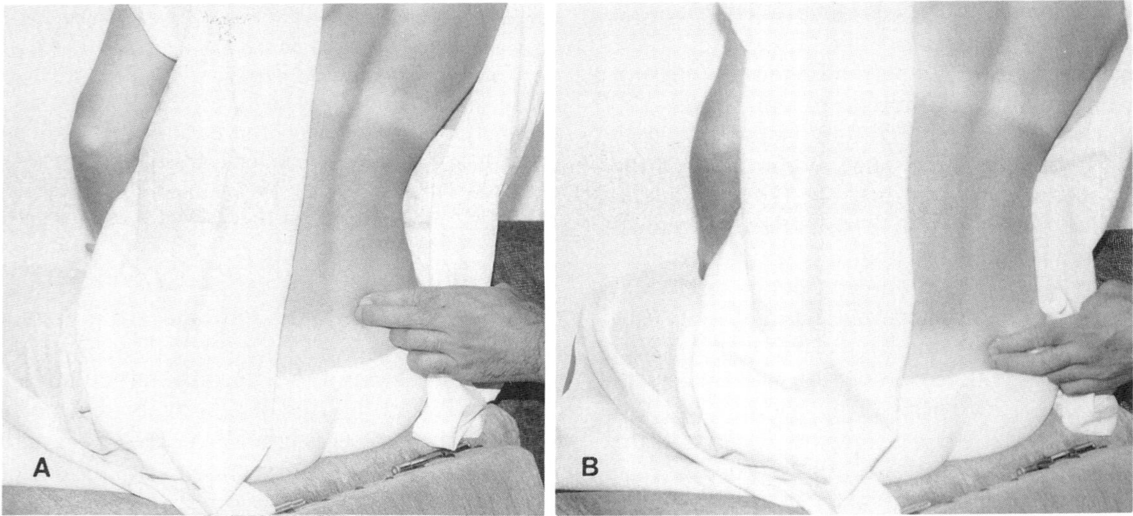

Figure 4.11. **A,** Motion palpation of the superior portion of the right sacroiliac joint during right lateral bending. **B,** Motion palpation of the inferior portion of the right sacroiliac joint during right lateral bending.

Chapter 7). This subtle movement is difficult to palpate and may be best evaluated with stress radiography because it normally involves about one degree of rotation at each segmental level. To palpate spinous movement on lateral bending, place the index finger in the interspinous space slightly favoring the side of lateral bending.

Extension motion is evaluated in the seated position (Fig. 4.13A-B). If a base posterior sacrum is present, the sacral base will appear not to nutate during extension. The spinous processes of the lumbar spine should move anteroinferior during extension. This arching forward of the lumbar spine for motion palpation is slightly different from the motion that occurs when the spine is extended from the neutral position for a stress radiograph. During the radiographic procedure the segments move in a posterior and inferior direction.

Flexion motion is evaluated by passively flexing the subject forward and noting separation of the spinous processes. The middle and upper lumbar segments are usually more easily evaluated for this motion because of the prominence of the spinous processes.

Thoracic Motion Palpation. Lateral bending of the thoracic spine can be evaluated similarly to the lumbar spine (Fig. 4.14). Lateral flexion is more difficult to eval-

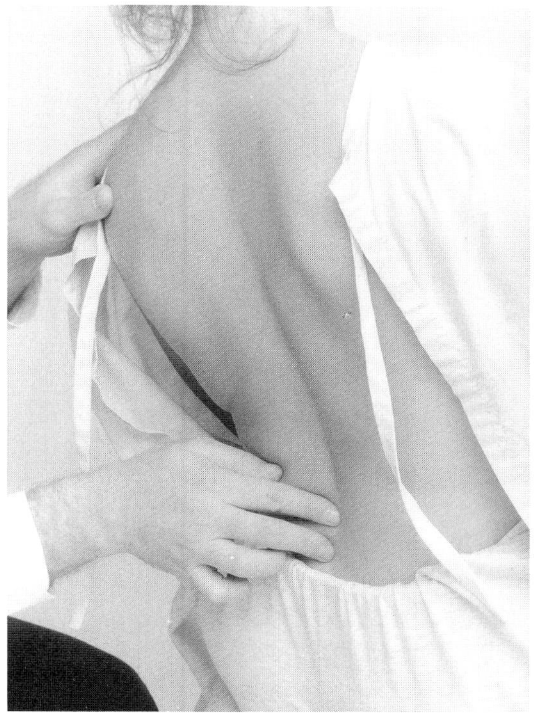

Figure 4.12. Motion palpation of L5 during left lateral bending. The first digit is at the inferior lateral margin of the L5 spinous process. During lateral flexion motion, there will be a relaxation of the soft tissue elements on the ipsilateral side of bend.

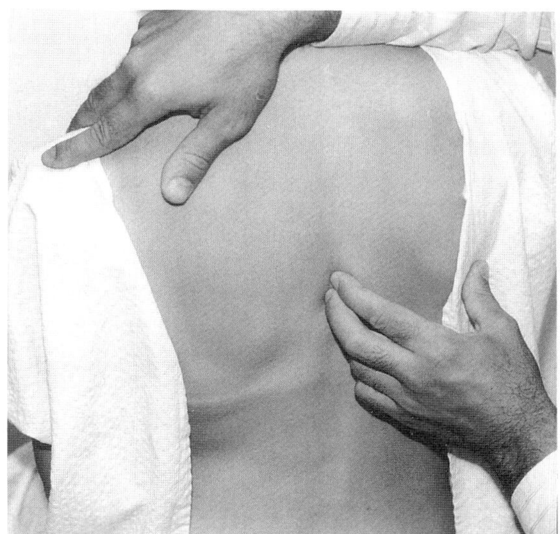

Figure 4.14. Motion palpation of the thoracic spine during left lateral flexion. The spinous processes approximate during bending and move toward the convexity of bend if normal coupling motion is present. This assessment can be accomplished while contacting either the ipsi- or contralateral interspinous spaces during lateral bending.

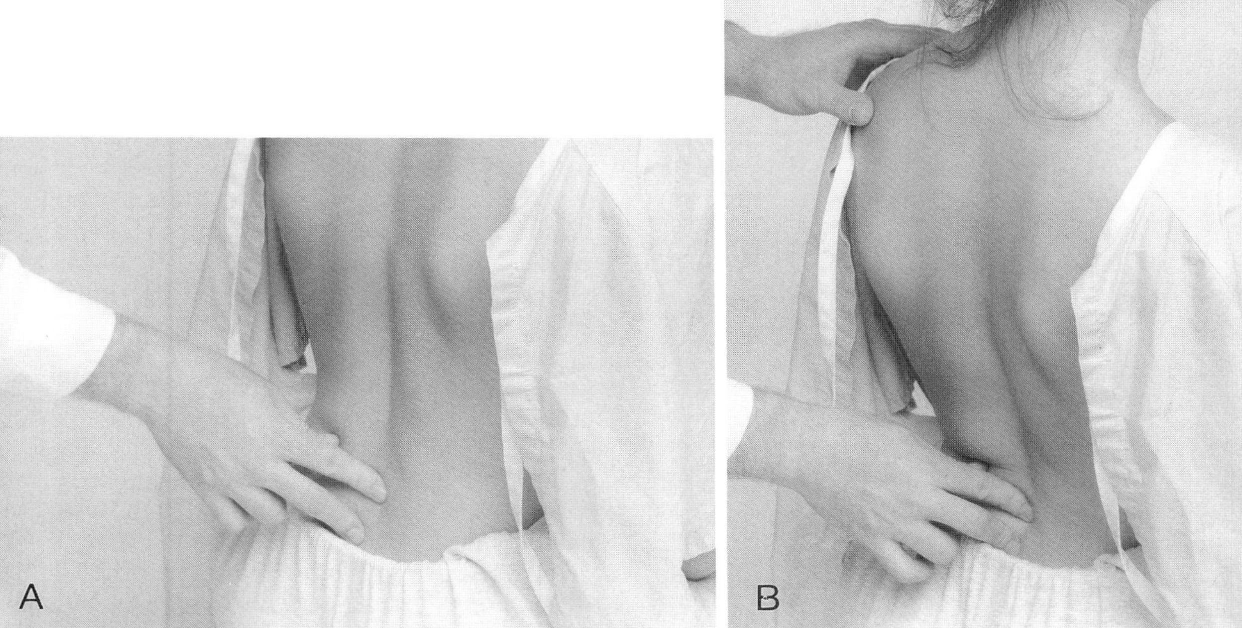

Figure 4.13. **A,** Motion palpation of lumbosacral movement. The examiner is contacting L5 and S1. **B,** Motion palpation of the lumbosacral junction. During extension, the examiner's finger approximate as L5 and the sacrum extend.

uate here because intersegmental motion is much less than the lumbar spine. Coupled motion of the segment involves rotation of the spinous process toward the convexity of bend, provided the thoracic spine is laterally flexed in isolation (See Chapters 2 and 8). Flexion-extension motion assessment is depicted in Figure 4.15. Rotational evaluation is demonstrated in Figure 4.16.

Cervical Motion Palpation. Motion palpation of the cervical spine is performed with the patient seated. A back support should be provided because this will facilitate the isolation of the region. Lateral bending and coupled motions of the spinous process toward the convexity of bend are assessed (Fig. 4.17A-C). The examiner may place one finger caudal to the segment in question and evaluate the suprajacent level. As the head and neck are laterally flexed, care should be taken to limit the lateral bending of the subjacent level. A relaxation of the soft tissues on the ipsilateral side of bending will be detected if normal motion is present. Lateral flexion is more difficult to assess than spinous rotation coupling. The movement of the spinous process toward the convexity of the bend can be palpated with the digit placed on the contralateral side of lateral flexion. Coupled motion in the mid cervical spine is greater than at the cervicothoracic junction (Fig. 4.18). These coupled motions, therefore, may be more easily evaluated here. Contacting the appropriate process may be difficult through the thick cervical musculature.

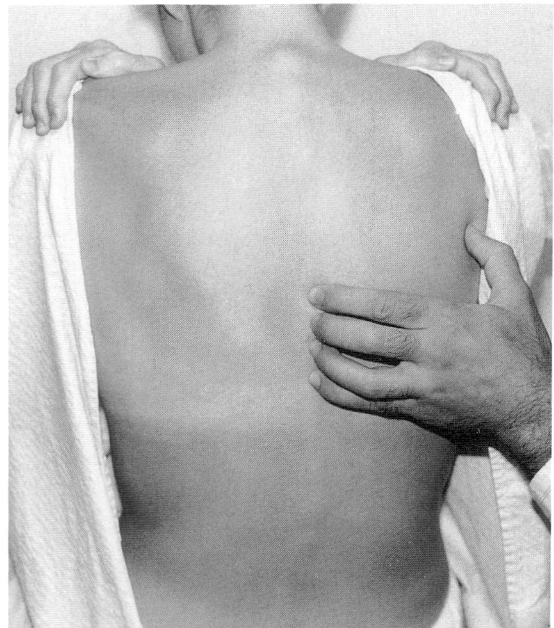

Figure 4.15. Motion palpation of the thoracic spine during flexion/extension. The patient crosses her arms and the examiner passively raises and lowers the thoracic spine by contacting the arms at the crossed elbows in front. The other hand is used to note separation of the spinous processes during flexion and approximation during extension.

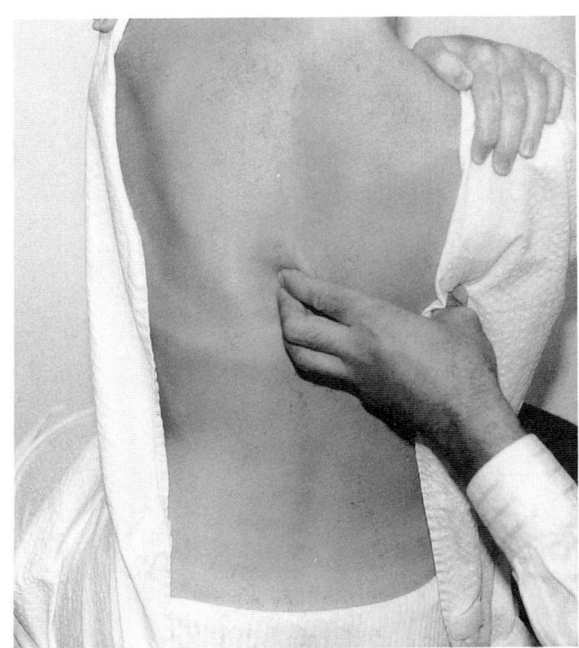

Figure 4.16. Motion palpation of the thoracic spine during axial rotation. The spinous processes should move toward the contralateral side of rotation if normal movement is present. Patient movement is guided with the non-contact hand as in Figure 4.15.

The hyperlordotic cervical spine is more difficult to evaluate in the mid cervical area.

During forward flexion, the spinous processes should separate and on extension, approximate. This movement can be detected by feeling the separation while the examiner contacts two adjacent spinous processes (Fig. 4.19). This movement is more difficult to evaluate in the mid-cervical area, where direct contact on the spinous process is more difficult to obtain. During extension, the spinous processes normally move closer together. If paradoxical motion is present (i.e., the segment flexes when extended), then approximation of the spinous process will not occur.

When extending the head, the C5 and C6 spinouses seem to "tuck away." Rather, the spinous moves posterior and inferior during extension and anterior superior during flexion. The sensation of the spinous disappearing during extension is likely due to the buckling of the posterior ligaments (i.e., ligamentum nuchae), thereby increasing the distance between the palpator's finger and spinous process (See Chapter 2: Landmark Identification).

Axial rotation is evaluated by noting movement of the spinous toward the contralateral side of axial rotation (Fig. 4.20). This movement is small in the lower cervical spine and greater in the upper cervical region.

Upper Cervical Motion Palpation. The atlantoaxial articulation is usually evaluated in lateral bending (Fig. 4.21) and axial rotation. The axis of rotation of the atlas on axis during lateral bending is toward the side of lateral bending (See Chapter 11). Rather than the atlas closing

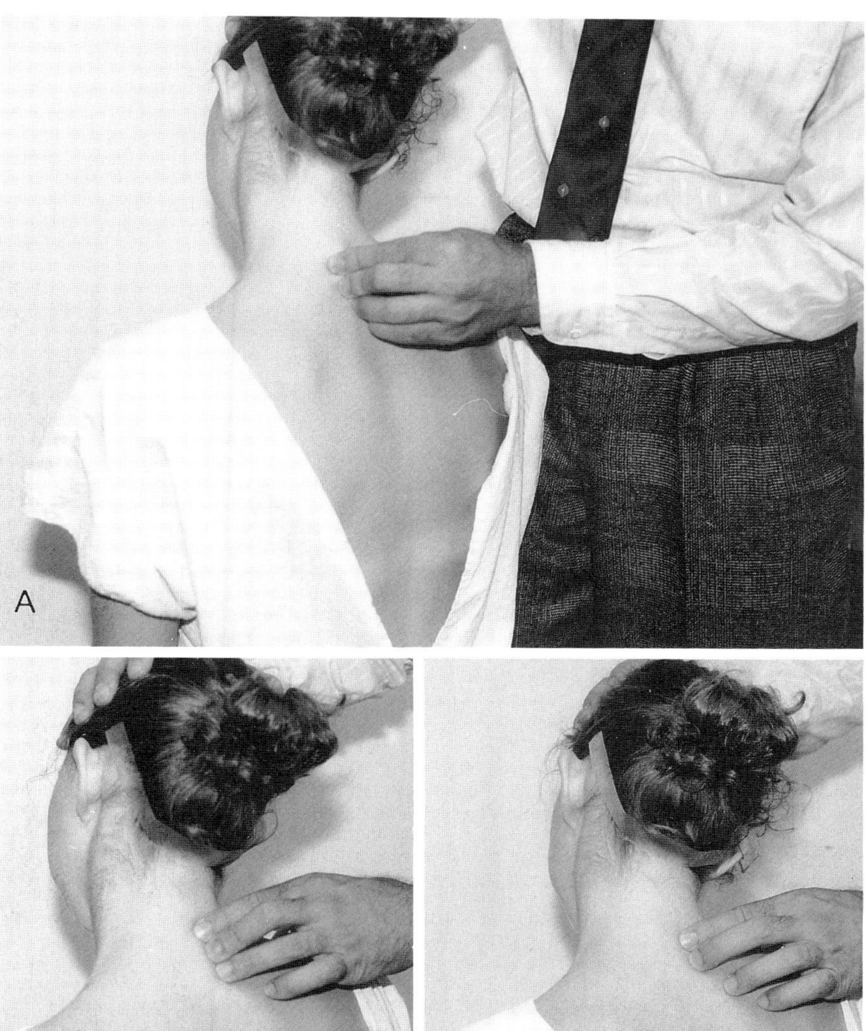

Figure 4.17. A, Motion palpation of the lower cervical spine during right lateral bending. The spinous process is between the thumb and first digit, while the second digit contacts the spinous below the level of assessment. The spinous process should move toward the contralateral side of bend if lateral flexion or normal coupling motion is present. **B,** Motion palpation of the lower cervical spine during right lateral bending. Contact is made over the spinous processes, especially the interspinous areas. **C,** Motion palpation of the lower cervical spine during right lateral bending. The examiner is contacting the right borders of the spinous processes on the ipsilateral side of bend.

down on the side of bend, it raises on the contralateral side. The Dvorak test may preferably be used to assess rotational fixation (See Fig. 4.7). The upper cervical spine is first isolated by having the patient flex the upper cervical spine followed with rotation of the head to each side. Palpation of C1-C2 rotation can be assessed with either the same contact as for lateral flexion assessment or by contacting the anterior intertransverse area between C1 and C2. The transverse process of C1 normally moves beyond that of C2 in the direction of the rotation. Flexion of C1-C2 may be evaluated with the same anterior intertransverse contact and slight flexion movement of the head.

The major motion for the occipitoatlantal motion segment is flexion extension. This movement can be evaluated by isolating each articulation in lateral flexion first by compressing the head into lateral bending followed with a rocking motion in flexion and extension. Anterior and posterior contacts similar to those of the C1-C2 assessment may be used.

Lateral flexion is evaluated by noting a relaxation of the soft tissue elements between the condyle and the transverse process of atlas on the ipsilateral side of bend. This motion is approximately 5° to each side. It is important that movement is not created at the mid and lower cervical spine during upper cervical motion assessments.

Instrumentation

PARASPINAL SKIN TEMPERATURE THERMOCOUPLE INSTRUMENTS

The main reasons for the use of skin temperature analysis are to obtain objective neurologic evidence of a VSC and to monitor the progress of patient care. Intersegmental

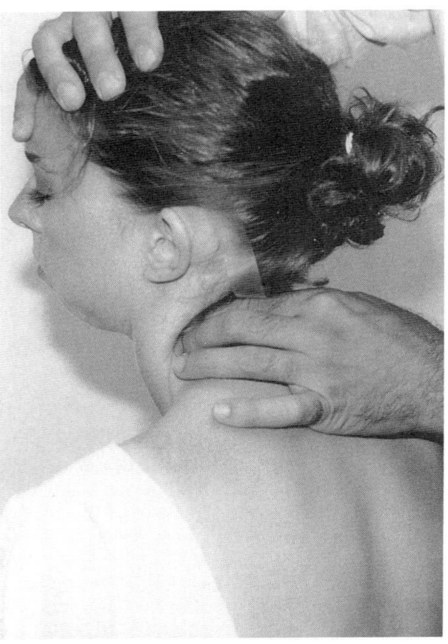

Figure 4.18. Motion palpation of the midcervical spine during left lateral bending. Notice how the soft tissue elements are moved anteriorward so that contact can be made at the lateral margins of the posterior articulations.

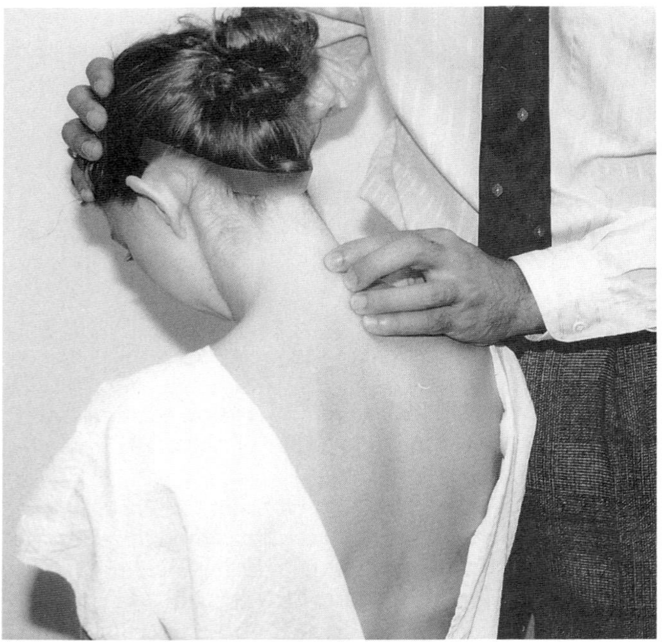

Figure 4.19. Motion palpation of the lower cervical spine during flexion. The examiner is noting separation of the spinous processes.

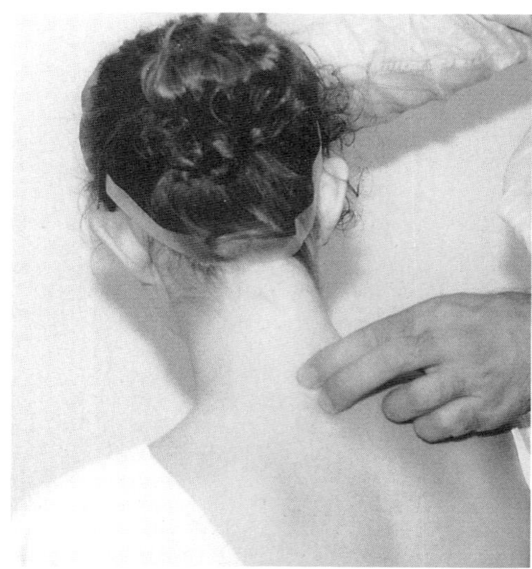

Figure 4.20. Motion palpation of the lower cervical spine during right axial rotation. The spinous processes should move toward the contralateral side of rotation.

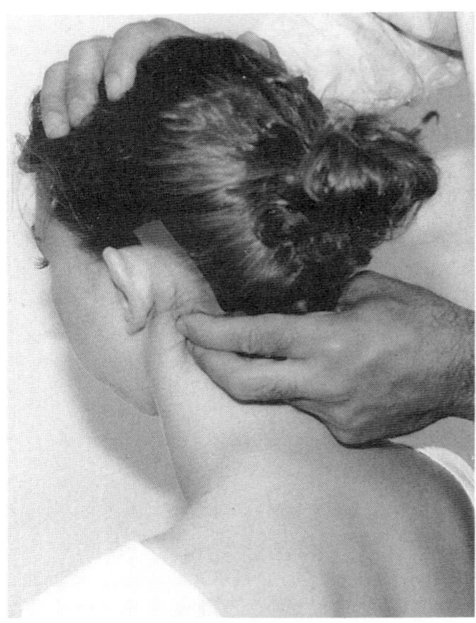

Figure 4.21. Motion palpation of C1-C2 during lateral bending. Notice how the soft tissue elements are moved forward in order that contact can be made just inferior to the atlas transverse processes and lateral to the C2 transverse process. If lateral flexion is present, there will be a relaxation of the soft tissue elements on the ipsilateral side of bend.

variations in skin temperature are a probable connection to nervous system phenomena related to the VSC.

Gonstead hypothesized that intersegmental variations in skin temperature were produced by inflammation from nerve root compression that radiated heat to the skin surface or from radiation of heat from the skin surface to the area of chronic nerve root compression (37). Heat exhibited on the surface of the skin is radiated from a maximum of 1 to 1.8 millimeters below the skin (53). The results of research into the mechanisms involved in the production of variations in skin temperature have provided more likely theories than the historical Gonstead hypotheses (54).

Thermographic findings are largely accepted as resulting from changes in underlying blood vascularity (55). Two main mechanisms thought to cause such blood vessel changes include Substance P release in response to dorsal sensory nerve stimulation and sympathetic nervous system activity. Sympathetic modulation is one of the more popular theoretical mechanisms of thermal dysfunction. Traditionally, preganglionic cell bodies were thought to be confined to the thoracic and upper lumbar levels (56), however, preganglionic sympathetic cell bodies have been identified at all levels of the spinal cord (57,58).

The recurrent meningeal (sinuvertebral) nerve innervates the articular capsule, PLL, and annulus. It has mixed sensory and sympathetic components and when stimulated may give rise to pain or thermal manifestations. Antidromic stimulation (propagation of an impulse in a reversed direction) of the dorsal root ganglion can raise skin temperature (59,60). The above has been termed the cutaneous axon reflex. It is possible that many different neural and myofascial mechanisms are involved in thermoregulation.

In the cervical and lumbar regions of the vertebral column there are large numbers of intersegmental connections between the nerves supplying contiguous spinal segments (51). The same is not true of the thoracic spine. Skin temperature alterations, therefore, may be more directly related to the segmental level involved in the thoracic region.

Thermocouple instruments, such as the Nervoscope (Fig. 4.22), consist of two thermal sensors composed of metal wires. When the sensors are at different temperatures, the voltage generated between them is roughly proportional to the difference in temperature because of the thermoelectric effect involving the drifting of free electrons in a metal from the warmer junction to the cooler junction (61). The low impedance thermocouples are connected in series with a micrometer to provide a differential measurement of temperature.

The Nervoscope and other similar instruments (Fig. 4.23) yield a qualitative assessment of thermal asymmetry. The temperature on one side of the spine is compared with that on the other. A scanning method is conducted whereby a bilateral skin temperature difference is depicted as a meter needle movement to one side or the other. A "reading" or temperature differential (TD) is considered significant if an abrupt "over and back" needle movement is seen over a one spinal segment distance during the scan (Fig. 4.24A-C). The magnitude of the TD (the amount of paraspinal temperature differential), is thought to be directly proportional to the amount of neurophysiologic involvement caused by the VSC. In the acute stage of spinal subluxation, large variations in heat are often seen. A gradual diminishment in the magnitude of the TD is interpreted as improvement in the aberrant neurophysiology. The monitoring of the intersegmental

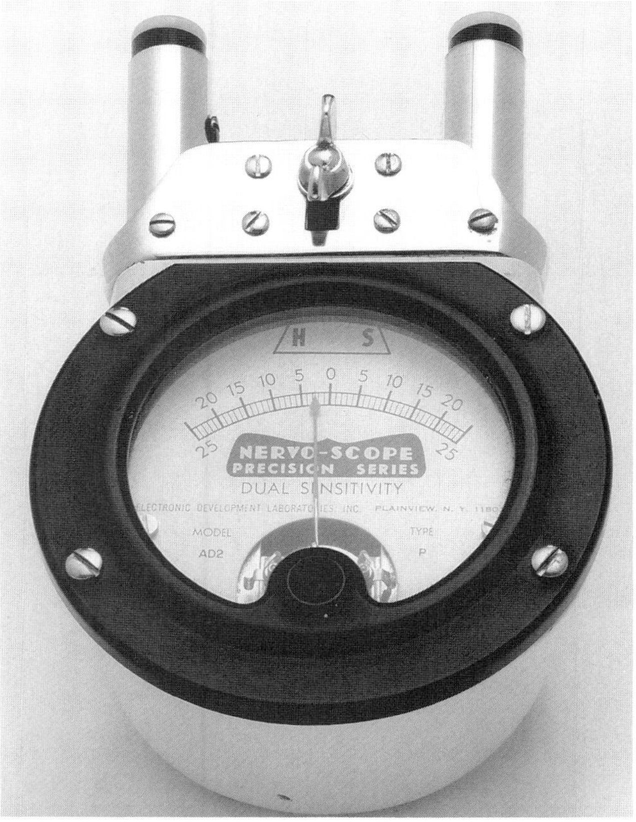

Figure 4.22. The Nervoscope.

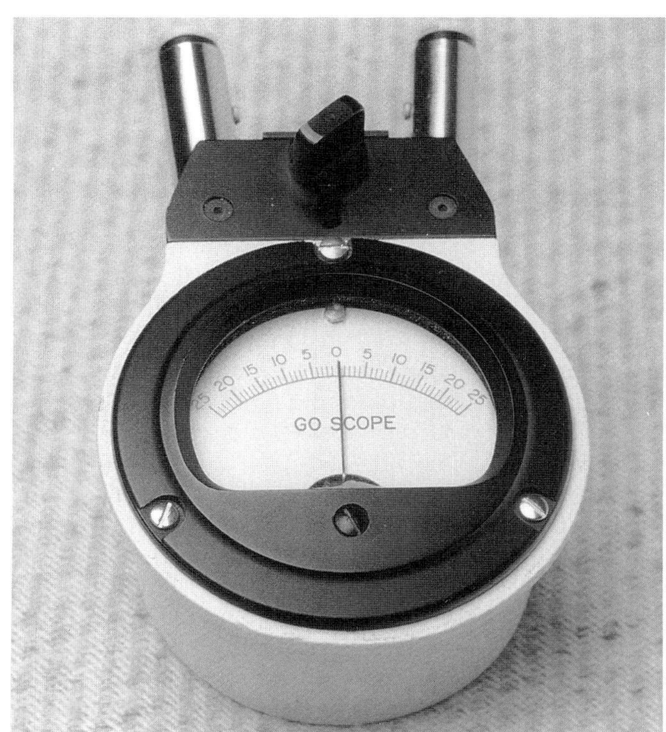

Figure 4.23. The GO scope.

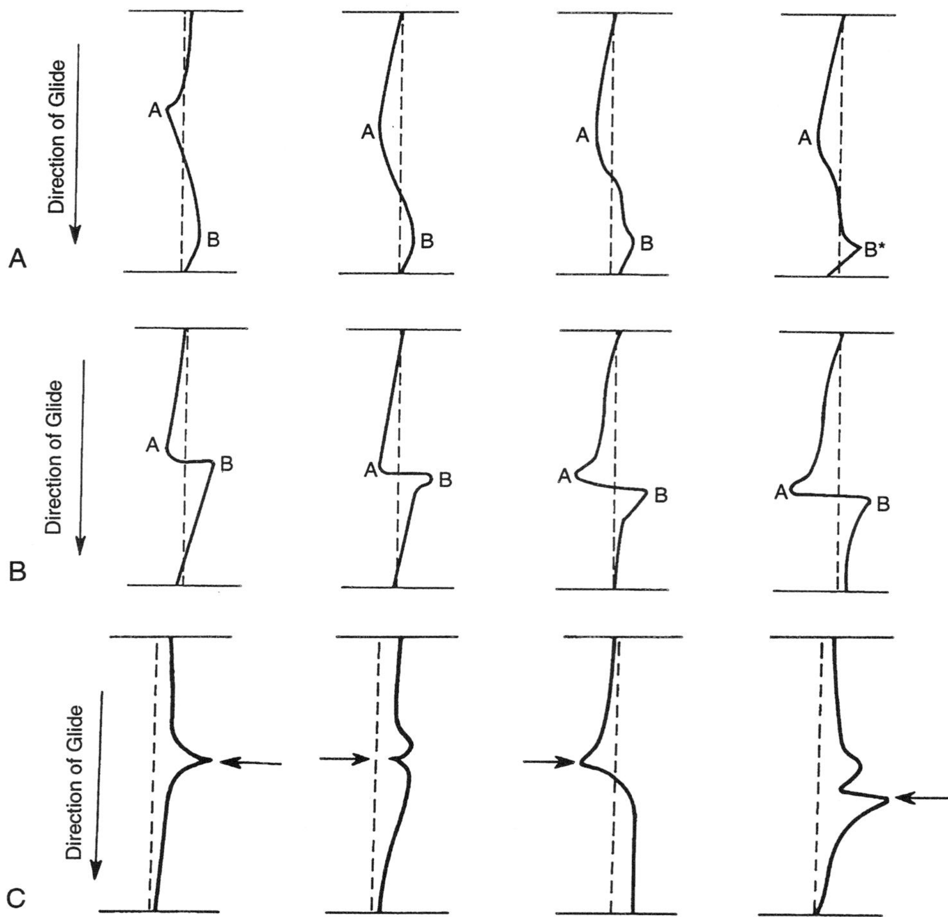

Figure 4.24. A, Successive scans with a cranio-caudal glide. B is recorded due to its accentuation after repeated glides. Modified from Plaugher G, Lopes MA, Melch PE, Cremata EE. The inter- and intraexaminer reliability of a paraspinal skin temperature differential instrument. J Manipulative Physiol The 1991;14:363. **B,** Successive scans with a caudal glide. In the fourth scan both A and B are of equal magnitude. In this case, two possible levels may be involved. Modified from Plaugher G, Lopes MA, Melch PE, Cremata EE. The inter- and intraexaminer reliability of a paraspinal skin temperature differential instrument. J Manipulative Physiol The 1991;14:363. **C,** Examples of four differential temperature differential patterns. Modified from Plaugher G, Lopes MA, Melch PE, Cremata EE. The inter- and intraexaminer reliability of a paraspinal skin temperature differential instrument. J Manipulative Physiol The 1991;14:363

heat differential is one of several parameters of assessment used to gauge patient progress in response to specific spinal adjusting.

The level of the TD is considered to be specifically associated with the functional spinal unit (FSU) underlying it. The location of the TD level relative to the bony landmarks helps to associate the temperature differential with a certain spinal nerve level. The relationship of the reading locations to the bony landmarks is mildly variable from patient to patient. The main factors influencing the relative reading location include the state of the sagittal curves and the presence of a scoliotic curve. The segmental nature of the spinal nerves, the posterior primary rami, and autonomic connections have led to the assumption that a local skin temperature differential will likely occur at the intersegmental level. For example, a C8 spinal nerve dysfunction that produces a paraspinal skin temperature differential will likely produce a differential at the C7-T1 disc space level. See Table 4.2 for a list of TD locations and their corresponding spinal levels.

There are some unanswered questions about reading locations and their significance. For instance, in the cauda equina region, a disc protrusion causing nerve root compression at one level most likely will affect the nerve root

Table 4.2.
Corresponding Segmental Levels for Temperature Differentials[a]

C0–C2	The TDs occur very close together. A condyle or atlas subluxation may create a differential at any location between C2 and C0.
C2–T3	The TD should be inferior to the spinous process.
T4	The TD should be at the same level of the spinous process.
T5–T9	The TD should appear in the interspinous space above the spinous process of the involved vertebra.
T10–T12	The TD should be at the level of the spinous process.
L1–L5	The TD should appear at the level of the lower one fourth of the spinous process.
Sacroiliac and inferior	The TD could appear anywhere between the superior boundaries of the sacroiliac articulation.

[a]Modified from Herbst RW. Gonstead chiropractic science and art. Mt. Horeb, WI:Sci-Chi Publications, 1968:167–168.

that exits the intervertebral foramen at the level below. In the case of a lumbar disc protrusion at L4, the L5 nerve root will more likely be compressed than the L4 nerve root.

The presence of an intersegmental temperature differential is not synonymous with the existence of VSC. Neurophysiologic involvement may exist at a specific spinal level without the concomitant presence of other subluxation parameters. Such a spinal level would not be considered a "subluxation." A hypermobile FSU may create aberrant nervous system activity. The hypermobile FSU can be a compensation for a restricted and subluxated FSU at another level, usually below the hypermobility (62).

It is possible that VSC induced skin temperature abnormalities may exist distally to the paraspinal region, or directly over the spine, without being revealed in the region of the skin scanned by the thermocouple. This phenomenon is one probable limitation of the exclusive employment of a bilateral thermocouple device for skin temperature analysis.

The reliability of the Nervoscope has been tested statically and in the dynamic scanning mode. The consistency in the measurement of the differential was determined to be excellent when tested by placing and then replacing the thermocouples statically on the same location on the skin (63). The statistical analysis methods used in the above study are suspect. In a study using the dynamic scanning mode, good intra and interexaminer reliability was seen in the thoracic region (kappa > 0.56), but not in the cervical region (6). Good intraexaminer correlation (ICC > 0.50) of the location marked for a temperature differential was found in the above study, once readings were detected in a given region. The same study yielded poor interexaminer concordance (ICC < 0.3) for temperature differential location in one series and good concordance (ICC $= 0.64$) for the second.

Caution must be taken in applying results from studies such as those above to the clinical setting. The dynamic scanning study must be repeated with more subjects and symptomatic patients. Other studies comparing the bilateral thermocouple to a more established reference test such as telethermography would be useful.

In summary, the bilateral thermocouple instrument is used to monitor skin temperature on each patient visit to aid in the location of neurologic dysfunction and to help determine the timing of and response to spinal adjustments.

SCANNING PROCEDURE

Typically, paraspinal skin temperature instruments are used to scan small sections of the spinal column, one after another (6). The probes are kept in perpendicular contact with the skin surface with sufficient pressure to prevent air gaps forming at the skin/thermocouple interface. The glide is caudocephalad for T2 to C0 and cephalocaudal for T2 to S2 (Fig 4.25A-B). Glide speed for nonamplified instruments should not exceed 0.5–1.0 cm/sec. If a temperature differential is suspected at a segmental level, the scan should be repeated several times to confirm the finding. Differentials that are accentuated with a repeat scanning procedure are considered more significant than those that diminish. The presence of moles or other lesions in the glide path lessens the validity of the procedure. If a scoliosis is present, then the scan and orientation of the instrument should follow the curvature. The newborn or toddler's loose skin will usually alter the scanning protocol (See Chapter 14).

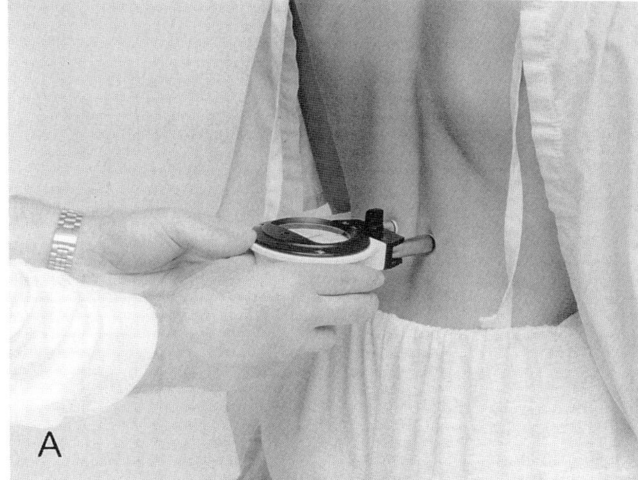

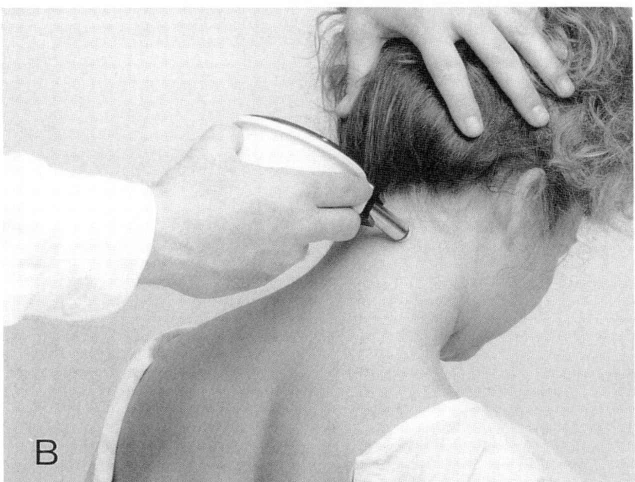

Figure 4.25. A, Temperature analysis of the lumbar spine. The glide should be cranio-caudal for the lumbar and thoracic spine. **B,** Temperature analysis of the upper cervical spine. The glide should be caudal-cranial for the cervical spine.

Leg Length Inequality

Prone measurement of leg length inequality (LLI) is common in the chiropractic profession. The procedure is likely most reliable when measured on a self-lowering table without altering the resting position of the legs before measuring. The patient is directed to stand on the platform of a table such as the hydraulic "hi-lo," with the patient's feet approximately six inches apart and heels even. The patient should then lean into the table as straight and as balanced as possible. Lower the table and instruct the patient not to move any part of his or her body. View the medial malleoli bilaterally, comparing the relative length of the legs without moving them. The thumbs can be placed on the inferior portion of the malleoli for comparison.

Measurements such as this are not likely reliable (64). The use of an apparent visually observed LLI as a sole indication of the need for treatment, or as a major outcome measure of the response to treatment, is likely invalid. Differentiation between functional and anatomical leg length inequality is presented in Chapter 6.

Plain Film Radiographic Examination

In this chapter, the discussion of the radiographic examination will focus on integrating the findings of radiographic analysis into the examination of the chiropractic patient. Historically, the use of radiography in chiropractic centered around the detection and quantification of the intervertebral misalignment. Stress radiography was added to the routine examination when ligament integrity was suspect. Such "bending views" have been proposed as valuable in determining intervertebral motion characteristics and can augment or replace motion palpation assessments.

As licensed x-ray supervisors, chiropractors usually expose and interpret their own radiographs, unlike the practicing medical doctor whose films are normally taken by a medical radiologist. For the above reason, chiropractors must differentially diagnose the results of the radiographic examination. The radiograph must be screened for pathology, fracture, and dislocation, as well as be interpreted for biomechanical relevance (See Chapter 5).

The minimal examination includes two views of the area of primary complaint, preferably perpendicular to each other (65). Other areas that might require adjustive intervention may be exposed. Additional projections, such as oblique radiographs, supplement the examination when indicated.

Adjustments given to aid the primary presenting complaint often result in the development of symptoms elsewhere, especially in chronic situations. These symptoms likely arise from compensation for the biomechanical changes resulting from adjustments at other spinal levels. The ability of some areas to respond to direct treatment often necessitates that other (symptomatically silent) areas be adjusted. The interdependency of the different spinal regions necessitates a full-spine examination (66). When the entire spine needs to be viewed, a properly exposed full-spine radiograph (See Chapter 5) will offer diagnostically useful information with comparatively less patient exposure than sectional analyses that require projectional overlap. For the above reasons and others, full spine visualization is preferable whenever possible in the chiropractic management of a VSC.

There are those in the profession that believe that chiropractic treatment is appropriate for pain relief only. Many chiropractors and some chiropractic institutions only take x-rays of a patient if fracture or pathology is suspected. It is the opinion of the authors that the application of the force required to cavitate an intervertebral articulation is a relatively invasive maneuver. It should be assumed that an individual presenting for treatment for spinal related pain or other symptoms is likely to have a history of paraspinal ligament damage. As was discussed in Chapters 2 and 3, the spinal ligaments are subject to the phenomenon of plastic deformation or creep. Previously injured ligaments will allow distortion of the alignment of the vertebra(e) they are meant to support. To introduce a force into the spine sufficient to produce abrupt intervertebral movement and cavitation, without previously determining the presence or absence and, most importantly, the direction of creep deformation at the level(s) being adjusted or manipulated, is to invite injury to the patient. The chiropractor has a responsibility to protect the patient at all times by ensuring that the treatment rendered is safe, as well as maximally effective.

Another important reason that radiographic examination is requisite for proper administration of the adjustment is that the symptomatic level is not necessarily the level to be adjusted. A hypermobile articulation may cause spinal related pain yet is not a candidate for spinal adjustment. Radiographic examination is the most useful tool for locating contraindications for the chiropractic adjustment. The use of stress radiographs appears to be far more accurate in assessing the intricacies of fixation dysfunction and abnormal coupling patterns, than other procedures. Because an adjustment is not a benign procedure, it is important that the force be directed where appropriate.

Spinal alignment characteristics are determined from qualitative inspection and the measurement of various anatomical configurations. The clinical significance of these measurements is controversial. To rely on static radiographic measurements as the primary criteria used to apply chiropractic care is to invite disaster. Clinical correlation of radiologically derived information is requisite for a complete evaluation. Generally, small measurements derived from radiographic marking systems must be suspect, especially if they are used to determine large postural asymmetries. Radiographic distortion and magnification will magnify slight changes such as those associated with scoliosis. If one focuses on intersegmental relationships, the significance of radiographic distortion reduces dramatically. The images of adjacent vertebrae will be projected and distorted similarly, producing relatively insignificant differences.

It is important to remember that plain film radiographs are static, two-dimensional instantaneous shadows of the patient. Often, the most misaligned motion segments are compensations for subluxations elsewhere. The freely movable areas compensate for the restricted areas when the individual is weight bearing and moving about. Global abnormalities in structural alignments may result from intersegmental fixed positional dyskinesia.

The lateral view is considered more important than the AP radiograph in spinal diagnosis. The disc space is most easily viewed on the lateral radiograph. Abnormalities in the integrity of the disc space may be suggestive of the physiologic age and state of health of the FSU (See Chapters 2 and 3).

FUNCTIONAL OR STRESS RADIOGRAPHY

The use of functional or stress radiography (bending views) is common for the purposes of the differential diagnosis of the presence or absence of ligament failure (65). The use of bending views for the differential diagnosis of the presence or absence of fixation dysfunction and abnormal coupling patterns is somewhat controversial, yet relatively common. The reliability of this measure to assess fixation dysfunction has not been determined. One review of the literature on lumbar functional radiography concludes that there may be a role for functional radiographs in ascertaining the physiologic age of the spine, disc protrusions, and instability (67).

Jirout (68) has demonstrated some of the intricate parameters of the three-dimensional nature of cervical lateral bending movement. The sagittal component of lateral bending varies considerably from deep inspiration to mid respiration to deep exhalation. The variability of all types of bending views must be determined to ascertain the indications and contraindications of their usage. Bending views aid in the visualization of intersegmental and global movement characteristics, and as such, often provide valuable insight into the nature of the presenting dysfunction.

All intervertebral articulations can be visualized with stress radiography in any single or combination of range(s) of motion(s). In the determination of fixation dysfunction, a very important factor to rule out is the presence of anatomical variation that may explain any apparent asymmetry in motion visualized on bending views. Equally important is the ruling out of projection distortion. It is also crucial that painstakingly diligent attempts are made to instruct the patient properly as to the movement desired and to observe that the patient has moved equally from side to side, when taking views of opposing movements.

A routine assessment of spinal movement includes the neutral position and extremes of movement to either side in the desired directions. One cannot adequately compare one direction with the other without the neutral view. Clinical experience has been that comparisons are best made from end-range to neutral on one side, then again on the other side. Analysis of intermediate movements of the FSU, determined through cineradiography, may prove to be a valuable method of assessment. Preliminary reports of interexaminer reliability in the mid cervical spine are encouraging (69). Possible indications of fixation dysfunction include an intersegmental decrease in one or more of the normal planes of motion for the articulation in question. The articulation in question is compared with those directly adjacent to it. Motion abnormalities consistent with the presence of fixation dysfunction may exist in singular or multiple planes.

Hypermobility dysfunction may occur secondarily to fixation dysfunction, primary ligament damage, or anomaly. Possible indications of hypermobility include an increase of intersegmental movement in one or more degrees of freedom. For a complete discussion of aspects of the functional radiographic examination, the reader is referred to Chapter 5.

ADVANCED DIAGNOSTIC PROCEDURES

In the past several years new developments in the area of sophisticated diagnostic procedures have contributed to a more complete illumination of the objective evidence associated with the VSC. Magnetic resonance imaging (static, functional and three-dimensional), thermography, and video fluoroscopy have and will continue to provide us with new insights into the nature of the VSC and its identification.

With the maturation of the chiropractic profession comes a sophistication in examination and treatment protocol. With an increase in the availability and understanding of special testing methods, those not routinely necessary, comes the opportunity to address the needs of the challenging patient more completely. An adequate understanding of the clinical value of special tests is necessary to avoid under or overutilization of any testing procedure.

Enthusiasm and criticism are often stimulated by new or popularized diagnostic tests. It is in the patient's best interests to develop the skill of filtering the emotional arguments of the critics and the promoters and rely on reason and available facts regarding the usefulness of any test. Historically, clinicians in all disciplines have developed their clinical protocols based on the workshops that they have attended, their instructor's views, trial-and-error experience, and their emotional bias toward treatment styles, rather than on scientifically validated protocols (70). It is refreshing to see a declining number of pseudo-religious practitioners that refuse to keep abreast of advances in the profession and incorporate them into their practices for the benefit of their patients. An increased emphasis is being placed on the development of standards of practice based on reason and the conclusions of scientific trials. Unfortunately, a number of the more progressive practitioners give up the principles and philosophy of chiropractic and in spite of a scientifically sound approach to their patient, ignore the reason for delivering chiropractic care. This approach sabotages the patient's right to the primary benefit of chiropractic care; the reduction or elimination of components of the vertebral subluxation complex which may contribute to or cause an alteration in homeostasis.

When considering special testing, one needs to consider whether an anatomic or a physiologic test is required. An anatomic test, as the name implies, gives information regarding a given structure and is helpful for viewing "visible" phenomenon. For example, an MRI can help the doctor "see" inside the spinal canal to assist in the evaluation of suspected disc herniation or other space occupying lesion. A physiologic test, such as an EMG or a thermogram, offers quite different information that may be of lesser or greater value depending on the specific information sought. The choice of a physiologic or anatomic test depends on the suspected diagnosis and the information required to progress with a modified treatment plan dependent on the results of the special test. When the results of a test, whether negative or positive, are not likely to affect the clinical course, a question arises regarding the need for the examination. The following discussion of specialized testing procedures is provided as a brief description of the possible applications available to the chiropractor.

Magnetic Resonance Imaging

Magnetic resonance imaging is generally regarded as an anatomic test, allowing the practitioner to "see" inside the involved area. An MRI is helpful to evaluate a suspected space occupying lesion in a patient with intractable headaches or suspected cord tumor. More commonly, an MRI assists in the characterization of a radicular lesion and verifies or negates the need for surgical consultation. MRI is useful for viewing changes resulting from chronic subluxations such as disc dehydration and protrusion and degenerative joint disease (71). These degenerative changes, commonly attributed to wear and tear due to old age, can be seen at levels of fixation dysfunction or at surrounding segments where hypermobility may occur.

Computerized Axial Tomography

Computerized axial tomographic (CT) scanning is an imaging tool quite similar in its application to MRI. Generally speaking, a CT scan is preferred for viewing bony changes and MRI is preferred for characterizing soft tissue lesions. Because hydrogen atoms found in high concentration in water assist in optimal MRI viewing, the cortical area of bone, which has a low water content, may be viewed better with CT than with MRI. Conversely, the medullary cavities of bone have a high hydrogen atom concentration and are viewed adequately with MRI scanning. Medullary tumors are sometimes best characterized with MRI (See Chapter 7). CT and MRI can offer much assistance, whether the results are positive or negative, in consideration of continued patient management, but caution is in order because of the fact that approximately 20 to 30% of "normal," asymptomatic individuals have positive findings on an MRI (35). Of course, what in fact constitutes normal has not yet been resolved.

Electromyographic Tests

Needle EMG is a functional test and is helpful for characterizing neural function. It verifies nerve damage as is often found as a result of components of the VSC, such as disc herniation, or peripheral neuropathies caused by carpal tunnel syndrome. A needle EMG is typically performed by neurologists and physiatrists and aids in the localization and characterization of neural involvements.

Needle EMGs are clinically useful when positive, but because of a high rate of false negatives, a negative test with high clinical suspicion should be followed by a thermogram or conduction velocity examination.

Conduction Velocity Tests

As implied by the name, these are tests used to measure the speed at which a nerve delivers an electrical signal. When the conduction velocity is altered in a section of or throughout the length of a nerve, this test assists in the location and presence of a lesion. This test is commonly performed by neurologists and physiatrists but also by some chiropractors.

Surface EMG

Paraspinal EMG has become popular within the chiropractic profession in recent years. Preliminary evidence (72–74) suggests that good levels of reproducibility can be obtained with surface EMG, provided technicians are adequately trained in the protocol of the examination, patient postures are controlled (75) and electrodes are of sufficient sensitivity.

Bone Scans

Bone scans are generally considered a physiologic test as they measure the amount of uptake of a radioactive isotope into bone. The injected isotope competes with blood calcium for absorption into bone and this phenomenon can help to identify areas of abnormal bone physiology as found with metastatic carcinoma and osteomyelitis.

Thermography

Thermography is a physiologic test considered sensitive for sensory/neural abnormalities and myofascial irritations (55). This test is typically used to characterize radicular pain patterns and soft tissue pain and differentially diagnose these conditions from vascular or referred etiologies for similar pain syndromes. Additionally, a negative thermogram is considered a strong indicator for the absence of an organic cause for a patient's pain complaints and is therefore an excellent test for malingering.

Liquid crystal thermography, where cholesterol esters change colors dependent on known temperature ranges, is used for all thermographic applications and is considered superior for breast and temporal mandibular joint (TMJ) studies. Much more research has been published regarding the use of electronic or telethermography and this method of thermographic analysis is generally preferred (55). This method uses an infrared detector that transfers the information to a computer for interpretation and visualization on a monitor. This information is often stored on video tape or stored on a hard disk for future interpretation.

Perhaps it is the sensitivity of the test which contributes to its suspected rate of high false positives. A large volume of research is now available in this field. Much of the skepticism regarding the validity of this procedure has diminished among informed investigators and clinicians. The insistence of established clinical protocol by thermographic societies has contributed greatly to the standardization and reliability of thermographic interpretation.

The worker's compensation system in California allows thermograms after sixty days of treatment, and the American Medical Association recently released an opinion on thermography classifying it as useful for a variety of neuromusculoskeletal disorders (76). It appears that overutilization of this procedure by a few has contributed to a widespread prejudice toward thermography. Future research should incorporate rigorous designs especially blinding and interpretation reliability. The use of thermography as an outcome measure following chiropractic care could also be a fruitful area for future research.

Computerized Musculoskeletal Analysis

Various manufacturers produce both similar and differing computerized instruments that measure muscular strength. These instruments seem to offer significant contributions in the diagnosis and management of musculoskeletal problems. The popularity and common use of these types of analyses will likely increase as the prices lower and physicians and physical therapists become more aware of the questionable reliability of manual muscle testing. These machines are designed to isolate a particular muscle or muscle group, assisting in correlating myologic weakness with other evidence of neuropathy in the diagnosis of a particular disorder.

Computerized testing units generally measure isometric, isotonic, and isokinetic muscular activity. Often, initial exercise rehabilitation is performed on these machines and this information assists in determining the need for endurance, strength, or power testing. Additionally, patterns of abnormalities can be diagnostically helpful as well.

Chiropractors typically use these instruments to determine the muscle weakness that may be correlated with nerve root pathology, and the determination of strength/body weight and agonist/antagonist muscular ratios. Specifically, a runner may have recurring knee injuries if the quadricepshamstring ratio is abnormal, as is commonly found. An optimal exercise rehabilitation, as can be properly determined from information obtained from this test may help a runner achieve a more desirable ratio of a hamstring with a muscular strength which is 75% that of the quadriceps. This balance will add to the stability of the knee and allow for a quicker rehabilitation, as well as protect against reinjury.

Studies suggest that extensor trunk strength is lost in the patient with back pain and bidirectional causal relationships have been discussed (See Chapter 7). The question still arises as to whether the low back pain contributes to the extensor muscular weakness or whether the extensor muscle weakness contributes to the development of low back pain, but most agree that the trunk extensor muscles should be 40% stronger than the trunk flexors. The term extensor weakness refers to either an actual muscular weakness as compared with body weight or a relative extensor weakness when compared with the strength of the trunk flexors.

It is suggested that muscular strength be accurately assessed before implementing a rigorous strengthening program in patients. The possibility exists of increasing a muscular ratio problem with low back patients that are given sit-ups to help assist in their management. It is likely that the extensors are weak in patients with low back pain. If computerized musculoskeletal analyses are not available, it is suggested that extensor strength always be prioritized in any trunk exercise program. McKenzie extension maneuvers have been shown to be more effective than the more traditional William's exercises in the management of low back patients (See Chapter 7).

Velocity measures for patients with impaired spine motion appears to be a valuable assessment. Velocity measures often show a greater ability to distinguish between symptomatic and pain-free subjects (77) (Fig. 4.26).

ORTHOPAEDIC AND NEUROLOGIC TESTING

A comprehensive physical examination includes orthopaedic tests. A properly executed orthopaedic evaluation

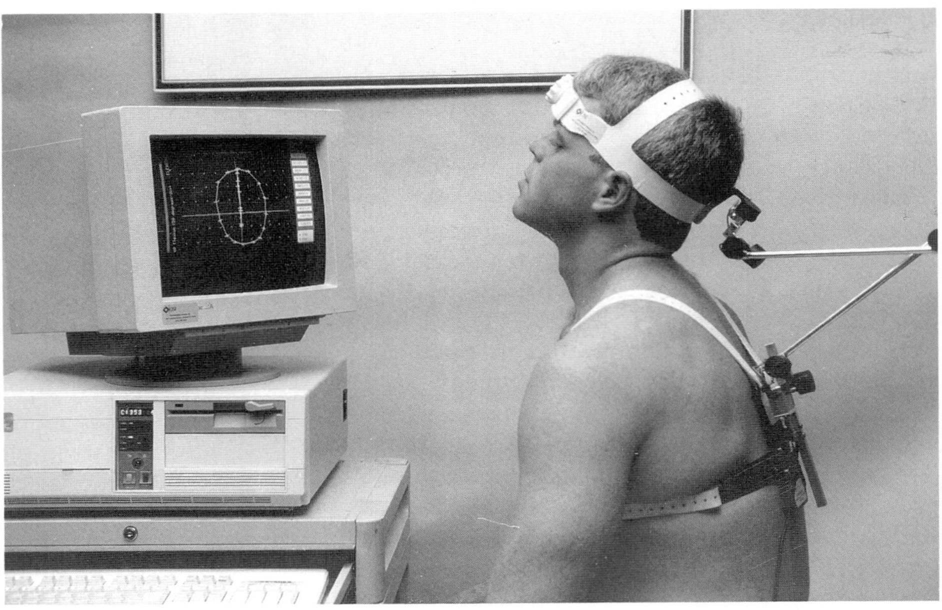

Figure 4.26. Computerized analysis of cervical spine range of motion and velocity. Courtesy of Orthopedic Systems Inc., Hayward, CA.

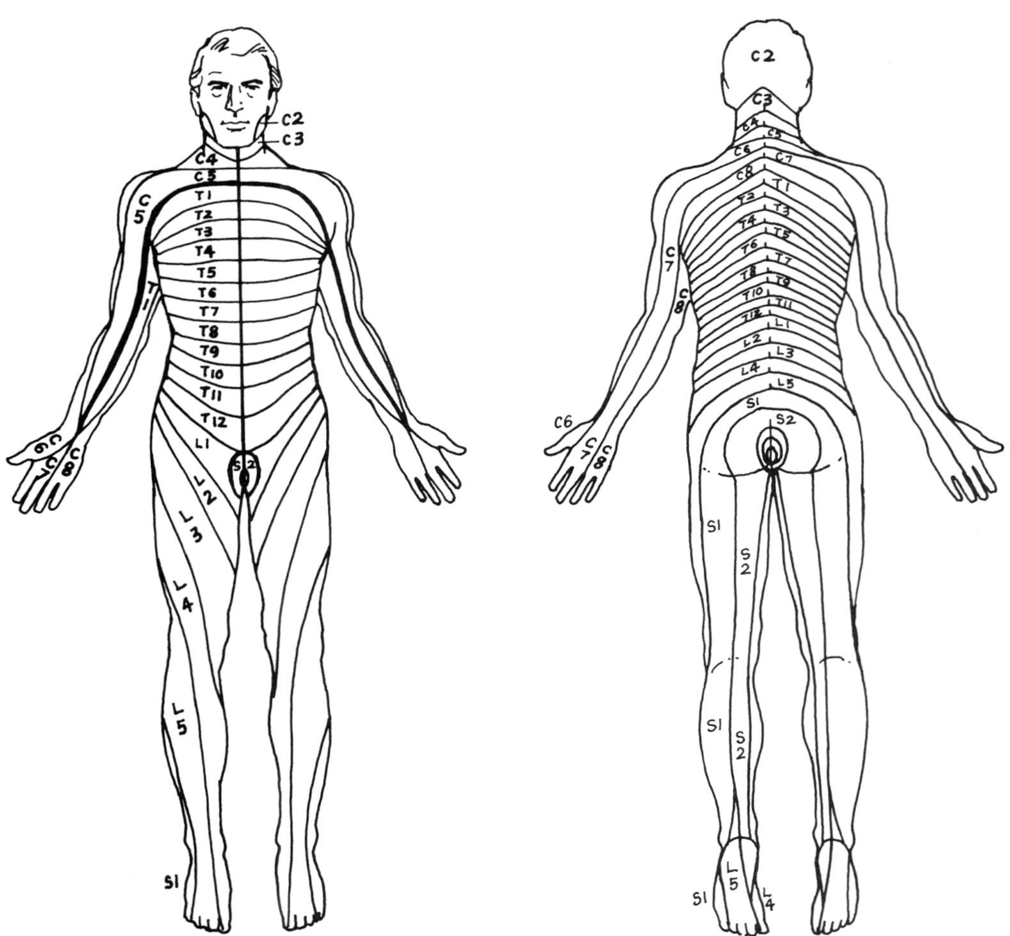

Figure 4.27. The dermatomes of the human. This distribution is based on hypalgesia from the compression of single nerve roots. Modified from Chusid JG. Correlative neuroanatomy and functional neurology. 19th ed. Los Altos, CA: Lange Medical Publishers, 1985:237.

can be complete, reliable, systematic, and practical. For assessment of components of the subluxation, the orthopaedic examination is relatively insensitive. For the purposes of localizing and reproducing the patient's experience of pain, the orthopaedic examination can be helpful. Spratt et al. (78) developed an assessment protocol for measuring outcomes for low back pain patients. A total of 21 physical examination tests were used. Interrater agreements were statistically high in the following areas: patient reported pain aggravation and pain location; rater observed dynamics of motion and degrees elevated in the straight leg raise; location of the most tender area; recording pain behaviors; test-retest comparisons. The above comprehensive examination was performed in an average of less than 14 minutes. This protocol is an example of a reliable and practical use for orthopaedic testing.

An alphabetical listing of orthopaedic tests that may be of use to the chiropractor is presented in Appendix 4B. This list is presented as a reference for the student or practicing doctor. It is expected that the individual will compile groups of tests from this list, and organize them into a flowing set of procedures for testing specific neuromechanically related, painful conditions.

Neurologic testing of dermatomes is very important, especially in the patient with a referred pain syndrome. Sensory evaluation can be performed with a pin wheel. In addition, reflex alterations and muscle strength loss will be indicative of impaired neural function. The human dermatomes are depicted in Figure 4.27.

REFERENCES

1. Shekelle PG, Adams AH, Chassin MR, et al. The appropriateness of spinal manipulation for low-back pain. Indications and ratings by a multidisciplinary expert panel. Santa Monica, CA: RAND, 1991.
2. Cassidy JD. Roentgenological examination of the functional mechanics of the lumbar spine in lateral flexion. J Can Chiro Assoc 1976;20:2.
3. Gunn CC, Milbrandt WE. Early and subtle signs in low back sprain. Spine 1978;3:267–281.
4. Keating JC. Inter-examiner reliability of motion palpation of the lumbar spine: a review of quantitative literature. Am J Chiro Med 1989;2:107–110.
5. Keating JC, Bergmann TF, Jacobs GE, Finer BA, Larson K. Interexaminer reliability of eight evaluative dimensions of lumbar segmental abnormality. J Manipulative Physiol Ther 1990;13:463–470.
6. Plaugher G, Lopes MA, Melch PE, Cremata EE. The inter- and intraexaminer reliability of a paraspinal skin temperature differential instrument. J Manipulative Physiol Ther 1991;14:361–367.
7. Browner WS, Newman TB, Cummings SR. Designing a new study: III. Diagnostic tests. In: Hulley SB, Cummings SR, eds. Designing clinical research. Baltimore: Williams & Wilkins, 1988:87–97.
8. Schalimtzek M. Functional roentgen examination of degenerated and normal intervertebral disks of the lumbar spine. Acta Radiol (Stockholm) 1954;116(suppl):300–306.
9. Parke WW. Applied anatomy of the spine. In: Rothman RH, Simeone FA, eds. The spine. 2nd ed. Philadelphia: WB Saunders Co., 1982:35.
10. Lehmann TR, Spratt KF, Tozzi JE, et al. Long-term follow-up of lower lumbar fusion patients. Spine 1987;12:97–104.
11. Triano JJ. The subluxation complex: outcome measure of chiropractic diagnosis and treatment. Chiropractic Technique 1990;2:114–120.
12. Zachman ZJ, Traina AD, Keating JC, Bolles ST, Braun-Porter L. Interexaminer reliability and concurrent validity of two instruments for the measurement of cervical ranges of motion. J Manipulative Physiol Ther 1989;12:205–210.
13. Million R, Hall W, Haavik Nilsen K, Baker RD, Jayson MIV. Assessment of the progress of the back-pain patient. Spine 1982;7:204–212.
14. Fairbank JCT, Couper J, Davies JB, O'Brien JP. The Oswestry low back pain disability questionnaire. Physiotherapy 1980;66:271–273.
15. Lacroix JM, Powell J, Lloyd GJ, et al. Low-back pain: factors of value in predicting outcome. Spine 1990;15:495–499.
16. White A. Back injury: prevention and rehabilitation. Paper presented via teleconference to the National Safety Council, May 18, 1983.
17. Adams AH. Methodological considerations in the selection of outcome measures for chiropractic practice. In: Proceedings of the 1991 international conference on spinal manipulation. Arlington, VA: FCER, 1991:9–11.
18. Sackett DL, Haynes RB, Tugwell P. Clinical epidemiology: a basic science for clinical medicine. Boston: Little, Brown & Co, 1985:14–49.
19. Barrows HS, Norman GR, Neufeld VR, Feightner JW. The clinical reasoning of randomly selected physicians in general medical practice. Clin Invest Med 1982;5:49–55.
20. Feinstein AR. Scientific methodology in clinical medicine: IV. Acquisition of clinical data. Ann Intern Med 1964;61:1162–1193.
21. Hall R, Horrocks JC, Clamps SE, et al. Observer variation in assessment of results of surgery for peptic ulcer. Br Med J 1976;1:814–816.
22. Wiesel SW, Tsourmas N, Feffer HL, Citrin CM, Patronas N. A study of computer-assisted tomography 1. The incidence of positive CAT scans in an asymptomatic group of patients. Spine 1984;9:549–551.
23. Frymoyer JW, Phillips RB, Newberg AH, MacPherson BV. A comparative analysis of the interpretations of lumbar spinal radiographs by chiropractors and medical doctors. Spine 1986;11:1020–1023.
24. Aoki N, Horibe H, Ohno Y, et al. Epidemiological evaluation of funduscopic findings in cerebrovascular diseases: III. Observer variability and reproducibility for funduscopic findings. Jpn Circ J 1977;41:11–17.
25. Gilbert JR, Evans CE, Haynes RB, Tugwell P. Predicting compliance with a regimen of digoxin therapy in family practice. Can Med Assoc J 1980;123:119–122.
26. Haynes RB, Taylor DW, Sackett DL, et al. Can simple clinical measurements detect patient noncompliance? Hypertension 1980;2:757–764.
27. Bakwin H. Pseudodoxia pediatrica. N Engl J Med 1945;232:691–697.
28. Stein J, ed. The random house college dictionary. Revised ed. New York: Random House Inc., 1980:131.
29. Herzog W, Read LJ, Conway PJW, Shaw LD, McEwen MC. Reliability of motion palpation procedures to detect sacroiliac joint fixations. J Manipulative Physiol Ther 1989;12:86–92.
30. Wiles MR. Reproducibility and interexaminer correlation of motion palpation findings of the sacroiliac joints. J Can Chiro Assoc 1980;24:59.
31. Plaugher G, Cremata EE, Phillips RB. A retrospective consecutive case analysis of pre-treatment and comparative static radiological parameters following chiropractic adjustments. J Manipulative Physiol Ther 1990;13:498–506.
32. Vernon H. Clinical note: S-O-R-E; A record-keeping system for chiropractic treatment visits. J Can Chiro Assoc 1990;34(2):93.
33. Gerow G. Osseous configurations of the axial skeleton: specific

application to spatial relationships of vertebrae. J Manipulative Physiol Ther 1984;7:33–38.
34. Panjabi M, White A, Brand R. A note on defining body part configurations. J Biomech 1974;7:385–87.
35. White A, Panjabi M, Brand R. A system for defining position and motion of human body parts. Med Biol Eng 1975;13:261–65.
36. White AA, Panjabi MM. Clinical biomechanics of the spine. 2nd ed. Philadelphia: JB Lippincott Co, 1990.
37. Herbst RW. Gonstead chiropractic science and art. Mt. Horeb: Sci-Chi Publications, 1968.
38. Hansen DT, Sollecito PC. Standard chart abbreviations in chiropractic practice. J Chiropractic Technique 1991;3:96–103.
39. Hogan WJ. Visceral causes of back pain: rules for the differential diagnosis of spinal pain [Abstract]. J Manipulative Physiol Ther 1991;14:277–278.
40. Plaugher G, Hendricks AH. The inter- and intraexaminer reliability of the Gonstead pelvic marking system. J Manipulative Physiol Ther 1991;14:Nov/Dec.
41. Plaugher G, Hendricks AH, Doble RW, Araghi HJ, Bachman TR, Hoffart VM. The effects of patient positioning and natural history on radiographically evaluated static configurations of the pelvis. In: Proceedings of the 1991 International Conference on Spinal Manipulation. Arlington, VA: FCER, 1991:194–196.
42. Lecture notes. Gonstead seminar of chiropractic. Mt Horeb, WI, 1991.
43. Warwick R, Williams PL, eds. Gray's anatomy. 35th British ed. Philadelphia: WB Saunders Co, 1973:584.
44. Panjabi MM, Yamamoto I, Oxland T, Crisco J. How does posture affect coupling in the lumbar spine? Spine 1989;14:1002.
45. Hadley LA. Anatomico-roentgenographic studies of the spine. Fifth printing. Springfield: Charles C Thomas, 1981:296–7.
46. Hurst HC. Chiropractic adjustive procedures vs mobilization exercises in kyphotic geriatric patients [Abstract]. Chiropractic Technique 1991;3:46.
47. Dvorak J, Dvorak V. Manual medicine: Diagnostics. New York: Thieme-Stratton Inc., 1984:6–11.
48. Magarey ME. Examination and assessment in spinal joint dysfunction. In: Grieve GP, ed. Modern manual therapy of the vertebral column. Edinburgh: Churchill Livingstone, 1986:481–97.
49. Dorland's illustrated medical dictionary. 24th ed. Philadelphia: WB Saunders Co, 1965:467.
50. Wright HM, Korr IM, Thomas PE. Local and regional variations in cutaneous vasomotor tone of the human trunk. Neural Transmission 1960;22:34–52.
51. Wyke B. The neurological basis of thoracic spinal pain. Rheumatol Phys Med 1970;10:356–367.
52. Jull G, Bogduk N, Marsland A. The accuracy of manual diagnosis for cervical zygapophyseal joint pain syndromes. Med J Aust 1988;148:233–236.
53. Hamilton BL. An overview of proposed mechanisms underlying thermal dysfunction. Thermology 1985: 1:81–7.
54. Buettner K. Effects of extreme heat and cold on human skin: 1. Analysis of temperature changes caused by different kinds of heat application. J Appl Physiol 1951;3:691–702.
55. Plaugher G. Skin temperature assessment for neuromusculoskeletal abnormalities of the spinal column: a review of the literature. J Manipulative Physiol Ther 1992;15:July/Aug.
56. Guyton AC. Textbook of medical physiology. Sixth ed. Philadelphia: W.B. Saunders Co., 1981:710.
57. Mitchell GAG. Anatomy of the autonomic nervous system. London: E and S Livingstone Ltd, 1955:116–118.
58. Randall WC, Cox JW, Alexander WF, Coldwater KB, Hertzman AB. Direct examination of the sympathetic outflows in man. J Appl Physiol 1955;7:688–698.
59. Howe JF, Loeser JD, Calvin WH. Mechanosensitivity of dorsal root ganglia and chronically injured axons: a physiological basis for the radicular pain of nerve root compression. Pain 1977;3:25–41.
60. Wall PD, Devor M. Sensory afferent impulses originate from dorsal root ganglia as well as from the periphery in normal and injured rats. Pain 1983;17:321–339.
61. Chang L, Abernathy M, O'Rourke D, Dittberner MK, Robinson C. The evaluation of posterior thoracic temperatures by telethermography, thermocouple, thermistor and liquid crystal thermography. Thermology 1985;1:95–101.
62. Cremata EE, Plaugher G, Cox WA. Technique system application: the Gonstead approach. Chiropractic Technique 1991;3:19–25.
63. Perdew W, Jenness ME, Daniels JS, et al. A determination of the reliability and concurrent validity of certain body surface temperature measuring instruments. Dig Chiro Econ 1976 May/June:60–65.
64. Falltrick DR, Pierson DS. Precise measurement of functional leg length inequality and changes due to cervical spine rotation in pain-free subjects. J Manipulative Physiol Ther 1989;12:369–73.
65. Yochum TR, Rowe LJ. Essentials of skeletal radiology. Baltimore: Williams & Wilkins, 1987.
66. Voutsinas SA, MacEwen GD. Sagittal profiles of the spine. Clin Orthop 1986;210:235–242.
67. Meeker WC. The role of functional radiographs of the lumbar spine. Proceedings: Current topics in chiropractic: reviews of the literature. Palmer College of Chiropractic West, 1984.
68. Jirout J. Significance of the time factor in the dynamics of the cervical spine. J Manual Med 1991: 6:59–61.
69. Antos JC, Robinson K, Keating JC, Jacobs GE. Interrater reliability of fluoroscopic detection of fixation in the mid-cervical spine. Chiropractic Technique 1990;2:53–55.
70. Barlow DH, Hayes SC, Nelson RO. The scientist practitioner: research and accountability in clinical and educational settings. New York: Pergamon Press Inc., 1984.
71. Crawshaw C, Kean DM, Mulholland RC et al. The use of nuclear magnetic resonance in the diagnosis of lateral canal entrapment. J Bone Joint Surg 1984;66B:711.
72. Komi P, Buskirk E. Reproducibility of electromyographic measurements with inserted wire electrodes and surface electrodes. Electromyography 1970;10:357.
73. Spector B. Surface electromyography as a model for the development of standardized procedures and reliability testing. J Manipulative Physiol Ther 1979;2:214.
74. Thompson J, Erickson R. EMG muscle scanning: stability of hand-held electrodes. Biofeedback Self Regulation 1989;14:55.
75. Mouton LJ, Hof AL, de Jongh HJ, Eisma WH. Influence of posture on the relation between surface electromyogram amplitude and back muscle moment: consequences for the use of surface electromyogram to measure back load. Clin Biomech 1991;6:245–251.
76. Council on Scientific Affairs. Thermography in neurological and musculoskeletal conditions. AMA Council Report. Thermology 1987;2:600–607.
77. Marras WS, Wongsam PE. Flexibility and velocity of the normal and impaired lumbar spine. Arch Phys Med Rehabil 1986;67:213–217.
78. Spratt KF, Lehmann TR, Weinstein JN, et al. A new approach to the low-back physical examination: behavioral assessment of mechanical signs. Spine 1990;15:96–102.

APPENDIX 4A. Chart Abbreviations

Chart abbreviations used in chiropractic practice. Modified from Hansen DT, Sollecito PC. Standard chart abbreviations in chiropractic practice. J Chiropractic Technique 1991;3:97–103.

A	assessment; anterior
abd	abduction

ACJ	acromioclavicular joint
add	adduction
adj	adjustment
agg	aggravated
am	morning
AP	antero-posterior
ASAP	as soon as possible
ASIS	anterior superior iliac spine
ASS	assisted
asym	asymmetrical
atr	atrophy
B	brisk; burning (pain)
B4	before
Ⓑ	bilateral
bog	bogginess of tissue
BP	blood pressure
BSE	bilaterally symmetrical and equal (DTRs)
BT	bitemporal
C	cervical
CC	chief complaint; cervical chair
chr	chronic
c/o	complains of
CP	cervical pillow; cold pack
crep	crepitation(s)
CSPT	cervical support
CT	cervico-thoracic; computerized tomography
cx	coccyx
D	dorsal
d	dull
/d	per day
dev	deviation (-ate)
DF	dorsiflex (-ion)
dim	diminish
distrx	distraction
DJD	degenerative joint disease
DOI	date of injury
DPAT	decreased pain after treatment
DTR	deep tendon reflexes
Dx	diagnosis
E	examination
EP	end play
ext	extension
exs	exercise(s)
fix/dys	fixation dysfunction
Fx	fracture
FS	full spine
GHJ	glenohumeral joint
GI	gastrointestinal
grd	grade
HA	headache
HBP	high blood pressure
hern	herniation
HNP	herniated nucleus pulposus
HT	hypertonus (-ic); hypertension
HE	hyperemia
Hx	history
IC	intercostal
ins	inspection
int	intermittent; internal
ISL	interspinous ligament
IVD	intervertebral disc
J	joint
KC	knee-chest table
L	lumbar
Ⓛ	left
Lat	lateral
LB	low back
LBP	low back pain
LC	lower cervical
LCUT	lower cervical-upper thoracic
LOD	line of drive
L/S, L-S	lumbosacral
MC	midcervical
MT	midthoracic
/m	per month
mm	muscles
mob	mobilize
MP	motion palpation
N	normal; negative
No△	no change
N & V	nausea and vomiting
N & T	numbness and tingling
O	objective
occ	occasional; occiput
OTJ	on the job
OV	office visit
P	pain; plan; procedure; posterior
PA	posterior-anterior
Pass	passive
PB	pelvic bench
PC	phone call
PDPR_%	patient describes pain reduction as _%
PE	physical examination; physical education
Pg, preg	pregnant
PI	personal injury; personal illness; posterior inferior
PIS	preinjury status
palp	palpation (-ate) (-atory) (-able)
pm	afternoon; physical medicine
PMS	premenstrual syndrome
Pn	pain
Pn→	radiating pain
PNF	proprioceptive neuromuscular facilitation
P 'n S	permanent and stationary
pos, +	positive
POT	pattern of thrust
PPD	permanent partial disability
PRAE	patient responding as expected
PSIS	posterior superior iliac spine
Pt	patient
PT	physical therapy
PTPW	patient tolerated procedure well
Ⓡ	right

rad	radiating; radial; radius
ref	refer (-red)
rel	relief (-ieved)
resp	respiration
ROM	range of motion
Rot	rotation
RTW	return to work
Rx	recommended therapy; prescription
S	subjective
sac	sacrum
SCJ	sternoclavicular joint
sev	severe
SI	sacroiliac
sl	slight
SLP	short leg, prone
SLS	short leg, supine
SLR	straight leg raise
SMT	spinal manipulative therapy
SO	suboccipital
SP	spine (-ous) (-al)
spondy	spondylolisthesis
Spr	sprain
str	strain
stim	stimulate (-tion)
sup	supine, supination
Sx	symptoms
T	thoracic; transverse
TD	temperature differential
TTD	total temporary disability
T-L	thoracolumbar
TMJ	temporomandibular joint
TP	trigger point
TPT	trigger point therapy
TTF	"taut-tender fibers"
Trx	traction
Tx	treatment
U	upper
UC	upper cervical
UT	upper thoracic
vert	vertebral
vis	visible, visual
VS	vital signs
w/	with
w/o	without
wk	week
WNL	within normal limits
WR	work restriction
/w	per week
x	times
yest	yesterday
Ø	none, no, restricted

Adjustment Grades (follow listing as a superscript, e.g., L5 PRS^{++}):

–	no joint movement
+	less than the appropriate movement
++	appropriate or good movement
+++	over adjusted

Pain Abbreviations:

Pn	pain
D	dull
S	sharp
B	burning

Pain Grades Visual Analog Scale (VAS) (1–10):

1	very mild
10	excruciating

Mobilization and Manipulation Grades:
Grade 1: Small amplitude movements performed at the beginning of the range of motion of an articulation
Grade 2: Large amplitude movements that do not reach the limit of the range
Grade 3: Large amplitude movements performed up to the limit of the range
Grade 4: Small amplitude movements performed at the limit of the range
Grade 5: Movement into the paraphysiologic range

APPENDIX 4B. Index of Tests

Accommodation Reflex

Description-Patient is asked to focus on practitioner's thumb that is held at arms length. Practitioner's thumb is brought close to the patient's nose to create eye convergence.

Significance-Positive; If pupils fail to constrict once eyes converge.

Indication-Afferent II, Efferent III, Center; occipital cortex.

Adam's

Description-Patient is standing and flexes forward. Observe the spine.

Significance-Positive; Scoliosis remains with hump on side of thoracic convexity.

Indication-Pathology, altered morphology, subluxation.

Adson's

Description-While the patient is sitting palpate the radial pulse while the patient's neck is rotated to the affected side, elevating the chin and holding the breath for 10–15 seconds.

Significance-Positive; Pain, paresthesia, decreased pulse.

Indication-Scalenus anticus syndrome, cervical rib, compression of brachial plexus, subluxation.

Allis

Description-Patient is supine with knees flexed to 90 degrees and toes kept level and equidistant caudally.

Significance-Disparity in knee height in cephalad-caudal plane indicates a short tibia. Disparity in lateral plane indicates short femur.

Indication-True short leg.

Anal Reflex

Description-Contraction of external anal sphincter, on stimulation of perineal skin.

Significance-Positive; No contraction

Indication-Lower motor neuron disorder; S2, S3, S4.

Ankle Clonus

Description-While the patient is supine the practitioner vigorously dorsiflexes the patient's ankle, then holds it in dorsiflexion.

Significance-Positive; Repeated, rapid, involuntary dorsiflexion of the ankle.

Indication-Upper motor neuron disorder; Central nervous system disease.

Apley's Compression

Description-Patient prone, with knee at 90 degrees flexion. Compression is applied to the plantar surface of the foot. The tibia is internally then externally rotated on the femur.

Significance-Positive; If pain is experienced on the medial aspect of the knee with external rotation, or lateral pain with internal rotation.

Indication-Medial or lateral Meniscus respectively.

Apley's Distraction

Description-Patient as above with practitioner's knee resting on patient's posterior thigh to hold femur to couch. Foot distracted and rotated on the femur.

Significance-Positive; If pain is experienced on the medial aspect of the knee with external rotation, or lateral pain with internal rotation.

Indication-Medial or lateral coronary ligaments. NOT meniscus.

Babinski Foot Sign

Description-While the patient is supine, stroke the lateral aspect of the plantar surface of the patient's foot from the heel to the big toe.

Significance-Positive; Extension of the large toe and flaring of the small toe.

Indication-Upper motor neuron disorder from central nervous system disease.

Babinski Pronation Sign

Description-Patient has eyes closed while sitting, arms elevated and forearm's supinated. Tap hands three times from underneath.

Significance-Positive; One or both hands pronate on downward movement.

Indication-Upper motor neuron disorder.

Beevor's Sign

Description-Patient sits up from a supine position.

Significance-Positive; When the naval deviates to one side.

Indication-Lower motor neuron disorder, T10-T12.

Bowstring Sign

Description-S.L.R. test is performed until pain is reproduced. Flex the knee and rest the lower limb on practitioner's shoulder. Place thumb in popliteal fossa over sciatic nerve. Apply firm pressure.

Significance-Positive; If the patient experiences pain in the back or down the leg.

Indication-Nerve root tension; Space occupying lesion; Nerve root compression.

Chaddock's

Description-Stroke down the ulnar side of the patient's forearm to the wrist.

Significance-Positive; Wrist flexion with flaring and extension of fingers.

Indication-Upper motor neuron disorder.

Compression Cervicals

Description-While the patient is sitting, apply downward pressure on the head.

Significance-Positive; Pain local or radiating.

Indication-Disc, Nerve root compression, Facet lesion, Arthritis, Adhesions, Altered morphology, Subluxation.

Consensual Light Reflex

Description-Shine light into one eye and wait for pupil of other eye to constrict.

Significance-Positive; If pupil of other eye fails to constrict.

Indication—Afferent II, Efferent III

Cough

Description-Patient holds breath and coughs.

Significance-Positive; Pain in the area of the space occupying lesion.

Indication-Disc, Space occupying lesion.

Cremasteric

Description-Superficially stroke medial aspect of thigh in a caudal direction.

Significance-Positive; If scrotum fails to elevate.

Indication-Lower motor neuron disorder.

De Kleyn's

Description-Patient is supine, neck is extended and rotated and held in that position for 15–30 seconds.

Significance-Positive; Nystagmus, loss of balance, nausea.

Indication-Basilar insufficiency.

Eden's

Description-While sitting the patient undergoes full active neck flexion with active shoulder depression and scapula approximation. Patient holds breath for 10–15 seconds.

Significance-Positive; Pain, paresthesia, decreased radial pulse.

Indication-Costoclavicular syndrome.

FABERE

Description-Patient lies supine with hip flexed, externally rotated and abducted to rest the lateral malleoli on the contralateral knee.

Significance-Positive; Pain in the hip.

Indication-Degenerative joint disease, Hip pathology, Subluxation.

Gaenslen's

Description-The patient is supine. Flex one knee and hold it to the patient's chest. Extend and drop the other leg over the side of the couch.

Significance-Positive; Pain in the sacroiliac region.

Indication-Sacroiliac lesion.

Glabellar Reflex

Description-Rapidly tap the supraorbital ridge several times.

Significance-Positive; The patient continues to blink when the tapping ceases.

Indication-Upper motor neuron lesion, VII CN.

Gordon's Squeeze

Description-Squeeze the patient's calf.

Significance-Positive; Extension of the large toes, and flaring of the small toes.

Indication-Upper motor neuron lesion from central nervous system disease.

Gower's Sign

Description-The patient is instructed to stand from prostrate to erect position.

Significance-Positive; When hands used step by step by pushing on legs as support.

Indication-Muscular dystrophy.

Hautant's

Description-The sitting patient's upper limbs are in an abducted forward position with both hands supinated. Eyes are closed, the neck is extended and rotated and held for 20–30 seconds.

Significance-Positive; If one or both arms drop into pronation.

Indication-Basilar insufficiency.

Hoffman's

Description-While the patient is sitting, the practitioner holds the patient's hand, which is supinated. The practitioner flicks the distal phalanx of the index finger into flexion.

Significance-Positive; Clawing of fingers and thumb.

Indication-Upper motor neuron disorder, Stroke, Parkinsonism.

Homan's

Description-Patient lies supine. The practitioner applies;
1. Forced dorsiflexion of the patient's foot.
2. Thumb pressure between medial and lateral gastrocnemius muscle.

Significance-Positive; Pain.

Indication-Deep Venous Thrombus (when accompanied by edema, heat). Subluxation of the tibio-fibula proximal joint.

Hoover's Sign

Description-1. Place palms under the patient's heels and ask the patient to press down. 2. The palm under the normal leg is placed on the dorsum of the foot and the patient is asked to lift that leg.

Significance-Positive; 1. Relatively little pressure is felt under the paralyzed leg in both tests (true organic paralysis as in hemiplegia). 2. Increased downward pressure is felt in the paralyzed leg as the normal leg is raised (Hysterical paralysis).

Indication-Upper motor neuron disorder.

Kemp's

Description-While the patient is standing, the lumbar spine is hyperextended in a posterolateral direction both left and right.

Significance-Positive; Gives pain in either the low back, buttocks or legs.

Indication-Disc, Synovial entrapment, Subluxation, Facet imbrication.

Lasegue's Rebound

Description-While lowering the patient's leg from a positive SLR, allow the limb to drop, forcing the patient to initiate a sudden active, instead of passive, limb lowering.

Significance-Positive; Causes a marked increase in pain.

Indication-Disc suspected.

L'Hermitte's Sign

Description-Soto Hall test in which a patient develops a sudden transient electric shock into the upper and lower extremities.

Indication-Spinal cord injuries, Cord degeneration, Multiple sclerosis.

Light Reflexes

Description-Shine light directly into one eye and wait for reflex.

Significance-Positive; If pupil fails to constrict.

Indication-Afferent II, Efferent III, Cortex, mid brain.

Lindner's

Description-While the patient is supine, the occiput is held and used as a lever to forcefully flex the neck, cervico-thoracic spine and upper thoracics. The patient is stabilized with the practitioner's caudad hand on the lower costo-sternal junction. The trunk is rounded into a large C shape curve.

Significance-Positive; If radicular pain is reproduced.

Indication-Space occupying lesion, Nerve root compression, Disc, Subluxation, Dural lesions, Fracture.

Maigne's

Description-The patient is sitting with the neck held in extension and contralateral rotation for 30 seconds on each side.

Significance-Positive; Nystagmus, loss of balance, nausea.

Indication-Basilar ischemia.

Mennell's

Description-1. The patient lies in the lateral decubitus position, with the inferior leg straight. The practitioner stands behind the patient and pulls the superior leg into forced hip extension with the caudad hand while the sacroiliac joint is stabilized with the cephalad hand. 2. Repeat the above procedure while the knee of the inferior leg is held to the chest.

Significance-Positive; 1. Pain in the sacroiliac joint, or lumbar spine. 2. Pain in the sacroiliac spine.

Indication-Sacroiliac joint or lumbar spine subluxation.

Minor's

Description-Patient rises from sitting position.

Significance-Positive; When the patient's weight is supported on the uninvolved side by placing the hand on the knee. The other hand is placed on the back on the involved side, while the hip joint is extended.

Indication-Sacroiliac subluxation, Disc, Fracture.

Oppenheim's Stroke

Description-The practitioner strokes the medial aspect of the patient's tibia.

Significance-Positive; Gives extension of the big toe and flaring of the small toes.

Indication-Upper motor neuron lesion from a central nervous system disease.

Patella Clonus

Description-With the patient's leg in extension, the practitioner rapidly and repeatedly pushes the patella distally.

Significance-Positive; Rapid involuntary contractions of the quadriceps giving rise to proximal distal movements of the patella when the stimulus ceases.

Indication-Upper motor neuron disorder due to central nervous system disease.

Phalan's

Description-While in a seated position, the patient approximates the dorsal aspects of both wrists to create forced, passive wrist flexion with active finger movements.

Significance-Positive; Pain, paresthesia or numbness in the median nerve distribution.

Indication-Carpal tunnel syndrome.

Romberg's

Description-Patient stands with feet together. First with eyes open then with eyes closed.

Significance-Positive; When patient sways and cannot right him or herself or falls to one side when both eyes are closed.

Indication-Cerebellar disorder, Posterior column, Atherosclerosis, Subluxation.

Scapular Approximation

Description-1. Bilateral abduction of arm to 90 degrees with extension from abducted position to create scapula approximation. 2. Flex neck to maximum.

Significance-Positive; Gives interscapular pain radiating to the axilla.

Indication-Thoracic subluxation.

Schaffer's Squeeze

Description-Squeeze the Achilles tendon.

Significance-Positive; Gives extension of the big toe.

Indication-Upper motor neuron disorder from a CNS disease.

Sign of the Buttock

Description-While the patient is supine, the hip is fully flexed while the knee is flexed. This is repeated with the knee extended (S.L.R.).

Significance-Positive; Gives pain when the knee is extended and pain when the knee is flexed.

Indication-Buttock lesion.

S.L.R. with Braggard's

Description-S.L.R. with forced dorsiflexion of the foot, at the leg position just below the level that elicits pain.

Significance-Positive; Gives an increase in pain.

Indication-Nerve root tension.

S.L.R. with External Rotation

Description-S.L.R. with external rotation of the femur. Externally rotate the femur just before the level of onset of pain with a normal S.L.R.

Significance-Positive; If there is an increase in the level of sciatic pain.

Indication-Piriformis syndrome.

S.L.R. with Kernig's

Description-S.L.R. with neck flexion. Flex the patient's neck at the leg position just before the onset of pain with a normal S.L.R.

Significance-Positive; Gives an increase in pain.

Indication-Space occupying lesion.

S.L.R. (Lasegue's)

Description-Supine: The patient raises an extended leg and bears the full weight of the limb. Hold the heel and maintain extension of the knee.

Significance-Positive; Gives pain in the back. Pain can be experienced in the buttock, hip or posterior thigh.

Indication-Sciatica; lumbosacral lesion; disc disease; spondylolisthesis; adhesions; intervertebral foraminal occlusion; subluxation.

Snout Reflex

Description-The practitioner gives a sharp tap to the patient's upper lip.

Significance-Positive; Gives a pouting of the lips.

Indication-Upper motor neuron lesion (C.N. VII).

Soto Hall

Description-While the patient is supine, the head and neck is passively flexed by the practitioner's cephalad hand. Flexion of the thoracic spine is prevented by the practitioner's caudad hand creating a slight downward pressure on the patient's sternum.

Significance-Positive, if pain occurs.

Indication-Fracture; disc disease; sprain; strain; subluxation.

Tandem Gait

Description-The patient is instructed to walk heel to toe, both forward and backward directions. The gait is observed for abnormality.

Significance-Positive; Abnormal balance

Indication-Cerebellar disease; posterior column; atherosclerosis; multiple sclerosis; CNS tumor; subluxation.

Trendelenberg

Description-The patient stands on one leg while the other leg is flexed at both the hip and knee to ninety degrees.

Significance-Positive; If the hip on the raised leg side drops lower than the standing leg side.

Indication-Hip disease; Gluteus medius weak on the weight-bearing leg.

Tromner's

Description-While the patient is sitting, the practitioner gives a sharp upward tap to the supinated middle finger and ring finger.

Significance-Positive; Finger flexion occurs.

Indication-Possible upper motor neuron disorder.

Underburger's

Description-The patient is instructed to march on the spot with both arms outstretched, eyes closed, and the head extended and rotated.

Significance-Positive; Loss of balance.

Indication-Basilar ischemia.

Valsalva

Description-The patient is instructed to hold their breath and bear down. This increases the pressure in the spinal canal, shunting the blood back to the paraspinal plexus, increasing the pressure near the space occupying lesion.

Significance-Positive; Gives pain in the area of the space occupying lesion.

Indication-Disc disease or other space occupying lesion.

Vertebral Artery Occlusion

Description-The patient lies supine with the neck in extension, rotation and lateral flexion.

Significance-Positive; If the patient turns pale, becomes dizzy, nauseated or suffers blurred vision within thirty seconds.

Indication-Basilar insufficiency.

Well Leg Raise

Description-S.L.R. with foot dorsiflexion on the asymptomatic side of a sciatic patient.

Significance-Positive; Reproduces pain on the symptomatic side.

Indication-Disc syndrome; space occupying lesion; sciatic nerve root involvement.

Wright's

Description-While the patient is sitting, abduct their arm above the head. Palpate the radial pulse through the arc of 180 degrees.

Significance-Positive; Decrease or obliteration of radial pulse.

Indication-Pectoralis minor involvement.

Wrist Clonus

Description-The practitioner vigorously applies quick, repeated extensions of the patient's wrist, then holds it in extension.

Significance-Positive; repeated, rapid, involuntary flexion/extension of the wrist.

Indication-Upper motor neuron lesion.

5 Plain Film Radiography in Chiropractic

STEPHEN H. ROWE with the assistance of STEPHEN G. RAY, ANTONI M. JAKUBOWSKI, and RONALD J. PICARDI

Since their contemporaneous discoveries in 1895, chiropractic and roentgenology have been linked in many of their technologic and applied advances (1,2). With the use of plain film radiography, chiropractic examination procedures changed from reliance solely on symptomatology and palpatory findings to include viewing of representations of underlying spinal and soft tissues. This new found ability advanced the science and art of chiropractic serving as an important tool in evaluating various clinical and theoretical approaches.

In 1932, Sausser, a chiropractor, took the first 14″ × 36″ anterior-to-posterior (AP) full spine radiograph. He later produced a 20″ × 72″ full body film in 1935 (3,4). The first X-ray machine west of the Mississippi was brought to Davenport, Iowa by B.J. Palmer in September of 1910. His X-ray research at the Palmer Research Center used thousands of patients and concluded that 64% of palpatory findings were in error, when compared to radiographic discoveries (5).

Gonstead (6) furthered the use of x-ray by developing a system of marking and analyzing the spine and pelvis for biomechanical misalignments. This system depends on strict patient positioning (7–9).

Today's chiropractors use radiographs to evaluate the acceptability of a patient for chiropractic care, uncover contraindications to chiropractic treatment, discover information that will alter the type, frequency, or force of treatment, assess the kinesiopathologic components of the vertebral subluxation complex and provide a teaching tool for patient education (Fig. 5.1).

Many texts (2,10) adequately cover the study and detection of those conditions that require allopathic intervention or alter the preferred biomechanical treatment. The purpose of this chapter is not intended to duplicate previous work, but instead to focus on the evaluation of the kinesiopathologic components of the vertebral subluxation complex through the appropriate use of plain film radiography.

Kinesiopathologies of the subluxation complex include positional dyskinesia, fixation dysfunction, hypermobility, instability, and changes in the axis of motion (11). As previously discussed (See Chapter 3), kinesiopathologic findings are only one component of the vertebral subluxation complex. The primary function of the doctor of chiropractic is the location and treatment of these biomechanical irregularities and their subsequent manifestations. It is imperative that examinations be performed with the highest degree of accuracy. The chiropractor should use all the readily available tools of inquiry to gain the most cost effective information to best evaluate each case.

When the findings of the history and physical examination indicate a need for an evaluation of the integrity and interrelationships of spinal structures, a roentgenologic examination should be performed.

The plain film radiograph is still the procedure of choice, in both time and cost effectiveness, for examinations of the skeleton (2). This is especially true when the diagnostic inquiry calls for a biomechanical analysis.

Risks of Ionizing Radiation

The relative risks of ionizing radiation must be considered whenever selecting the appropriate views for each radiographic examination. It has been well documented that there are potential negative biologic effects of human exposure to ionizing radiation (1,12). Because the biologic consequences of irradiation are cumulative, it is important to consider the risks and make every reasonable attempt to minimize exposure without sacrificing the quality of information obtained (1).

Biologic effects are both dosage and tissue dependent. The radiosensitivity of different tissues necessitates safety standards during a radiographic examination. Tissues that are more differentiated, more mature, and less likely to divide are less radiosensitive than those that are primitive, nondifferentiated, and more likely to divide. The biologic effects of radiation can be divided into two categories: somatic and genetic.

SOMATIC

Somatic effects can be subdivided into two groups, local and general. Local injuries were more common early in the study of diagnostic x-rays as experimentation using multiple exposures on various body parts were performed. The frequency of these injuries was reduced as proper usage of radiographic equipment became the norm (2).

Few general effects of exposure have been docu-

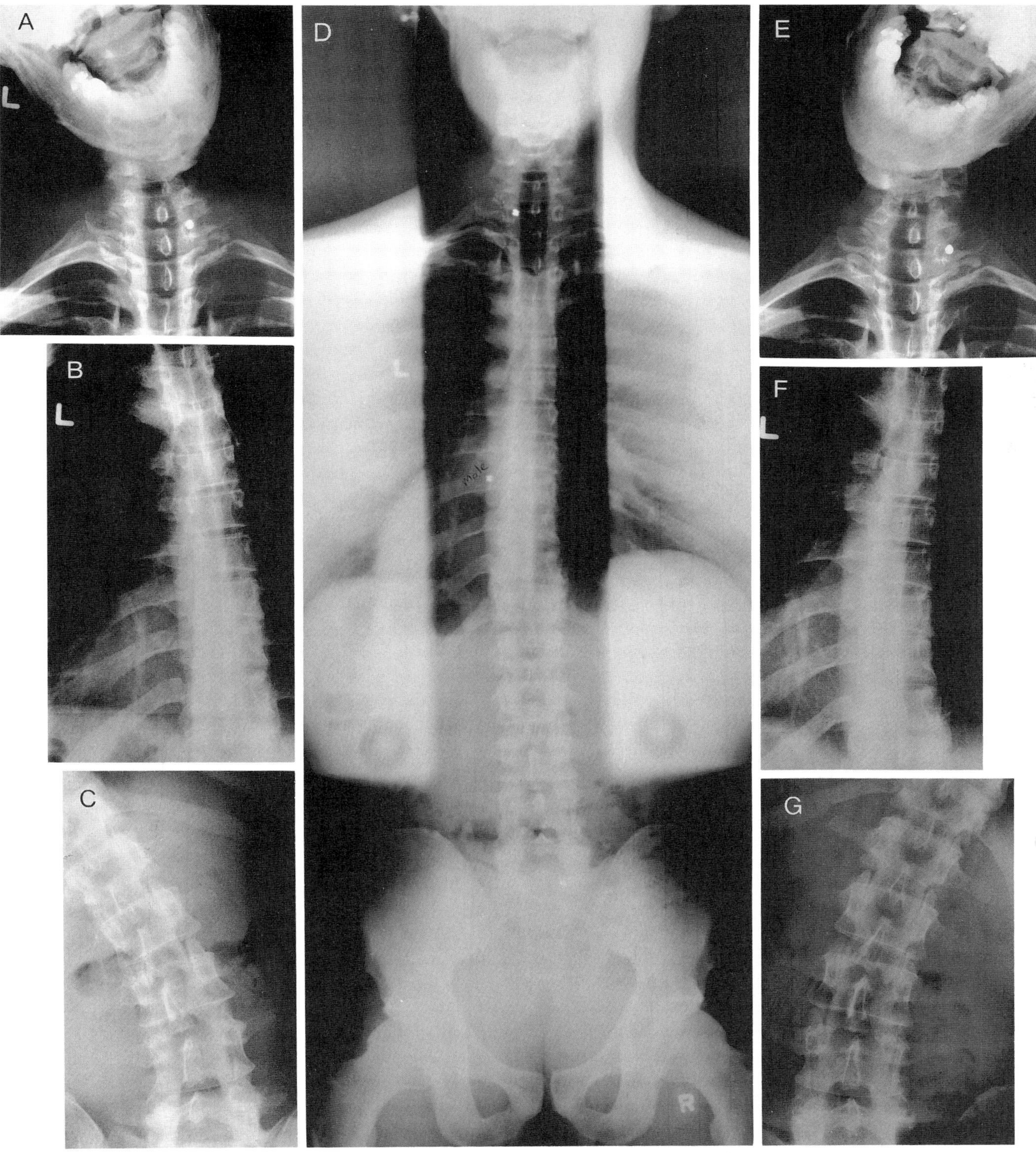

Figure 5.1. AP full spine with cervical, thoracic, and lumbar stress radiographs for analysis of the coronal plane kinesiopathologic components of the motion segment.

mented in humans as a result of diagnostic x-rays. Although there are some data which suggests a doubling of the incidence of leukemia in children whose mothers had roentgen pelvimetry performed during pregnancy. After the atomic bomb was dropped on Hiroshima and Nagasaki, the incidence of leukemia was increased proportional to the distance from the hypocenter. There also exist data suggesting an increase in cancer of the thyroid in patients who received therapeutic radiation of the thymus in infancy (10).

Animal experimentation demonstrates that with enormously high levels of whole body exposure, life-span is shortened. There are no data that suggest a shortened life span in radiology technicians who are exposed to increased levels of radiation throughout their lifetime (10).

GENETIC

The genetic effect of radiation is primarily the production of mutations. The gonadal dose seems to be directly proportional to the number of mutations, regardless of the time lapse between exposures. According to Crow (13), 100 R in one dose has the same genetic effect as the same dose given over a longer period of time.

A total dose of 30 to 80 R to the gonads of the entire population would double the existing mutation rate of humans (10,14). The National Academy of Sciences committee on genetic effects of atomic radiation suggests that up to 30 years of age, no more than 10 R be received by an individual, excluding natural causes (10). Because the gonadal effect is of the greatest importance to the entire population in the long term, it is crucial to use diagnostic x-rays judiciously and to apply gonadal shielding whenever possible. An exception would be when shielding obscures a suspected abnormality.

To put into perspective the amounts of radiation required to increase the risk of genetic mutation, the following comparison is made. In 1988, the conference of Radiation Control Program Directors set guidelines for different diagnostic studies performed (15). An AP full spine view using a 400 film screen speed combination yields about 145 mR of total body exposure (16). Gonadal dose would be approximately 20% or about 30 mR. This would mean that a 30-year-old man would have to receive a minimum of 333 AP full spine exposures at 400 speed before the National Academy of Science guidelines would be met. A 1200 speed system with gonadal shielding would require more than 1000 AP full spine exposures to double the risk of the genetic mutation rate. It becomes clear that even pre and post full spine views create a minimal overall risk of genetic mutation.

When assessing radiation from full spine views in comparison with occupational limits set forth by the National Council on Radiation Protection, an individual would be allowed a yearly exposure of the equivalent of 34 AP full spine views taken with a 400 speed system. Using a 1200 speed system would allow for additional exposures. Of course medical exposure risk assessment is different from occupation exposure risk assessment. The comparison is made only to put into perspective the relative risk of diagnostic exposure. Exposure to ionizing radiation causes biologic effects and must always be treated judiciously. The clinical benefit must be weighed and balanced with any potential negative effects.

The use of nutritional measures to counter the effects of ionizing radiation is somewhat controversial. There is some evidence that ingestion of vitamin E, or other antioxidants, may provide some protection from low-dose irradiation (17). This is based largely on work with laboratory animals.

TECHNICAL CONSIDERATIONS

The taking of high quality diagnostic radiographs requires that proper equipment, technique and patient preparation be used.

Equipment

ALIGNMENT

To reduce film distortion, the x-ray equipment should be aligned so that the central ray passes through the center of the grid at exactly 90° to the grid cabinet and the film. To ensure this, the bucky should be held in a vertical position with the cassette and film centered to the primary x-ray beam. The tube should be positioned so that the beam travels horizontally and strikes the bucky and film in a perpendicular fashion at all heights and distances.

COLLIMATION

The use of a field restricting collimator is one of the most effective means of reducing the amount of radiation the patient and the operator are exposed to during a radiologic examination (1). The collimator can restrict the beam to a chosen area of the body. Most collimators are equipped with a light localizer that provides a visual indication of the size and location of the x-ray field. It is imperative that the x-ray beam be restricted to the area of clinical interest and not exceed the size of the film. When the area of interest is smaller than the film, the x-ray beam should be further restricted to only involve that area. It is essential that the patient's eyes be collimated out of the exposure field during a radiographic examination.

In addition to protecting the patient and the technician from excessive dosage, collimation also increases the quality of the radiograph by improving contrast and detail of the film by reducing the amount of scatter radiation during the exposure.

RADIOGRAPHIC GRIDS

Radiographic grids are devices comprised of vertically aligned thin strips of lead that are placed in front of the cassette for the purpose of minimizing the amount of scatter radiation striking the film (1). Scatter radiation, radiation that has already struck an object and has changed direction, is often no longer oriented with the primary beam, and therefore cannot pass through the thin spaces between the grid strips. This reduces the amount of secondary exposure and improves the film quality. Grids are coordinated with the x-ray unit depending on the highest kVp usually used (Table 5.1).

FILM-SCREEN COMBINATION

With the development of film that is more radiosensitive and with increased illumination from intensifying screens, the amount of radiation required to create an acceptable image, and thus expose the patient has been greatly decreased (Table 5.2). These faster film-screen combinations may result in a slight loss of detail (1), although this is usually not significant enough to affect the quality or amount of information gained from the study.

At the time of this writing, the fastest film-screen combination commercially available for adequate diagnostic study is the ultra high speed Kodak TMH film used with Fast Lanex Rare Earth Screens (18). The result is a 1200 speed system.

Conditions exist where changing the type of film used with a set of intensifying screens can drastically affect the amount of radiation required to obtain a diagnostic film image. For example, when using DuPont Quanta III rare earth screens with Cronex 7 film, a 400 speed system is produced. By only changing to Cronex 4 film, the system is converted to an 800 speed system, greatly reducing patient exposure (19). Practitioners currently using rare earth Lanex fast screens with older film can cut overall MAS by up to 50% just by using Kodak TMH film. These changes do not significantly increase the difficulty in obtaining high quality films and are probably the most cost effective, high patient benefit, radiation safety measures the clinician can implement.

Table 5.1.[a]
Recommended Grid Ratios for Various kVP[a]

Highest kVp	Recommended Grid Ratio
80	8:1
100	10:1
110	12:1
120	16:1

[a]From Hildebrandt RW. Chiropractic spinography. 2nd ed. Baltimore: Williams & Wilkins, 1985:35.

Table 5.2.
Comparative ESE Values in mR per Exposure Between 1200 Speed Systems at 80″ and 40″[a]

View ('86)	1200 Speed @ 40″	1200 Speed @ 80″	NCRP ('89) Median Values	CDRH
AP Cervical 23 cm.	8 mR	10 mR	260 mR	162 mR
AP Thoracic 24 cm	23 mR	26 mR	663 mR	465 mR
AP Lumbar 24 cm	71 mR	67 mR	884 mR	448 mR

[a]Dosimetry by Upstate Medical Physics, Inc. Rochester, NY 14609, "Average ESE Exposure to US Population from Diagnostic Medical Radiation," NCRP report #100, 1989, and "Recommendations for Evaluation of Medical Exposure from Diagnostic Exams" values are from the median ESE, CDRH HHS Pub (FDA) 85-8247.

There are situations, such as a potential spinal or extremity fracture, when the need for detail outweighs the benefits of reduced patient exposure. The use of lower speed screens may be more appropriate in these circumstances. It is therefore recommended that a chiropractor have more than one screen/film combination set available, one high speed system of 800–1200 for spinography and one slower speed system, of 200–400, for fracture or pathology evaluation.

PREPATIENT FILTRATION SYSTEMS

Shielding. Because of the high radiosensitivity of certain body parts, such as the eyes, thyroid, breasts and especially the gonads, shielding systems have been developed to guard these structures from exposure whenever possible. It is imperative that these tissues be excluded from the exposure field, unless doing so would obscure an area of interest. When it is necessary that these tissues be irradiated, all efforts should be made to reduce their exposure. This is often accomplished by the use of specialized patient shielding.

Shields are made of lead, copper, aluminum, or combinations of these and are intended to block specific tissues from the x-ray field. Shields fall into two major categories: contact and shadow shields.

The contact shields are placed directly on the patient, especially in front of the eyes or gonads, and are usually held on with straps, velcro, or clips (Fig. 5.2A-B). Shadow shields are either collimator mounted, such as those provided with the Nolan (20,21) (Fig. 5.3) or Sportelli Systems (21,22), or can be side mounted with shields that swing out in front of the patient, like those of the Bolin wedge filter system (Fig. 5.4) (23). Studies have demonstrated that the degree of protection offered by shadow shields is approximately equal to that of shaped contact

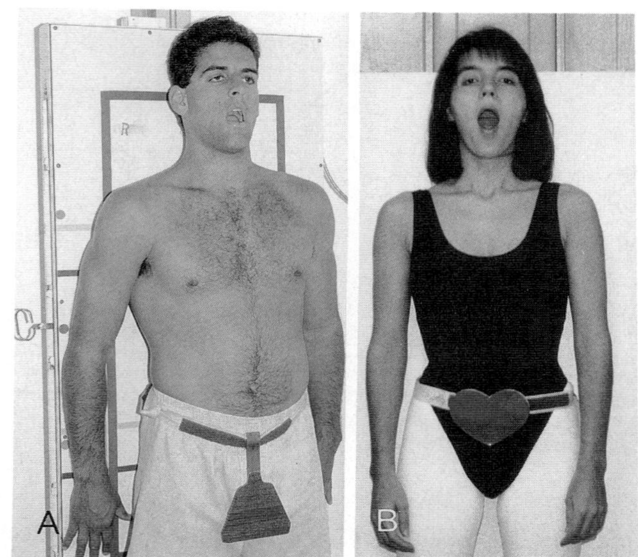

Figure 5.2. **A,** Male contact gonadal shielding. **B,** Female contact gonadal shielding.

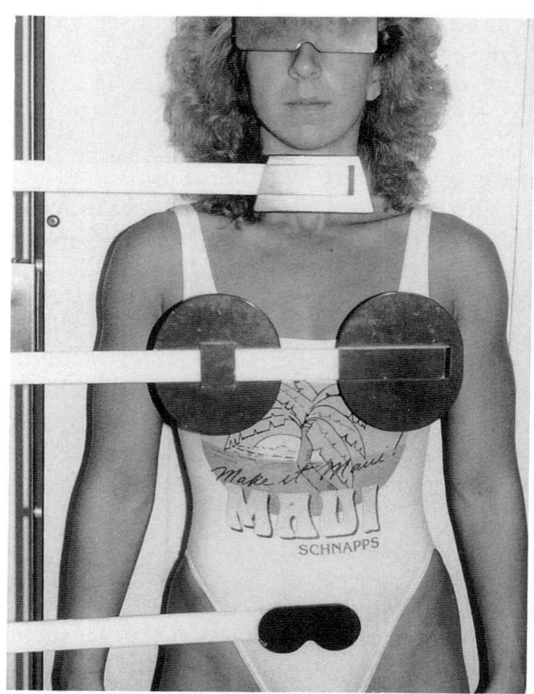

Figure 5.4. Side mounted shadow shielding for gonads, breasts, thyroid, and eyes.

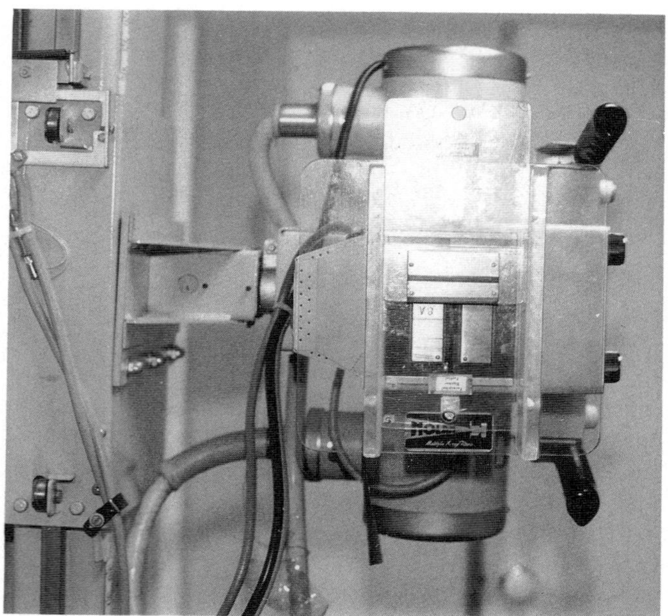

Figure 5.3. Collimator mounted breast shadow shielding, with cervical compensating filter.

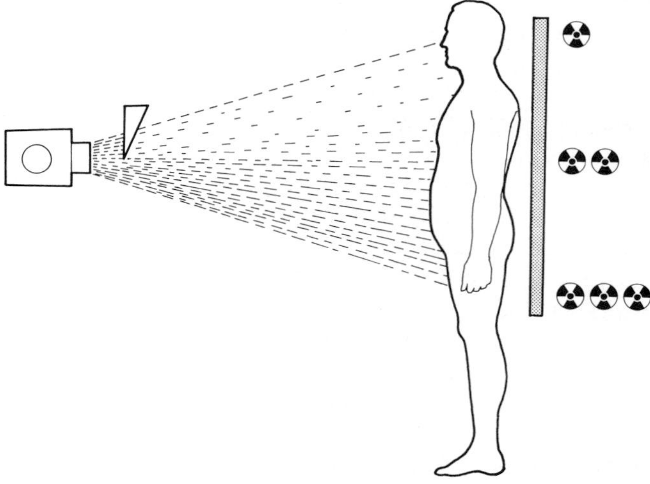

Figure 5.5. Pre-patient filtration reduces the amount of radiation before penetrating the patient and thus reduces exposure.

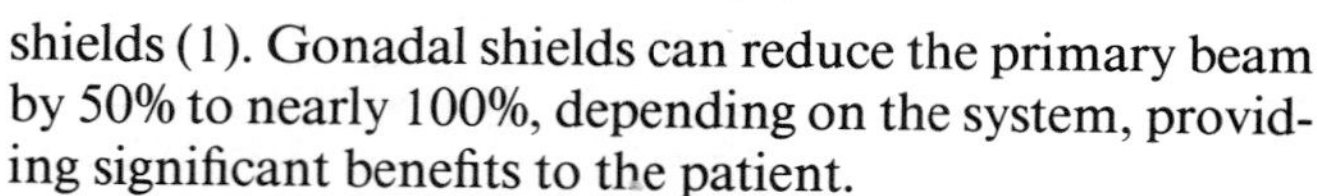

shields (1). Gonadal shields can reduce the primary beam by 50% to nearly 100%, depending on the system, providing significant benefits to the patient.

Compensating Filters. There are pretarget filtration systems that regulate the amount of radiation striking the patient (20–24) (Fig. 5.5). They are adaptable for taking full-spine or sectional radiographs. These filters, usually aluminum or aluminum copper combinations, attach to the front of the collimator. The aim is to create equal radiodensity of all body parts during the exposure. This allows for specific modifications for different body types and sizes, and reduces patient exposure. These systems may be slightly more time consuming in their application than those with less flexibility, but they produce higher quality radiographs with less patient exposure.

The cervical spine is typically 20 to 30% of the lateral thoracic measurement. Prepatient filtration of this area should provide for satisfactory imaging of the C7, T1 and the upper thoracic area, without overexposing the cervical spine.

When taking an AP view, the doctor may want to place the top of a prepatient filter to the bottom of the open jaw, this will approximately equalize the density of the lower occiput, mandible and lower cervical areas. The limitations on the quality of the radiograph produced are limited by the skill of the technician instead of equipment restrictions.

LONG WAVELENGTH FILTRATION

The U.S. Food and Drug Administration recently approved a prepatient filter known as the Niobi-x (25). Made from the element Niobium, previously known as Columbium, the filter is placed in the beam at the x-ray tube port. The physical characteristics of Niobium remove low energy x-rays that are of the harmful long wavelengths. Low energy x-rays contribute little to diagnostic quality while increasing patient dose. Scatter radiation is reduced and film quality may also be enhanced.

ULTRA HIGH FREQUENCY X-RAY GENERATORS

In contrast to single phase systems, ultra high frequency generators provide a decrease of 50% in exposure time, lower overall patient dose, as well as increased technical accuracy and consistency of imaging. This technology produces a higher quality image with greater detail and contrast. The high frequency wave consists of sustained penetrating waves. The soft or inefficient radiation is reduced in high frequency generation (26).

X-ray Technique Variables

The most important factors affecting image quality and patient dose are milliamperage, kilovoltage and focal film distance. Milliamperage is the variable that determines the quantity of x-rays produced (1). As the milliamperage is raised, the number of x-ray photons produced increases. The longer the current is sustained, the greater the total dose of radiation absorbed by the patient. The current produced (milliamperage) multiplied by the time (seconds) determines total MAS. Overexposure causes unnecessary risk to the patient. Underexposure also increases risks if the radiograph is not of diagnostic quality and requires a retake. Ideally, the clinician should use the smallest MAS possible to obtain an image of diagnostic quality.

The kVP, or kilovoltage potential, determines the quality or energy of the X-rays produced. High kVP techniques create an x-ray beam with a high percentage of high energy, penetrating photons. These high energy photons are of shorter wavelengths which are generally considered safer for the patient. The higher power reduces patient skin dose, although the higher energy photons do travel further in the body and result in a slight increase in the internal organ dose (27).

High kVP results in a long gray scale of contrast. Osseous detail may be reduced if kVP is beyond an optimal range. The highest kVP technique that yields an acceptable diagnostic image with appropriate contrast is recommended. This is generally 80–110 kVP for the spine and pelvis.

Focal film distance (FFD) or source image distance (SID) affects image quality. As the distance between the tube and patient is increased there is less angulation, or angle of inclination, between the focal spot and the object. This results in a sharper radiographic image by reducing the amount of distortion and magnification (1).

Patient Preparation

The patient is prepared for a radiographic examination by removing all metal, jewelry, hair clips, and dentures if applicable. Trousers with metallic zippers and bras with metal clips or stays are also removed. The patient should be provided with a gown and instructed to put it on with the opening in the back. The patient should be without shoes, unless a heel lift or other orthotic insert is worn.

For females of childbearing age, inquiry must be made as to whether the patient is pregnant. This is best done on the initial history form, again verbally during the preradiographic consultation, and again with a sign in the x-ray room (28). If the patient is unsure as to her pregnancy status, then the "10-day rule" should apply. The 10-day rule excludes the taking of all but emergency films at any time during the menstrual cycle except for the first 10 days after the onset of menses. This rule should be followed to reduce the risk of first trimester fetal irradiation, when the fetus is most susceptible to exposure. The exception to this rule is when the ramifications of not taking the film puts the mother at serious risk (29).

Recent reports concerning the application of the "10-day rule" suggest that when recommended safety precautions are used the risk of injury to the patient or to her progeny from irradiation of diagnostic x-ray, even during the first trimester, is so minimal that pregnancy termination is rarely justified (30).

Many doctors tape metallic objects (BBs or lead shot) onto the patient at landmarks such as the vertebral prominence, L5-S1, superficial marks such as moles and scars or areas of positive clinical findings. This helps to compare apparent relationships accurately between osseous structures and examination findings (Fig. 5.6A-B). If a BB is placed at the inferior aspect of the vertebral prominence, assuming it is C7, and the doctor finds that on the lateral film the BB is viewed at the inferior aspect of C6 instead, a more accurate reference point for palpation can be used. The doctor should take all efforts to minimize the chance of obscuring crucial structures.

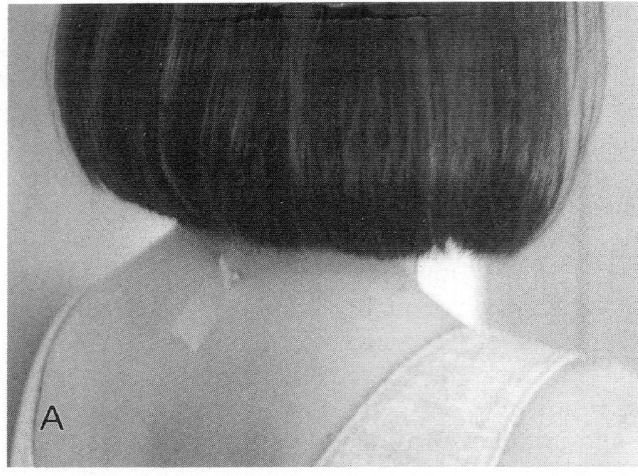

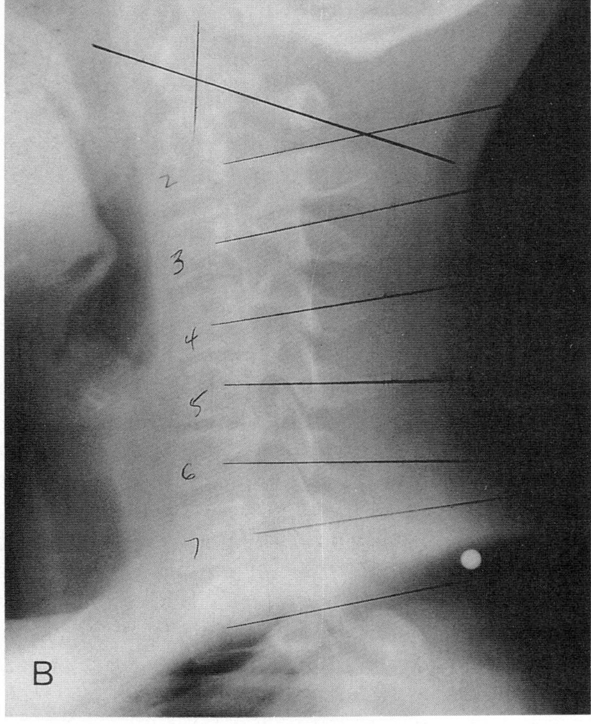

Figure 5.6. **A,** Attachment of a metallic marker to the patient. **B,** The lateral view should be used for comparison because projection of the metallic object on the AP view may distort the relationship between the skin and underlying spinal structures, unless it is placed close to the central ray.

RADIOGRAPHIC EXAMINATION

Following a thorough history and physical examination, the chiropractor may conclude that the patient is indeed a potential candidate for care. After ascertaining that there are no contraindications for the patient to be exposed to ionizing radiation, a determination may be made that the benefits in gaining this information, outweigh the potential risks. The doctor's professional judgment must be used in the proper selection of the type of film studies required to obtain the information necessary while eliminating both unnecessary and excessive exposure (31). It is important to only take views that have the potential to provide information that will determine or alter treatment (32). To base the radiographic examination on convention or on a predetermined view choice seems imprudent. The view selection should be based on the specific findings of the history and physical examination (See Chapter 4) and should be focused on obtaining information that will determine treatment.

Full Spine Radiography

When a spinal assessment is called for based on the results of the history and physical examinations, full spine weight-bearing films are the views of choice (Fig. 5.7) (24,33). There has been significant controversy about the comparative value of full spine and sectional radiographs. It has been repeatedly recounted that there are inherent drawbacks in full spine films, especially in the areas of film distortion, increased patient exposure, and the difficulty in producing quality films (34). Although these criticisms have been propagated for years with a great degree of emotional devotion, the current scientific literature has found these concerns to be greatly overstated. Phillips' study (35) involving Diplomates of the American Chiropractic College of Roentgenology evaluating sectional and full spine radiographs concluded that although there may be some slight reduction in image quality, the diagnostic value of full spine x-rays appears to be equal to that of sectional views.

The 14″ × 36″ AP film is probably the single most commonly taken view that provides the greatest amount of information (24) (Fig. 5.8). The obvious advantage of seeing the entire spine and viewing the postural relationships of articular and noncontiguous structures at once, gives the practitioner the benefit of understanding distant effects of spinal dysfunction on the whole spine. If one were only able to view a 8″ × 10″ of a compensated curve, the cause of the problem could easily go undetected, especially in the case of a patient with a global lateral list.

With the technologic advances in taking full spine radiographs, the patient is exposed to less radiation than standard sectional views when the entire spine must be visualized (1,34,36). To include all vertebral segments during a sectional examination, it is necessary to overlap areas. Consequently, this increases the received skin dosage in those areas caused by the projectional overlap (Fig. 5.9A-B). This is particularly relevant when one considers that the radiosensitive thyroid gland falls within one such area, between C6 and T1, at the overlap of the cervical and thoracic views (1).

In the ongoing effort to achieve specificity when examining and adjusting the spine, the doctor must be certain as to which motion segment is being evaluated or treated. The doctor must first be sure of the number of spinal segments. This information is then correlated with superfi-

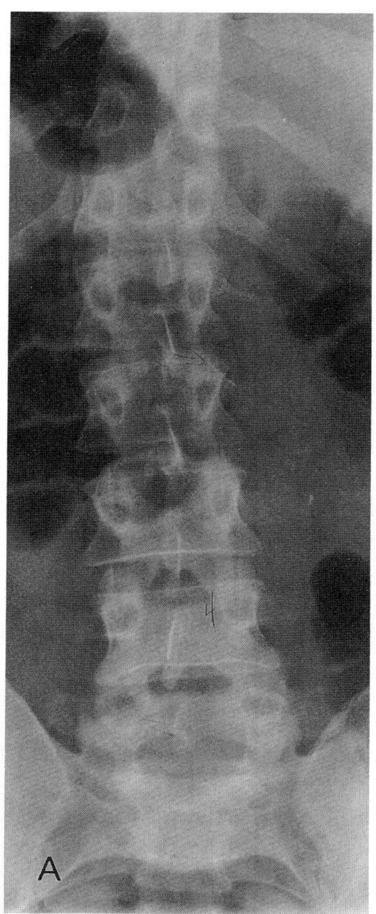

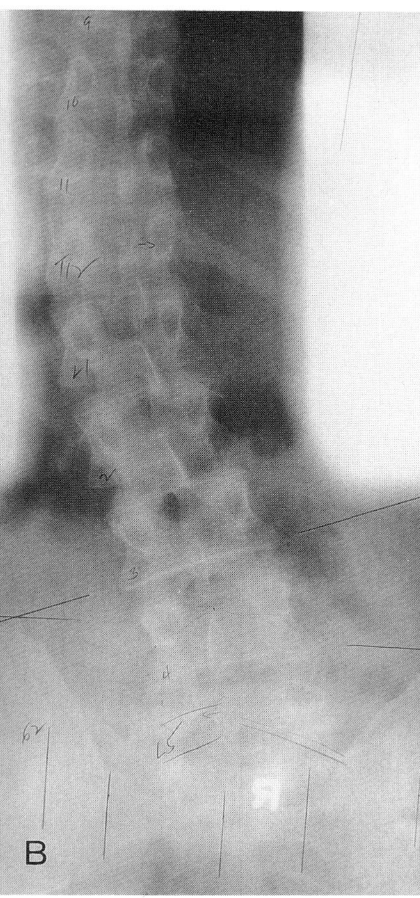

Figure 5.7. A, Radiograph was taken with the patient recumbent and was interpreted as normal by a medical radiologist. **B,** Radiograph was taken shortly after with the patient in a weight-bearing position. These radiographs illustrate the importance of a weight-bearing assessment when biomechanical information is needed.

cial bony landmarks. Because of the anomalous variations in individual spines and the reality of missing or overlapping areas when taking sectional views, the AP full spine radiograph is the only sure way to determine the number of spinal segments.

Most full spine films should be taken at a FFD of 84″. This distance is recommended for all those taking 14″ × 36″ films to reduce distortion and magnification and to increase film quality (3,31). Obviously, space limitations or state regulations in some offices may preclude this focal film distance.

DISTORTION, DISTANCE, AND FILM SIZE

The angle of incidence (AI) of the furthest ray penetrating the patient and exposing the film creates the most distortion in the image. The quality of the radiograph is improved when the angle of incidence is minimized, producing less projectional distortion (PD). This is done primarily by increasing the focal film distance. Table 5.3 provides the angles of incidence for common radiographic situations. The angle of incidence at the periphery of an 8″ × 10″ film taken at 40″ is 7.2°. To achieve this same angle on a 14″ × 36″ radiograph the FFD would have to be 144″. The AI for a 14″ × 17″ film taken at 40″ is 12.0°. A 14″ × 36″ full spine radiograph taken at 84″ will provide the same AI. Although the shorter FFD normally used for full spine spinography, 72″ to 84″, does increase the PD to some extent, its effect on the usefulness of the film is minimal. Adjacent structures have similar PD and therefore will illustrate dyskinetic relationships when present (6,37,38).

SPLIT SCREENS

It has been long thought that with 14″ × 36″ full spine films there was an inherent sacrifice in film quality. This resulted primarily from the difficulty in exposing body

Table 5.3.
Angle of Incidence for Common FFDs and Film Sizes

View	Distance	Angle of Incidence
8 × 10	40″	7°
8 × 10	72″	4°
14 × 17	40″	12°
14 × 17	60″	8°
14 × 17	72″	6.7°
14 × 36	72″	14°
14 × 36	80″	12.6°
14 × 36	84″	12°

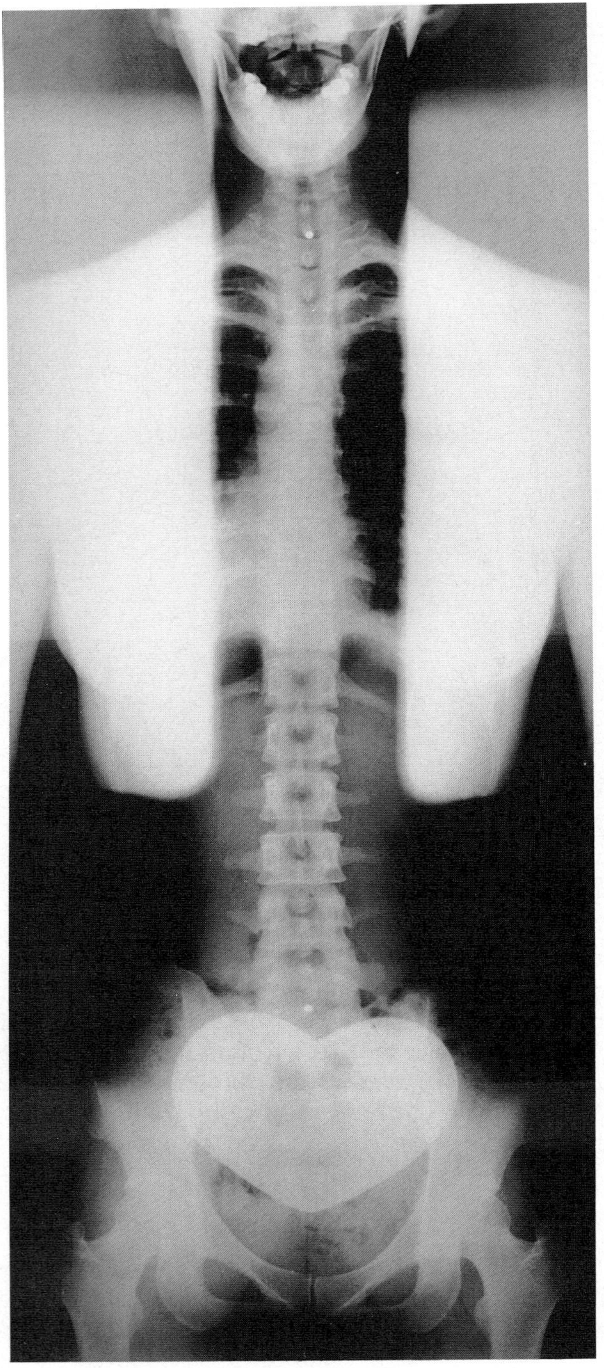

Figure 5.8. Anteroposterior full spine for biomechanical analysis.

parts of varying thickness and varying densities on the same film. An early effort to remedy this was to use "split screen" speed intensifying screens (24) to equalize the radiographic image produced by the varied amounts of ionizing radiation passing through the different body parts. Slower screens were used behind thinner body parts, with faster screens behind thicker or more dense parts. This attempt improved film quality significantly, although there were still inherent drawbacks. These "spilt screens" made it difficult to get diagnostic views of certain areas of the spine because of individual size and body types. Clear visualization of the vertebral prominence area, for example, is made more difficult with split screens. Because split screens regulate the amount of illumination of the intensifying crystals after the x-rays have passed through the patient, they require exposing the patient to added radiation (Fig. 5.10).

With improvements in equipment and techniques for taking high quality full spine radiographs without "split intensifying screens," the use of these screens, with their added patient exposure, is outdated (6,34).

HOMOGENEOUS SCREENS

A system that uses homogeneous, or uniform, intensifying screens is now in common use by the profession (24). This system uses one, usually ultra high speed screen set, for the entire 14″ × 36″ cassette. It is necessary to use a prepatient filtration system (See Pre Patient Filtration) with these cassettes to produce a radiograph of high quality. Although these systems may be slightly more time consuming in their application, they have the advantages of reducing patient exposure and providing increased flexibility for different body types. As previously discussed, by regulating the x-ray beam *before* the patient rather than at the intensifying screens, exposure is significantly reduced (See Fig. 5.5). These systems allow for adequate alterations for most body types and usually result in higher quality radiographs.

PATIENT MEASUREMENT

The patient should be measured with accurate calipers. Measurements are made at the following locations for the full spine lateral view; the greater trochanters, the thinnest area of the waist, the chest under the axillae, and the neck (Fig. 5.11A-C). For the AP view, measurements should be made at the neck, sternum, and the largest part of the abdomen (Fig. 5.12A-C). Most importantly, the doctor should follow a consistent measuring procedure that is accurate and correlated with the technique chart used. There are sophisticated calipers that when properly calibrated will provide exposure factors during measuring and reduce the set-up time for the examination (Fig. 5.13) (39).

PATIENT POSITIONING

The patient is positioned in a weight-bearing position to properly assess the spine and pelvis at interface with gravity (33,40,41).

AP Full Spine. For the AP radiograph, the patient should be in the center of the bucky with heels parallel to the bucky and perpendicular to the beam. A scribed line, that repeated trauma and continuing stress on the three joint complex causes stretching or attenuation of the capsular ligament and increased damage to the intervertebral disc, thus causing laxity of the capsule and bulging of the disc. This leads to an increase in the abnormal biomechanics of the joint. The wide range of definitions regarding this subject makes evaluation more difficult because any test must be definition specific.

Of the tools used for determining instability, static and stress radiographs and cineradiography are most common (34,46). Cineradiographic studies are valuable in that they allow the clinician to visualize the functional spinal unit in a dynamic manner and allow for predictions of the physiologic and anatomic changes associated with dysfunction. A retrospective study (47) demonstrated videofluoroscopy (VF) to be more accurate or superior in detecting cervical spine instability than plain film. This study suggested early use of VF in evaluation and management of cervical spine injuries. Cost considerations, however, usually place this procedure out of the realm of most evaluations.

Plain film radiographs, both neutral and stressed, can be used in the evaluation of instability. Consideration must be made for projectional distortion (PD), the quality of the radiographic image, and the experience of the clinician.

The accuracy of instability evaluation can be adversely affected by PD that can give the evaluator the impression that the continuity of the ligamentous structures has been lost, when no damage has in fact occurred. It is therefore recommended that a FFD of at least 72″ or greater be used when evaluating for instabilities. At these longer distances, PD is greatly reduced and the accuracy of evaluation is increased (43).

Relative Considerations

Conditions that require alteration in the force, frequency, or osseous site of contact can also be uncovered from the plain film radiograph. Osteoporosis (viewed as osteopenia) may require an alteration in the magnitude of force applied during a treatment, providing that if the severity does not contraindicate chiropractic adjustments entirely. Decreased bone mass associated with osteoporosis weakens the bone. To be observable on a radiograph, at least 30 to 50% loss of bone tissue must occur (2). In the osteoporotic spine, the chiropractor should avoid using the weakened transverse, mamillary processes or ribs as lever arms, and relocate the force of the adjustment to more stable structures, such as the spinous process or spinolaminar junction.

ANALYZING THE FULL SPINE FILM

Before discussing the marking procedure used with the Gonstead full spine approach, it is important to reiterate that this marking system should not be used as the sole criteria for locating the dysfunctional motion segment. This determination is made after a comprehensive history and physical examination (See Chapter 4). The marking system is used to determine the positional dyskinesia of the affected motion segment. Combined with motion palpation and dynamic stress radiographs, the kinesiopathologic components of the subluxated vertebra are determined, and the pattern of thrust during the adjustment can be ascertained.

Marking the AP Radiograph

GONSTEAD PELVIC MARKING SYSTEM

This system for full spine x-ray analysis provides a method of measuring innominate length and width, femoral head height (leg length inequality), and sacral rotation (6). Recent investigations (7,8) have found excellent levels of reliability and time-course stability for these procedures (Fig. 5.18A).

Using a standard x-ray marking pencil, the doctor places small dots at the top and bottom portions of the innominate. Then, similar dots are placed at the upper edge of each femur head. Another dot is placed at each junction of the articular processes of the sacrum and the alae (Fig. 5.18B). Dots are also placed at the center of the S2 tubercle (or S3 if S2 is not visible or is congenitally absent). A small dot is placed at each lateral border of the sacral alae, and at the center point of the pubic symphysis. A dot is placed on the lateral and medial borders of each ilium.

A rolling parallel ruler is used to draw a line connecting the femoral head points. This line is called the femoral head line (FHL) (Fig. 5.18B, Line A). The parallel is then rolled from the FHL upward, stopping at the cephalad innominate point first encountered. A 3-inch line parallel to the FHL is drawn (Fig. 5.18B, Line B), and the ruler is rolled upward to the second innominate, where a similar line is drawn (Fig. 5.18B, Line C). The parallel is then turned 180°, realigned with the FHL, and rolled down to the first point of the caudal innominate, a 3-inch line is drawn (Fig. 5.18B, Line D). The ruler is then rolled down to the dot on the other innominate, where a similar line is inscribed (Fig. 5.18B, Line E).

Innominate measurements are made by placing the left hand edge of the ruler on the line at the top of the ilium and recording the length to the nearest 0.5 mm at its intersection with the line at the bottom. This procedure is repeated on the opposite side. The longer innominate is considered to have deviated in a PI (posteroinferior or $-\theta X$) direction. The shorter innominate is listed as an AS (anterosuperior or $+\theta X$). The innominate misalignments are determined in relationship to their articulation with the sacrum.

The shape of the obturator foramina will also appear

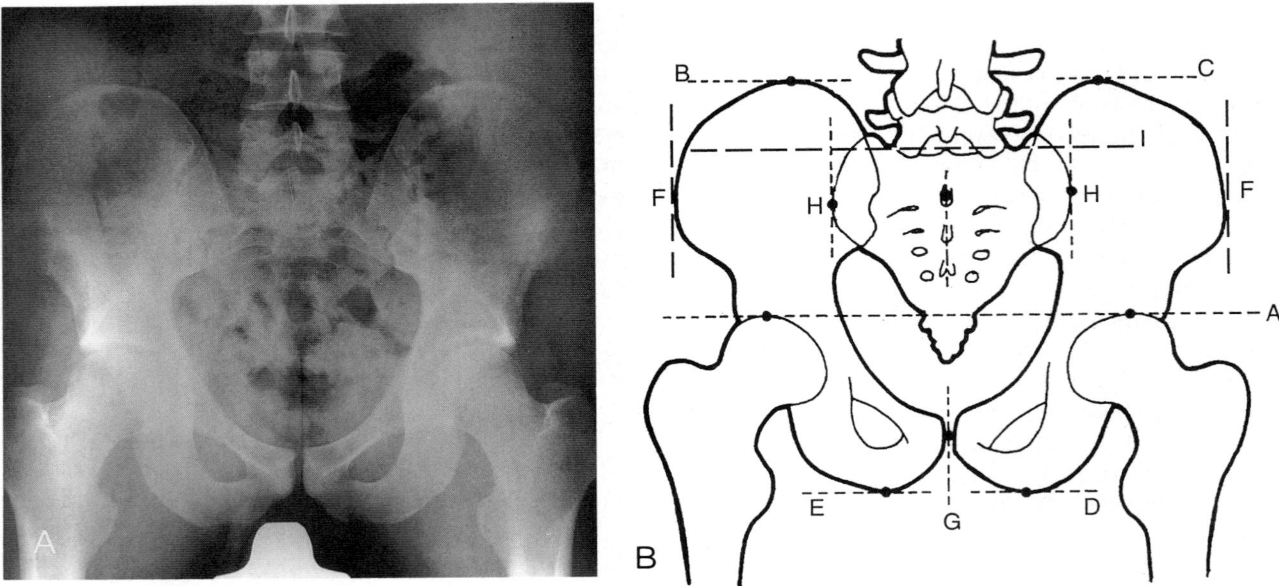

Figure 5.18. **A,** AP pelvic radiograph. **B,** Line drawing of the same pelvis as in **A.**

changed with a PI or AS ilium misalignment. On the side of the PI, the obturator will appear to be longer diagonally, and shorter on the side of an AS (6).

The ruler is turned so that it is perpendicular to the FHL and is rolled laterally until it intersects with the medial and lateral border marks on each ilium. A 2-inch line is drawn at each of these dots (Fig. 5.18B, Line F). The parallel is then rolled to the S2 (or S3) point, a perpendicular line is inscribed 3 inches caudally, and continued near the pubic symphysis (Fig. 5.18B, Line G).

The innominate rotational component can then be determined in a number of ways. The most common method is by measuring the distance that the pubic symphysis deviates from the perpendicular line drawn from S2 or S3. This represents ilium rotational misalignment around the Y axis. The side of pubic symphysis deviation is the side of the internal (In) misaligned ilium. The opposite side would be listed as an external (Ex) ilium misalignment. The distance in millimeters between the vertical line and the symphysis deviation should be measured. The listing for the ilium misalignment is by convention listed on the side of L5 body rotation.

An alternative method to determine In or Ex misalignment is to observe the shape of the obturator foramina. The shape of the obturators will change with ilium misalignments. The obturator on the side of the Ex ilium misalignment will increase in length at its base, while it will appear narrower on the side of In misalignment (6).

A third method for determining the rotational ($\pm\theta Y$) component of ilium misalignment is to measure the width between the medial and lateral borders of the ilium. The parallel ruler is placed on the FHL with the left edge on the medial line of the right ilium. The distance is measured to where it intersects the lateral line. Then, with the ruler parallel to the FHL and with the left edge on the lateral edge of the left ilium, the measurement is made to the medial border line. Each measurement is marked on the lateral aspect of the ilium. The larger measurement represents the In ilium, the smaller the Ex. This procedure is usually used when necessary anatomic structures are not clearly visible.

The edge of the ruler is then placed at the two dots at the superior portion of the sacrum, and a 5-inch line is drawn (Fig. 5.18B, Line I). This represents the sacral horizontal plane line (SHPL) and illustrates whether the sacral base is level or has misaligned inferiorly on one side. The ruler's leading edge is then aligned with the FHL and rolled upward until it touches the higher of the two sacral points. A 1-inch line is drawn above the lower dot. If this line is not parallel to the FHL, it must be determined if this is caused by an inferior sacral misalignment ($\pm\theta Z$) or from malformation of the sacrum (6) (See Chapter 6). To do this, the doctor locates bilateral points, such as the center of the sacral foramina or the sacral crests, and connects them with lines. Lines drawn through these points are parallel if the sacrum is symmetrical and would not be the cause of the discrepancy between the FHL and SHPL. In this case, the parallel ruler is placed perpendicular to the SHPL and advanced laterally to the dots on each edge of the sacrum. A 2-inch line is then drawn through each of these dots. Along with any sacral rotational misalignment, an inferior sacral listing would be included.

If the sacrum is shown to be malformed, or if the SHPL and FHL are parallel, then the ruler is placed perpendicular to the femur head line and the lines drawn through the dots on the lateral borders of the sacrum are so oriented.

Sacral rotational misalignment (Y axis) is determined by measuring the distance from the S2 or S3 center to the lateral borders of the sacral alae (Fig. 5.18B, Line H). The ruler is placed at the center of the sacrum (S2), and the distances are measured to the nearest 0.5 mm. Distances greater than 7 mm are usually considered significant, although misalignment of any magnitude can be important if clinical findings such as fixation and swelling at the joint are present (6). The greater measurement represents a potential axial rotational dyskinesia in relationship to the ilium, such that one alae has rotated posterior. The sacrum is listed as a P-L or P-R. Rotation of all lumbar segments to the same side is further suggestion of a rotated sacrum (6).

Sacral inferiority is only considered valid if the side of inferiority is not associated with sacral malformation as previously discussed. If there is no evidence of sacral malformation and the SHBL is not parallel to the FHL, then the sacral listing includes the inferior subscript and the listings would be noted PI-R or PI-L.

To evaluate leg length inequality, the lateral edge of the ruler is placed at the edge of the film and is rolled upward until it contacts the more cephalad femoral head. A 2-inch line is then drawn above the lower femoral head.

Leg length inequality is measured by placing the lateral border of the ruler at the lowest femoral head and recording the distance between this point and the line directly above it in millimeters. This is the measured difference (MD) the femoral head has deviated from horizontal but may not be a true measurement of leg length deficiency. Misalignments of the innominate can influence the apparent leg length measurements. Gonstead developed the following procedures for determining the actual anatomic leg length differences and for differentiating them from the apparent physiologic leg length differences; for every 5 mm of AS ($+\theta X$) or In misalignment the femur head height will be raised by 2 mm; for every 5 mm of PI ($-\theta X$) or Ex misalignment, the femur head height will be lowered 2 mm (6). Combinations of compound ilium misalignments are either cumulative or can neutralize each other, depending on the particular coefficients of misalignment.

A correction of ilium misalignment will improve the apparent leg length discrepancy by the same 1:0.4 ratio. For each 5 mm of AS or In correction, the femur length will be lowered by 2 mm. For every 5 mm of PI or Ex correction the femur length will be raised by 2 mm. To compute this, multiply the ilium correction by 0.4 to determine the leg length change (6). This formula becomes very important when considering the use of a heel or shoe lift (See Chapter 6).

MARKING THE SPINAL SEGMENTS

The purpose of the anteroposterior evaluation is to gather important information concerning scoliosis, intervertebral disc wedging ($\pm\theta Z$) and vertebral rotation ($\pm\theta Y$) (6,37,38). It also allows visualization of the areas of compensation and helps in the determination of how a particular segment may be adjusted (6) (Fig. 5.19).

The marking of the AP film continues by numbering each segment (Fig. 5.20). The leading edge of the parallel ruler is then placed on the femur head line (FHL) and rolled cephalad to the inferior portion of the L5 facets or to like points at the intersection of the intervertebral

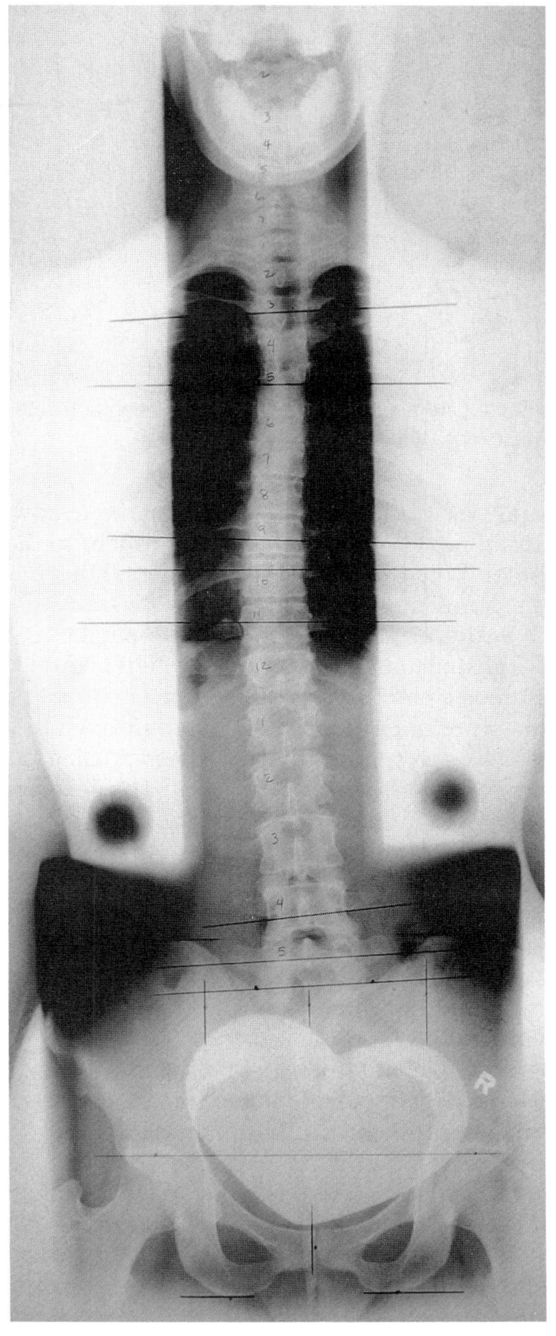

Figure 5.19. AP full spine radiograph allows for pathological and kinesiopathological analysis of the spine and pelvis.

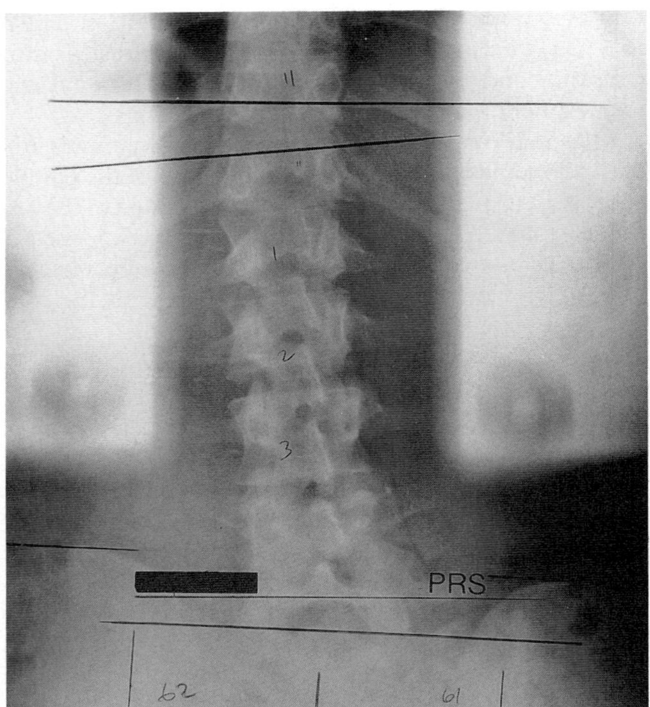

Figure 5.20. AP lumbar from a full spine radiograph with roentgenometric lines included.

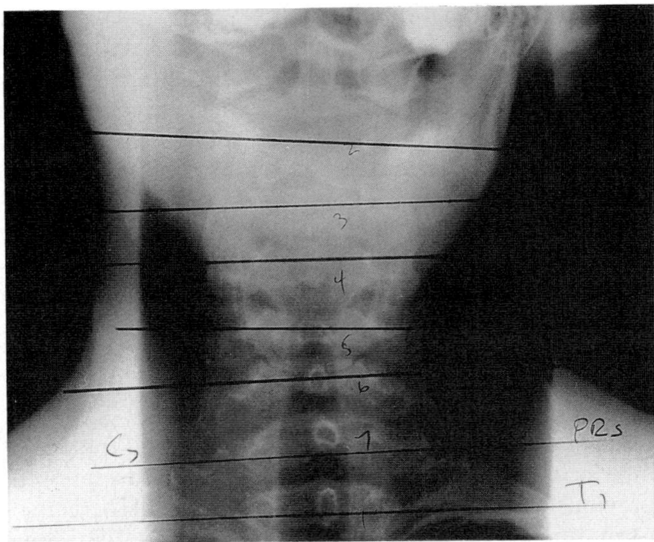

Figure 5.21. AP cervical from a full spine radiograph with roentgenometric lines included.

body-transverse shadows. The ruler is then advanced upward on the film comparing each segment to the true horizontal. When a segment is encountered that deviates from the horizontal, it is marked along the transverse axis for the entire length of the ruler. The parallel is again rolled cephalad until a vertebral segment is identified that has resumed a horizontal position.

This procedure is followed upward through the lumbar and thoracic spine with each vertebra being marked that has deviated from the horizontal. The next segment that returns to a horizontal orientation is also marked. Once the thoracic area has been marked, dots are placed on all the uncinate processes of C7 through C3, and at the laminar junctions of C2 (Fig. 5.21). The edge of the ruler is then aligned to the dots placed on the uncinate processes of C7 and rolled caudally to the lower third of the vertebral body and a line is drawn the entire length of the parallel. Similar lines are drawn successively at C6 through C2. If lateral wedging ($\pm \theta Z$) exists, the two lines will diverge laterally to one side or the other. This represents wedging of the motion segment.

The next step in the AP film analysis is the determination of rotation (Y axis). The side of the vertebral body that misaligns posteriorly will exhibit a pedicle shadow that widens horizontally and appears to migrate toward the center of the body. The pedicle on the opposite side will appear to narrow and will appear displaced to the lateral margin of the vertebral body. The inferior articular processes can also be used to help determine body rotation. As the vertebral body rotates, the width of the inferior articular process will appear narrowed on the side of spinous laterality and widened on the side of posterior body rotation (6, 48).

As a check for vertebral rotation, it is often helpful to place a dot at each superior and inferior corner of the body. Lines are then drawn connecting the left upper to the right lower and the right upper to the left lower. The position of the spinous process is compared with the intersection of these two lines. A rotated spinous will deviate towards the lateral border of the body on the same side. Because the long spinous processes are often anomalous, this method can be misleading and should be used only as a check (49). It is important that each segment be analyzed relative to the segment below.

MARKING THE UPPER CERVICAL SPINE

Because of the anatomic and biomechanical differences in the upper cervical spine, the roentgenometric line drawing system is unique to this area (See Chapter 11) (Fig. 5.22). Dots are placed at the intersections of the transverse processes-lateral masses of atlas, bilateral points on the axis body, and at like points on the occiput. The edge of the ruler is placed on the dots of the C2 body, and a line is then drawn the entire length of the ruler (axis transverse plane line). This procedure is followed for the atlas by placing the leading edge of the ruler on the dots made at the lateral mass-transverse process intersection, and drawing a line, the transverse plane line (TPL), the entire length of the ruler. The transverse condyle line (TCL) is then drawn at the two points on the occiput (6).

In the optimally aligned spine these lines should all be relatively parallel. If the TPL and the ATPL diverge in

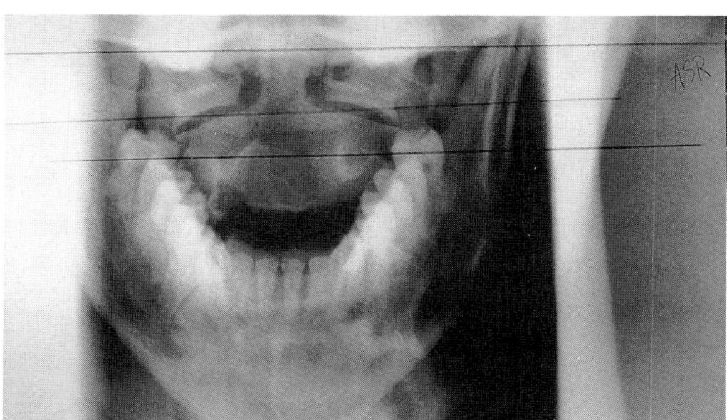

Figure 5.22. AP upper cervical spine from a full spine radiograph with roentgenometric lines included.

either direction, it indicates that the atlas may have misaligned laterally (i.e., $\pm\theta Z$) toward that side with respect to axis.

If the TPL and TCL are not parallel, it indicates that the occiput has misaligned (i.e., $\pm\theta Z$) on that side with respect to atlas. Generally, the TPL and ATPL would be parallel in a case where the occiput is subluxated, because it is rare that the atlas and occiput would both be subluxated.

Rotation of atlas can be determined in a number of ways. The most common is to compare the widths of the lateral masses of C1. The lateral mass that exhibits a wider measurement has rotated anteriorly, whereas the posteriorly rotated lateral mass will appear narrower. This is due to the "kidney bean" shape of the lateral mass and how they appear on the radiograph in different orientations (See Chapter 11) (43).

An alternative method for determining rotation of atlas is to view the space between the odontoid process and the lateral mass on each side. When the atlas rotates posteriorly, the odontoid-lateral mass space widens, whereas the opposite side narrows (6).

To determine the rotation of an occipital condyle subluxation, the rotation of the atlas is noted, since the atlas should compensate opposite the rotational coefficient of occipital misalignment. Occipital rotation therefore is indirectly determined relative to atlas rotational misalignment (6). Other systems of upper cervical x-ray marking have demonstrated good levels of interexaminer reliability (50).

Marking the Lateral Full Spine Radiograph

CERVICAL-THORACIC PORTION

To mark the lateral cervicothoracic view, a standard x-ray marking pencil is used to number the segments to match the numbering on the AP film (Fig. 5.23). Dots are then placed on the inferior portion of the vertebral bodies of C2 through T1, at the anterior and posterior body margins.

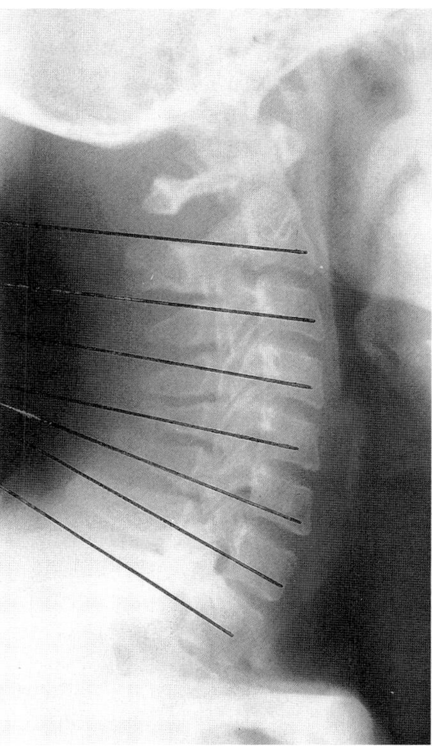

Figure 5.23. Lateral cervicothoracic view from FS radiograph with roentgenometric lines included.

Using the parallel ruler, the edge is placed so it aligns with each of the two dots on the vertebral body. The ruler is then rolled upward into the inferior third of the body and a line is drawn along its entire length. This procedure is repeated from T1 through C2. These lines represent the intervertebral disc plane lines.

Analysis of the lateral cervical spine begins with evaluation for spinal instability. A systematic approach is initiated as previously discussed. The soft tissues must be evaluated for increases in the retropharyngeal and retrotracheal spaces. Although some disagreement exists as to normal measurements, the latter should not exceed 22 mm, whereas the former should not exceed 7 mm (2). Increases in either or both of these spaces may indicate the presence of a space occupying lesion, osteophytic spurring, or posttraumatic edema from contusion or fracture.

The presence of anterolisthesis or retrolisthesis will be apparent on the lateral view and may suggest a loss of ligamentous integrity, a partial or complete dislocation, a fracture, positional dyskinesia or spinal instability. It should be noted that malposition by itself does not alone indicate spinal instability, confirmation is by flexion/extension views.

After an evaluation for spinal instability, analysis of cervical spine alignment is made. Working with the concept that optimal spinal function depends on optimal vertebral alignment, the relationships of the vertebral bodies should be checked. In the normal cervical spine, the lordotic physiologic curve should be a smooth, uninterrupted arch and is represented by a line (George's line) drawn along the posterior aspects of the vertebral bodies. Interruption of this line indicates misalignment of one or more of the cervical segments. The "perfectly" aligned cervical spine would exhibit intervertebral discs that are slightly wedged in the posterior, without anterior or posterior displacement of the vertebral bodies. Thus, the "normal" cervical lordosis would be maintained. This lordotic curve is extremely important in that it helps to maintain the upright posture of the head by balancing the skull over the torso, improves the flexibility of the neck, and helps dissipate the shock of walking, running, and impact trauma (44,51).

In the optimal cervical spine, the IVD plane lines will converge posteriorly at a single point (6). The cervical spine must accommodate the head in a neutral position, and it is here that major compensatory factors cause the cervical spine to deviate from normal. The proprioceptive, visual, and vestibular systems work in concert to assure that the head is kept in an upright posture and body balance is maintained, but in doing so, strength and stability in local and distant areas of the spine may be sacrificed (6,44). In cases of single or repeated hyperextension injuries, or in individuals whose work activity causes prolonged hyperextension of the neck, the cervical physiologic curve may become hyperlordotic. This will present radiographically when the IVD plane lines converge very close to the vertebral bodies.

The most frequently seen cervical physiologic compensatory mechanism is the hypolordotic or kyphotic cervical spine (44,46) (Fig. 5.24). The lower IVD plane lines

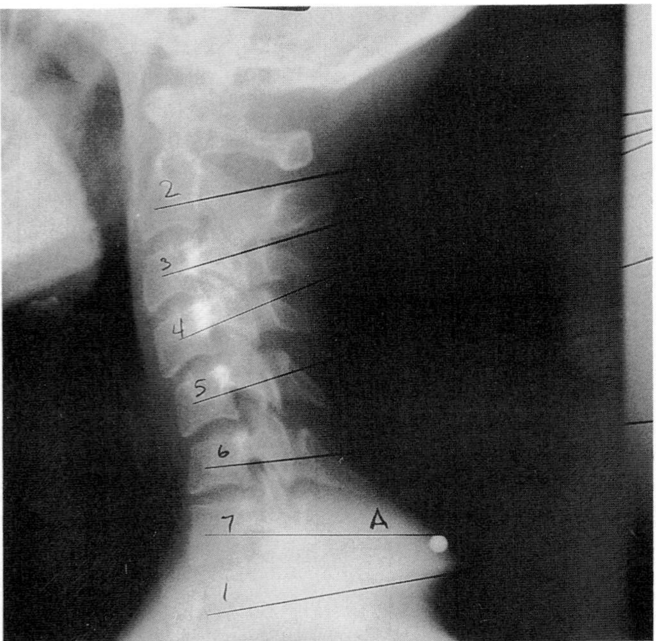

Figure 5.24. Kyphotic cervical spine from a full spine radiograph, note convergence of IVD plane line (Line A) representing a posterior inferior seventh cervical segment.

converge close to the vertebral bodies, whereas the middle and upper plane lines diverge posteriorly. This phenomenon is exaggerated in the kyphotic cervical spine.

The classical interpretation of the lateral cervical marking system is that the line that crosses the closest to the bodies is considered to have misaligned posteriorly and inferiorly ($-Z$, $-\theta X$) (Fig. 5.24, Line A). The greater the degree of inferiority, the closer to the bodies the two lines will intersect (6). The disc plane lines above the posterior-inferior segments will diverge to the posterior and are considered compensatory to the suspected subluxation below. Herbst (6) states that, "there is an extremely high correlation between the actual subluxation and the inferior vertebra in that vicinity—in fact, they correspond almost 100% of the time." This statement is not always borne out on motion radiographs, which at times demonstrate an inferior segment to be mobile. The neutral radiographic exam should be supplemented with stress x-rays in flexion and extension to determine the motion characteristics of the segment.

MARKING THE LATERAL UPPER CERVICAL SPINE

Analysis of the upper cervical spine is initiated with an evaluation for spinal instabilities similar to other areas of the spine (Fig. 5.25). Special attention must be given to any increased width of the atlanto-dental interval. Here again, there is some disagreement as to what constitutes "normal," but most authorities indicate that the ADI should not exceed 3 mm in the adult, and 5 mm in children (2). Approximately 20% of individuals with Down's Syndrome have a congenital absence of the transverse ligament and usually present with an increased ADI. Other factors, such as degenerative diseases and collagen disorders can also cause an increase. The lateral neutral view should not be used exclusively to determine the ADI, because a torn transverse atlas ligament may not cause an apparent increase until the joint is stressed during flexion (46).

The lateral cervical analysis is concluded by placing two dots on the C2 odontoid process, one centrally at its base, and the other at its superior margin (See Chapter 11). The line drawn through these points is called the "odontoid line." Another line is drawn perpendicular to the odontoid line and is placed through the middle portion of the C2 body and is designated the "odontoid perpendicular line" (6).

The atlas A-P plane line is formed by a line drawn through two dots placed at the anterior tubercle and posterior arch of C1. If the posterior ring of atlas is viewed on the radiograph as divided, then the dot is placed in the middle of the broadened image of the posterior arch (6).

Two dots are placed at the anterior and posterior borders of the foramen magnum, and a line is drawn through these points. This line depicts the occipital "foramen magnum" line and represents the position of the skull. Because it can be very difficult to determine this line, the

Table 5.5A.
Mean and Range in Degrees for Ranges of Motion of the Lumbar Functional Spinal Units During Flexion-Extension Motion[a]

FSU	Mean	Lower	Upper
		Flexion-Extension	
L1–L2	12.0	9.0	16.0
L2–L3	14.0	11.0	18.0
L3–L4	15.0	12.0	18.0
L4–L5	17.0	14.0	21.0
L5–S1	20.0	18.0	22.0

[a]From White AA, Panjabi MM. Clinical biomechanics of the spine. Philadelphia: JB Lippincott, 1978.

Table 5.5B.
Mean and Range in Degrees for Ranges of Motion of the Lumbar Functional Spinal Units During Lateral Bending[a]

FSU	Mean	Lower	Upper
		Lateral Bending (One Side)	
L1–L2	6.0	3.0	8.0
L2–L3	6.0	3.0	9.0
L3–L4	8.0	5.0	10.0
L4–L5	6.0	5.0	7.0
L5–S1	3.0	2.0	3.0

[a]From White AA, Panjabi MM. Clinical biomechanics of the spine. Philadelphia: JB Lippincott, 1978.

Table 5.5C.
Mean and Range in Degrees for Ranges of Motion of the Lumbar Functional Spinal Units During Axial Rotation[a]

FSU	Mean	Lower	Upper
		Axial Rotation (One Side)	
L1–L2	2.0	1.0	3.0
L2–L3	2.0	1.0	3.0
L3–L4	2.0	1.0	3.0
L4–L5	2.0	1.0	3.0
L5–S1	5.0	3.0	6.0

[a]From White AA, Panjabi MM. Clinical biomechanics of the spine. Philadelphia: JB Lippincott, 1978.

ing on the size of film, different alignment procedures are used. The most important factor is that the patient's entire spine is projected onto the film.

The patient is instructed to flex laterally to the maximum. Ensure that no rotation ($\pm\theta Y$) of the lumbar spine or pelvis has occurred, that the patient's mid sagittal plane is centered and perpendicular to the bucky, and that the patient is positioned so that the lumbar spine in the stressed posture will project onto the film. Appropriate shielding should be used to protect the patient. The exposure should be made during suspended expiration (Fig. 5.33).

NORMAL LUMBAR LATERAL FLEXION

The general outline of the vertebral bodies should maintain constant relationships to one another. The normal coronal coupling pattern of the lumbar spine involves lateral flexion ($\pm\theta Z$) with axial rotation ($\pm\theta Y$). As the lumbar spine is laterally flexed, axial rotation is combined with lateral bending such that the spinous processes rotate towards the ipsilateral side of lateral bend ($+\theta Z$ with $+\theta Y$, and $-\theta Y$ with $-\theta Z$.) Rotation ($\pm\theta Y$) proceeds smoothly from the lumbosacral junction upwards as evidenced by progressive migration of the pedicular image

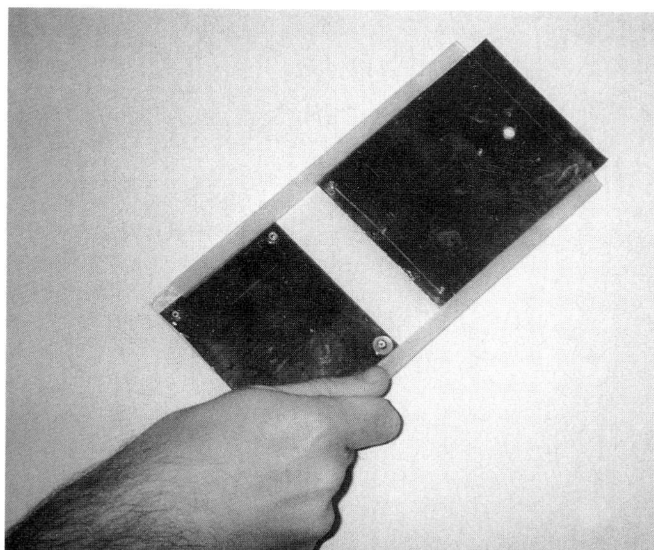

Figure 5.32. Lead blockers are used to reduce the x-ray field to the film size, thus allowing for a constant central ray height.

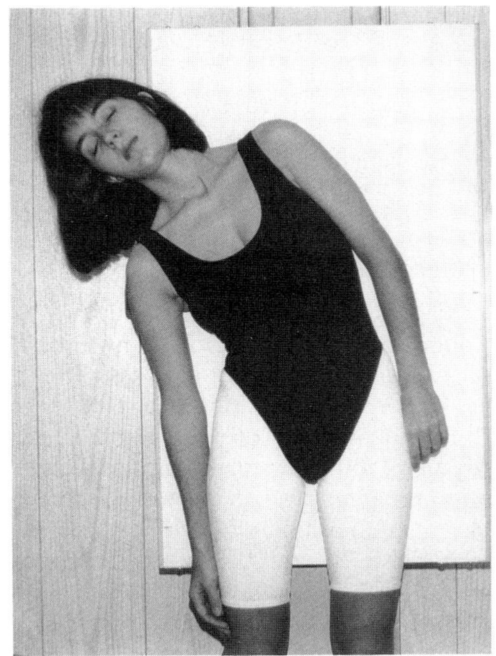

Figure 5.33. Patient positioning for the AP lumbar lateral bending exposure.

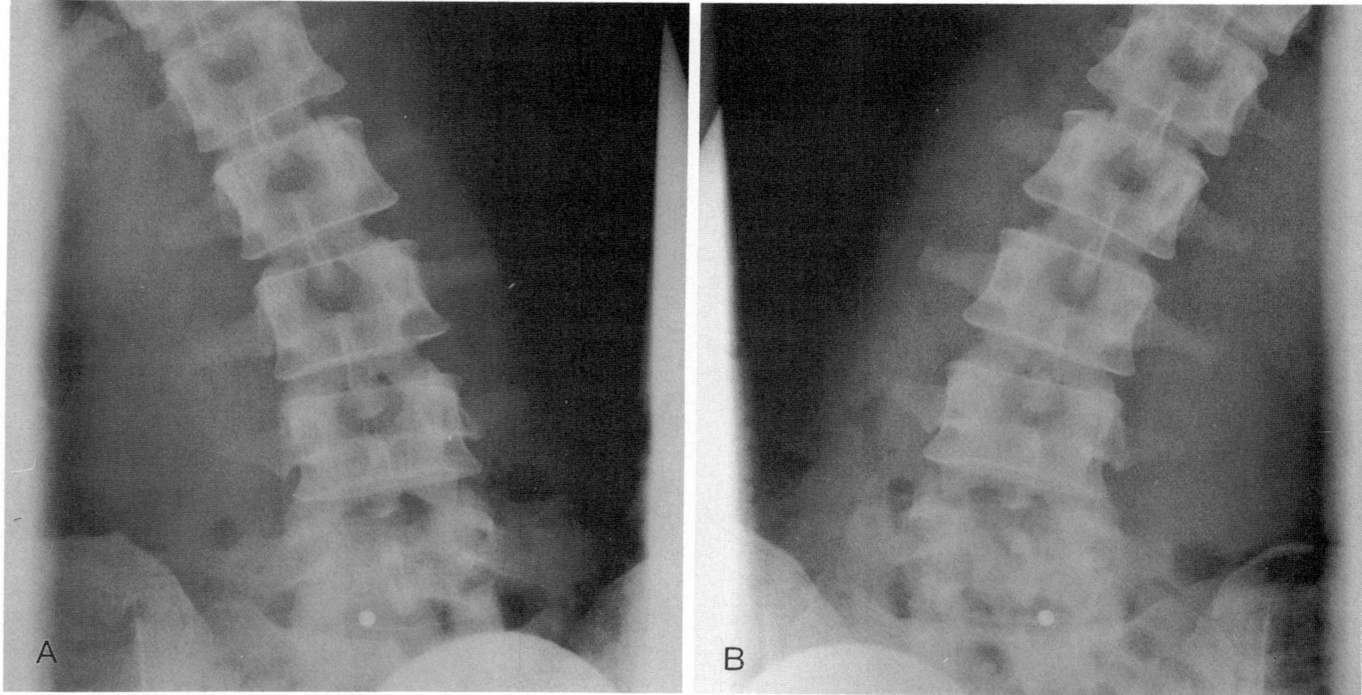

Figure 5.34. **A**, Near normal AP lumbar left lateral bending radiograph. **B**, Near normal AP lumbar right lateral bending radiograph.

relative to the general outline of the vertebral body (43) (Fig. 5.34A-B).

DYSFUNCTIONAL LATERAL FLEXION

A lumbar FSU is considered to be dysfunctional when it exhibits abnormal movement. This movement can be abnormal in quality (coupling patterns) or in quantity (increased or decreased motion). It can be either unilateral or bilateral and can occur along a single axis of motion or along multiple axes of motion. This dysfunctional motion may involve an increase, decrease or complete lack of vertebral body lateral flexion ($\pm\theta Z$) or can involve paradoxical lateral flexion to the opposite side. Rotation ($\pm\theta Y$) may also be affected and can be manifested as increased, decreased, paradoxical, or complete lack of spinous rotation (See Chapter 7). These deficits may occur singularly or in combination.

ANALYZING THE AP LATERAL FLEXION RADIOGRAPH

A standard X-ray pencil is used for the marking of this film. It begins by numbering each segment. Dots are then placed on like points on the right and left of each vertebra. The X axis is determined for each vertebra by connecting these points with a line. The spaces between these lines represent the shape of the disc during lateral flexion.

Rotation is determined by a comparison of the pedicular shadows. The pedicles are compared first right to left and then to those of the vertebra below. The degree of rotation is determined by the shape and position of the pedicles as discussed for the AP static radiograph. Rotation can be checked by placing dots at the far right and left corners of the superior and inferior end-plates. These dots are then connected, the upper right with the lower left, and the upper left with the lower right. The intersection of these lines designates the midpoint of the vertebra. The point of the spinolaminar junction can be compared with this midline to determine the direction of spinous rotation. It is important to understand that the spinous processes are often anomalous making this method suspect (49).

The comparison of stress lateral flexion radiographs to the static film helps to evaluate the static listing and provides additional information regarding the significance of the static misalignment. When the dynamic radiographic findings are in agreement with those on the static film, then treatment may proceed with confidence. If, for example, a lumbar segment is found to be deficient in both $+\theta Z$ and $+\theta Y$ during right lateral bending, and if on static comparison a misalignment of PLI is found, then the chiropractor can proceed with an adjustment of a PLI. A lumbar segment that demonstrated a decreased $+\theta Z$ during right lateral bending and showed a deficit in $-\theta Y$ in left lateral bending would support a static misalignment of PRS. Treatment with an adjustive thrust can follow (Fig. 5.35A-B). If, however, a lumbar vertebra were

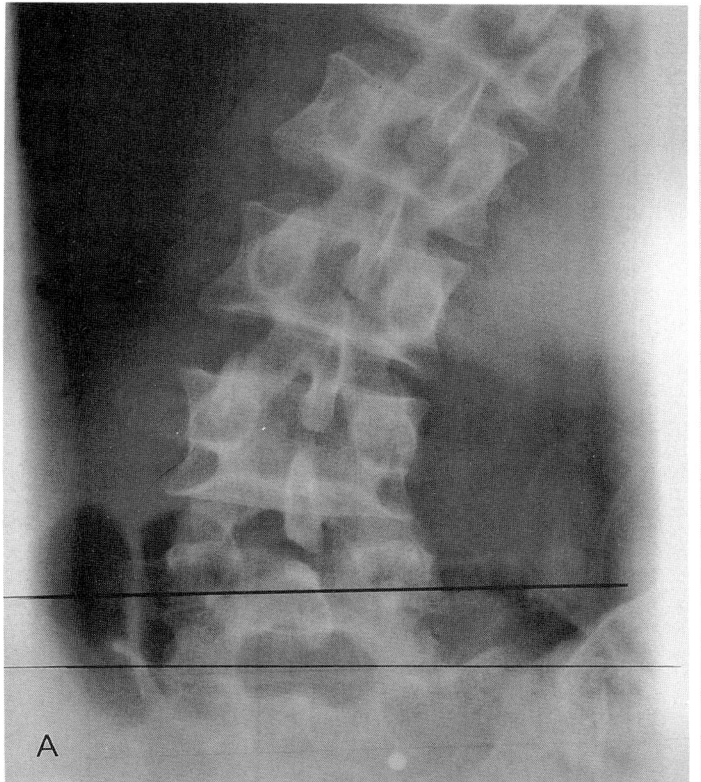

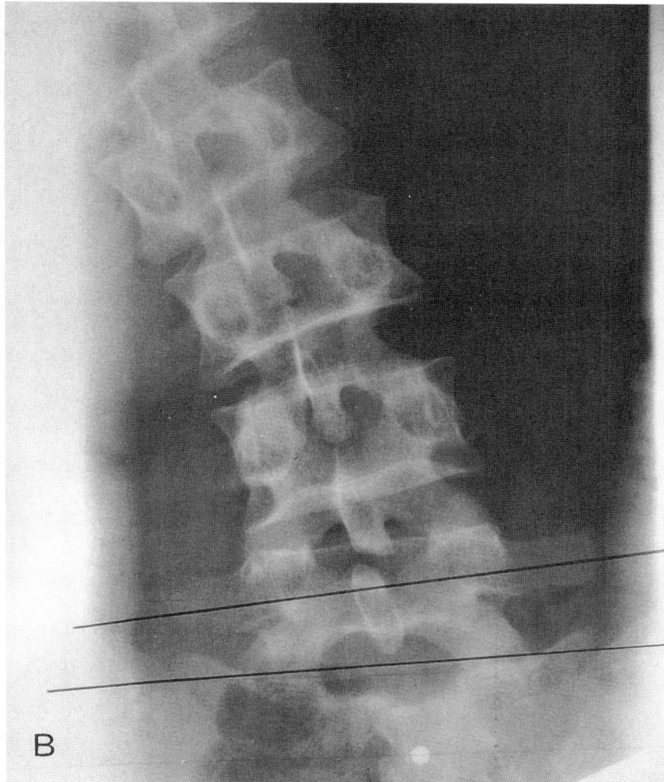

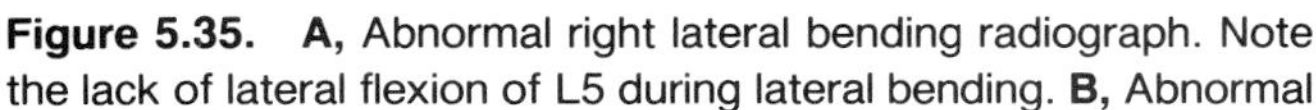

Figure 5.35. **A,** Abnormal right lateral bending radiograph. Note the lack of lateral flexion of L5 during lateral bending. **B,** Abnormal left lateral bending. Note the lack of left spinous rotation of L4 (coupled motion) during lateral flexion.

to be viewed in a static misaligned position but during stress evaluation demonstrated normal or hypermobile motion, it would indicate a compensation and is consequently a contraindication for manipulation.

The sacrum can also be evaluated during lateral bending. The sacrum should rotate around the $\pm\theta Y$ axis during lateral flexion, with the sacral ala on the side opposite of the lateral bending rotating posterior. This can be analyzed by measuring the distance between the lateral borders of the sacrum and the center of S2 during lateral flexion. This should be compared to the measurements on the static radiograph and during opposite side lateral bending. If the measurement on the side of lateral flexion does not decrease, then the sacrum can be considered to be fixated in a posterior position (P-L, P-R) on the side of lateral flexion (See Chapter 6).

LUMBAR FLEXION/EXTENSION

The lumbar flexion or extension radiograph may be taken on a 14″ × 17″ film or on a horizontally placed smaller film. For the best comparison, the FFD should be the same as the static lateral, whether a full spine or sectional view was performed. The FFD should be a minimum of 72″. The central ray can be left in the same position as for the full spine, if external lead blockers are used.

PATIENT POSITIONING FOR LUMBAR FLEXION/EXTENSION

While in the upright posture, the patient should be instructed to assume the desired stressed posture. The doctor should ensure that the entire lumbar spine will be projected onto the film.

The pelvis can be stabilized with a compressive device or the patient's pelvis can be supported against the bucky. Appropriate shielding should be used. The patient is instructed to remain perfectly still and suspend respiration during the exposure (Fig. 5.36–5.37).

NORMAL LUMBAR FLEXION/EXTENSION

In the sagittal plane, flexion/extension coupling patterns of the lumbar spine consist of rotation about the X axis ($\pm\theta X$) and should not normally involve any anterior or posterior translation ($\pm Z$). Failure of the motion segment in shear indicates disc disruption (See Chapter 2).

During flexion of the lumbar spine, each segment should rotate in a $+\theta X$ direction. There will be a fanning of the spinous processes and an anterior wedging of each IVD. There should be a smooth and even anterior curve with no anterior or posterior displacement (Fig. 5.38A).

During extension, each segment will rotate in a $-\theta X$ direction. There should be an approximation of the spi-

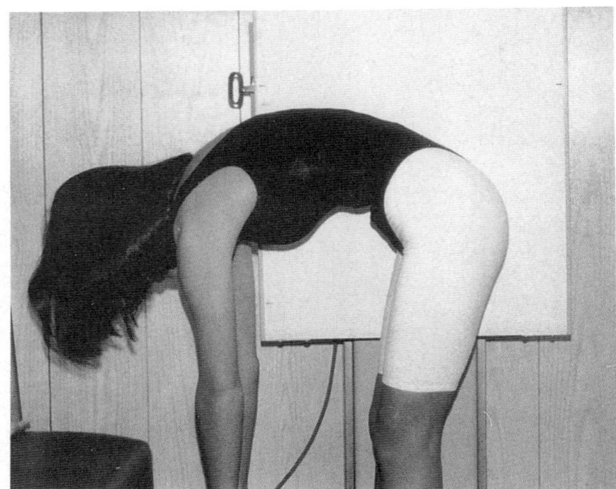

Figure 5.36. Patient positioning for lumbar sagittal flexion.

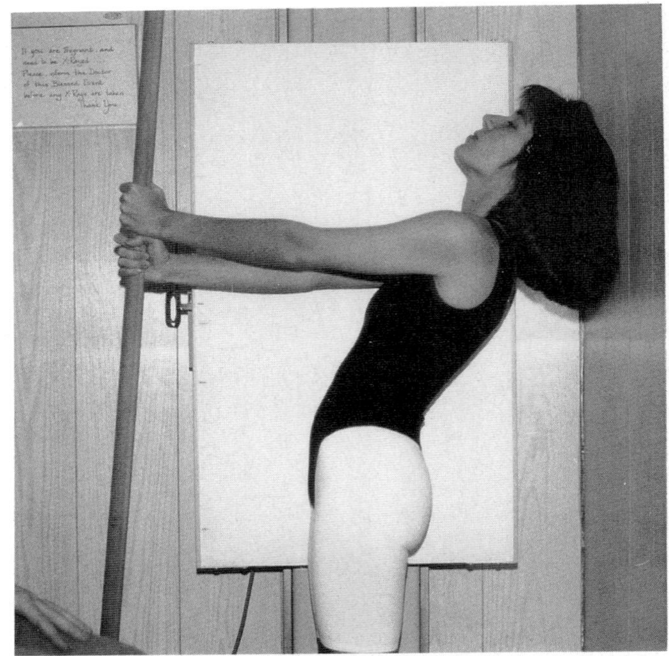

Figure 5.37. Patient positioning for lumbar sagittal extension.

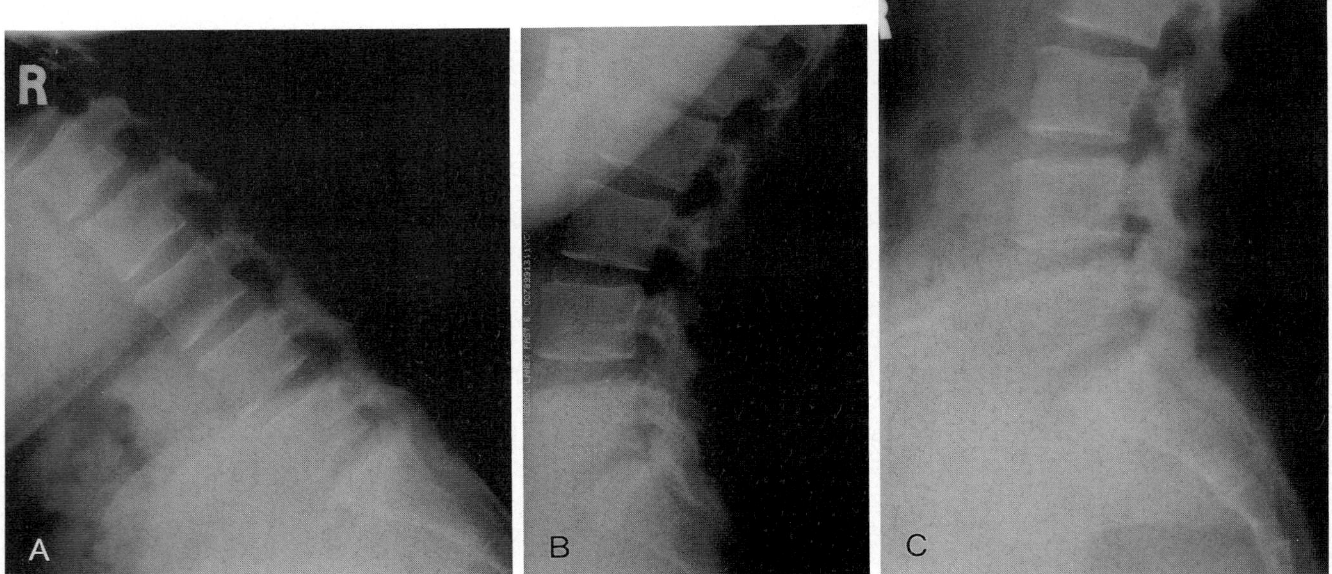

Figure 5.38. **A,** Near normal radiograph of lumbar sagittal flexion. **B,** Near normal radiograph of lumbar sagittal extension. **C,** Near normal sagittal neutral radiograph of the same patient as in **A** and **B**.

nous processes and a posterior wedging of the IVDs. A smooth and even posterior curve should be produced with no anterior or posterior translation (Fig. 5.38B-C).

ANALYSIS OF DYSFUNCTIONAL LUMBAR FLEXION/EXTENSION RADIOGRAPH

The spine should be evaluated qualitatively because there is not significant agreement as to the quantitative parameters of lumbar flexion or extension. The function of each segment should be compared with the motion of the segments above and below, keeping in mind that flexion and extension decreases incrementally from L5-S1 up through L1-L2. Each segment should be observed for increased or decreased motion, altered axis of rotation and anterior or posterior translation.

During lumbar flexion, if a particular segment does not move in a $+\theta X$ direction, then it can be considered to be fixated in a posterior inferior position and is a candidate for an adjustment (Fig. 5.39A-B). If, however, a segment demonstrated excessive $+\theta X$ motion during lumbar flexion, then that FSU would be considered a compensation and is contraindicated for an adjustment.

During lumbar extension, if a segment does not move in a $-\theta X$ direction or exhibits an increase in retrolisthesis, then that FSU is considered fixated and is a candidate for adjustments (70) (Fig. 5.39C and 5.40A-B).

Lumbar flexion/extension studies serve as important confirmation of spinal instability. The motion between segments effected will increase proportionately to the degree of ligamentous and disc damage. In the lateral view, those segments with severe instability may exhibit paradoxical motion when stressed (70).

Thoracic Spine

PATIENT POSITIONING FOR THORACIC LATERAL FLEXION

Lateral flexion. The AP thoracic lateral flexion radiographs should be taken on an 8″ × 10″, 10″ × 12″, or a 14″ × 17″ film. The x-ray field is collimated to the area of interest. The FFD should be at least 72″ and replicate the FFD of the AP neutral.

The patient is asked to stand with the mid sagittal plane perpendicular to the bucky, chin slightly elevated,

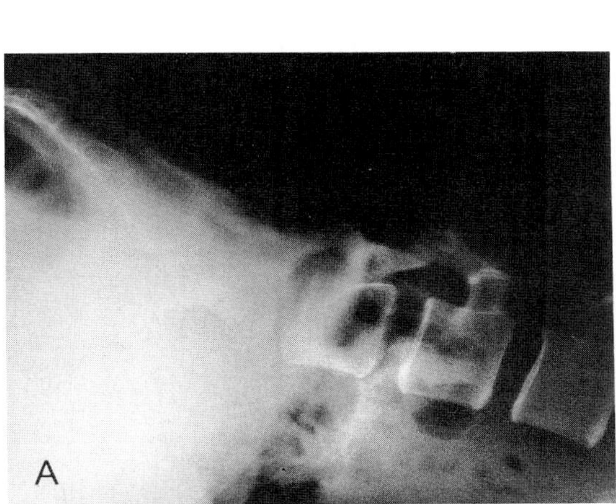

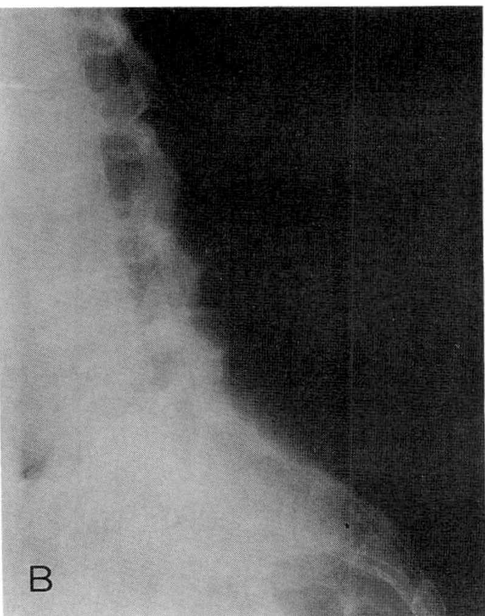

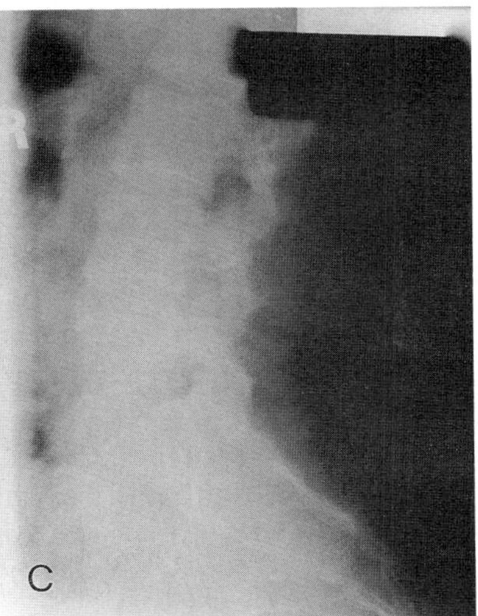

Figure 5.39. **A,** Dysfunctional radiograph of lumbar sagittal flexion. Note the posterior displaced L5 vertebra. **B,** Abnormal lumbar flexion. Notice the fixated posterior and inferior L5 vertebra. **C,** Abnormal lumbar extension. Notice the retrolisthesis at L5.

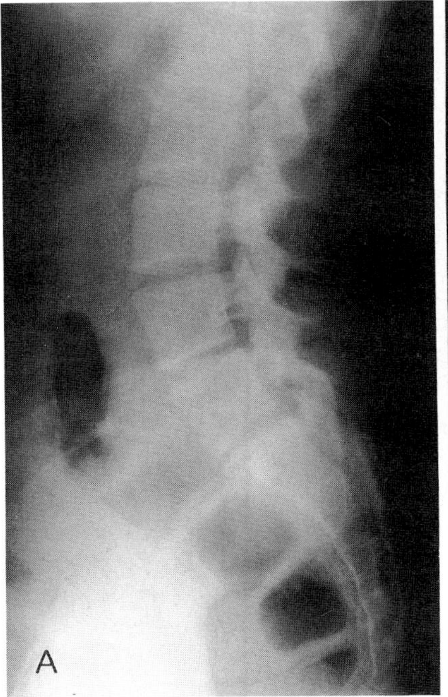

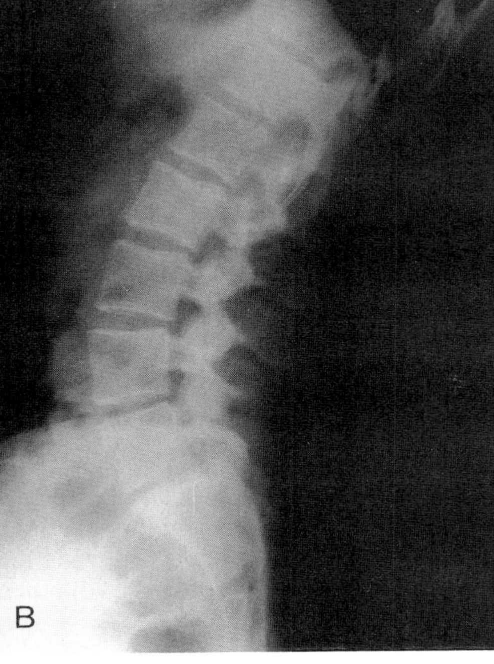

Figure 5.40. **A,** Neutral position. Notice the posteriorly wedged disc at L5-S1, indicative of a base posterior sacrum (See Chapter 7). **B,** Abnormal radiograph of lumbar sagittal extension of patient in **A**. Notice failure of the L5-S1 motion segment to extend ($-\theta X$).

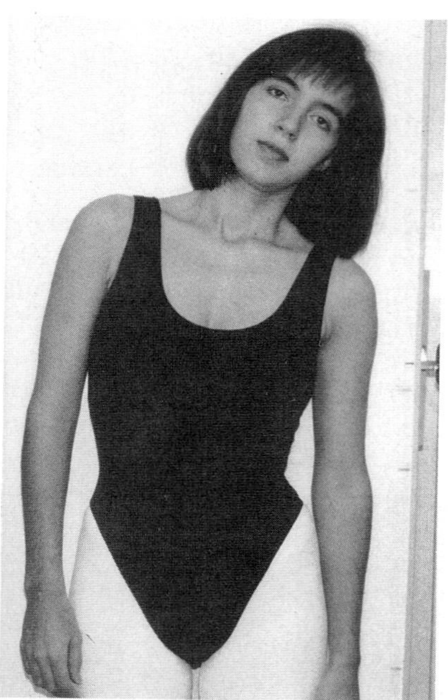

Figure 5.41. Patient positioning for the thoracic AP lateral flexion radiograph.

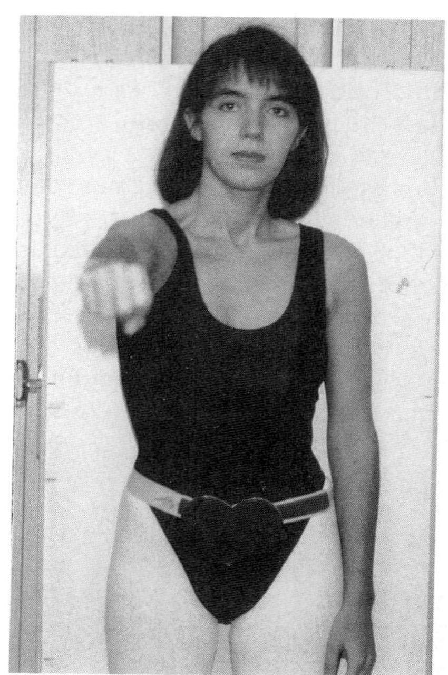

Figure 5.42. Patient positioning for AP thoracic axial ($\pm\theta Y$) rotation.

and arms to the sides. The doctor instructs the patient to bend the thoracic spine laterally, ensuring that no lumbar lateral flexion or pelvic rotation occurs. The patient is instructed to hold this position (the palmar surface of the lower hand should be approximating the lateral surface of the ipsilateral knee) and suspend full expiration (Fig. 5.41).

Rotation. For rotation, the patient begins in the same static position and then rotates the thorax by bringing a shoulder and/or arm forward, ensuring that the pelvis remains parallel to the bucky (Fig. 5.42).

ANALYSIS

Lateral bending. The thoracic spine is analyzed primarily during lateral bending and rotation. Lateral flexion of each FSU should occur similarly as in other areas of the spine. When the patient isolates thoracic movement, so that no lumbar lateral flexion occurs, the normal coupling motion involves contralateral spinous rotation during lateral bending.

The spinous processes should rotate in a $+\theta Y$ direction during left lateral flexion and in a $-\theta Y$ direction during right lateral flexion. Rotation should progress as one moves cephalad. The mortise-like configuration of the thoracolumbar zygapophyseal joints severely limits axial rotation (71) (Figs. 5.43, 5.44A-B).

If lateral bending is not isolated to the thoracic spine, then the lower thoracic segments will follow the lumbar pattern of ipsilateral spinous rotation. The upper thoracic segments should follow a contralateral pattern. Generally, this transition occurs at the mid thoracic area.

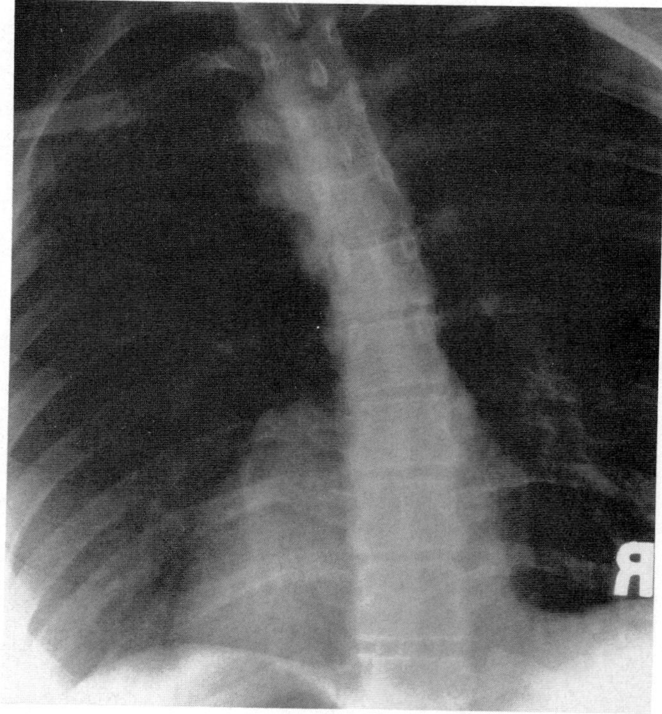

Figure 5.43. AP radiograph of near normal thoracic AP lateral flexion.

Rotation. If a question involving thoracic rotation remains, it can be evaluated further by inducing thoracic rotation without lateral bending. The spinous processes should move in the same direction as the rotation of the thorax, again progressively, as one moves cephalad (Figs. 5.45–5.46).

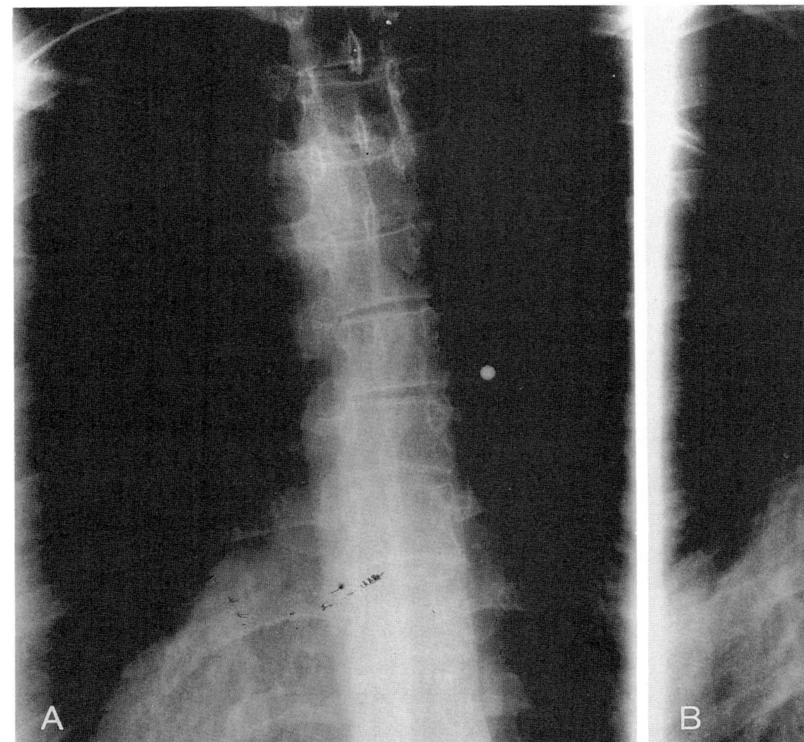

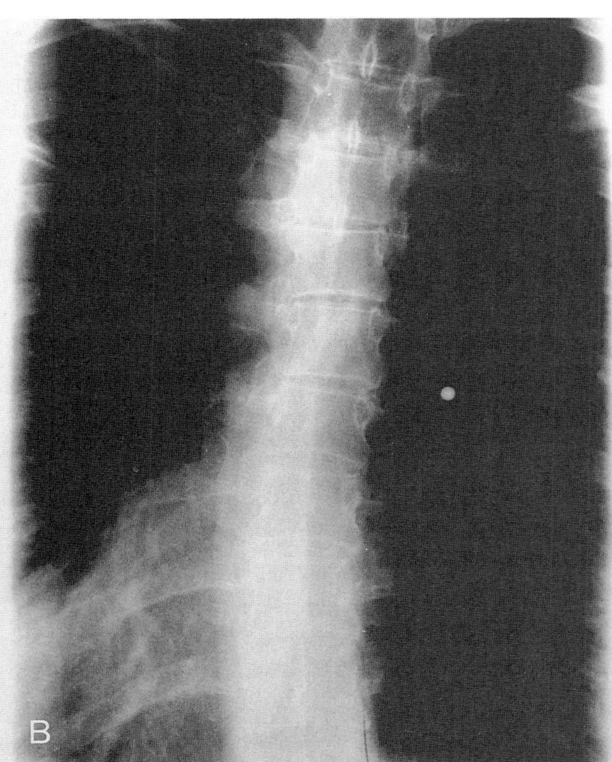

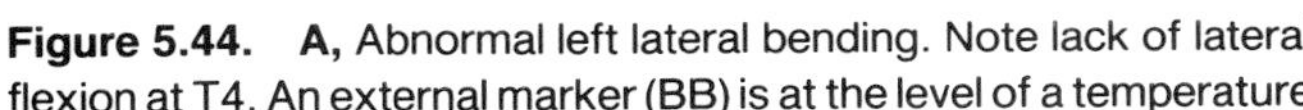
Figure 5.44. **A,** Abnormal left lateral bending. Note lack of lateral flexion at T4. An external marker (BB) is at the level of a temperature differential. **B,** Right lateral bending. Note severe dysfunction in lateral flexion ($+\theta Z$) of T6 during bending.

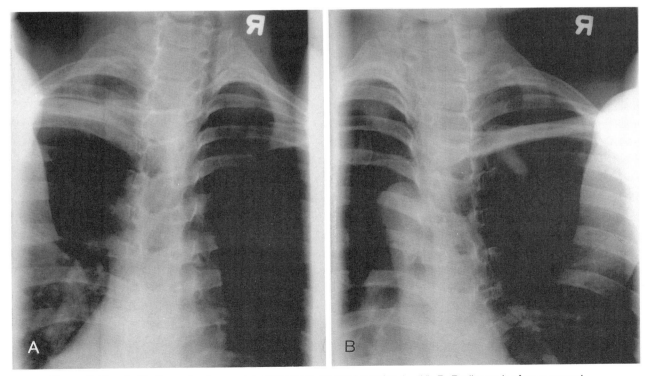

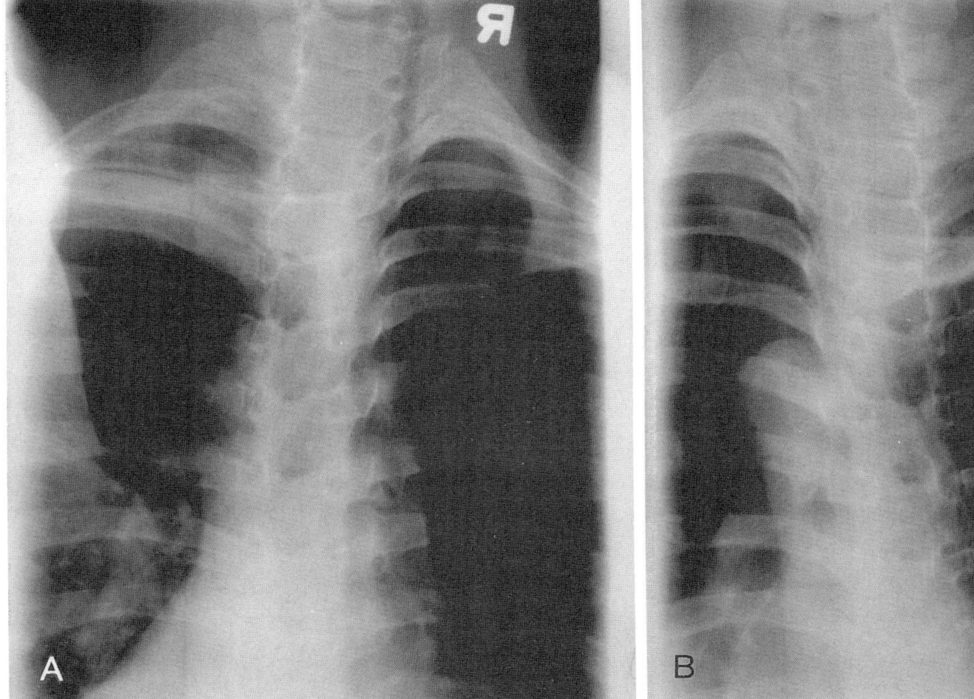

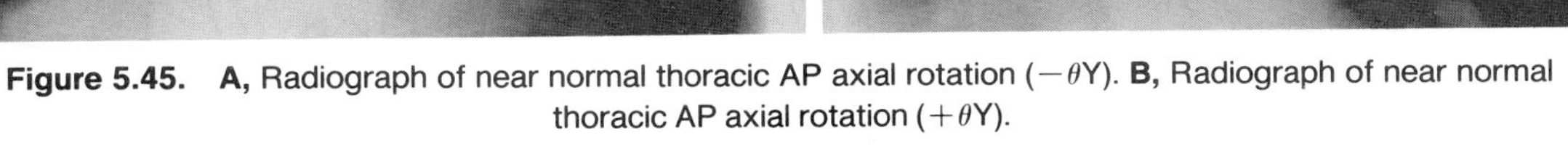
Figure 5.45. **A,** Radiograph of near normal thoracic AP axial rotation ($-\theta Y$). **B,** Radiograph of near normal thoracic AP axial rotation ($+\theta Y$).

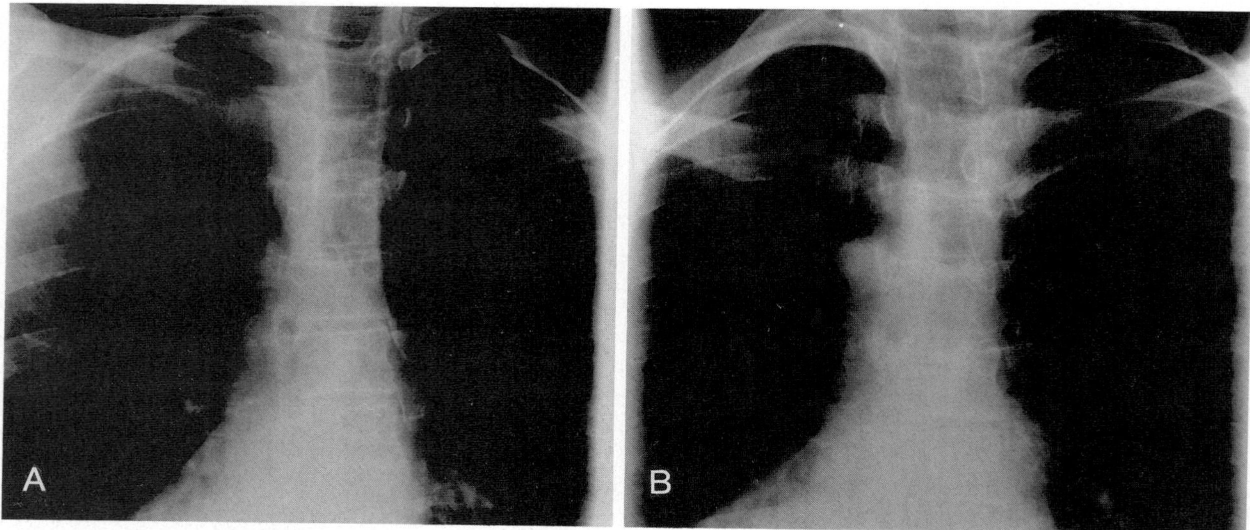

Figure 5.46. **A,** Radiograph of dysfunctional thoracic axial rotation ($-\theta Y$). Note the lack of $-\theta Y$ of T4 and T5 during right body rotation. **B,** Thoracic axial rotation ($+\theta Y$).

Cervical Spine

The biomechanical functions of the cervical spine include the support of the head, allowance of complex motion, and the protection of neural elements. Support is achieved through ligamentous and muscular forces along with an ingenious set of anatomic structures (33). The resultant structure has the capacity to sustain and attenuate many different loads while allowing a wide range of movements (72).

The functional examination of the cervical spine during flexion, extension, and lateral bending is a valuable method to determine pathologic joint conditions. The representative values of the range of motion of the cervical spine have been provided (Table 5.6A-C).

Table 5.6A.
Mean and Range in Degrees for Ranges of Motion of Cervical Functional Spinal Units During Flexion-Extension Motion

FSU	Mean	Lower	Upper
		Flexion-Extension	
C0–C1[a]	24.5	9.9	37.4
C1–C2[b]	15.0	8.0	22.0
C2–C3[b]	12.0	6.0	17.0
C3–C4[b]	17.0	10.0	24.0
C4–C5[b]	21.0	14.0	28.0
C5–C6[b]	23.0	16.0	31.0
C7–T1[c]	6.0	4.0	17.0

[a]Panjabi M, Dvorak J, Duranceau J, et al. Three-dimensional movements of the upper cervical spine. Spine 1988;13:728.
[b]Dvorak J, Froehlich D, Penning L, Baumgartner H, Panjabi M. Functional radiographic diagnosis of the cervical spine: flexion/extension. Spine 1988;13:748.
[c]White AA, Panjabi MM. Clinical biomechanics of the spine. Philadelphia: JB Lippincott, 1978.

Table 5.6B.
Mean and Range in Degrees for Ranges of Motion of Cervical Functional Spinal Units During Lateral Bending[a]

FSU	Mean	Upper	Lower
		Lateral Bending (One Side)	
C0–C1[a]	5.0		
C1–C2[b]	6.7	0.8	16.5
C2–C3[a]	6.0		
C3–C4[a]	6.0		
C4–C5[a]	6.0		
C5–C6[a]	6.0		
C6–C7[a]	6.0		
C7–T1[a]	6.0		

[a]Penning L. Normal movements of the cervical spine. Am J Roentgenol 1979;130:317.
[b]Panjabi M, Dvorak J, Duranceau J, et al. Three-dimensional movements of the upper cervical spine. Spine 1988;13:728.

Table 5.6C.
Mean and Range in Degrees for Ranges of Motion of Cervical Functional Spinal Units During Axial Rotation[a]

FSU	Mean	Upper	Lower
		Axial Rotation (One Side)	
C0–C1	1.0	−2.0	5.0
C1–C2	40.5	29.0	46.0
C2–C3	3.0	0.0	10.0
C3–C4	6.5	3.0	10.0
C4–C5	6.8	1.0	12.0
C5–C6	6.9	2.0	12.0
C6–C7	5.4	2.0	10.0
C7–T1	2.1	−2.0	7.0

[a]From Penning L, Wilmink JT. Rotation of the cervical spine. Spine 1987;12:732.

PATIENT POSITIONING FOR AP CERVICAL LATERAL FLEXION

The cervical lateral bending radiographs should be taken on an 8″ × 10″ film at the same FFD and central ray height as the neutral AP. The minimal FFD is 72 inches.

The patient is asked to stand with the mid sagittal plane perpendicular to the bucky and aligned with the vertical component of the central ray. The patient is instructed to flex the head laterally, making sure the contralateral shoulder does not rise. Ensure that no rotation ($\pm\theta$Y) or sway has been introduced and that the cervical spine will be projected onto the film. The patient is instructed to suspend respiration and remain perfectly still. A filtration system should be used to protect the patient and improve film quality. The exposure is taken during suspended respiration (Fig. 5.47).

LATERAL FLEXION OF THE CERVICAL SPINE

During lateral flexion, the vertebral bodies should maintain constant relationships to one another. The normal coronal coupling patterns in the lower cervical spine (C2-C7) are attributed to soft tissue tensions as well as the spatial orientations of the facets (43,51). Lateral flexion is limited by the uncinate processes at the end-range.

The normal coupling motion of lateral flexion ($\pm\theta$Z) in the cervical spine is similar to the patterns in the normal thoracic spine. The spinous processes migrate to the convexity of the curve during lateral flexion. Therefore, in right lateral bending ($+\theta$Z), the spinous processes rotate to the left ($-\theta$Y) and in left lateral bending ($-\theta$Z), there is an associated axial rotation of the spinous processes to the right ($+\theta$Y) (73). Rotation ($\pm\theta$Y) should proceed smoothly from the upper thoracic spine evidenced by progressive spinous process migration relative to the general outline of the vertebral body (Fig. 5.48).

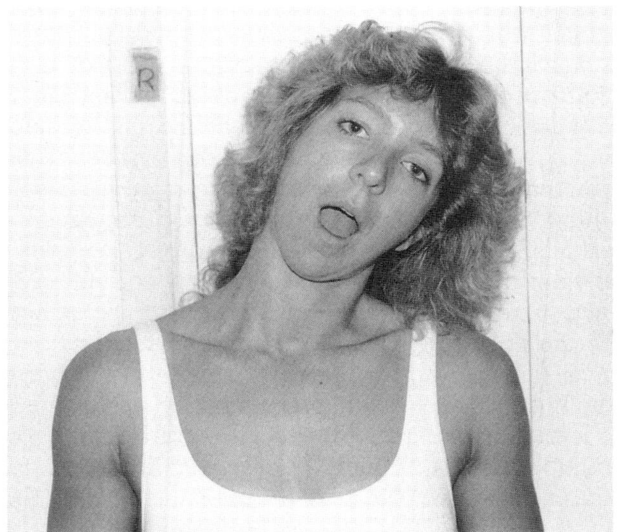

Figure 5.47. Patient positioning for the cervical AP lateral flexion radiograph.

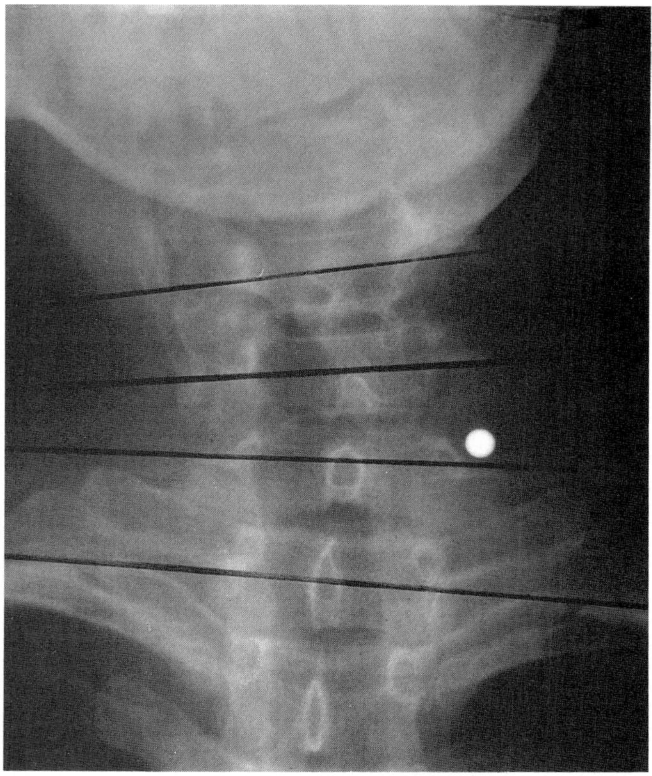

Figure 5.48. Radiograph of near normal cervical AP lateral flexion.

Lysell et al. (73) have studied the coupling mechanism of axial rotation occurring simultaneously with lateral flexion. There is a gradual increase in coupling as one moves cephalad:

> C2; For every 3° of lateral flexion there is 2° coupled axial rotation (ratio of 2:3)
>
> C7; For every 7.5° of lateral flexion there is 1° coupled axial rotation (ratio of 1:7.5)

Lysell et al. (73) hypothesize that the decrease in axial rotation in the lower cervical spine, is due to facet geometry.

Because of the unique anatomical and physiologic make-up of the upper cervical spine, special consideration must be taken during analysis of this area. Little normative data exist regarding the intricate biomechanics of this region during lateral bending. During lateral flexion of the normal upper cervical spine, there should be little or no side slippage of C1 on C2 (Fig. 5.49A-C). Excessive laterolisthesis (>4 mm) of this area is a sign of ligamentous damage. Because the lateral atlantoaxial joints have biconvex surfaces, when axial rotation occurs, there is a −Y translation of the atlas. The horizontal plane lines of the atlas and axis should converge on the side of lateral bend.

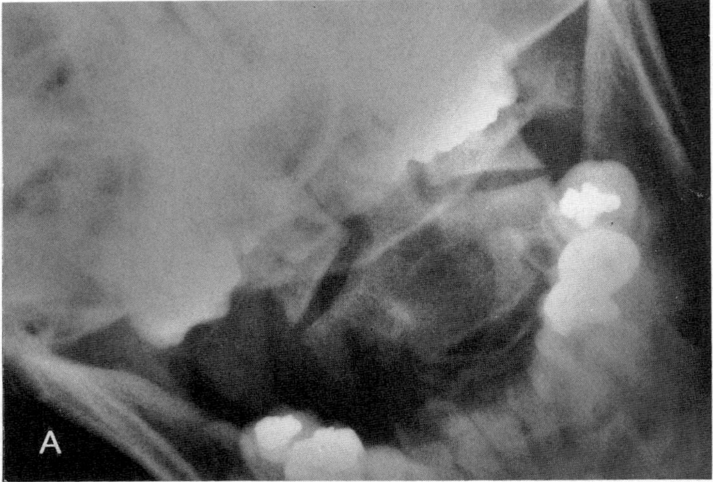

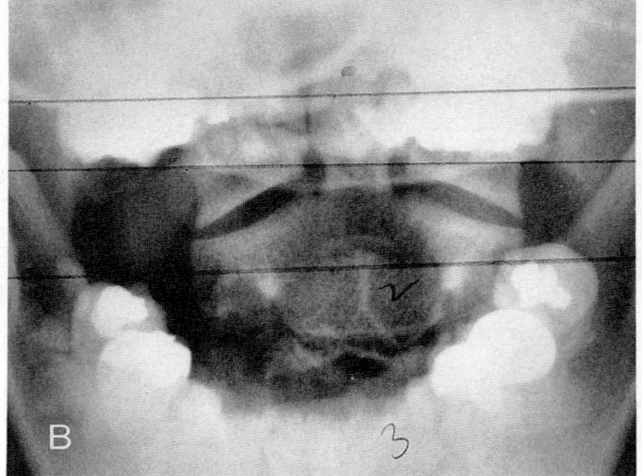

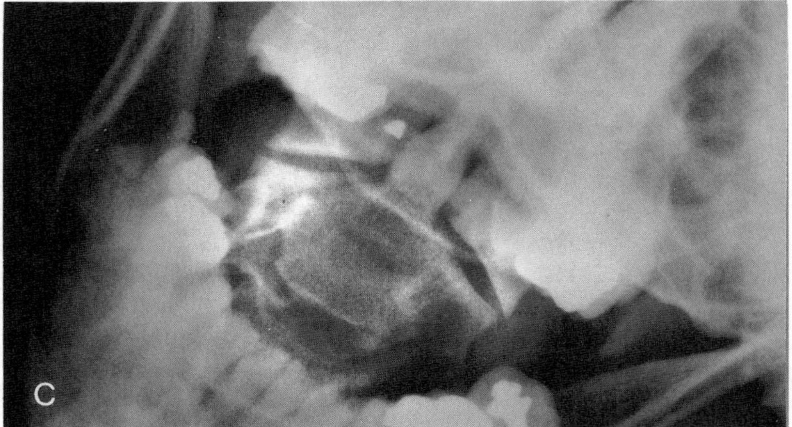

Figure 5.49. **A,** Upper cervical left lateral flexion. **B,** The neutral radiograph of the patient in **A** and **C**. **C,** Right lateral bending.

DYSFUNCTIONAL CERVICAL LATERAL FLEXION

Radiographs of the lower cervical spine are analyzed similarly to other spinal lateral flexion radiographs. Normal coupling action of the cervical spine is taken into consideration. When there is a reduced movement at a motion segment in the cervical spine because of injured tissues, there is often a compensatory increase in the motion of adjacent segments. These compensations may be displayed as misalignments on a static radiograph, and it will be very difficult to differentiate from misaligned fixated segments. It is essential that they be distinguished to determine the proper course of treatment. This can best be done with stress radiographs. If on assuming a stressed posture, the movement of the segment agrees with the static misalignment and demonstrates decreased motion, that FSU is a good candidate to be adjusted. If the segment is shown to be a hypermobile compensation, then manipulation is contraindicated.

If a segment shows decreased motion in both $+\theta Z$ and $-\theta Y$ during right lateral bending, and a check of the static misalignment demonstrates a PRS, then a fixated motion segment would be substantiated and a course of adjustive therapy indicated. A segment that shows a PLI static misalignment and displays a decrease in $+\theta Z$ during right lateral bending and a decrease in $+\theta Y$ during left lateral bending would substantiate the accuracy of the static misalignment. This can provide additional evidence in determining the directional vectors of an adjustment thrust (Fig. 5.50). If, however, the FSU demonstrates hypermobility during a stressed posture and shows no fixation dysfunction, then that segment should not be adjusted regardless of any apparent static misalignment.

Carrick (66) noted that deviations from the normal coupling mechanism in the cervical spine were related to the level of clinical radiculopathy. Aberrances in the coupling mechanism of the FSU of the cervical spine were reduced through chiropractic adjustments, and post adjustive examination revealed improvements in sensation, motor power, and deep tendon reflexes, as well as symptoms.

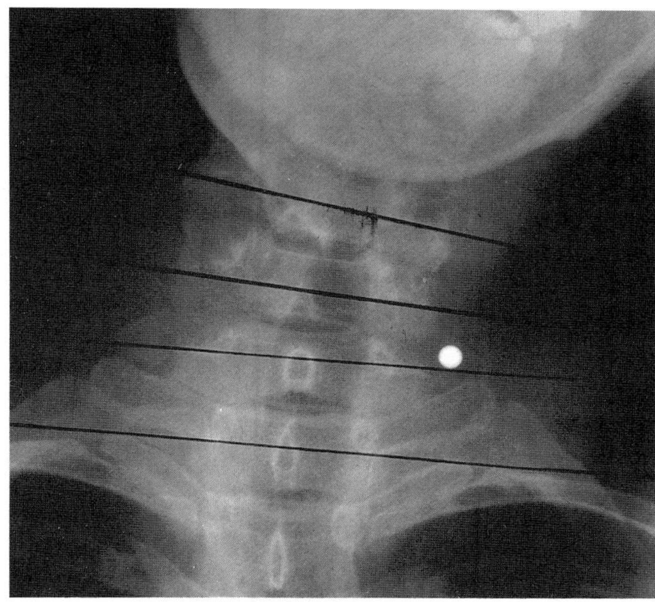

Figure 5.50. Radiograph of a dysfunctional cervical AP lateral flexion. Note the lack of lateral flexion of C7 in $+\theta Z$. The marker represents the site of a temperature differential.

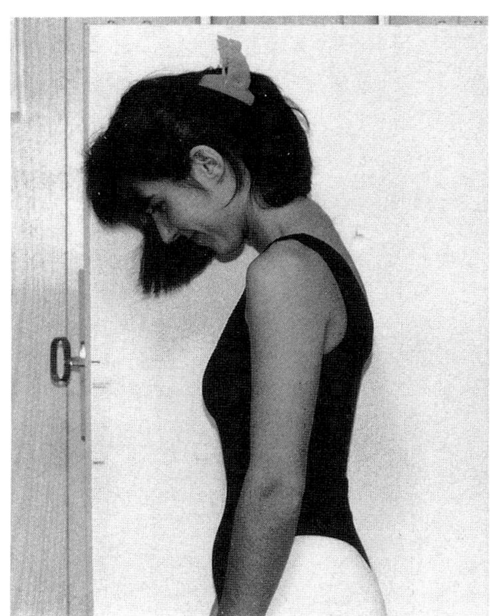

Figure 5.51. Patient positioning for sagittal cervical flexion.

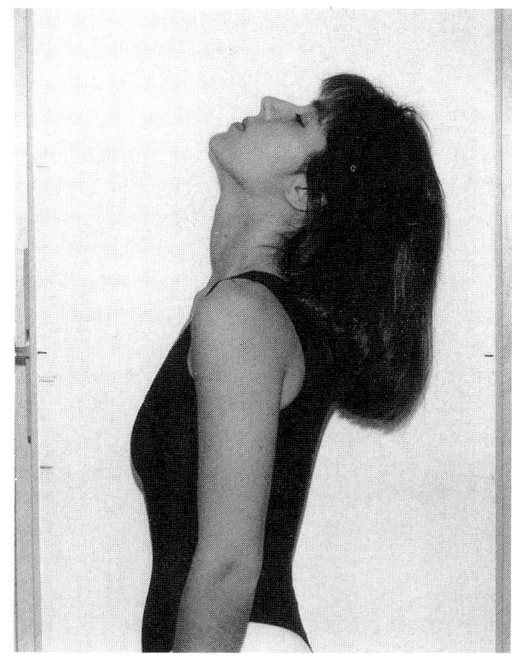

Figure 5.52. Patient positioning for sagittal cervical extension.

PATIENT POSITION FOR CERVICAL FLEXION/EXTENSION RADIOGRAPHS

A cervical flexion or extension radiograph should be taken on a 8″ × 10″ at the same FFD as the neutral AP, a minimum of 72″. The patient is instructed to stand with the mid coronal plane perpendicular to the bucky and aligned with the vertical component of the central ray. The patient is instructed to assume the desired stressed position. The doctor must check to ensure that no rotation ($\pm\theta Y$) or lateral flexion ($\pm\theta Z$) has been introduced and that the cervical spine will be projected onto the film. A filtration system should be used to protect the patient and improve film quality. The patient is instructed to suspend respiration and remain perfectly still during the exposure (Figs. 5.51–5.52).

CERVICAL FLEXION/EXTENSION ANALYSIS

Sagittal plane dynamic stress studies of the cervical spine offer additional information that the neutral lateral does not. These radiographs allow for visualization of the FSU and aberrations in intersegmental motion and also provide confirmation of ligamentous, IVD, and suspected fracture instabilities (46).

Extension/flexion movements of the cervical spine are similar to those of the lumbar spine and are analyzed accordingly (Fig. 5.53A-B). In the flexion view ($+\theta X$), the facet joints and their ligamentous supports are stretched (Fig. 5.54A-B). Damage to these ligaments become more apparent as they are called on to limit the extent of motion. Posterior ligament damage will allow an increase in the posterior height of the IVD and a corresponding decrease at its anterior aspect during motion. The spinous processes will exhibit a "fanning" effect caused by the instability of the posterior spinal ligaments, that exceeds normal fanning. Instability of the transverse ligament is indicated when the ADI increases by 5 mm or more and is not only a contraindication to chiropractic adjustments but also an indication for neurosurgical referral (2,46).

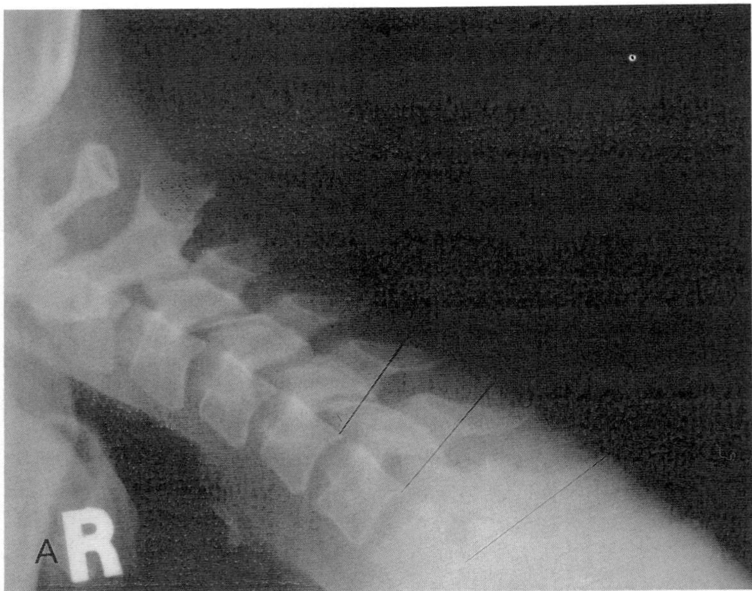

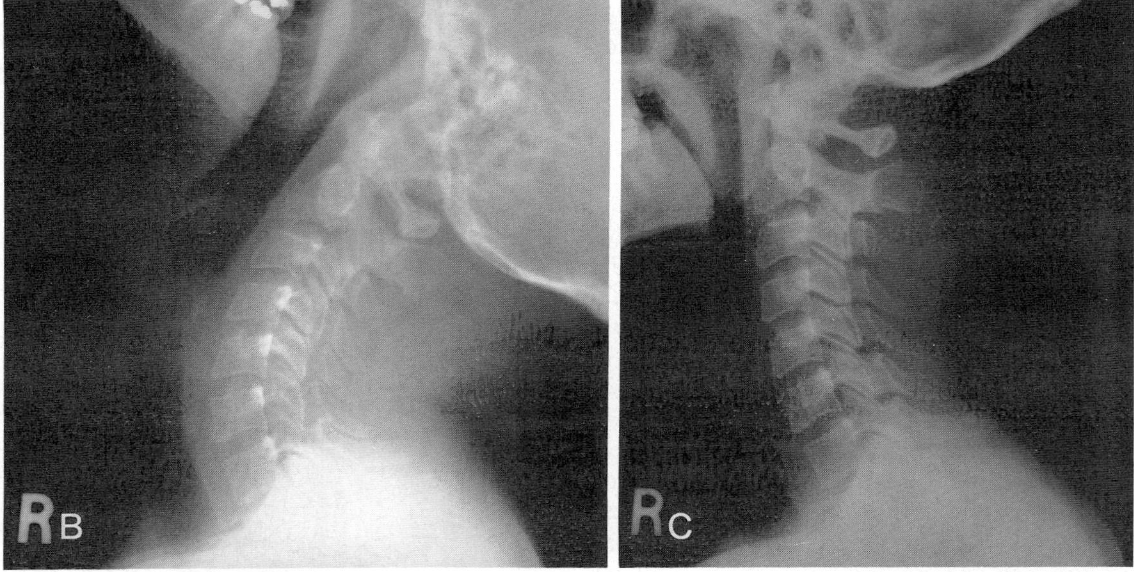

Figure 5.53. **A,** Near normal radiograph of cervical flexion. **B,** Near normal radiograph of cervical extension. **C,** Near normal neutral lateral radiograph of the same patient as in **A** and **B**.

An important additional consideration is the comparison of the occipital-atlanto-axial (OAA) interspaces. The space between the posterior tubercle of atlas and the spinous process of axis should be approximately equal to the interspace between the posterior tubercle of atlas and the occiput. This relationship, although quantitatively changed, should maintain a relative ratio in the neutral lateral, flexion, and extension radiographs. Lack of normal translation may indicate fixation, but excessive motion should be regarded with a great deal of caution, especially in the child, because this area may be relatively less stable because of its anatomic configuration (43).

In the sagittal extension view ($-\theta X$), the anterior cervical structures are stretched, while the posterior elements are compressed. Damage to the ALL, the anterior portion of the IVDs, and avulsion fractures of the anterior vertebral bodies may become more visible as increased motion or osseous displacement occurs. The facets are evaluated for proper posteroinferior glide, with associated approximation of the spinous processes (Fig. 5.55).

To complete the analysis of the lateral cervical views, templating of the segments in the neutral, flexed and extended positions may provide evidence of instability. Acetates are used to compare the cervical spine as it translates between the neutral position and the extremes of flexion/extension. The reader is directed to a method developed by Henderson and Dorman (74).

Other useful methods of analysis for the presence of

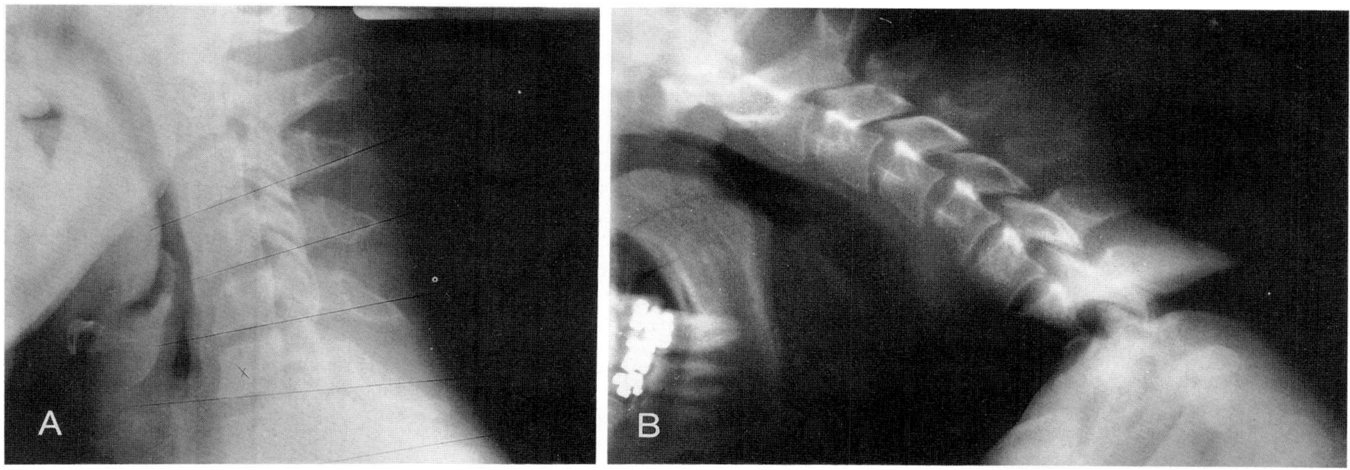

Figure 5.54. **A,** Radiograph of dysfunctional cervical flexion. Note failure of C6 to flex. **B,** Abnormal cervical flexion. Note failure of C7 to flex.

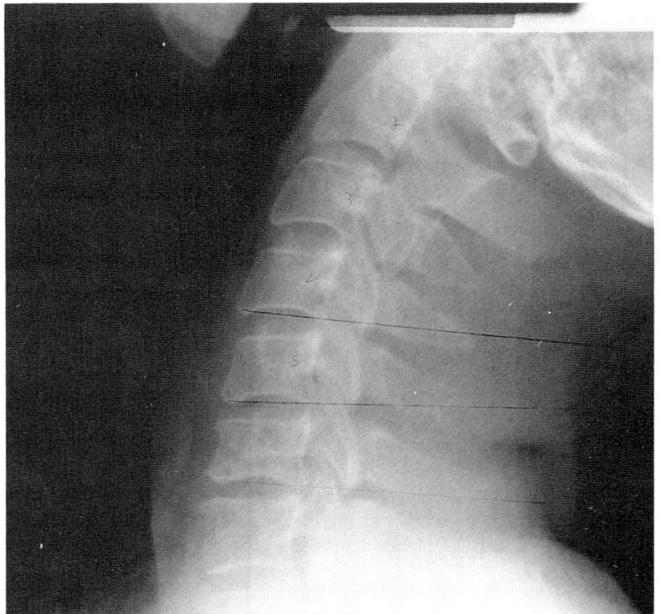

Figure 5.55. Radiograph of abnormal cervical extension. Note failure of C5-C6 to extend.

fracture and ligament damage are magnetic resonance imaging (MRI), tomography, and computerized axial tomography (CT).

Posttherapeutic Radiologic Examinations

Posttherapeutic radiologic examinations provide an assessment of the effectiveness of treatment in altering kinesiopathologies. Desired and undesired changes in positional dyskinesia, fixation dysfunction, altered axis of rotation or hypermobility can be monitored through comparative radiography. With the advances in equipment and technology, exposure levels have decreased significantly for radiologic examinations. As the risks decrease, the application of post radiographs becomes more acceptable. The findings from these post radiographs provide information that can affect the clinical management of the patient and thus may be justified when clinical findings indicate the need for reevaluation.

Indications for the Comparative Examination

It is important to only take views that have the potential to provide information that will alter future treatment. The view selection should be based on the most recent physical examination findings and information derived from the initial radiographs. In general, full spine or sectional comparative radiography is justified by the attending physician if such information would alter the course of treatment. Examples of indications include, but are not limited to the following:

1. When clinical examination procedures (e.g. pain questionnaires, motion palpation findings, instrumentation findings, etc.) do not correlate with the information from the most recent radiographic examination;
2. If the patient was initially x-rayed in an acute or antalgic position, since changes in tonicity of the paraspinal musculature would alter the postural configuration of the spinal column;
3. If the patient's clinical symptomatology does not improve within a four to six week period. There may be instances where comparative radiographs would be required prior to this time period. The major determining factor would be if physical findings do not correlate with the initial radiographs. A second chiropractic opinion is often helpful, if the attending physician is contemplating a comparative examination;
4. If there has been the introduction of a foot orthotic (e.g. heel lift) and the physician needs to determine the postural adaption to the device;

5. There is an alteration in the orthopedic or neurological findings unexplainable without a radiograph. In many instances additional diagnostic tests, such as electronic thermography or electromyography, may be more appropriate for gaining the necessary information critical to case management;
6. There has been a traumatic insult since the initial radiograph;
7. To monitor a potentially progressive scoliosis;
8. To follow a pathological process such as degenerative joint disease, fracture healing or post-traumatic ligamentous laxity or creep;
9. If initial radiographs were not performed in an upright weight-bearing position.
10. To monitor response to treatment in terms of biomechanical parameters, if the information derived from the radiograph is likely to alter case management.

Contraindications for Comparative Examinations

Comparative radiographic examinations should not be performed in the following circumstances:

1. When there is any possibility of pregnancy (unless not performing the procedure would place the mother at risk);
2. In the absence of objective clinical findings indicating the need for comparative examination;
3. When no possible change in treatment procedures would be anticipated from the examination;
4. When appropriate filtration, shielding and high speed screen/film (e.g. 1200 speed) are not being used.

PATIENT EDUCATION

The radiograph serves as an important aid in educating patients about their spinal condition and how that condition deviates from normal. The old adage "to see is to know, and not to see is to guess," holds for the patient as well as the doctor. Enabling the patient to view the kinesiopathologic components of the vertebral subluxation complex (See Chapter 3) with a proper explanation from the doctor helps the patient understand the important underlying evidence of the condition. This not only helps the patient to appreciate that, like degenerative manifestations themselves, symptomatology is a result of the causative condition and is not the disease itself. This comprehension by the patient tends to foster improved involvement and compliance towards a more complete resolution of the malady beyond the initial symptomatic improvement. This alone is not justification for performing a radiographic examination but can serve as an additional benefit should a radiographic examination be required.

REFERENCES

1. Hildebrandt RW. Chiropractic spinography. 2nd ed. Baltimore: Williams & Wilkins, 1985.
2. Yochum TR, Rowe LJ. Essentials of skeletal radiology. Baltimore: Williams & Wilkins, 1987.
3. Howe JW, Buehler MT, Palmateer DC, Hollen WV. Research on several parameters relating to full spine radiography. ACA J Chiro 1970;Sept:S57–64.
4. Hildebrandt RW. Chiropractic spinography and postural roentgenology-part I: history of development. J Manipulative Physiol Ther 1980;4:87–92.
5. Palmer BJ. Bigness of the fellow within. Davenport: BJ Palmer Publisher, 1949:196.
6. Herbst RW. Gonstead chiropractic science and art. Mt. Horeb, WI: Sci-Chi Publications 1968.
7. Plaugher G, Hendricks AH. The inter- and intraexaminer reliability of the Gonstead pelvic marking system. J Manipulative Physiol Ther 1991;14:503–508.
8. Plaugher G, Hendricks AH, Doble RW, Araghi HJ, Bachman TR, Hoffart VM. The effects of patient positioning on radiographically evaluated static configurations of the pelvis. Proceedings of the 1991 Conference on Spinal Manipulation. Arlington, VA, 1991.
9. Schram SB, Hosek RS, Silverman HL. Spinographic positioning errors in Gonstead pelvic x-ray analysis. J Manipulative Physiol Ther 1981;4:179–181.
10. Paul LW, Juhl JH. The essentials of roentgen interpretation. 3rd ed. New York: Harper & Row, 1972.
11. Cremata EE, Plaugher G, Cox WA. Technique system application: the Gonstead approach. Chiropractic Technique 1991;3:19–25.
12. Sinclair WK. Effects of low-level radiation and comparative risk. Radiol 1981;138:1–9.
13. Crow JF. Genetic considerations in establishing radiation doses. Radiol 1957;69:18.
14. National Council on Radiation Protection, Report No. 17,33, 34. NCRP Publications, Washington D.C., 20008.
15. Committee on Quality Assurance in Diagnostic Radiology (H-7); average patient exposure guides. CRCPD Publication 88–5, 1988:3.
16. Plaugher G, Cremata EE, Phillips RB. A retrospective consecutive case analysis of pretreatment and comparative static radiological parameters following chiropractic adjustments. J Manipulative Physiol Ther 1990;13:498–506.
17. Hecht AI, Mohrmann K. Vitamin E and low dose irradiation. ACA J Chiro 1980;14:S89–91.
18. Eastman Kodak Company. Rochester, NY 14650
19. DuPont Co. Burbank, CA 91505.
20. Gatterman B. Filtration in chiropractic. Int Rev Chiro 1985;Winter:62–63.
21. Merkin JJ, Sportelli L. The effects of two new compensating filters on patient exposure in chiropractic full spine radiography. J Manipulative Physiol Ther 1982;5:25–29.
22. Webster LL. Sportelli Wedge critique. Today's Chiro 1983;Sept/Oct:58.
23. Buehler MT, Hrejsa AF. Application of lead-acrylic compensating filters in chiropractic full spine radiography: a technical report. J Manipulative Physiol Ther 1985;8:175–180.
24. Nelson RD. The APFS x-ray view. ACA J Chiro 1980;14:S39–41.
25. Rad/Red Laboratories Inc. Oakville, Ontario.
26. Yochum TR. Evolution to revolution. Am Chiro 1990;(Sept):25–28.
27. Syllabus on diagnostic x-ray radiation protection for certified x-ray supervisors and operators. State of California Department of Health Services. Sacramento, CA, 1982:Jan.
28. Hunt D. Better ways to shield patients from radiation. Dig Chiro Econ 1981 Mar/Apr:51,125.
29. American Chiropractic College of Radiology. Radiographic guidelines for use in chiropractic. American Chiropractic College of Chiropractic Organizational Policy, 1984.
30. Howe JW, Yochum TR. X-ray, pregnancy, and therapeutic abortion: a current perspective. ACA J Chiro 1985;19(4):76–80.
31. Field TJ, Buehler MT. Improvements in chiropractic full spine radiography. J Manipulative Physiol Ther 1981;4:21–25.
32. Maurer EL. Biologic effects of x-ray exposure: an update of princi-

ples, revised maximum permissible dose recommendations and new patient protection legislation. J Am Chiro Med 1988;1:115–118.
33. Hildebrandt RW. Chiropractic spinography and postural roentgenology-part II: history of development. J Manipulative Physiol Ther 1981;4:191–201.
34. Peterson C, Gatterman MI, Wei T. Chiropractic radiography. In: Gatterman MI, ed. Chiropractic management of spine related disorders. Baltimore: Williams & Wilkins, 1990:90–110.
35. Phillips RB. An evaluation of chiropractic x-rays by the diplomate members of the American chiropractic college of roentgenology. ACA J Chiro 1980;14:S80–88.
36. Hardman LA, Henderson DJ. Comparative dosimetric evaluation of current techniques in chiropractic full-spine and sectional radiography. J Can Chiro Assoc 1981;25:141–145.
37. Zengel F, Davis BP. Biomechanical analysis by chiropractic radiography: part II. Effects of X-ray projectional distortion on apparent vertebral rotation. J Manipulative Physiol Ther 1988;11:380–389.
38. Zengel F, Davis BP. Biomechanical analysis by chiropractic radiography: part III. Lack of effect of projectional distortion on Gonstead vertebral endplate lines. J Manipulative Physiol Ther 1988;11:469–473.
39. Accurad. Nolan x-ray filters. Wanganue, New Zealand.
40. Hildebrandt RW. The chiropractic spinography issue [Editorial]. J Manipulative Physiol Ther 1981;4:171–172.
41. Denslow JS, Chace JA, Gutensohn OR, Kumm MG. Methods in taking and interpreting weight-bearing x-ray films. J Am Osteopath Assoc 1955;54:663–670.
42. Shar-Tek. c/o Sharon Logan. Life Chiropractic College West, 22336 Main St. Hayward, CA 94541.
43. White AA, Panjabi MM. Clinical biomechanics of the spine. Philadelphia: J.B. Lippincott, 1978.
44. Jackson R. The Cervical Syndrome. 4th ed. Springfield: Charles C Thomas, 1977:212–222.
45. Kirkaldy-Willis WH. Managing low back pain. New York: Churchill Livingstone, 1988.
46. Foreman SM, Croft AC. Whiplash injuries; the cervical acceleration/deceleration syndrome. Baltimore: Williams & Wilkins 1987.
47. Bailey DN. Plain film vs. videofluroscopy. ACA J Chiro 1991;28(July):59–62.
48. Russell GG, Raso VJ, Hill D, McIvor J. A comparison of four computerized methods for measuring vertebral rotation. Spine 1990;15:24–27.
49. Van Shaik JPJ, Verbiest H, Van Schaik FDJ. Isolated spinous process deviation a pitfall in the interpretation of AP radiographs of the lumbar spine. Spine 1989;14:970.
50. Jackson BL, Barker W, Bentz J, Gambali AG. Inter- and intra-examiner reliability of the upper cervical x-ray marking system: a second look. J Manipulative Physiol Ther 1987;10:157–163.
51. Kapandji I. The physiology of the joints. Vol. 3. New York: Churchill-Livingstone, 1974.
52. Shaffer WO, Spratt KF, Weinstein J, Lehmann TR, Goel V. The consistency and accuracy of roentgenograms for measuring sagittal translation in the lumbar vertebral motion segment. Spine 1990;15:741–750.
53. Saraste H, Brostrom LA, Aparisi T, Axdorph G. Radiologic measurement of the lumbar spine. Spine 1985;10:236–241.
54. Banks SD. The use of spinographic parameters in the differential diagnosis of lumbar facet and disc syndromes. J Manipulative Physiol Ther 1983;6:113–116.
55. Dupuis PR, Yong-Hing K, Cassidy JD, Kirkaldy-Willis WH. Radiologic diagnosis of degenerative lumbar spinal instability. Spine 1985;10:262–286.
56. Bronfort G, Jochumsen OL. The functional radiographic examination of patients with low-back pain: a study of different forms of variations. J Manipulative Physiol Ther 1984;7:89–97.
57. Dvorak J, Panjabi MM, Chang DG, Theiler R, Grob D. Functional radiographic diagnosis of the lumbar spine. Spine 1991;16:562–571.
58. Weitz EM. The lateral bending sign. Spine 1981;6:388–397.
59. Duncan W, Hoen TI. A new approach to the diagnosis of herniation of the intervertebral disc. Surg Gynecol Obstet 1942;75:257–267.
60. Cassidy JD. Roentgenological examination of the functional mechanics of the lumbar spine in lateral flexion. J Can Chiro Assoc 1976;July:13–16.
61. Haas M, Nyiendo J, Peterson C, et al. Interrater reliability of roentgenological evaluation of the lumbar spine in lateral bending. J Manipulative Physiol Ther 1990;13:179–189.
62. Dvorak J, Froehlich D, Penning L, Baumgartner H, Panjabi MM. Functional radiographic diagnosis of the cervical spine: flexion/extension. Spine 1988;13:748–755.
63. Dimnet J, Fischer LP, Gonon G, Carret JP. Radiographic studies of lateral flexion in the lumbar spine. J Biomech 1978;11:143–150.
64. Henderson DJ, Dormon TM. Functional roentgenometric evaluation of the cervical spine in the sagittal plane. J Manipulative Physiol Ther 1985;8:219–227.
65. Speiser RM, Aragona RJ, Heffernan JP. The application of therapeutic exercises based upon lateral flexion roentgenography to restore biomechanical function in the lumbar spine. Chiro Res J 1990;1(4):7–16.
66. Carrick FR. Cervical radiculopathy: the diagnosis and treatment of pathomechanics in the cervical spine. J Manipulative Physiol Ther 1983;6:129–135.
67. Carrick FR. Treatment of pathomechanics of lumbar spine by manipulation. J Manipulative Physiol Ther 1981;4:173–178.
68. Panjabi MM, White AA. Basic biomechanics of the spine. Neurosurgery 1980;7:76–93.
69. Kirkaldy-Willis WH, Farfan HF. Instability of the lumbar spine. Clin Orthop 1982;165:110–123.
70. Lopes MA, Plaugher G, Ray SG: Closed reduction of retrolisthesis: a report of two cases. Proceedings of the 1991 International Conference on Spinal Manipulation, 1991:110–114.
71. Singer KP, Giles LGF. Manual therapy considerations at the thoracolumbar junction: an anatomical and functional perspective. J Manipulative Physiol Ther 1990;13:83–88.
72. White AA, Southwick WO, Panjabi MM, Johnson DM. Practical biomechanics of the spine for orthopedic surgeons. Instructional course lectures. American Academy of Orthopedic Surgeons. St. Louis: CV Mosby Co., 1974
73. Lysell E. Motion in the Cervical Spine. Acta Orthop Scand 1969;123 .
74. Henderson DJ, Dorman TM: Functional roentgenometric evaluation of the cervical spine in the sagittal plane. J Manipulative Physiol Ther 1985;8:219–227.

6 Pelvis

PETER J. WALTERS

The pelvis is the means by which the weight of the erect posture is transferred to the lower limbs. Its shape and function enables the individual to perform a range of activities, such as sedentary sitting and standing, walking and running. These activities distinguish humans from their relatives on the ancestral tree, yet the literature tends to discuss the components of the pelvis in isolation.

There is considerable controversy as to the types of joints that exist in the pelvis, as well as the number of ligaments. In addition, there is debate over joint dysfunction, axes of rotation and translation, unilateral joint dysfunction, short leg syndromes, asymmetry of bones, joint innervation, accessory joints, patterns of pain, and the role of the muscles spanning the joint.

The pelvis has been overlooked by many as a potential site of dysfunction causing low back pain. During the dynasty of the disc, for most of this century, the sacroiliac articulation was virtually ignored. For many years the joint was considered immovable. When Gonstead graduated as a chiropractor in 1923, the pelvis was not considered movable or regarded as a potential site for a subluxation. Repeatedly, he observed patients with pain and edema over the sacroiliac joints after falls and lifting strains. By observing and correlating observations with x-ray findings, he developed the concept of pelvic listings to confirm the clinical observation of a sacroiliac subluxation. Indeed, Gonstead was the first to describe pelvic listings and the adjustments for their correction.

The following presentation will summarize the generally accepted view of the pelvis anatomically, functionally and clinically. More importantly, it will outline a thorough approach to what is regarded by many as the most common site for the origin of back pain.

ANATOMY

The pelvis is made up of the sacrum, two innominate bones, the coccyx, and connective tissues. It serves as a support for the vertebral column and as such, is strongly constructed to withstand the compressive forces of the trunk via the fifth lumbar vertebra. The pelvis supports and protects to some degree the viscera of the region, such as the uterus, ovaries and lower intestines, and acts as the means by which the trunk articulates with the lower limbs, thus absorbing the ground reaction forces via the acetabulae (1). The pelvis includes all structures between the fifth lumbar vertebra and the femoral heads (2) (Fig. 6.1).

In a normal fully functional pelvis, the trunk weight passes through the body of the fifth lumbar vertebra (L5) via the alae of the sacrum to the acetabulum. Ground reaction forces are transferred via each femur to its acetabulum, with some of the force passing horizontally to the pubic ramus, meeting at the pubic symphysis (3,4). The ability of the pelvis to function in this manner and provide mobility for upright movements, depends on the strength and stability of both sacroiliac joints and the pubic symphysis. The latter is universally regarded as an amphiarthrodial joint where the two osseous surfaces are connected by an elastic fibrocartilage. This allows very slight movement in all directions, depending on the elasticity of the cartilage (1,2,5).

Sacroiliac Joint

The sacroiliac joint has undergone a checkered history of description. It has been described as being amphiarthrodial and diarthrodial. The diarthrodial joint is a true synovial joint. These joints possess a cavity and are specialized to permit movement (5).

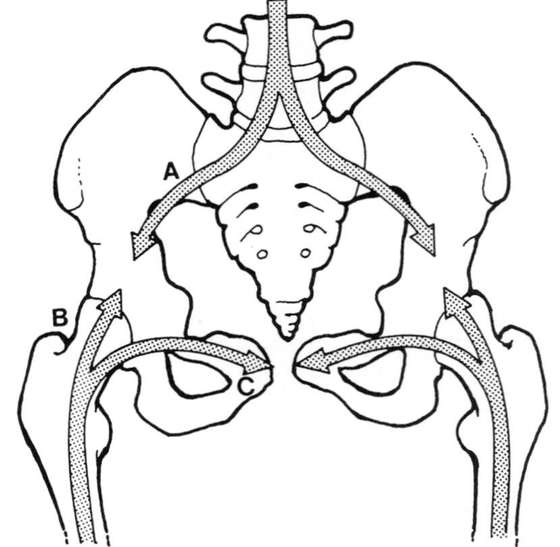

Figure 6.1. **A,** The trunk weight passes through the body of the fifth lumbar via the alae of the sacrum to the acetabulum. **B,** Ground reaction forces are transferred by each femur to its acetabulum. **C,** Some of the force passes horizontally to the pubic ramus, meeting at the pubic symphysis. Modified from Kapandji IA. The physiology of the joints. Vol 3. Edinburgh: Churchill Livingstone 1978:57.

The articular surfaces of the bones are covered with hyaline cartilage and united by an articular capsule. The inner surface of the capsule is lined by a synovial membrane that produces synovial fluid for lubrication of the joint cavity.

According to Cichoke (6), the sacroiliac joint was regarded as a diarthrodial joint in the 18th and 19th centuries by at least six authors and only regarded as amphiarthrodial in the 20th century. By the mid 20th century the joints were being described as diarthro-amphiarthrodial.

Currently, there is a consensus that the sacroiliac joint is a true diarthrodial joint. The shape has been described as auricular, facing posterolaterally on the cephalad half of the sacrum. It has an upper vertical and lower horizontal portion. The latter approaches the posterior border of the sacrum directly medial to the posterior superior iliac spine (PSIS) (7) (Fig. 6.2)

The hyaline cartilage on the sacral surface is three times as thick as the fibrocartilage on the iliac surface (8). The joint cavity is formed during the second fetal month. Grooves and ridges develop on the articular surfaces of the sacrum first, and then the ilium after puberty. The joints of the male are built for strength and have extra and intraarticular tubercles (ridges), whereas the female articulation is for mobility and parturition (6,9). Modelling of the joint progressively occurs with age. Stability increases with the hypolordotic lumbar spine. The hyperlordotic lumbar spine and female pelvis is regarded as being more diarthrodial and therefore more mobile (7,10) (Fig. 6.3).

The ventral or anterior portion of the joint (the lower two thirds) is lined by synovial membrane. The dorsal or posterior portion of the joint (the upper third) is joined by fibrous attachments and does not contain synovial tissue. The most common sacral segments articulating with the ilium are S1, S2, and S3 (11).

Bowen and Cassidy (8) demonstrated that degenerative changes occur early in life and progress with age, until by the fourth and fifth decade, the groove on the sacrum has deepened, and marginal osteophytes have developed.

Otter (3) concluded that asymmetry of the joints intrapelvically is common, and changes in the joint occur in response to imposed stress with age. He adds that during a lifetime, the sacroiliac joint probably displays a spectrum of diarthrosis, amphiarthrosis and ankylosis. The latter being rare (8). Denton (3,12) studied A-P plain radiographic films of the sacro-iliac joints and put them into 5 broad categories (Fig. 6.4 A-E).

Ligaments

The ventral sacroiliac ligament is a thickening of the anterior and inferior parts of the fibrous capsule. It is thickest where it connects the sacrum and ilium at the third sacral segment.

The interosseous sacroiliac ligament is the main connecting ligament. Its fibers are short, very strong, and run from bone to bone within the confines of the narrow cleft. Illi's ligament has been confirmed by Janse (13) and most recently by Freeman et al. (14). It courses from a posterosuperior attachment on the ilium to an anteroinferior attachment on the sacrum and is considered an anterior

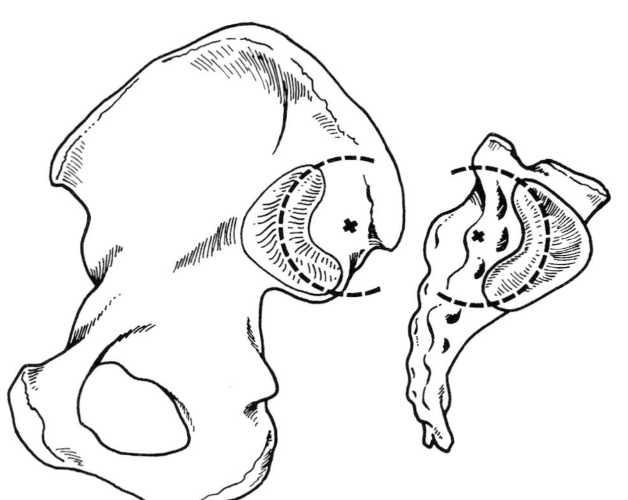

Figure 6.2. The sacroiliac joint is auricular in shape when viewed laterally having an upper vertical and lower horizontal portion. It faces postero-laterally on the cephalad half of the sacrum. The lower horizontal portion approaches the posterior border of the sacrum medial to the PSIS. Modified from Kapandji IA. The physiology of the joints. Vol 3. Edinburgh: Churchill Livingstone 1978:59.

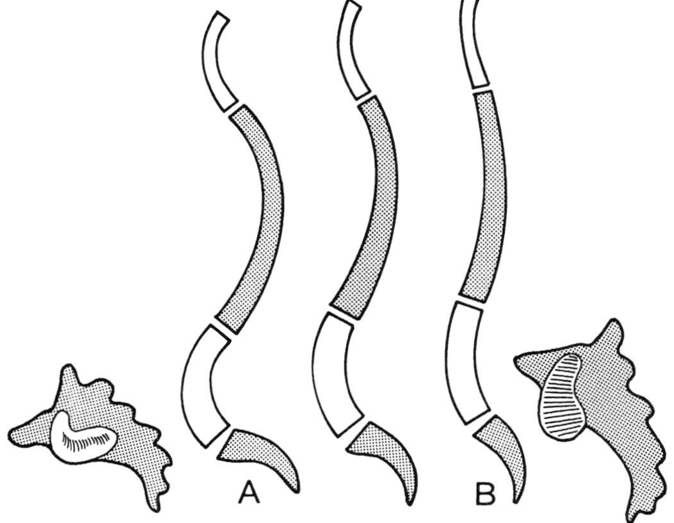

Figure 6.3. **A,** The more mobile, female sacroiliac joint is associated with a hyperlordotic lumbar spine. **B,** The stronger, less mobile, male sacroiliac joint has extra and intra articular ridges and is associated with a hypolordotic lumbar spine. Modified from Kapandji IA. The physiology of the joints. Vol 3. Edinburgh: Churchill Livingstone 1978:61.

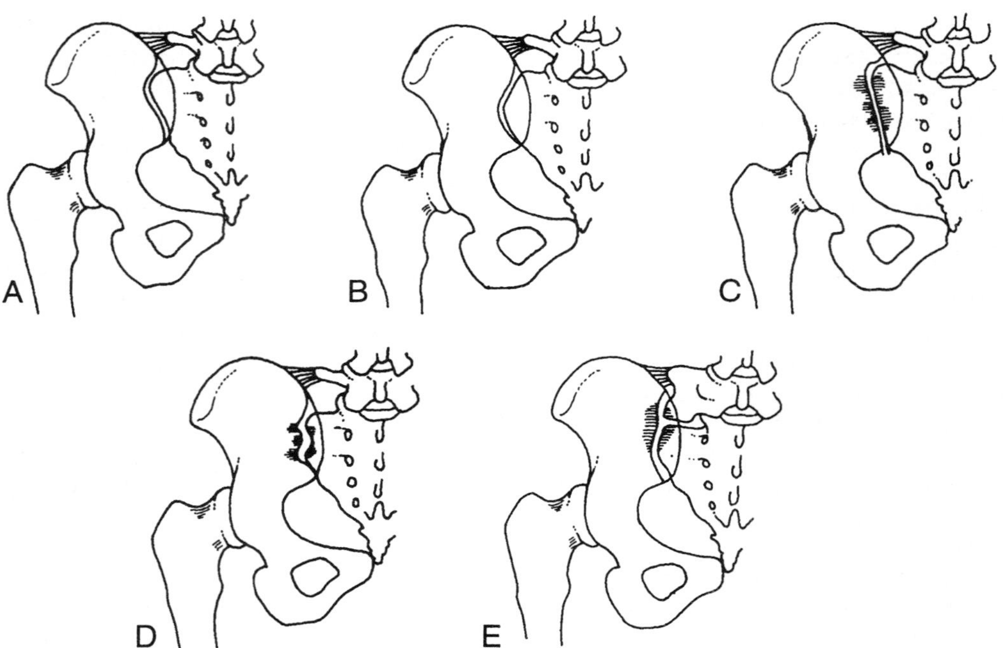

Figure 6.4. **A,** An S-shaped, normal joint. This configuration is strong and allows good mobility. **B,** A C-shaped sacroiliac joint. This configuration tends to be less stable. **C,** A straight sacroiliac joint. This joint tends to be less stable. Reactive sclerosis caused by joint stress is a common radiographic finding. **D,** This configuration has been described as an inverted "S" with a tuberous projection. It is believed to be an attempt by the structure to compensate and stabilize a prepubescent injury. **E,** Transitional articulation. Because weight-bearing ligaments are attached to the mobile transitional segment, this leads to an unstable joint. Modified from Denton D. Biomechanics of the pelvis. The Denver conference of the A.C.A Council on Technic 1980.

extension of the interosseous ligament. It limits anterior inferior movement of the sacrum.

The dorsal sacroiliac ligament overlies the interosseous ligament and between them lie the sacral spinal nerves and vessels. The upper fibers pass from the intermediate and lateral crests of the sacrum to the posterior superior iliac spine. The lower fibers pass from the third and fourth segments of the sacrum, and divide and travel obliquely to the posterior superior iliac spine, and laterally with fibers of the sacrotuberous ligament.

The sacrotuberous ligament extends from the posterior iliac spine (blends with the dorsal sacroiliac ligament) to the lower transverse tubercles of the sacrum and coccyx, and runs caudally and laterally to insert on the medial aspect of the ischial tuberosity. The falciform process is an anterior extension from this insertion along the ramus. The ligament is pierced by the coccygeal branches of the inferior gluteal artery and perforating cutaneous nerve. Vleeming et al. (15) note that gluteus maximus, piriformis, and the long head of biceps femoris attach to the sacrotuberous ligament and conclude therefore, that these muscles, via the sacrotuberous ligament, may influence movement of the sacroiliac joint.

The sacrospinous ligament is anterior to the sacrotuberous ligament. It extends from the lateral margins of the apex of the sacrum and the base of the coccyx to the spine of the ischium.

The iliolumbar ligament is attached to the tip and anterior and inferior portions of the transverse process of the fifth lumbar vertebra (with a weak attachment to the fourth lumbar vertebra transverse process) and extends via two main bands. The upper band attaches to the iliac crest and forms part of the origin of the quadratus lumborum muscle. The lower band attaches to the anterior part of the upper surface of the lateral part of the sacrum and blends with the ventral sacroiliac ligament. This ligament is actually the iliocostalis lumborum muscle in the young and gradually differentiates into a ligament (16).

The ventral, interosseous, and dorsal sacroiliac ligaments are called capsular ligaments. The iliolumbar, sacrotuberous and sacrospinous ligaments are termed accessory ligaments (3).

Innervation

Sacroiliac joint innervation is derived from the sacral and lumbar plexuses (3). Asymmetry in supply is common (17).

Lumbosacral facet joint capsules are supplied by the L5 posterior primary division, which also supplies the multifidus muscle.

The anterior aspects of the sacroiliac joint are supplied by L2–4. The actual branch, which supplies the joint, has not been identified.

Posterior and interosseous ligaments and the posterior joint are supplied by the posterior rami of S1, S2, and branches from the superior gluteal nerve (L4-S1). A plexiform network from the posterior primary rami of S1 and

S2, plus L5 and S4, covers the posterior aspect of the joint and is embedded in the dense ligamentous mass (3,18).

The sacrotuberous and sacrospinous ligaments receive fibers from S1–3. The sacrotuberous ligament receives additional branches from the anterior division of S4, from the gluteal nerve (L5-S2), and from the branches to the piriformis muscle (S1–2) and lateral head of biceps femoris (S1–2).

The iliolumbar ligament is supplied by L1 (15) with the posterior aspect supplied by the L4 lateral posterior primary division and possibly L5 (14). In summary, the sacroiliac joint innervation includes origins from L1 to S4.

PUBIC SYMPHYSIS

There are three joints in the pelvic ring; the two sacroiliac joints plus the pubic symphysis. Malfunction in one will have a destabilizing effect on the other two.

As mentioned earlier, the pubic symphysis is an amphiarthrodial joint. Under weight bearing, Kapandji (4) states that its role is to maintain the hold of the iliac bones on the sacrum via a pincer movement. The sacrum is fitted into the pelvic ring under considerable tension by the interosseous ligaments and the ligaments of the pubic symphysis (10) (Fig. 6.5).

There are arguments to suggest that the pubic symphysis is actually under traction forces during weight bearing (10). Sandoz (10) postulates that traction forces would be at a maximum when supine and that this traction force would be partially counteracted by a compression force transmitted from the ground, laterally from the femoral heads when standing.

Sandoz further points out that an uneven leg length can cause unilateral torsion to the pelvic ring, thus resulting in a posterior rotation of the innominate on the long leg side, which is evidenced by an elevated pubic bone on the A-P plain film radiograph.

Innervation

The pubic symphysis receives its innervation from L1-S4.

BIOMECHANICS

The sacroiliac joints allow an independent movement of the ilia and sacrum. It is this movement that distinguishes humans from other animals and allows them to walk upright and hold their head relatively stationary in the anteroposterior projection. The pelvis is a three joint complex, with the symphysis pubis anteriorly and the sacroiliac joints posteriorly. Because L5 is so intimately connected with the sacrum and ilium, it must also be considered when discussing the biomechanics of the pelvis.

Lumbosacral Motion

As stated previously, the coronally orientated facets, combined with the iliolumbar ligaments, allow, but control lateroflexion and rotation between L5 and sacrum and results in the hinge disc being L4–5. During flexion and extension, the hinge disc is L5-S1. If the sacrum rotates anteriorly and inferiorly on one side with the ilia, the L5 vertebral body rotates in the opposite direction. This is largely due to the restraint of the iliolumbar ligaments. Congenital anomalies, such as asymmetrical facets and transitional vertebrae, have a destabilizing influence on the pelvis and lumbar spine (3).

Sacroiliac Motion

The sacrum approaches static equilibrium in the slightly flexed, prone position (19,20). In this position, inferior and superior forces are removed.

When sitting or standing, forward flexion of the trunk causes the sacral base to pivot anteriorly and inferiorly, while the apex moves posteriorly and superiorly. At the same time, the posterior superior iliac spines move pos-

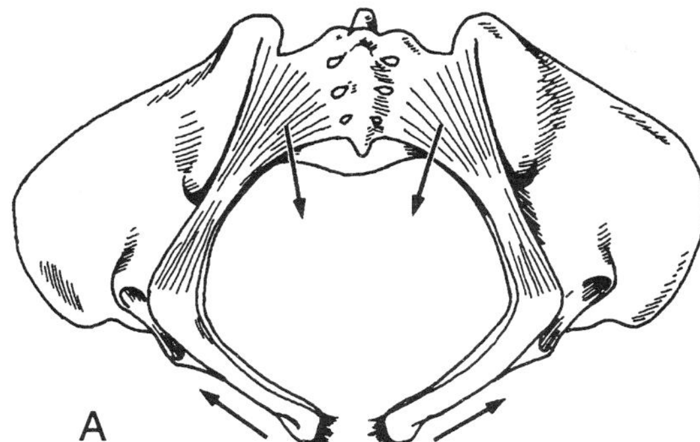

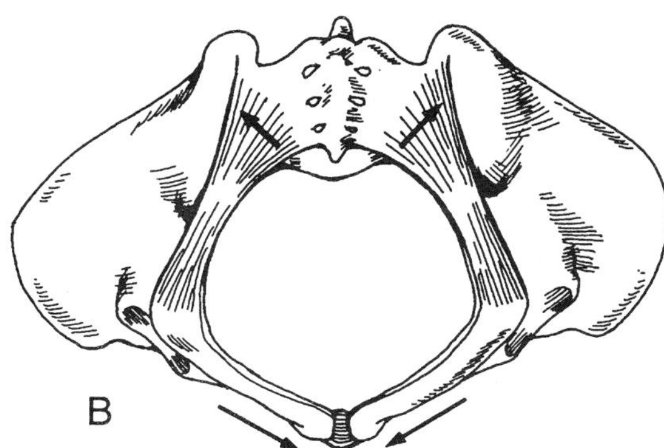

Figure 6.5. The sacrum is fitted into the pelvic ring under considerable tension by the interosseous ligaments and the ligaments of the pubic symphysis. **A,** While supine, the pubic symphysis is under traction forces. If severed, it separates and the sacrum tends to subluxate posterior to anterior (+Z). **B,** Ground reaction forces create a counteracting compression force. Modified from Kapandji IA. The physiology of the joints. Vol 3. Edinburgh: Churchill Livingstone 1978:57.

teriorly, inferiorly, and medially, relative to the sacrum. The ischia move anteriorly, superiorly and laterally. Extension induces exactly the opposite motion (19–21).

While sitting, the weight-bearing ground reaction force is essentially via the ischial tuberosities. The ischia separate and the iliac crests approximate. This induces an anterior inferior glide of the sacral base and a simultaneous posterior superior glide of the sacral apex.

On rising to the standing position, ground reaction forces now act through the femoral heads to counteract the weight bearing forces through the sacrum. This brings the ischia closer together, the iliac crests flare, the sacral base moves posteriorly, while the apex rotates anteriorly.

While in the standing position, unilateral hip flexion past 90° will result in the ipsilateral ilium rotating anterior to posterior about a horizontal axis of rotation. Whether the transverse axis is at the level of S2, symphysis pubis or is a shearing mechanism, is discussed later. This will lift the pubis upward in relation to the contralateral pubis. The posterior superior iliac spine can be palpated to move posteriorly and inferiorly in relation to the sacrum. The sacrum can be palpated to move posteriorly and inferiorly to the contralateral ilium. If hip flexion continues, the contralateral sacroiliac joint will reach its limit of movement and the whole pelvis will rotate posteriorly (19–21).

In the standing position, lateroflexion (sidebending) will induce a flaring away of the contralateral ilium.

According to Grice (22) and Faye (19), the above parameters are invoked in the following manner. On right step, as the heel strikes, the right ilium rotates posteriorly and inferiorly, the sacral base rotates anteriorly and inferiorly on the right and the right transverse process of L5 is pulled back by the connection of the iliolumbar ligament (19,20). Greenman (23) states that the lumbar spine alternates with sidebend and rotation during gait. He points out that with right heel strike, the sacrum and L5 have undergone $+\theta Y$ axial rotation. Faye, in contrast, claims that the lumbars remain relatively stable when walking, unless the pelvic biomechanics are hypomobile and further states that sacroiliac dysfunction in the young leads to abnormal gait and muscle development (19,20). Cichoke (6) reports that the strongest ligaments over the sacroiliac joint run in such a direction that the fibers tightened when the innominate rotates posteriorly and become loose when the innominate rotates anteriorly.

Gracovetsky (16), however, regards the spine as an engine transferring potential energy (from gravitational forces and that stored in muscles) plus elastic energy (in ligaments) to kinetic energy and thus forward motion during walking. This is achieved through the lordosis in the lumbar spine, producing an axial torque in side bending, called the coupled motion (See Chapter 2). This occurs at heel strike with the ground. The combination of cervical lordosis, thoracic kyphosis, and lumbar lordosis provides the axial torque that drives the pelvis, counter-rotates the shoulders, and maintains the head in a steady and neutral position. Gracovetsky concludes that the reaction of the joints in the spine and the pelvis distributes the power generated by the spinal engine. The redistribution of power caused by subluxation fixations (joint dyskinesia) is of paramount importance to chiropractors. Gracovetsky's spinal engine theory lends further credence to the chiropractic theory that subluxations will affect nerve supply to muscles which in turn will affect spinal balance and gait patterns. His theory supports the approach that emphasizes full spinal assessment in patient care (16).

In spite of the above known biomechanics of the pelvis, controversy and confusion remains as to the axis of rotation to enable the sacroiliac joint movement yet maintain pubic symphysis stability. Great confusion and debate has resulted in numerous transverse axes of rotation being identified ranging from the symphysis pubis to the S2 sacral segment, and anywhere in between.

An analysis of the methods used in trying to determine the axis of rotation clarifies the subject to a degree. Egund (24) summarized much of the research in the 19th century plus his own findings as related to sacral nutation and counternutation in trunk flexion and extension and found the transverse axis of rotation to be located at the level of S2 at the iliac tuberosity. Kapandji (4) confirms this finding, stating that the axis of rotation is immediately posterior to the sacroiliac joint. Weisl (25) found that the sacrum did not rotate about a fixed horizontal axis and described it as an angular dynamic axis 5 to 10 cm vertically below the sacral promontory. It varied for different movements of the same individual. Dontigny (26) says that in standing trunk flexion, sacral nutation occurs around a transverse axis near the central aspect of the sacroiliac joint while the innominate rotates around a transverse axis through the acetabulum.

During walking, there is a vertical, horizontal and oblique axis of rotation described. Greenman (23) and Gracovetsky (16) describe a vertical axis of rotation about which the pelvis and shoulder girdle counter-rotate providing the cross pattern upright gait. The horizontal axis of rotation when walking is described at the transverse axis of the symphysis pubis (23,27,28,29). In fact, Wells cites Pitskin and Pheasant who point out that if the transverse axis of rotation during walking was through the sacrum or hip joints, the pubic symphysis would rupture (30). Greenman (23) describes the pubic symphysis during walking as having an up and down oscillation in a sinusoidal curve with very little translation. It is the most stable point within the pelvic girdle during walking.

White and Panjabi (27) describe sidebend and rotation of the sacrum as coupled movements. They point out that a coupled motion will bring about a change in the axis of rotation and argue that at any one moment, therefore, there is an instantaneous axis of rotation.

Dontigny cites McConnell and Teall who describe a position where the ilium is forward, the ischium is backward and the innominate is thrown downward causing an apparent lengthening of the limb when the patient is prone (26). Greenman (28) describes a superior and inferior innominate shear mechanism that is caused by trauma and is related to an iliac rotation either forward or backward with concomitant alteration of each pubic bone at the symphysis. In a later paper (23) he describes how if sacroiliac joint surfaces are parallel or have a flattened convex-concave relationship, a superior to inferior translatory movement results. In addition, if the convex-concave relationship is reversed, the innominate rotates around a vertical axis resulting in medial or lateral rotation termed an in-flare or an out-flare dysfunction.

Mitchell et al. (31) summarized that there was a sacral respiration transverse axis through the PSIS, a standing sacral transverse axis through S2 with flexion and extension, and four walking axes. These were a transverse axis through S3, a transverse axis through the pubic symphysis and two diagonal axes. One from the upper left to the lower right and vice versa.

MYOFUNCTION OF THE PELVIS

The joint movement described above is the end result of leverage forces supplied by muscle action. We will use Faye's right forward step mechanism to explain this further (19,22).

In taking the right forward step, the hip flexes mainly as a result of the action of rectus femoris. Body weight transfers to the left limb and is stabilized by the left gluteus minimus and medius. This results in the right pelvis raising to a higher level (2) (as seen in Trendelenberg test). The right ilium rotates posteriorly, while the right side of the base of sacrum rotates anteriorly and inferiorly and vica versa with the left ilium. The upper sacroiliac joint on the right side is closed by the sacrospinalis muscle. The left iliopsoas contracts to counteract the right sacrospinalis contraction. The action of the posterior movement of the right ilium and support by the left gluteus minimus muscle produces a lateral pelvic shift to the left. This is allowed by the mobility of the left hip joint. Stabilization is by the action of the left piriformis muscle, which closes the left side lower sacroiliac joint and induces an external rotation of the femur. With the right ilium moving posterior and inferior, the normal coupled movement is for the ilia to externally rotate while the piriformis relaxes. This induces a medial rotation in the right femur. The forward thrust in the step by the left leg is induced by gluteus maximus and hamstring contraction on the left side. The left gluteus maximus counteracts flexion of the left hip in the above right forward step action (2).

The clinical significance of the above muscle actions is that shortened, hypertonic muscles, with an inability to relax when necessary, will induce functional dyskinesia to the pelvis. Fixation in joints result, causing a shift in the axis of rotation leading to a subluxation complex. The nerve supply to some of these muscles originates in the thoracolumbar and lumbar spine Table 6.1. The clinical significance of this will be discussed later.

Table 6.1.
The Nerve Supply (N), Segmental Derivations (S), Origins (O), and Insertions (I) of Some Key Pelvic Muscles

Gluteus Minimus
- N: Superior gluteal nerve
- S: L5-S1
- O: Outer surface of the ilium
- I: Greater trochanter

Gluteus Medius
- N: Superior gluteal nerve
- S: L5-S1
- O: Outer ilium
- I: Oblique ridge on the lateral surface of the greater trochanter

Gluteus Maximus
- N: Inferior gluteal nerve
- S: L5-S2
- O: Lateral lip of the iliac crests plus the lower lateral borders of the sacrum and coccyx
- I: Iliotibial band over the greater trochanter

Psoas Major
- N: Lumbar plexus
- S: L1-L3
- O: Transverse processes, bodies and discs of all lumbar segments
- I: Lesser trochanter of the femur

Iliacus
- N: Femoral nerve
- S: L2-L3
- O: Sacrum, iliac crest and iliac fossa
- I: Femur

Piriformis
- N: Sacral plexus
- S: L5-S2
- O: Pelvic surface of the sacrum at foramen 1-4 and margin of the greater sciatic foramen
- I: Greater trochanter of the femur

Rectus Femoris
- N: Femoral nerve
- S: L2-L4
- O: Anterior inferior iliac spine above the rim of the acetabulum
- I: Proximal border of the patella and the tibial tuberosity

Sacrospinalis (Erector Spinae)
- N: Dorsal rami from adjacent spinal segments
- S: T11-L5
- O: Medial and lateral sacral crest, medial iliac crest, dorsal sacrotuberous and sacroiliac ligaments
- I: Spinous processes of the lumbar segments plus the 11th and 12th thoracic spinous processes

Two other major muscle groups, the hamstrings and the quadriceps, need to be listed in the function of the pelvis. In forward flexion, the paravertebrals support the trunk and lumbar spine for the first 30° until ligaments take over that role (32). Beyond this, the pelvis rotates around the hip joints to allow further flexion. The degree of flexion attained now depends on the ability of the hamstrings to relax and stretch. If this is limited, greater strain is placed on spinal and pelvic ligaments leading to back strain. Shortened, hypertonic hamstrings leads to a more posterior inferior position adopted by the ilium.

Shortened hypertonic quadriceps muscles may cause a more anterior superior position being adopted by the ilium and subsequent loss of lordosis of the lumbar spine and posterior superior movement of the sacral base.

DEGENERATIVE JOINT DISEASE

The sacroiliac joint, being a diarthrodial joint with articular facets, hyaline cartilage, synovial lining and capsule, is subject to the pathologic changes that might occur in any joint, such as tuberculosis, and pyogenic and nonpyogenic arthritides (6,7).

Age-associated degenerative changes in the sacroiliac joint are common and appear around the fourth decade (33). Premature degenerative changes are seen after trauma or altered-weight bearing phenomena, such as scoliosis or leg length inequality. The radiographic signs are limited to the lower two-thirds of the joint (the synovial compartment). These include loss of joint space, subchondral sclerosis, and osteophytes (33). The vacuum phenomena, occasionally seen, is not diagnostic of degenerative joint disease in the sacroiliac joint (33) (Fig. 6.6).

Accessory sacroiliac articulations occur in 10 to 36% of population samples studied (34,35). They have been identified as arising from two possible sites (34). The more common superficial accessory sacroiliac joint is seen on the anteroposterior plain radiograph between the posterior superior iliac spine and the lateral crest of the sacrum opposite the second posterior sacral foramen. The deeper accessory sacroiliac joint is less common and is found between the large roughened tuberosity of the ilium and the smaller sacral tuberosity opposite the first posterior sacral foramen.

A small study by Bull (35) revealed that accessory sacroiliac joints are more prevalent in the more mobile sacroiliac joints, where there is an anterior inferior sacral base and an increased lumbar lordosis and sacral base angle. He postulates that it may be an attempt at stabilization in response to environmental stress in adulthood.

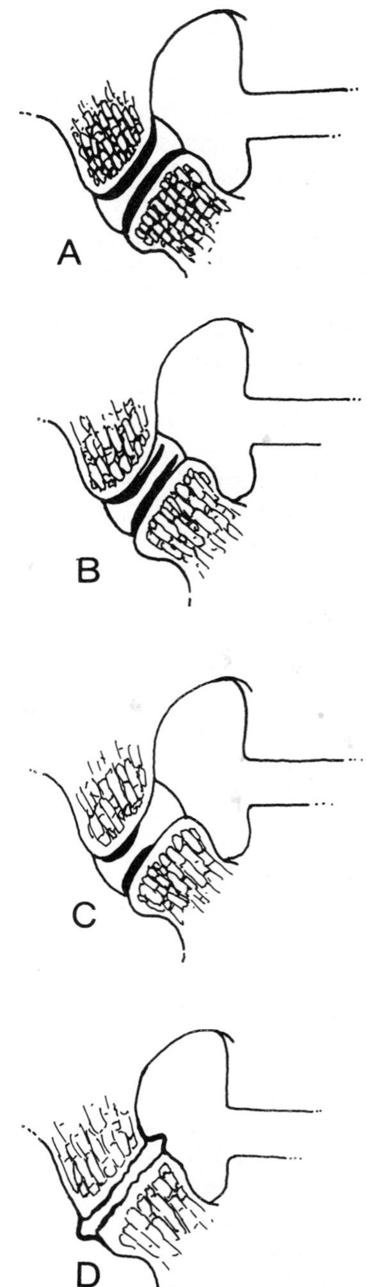

Figure 6.6. The radiographic signs in age related degenerative changes in the sacroiliac joint are limited to the lower two-thirds of the joint. **A,** Normal joint. **B, C,** Erosion of the cartilage and pseudowidening of the joint space. **D,** Narrowed joint space.

SACROILIITIS

Inflammation of the sacroiliac joint can arise from infection or by one of the inflammatory arthritides. It can be unilateral or bilateral.

The earliest sign, radiographically, is widening of the joint space and loss of the normally sharp cortical margin, due to the demineralization of the articulating bony surfaces. Narrowing of the joint space and bony ankylosis are expressions of healing and occur late in the course of inflammatory arthritis (33,35,36).

Infection is the most common cause of unilateral sacroiliitis. It occurs either by a hematogenous route or by spreading from a contiguous source (35,36). There is usually pain, tenderness, and heat in the joint area. The patient may be febrile, have an elevated erythrocyte sedimentation rate (ESR) and raised white blood cell count.

ANKYLOSING SPONDYLITIS

Ankylosing spondylitis is the most common cause for bilateral sacroiliitis. This painful condition affects predominantly young men between the ages of 15 and 35 (mostly in the third decade). The onset of symptoms is confined primarily to the low back and pelvis. HLA-B27 blood antigen is present in 90% of cases.

The sacroiliac joint involvement is best seen on plain radiographs with angulated A-P views (33). Even at its earliest clinical stages, radiographic signs are present (33,35,36). Further changes can be detected 3 to 6 months

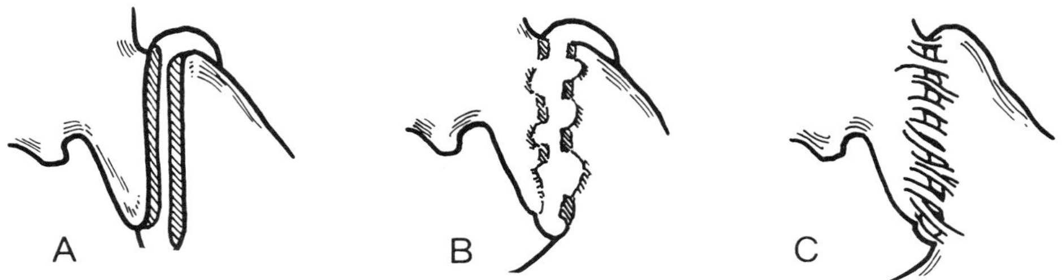

Figure 6.7. Radiographic signs in ankylosing spondylitis. **A,** Normal joint. **B,** Inflammation and erosion of the hyaline cartilage leading to the pseudowidening of the joint. **C,** Narrowed joint space and ankylosis. Modified from Yochum TR, Rowe LJ. Essentials of skeletal radiology. Baltimore: Williams & Wilkins 1987:616.

later (33). Alterations are more prevalent in the lower two-thirds of the joint, which corresponds to the synovial portion (33,35,36).

The first stage seen on the radiographs is the initial pseudowidening of the sacroiliac joint because of the inflammatory erosion of the hyaline cartilage. This occurs predominantly on the iliac side of the joint. This is followed by reactive sclerosis and bony bridging. The final stage is seen as a narrowing of the joint space. The sclerosis gradually disappears and is replaced by a generalized osteoporosis. Ossification of the ligaments occurs, leading to ankylosis of the joint (33,35,36). The time span for the three stages takes from 7 to 23 years, with a mean of 14 years (33) (Fig. 6.7).

OSTEITIS CONDENSANS ILII

This condition should be called osteosis condensans ilii because the process has been shown to be noninflammatory (10). The general consensus is that it is a direct result of a reaction to mechanical stress (10,33,35,36). Radiographically, there is bilateral, symmetrical, well defined, triangular sclerosis on the inferior portions of the iliac sides of the sacroiliac joint (35). The symptomatic patient is typically a multiparous female between 20 and 40 years of age (33). The symptoms begin during the last trimester of pregnancy and coincide with the greatest gain in weight. Sandoz (10) speculates that functional radiographs made in alternate monopodal stance shows the absence of pelvic instability. This confirms clinical examination findings of a normal Trendelenberg test (10,33). Sandoz speculates that the increased weight forces the sacrum into a $+\theta X$ rotation. This is restricted by the sacrospinous and sacrotuberous ligaments and by a bony lock constituted by the forward thrust of the first sacral segment against the ilia at the linea terminalis. In the upright position, the articular cartilage and the ilium are submitted to a constant compression and, in accordance with Wolf's law of adaptation, there is a reactive condensation of the bone (10).

The bony sclerosis is located on the ilium at the level of the linea terminalis (10) and is best depicted with an anterior posterior, 30° cephalad angulated tube projection (33).

PSORIATIC ARTHRITIS

Between 30 and 50% of individuals with psoriatic arthritis will have sacroiliac joint changes. Bilateral asymmetrical sacroiliitis is the most common presentation (33). Radiographic changes include erosions, initial widening of the joint space, hazy joint margins and sclerosis, predominantly along the length of the iliac surface (33,35). HLA-B27 antigen is present in 75 to 90% of patients with sacroiliac involvement (33,35). Clinically, the onset of sacroiliac joint changes occurs in the fourth decade.

REITER'S SYNDROME

Sacroiliac involvement is common and is usually the earliest manifestation of Reiter's syndrome. Only 50% of patients will show radiographic signs, most during the later years of the course of the disease (33,35). Radiographic signs of this disease have a tendency to be bilateral and asymmetrical. They can present as unilateral in the early stages and bilaterally symmetrical in the later stages. Radiographic signs include erosions, altered joint space and sclerosis, predominantly on the iliac side of the joint. Symptoms and signs appear from 15 to 30 years of age, accompanied by the triad of sacroiliitis, uveitis and urethritis. The blood antigen HLA-B27 is present in 75 to 90% of patients (33,35).

LEG LENGTH INEQUALITY

A short leg can be due to congenital factors, the direct result of a slipped femoral capital epiphysis, a fracture in either the femur or tibia, or paralysis from disease such as polio. Surgical alteration from hip prosthesis can cause leg length inequality as well. Sandoz (37) reports that between ⅔ and ¾ of all humans present with a difference in leg length.

The mechanism and method of treatment of LLI will be dealt with later. The biomechanical stresses and muscle imbalances caused by LLI become a complex of static forces while standing, and dynamic forces during normal gait patterns. The increased ground reaction force on the side of the long leg can cause the ipsilateral ilium to rotate posteriorly. This puts a vertical strain on the ipsilateral pubic bone, resulting in its elevation relative to the contralateral pubic bone at the symphysis. There tends to be a lumbar scoliosis convex on the short leg side. This is aggravated when the short leg moves into posterior stance during walking (10). Sciatica and unilateral hip symptoms are much more common on the side of the long leg (38).

Sandoz (10) has observed that a considerable LLI can induce a pelvic distortion. The long leg tends to rotate the innominate backwards (PI), resulting in an elevated ipsilateral pubis. This fixed posterior rotation on the ipsilateral (long leg) ilium, may favor the development of a superficial accessory sacroiliac joint.

Klein (39) observed that a compensatory mechanism, foot pronation, occurred on the side of the short leg. This resulted in genu valgus and medial collateral ligament strain and undue sacroiliac stress on the same side. Lawrence (38) reports that the short leg has overall weakness of muscle strength when compared to the long leg. Sandoz (37) cites studies that demonstrate increased activity occurring in erector spinae, gluteus maximus, anterior thigh and calf muscles on the side of the long leg, if the discrepancy is 2 cm or more.

The physical presentation of LLI, according to Sandoz (10), is that a horizontal line through the posterior superior iliac spines will show one side to be lower, whereas a line through the anterior superior iliac spines will show the situation in reverse. Altered biomechanics will lead to altered pathophysiology (10). There is considerable debate as to the significance of LLI in creating pathological states. Some authors claim 5 mm or less has a definite significance in mechanically related dysfunctions around the hips, pelvis and spine (40,41). Other investigators say less than 12.7 mm (half an inch) is not significant and has no pathologic implications (42). Giles (41) performed a study that demonstrated that a LLI of more than 9 mm induced changes in lumbar facet joint symmetry more commonly than a LLI of less than 4 mm.

Measurement of LLI can be performed via radiographic or clinical analysis. Radiographic analysis is regarded by most authors to be the most accurate. Of the clinical methods used, the most accurate assessment is to palpate the iliac crests and add lifts under the foot on the short leg side until the iliac crests are level. Of the tape measurement systems, the most accurate was the measurement from the anterior superior iliac spine to the lateral maleolus (42). The difficulty with clinical methods is in obtaining reliable, reproducible results. This can be hampered by factors such as obesity, scoliosis, and severity of back pain (38,42).

Clinical assessment of the presence of a true short leg is by Alli's test, which differentiates femoral from tibial shortness. With the patient supine and knees flexed to 90° and toes level, a disparity in knee height in the cephalad-caudal plane indicates a short tibia. Disparity in the lateral plane indicates a short femur.

Commonly seen, is the situation in which leg lengths are equal in the presence of a pronated foot. This results in a functional short leg. For ease of description, consider a right-sided congenital foot pronation. This is where the medial head of the talus has rotated internally, leading to the unlocking of the midtarsal joint (naviculo-talus joint), and a flattening of the longitudinal arch of the foot. At the same time, this induces an artificial shortening of the right leg (as the foot support collapses lower to the ground) of up to half a centimeter (43). The distal tibia follows its base (the talus) resulting in an internally rotated tibia that induces an internally rotated femur and hip joint. This adds tension to the ipsilateral iliopsoas and internal hip rotator muscles as they are stretched (43). An increased lumbosacral angle is induced, leading to hyperlordosis and a scoliosis with lumbar convexity on the ipsilateral side.

In a study of 25 patients, Smith and Markham (Personal Communication, In Shoe Systems, Bellingham,WA) found that foot pronation lead to a difference in femoral head height by up to 5 mm (average 2.2 mm) and increased the lumbosacral angle by up to 25° (average 4.1°).

GONSTEAD METHOD FOR THE PELVIS

The Gonstead technique is a system of meticulously analyzing the patient, and on the basis of all information acquired, deciding what corrective steps to take. The basic premise for this system revolves around:

i. Level Foundation
ii. Intervertebral Disc
iii. Compensation
iv. Fixation/Subluxation
v. Listing

It is the pelvis that the level foundation refers to. When level, the pelvis allows the forces of gravity to maintain the chiropractic adjustment and not work against it. In no way does this imply that the objective is for the chiropractor to straighten the spine especially if the deviation is due to malformation of the soft or hard tissue elements.

After all other tests have been performed, the radiographic line drawings and listings show the way in which the vertebra and joints have been "twisted and jammed" (fixated). This then informs the practitioner of the specific contact and direction of thrust required to reverse the positional dyskinesia and to prevent further ligamentous damage during the thrust. The adjustment restores normal function to the motion segment, thus removing neurologic dysfunction. In many instances, positional dyskinesia as indicated by listing measurements on radiographic films is reduced. If the condition is extremely chronic, there may be no positional change on re-evaluation.

Examination

The spinal examination chapter details the comprehensive approach. The following section will deal with particular topics relevant to the pelvis. Some of the topics under each heading will have relevance to previous sections on biomechanics, pathologic states, innervation, and muscle actions. The relevance of others will be seen in the clinical presentation section.

HISTORY

A standard health history should be taken to enable a thorough differential diagnosis. While this chapter is not designed to describe systems analysis, the following are a few examples designed to outline some relevant questions regarding the pelvis. For the female, of particular relevance is the number of children. This provides the practitioner with clues as to the total amount of strain on the mother's pelvis because of parturition and from bending and lifting in the first year of each child. Previous illnesses, such as abdominal disease, that could cause viscerosomatic pain, abdominal surgery, pelvic infections, joint disorders, or diseases such as osteitis condensans ilii, should be determined. Disease states such as ankylosing spondylitis, inflammatory diseases such as Reiter's, infection in blood, joints or bones, psoriasis, arthritis etc., should be queried. It is necessary to identify accidents that have caused low back pain, such as lifting strains, sporting injuries, motor vehicle accidents, sneezing or coughing fits. Fractures of the leg or pelvis can cause a shortening of the leg or hip dysfunction.

Hip prostheses can affect the function of the pelvis. The history of surgery for cancer of the bowel, kidney, prostate or uterus must be queried as these cancers can metastasize. Occupations that involve prolonged standing, bending, driving, sitting, lifting and digging can all cause postural and repetitive strain to the spine and pelvis. Age and weight can help categorize the probability of a certain condition, such as Perthe's in young teenage males, osteitis condensans ilii in multiparous females, loss of muscle tone and spinal protection in overweight unfit middle aged males, and osteoporosis in post menopausal females.

A detailed description of the pathomechanics of all micro/macro traumatic episodes that the patient has experienced should be taken. This should include the site of the symptoms as well as aggravating and relieving factors. A sacroiliac subluxation is usually aggravated with prolonged standing and walking and is relieved with sitting. Disc problems in the lumbar spine will be aggravated with sitting.

POSTURAL ANALYSIS

Postural analysis is conducted to determine abnormal postural and gravitational stresses on the spine. Of particular importance in the coronal plane is the relative levels of the posterior-superior iliac spines, the iliac crests, greater trochanters, gluteal folds and anterior-superior iliac spines. These observations provide initial indications of a level foundation, possible pelvic subluxations, and anatomic LLI. The spine is examined for scoliosis, and differentiation of functional or structural scoliosis is determined with Adam's test (See Chapter 9). Foot pronation and the integrity of the longitudinal arch is investigated because this may contribute to LLI. Laterally, observation is made of the spinal curves, particularly the degree of lumbar lordosis, pelvic tilt and abdominal muscle tone is noted. Included in this examination is an analysis of gait. A shorter stride on one side may indicate a short leg or a fixation dysfunction at the sacroiliac joint. Foot pronation must also be observed for during this procedure.

PHYSICAL EXAMINATION

A thorough orthopedic and neurologic examination is required, including vital signs. Of particular relevance is the differential diagnosis of disc herniation, nerve root inflammation, and myofascial trigger point pain referral patterns. In addition, relative shortening and weakness of the iliopsoas, quadriceps, and hamstring muscles should be investigated.

STATIC PALPATION

Attention should be directed to locate areas of tenderness, edema (e.g. PI has edema in the posterior superior area of the sacroiliac joint, AS in the posterior inferior area of the sacroiliac joint and Ex in the entire posterior area of the joint), heat, and hypertonic muscle changes. This provides vital clues as to the histopathologic, myopathologic and biochemical components of the subluxation complex.

MOTION PALPATION

The pelvis is a closed kinematic system. To locate and isolate joint fixation dysfunction and compensatory hypermobility, the motion of the sacroiliac joints, pubic symphysis, and lumbosacral joints require examination. It is clinically accepted by many authors (19,20,21,32,44, 45,46) that the motion of sacroiliac joints can be palpated and observed. As such, fixations can be located based on both the aberrant patterns of motion and the juxtaposition of two opposing bones at the joint surface. There are thirteen methods for motion palpating sacroiliac joints currently described.

Sitting Sacroiliac Motion Palpation of Axial Rotation. To palpate the left sacroiliac joint, the practitioner stands on the left side of the seated patient, facing them obliquely. The left hand is placed on the patient's right shoulder. The tip of the right middle finger is placed on the patient's left posterior superior iliac spine, while the tip of the index finger rests on the immediately adjacent sacrum. The practitioner actively rotates the patient's slightly flexed trunk to the left. This movement will create motion at the sacroiliac joint and the fingers will separate. The practitioner moves to the right side to palpate the right sacroiliac joint.

Prone Sacral Push. The practitioner applies firm vertical, downward pressure to the sacrum of the prone patient. The patient's feet should be extending comfortably over the end of the pelvic bench. With normal sacroiliac motion, the feet will externally rotate when the pressure is applied. They return to neutral when the pressure is released. If there is a sacroiliac fixation, the foot on the fixated side will either move sideways or lift slightly.

Sitting Side Bend. The practitioner is positioned behind the seated patient and places each thumb on each of the patient's posterior superior iliac spines. The patient is asked to actively sidebend while maintaining both buttocks firmly in contact with the surface on which they are seated. The normal motion is for both posterior superior iliac spines to stay level. If one joint is fixated, the PSIS on the fixated side will ride up with contralateral side bend.

Knee Chest Push Pull. With the patient positioned correctly on the knee chest table, the practitioner's thumbs are placed over the posterior superior iliac spines of the patient with each hand wrapping around toward the anterior superior iliac spine. A series of counteracting, alternating push pull moves are made, feeling for motion in each of the sacroiliac joints.

Knee Chest Rocking. With the patient positioned correctly on the knee chest table, the practitioner places the right thumb on the second sacral tubercle and the tip of the index finger on the posterior superior iliac spine. The patient is rocked alternately left, then right. As the patient rocks to the left, the thumb and index finger should approximate. They then separate with rocking to the right. In a fixated segment, no gliding action occurs when rocking to that side.

Standing Flexion. The practitioner is located behind the standing patient with the right thumb placed on the apex of the patient's sacrum and the tip of the right index finger placed on the right posterior superior iliac spine. As the patient flexes forward, the thumb and index finger separate with a normally functioning sacroiliac joint. This test is repeated as for the left side.

Sitting Flexion. The practitioner is located behind the seated patient and places each thumb on each of the patient's posterior superior iliac spines. The patient is asked to actively flex their trunk while maintaining both buttocks firmly in contact with the surface of the couch. During this action both thumbs should remain level. If one segment is fixated, the thumb over the PSIS on the fixated side will ride up.

Standing Side Bend. Contact as in Sitting Side Bend Test and the patient is asked to actively side bend, keeping both feet firmly in contact with the ground. The normal motion is for the posterior superior iliac spines to glide naturally but remain level. If one joint is fixated, the segment on the fixated side will ride up with contralateral side bend.

Standing Knee Bend PSIS Contact. The contact is the same as in standing side bend. The patient flexes the knee and elevates it as high as possible, in a smooth action achieving maximal active hip flexion. With normal motion, the posterior superior iliac spine on the side of hip flexion moves inferiorward while the contralateral side remains higher. The degree of inferiorward excursion should be compared bilaterally.

Standing Knee Bend PSIS-Sacrum Contact

A. *Flexion Component of the Upper Sacroiliac Joint:* The practitioner is located behind the standing patient. To test the right sacroiliac joint, the right thumb is placed on the right posterior superior iliac spine of the patient. The left thumb is placed on the second sacral tubercle. The patient flexes the right knee and elevates it as high as possible in a smooth action achieving maximal active hip flexion. In normal movement, both thumbs approximate as the ilium moves posteriorly and inferiorly and the sacrum moves anteriorly and inferiorly. If the joint is fixated, both thumbs move as one unit and fail to approximate. This theoretically tests the upper sacroiliac joint flexion component.

B. *Extension Component of the Upper Sacroiliac Joint:* Contact as in (a). The patient flexes the left knee and elevates it as high as possible in a smooth action, achieving maximal active hip flexion. In normal movement, both thumbs separate as the ilium moves anteriorly and superiorly and the sacrum moves posteriorly and superiorly. If the joint is fixated, both thumbs move as one unit and fail to approximate. This tests the upper sacroiliac joint extension component.

C. *Flexion Component of the Lower Sacroiliac Joint:* The practitioner's left thumb contacts the sacral apex, while the right thumb contacts the inferior aspect of the sacroiliac joint on the ischium. For the right joint, the patient flexes the right knee as in (a). When movement is normal, the practitioner's right thumb moves laterally. When the joint is fixated, the practitioner's right thumb moves slightly upward as the patient elevates the right knee.

D. *Extension Component of the Lower Sacroiliac Joint:* The contact is the same as in (c). The patient elevates the left knee. When movement is normal, the practitioner's right thumb moves upward. If the joint is fixated, no movement is discernible.

INSTRUMENTATION

The subject of the use of the bilateral temperature differential instruments such as the Nervoscope for measuring temperature asymmetries of the spinal column has been dealt with earlier in Chapter 4. Although criteria have been set down for conducting and interpreting readings over the spinal column, the interpretation for the pelvis remains poorly defined. The Nervoscope can register for a sacroiliac subluxation. This occurs more reliably when the subluxation is in the acute, inflammatory state. Chronic fixations may or may not register a temperature differential. To obtain a reading it helps to "tilt" the Nervoscope from side to side (i.e., $\pm\theta Z$ movement).

A PIEx subluxation will tend to give a temperature differential at the upper sacroiliac joint, presumably because this is the area of inflammation (44).

An ASIn subluxation will tend to give a temperature differential at the lower sacroiliac joint, presumably because this is the area of inflammation.

A base posterior sacrum will usually cause a temperature differential at the lumbosacral junction. For an acute condition, a significant change in the instrument reading after the adjustment can take at least 6 hours.

As presented in the section on innervation of the sacroiliac joint, the segmental innervation extends from L1 to S4. Additionally, the innervation of the anterior and posterior aspects of the amphiarthrodial and diarthrodial portions of the joint at the same level differs. Further work needs to be done in this area to lay down firm criteria for conducting and interpreting the use of the Nervoscope on the pelvis. Therefore, at this stage, observation and palpatory assessments are the preferred examinations, supported with plain film radiography (44,46).

Clinical Presentations and Management

The sacroiliac joint can present with a diversity of symptoms and signs that require very careful analysis. Researchers have found that pain in the sacroiliac joint was associated with either marked increases or decreases in mobility of the joint (47). Sacroiliac joint fixation was found in 28.1% of school age children 6 to 17 years of age. In the same study, low back pain was present in 23.5%. This gave a significant association between sacroiliac hypomobility and a history of low back pain (48).

Sacroiliac pain may be characterized by low back pain plus pain and localized tenderness over the joint, extending to the buttock, groin, genitalia, trochanteric region, mainly posterior, but also medial and anterior. It may also cause thigh pain, pain that extends to the heel, and lateral border of the foot (3,7,20,21,32,45,48,49). It is commonly referred and the extent of the referral is regarded as an indication of the severity of the nerve root inflammation (49). In a literature review by Otter, the peripheral nociceptive system is classified into interstitial and perivascular nociceptive receptors (3). The systems are activated by sufficiently severe degrees of mechanical tissue distortion or marked chemical alteration of the tissue fluid. Thus, he describes mechanical changes as giving rise to pressing, stabbing, bursting or vise-like sensations and chemical alterations as scalding or burning sensations.

If we can generalize about the complex pelvic area in relation to the sacroiliac joint then, typically, the patient has hurt the sacroiliac joint with a lifting and twisting action. This results in a grabbing sensation in the back which worsens to the point of the patient experiencing difficulty rising from the bed the next morning. There is unilateral pain and no neurologic signs. Difficulty is experienced rising from a prolonged sitting position and can be aggravated by walking. Stabbing pain is experienced with certain movements, particularly ipsilateral side bending when standing.

Management of an inflamed sacroiliac subluxation requires that ice be applied after the adjustment for 10 to 15 minutes every hour, as is practicable, for at least 24 hours. After the adjustment, the patient should go for a 5- to 10-minute walk. This is of utmost importance in the pelvis, because walking will help mobilize the pelvic joints. To get straight into a car, either to drive or be driven home, is contraindicated. Under no circumstances is heat applied to an acute inflammatory low back condition.

The chronic degenerative condition will usually undergo a more gradual improvement. Because of chronic ligamentous contracture, it may not be possible to obtain an audible set initially. These patients need a number of adjustments to restore normal joint function.

The Pelvic Bench

The patient lies on their side, on the third of the table nearest to the doctor, who is standing at the side of the pelvic bench (Fig. 6.8) (50). The patient's down side leg is pushed to a straight position so that the foot extends over the end of the bench corner (for ease of rolling). The head is on its side, facing the side the doctor is standing on, with the neck in a neutral position. The patient's shoulders are positioned in a vertical plane with the downside shoulder being drawn slightly caudally. The patient's hands are approximated in a comfortable position near the trunk. The high side leg is flexed at the hip and knee so that the foot is hooked behind the knee of the low side leg.

The doctor stands facing the patient approximately at the level of their pelvis. Skin on skin contact is made so that the joint is palpated with the doctor's cephalad hand and slack tissue pulled in the direction of the intended adjustment. The pisiform or finger of the caudad hand is then applied to the joint being adjusted. The patient's

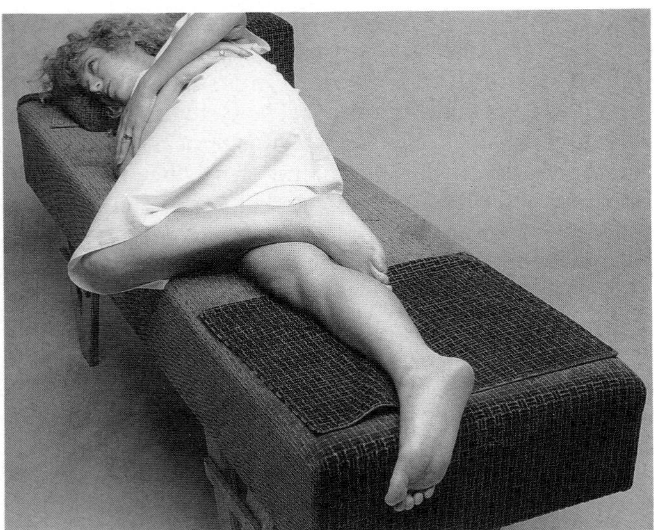

Figure 6.8. Basic position on the pelvic bench.

high side knee is straddled and moved cephalad until the joint is felt to move back into the pisiform contact hand. The knee is then brought back to reduce the tension in the sacroiliac joint.

The cephalad hand cups the anterior inferior aspect of the acromioclavicular portion of the shoulder joint and applies a slight pressure in a cephalad direction. The doctor maintains shoulder and pisiform contact and steps back slightly from the bench. The patient is rolled to the side towards the doctor who then places the anterior thigh of the caudad leg gently along the side of the patient's thigh. The cephalad leg is positioned approximately level with the patient's lower rib cage while the same foot is pointing toward the shoulder contact.

The end result is that the doctor's caudad leg should be straight. It should be making ground contact with the ball of the foot, inducing a straight back and comfortable preadjustment stance, resulting in no spinal strain to the doctor and the patient.

The adjustment is executed by lowering the caudad elbow to enable the forearm to point in the direction of the thrust. The push move adjustment is executed by dropping to set the joint followed with a holding for two seconds. There should be no recoil or rebound. No thrust should be applied to the patient's shoulder. In essence, the doctor will roll the patient over, get him or her to relax, then thrust and hold.

The Knee Chest Table

The patient kneels and rests both head and upper anterior chest on the head rest section while holding onto the side hand grips. Both knees are separated sufficiently to be as wide as both hip joints. Both femurs should be sloping 5–10° caudad from the vertical. The ankles have the same separation distance as the knees. The shoulders should be the same height as the hip and pelvic joints (See Chapter 7).

PI Ilium

The ilium portion of the innominate articulates with the sacrum. A posterior inferior ilium is one that has rotated about the center of axis and juxtapositioned itself in a posterior and inferior position relative to the sacrum. In fact, it has rotated counter clockwise around the X axis ($-\theta X$) and posterior on the Z axis (-Z). It is relatively fixated in this position.

AP FILM ANALYSIS

The vertical height of the innominate from the iliac crest to the ischial tuberosity increases (Fig. 6.9). This also occurs on the lateral film. The size of the obturator foramen increases, in vertical and diagonal length. The PI ilium causes the femoral head to appear lower. This creates a functional shortening of the leg length.

LATERAL FILM ANALYSIS

There may be an increased lumbar lordosis on the lateral film or an increased sacral base angle.

CLINICAL FINDINGS

For a PI ilium, the posterior superior aspect separates and becomes edematous (Fig. 6.10). The posterior superior aspect can be statically palpated for edema and tenderness. A PI ilium induces a relative anterior inferior shift of the ipsilateral sacral base.

An increased lumbar lordosis may result from a PI ilium subluxation. The gluteal fold is lower on the side of the PI ilium. The leg length check will likely reveal a short leg on the PI side, unless an anatomical discrepancy is present.

Name of technique: Gonstead

Name of technique procedure: Side posture PI ilium push adjustment (Fig. 6.11).

Indications: PI subluxation.

Contraindications: All other listings, hypermobility, instability, lytic metastasis in the region, inability to lie in the side posture position, previous hip replacement surgery.

Patient position: The patient lies in the side posture position on the pelvic bench. The PI ilium is on the high side.

Doctor's position: The doctor adopts the side posture position for the pelvic bench.

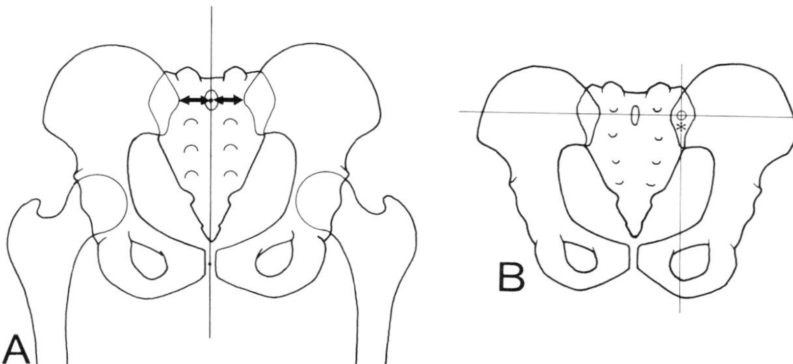

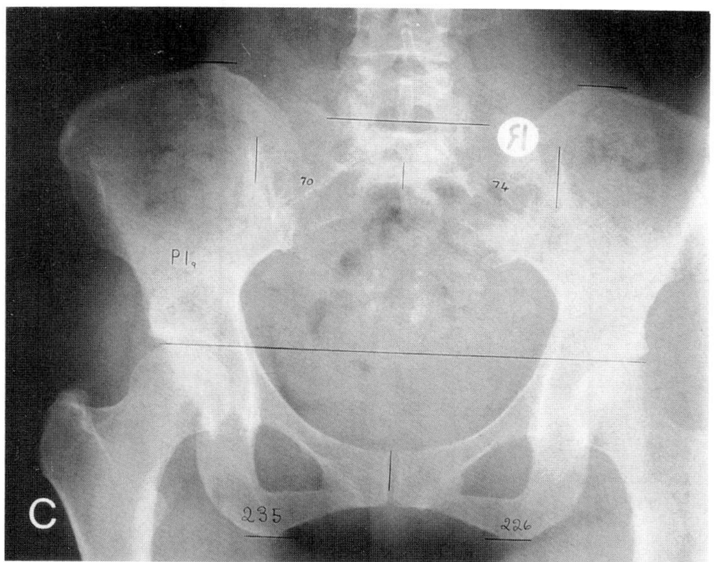

Figure 6.9. **A,** Normal AP pelvis. **B,** Right PI ilium with increased vertical height of the innominate and increased diagonal and vertical length of the obturator foramen. **C,** Plain film of left PI ilium.

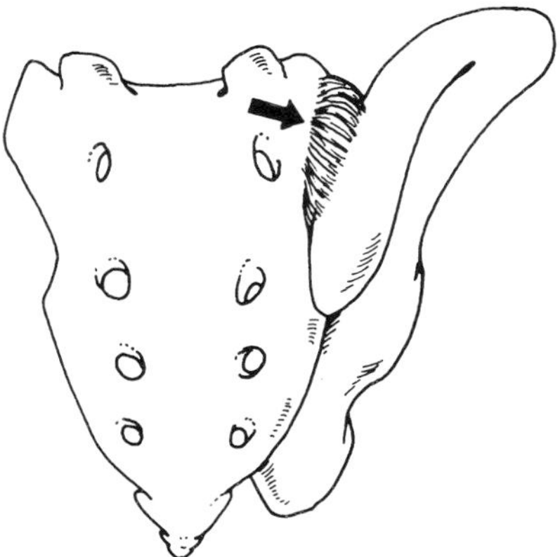

Figure 6.10. A PI ilium showing the palpable edematous and tender area of the sacroiliac joint.

Contact Point: Skin on skin contact is made so that the doctor's cephalad hand takes up slack tissue in a cephalad direction over the high side PSIS. The pisiform of the caudad hand is applied to the posterior inferior border of the high side PSIS. The patient's high side knee is straddled and moved cephalad until the PSIS is felt to move back into the pisiform contact hand. The knee is then brought back slightly until the tension in the joint is felt to release.

Supporting hand: The doctor supports the anterior shoulder as described in the side posture position for the pelvic bench.

Pattern of thrust: The doctor lowers the caudad elbow to the level of the contact point to allow the direction of thrust to be posterior to anterior ($+Z$) and inferior to superior ($+\theta X$) in the direction of the plane of movement of the sacroiliac joint.

Name of technique: Gonstead

Name of technique procedure: Hi-lo prone PI ilium push adjustment.

Indications: PI subluxation.

Contraindications: All other listings, hypermobility, instability, lytic metastasis in the region, inability to lie prone.

Patient position: The patient lies prone, with both arms resting over the side of the table.

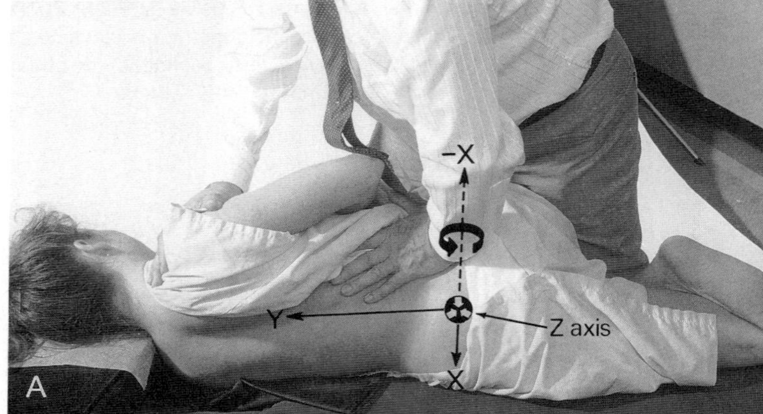

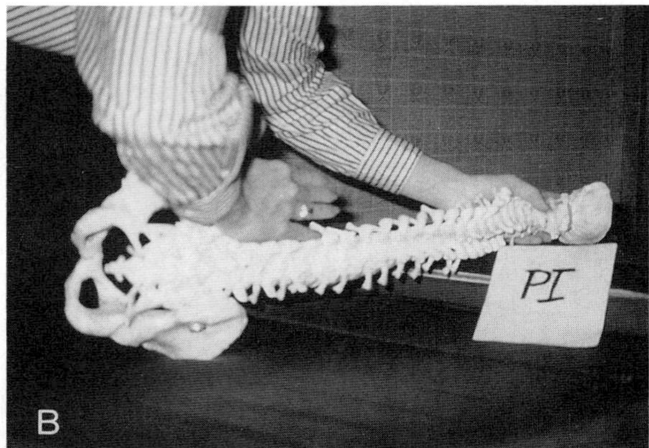

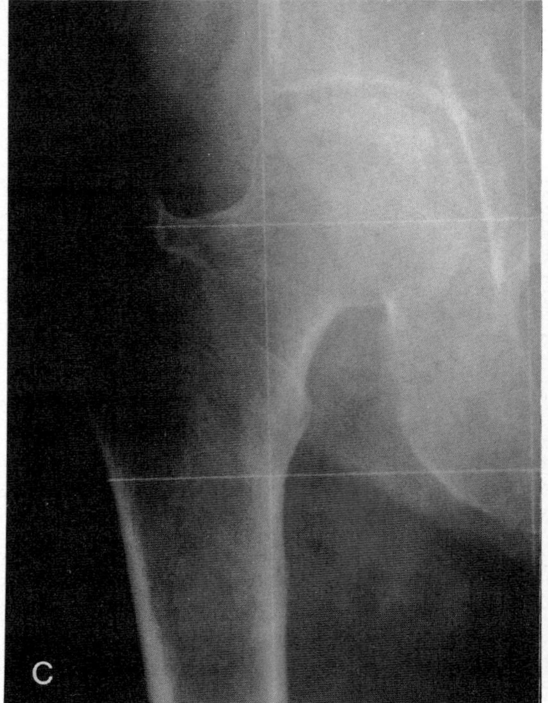

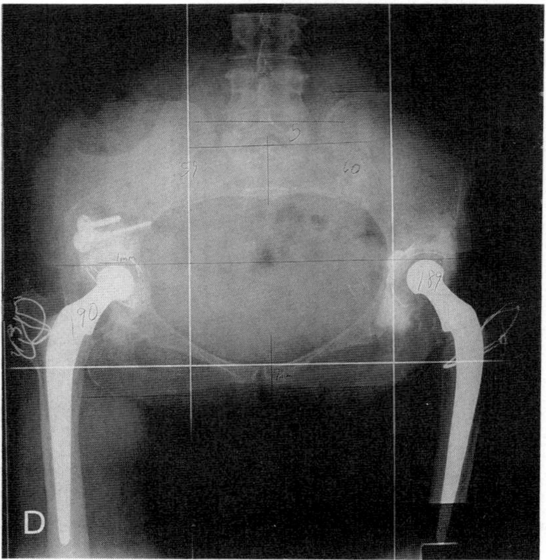

Figure 6.11. **A,** Correct set up for a side posture right PI ilium push adjustment. **B,** Left PI set-up on an anatomic model. **C,** Lytic metastasis of the proximal femoral shaft—a contraindication for side posture adjustments. This patient died one month after the radiograph was taken. **D,** Bilateral hip prostheses. A contraindication for side posture adjustments.

Doctor's position: The doctor stands on the opposite side of the patient's PI ilium at the level of the patient's thigh and as close to the table as possible with the outside foot placed directly in front of the inside foot.

Contact point: The contralateral PI ilium is skin to skin contacted with the heel of the doctor's inside hand just inferior to the PSIS.

Supporting hand: The doctor's outside hand stabilizes the near side AS ilium at the ischial spine with the heel of the hand.

Pattern of thrust: The adjustment is made by applying pressure to take up tissue slack and thrusting with a straight arm in a posterior to anterior direction ($+Z$) and inferior to superior ($+\theta X$) in the plane of movement of the joint. The joint is set and held for 2 seconds. No rebound is made. No thrust is made with the stabilizing hand.

Name of technique: Gonstead

Name of technique procedure: Knee chest PI ilium push adjustment.

Indications: PI subluxation.

Contraindications: All other listings, hypermobility, instability, lytic metastasis in the region, inability to kneel or extend the lumbar spine.

Patient position: The patient assumes the basic position.

Doctor's position: The doctor stands behind the patient and straddles their ankles.

Contact point: The heel of one hand contacts inferior to the PSIS of the PI ilium.

Supporting hand: The AS ilium is stabilized by contacting the ischial spine with the heel of the hand.

Pattern of thrust: The adjustment is made by applying pressure to take up tissue slack and thrusting in a posterior to anterior (+Z) and inferior to superior (+θX) direction in the plane of movement of the joint. The joint is set and held for 2 seconds. There is no rebound. No thrust is made with the stabilizing hand. Care should be taken that the patient's pelvis is balanced centrally over the knees before the adjustment.

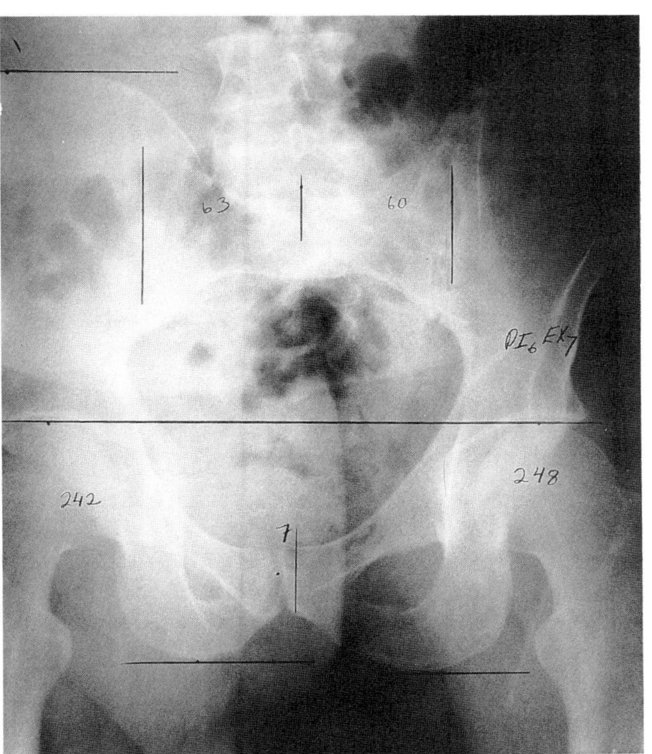

Figure 6.12. Plain film line drawing of a right PIEx ilium with increased vertical height of the innominate and increased diagonal measurement and width of the obturator foramen.

PIEx Ilium

In rotating counterclockwise to assume a posterior inferior (PI) position (−Z, −θX), the ilium may flare away from the sacrum in a −θY rotation on the left or a +θY on the right, and is thus listed as having moved externally (Ex).

AP FILM ANALYSIS

The vertical height of the innominate from the iliac crest to the ischial tuberosity increases (Fig. 6.12). The size of the obturator increases. The PI increases the diagonal measurement. The Ex increases the width. The femoral head is lower. The PI lowers the femoral head. The Ex also lowers the femoral head.

LATERAL FILM ANALYSIS

There may be an increased lumbar lordosis on the lateral film. The PI increases the lumbar lordosis. The Ex may also increase it.

CLINICAL FINDINGS

The PI opens the joint space at the posterior superior and anterior inferior margins. The Ex opens the posterior joint space. The combined result is an increased opening of the posterior superior joint space creating a palpable, tender and edematous region.

Name of technique: Gonstead

Name of technique procedure: Side posture PIEx ilium push adjustment (Fig. 6.13).

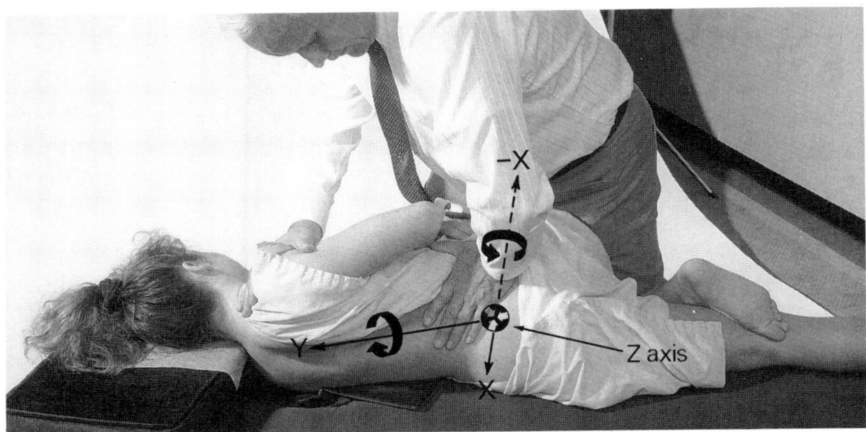

Figure 6.13. Side posture right PIEx ilium push adjustment.

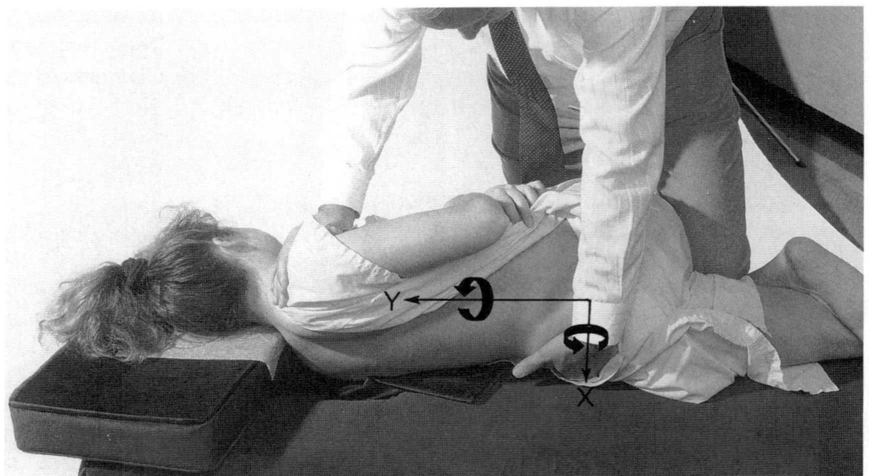

Figure 6.14. Side posture PIEx pull adjustment.

Indications: PIEx subluxation.

Contraindications: All other listings, hypermobility, instability, lytic metastasis in the region, inability to lie in the side posture position, previous hip replacement surgery.

Patient position: The patient adopts the side posture position on the pelvic bench. The PIEx ilium is on the high side.

Doctor's position: The doctor adopts the side posture position for the pelvic bench.

Contact point: The pisiform of the caudad hand is applied to the inferior and lateral border of the PSIS. The patient's high side knee is straddled and moved cephalad until the PSIS is felt move back into the pisiform of the contact hand. The knee is then brought back slightly until the tension in the joint is felt to release.

Supporting hand: The doctor supports the anterior shoulder as described in the side posture position for the pelvic bench.

Pattern of thrust: The doctor lowers the caudad elbow to a level that is higher than the contact point, ensuring that the direction of thrust is posterior to anterior ($+Z$), inferior to superior ($+\theta X$), and lateral to medial ($-\theta Y$ on right, $+\theta Y$ on left). The contact hand is torqued clockwise to induce $-\theta Y$ movement if the patient is right side up, and anticlockwise to induce $+\theta Y$ motion if the patient is left side up.

Name of technique: Gonstead

Name of technique procedure: Side posture PIEx pull adjustment (Fig. 6.14).

Indications: PIEx subluxation.

Contraindications: All other listings, hypermobility, instability, lytic metastasis in the region, inability to lie in the side posture position, previous hip replacement surgery.

Patient position: The patient lies in the side posture position for the pelvic bench with the PIEX ilium on the down side.

Doctor's position: The doctor adopts the side posture position for the pelvic bench with some slight modification for the contact point.

Contact point: The doctor's cephalad hand lifts the patient's pelvis to enable the caudad hand to slide under the ilium so that the fingers extend around to the ASIS. The pelvis is released by the cephalad hand and allowed to rest totally on the doctor's caudad contact hand. The contact hand is drawn supero-medial to take up tissue slack and bring the pisiform inferior and lateral to the PSIS. At this point the fingers of the contact hand are inferior to the PSIS. If the Ex is a greater component, the fingers are moved to a more lateral position. If the PI is a greater component, the fingers are moved to a more inferior position.

Supporting hand: The doctor supports the anterior shoulder as described in the side posture position for the pelvic bench. The patient's pelvis is stabilized by the doctor resting the caudad knee against the posterior thigh of the patient's flexed high side leg.

Pattern of thrust: The thrust is posterior to anterior ($+Z$) in an inferior to superior ($+\theta X$) and lateral to medial ($+\theta Y$ on left $-\theta Y$ on right) direction via the pisiform contact. No thrust is given by the doctor's knee.

Name of technique: Gonstead

Name of technique procedure: Hi-lo prone PIEx ilium push adjustment.

Indications: AS ilium.

Contraindications: All other listings, hypermobility, instability, lytic metastasis in the region, inability to kneel or extend the lumbar spine.

Patient position: The patient assumes the basic position.

Doctor's position: The doctor stands behind the patient and straddles their ankles.

Contact point: The heel of the adjusting hand contacts the ischial spine of the AS ilium.

Supporting hand: The PI ilium is stabilized by contacting the PSIS with the heel of the hand.

Pattern of thrust: The adjustment is made by applying pressure to take up tissue slack. The thrust is made with a straight arm in a posterior to anterior direction, indicated by the shaft of the femur on the AS ilium side, to create a $-\theta X$ movement. Care must be taken not to thrust with the stabilizing hand.

ASIn Ilium

In rotating clockwise around the X axis to assume an anterior superior position (AS), the ilium may move toward the sacrum in a $+\theta Y$ direction on the left or a $-\theta Y$ on the right and is thus listed as having also moved internally (In).

AP FILM ANALYSIS

The vertical height of the innominate from the iliac crest to the ischial tuberosity decreases (Fig. 6.20). The size and shape of the obturator foramen decreases. The AS decreases the diagonal measurement. The In decreases the width. The femoral head height is raised. The AS raises the femoral head height. The In raises the femoral head height. This occurs, assuming no other factors are involved that affect leg length inequality.

LATERAL FILM ANALYSIS

The lumbar lordosis decreases. The AS decreases the lumbar lordosis. The In also decreases the lumbar lordosis.

CLINICAL FINDINGS

The AS opens the sacroiliac joint at the posterior inferior aspect. The In opens the anterior joint space. The combined result is an increased opening in the anterior superior sacroiliac joint space. Palpable edema and tenderness may not be present. There may be groin pain associated with damage to the anterior ligamentous elements of the sacroiliac joint.

Name of technique: Gonstead

Name of technique procedure: Side posture ASIn ilium push move adjustment (Fig. 6.21).

Indications: ASIn subluxation.

Contraindications: All other listings, hypermobility, instability, lytic metastasis in the region, inability to lie in the side posture position, previous hip replacement surgery.

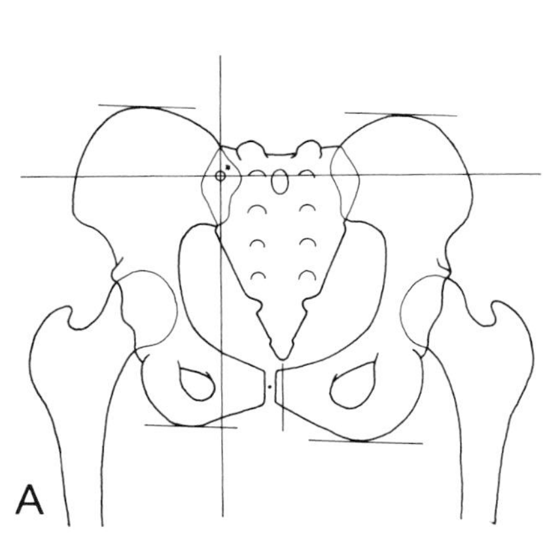

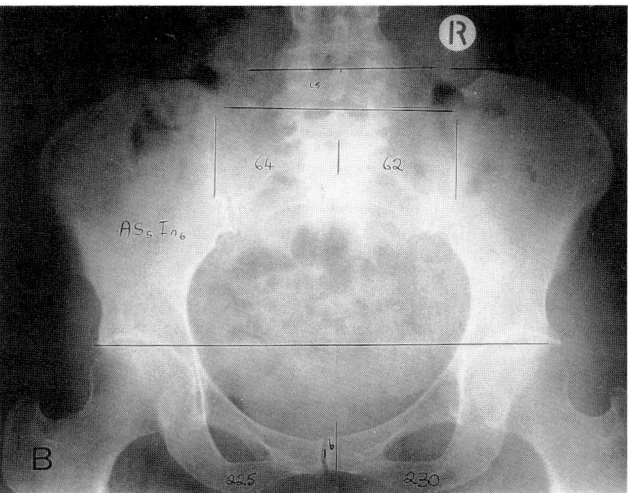

Figure 6.20. **A,** Left ASIn ilium with decreased vertical height of the innominate and decreased diagonal measurement and width of the obturator foramen. **B,** Plain film of a left ASIn ilium.

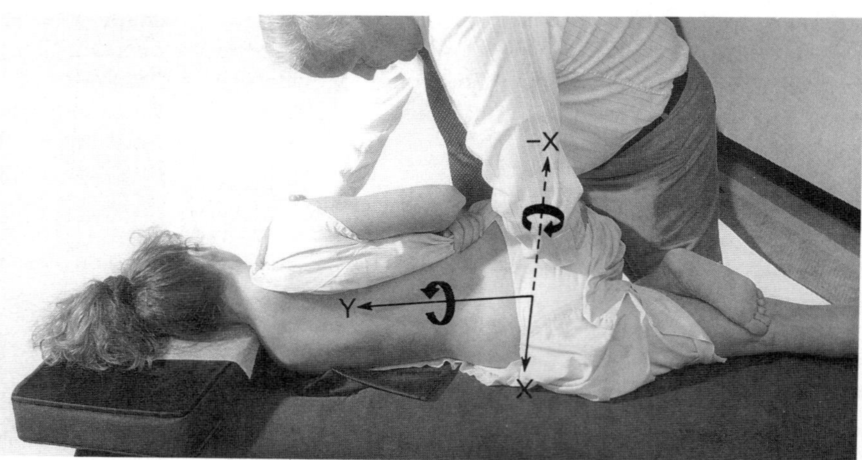

Figure 6.21. Side posture right ASIn ilium push move.

Patient position: The patient lies in the side posture position on the pelvic bench. The ASIn ilium is on the high side.

Doctor's position: The doctor adopts the side posture position for the pelvic bench.

Contact point: The contact point is medial to the rim of the acetabulum, over the ischial spine.

Supporting hand: The doctor supports the anterior shoulder as described in the side posture position for the pelvic bench. Skin on skin contact is made, so that the cephalad hand of the doctor takes up slack tissue towards the shaft of the femur. The pisiform of the caudad hand is applied to the contact point. The patient's high side knee is moved cephalad until tissue pull is felt under the contact hand. The knee is brought back slightly to release tension. The patient is rolled, the contact arm bent further at the elbow depending on the degree of In.

Pattern of thrust: The adjustment is made by thrusting in the direction indicated by the shaft of the femur, generally toward the doctor's symphysis pubis. The direction is superior to inferior, creating a $-\theta X$ movement, and medial to lateral for the In component. A torque action is included with the thrust; clockwise for the left ilium ($-\theta Y$) and anticlockwise for the right ilium ($+\theta Y$).

Name of technique: Gonstead

Name of technique procedure: Hi-lo prone ASIn ilium push adjustment (Fig. 6.22).

Indications: ASIn subluxation.

Contraindications: All other listings, hypermobility, instability, lytic metastasis in the region, inability to lie prone.

Patient position: The patient lies prone, with both arms resting over the side of the table.

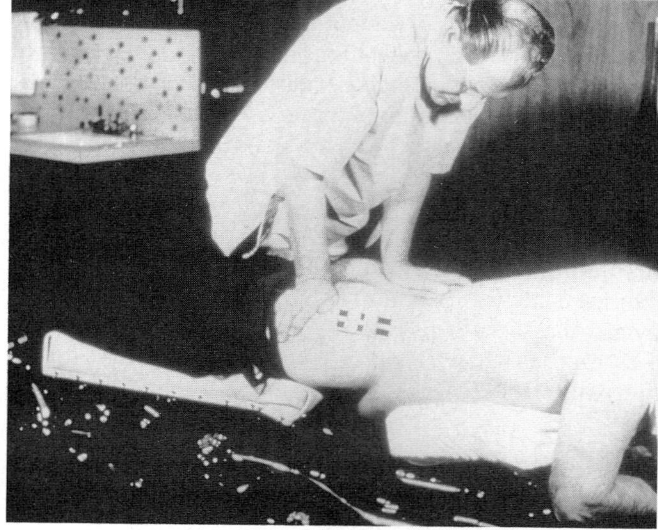

Figure 6.22. Prone right ASIn ilium adjustment.

Doctor's position: The doctor stands on the contralateral side of the ASIn ilium at the level of the patient's thigh and as close to the table as possible with the outside foot placed directly in front of the inside foot.

Contact point: The contralateral ASIn ilium is contacted skin to skin with the heel of the doctor's inside hand over the ischial spine, taking up tissue slack in a superior to inferior and medial to lateral direction.

Supporting hand: The doctor's outside hand stabilizes the near side PSIS.

Set up: The doctor achieves the correct line of correction by positioning the contact arm's shoulder vertically over the S2–3 sacral tubercles.

Pattern of thrust: The thrust is with a straight arm in a posterior to anterior, slightly superior to inferior ($-\theta X$), and medial to lateral ($-\theta Y$ on the left and $+\theta Y$ on the right) direction.

Name of technique: Gonstead

Name of technique procedure: Knee chest ASIn ilium push adjustment.

Indications: ASIn subluxation.

Contraindications: All other listings, hypermobility, instability, lytic metastasis in the region, inability to kneel and extend the lumbar spine.

Patient position: The patient assumes the basic position on the knee chest table.

Doctor's position: The doctor stands behind the patient and toward the contralateral side of the ASIn ilium while straddling the patient's ankles.

Contact point: The heel of the adjusting hand contacts the ischial spine of the ASIn ilium.

Supporting hand: The near side ilium is stabilized by contacting the ischial spine with the outside hand.

Pattern of thrust: The adjustment is made by applying pressure to take up tissue slack and thrusting with a straight arm in a posterior to anterior direction and slightly superior to inferior ($-\theta X$) direction down the shaft of the femur and in a slightly medial to lateral ($-\theta Y$ on the left, $+\theta Y$ on the right) direction, depending on the degree of In present.

ASEx Ilium

In rotating $+\theta X$ around the X axis to assume an anterior superior position (AS), the ilium may move away from the sacrum in a $-\theta Y$ direction on the left or a $+\theta Y$ on the right and is thus listed as having moved externally (Ex).

AP FILM ANALYSIS

The vertical height of the innominate from the iliac crest to the ischial tuberosity decreases (Fig. 6.23). The size and shape of the obturator foramen change. The AS decreases the diagonal measurement. The Ex increases the width. The femoral head height changes. The AS raises the femoral head height. The Ex lowers the femoral head height. The combined result either raises or lowers the femoral head height depending on which one predominates, if no other factors are involved.

LATERAL FILM ANALYSIS

The lumbar lordosis can change. The AS decreases the lumbar lordosis. The Ex increases the lumbar lordosis. The combined result depends on whether the As or Ex predominates.

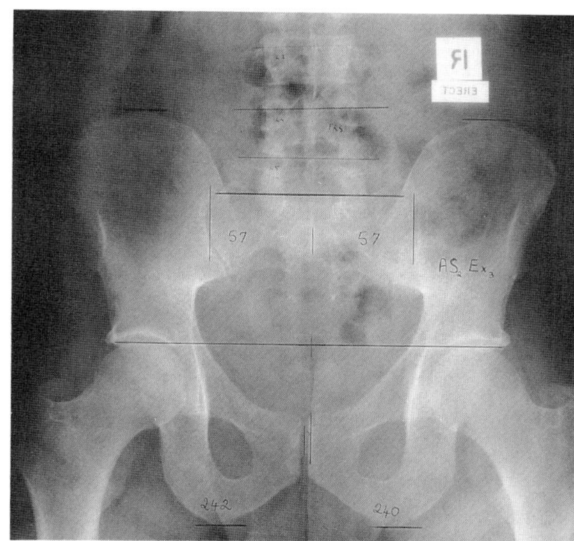

Figure 6.23. Plain film of right ASEx ilium.

CLINICAL FINDINGS

The AS opens the sacroiliac joint at the posterior inferior aspect. The Ex opens the posterior joint space. The combined result is an increased opening in the posterior inferior sacroiliac joint space, creating a palpably tender, inflamed and edematous region.

Name of technique: Gonstead

Name of technique procedure: Side posture ASEx ilium push adjustment.

Indications: ASEx subluxation.

Contraindications: All other listings, hypermobility, instability, lytic metastasis in the region, inability to lie in the side posture position, previous hip replacement surgery.

Patient position: The patient lies in the side posture position on the pelvic bench. The ASEx ilium is on the high side.

Doctor's position: The doctor adopts the side posture position for the pelvic bench.

Contact point: Skin on skin contact is made so that the cephalad hand of the doctor takes up slack tissue in an inferior direction towards the posterior shaft of the femur. The pisiform of the caudad hand is applied to the contact point, which is medial to the rim of the acetabulum, over the ischial spine.

Supporting hand: The doctor supports the anterior shoulder as described in the side posture position for the pelvic bench.

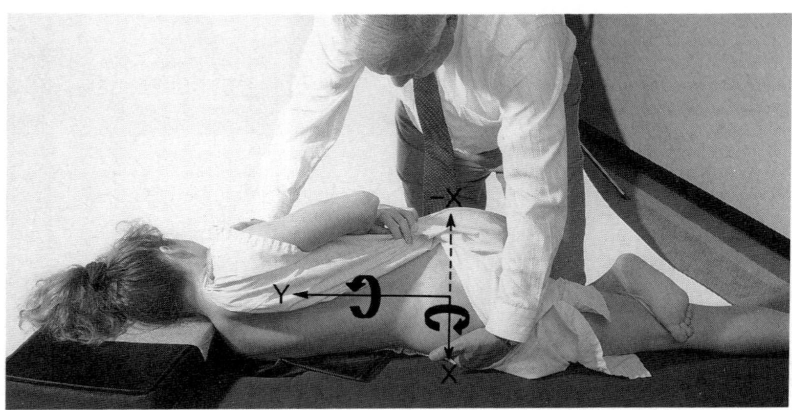

Figure 6.24. Side posture left ASEx ilium pull move adjustment.

Set up: The patient's high side knee is moved cephalad until tissue pull is felt under the contact hand. The knee is brought back slightly to release the tension. The patient is rolled slightly with the contact elbow being relatively higher than the contact point depending on the degree of Ex.

Pattern of thrust: The adjustment is made with a thrust in a posterior to anterior and superior to inferior ($-\theta$X) direction, down the shaft of the femur, and slightly lateral to medial ($+\theta$Y on the left, $-\theta$Y on the right) with a slight torque. The contact hand is torqued anticlockwise for the left side and clockwise for the right side up.

Name of technique: Gonstead

Name of technique procedure: Side posture ASEx ilium pull move adjustment (Fig. 6.24).

Indications: ASEx subluxation.

Contraindications: All other listings, hypermobility, instability, lytic metastasis in the region, inability to lie in the side posture position, previous hip replacement surgery.

Patient position: The patient lies in the side posture position on the pelvic bench. The ASEx ilium is on the down side.

Doctor's position: The doctor adopts the side posture position for the pelvic bench, but stands more cephalad and slightly further away from the pelvic bench.

Contact point: The doctor's cephalad hand lifts the patient's pelvis to enable the caudad hand to slide under the ilium so that the fingers extend around and under the ASIS. The pelvis is released by the cephalad hand and allowed to rest totally on the doctor's caudad (contact) hand. The contact hand is drawn infero-medial to take up tissue slack and bring the pisiform just medial to the rim of the acetabulum and lateral to the ischial spine.

Supporting hand: The doctor supports the anterior shoulder as described in the side posture position for the pelvic bench. The patient's pelvis is stabilized by the doctor resting the caudad knee against the posterior thigh of the patient's flexed high side leg.

Pattern of thrust: The thrust is posterior to anterior and superior to inferior ($-\theta$X), plus lateral to medial ($+\theta$Y on the left, $-\theta$Y on the right) direction. The thrust is achieved by rapidly straightening the flexed wrist of the contact hand while the doctor's caudad knee stabilizes the patient's pelvis with a positive contact against the posterior thigh of the patient. No thrust is given by the doctor's knee.

Name of technique: Gonstead

Name of technique procedure: Hi-lo prone ASEx ilium push adjustment.

Indications: ASEx subluxation.

Contraindications: All other listings, hypermobility, instability, lytic metastasis in the region, inability to lie in the prone position.

Patient position: The patient lies prone, with both arms resting over the side of the table.

Doctor's position: The doctor stands on the side of the ASEx ilium at the level of the patient's thigh and as close to the table as possible with the outside foot placed directly in front of the inside foot.

Contact point: The ipsilateral ASEx ilium is contacted skin to skin with the heel of the doctor's outside hand lateral to the ischial spine.

Supporting hand: The doctor's inside hand stabilizes the far side PSIS.

Pattern of thrust: The adjustment is made by applying pressure to take up tissue slack and thrusting with a straight arm in a posterior to anterior, superior to inferior ($-\theta$X) and lateral to medial ($+\theta$Y on the left, $-\theta$Y on the right) direction. This is achieved by the doctor positioning the contact arm's shoulder vertically and laterally to the ipsilateral ilium's PSIS.

Name of technique: Gonstead

Name of technique procedure: Knee chest ASEx ilium push adjustment.

Indications: ASEx subluxation.

Contraindications: All other listings, hypermobility, instability, lytic metastasis in the region, inability to kneel and extend the lumbar spine.

Patient position: The patient assumes the basic position for the knee chest table.

Doctor's position: The doctor stands behind and to the ASEx side of the patient and straddles the ankles.

Contact point: Skin on skin contact is made by the heel of the adjusting hand over the lateral edge of the ischial spine, medial to the rim of the acetabulum, of the ASEx ilium.

Supporting hand: The opposite ilium is stabilized by contacting the PSIS.

Pattern of thrust: The adjustment is made by applying pressure to take up tissue slack. The thrust is made with a straight arm in a posterior to anterior direction down the shaft of the femur, creating a $-\theta X$ movement, and lateral to medial ($+\theta Y$ on the left, $-\theta Y$ on the right),direction. The greater the Ex component, the greater the degree of lateral to medial thrust.

In and Ex

The ilium can torque lateral to medial (a $+\theta Y$ rotation on the left, $-\theta Y$ on the right) to assume an In position, i.e., internally toward the sacrum. It can also torque medial to lateral (a $-\theta Y$ rotation on the left, $+\theta Y$ on the right) to assume an Ex position, i.e., externally away from the sacrum. Because they are joined at the symphysis pubis, if one side is In, the other side is Ex. Only one of the ilia is actually in a fixated and subluxated condition. The other is the compensation.

AP FILM ANALYSIS

The vertical height of the innominate from the iliac crest to the ischial tuberosity remains unchanged for both the In and Ex (Fig. 6.25). The size and shape of the obturator foramen changes. The In has a more narrow width. The

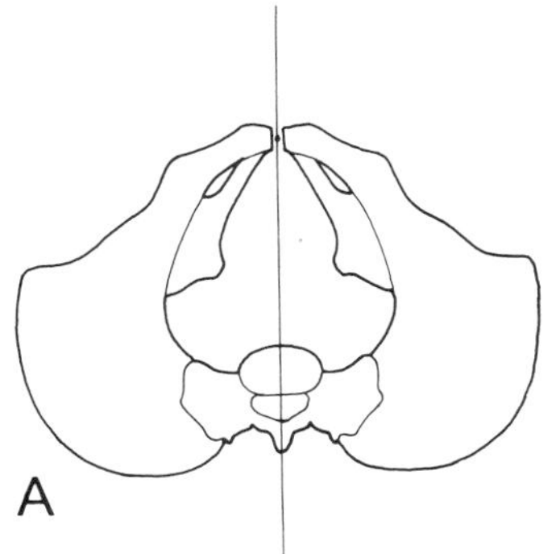

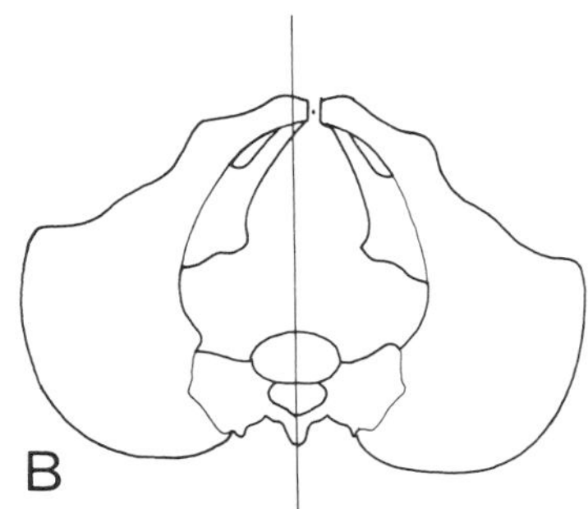

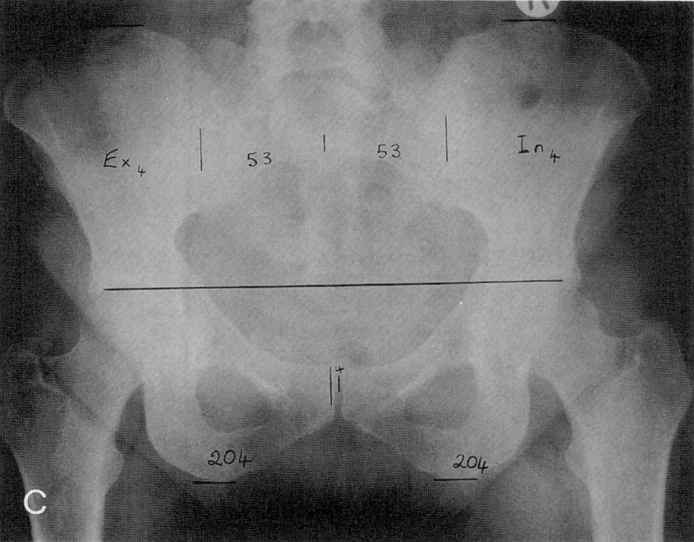

Figure 6.25. **A,** Transverse view of a normal pelvis. **B,** Left Ex and right In ilium. **C,** Plain film of left Ex and right In ilium.

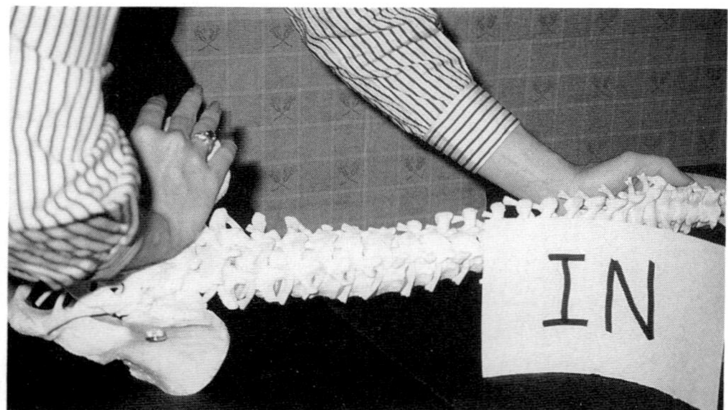

Figure 6.26. Side posture In ilium push move adjustment set-up on an anatomic model.

Ex has a wider width. The femoral head height changes. The In tends to raise the femoral head height. The Ex tends to lower it.

LATERAL FILM ANALYSIS

The lumbar lordosis may change. The In tends to decrease the lumbar lordosis and the Ex increases it.

CLINICAL FINDINGS

The In opens the joint at the anterior aspect creating an edematous area. The Ex opens the joint at the posterior aspect, creating a palpable, tender, edematous area. In the supine patient the In ilium will tend to cause the ipsilateral foot to flare away from the median line, while the Ex ilium will tend to cause the ipsilateral foot to converge toward the median line. This may also be visible in the standing position.

Name of technique: Gonstead

Name of technique procedure: Side posture In ilium push move adjustment (Fig. 6.26).

Indications: In ilium.

Contraindication: All other listings, hypermobility, instability, lytic metastasis in the region, inability to lie in the side posture position, previous hip replacement surgery.

Patient position: The patient lies in the side posture position on the pelvic bench. The In ilium is on the high side.

Doctor's position: The doctor adopts the side posture position for the pelvic bench.

Contact point: Skin on skin contact is made so that the cephalad hand of the doctor takes up slack tissue in a medial to lateral direction near the center of the sacroiliac joint. The pisiform of the caudad (contact) hand is applied just medially to the PSIS.

Supporting hand: The doctor supports the anterior shoulder as described in the side posture position for the pelvic bench.

Pattern of thrust: The elbow is lowered to enable the thrust to be made in a medial to lateral ($-\theta$Y on the left, $+\theta$Y on the right) direction.

Name of technique: Gonstead

Name of technique procedure: Side posture In ilium pull adjustment.

Indications: In subluxation.

Contraindications: All other listings, hypermobility, instability, lytic metastasis in the region, inability to lie in the side posture position, previous hip replacement surgery.

Patient position: The patient lies in the side posture position on the pelvic bench. The In ilium is on the high side.

Doctor's position: The doctor adopts the side posture position for the pelvic bench, standing slightly further away from the pelvic bench.

Contact point: The finger tips of the caudad hand are applied medially to the center of the sacroiliac joint.

Supporting hand: The doctor supports the anterior shoulder as described in the side posture position for the pelvic bench.

Pattern of thrust: The doctor remains more upright and thrusts by pulling the ilium in a medial to lateral direction.

Name of technique: Gonstead

Name of technique procedure: Side posture Ex ilium pull adjustment (Fig. 6.27).

Indications: Ex subluxation.

Contraindications: All other listings, hypermobility, instability, lytic metastasis in the region, inability to lie in the side posture position, previous hip replacement surgery.

Patient position: The patient lies in the side posture position on the pelvic bench. The Ex ilium is on the down side.

Doctor's position: The doctor adopts the side posture position for the pelvic bench, with some slight modification for the contact point.

Contact point: The doctor's cephalad hand lifts the patient's pelvis to enable the caudad hand to slide under the ilium so that the fingers extend around the ASIS. The pelvis is released by the cephalad hand and allowed to rest totally on the doctor's caudad (contact) hand. The contact hand is drawn medially to take up tissue slack and bring the pisiform to the lateral border of the PSIS.

Supporting hand: The doctor supports the anterior shoulder as described in the side posture position for the pelvic bench.

Pattern of thrust: The patient's pelvis is stabilized by the doctor resting their caudad knee against the posterior thigh of the patient's flexed high side leg. The thrust is lateral to medial ($+\theta Y$ on the left, $-\theta Y$ on the right) via the pisiform contact. This is achieved by extending the flexed wrist of the contact hand. It is stabilized by a gentle but positive contact by the doctor's knee against the posterior thigh of the patient. No thrust is given by the doctor's knee.

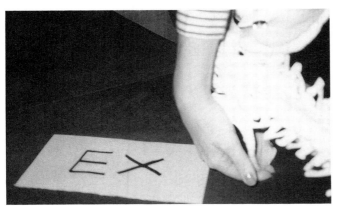

Figure 6.27. Side posture right Ex ilium pull move adjustment setup on an anatomic model.

In-Ex Ilium

It is possible to have both left and right ilia fixated and subluxated. This occurs when there is no AS or PI component and no lumbar axial rotation. When this occurs, both listings are recorded, the left listing first, followed by a hyphen before the right listing.

Name of technique: Gonstead

Name of technique procedure: Side posture In-Ex ilium pull adjustment (Fig. 6.28).

Indications: In-Ex subluxation.

Contraindications: All other listings, hypermobility, instability, lytic metastasis in the region, inability to lie in the side posture position, previous hip replacement surgery.

Patient position: The patient lies in the side posture position on the pelvic bench. The In ilium is on the high side, the Ex is on the down side.

Doctor's position: The doctor adopts the side posture position for the pelvic bench with some slight modification for the contact point.

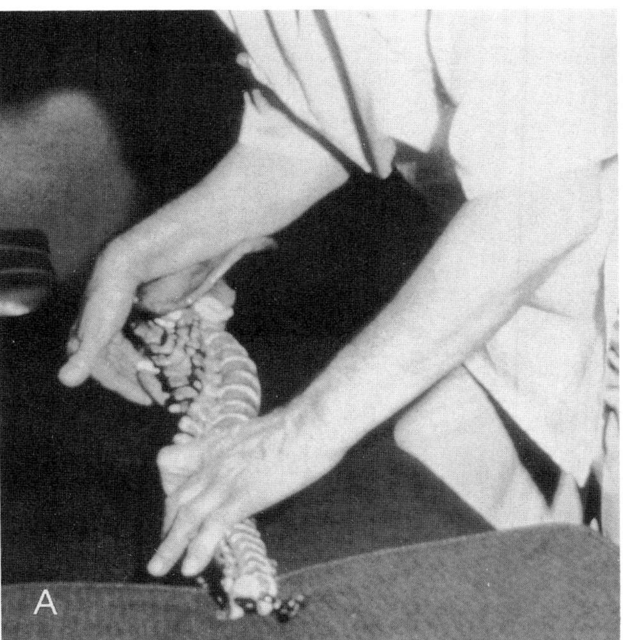

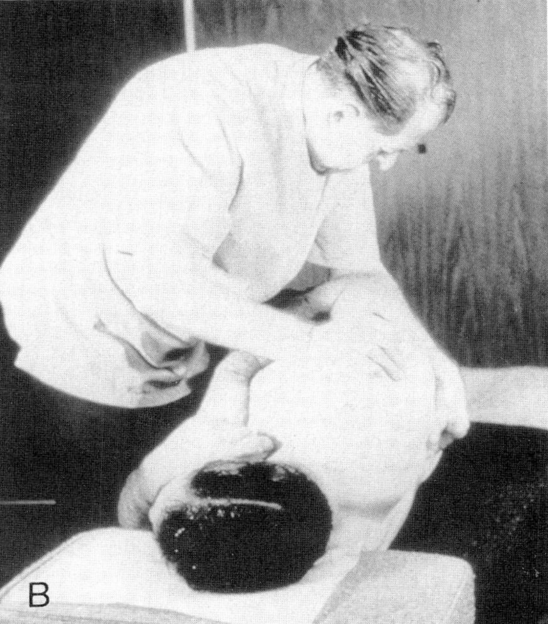

Figure 6.28. A, Side posture In-Ex ilium pull adjustment on an anatomic model. **B,** Side posture adjustment for an In-Ex listing.

Contact point: The doctor's cephalad hand lifts the patient's pelvis to enable the caudad hand to slide under the ilium so that the fingers extend around to the ASIS. The pelvis is released by the cephalad hand and allowed to rest totally on the doctor's caudad contact hand. The contact hand is drawn superomedial to take up tissue slack and bring the pisiform caudad and lateral to the PSIS. Along with the pisiform contact, the doctor's forearm contacts the caudad and medial border of the PSIS of the In ilium on the high side.

Supporting hand: The doctor supports the anterior shoulder as described in the side posture position for the pelvic bench.

Pattern of thrust: The thrust is directed through the sacroiliac joints by the pisiform and forearm, to achieve a simultaneous bilateral correction of the Ex and In ilia.

SACRUM

The sacrum articulates at three joints (the left and right sacroiliac joints and the lumbosacral junction). As a result, the sacrum is regarded as moving in rotation about the X axis and the Y axis. As reviewed earlier in this chapter, the sacroiliac joint is made up of an upper amphiarthrodial section and a lower diarthrodial (synovial) section. The female sacroiliac joints are built for mobility, whereas the male joints are built for strength and contain articular ridges. The joints are asymmetrical in individuals and changes in the joint occurs in response to imposed stress with age. The sacral segments articulate before fusing at approximately 10 years of age. It is logical to assume therefore that the sacrum can have more complex fixation subluxation complexes within each sacroiliac joint.

P-R, P-L, PI-R, PI-L

The sacrum may undergo a clockwise rotation about the Y axis and is listed as having moved posterior on the left, P-L, $(+\theta Y)$. An anticlockwise rotation is listed as posterior on the right, P-R $(-\theta Y)$. The sacrum may undergo a clockwise rotation about the Z axis and is listed as having moved inferior on the right $(+\theta Z)$. An anticlockwise rotation is listed as inferior on the left $(-\theta Z)$ (Fig. 6.29).

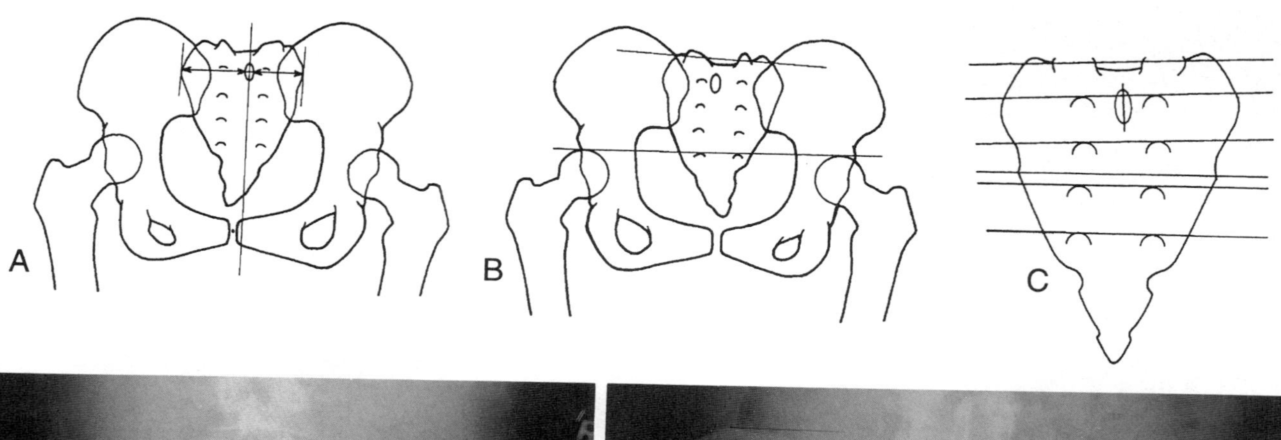

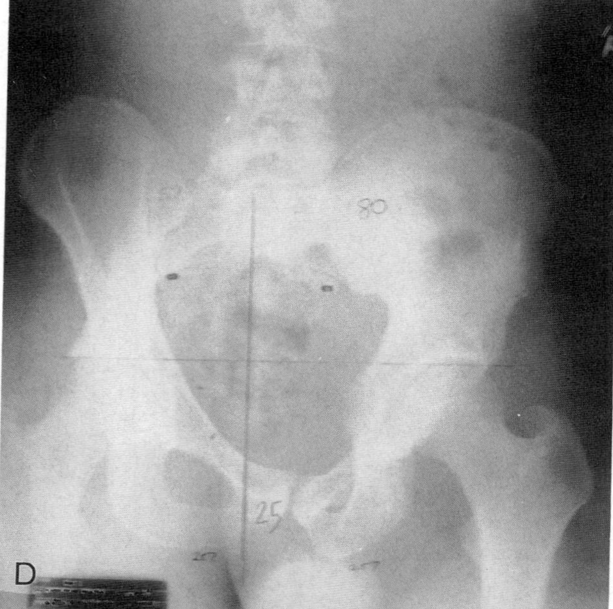

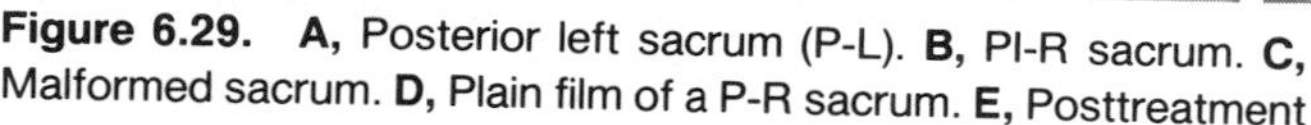

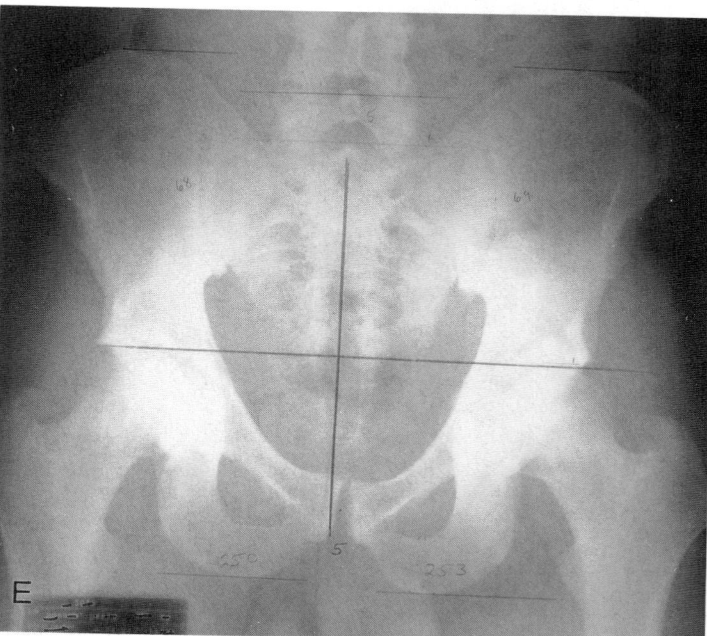

Figure 6.29. **A,** Posterior left sacrum (P-L). **B,** PI-R sacrum. **C,** Malformed sacrum. **D,** Plain film of a P-R sacrum. **E,** Posttreatment radiograph of patient depicted in **D**. This radiograph was performed 6 hours after the original.

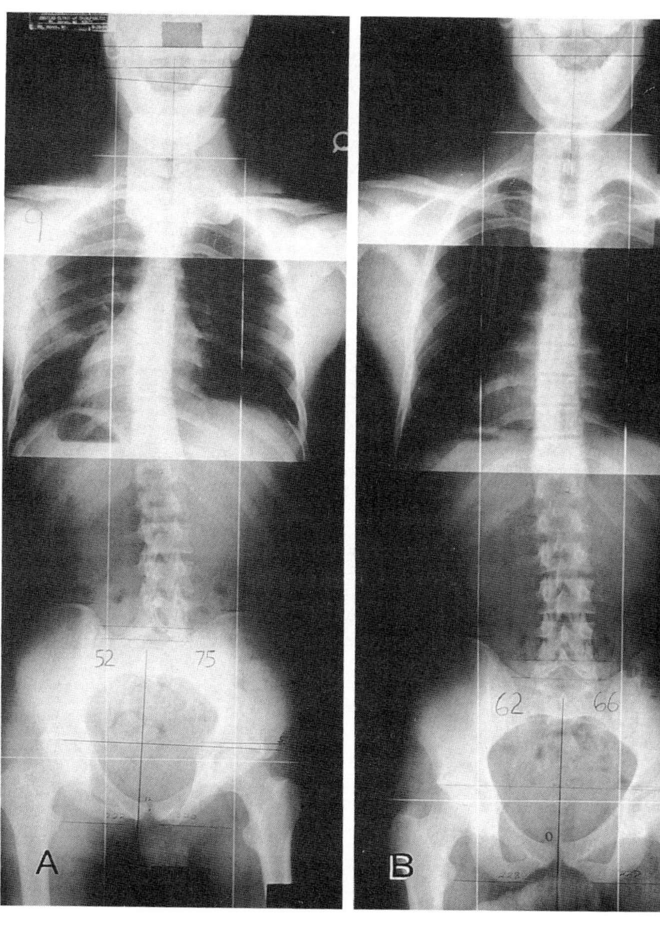

Figure 6.30. **A,** Pretreatment radiograph of a P-R sacrum. **B,** Posttreatment radiograph of **A**.

AP FILM ANALYSIS

Because the posterior surface of the sacrum is convex, the distance from the second sacral tubercle to the left lateral border of the sacrum on the AP radiographic film is greater for a P-L listing than the distance to the right lateral sacral border.

In the majority of cases, sacral inferiority is due to malformation of the sacral plateau. This is best confirmed by drawing a series of connecting horizontal lines through like points (Fig. 6.29C). The lumbar spine will rotate with the sacrum.

CLINICAL FINDINGS

Motion palpation reveals a restriction in motion in the sacroiliac joint on the side of sacral posteriority. The joint becomes edematous and tender on palpation along the posterior aspect (Fig. 6.30–6.33).

Name of technique: Gonstead

Name of technique procedure: Side posture sacral push adjustment, subluxation side up (Fig. 6.34).

Indications: P-R, P-L, PI-R, and PI-L subluxations.

Contraindications: All other listings, hypermobility, instability, lytic metastasis in the region, inability to lie in the side posture position, previous hip replacement surgery.

Patient position: The patient lies in the side posture position on the pelvic bench. The subluxation is on the high side.

Doctor's position: The doctor adopts the side posture position for the pelvic bench.

Contact point: The doctor's caudad hand makes a skin on skin contact via the pisiform on the sacral alar, as lateral as possible, yet medial to the posterior superior iliac spine so as to avoid contact with it. The contact hand's fingers should point downward to the floor (i.e., they should be resting across the sacrum and contralateral PSIS). A thenar contact can also be made.

Supporting hand: The doctor supports the anterior shoulder as described in the side posture position for the pelvic bench.

Pattern of thrust: The doctor leans over the patient to lower the elbow to the level of the plane of the sacroiliac joint. The adjustment is made by thrusting through the plane of the sacroiliac joint posterior to anterior, $-\theta Y$ for a P-L and $+\theta Y$ for PR. If there

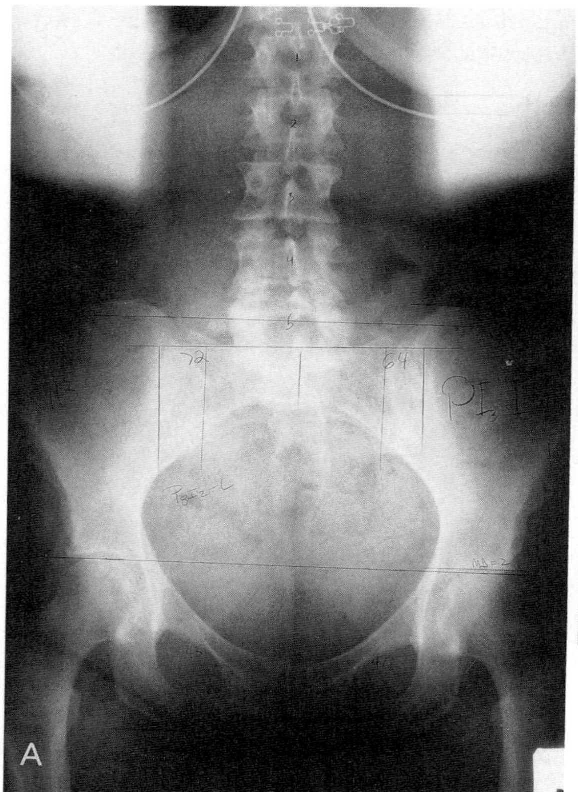

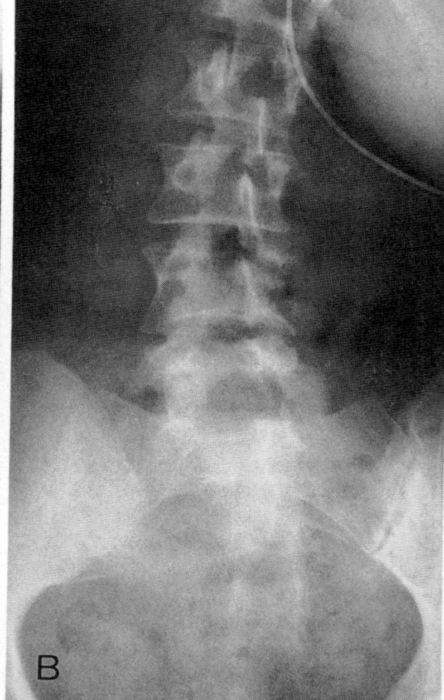

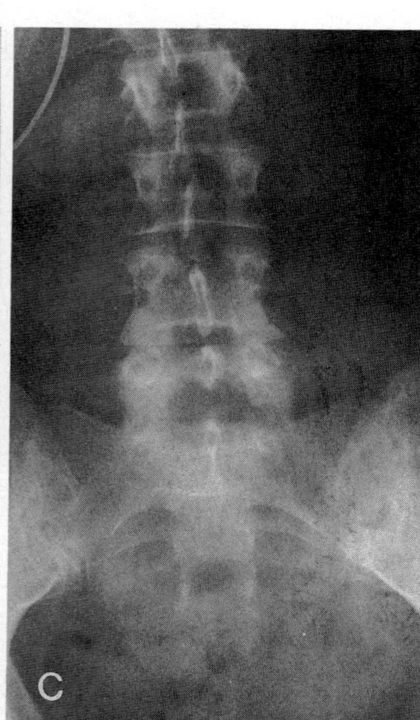

Figure 6.31. **A,** AP radiograph of a PI-L sacrum. **B,** Right lateral bending demonstrates normal rotation of the lumbar spine and sacrum. **C,** Effect of PI-L sacral rotation on the lumbar spine and sacrum during left side bending. Note the decreased $-\theta Z$ and $-\theta Y$ on the side of sacral posteriority when in left side bend.

is an inferiority of the sacrum, a torque is applied through the pisiform during the thrust. The torque is clockwise for a PI-L, ($+\theta Z$), and anticlockwise for a PI-R, ($-\theta Z$).

Name of technique: Gonstead

Name of technique procedure: Side posture sacral push adjustment, subluxation side down (Fig. 6.35).

Indications: P-R, P-L, PI-R, and PI-L subluxations.

Contraindications: All other listings, hypermobility, instability, lytic metastasis in the region, inability to lie in the side posture position, previous hip replacement surgery.

Patient position: The patient lies in the side posture position on the pelvic bench. The subluxation is on the down side.

Doctor's position: The doctor adopts the side posture position for the pelvic bench.

Contact point: The doctor's caudad hand makes skin on skin contact via the pisiform on the sacral ala as lateral as possible, yet medial to the PSIS so as to avoid contact with it. The contact hand fingers should point cephalad, with the index finger resting near the lumbar spine.

Supporting hand: The doctor supports the anterior shoulder as described in the side posture position for the pelvic bench.

Pattern of thrust: The doctor leans over the patient to align the forearm to the level of the plane of the sacroiliac joint. The adjustment is made by thrusting through the plane of the sacroiliac joint posterior to anterior ($-\theta Y$ for P-L and $+\theta Y$ for P-R). If there is an inferiority of the sacrum, a torque is applied through the pisiform during the thrust. The torque is clockwise for a PI-L, ($+\theta Z$), and anticlockwise for a PI-R, ($-\theta Z$).

Name of technique: Gonstead

Name of technique procedure: Hi-lo prone sacrum push adjustment.

Indications: P-R, P-L, PI-R, and PI-L subluxations.

Contraindications: All other listings, hypermobility, instability, lytic metastasis in the region, inability to lie prone.

Patient position: The patient lies prone, with both arms resting over the side of the table.

Doctor's position: The doctor stands facing the patient on the contralateral side of the posterior sacral subluxation at the level of the middle of the sacroiliac joint.

Contact position: Skin on skin contact is made with the caudad hand on the lateral border of the sacrum, immediately medial to the PSIS.

Supporting hand: Stabilization occurs by gripping the contact hand wrist with the cephalad hand. The caudad arm is locked at

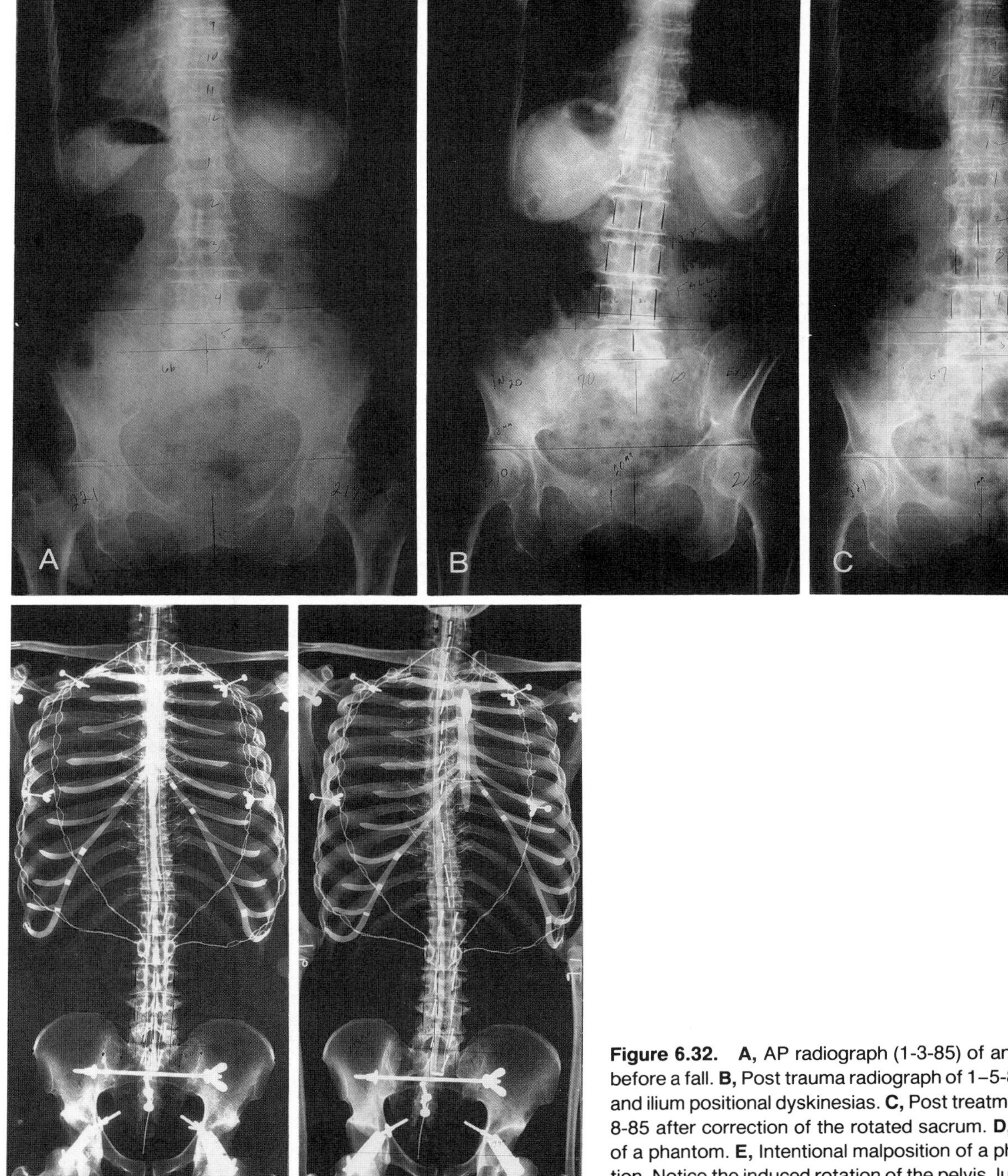

Figure 6.32. **A,** AP radiograph (1-3-85) of an 82-year-old female before a fall. **B,** Post trauma radiograph of 1–5-85. Notice the sacral and ilium positional dyskinesias. **C,** Post treatment radiograph of 4-8-85 after correction of the rotated sacrum. **D,** Normal positioning of a phantom. **E,** Intentional malposition of a phantom in axial rotation. Notice the induced rotation of the pelvis, lumbar spine and thorax. Compare to the radiograph in **B** in which pelvic positional dyskinesia has little effect on the rotational coefficients of the lumbar spine.

the elbow and the forearm aligned with the plane of the sacroiliac joint.

Pattern of thrust: The patient exhales, tissue slack is removed with increasing downward pressure. The adjustment is made by thrusting posterior to anterior and slightly laterally through the plane of the sacroiliac joint, ($-\theta Y$ for P-L, and $+\theta Y$ for P-R). If there is an inferiority of the sacrum, a torque is applied through the pisiform during the thrust. The torque is clockwise for a PI-L, ($+\theta Z$), and anticlockwise for a PI-R, ($-\theta Z$).

Management

The choice of adjusting subluxated side up versus side down depends on clinical results with that individual patient. There are no strict guidelines. Sometimes obese patients are easier to adjust with the subluxated side down because it locks the ilium and enables easier movement of the sacrum. In some instances, the patient may experience increased discomfort one way, hence the choice for the alternative approach. Hip and knee problems resulting in pain or limitation in movement may dictate a certain approach.

The preferred approach is with the patient in side posture on the pelvic bench. If the patient is too obese to adjust, the second choice is the knee chest table. The reason that the knee chest table is not the preferred approach is that the sacroiliac joints are weight bearing and hence are not completely relaxed (Personal Communication, Dr. Alex Cox).

Clinical observations of a sacroiliac syndrome alone make it difficult to determine if the patient is suffering from an ilium or a sacral subluxation. Clinical observations suggest that the patient will respond more favorably if the outlined protocol is followed (50). An analysis of the AP plain film radiograph will determine which short lever arm to contact for the adjustment.

A posteriorly rotated sacrum is generally regarded as clinically significant if the difference between the left and right measurements is 7 mm or greater.

The decision as to whether to adjust the sacrum or the ilium depends on the following three rules:

1. If there is no ilium listing, the sacrum is adjusted.
2. If the ilium on the side of sacral posteriority has a listing of AS, In, or any compound listing in which AS or In are the dominant factors, the sacrum is adjusted to the ilium. This should correct the sacral rotation and the AS and In ilium components simultaneously.
3. If the ilium on the side of sacral posteriority has a listing of PI, Ex, or any compound listing in which PI or Ex are the

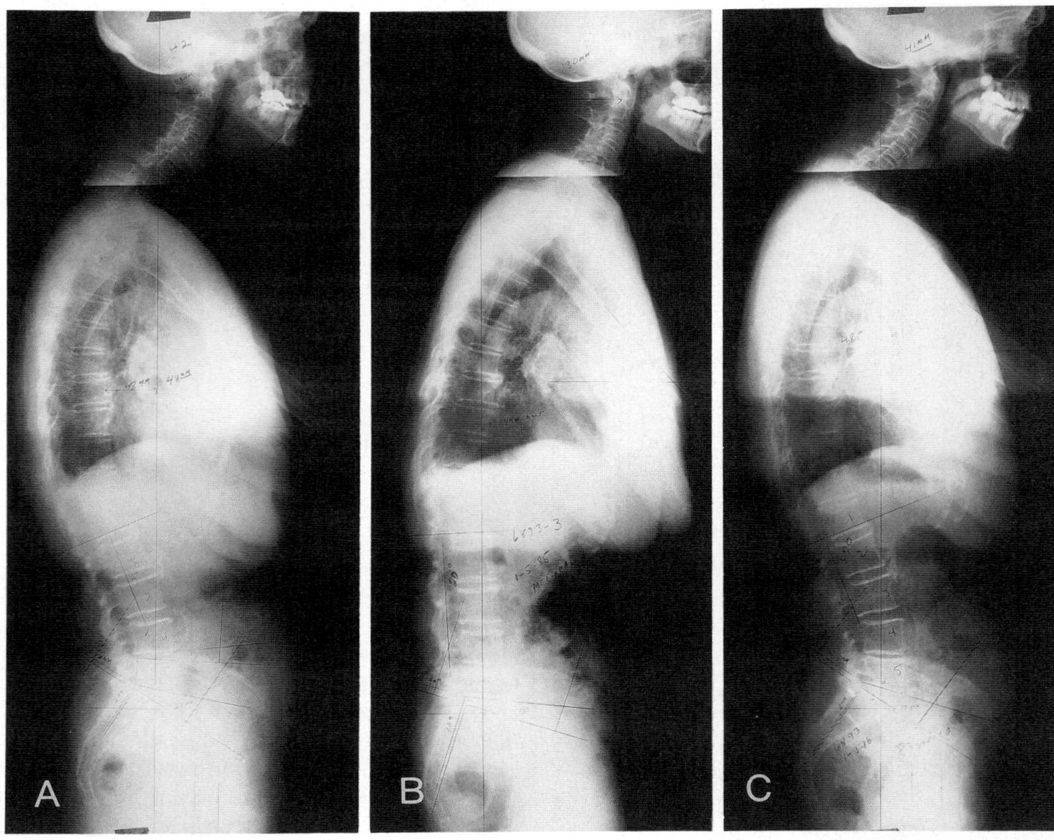

Figure 6.33. **A,** Pretrauma lateral radiograph of the patient in Figure 6.32A. **B,** Post trauma radiograph of patient in Figure 6.32A. Notice loss of the normal lumbar lordosis. **C,** Posttreatment lateral radiograph of patient in Figure 6.32A.

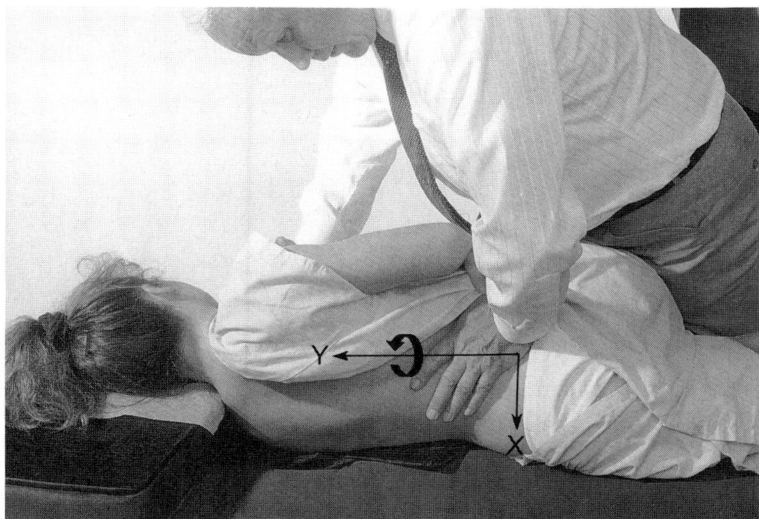

Figure 6.34. Side posture sacral push adjustment, subluxation side up.

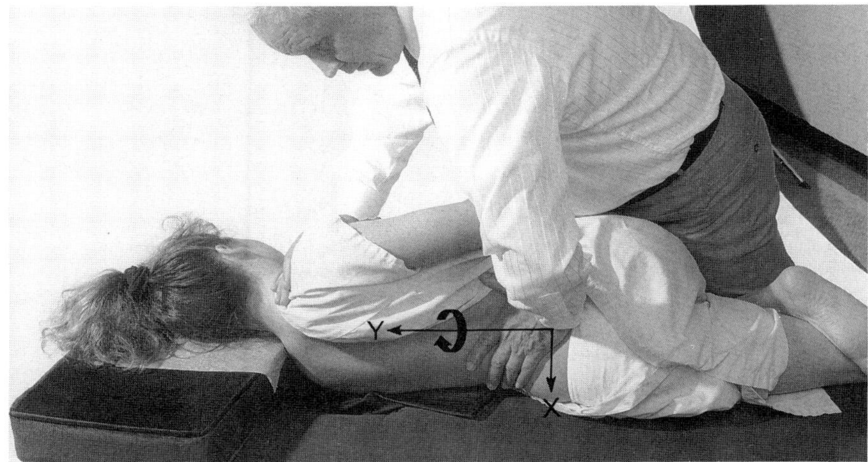

Figure 6.35. Side posture sacral push adjustment, subluxation side down.

dominant factors, the ilium is adjusted to the sacrum. If the sacrum were adjusted to the ilium it would increase the PI and exacerbate the already inflamed joint capsule.

4. With an AS or In ilium listing, the sacrum needs to be adjusted if the ipsilateral leg is shorter (supine leg check) and no anatomic deficiency is present. This is recorded as an S-ASIn. The ilium needs to be adjusted if the ipsilateral leg is longer.
5. If there is an AS, In, or ASIn, and no pain is palpable, set the ilium to the sacrum. If an AS, In, or ASIn is present and there is palpable pain and edema, set the sacrum to the ilium.

Segmental Sacral Subluxations

Sacral segments fuse in children at approximately 10 years of age. Before this, they have a degree of articulation with a disc space separating each segment. A condition often seen in children is a posterior open wedge shaped disc between S1 and S2. This is often accompanied by a posterior (−Z) movement of S2 relative to S1. In the child, this displacement may be associated with enuresis. If left uncorrected, this condition is seen in adults as a thickened rudimentary posterior open wedge disc. The second sacral segment may appear in a posterior position (−Z) relative to S1. The following is a brief summary of the work of Dr. Max Joseph. It details some of the more salient points required to recognize this condition (Unpublished data, Dr. Max Joseph, Mornington, Vic., Australia).

AP FILM ANALYSIS

Repeated observations of the S2 congenital asymmetry has revealed a high frequency of other abnormalities occurring; spina bifida S1 or L5, transitional L5 or S1, failure of the iliac crest line to pass through the L4–5 disc space, asymmetrical sacroiliac joint shapes.

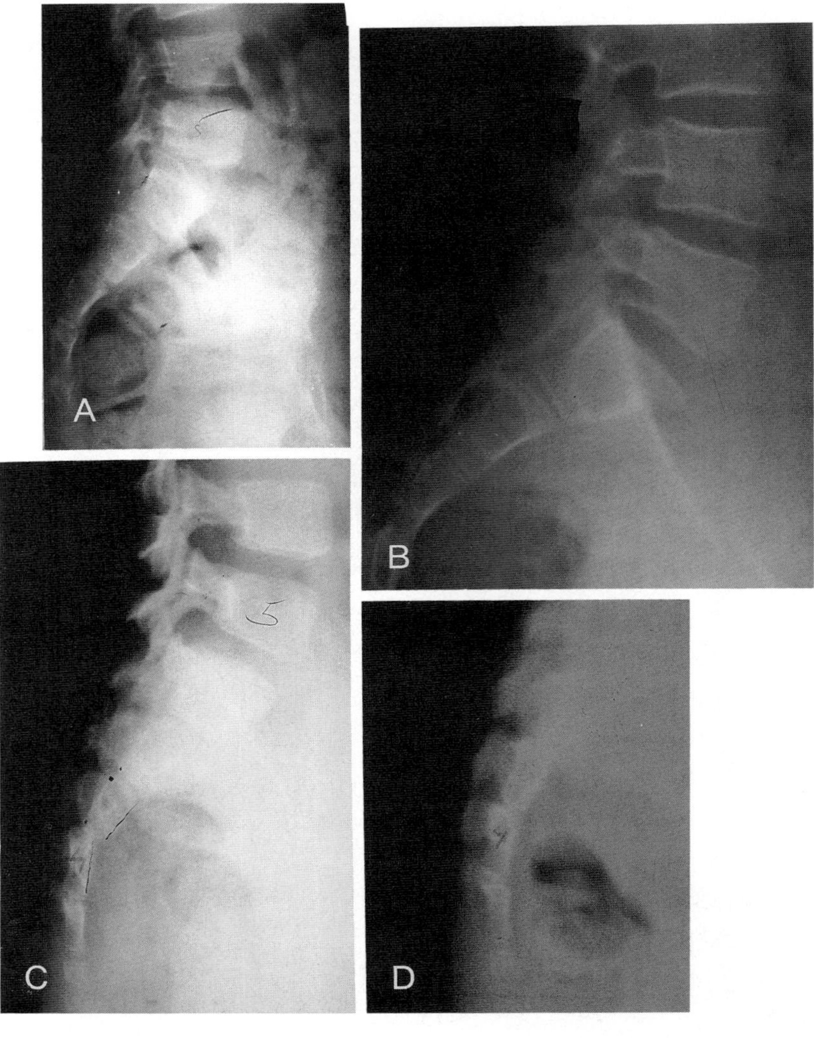

Figure 6.36. **A,** Plain film lateral view showing posteriorly open wedge between S1 and S2 in a child. **B,** S2 subluxation of a young adult. **C,** S4 subluxation of a child. **D,** Posttreatment radiograph of patient depicted in **C**.

LATERAL FILM ANALYSIS

There may be a posterior L5, S1-S2 rudimentary disc with or without "gibbus type" contour, or a posterior open wedge rudimentary disc between S1 and S2 (Fig. 6.36).

CLINICAL FINDINGS

There is usually no temperature differential present. The patient may complain of chronic unilateral or bilateral hip pain (with associated hip pathology). In general, the patient can have any symptoms associated with the lumbar or sacral plexuses. There is usually tenderness present at the tubercle of the involved segment.

Name of technique: Gonstead

Name of technique procedure: Side posture S2 sacral push adjustment.

Indications: S2 subluxation.

Contraindications: All other listings, hypermobility, instability, lytic metastasis in the region, inability to lie in the side posture position, previous hip replacement surgery.

Patient position: The patient lies in the side posture position on the pelvic bench.

Doctor's position: The doctor adopts the side posture position for the pelvic bench.

Contact point: Skin on skin contact is made by the pisiform of the caudad hand on the inferior border of the second sacral tubercle.

Supporting hand: The doctor supports the anterior shoulder as described in the side posture position for the pelvic bench.

Pattern of thrust: Posterior to anterior ($+Z$) and inferior to superior ($+\theta X$).

Name of technique: Gonstead

Name of technique procedure: Prone S2 sacral adjustment.

Indications: S2 subluxation.

Contraindications: All other listings, hypermobility, instability, lytic metastasis in the region, inability to lie prone, abdominal aortic aneurysm, severe osteoporosis.

Patient position: Prone on the hi-lo table.

Doctor's position: At the level of the sacrum, standing facing the hi-lo.

Contact point: Skin on skin contact with the pisiform of the cephalad hand on the inferior border of the second sacral tubercle. The fingers pointing caudad and resting on the buttocks.

Supporting hand: The caudad hand clasps the wrist of the contact hand.

Pattern of thrust: Posterior to anterior ($+Z$) and inferior to superior ($+\theta X$). If the patient is very obese or otherwise cannot be adjusted with the preceding maneuvers, a table with a drop mechanism may be used.

COCCYX

The coccyx sits at the apex of the sacrum and can undergo a $-\theta X$ rotation and is listed as anterior (A). This may be combined with either a $-\theta Z$, or $+\theta Z$ rotation and is listed as an anterior right (AR) or anterior left (AL) lateral deviation (Fig. 6.37).

CLINICAL FINDINGS

The coccyx subluxation usually presents following trauma. This generally involves falling onto the buttocks creating the anterior and/or lateral deviation. There will usually be edema and severe tenderness to palpation. Localized pain is experienced when sitting, rising from sitting, and on defecation.

Name of technique: Gonstead

Name of technique procedure: Hi-lo prone coccyx pull/thrust adjustment (Fig. 6.38).

Indications: A, AR, and AL coccyx.

Contraindications: All other listings.

Patient position: The patient lies prone, with both arms resting over the side of the table. The pelvic support is raised to elevate the coccyx.

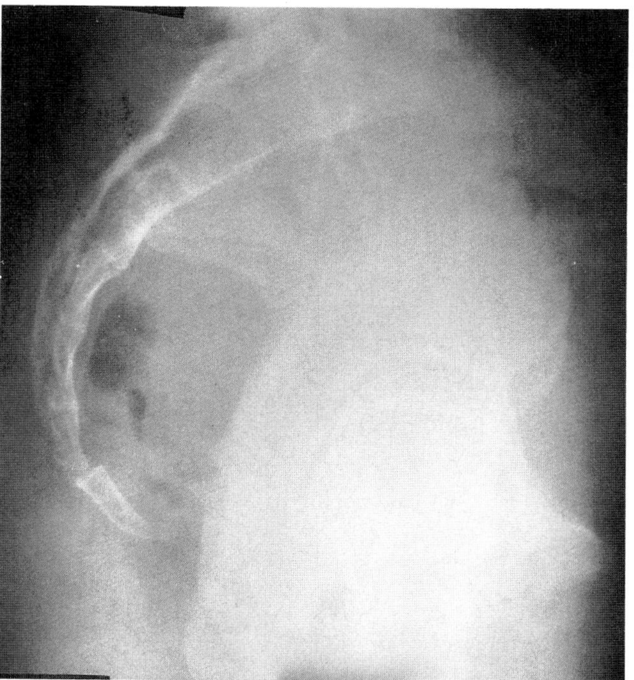

Figure 6.37. Lateral radiograph of an anterior coccyx.

Doctor position: The doctor stands facing the patient at the level of midthigh on the side of lateral deviation. If no lateral deviation is present, either side is suitable.

Contact Point: The cephalad thumb of the doctor contacts the coccyx approximately two to three centimeters inferior to the sacrococcygeal junction. Thin cotton cloth separates the skin on skin contact.

Supporting hand: The caudad hand makes a pisiform contact distal to the contact thumb's metacarpophalangeal joint and grips the contact hand for improved stabilization.

Pattern of thrust: Tissue slack is removed by the stabilization hand applying slight pressure in a posterior to anterior and inferior to superior direction. The adjustment is made by applying a thrust in an inferior to superior, ($+\theta X$) direction.

SHORT LEG SYNDROME

The Gonstead system pays particular attention to the level foundation concept as a basic premise for spinal column integrity. When completing line drawings on an AP plain radiograph of the lumbar-pelvis, it is frequently noted that the femoral head line is not horizontal. In other words there is an obvious difference in femoral head heights. This denotes a leg length inequality, (LLI) or short leg.

This LLI may be due to pelvic subluxations or foot pronation and is referred to as either a functional short leg, or a physiologic short leg. When the LLI is due to an

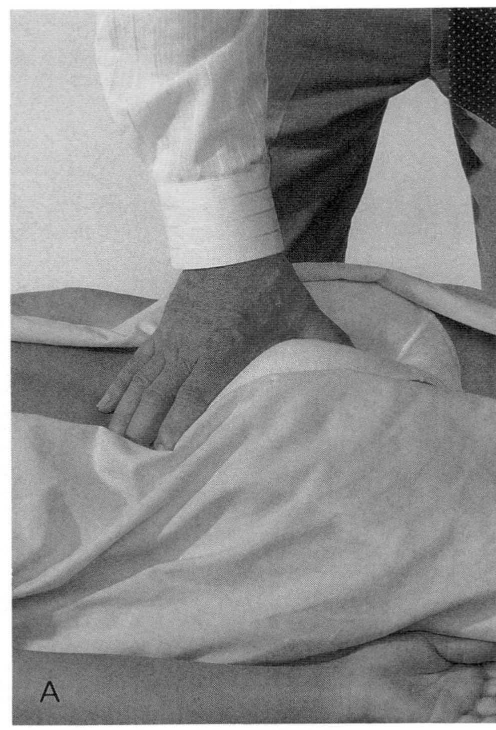

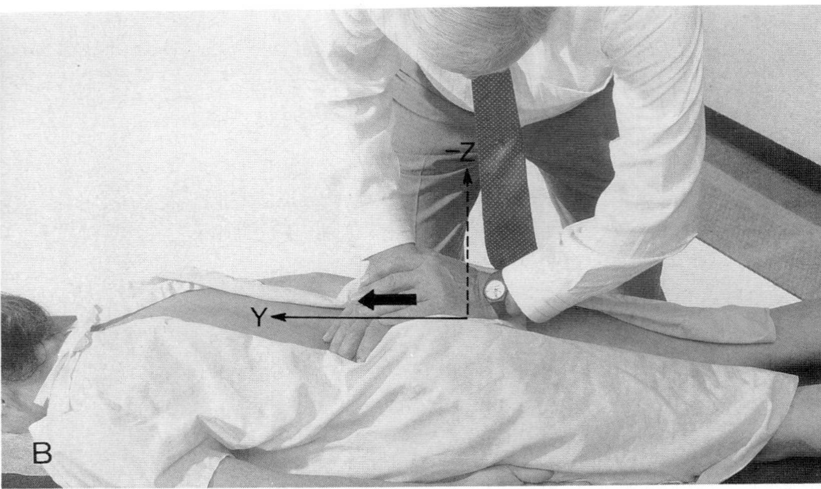

Figure 6.38. **A,** Contact point for the prone coccyx pull-thrust adjustment. **B,** Pattern of thrust for the anterior coccyx.

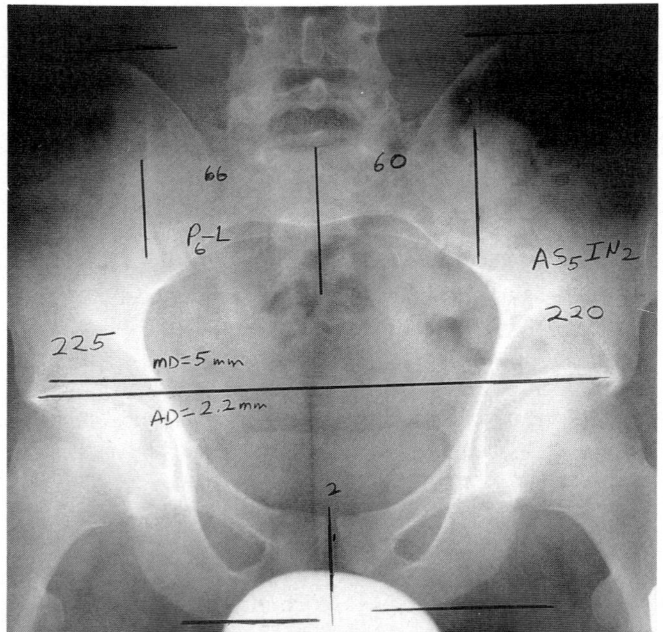

Figure 6.39. AP plain film demonstrating pelvic listings, discrepancy in femoral head height measurements and the actual difference after applying the 5:2 rule.

actual difference in leg length, it is referred to as either a true short leg, or an anatomic short leg.

Distinguishing the cause of LLI is paramount in determining the correct management of the patient. This is particularly important in deciding on the prescription of a heel lift or other orthotic insert.

Functional Leg Length Inequality From Pelvic Subluxation

A posterior-inferior (PI) and an external (Ex) ilium causes the acetabulum to move in an anterior and superior direction. For heel contact to be maintained on the ground, the acetabulum is lowered and hence appears on the AP film as a lowered femoral head.

An anterior-superior (AS) and an internal (In) listed ilium causes the acetabulum to move in a posterior and inferior direction. Heel contact forces the acetabulum to raise and hence appears on the AP film as a raised femoral head line (Fig. 6.39).

Plaugher and Hendricks have demonstrated a high level of inter- and intraexaminer reliability for line drawings of the pelvis using the Gonstead method (46).

After many years of extensive investigation, using pre- and postadjustment radiography at the Gonstead clinic, the 5:2 (i.e., 1.0:0.4) rule was formulated (Personal Communication, Dr. Alex Cox). The effect of ilium correction on the ipsilateral femoral head height projection on the AP film is as follows:

1. For every 5 mm of PI, or Ex correction, the femoral head height will be raised 2 mm.
2. For every 5 mm of AS, or In correction, the femoral head height will be lowered 2 mm.

Examples:

A PI_5 will result in the ipsilateral femoral head being 2 mm lower on the AP film.

A PI_{10} Ex_5 will result in the ipsilateral femoral head being 6 mm lower on the AP film.

An AS_5 will result in the ipsilateral femoral head being 2 mm higher on the AP film.

A PI_{10} In_5 will result in the ipsilateral femoral head being 2 mm lower on the AP film.

An AS_3 In_2 will result in the ipsilateral femoral head being 2 mm higher on the AP film.

CLINICAL FINDINGS

The subluxated ilium results in ipsilateral symptoms such as buttock, hip, leg and groin pain. This type of LLI is managed by adjusting the subluxated ilium. The short leg side ilium is either PI or Ex. The psoas, piriformis and gluteals are generally tender on the short leg side.

Functional Leg Length Inequality From Foot Pronation

A pronated foot is recognized by a flattened longitudinal arch. This occurs when the subtalar joint pronates, because of the talus rotating medially. When this occurs the entire lower limb internally rotates. This results in an ipsilateral iliopsoas muscle stretch and subsequent increased sacral base angle. It also results in a functional shortening of that limb and a lowered femoral head height on the AP film.

Brown, Markham and Smith (In Shoe Systems, Bellingham, WA., Personal Communication) in a study of 25 patients using Gonstead line drawings on A-P films demonstrated that by correcting foot pronation, femoral head height increased on average, 2.2 mm (maximum 5 mm).

CLINICAL FINDINGS

Foot pronation results in ipsilateral internal hip rotator muscle tenderness and ipsilateral sacroiliac tenderness. A further test was described by Brown (Personal Communication) to distinguish LLI caused by foot pronation or anatomic short leg. With the patient standing, the ASISs are palpated bilaterally, noting which is higher. The PSISs are then palpated noting which is lower. For a pronated foot, the lower PSIS will be on the same side as the higher ASIS. Without moving the patient, externally rotate the lower limb so as to place the subtalar joint in the neutral position. It will be noted that the ASISs and PSISs will approximate a more level position. If a true anatomic LLI is present, both the ASIS and PSIS will be high (or low) on the same side.

MANAGEMENT

If the foot pronation is prominent when observing the patient's gait and standing posture, and in addition to this the patient's condition remains unstable after adjustments, orthotics should be prescribed.

The orthotic should be molded with the patient's foot aligned to bring the talus to the neutral position. With the subtalar joint in a neutral position, the mid-tarsal joint is further stabilized. Precision vacuum-molded orthotics are available for chiropractors, or the patient can be referred to a podiatrist.

Anatomic Leg Length Inequality

After applying the 5:2 rule and ruling out any other predisposing factors to LLI, an anatomic true short leg is often observed. This difference can be quantified. An example would be a difference in femoral head height of 10 mm with a PI_3Ex_2 on the short leg side. After applying the 5:2 rule, the PIEx subluxation correction would still leave an LLI of 8 mm.

CLINICAL FINDINGS

Although there are exceptions to the rule, in a series of 50 cases with true short leg the author has observed that the majority of patients complained of pain on the contralateral side. They experienced pain on the long leg side in the buttock, and sacroiliac joint. Also observed was ipsilateral long leg psoas contraction, with tenderness, plus gluteal and piriformis tenderness. The sacrum drops inferiorward on the short leg side.

MANAGEMENT

Once a true short leg has been established, the doctor must first establish if it is significant and if so, whether a heel lift or orthotic is required. The patient's subluxation(s) must first be treated (Fig. 6.40). If the subluxation proves to be unstable and matches a history of recurring episodes, then a heel lift may well be indicated. If the patient responds to adjustments and remains stable in spite of a large LLI, then this patient does not require a heel lift.

Author opinions about the amount of LLI tolerated vary. As a general guide, 5 mm LLI or greater is significant if the subluxation is unstable after correction.

A heel lift raises the ipsilateral head height and induces an ipsilateral side bend in the lumbar spine. The coupled movement is for vertebral body rotation to the opposite side. Therefore a heel lift should only be prescribed if L5 vertebral body rotation is to the short leg side and the lumbar spine convexity is on the short leg side.

The foundation for the spine is the sacrum, not the femoral heads. If the sacral groove line is level, then a heel lift for a true short leg is contraindicated. A malformed sacrum, inducing an unlevel sacral groove line, may well need a heel lift to create a level foundation.

In some situations, age and the degree of chronicity

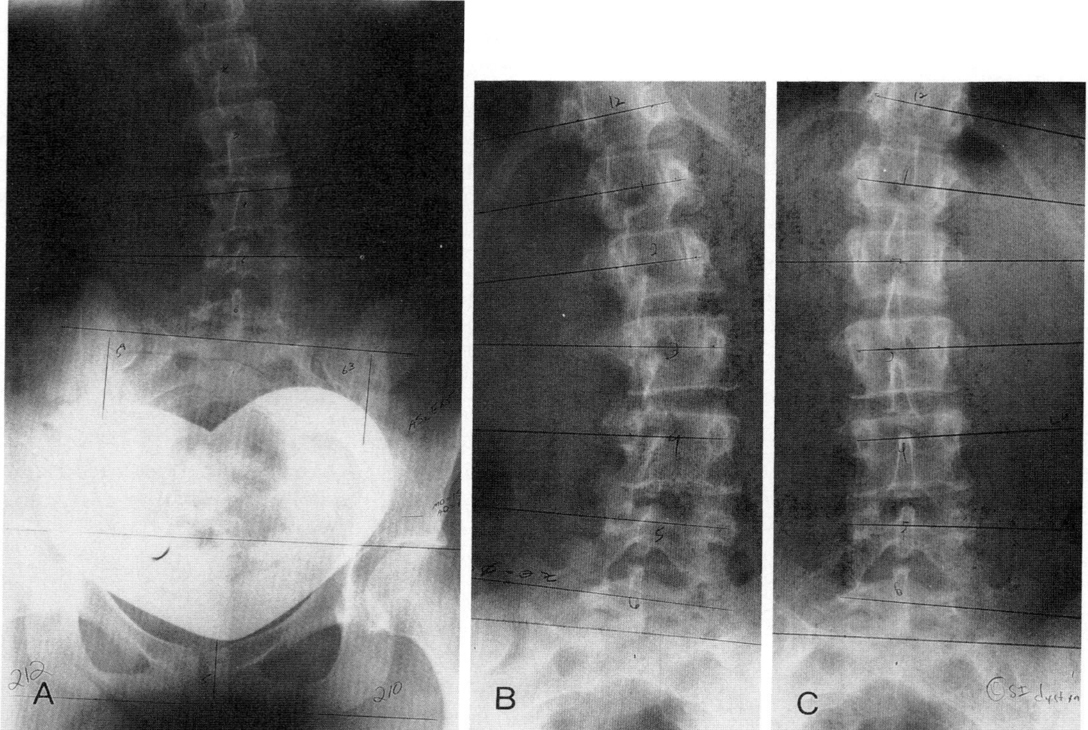

Figure 6.40. **A,** A right anatomic short leg of 13 mm has induced a lumbar convexity to the right. **B,** Left side bend allows for $-\theta Z$ and $-\theta Y$ motions. **C,** Right side bend has decreased $+\theta Z$ and $+\theta Y$ movements. This is an example of the need to address the fixation dysfunction of the spine above before adding a heel lift.

and even degenerative changes in the spine may prevent adaptation to a heel lift. These changes must be investigated in the lumbosacral region as well as the thoraco-lumbar region before prescribing.

In adults, the ability for the spine to adapt and the amount of heel lift required, determines whether to fit the full amount all at once or increase the amount of lift gradually over several weeks or months. Heel lifts are never prescribed while the patient is in an acute inflamed condition.

After the application of a heel lift, the patient will need periodic treatment to ensure that full spine functional adaptation occurs. Some of the greatest changes occur at the thoraco-lumbar junction and the upper cervical region.

Once a heel lift has been successfully prescribed, patients use them for the rest of their lives.

REFERENCES

1. Taber's Cyclopedic Medical Dictionary. Philadelphia: FA Davis, 1977.
2. Warwick R, Williams P, eds. Grays Anatomy 35th ed. Norwich, England: Longman, 1973.
3. Otter R. A review study of the differing opinions expressed in the literature about the anatomy of the sacroiliac joint. Euro J Chiro 1985;33:221–242.
4. Kapandji IA. The physiology of the joints. Vol.3. Edinburgh: Churchill Livingstone, 1978.
5. O'Rahilly R, ed. Anatomy. A regional study of human anatomy. 5th ed. Philadelphia: WB Saunders Company, 1986.
6. Cichoke AJ. Anatomy and function of the sacroiliac articulations: A review of the literature. Chiropractic 1989;2:65–70.
7. Steindler A. Kinesiology of the human body. Springfield: Charles C Thomas, 1970.
8. Bowen V, Cassidy JD. Macroscopic and microscopic anatomy of the sacroiliac joint from embryonic life until the eighth decade. Spine 1981;6:620–628.
9. Brooke R. The sacroiliac joint. J Anat 1924;58:299–305.
10. Sandoz RW. Structural and functional pathologies of the pelvic ring. Ann Swiss Chiro Assoc 1981;VII:101–160.
11. Bellamy N, Park W, Rooney PJ. What do we know about the sacroiliac joint? Semin Arthritis Rheum 1983;12:282–307.
12. Denton D. Biomechanics of the pelvis. From "The biomechanics of the pelvis," The Denver conference of the A.C.A. Council on Technic, 1980.
13. Janse J. The concepts and research of Dr. Fred Illi. National College Journal of Chiropractic 1956;28:10–34.
14. Freeman MD, Fox D, Richards T. The superior capsular ligament of the sacroiliac joint: presumptive evidence for confirmation Of Illi's ligament. J Manipulative Physiol Ther 1990;13:384–390.
15. Vleeming A, Stoeckart R, Snidjers CJ. The sacrotuberous ligament: a conceptual approach to its dynamic role in stabilizing the sacroiliac joint. Clin Biomech 1989;4:201–203.
16. Gracovetsky S. The spinal engine. Wien: Springer-Verlag, 1988:286–329.
17. Solonen KA. The sacroiliac joint in the light of anatomical and roentgenological and clinical studies. Acta Orthop Scand 1958; VII:160–162.
18. Homewood AE. The neurodynamics of the vertebral subluxation. Ontario: Chiropractic Publishers, 1973.

19. Schafer RC, Faye LJ. Motion palpation and chiropractic technique: principles of dynamic chiropractic. Huntington Beach, USA: Motion Palpation Institute, 1989.
20. Schafer RC. Clinical biomechanics: musculoskeletal actions and reactions. 2nd ed. Baltimore: Williams & Wilkins, 1987.
21. Faye LJ. Spinal biomechanics. Motion Palpation Institute. Seminar notes, 1985.
22. Grice A. Mechanics of walking, development and clinical significance. J Can Chiro Assoc 1972;16:15–23.
23. Greenman PE. Clinical aspects of sacroiliac function in walking. Manual Med 1990;5:125–130.
24. Egund N, Olssen TH, Schmid H, Selvik G. Movements in the sacroiliac joints demonstrated with roentgen stereophotogrammetry. Acta Radiol Diagn 1978;19:833–846.
25. Weisl H. The movements of the sacroiliac joint. Acta Anat 1955;23:80–91.
26. Dontigny RL. Anterior dysfunction of the sacroiliac joint as a major factor in the aetiology of idiopathic low back pain syndrome. Phys Ther 1990;70:250–262.
27. Gatterman MI. Disorders of the pelvic ring. In: Gatterman MI, ed. Chiropractic management of spine related disorders. Baltimore: Williams & Wilkins, 1990:111–128.
28. Greenman PE. Innominate shear dysfunction in the sacroiliac syndrome. Manual Med 1986;2:114–121.
29. Frigerio N, Stowe RR, Howe JW. Movement of the sacroiliac joint. Clin Orthop 1974;100:370–377.
30. Wells PE. Movements of the pelvic joints. In: Grieve GP, ed. Modern manual therapy of the vertebral column. New York: Churchill Livingstone, 1986:176–181.
31. Mitchell FL, Moran PS, Pruzzo NA. An evaluation and treatment manual of osteopathic muscle energy procedures. 1st ed. Missouri: Mitchell, Moran and Pruzzo, Associates, 1979.
32. Cailliet R. Low back pain syndrome. 3rd ed. Philadelphia: F.A. Davis, 1981.
33. Yochum TR, Rowe LJ. Essentials of skeletal radiology. Baltimore: Williams & Wilkins, 1987.
34. Bull PW. Accessory sacroiliac articulations. J of U.C.A. of Australasia, Ltd. 1984;4:12–16.
35. Bull PW. Radiological manifestations of diseases of the sacroiliac joints. J of U.C.A. of Australasia Ltd. 1985;5:23–26.
36. Forrester DM, Nesson JW. The radiology of joint disease. Philadelphia: WB Saunders, 1973.
37. Sandoz R. Principles underlying the prescription of shoe lifts. Ann Swiss Chiro Assoc 1986;IX:49–89.
38. Lawrence DJ. Chiropractic concepts of the short leg: a critical review. J Manipulative Physiol Ther 1985;8:157–161.
39. Klein KK. Developmental asymmetries of the weight bearing skeleton and its implications in knee stress and knee injury: a continuing report. Athletic Training 1982;18:207–208.
40. Stoddard A. Manual of osteopathic technique. 2nd ed. London: Hutchinson Co. 1959:39–41, 211–214.
41. Giles LGF, Taylor JR. Lumbar spine structural changes associated with leg length inequality. Spine 1982;7:159–162.
42. Woerman AL, Binder-Macleod A. Leg length discrepancy assessment: accuracy and precision in five clinical methods of evaluation. J Orthop Sports Phys Ther 1984;5:230–239.
43. Dishman RW. Chiropractic Foot Orthotics. Huntington Beach, CA: Motion Palpation Institute, 1988.
44. Lecture Notes. Gonstead Seminar of Chiropractic. Mt Horeb, WI, 1989.
45. Kirkaldy-Willis WH. Managing low back pain. New York: Churchill Livingstone, 1983.
46. Plaugher G, Hendricks AH. The inter- and intraexaminer reliability of the Gonstead pelvic marking system. J Manipulative Physiol Ther 1991;14:503–508.
47. Mierau DR, Cassidy JD, Hamin T, Milne RA. Sacroiliac joint dysfunction and low back pain in school aged children. J Manipulative Physiol Ther 1984;7:81–84.
48. Diakow PRP, Cassidy JD, DeKorompay VL. Post surgical sacroiliac syndrome: a case study. J Can Chiro Assoc 1983;27:19–23.
49. Sandoz R. The choice of appropriate clinical criteria for assessing the progress of a chiropractic case. Ann Swiss Chiro Assoc 1985; VIII:53–74.
50. Herbst RW. Gonstead chiropractic science and art. Mt Horeb, WI: Sci-Chi Publications, 1968.

7 Lumbar Spine

GREGORY PLAUGHER

Knowledge gained from studying the spinal column in sections is inherently weak. The spine exists and functions as one integrated whole, one area of the spine often being affected by other more distant regions. Similarly, the spinal column and pelvis are supported and acted on by the lower and upper extremities, thus influencing them in diverse and complex interactions.

The lumbar spine is unique for a variety of reasons. Because each region of the spine supports the weight of the body in increasing amounts as one moves caudal, the lumbar column is especially susceptible to extreme axial loads and external bending torques or moments. This may be the reason there is an increase in lumbar spinal dysfunction among truck drivers and hard laborers (1,2). The lumbar spine is a point of transfer of forces from the strong bony pelvis to the flexible axial motion segments.

As with the more caudal structures of the body, dysfunction in the lumbar spine will have direct mechanical reactions in the joints above, a continuation of the foundation principle discussed in Chapter 6. This is the reason a pronated foot can influence pelvic list and the posture of the torso, or an increase in the lumbar lordosis with hyperextension of the upper lumbar motion segments, may reduce the cervical lordotic curve (Fig. 7.1).

This chapter covers the dysfunction and management of disorders afflicting the vertebral joints of L1 to S1. The mechanical lesion is emphasized, although some attention is given to organic and visceral conditions that may impact on the decision making processes of the astute clinician. A few aspects of the clinical anatomy and biomechanics of the lumbar spine are presented here. This subject, however, is covered in more detail in Chapter 2, which the reader is encouraged to review before proceeding. The pathomechanics of the lower spine and its relationship to the vertebral subluxation complex is covered. The chiropractic management of mechanical disorders of the low back is thoroughly discussed.

CLINICAL ANATOMY AND BIOMECHANICS

Central Joint

The central joint is composed of two vertebral bodies, their associated end-plate structures and their common intervertebral disc, which is composed of the annulus fibrosis and the nucleus pulposus.

END-PLATE

The hyaline cartilage end-plate acts as the transition zone from vertebra to disc. Rather than herniate the intervertebral disc, a compressive overload will fracture the end-

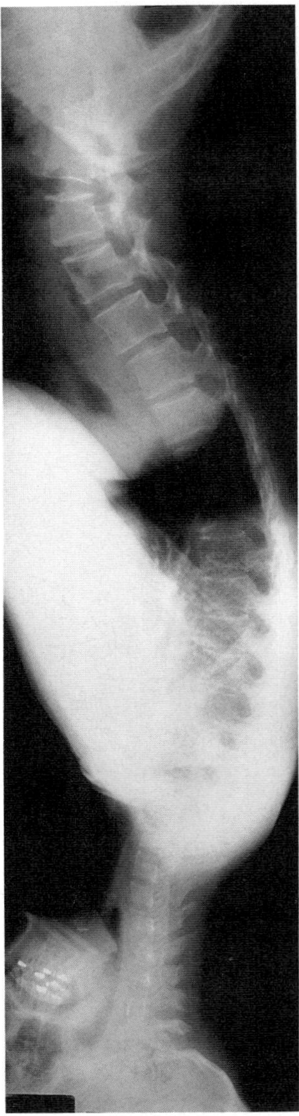

Figure 7.1. Lateral full spine radiograph (two exposures) illustrating how reduction of the cervical lordosis can occur in compensation for abnormalities (e.g., hyperextension of the upper lumbar spine) in the lower spine.

plate. Fractures of this structure are one of the most common findings on cadaver dissection (3). Callous formation in the area after injury will inhibit diffusion of nutrients to the avascular disc, thus leading to degeneration. Compression overload, causing fracture and eventual degeneration of the soft tissue elements with bone proliferation, can lead to central canal stenosis. Instability is rare however, unless it is combined with torsional injuries of the annulus.

ANNULUS FIBROSIS

The annulus is composed of concentric lamellae that tend to resist various loads applied to the motion segment. There is great resistance to compression and shear. Resistance to flexion and extension is also high. Because of the anisotropic properties of the annulus (See Chapter 2) however, it cannot resist all loads in an equal manner. Applications of axial torque will tend to compromise the annular fibers, especially if they are distracted, as happens in the forward bent position. Micro-failure of the annulus begins to occur at approximately 3° of axial rotation. Torsional loads will affect the posterior joints as well, leading to synovitis and degeneration. With time, torsional injuries can cause instability of the motion segment.

NUCLEUS PULPOSUS

The nucleus pulposus has a high water content that tends to decrease with age. In the nondegenerated disc, the nucleus is a highly pressurized structure that will deform when loaded. When compressed, the nucleus will bulge peripherally transferring forces to the annulus. During forward flexion, the nucleus bulges posteriorly.

The disc's ability to swell is great in the lumbar spine. In the degenerated disc, where it is difficult to differentiate the annulus from the nucleus, the disc's ability to swell is reduced. Schmorl's nodes are a result of nuclear protrusion into the end-plate from compressive overload.

Disc Pressure

The pressure within the intervertebral discs of the lumbar spine has been studied by Nachemson (4). Table 7.1 demonstrates the different forces that develop within a lumbar L3 disc during different activities and postures. This table is of help in managing the patient who has disc trauma because certain activities will most likely cause further injury. It must be kept in mind however, that these measurements are taken with the subject in a quasistatic position. This may not be reflective of how pressures would develop in a person executing a dynamic lift (See Chapter 2). Nonetheless, they are important for understanding relative differences in disc pressure.

Table 7.1.
Approximate Load on the L3 Disc in a 70-kg Subject[a]

Position or Activity	Newtons of Force (N)
Supine, traction of 500 N	0
Supine, semi-Fowler position	100
Supine	250
Supine, tilt table at 50°	400
Sitting, with lumbar support, 110 degree inclination	400
Supine, arm exercises	500
Standing, at ease	500
Coughing	600
Straining	600
Forward bend, 20°	600
Upright sitting, without support	700
Bilateral leg lift	800
Forward bend, 40°	1000
Forward bend, 20° while holding 20 kg	1200
Sit-up exercises	1200
Lifting 10 kg with back straight and knees bent	1700
Lifting 10 kg with back bent	1900
Holding 5 kg with arms extended	1900
Forward flexed and rotated 20° while holding 10 kg	2100

[a]From Nachemson AL. Disc pressure measurements. Spine 1981;6:93–97.

Posterior Joints

ORIENTATION

The anatomy of the facet joints is important in understanding the biomechanical function of the three joint complex. Dysfunction at the posterior joints usually occurs secondary to, or simultaneously with injury at the central joint (5). The zygapophyseal joints are richly innervated with pain fibers (6) and can be a source of pain if inflammation is present, or a synovial fold becomes entrapped between the two facet surfaces.

Radiographic methods have been used to determine the spatial orientation of the lumbar facet planes. The AP radiograph is helpful in determining the facet planes but the CT scan is preferred, because of its cross sectional capability. From L1 to L4 the facets are "J" shaped. Posteriorly, they begin in the sagittal plane while turning medialward at the anterior (Fig. 7.2A). This configuration limits Y axis rotation (7) and provides some resistance to anterior shear. At L5-S1 the facets can best be described as being in the coronal plane. This orientation is present to counteract the tremendous anterior shear component at that level (Fig. 7.2B).

Although the facet orientation at L5-S1 would seem to allow more rotation around the Y axis, this is controlled by the strong iliolumbar ligaments that tend to inhibit the amount of Y axis rotation the joint actually undergoes. The maximal amount of axial rotation (Y axis) is approximately 1° to each side at L1 through L4 and 2° in each direction at the lumbosacral junction (8). Keep in mind, however, that this is axial rotation of joints without posterior displacement. When a large amount of retrolis-

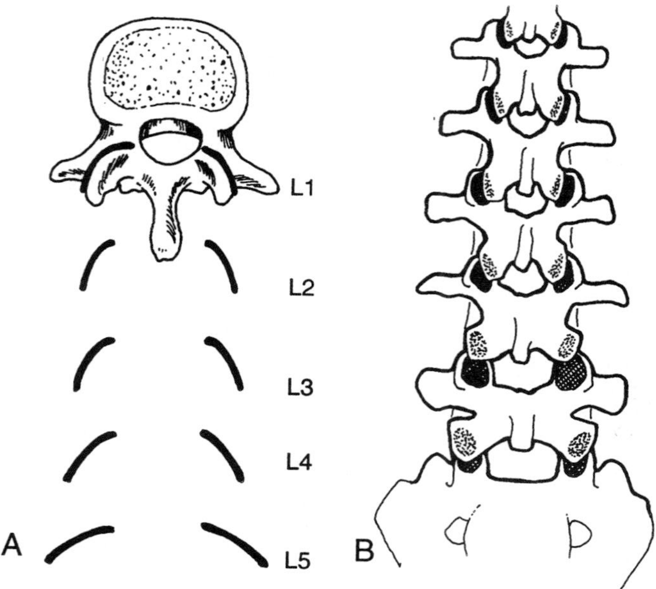

Figure 7.2. **A,** Facet planes of the lumbar spine. Horizontal (X-Z) plane. **B,** Frontal (X-Y) plane.

thesis is present, as is often the case in a torsionally injured lumbar spine, the subsequent separation of the facets allows more intersegmental axial rotation to occur. Correction of the axially rotated segment with an adjustment often will not occur if the doctor fails to consider the posterior displacement.

TROPISM

The incidence of asymmetry of the articular processes is quite high. In their investigation, Ho and Chace (9) report that asymmetries in at least one lumbar spine facet occurred in 58% of the subjects tested. The asymmetry is lowest at L1. The total asymmetrical frequency rises in the lower segments, reaching a peak at L4 and then decreasing at L5. Hagg and Wallner (10) similarly found a high incidence of facet asymmetry, occurring in about 50% of patients with lumbar disc herniation.

Farfan and Sullivan (11) report an apparent correlation between facet joint asymmetry and dysfunction of the intervertebral disc. The more oblique facet often is associated with the side of sciatica in patients presenting with radicular pain into the lower extremity. The study by Hagg and Wallner (10),however, found no correlation between the side of asymmetry and protrusion of lumbar intervertebral discs.

The high incidence of facet asymmetry illustrates the importance of analyzing the kinematic behavior of the motion segment from a structural standpoint. Any examination that analyzes lumbar spine motion, radiographic or palpatory, must be supplemented with a static anteroposterior radiograph, unless contraindicated (See Chapter 5), to determine facetal geometry qualitatively.

COMPRESSION LOADS

The angle of the facet joints enable them to respond to external forces and at the same time guide the type of motion the spine is able to perform. Compression forces (Y axis) are counteracted in part by the facets. Approximately 16% of this compressive load is taken up by the facetal pillars themselves when in the standing position. The facets at the L2-L3 level share a higher percentage of the axial compressive loads than the facets at the L4-L5 level (12). As the spine is flexed, such as occurs in the sitting posture, the facets resist little compressive load (13). Facet load remains relatively constant with increasing segmental compressive loads, such that the facet load expressed as a percent of load applied to the segment, decreases with increasing axial forces (12). When compressive loads become great, the end-plate is the first to fail (5). Very little injury is sustained by the facet joints or the annulus.

Miller (14) summarizes the role of the apophyseal joints in various loads. During axial compression (Y axis) and lateral flexion (Z axis), the facets are not heavily burdened. However, the facets can be more stressed during shear forces. When the motion segment is flexed, extended or anteroposteriorly sheared, the facet joints relieve some of the load taken by the disc. The facet joints resist approximately ⅓ of the shear force of the motion segment with the disc resisting the remaining ⅔ (15).

Motion Patterns

CORONAL (X-Y) PLANE

The coupling pattern of the lumbar spine is axial rotation (Y axis) with lateral flexion (Z axis). As the spine is laterally flexed, the spinous process of that segment rotates towards the same side (Fig. 7.3A-B). Coupling of the lumbar spine occurs in three dimensions. A slight amount of flexion occurs in addition to the axial rotation. This is true however, only when the lumbar lordosis is present. If the lordosis is flattened such as during the sitting posture, then a slight amount of extension occurs at the joint in addition to the axial rotation (16).

It is important to analyze both lateral flexion and axial rotation motions when studying the kinematics of the spine with stress radiography. Lateral bending radiographs can show a joint that is laterally flexing normally but is not exhibiting proper coupling characteristics. Normal lateral flexion behavior is called Type 1 (Fig. 7.4). Type 2 indicates the spine is laterally bending but not axially rotating. Type 3 motion describes a motion segment that is not laterally flexing but has normal coupling of

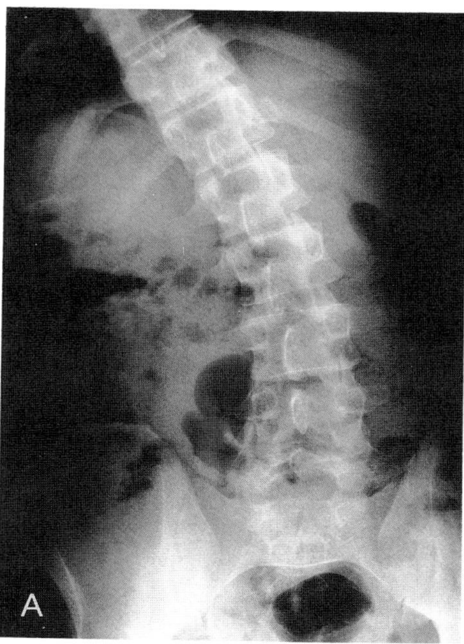

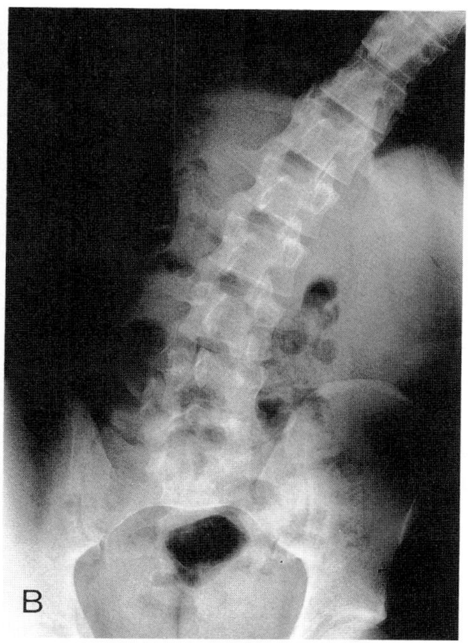

Figure 7.3. **A,** Normal lateral bending of the lumbar spine with coupling of the spinous processes towards the concavity of bend. **B,** Abnormal coupling of the spinous processes towards the convexity of bend. This patient also has a spondylolisthesis of L5.

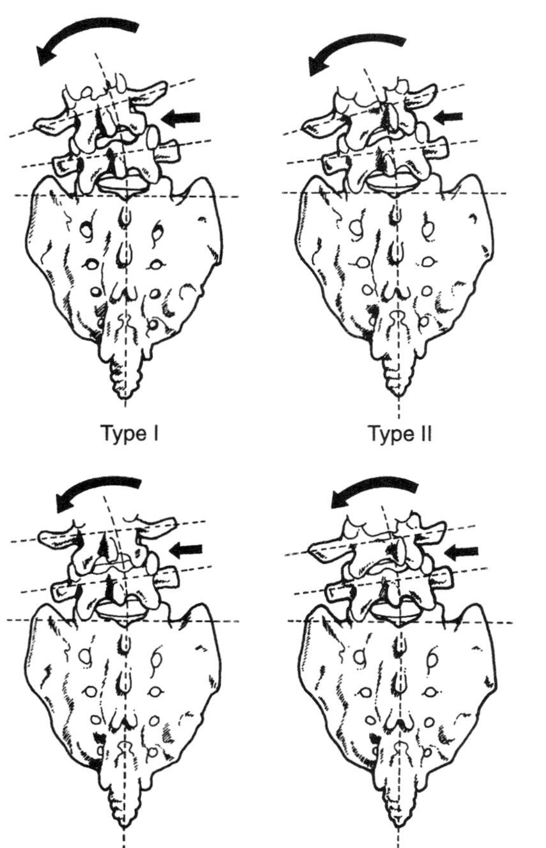

Figure 7.4. Lateral bending of the lumbar spine; Types 1–4.

axial rotation (17). Type 4 dysfunction describes a motion segment that is not laterally bending nor axially rotating during lateral flexion of the lumbar spine. Figure 7.4 illustrates the various motion patterns of the lumbar spine during lateral bending.

The amount of lateral flexion at a motion segment is dependent on the level. Two to three degrees are allowed at L5-S1; five to ten at L3-L4; three to nine at L2-L3 and from three to eight at L1-L2 (8). The ranges cited represent common ranges of motion. Many studies are in vitro analyses. They are not necessarily reflective of an in vivo normal motion segment (i.e., absence of degeneration).

SAGITTAL PLANE

Flexion and extension (X axis rotation) is quite large when compared with the other degrees of freedom. The average (mean) amount of combined flexion and extension for the lumbar motion segments are as follows: L1-L2, 7.5°; L2-L3, 7.5°; L3-L4, 18°; L4-L5, 22°; L5-S1, 18° (18). Maximal flexion is restricted by the posterior soft tissues and extension is restricted by the anterior soft tissues.

The analysis of patterns of motion during flexion and extension has only been performed on patients with low back pain. In a study by Putto and Tallroth (19), they found that during flexion all segments rotated forward ($+\theta X$) but that coupling of translation along the Z axis varied depending on the level. From L1 to L4 there was a slight anteriorward translation (0.85–2.8 mm) but at L5 the translation is posteriorward. This is due to the pull of the lumbodorsal fascia when there is a small spinous process at L5 (See Chapter 2). Translation, either anterior or posterior, is most likely a reflection of disc injury at the motion segment. The patient with lumbar spine injury should always be cautioned against any activities that cause flexion of the low back. The exact amount of in vivo translation that is possible is difficult to determine from the study by Putto and Tallroth of patients with chronic low back pain because no details of the radiographic technique (i.e., film focal distance) are provided. It is known that radiographic magnification varies with the focal film distance and the object film distance, and that this would effect millimetric measurements. Normal lumbar flexion is illustrated in Figure 7.5.

A study by Yoshioka et al. (20) determined the motion characteristics of the lumbar spine in the sagittal spine in a group of pain-free young Japanese adults. Of interest was the fact that during sagittal plane motion the L4 segment showed primarily a translational strategy ($\pm Z$), and the L5 segment, a predominantly rotational ($\pm \theta X$) motion characteristic. The reduced amount of translation at L5 could be due to the restraining aspect of the iliolumbar ligaments (20). The increased translation at the L4-L5 level may be due to early disc degeneration. There is no way to know however, because the radiologic analysis was not correlated with MRI findings. The average ranges of motion (θX) from maximal extension to maximal flexion for each lumbar level were as follows (20):

L1 = 12.7°
L2 = 16.6°
L3 = 16.7°
L4 = 18.3°
L5 = 19.6°

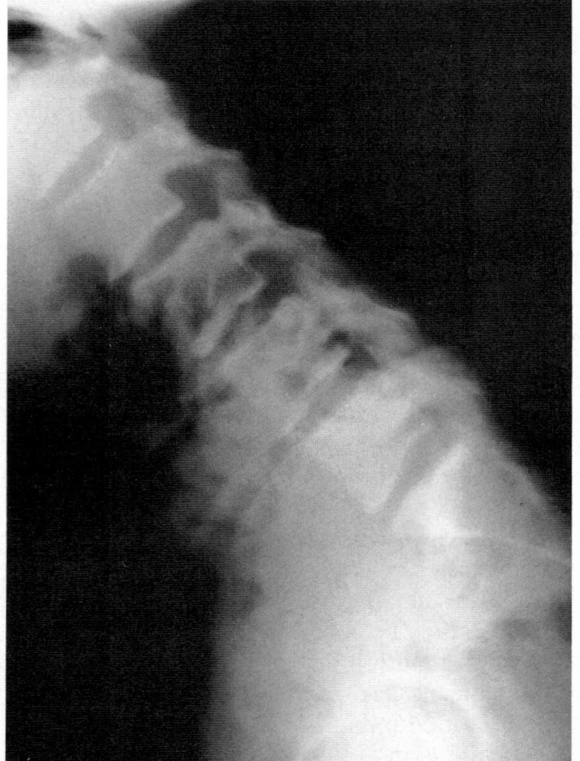

Figure 7.5. Normal lumbar flexion. Notice the lack of anterior translation, which would indicate pathology of the disc and facet joints.

Posture

The posture of the lower spine in the sagittal plane is a lordotic configuration (Figures 7.6A-B). The curve is acquired and is developed when the toddler begins to walk. The wedge shape of the intervertebral discs and the vertebral bodies, especially L5, primarily form the lumbar lordosis. The human lordosis is vital to providing the maximal strength vs. flexibility compromise. It represents a highly evolved structure and is responsible for the body's ability to lift great loads, in contrast to other primates (21). There are many anatomic factors that determine the extent of the lumbar curve.

It is generally agreed that the L3 vertebral body should be the most anterior vertebra in the lumbar lordosis. Many investigators have attempted to quantify the normal lumbar curve. While most investigations have been performed with the subject in the recumbent position, one report (22) used patients who had films taken in the standing position. These patients were considered to have relatively normal static radiographic posture. The range of the lumbar lordosis was 35° to 54°. The lordosis angle was constructed with L1 and L5 used as the end vertebrae. In another study (23), the standing lumbar lordosis was evaluated in a series of patients presenting to an outpatient chiropractic clinic. The lumbar lordosis angle was found to have a mean of 59.4° (SD: 10.4). This measurement however, used L1 and S1 for the end vertebrae. Lumbar curves outside of the ranges cited should be considered either hypo or hyperlordotic. The patient's posture can then be compared to the clinical assessment. It is important to keep in mind that the lumbar lordosis is a compound curve with the steepest angulation at the lumbosacral junction. It may be unlikely that a single angle is best representative of the lumbar lordosis (18).

LUMBAR SPINE DYSFUNCTION

Risk Factors

Heliovaara (24) found that obesity and increased body height (men; > 180 cm; women; > 170 cm) increased an individual's risk for development of a lumbar disc herniation. Genetic factors are also at work in the etiology of this disorder. The relative risk of developing a disc herniation before the age of twenty-one is approximately five times greater in patients with a family history (25).

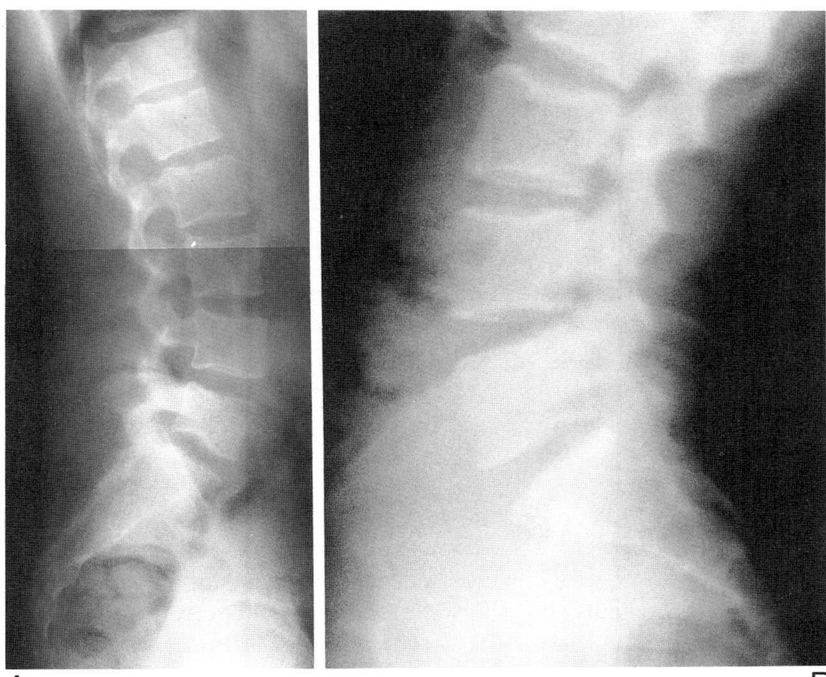

Figure 7.6. **A,** Example of a relatively normal lumbar lordosis. Notice particularly the normal disc height present at L5-S1. Abnormalities are present, such as end-plate nuclear depressions. **B,** A relatively normal lumbar lordosis of an athlete. Notice the wedge-like appearance of the intervertebral discs at all levels. The same individual is pictured in Figure 7.5.

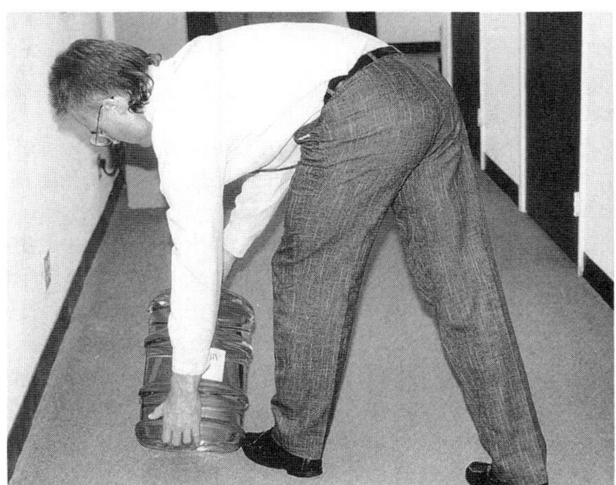

Figure 7.7. Pathomechanics of lumbar spine injury. Torsion, lateral bending, flexion, and compression loads are depicted.

Patients with a history of a traumatic back injury had a 2.5-fold risk of having sciatica or low back pain in a large survey conducted in Finland (26). Smoking also appears to be a risk factor for developing low back pain.

Pathomechanics

The relaxation phenomenon is seen when the lumbar spine and pelvis are forwardly flexed 45° or more (27). The paraspinal muscles become myoelectrically silent in this posture. Freefall is prevented because of the tension in the midline ligaments and the lumbodorsal fascia. The relaxation phenomenon also exists on maximal lateral bend (28). It is easy to see why most lumbar spine injuries occur when the spine is flexed forward and laterally bent. In this posture, the ligaments take the majority of any load applied, which usually leads to failure of the system.

Most injuries to the lumbar spine happen because of a failure in the ligamentous and muscular systems in providing a sufficient response to external forces or moments. These are usually either of a compressive nature (Y axis translation) or torsional (Y axis rotation). A macro-traumatic event often precipitates lumbar spine injury. Certain situations may arise however, where an accumulation of micro-traumatic episodes leads to a failure of the joint. The classic example of this is the truck driver. The driver is subjected to repeated compression and vibratory forces with the spine in a relatively flexed position. It is widely known that truck drivers suffer from a higher incidence of low back pain when compared to the population as a whole (29). The posture of the single traumatic injury is most often associated with flexion (compression) in combination with lateral bending and axial rotation (Fig. 7.7) (8,30–32). In vitro hyperflexion of motion segments results in 43% of the discs sustaining prolapse (33).

COMPRESSION OVERLOAD

Purely compressional overload ($\pm$Y) results in damage or fracture of the end-plate. The annulus and the facet joints receive little injury during compressional overload (3). The fractured end-plate is one of the most common pathologic findings during lumbar dissections (3). Farfan lists four different types of laboratory injuries that can occur at the end-plate (Fig. 7.8):

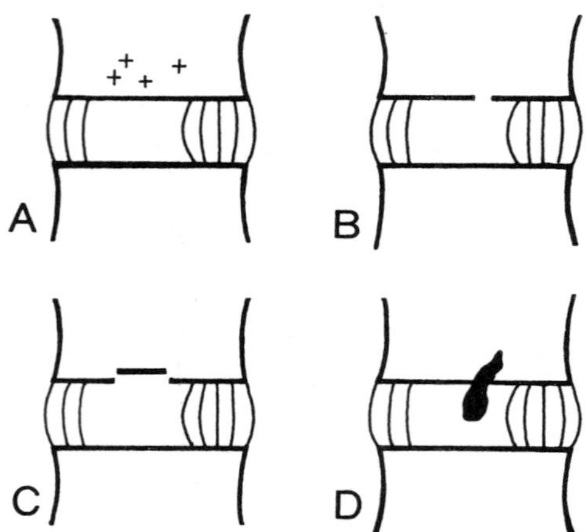

Figure 7.8. End-plate injuries of the lumbar spine. **A,** Subchondral fracture. **B,** Fissure fracture of the end-plate. **C,** Depressed fracture. **D,** Fracture with disc material forced into the vertebral body. Modified from Farfan HF. Symptomatology in terms of the pathomechanics of low-back pain and sciatica. In: Haldeman S, ed. Modern developments in the principles and practice of chiropractic. East Norwalk, CT: Appleton-Century-Crofts, 1980:173.

1. Sub-endplate compression fractures of cancellous bone. The overlying end-plate and cartilage are intact and still maintain the normal fluid barriers between disc and vertebral body.
2. Fractures of the end-plate and cartilage which open a communication between the disc and vertebral body. These fractures are of three types:
   a. fissure fractures of the end-plate
   b. depressed fractures of the end-plate
   c. fissure or depressed fractures with disc material forced into the vertebral body

Once the end-plate has been fractured, a significant weakness exists in the central joint. Normally the end-plate can withstand high intradiscal pressures. The fractures however, greatly decrease the end-plate's ability to support these high pressures (18). The vertebral body is the structure that acts as the great shock absorber for the spinal column. This is accomplished through a sensitive hydraulic system that depends on the rate of loading (5) (See Chapter 2). With fractures of the end-plate or the peripheral cortex, this hydraulic shock absorbing function is impaired (3).

TORSIONAL OVERLOAD

Torsional overload usually occurs when the spine is anteriorly flexed. During flexion, the posterior annulus becomes stretched (See Chapter 2). There is a more vertical arrangement of the collagenous fibers in the outer annulus when the joint is flexed. The strength of collagen is greatest along the orientation of the fibers. This arrangement is present so that the spine can resist the force of flexion and extension and lateral bending. This distribution is least suited to resistance of forces perpendicular to it, such as axial torsion. Additionally, the facets become separated to some extent during flexion, allowing more axial rotation at the joint (34). Torsional forces damage simultaneously both the facets and the annulus (35), because they are the elements that resist this motion (36). Rotations greater than 3.0° begin tearing the outer fibers of the annulus (18). Subchondral fractures occur at the posterior joints with resultant effusion, synovitis and motion limitation after forced rotation (3).

Repeated torsional overloads gradually damage inner fibers of the annulus until eventually a communication will exist between the nucleus and annulus. These tears are most often at the posterolateral angles and are called radial fissures.

RADIOGRAPHIC EVALUATION

After the joint has been injured in torsion, the radiograph usually shows a posterior displacement (retrolisthesis) on the segment below (18). This −Z translation of the vertebra on the segment below is a common radiographic and dissection finding in the lumbar spine (23,37–39) (Fig. 7.9A-F). Accompanying the −Z displacement, the A-P radiograph may also show rotational (Y axis) distortions, and/or lateral flexion positional dyskinesias (Z axis rotation) (Fig. 7.10) (37,38).

As the intervertebral disc and other soft tissues are moved beyond their physiologic range, two things occur simultaneously. The ligaments fail (disc, articular capsules, paravertebral ligaments) and the joint assumes a position outside of its physiologic range (40). The amount of displacement is usually quite small, but as the ligaments become more stressed from repeated injuries, and as the creep properties of the joint increase, the amount of positional change can be quite large.

Torsional force, with its concomitant rotational deformity of the intervertebral joint, is capable by itself of causing nerve root dysfunction. As the pedicle is moved medially on the opposite side of the torsional movement, the nerve root is deformed. With a rotation of 9°, the nerve root can be stretched approximately one centimeter. By reversal of the rotational deformity through spinal adjustments, the nerve root can be restored to a less tensile state (3). Adjustments can also be made to reduce retrolisthesis if present (23).

Disc Nomenclature

The names that have been ascribed to different dysfunctional states of the intervertebral disc are numerous. There seems to be little consistency among authors when describing identical lesions. To clarify the terminology problem, illustrations have been provided (Fig. 7.11A-D). The different types of disc pathologies are not necessarily progressive stages of injury. One dysfunctional state may not lead into the next.

Pain can arise from just about any injured area in the lumbar spine except the nucleus pulposus (Fig. 7.12). The outer annulus, facet joints, periosteal structures, muscle and fascial elements, are all richly innervated with pain fibers (8).

Rydevik et al. (41) determined that a herniated lumbar disc might be expected to reduce blood flow to the sensory cell bodies in the dorsal root ganglion, which may produce pain. This is a relatively new theory on the production of pain in patients with lumbar disc herniation.

Mechanisms of the Positional Dyskinesia

A positional dyskinesia of the motion segment is that situation where a vertebra has moved into a position that is not within the physiologic range of the joint. This malalignment, when present, is usually visible on standard plain film radiographs.

When the ligaments of the three-joint complex are damaged, one can assume that the vertebra was moved beyond its physiologic range (40). Torsional injuries may produce rotation (θY), wedging (θZ), inferiority ($-\theta X$) and posteriority ($-Z$). Because the positional state of the joint is reflective of the injury to the soft tissues, great care must be exercised when introducing a force into the motion segment. Already damaged ligaments should not be compromised further, as this will precipitate an inflammatory reaction, accelerating the degenerative process. The pattern of thrust of the adjustment should be exactly opposite the direction of ligamentous damage.

The adjustment is designed to reduce the dyskinesiologic position of the segment. This will normalize the axis

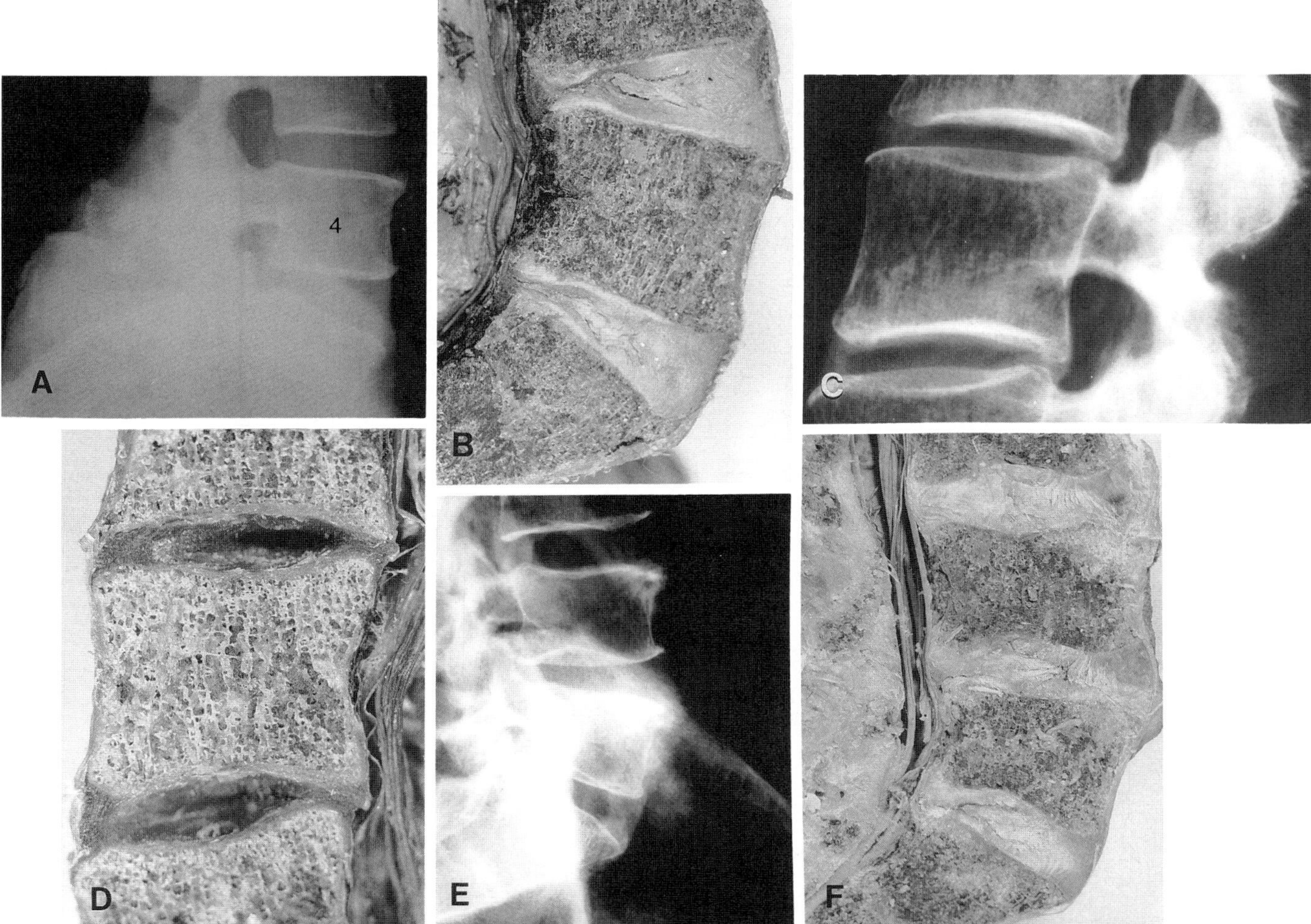

Figure 7.9. **A,** Radiograph of cadaver specimen. Notice the retrolisthesis at the L4 level. **B,** Cadaver specimen of **A**. There is internal disc disruption at the L4-L5 and L5-S1 interspaces. **C,** Radiograph demonstrating retrolisthesis and the vacuum phenomenon (See Chapter 5). **D,** Specimen showing signs of internal disc disruption at both levels. **E,** Radiograph demonstrating retrolisthesis at L4 and L5. Traction osteophytes indicateive of instability are present at the anterosuperior margin of L5 and the anteroinferior margin of L4. **F,** Specimen showing annular bulging at multiple levels with retrolisthesis of the vertebral bodies.

of motion around which joints move and decrease tension in the stressed soft tissues.

Normalization of position of individual segments may have an effect on the posture of the lumbar spine as a whole. A return to the normal range of lordosis of the lumbar spine will logically place less stress on individual segments of the curve. Similarly, normalization of the posture of the lower spine will have a positive effect on the thoracic and cervical sagittal curves. The sagittal curves of the spinal column are all interdependent (42).

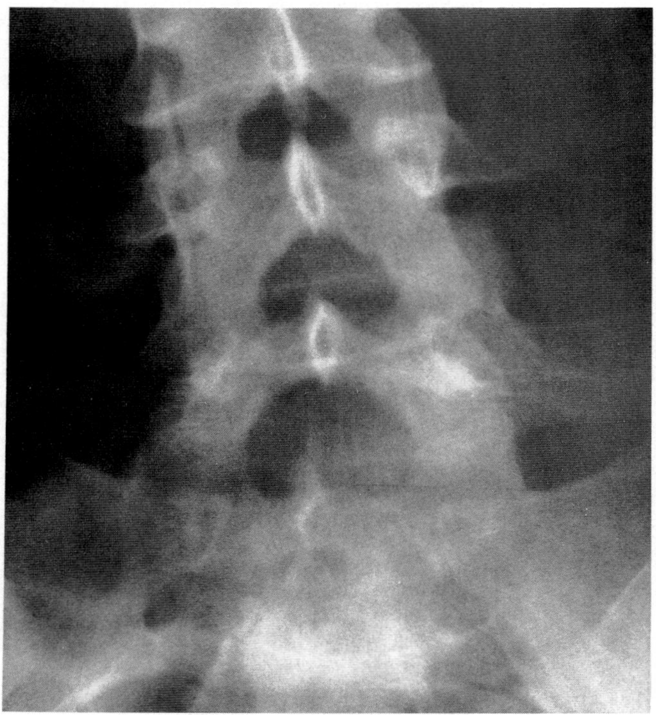

Figure 7.10. Neutral AP radiograph demonstrating a lateral flexion positional dyskinesia at L5-S1 and L4-L5.

Mechanisms of Fixation Dysfunction

Fixation dysfunction is that state of restricted motion at the pathologic joint. Hypomobility is a nonspecific term that may or may not indicate a pathology. For example, asymmetry of the articular pillars and other anomalies can restrict motion in one or more directions, but by itself is not reflective of a pathomechanical process occurring at the motion segment. Anomaly of the zygapophyseal joints of the lumbar spine, especially L4-L5, is common. Plain film radiography should be used to assess the presence of facetal anomaly, although CT is preferred.

Patients with low back pain often have absence of motion (43) or abnormal coupling patterns of the lower lumbar spine. The etiology of fixation dysfunction is most likely multi factorial (44). An entrapped meniscoid within the facet joint that causes pain has been proposed as a mechanism that reduces motion at a joint via a secondary reflexive muscular contraction. Other mechanisms include displacement of the nucleus and hard annular fragments, periarticular connective tissue adhesions and segmental muscular contraction (44). Disc displacement and dysfunction is most likely a major cause of fixation dysfunction in the lumbar spine. An adjustment may be able to move displaced nuclear or annular material (Fig. 7.13).

Regardless of the mechanism by which the joint becomes fixated, a restriction of mobility is pathologic and should be remedied. In the acute stage of injury, both the facets and disc may restrict motion at the joint because of swelling within the capsule or disc. A joint that is left in an immobilized state will show the following changes under biochemical assessment (45):

1. A reduction in glycosaminoglycans and water
2. An increase in intermolecular cross-linkages

Collagen cross-linkages may be broken with an adjustment, thus restoring mobility. The reduction of inflammatory edema within the disc or apophyseal joints would

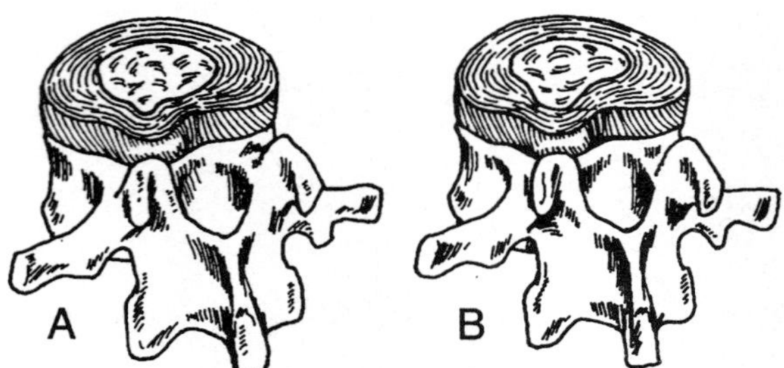

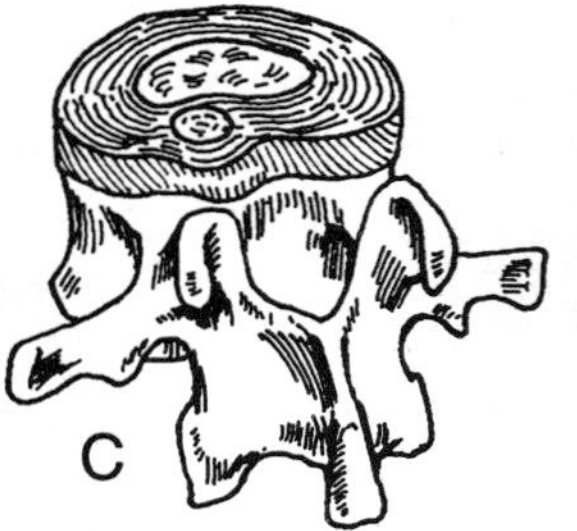

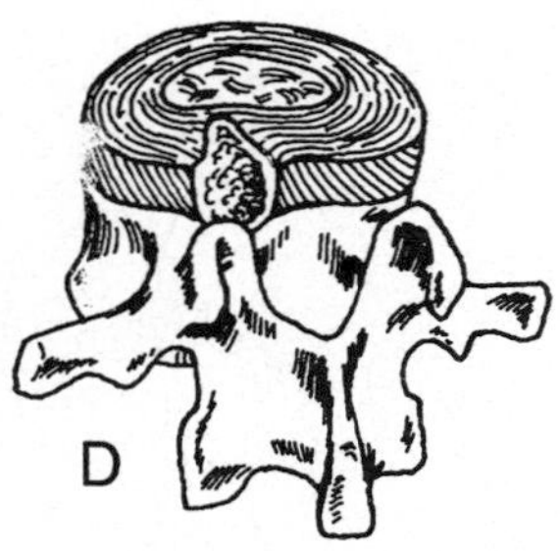

Figure 7.11. Disc injuries. **A,** Disruption of the posterolateral annulus with minor bulging. **B,** Moderate disc bulge. The *dotted line* represents the original position of the annulus. The patient may be experiencing sciatica. **C,** A sequestered fragment. **D,** A ruptured disc. The sequestered fragment is still anchored somewhat to the remainder of the disc. This type of pathology is unlikely to respond favorably to manipulative procedures. Modified from White AA, Panjabi MM. Clinical biomechanics of the spine. 2nd ed. Philadelphia: JB Lippincott, 1990:393–394.

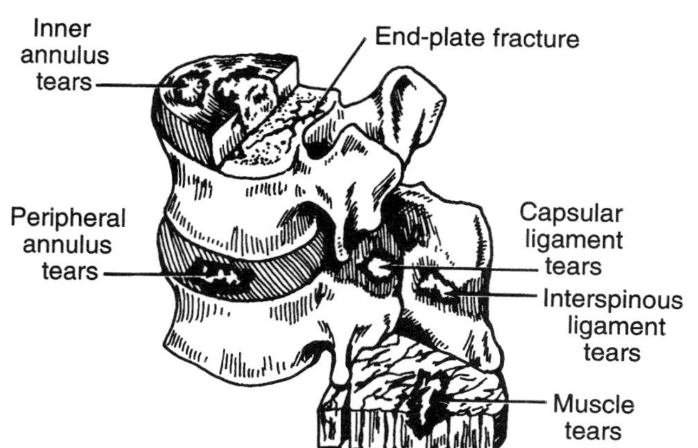

Figure 7.12. Back injury may result in damage to a variety of structures, all of which can give rise to pain, directly or indirectly. Modified from White AA, Panjabi MM. Clinical biomechanics of the spine. 2nd ed. Philadelphia: JB Lippincott, 1990:392.

likely increase mobility and decrease pain by decreasing tension on the pain sensitive periphery of the disc and the pain sensitive articular capsule. A global decrease in mobility is relatively common in patients with low back pain. Mellin (46) suggests that this is due to ligamentous or capsular stiffness of the involved articulations. Range of motion exercises for the lumbar spine should be encouraged as the patient begins to regain function from improvement in the intersegmental fixation dysfunction. Stokes et al. (47) found that movement in laboratory animals tended to help the joint to recover from experimental injury.

ADJUSTMENT EFFECTS

Pearcy et al. (48) showed that conservative measures (abdominal strengthening exercises, pelvic tilt exercises and back school) were unable to normalize abnormal coupling patterns of the lumbar spine. Carrick (49) however, has shown that lateral flexion fixation dysfunction and abnormal coupling patterns of the lumbar spine respond readily to spinal manipulation.

Bronfort and Jochumsen (50) documented increased intersegmental motion in patients with fixation dysfunction after a course of specific spinal manipulation. In their study on radiographic analysis of vertebral motion disturbances, they found a high correlation between plain film assessment and the cineradiographic procedure. Their recommendations were that stress plain film analysis be used to evaluate accurately, motion dysfunction of the lumbar spine.

Because the adjustment introduces motion at the joint, a reduction in the fixation dysfunction may occur (7.14A-D). An acute subluxation can cause global restrictions in motion (Fig. 7.14E-G). Fixation caused by chronic mechanisms, such as periarticular adhesions may

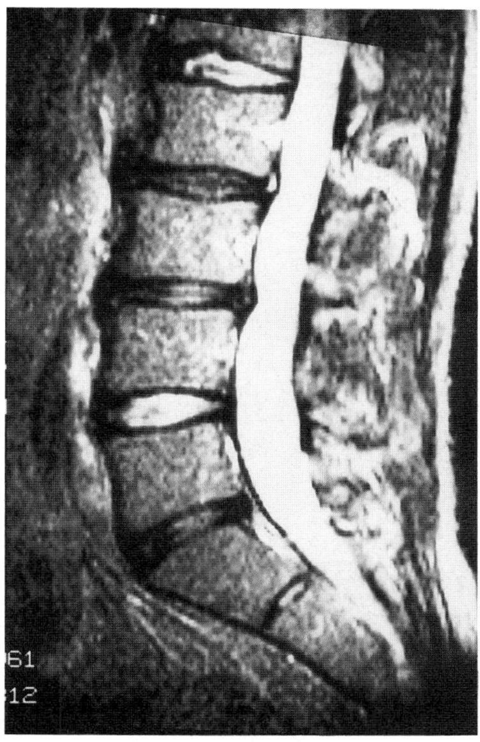

Figure 7.13. A MRI of a disc protrusion at L5 with concomitant retrolisthesis. A posterior to anterior adjustment could move the displaced disc material away from the nerve root.

take multiple adjustments to remedy. Adjustments can be supplemented with specific postural isometric exercises or maneuvers (51). In situations where the extent of degenerative processes in the joints is severe, a complete normalization of mobility seems unlikely (Fig. 7.15). This may also be true of the positional state of the segment. The more damaged the ligaments are, the less likely they will be able to shorten and heal, thereby countering progressive creep properties of the articulation.

Degeneration

Degeneration has been covered extensively elsewhere (See Chapter 2). Disc degeneration of the lumbar spine occurs in response to trauma. These traumatic injuries (compressive and torsional overload) most likely occur at a very early age. Paajanen et al. (52) used magnetic resonance imaging to study disc degeneration in young low back pain patients. The average age of the patients was 20 years. Fifty-seven percent of those suffering from low back pain had one or more abnormal lumbar discs. A control group of pain-free individuals was also analyzed with MRI. Approximately 35% of these individuals showed signs of degeneration. End-plate changes, detected radiographically, were clearly associated with disc degeneration. Therefore, damaged end-plates are likely one etio-

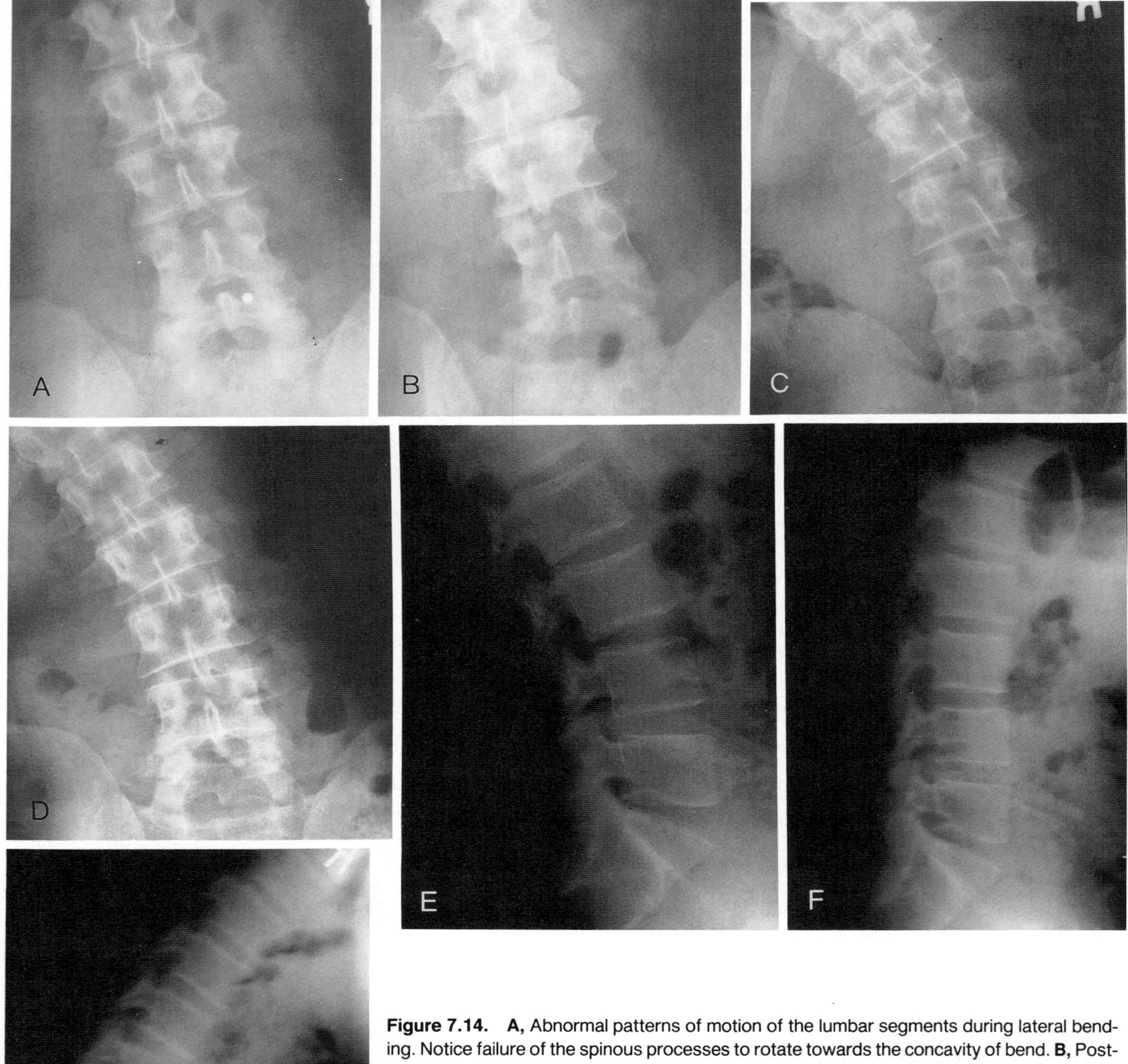

Figure 7.14. **A,** Abnormal patterns of motion of the lumbar segments during lateral bending. Notice failure of the spinous processes to rotate towards the concavity of bend. **B,** Post-treatment radiograph. **C,** Radiograph demonstrating abnormal coupling patterns. **D,** Post-treatment radiograph demonstrating a more normal coupling pattern. The two patients in Figures 7.15A-D received a combination of spinal adjustments to the lower lumbar level(s) and specific isometric exercises or maneuvers. **E,** Neutral radiograph demonstrating retrolisthesis at L5 with slight disc thinning at that level. **F,** Flexion showing marked limitation in forward bending. **G,** Post (30 min.) radiograph after an L5 adjustment.

logic and/or associated factor in the development of disc degeneration. Many of the MRI detected abnormal joints had no radiographic changes. Early degenerative disc disease may exist long before there is loss of disc height or other obvious radiographic findings of degenerative joint disease (53). MRI is an excellent clinical and research tool for identifying early biochemical changes in the intervertebral disc (Fig. 7.16). These changes are likely to occur even before there is histologic evidence of degeneration (54).

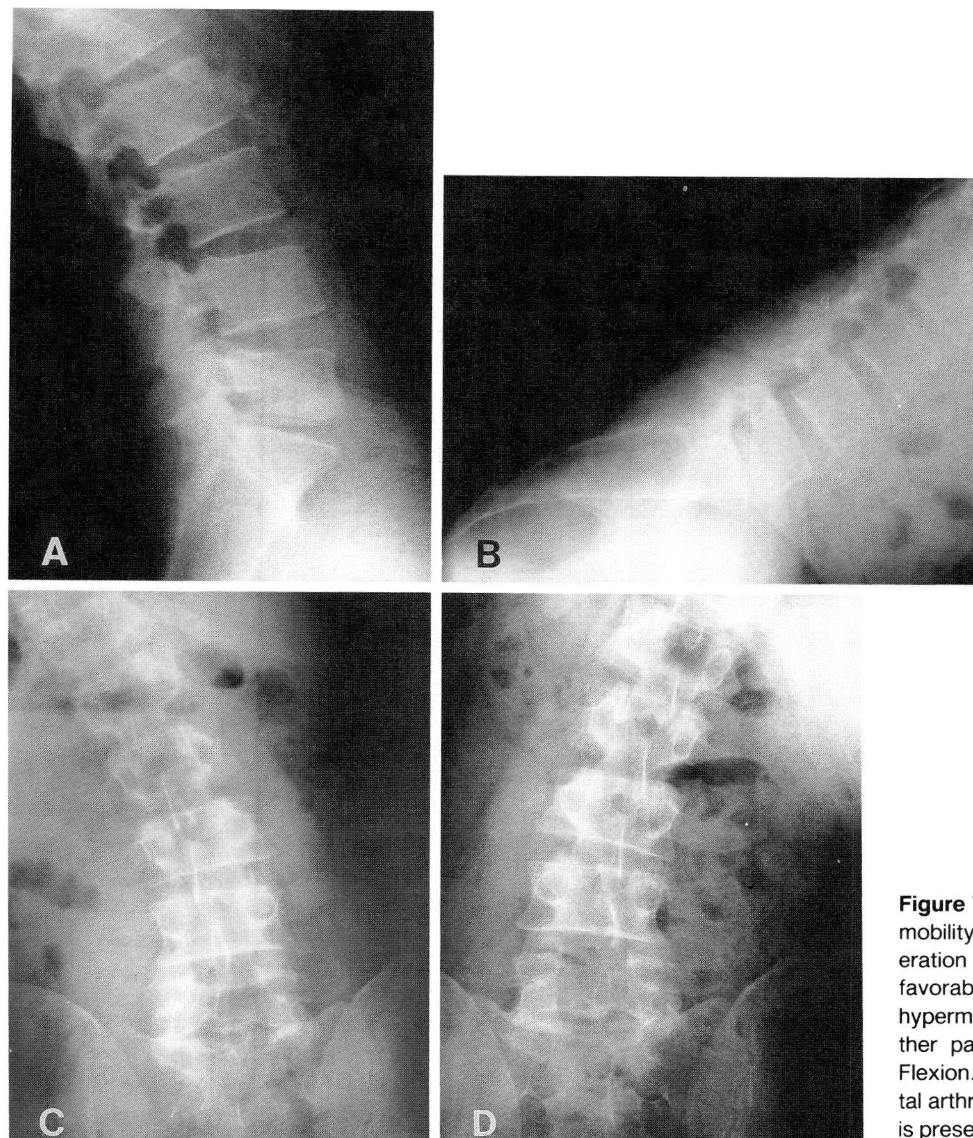

Figure 7.15. Disc degeneration leads to less mobility at the affected level. The more degeneration that is present at that level, the less favorable the prognosis should be. Ultimately, hypermobility at adjacent levels will lead to further pathology. **A,** Extension radiograph. **B,** Flexion. **C,** Left lateral bending. Notice the facetal arthrosis at L5-S1. Relatively normal motion is present. **D,** Right lateral bending. There is fixation dysfunction for $+\theta Z$ motion at L5-S1.

Disc degeneration at the central joint will lead to greater loads borne by the posterior joints. A consequence of this high stress may be pain from subchondral bone, or soft tissue nipped between the facets (31). The pattern of disc degeneration begins with nuclear dehydration, followed by greater and greater internal disruption. Resorption of disc material occurs in the late stage. Osteophytic ridges also narrow the contents of the lateral recess and IVF (55).

Compensation Reactions

Gonstead was one of the first chiropractors to recognize compensation as a reaction to the subluxation (56). Static and dynamic reactions to primary lesions of the lumbar spine are termed compensation reactions. When a motion segment becomes restricted in a particular direction of motion, adjacent articulations will compensate with increased mobility, in order that the total global range is preserved. This hypermobile compensation is usually benign and a normal reaction to a fixation. If the primary lesion is allowed to be present for an unnecessary length of time, the secondary reaction can become pathologic. The hypermobile state can induce injury to the supportive tissue and neurovascular bundles. The signs of inflammation and altered neurologic function may be present at the secondary lesion and can be a primary source of symptomatology for the patient. Because the secondary lesion can often times be more symptomatic than the primary lesion, objective criteria, such as stress radiography should be used exclusively to identify the primary site. Management protocols based on the symptom-

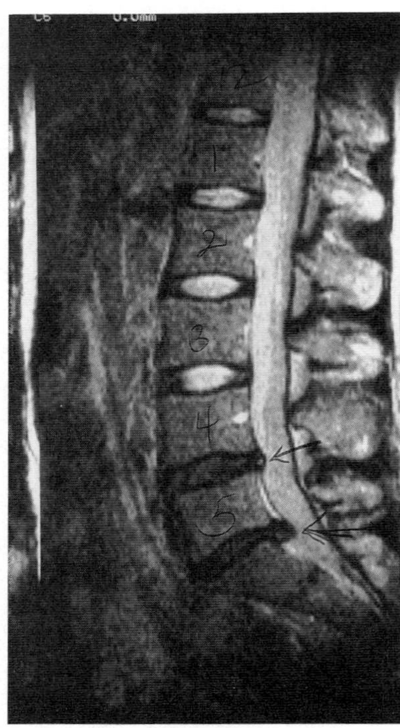

Figure 7.16. Herniation of the disc at L5 and L4. There is decreased signal intensity at L5, L4 and L1.

atic picture often lead to inappropriate treatment by the inexperienced clinician. Adjustments to hypermobile or normal articulations are contraindicated.

INSTABILITY

Instability can be defined as the hypermobile state of a joint which begins to cause neurologic impairment (57). In addition to low back pain, the patient may experience a feeling of weakness or vulnerability in the lumbar spine, or give an account of a "catch" in the back when moving from a stooped to an upright position. Compression overload rarely will lead to instability unless combined with a torsional injury. When experimental end-plate injuries are created, the joint still maintains its capacity to support axial load (57). Torsional overload is more likely to cause instability because when failure occurs at the annulus and facets, there is no back-up system to provide support.

Dupuis et al. (58) define instability as not only increased movement above normal, but also movements that are in abnormal directions, such as abnormal coupling patterns. If this definition is followed, most dysfunctional states of the lumbar spine would be classified as biomechanically but not necessarily neurologically unstable. Abnormal coupling patterns could make the patient more vulnerable to future injury, because the motion segment will be loaded asymmetrically even when the individual moves in a symmetrical manner.

There is some controversy regarding the usefulness of plain radiographs in identifying instability, because of the fact that many pain-free individuals exhibit somewhat large translational displacements during sagittal plane motion (59). It is regarded however, as the examination of choice. The controversy mostly stems from categorizing pain-free individuals as normal without regard to underlying silent pathology that may be present.

Traction compression radiography appears also to be a useful indicator of lumbar segmental instability (60). In this procedure, lateral radiographs are taken with the patient under traction (hanging from a horizontal bar) and under compression (addition of a 44 lb rucksack or backpack in the standing position).

Weiler et al. (61) have used a computerized analysis that appears to be more sensitive in identifying individuals with instability. Bi-planar radiography can also be used, but because of equipment requirements, this has been primarily confined to the research setting. The plain radiographic analysis provided, describes instability of the lumbar spine at its most common level of involvement, the L4-L5 motion segment (Fig. 7.17A-B).

The vacuum phenomenon, from severe internal disc disruption is a sign that instability is present. The extension radiograph displayed the vacuum phenomenon in about half of the 52 symptomatic patients studied by Goobar et al. (62). The author hypothesizes that in the absent of a precipitating singular traumatic episode at the L4-L5 level, instability begins as a relatively benign hypermobility caused by fixation dysfunction below (Fig. 7.17C-G). In this respect, instability can be thought of as a chronic condition.

Some discussion must be given here to the "Three Phases of Degeneration" outlined by Kirkaldy-Willis (55,63). Dysfunction, the initial phase, is characterized by hypomobility and/or abnormal coupling patterns of the spine. The second phase is termed instability. Here, the motion segment has increased translational movement caused by internal disc disruption. The final phase of the process is termed stabilization. The motion segment gradually is stabilized through a decrease in disc space height and other signs of degenerative joint disease, such as osteophyte formation. While Dr. Kirkaldy-Willis does not state that each phase runs serially into the other at the same segmental level, this notion is somewhat implied, leading to some confusion in the literature (64). If hypomobility were to lead to instability, the joint would necessarily have to pass through a stage of normal movement. There would clearly be no need to adjust these patients. Their fixation dysfunction will normalize as time passes. This is not the case however. The dysfunction phase at one level more likely leads to hypermobility at another level that then becomes unstable. This unstable articulation, then gradually restabilizes with time. The fixated joint as well will undergo degeneration and stabilization,

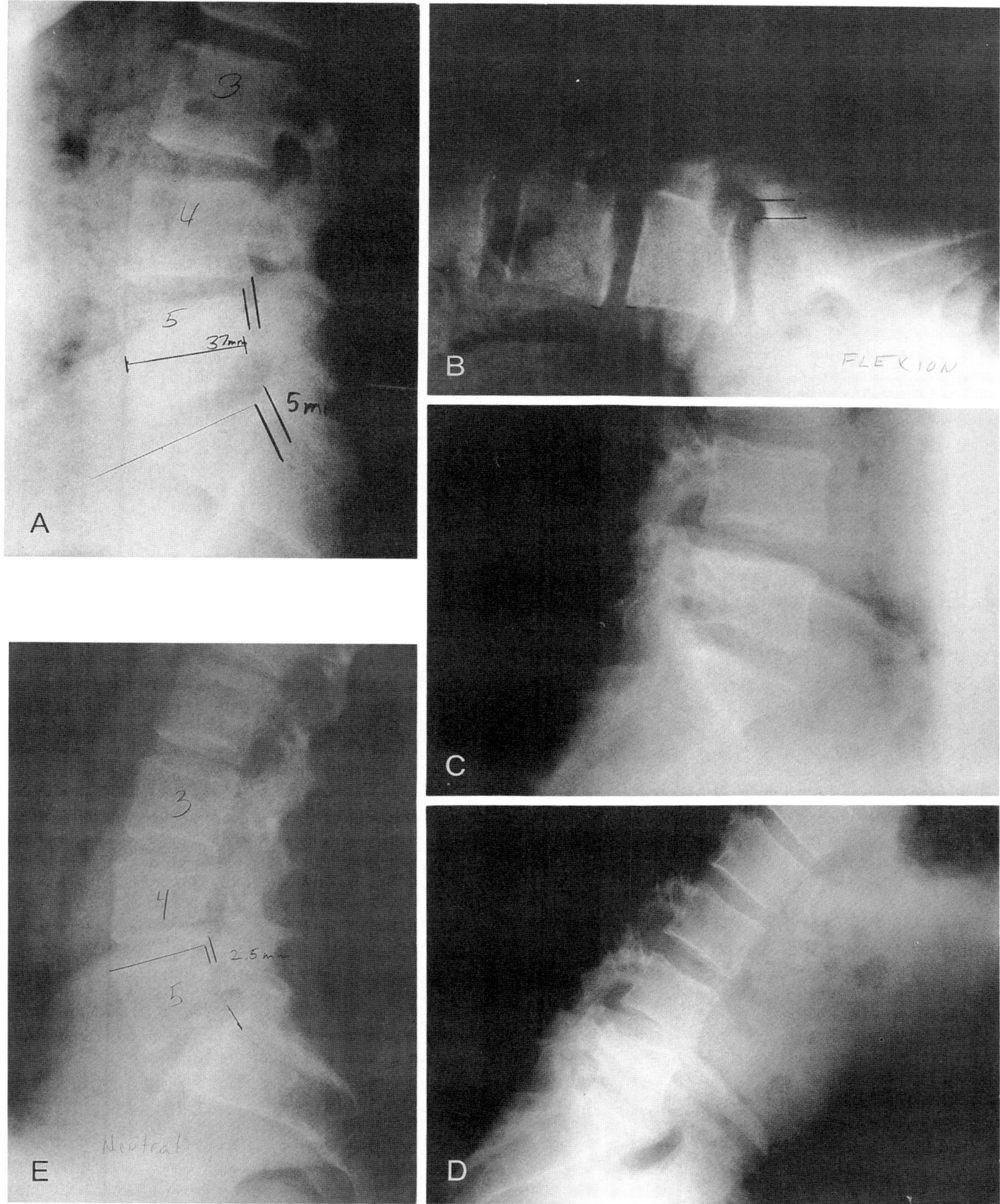

Figure 7.17. Instability combined with fixated or persistent retrolisthesis. **A,** Neutral. Retrolisthesis of L5 and L4. **B,** Flexion. Notice the reduction of retrolisthesis at L4. **C,** Neutral. Retrolisthesis at L5. **D,** Flexion. There is hyperflexion ($+\theta X$) at L4. The dot represents the George's line of S1, demonstrating the retrolisthesis at L5. **E,** Neutral. Retrolisthesis at L4 only. Notice the traction osteophyte at the anterosuperior margin of L4, indicative of instability at L3-L4. **F,** Flexion. There is persistent retrolisthesis at L4 and hyper flexion at L3. **G,** MRI of patient in Figures 7.17E-F One year later. The patient now has acute symptomatology. There are annular protrusions at multiple levels. Notice also the decreased signal intensity of the nucleus, especially L4-L5.

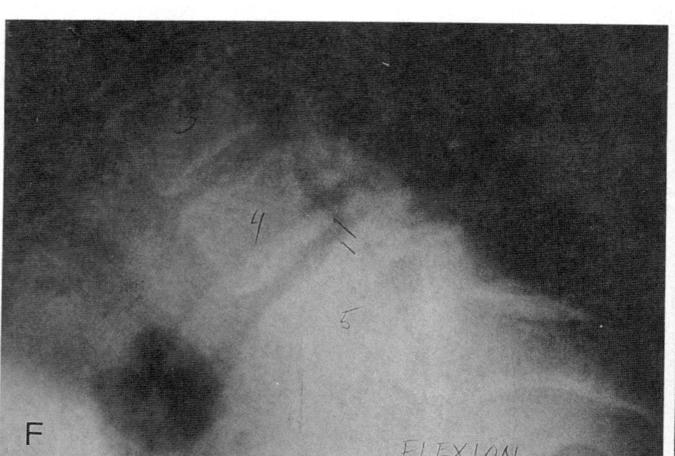

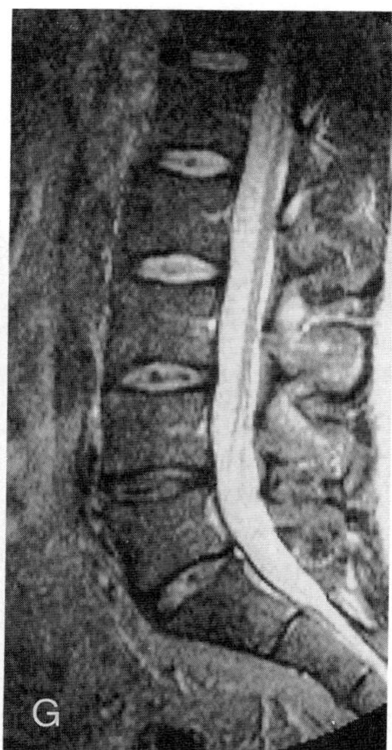

Figure 7.17. *Continued*

primarily because of the loss of motion (See Fixation Dysfunction). It may not pass through an unstable phase during this process.

TREATMENT

Frymoyer and Selby (65) have advocated surgical fusion with the joint in flexion as the treatment for lumbar retrolisthesis. This treatment is not valid in light of conservative measures that have shown merit. Plaugher et al. (23), in a retrospective consecutive analysis of 49 patients, demonstrated that lumbar retrolisthesis was reduced an average of 34% while the patient was under chiropractic care. Assessments were made after an average of eight treatments. The adjustments were performed in the side posture position, emphasizing a posterior to anterior (+Z) pattern of thrust followed by a "holding" of the segment for 1–2 seconds.

Lehmann et al. (66) evaluated the long-term results in patients undergoing lower lumbar fusion. Follow-up ranged from 21 to 52 years; the median was 33 years. Forty-four percent of the patients were still experiencing low back pain and 57% had had low back pain in the past year. Fifty-three percent were using medication to control pain. Segmental instability above the level of fusion occurred in 45%, and 42% had developed central spinal canal stenosis. The interesting aspect of this study was that most patients were generally satisfied with the results of their surgery. Perhaps their expectations were not high from the onset.

Lopes et al. (67) report two cases with lumbar retrolisthesis which were reduced after a +Z thrust technique. In one of the cases, motion studies were performed in flexion and extension. Improvement in fixation dysfunction and paradoxical motions were also observed. The other case showed a reduction of approximately 35% after one treatment. Prospective studies are needed in the area of closed reduction of lumbar retrolisthesis. The practitioner needs to know how many adjustments are required to effect a reduction and when should treatment be tapered. More study is needed to determine the effects of retrolisthesis and its amelioration on the neurophysiology of the individual, and their future level of degeneration at that level and adjacent segments. Preliminary evidence thus far is promising.

No adjustive thrusts should be administered to the hypermobile segment, and if performed, may be a cause for increased symptomatology in the patient. Because the hypermobility usually occurs above the fixated level, an adjustment at the segment above the fixation may cause the patient's condition to remain unchanged or temporarily worsen symptomatically. The primary lesion should be addressed and once mobility is restored or improved at the restricted level, the hypermobile compensation reaction hopefully will begin to restabilize.

Static Compensation Reaction in the Sagittal Plane

Static compensation reactions of the lumbar spine are common. A change in the lordotic configuration of the lumbar spine can often be detected by x-ray. It is important to remember that the lumbar lordosis is a compound curvature. One angle for the entire lordosis does not adequately describe the static mechanical configuration of the region. Normally, there is a steeper angle between L4, L5 and S1. The lordosis diminishes in the upper lumbar segments as the lordosis turns to kyphosis in the thoracolumbar and thoracic regions of the spine.

An increase in the lower angle of the lordosis is usually best described by Fergusen's sacral base angle measurement. When posteriority (retrolisthesis) of a lower lumbar segment, especially L5, is accompanied by an extreme inferiorward tipping of the vertebral body ($-\theta X$), an increase in the sacral base angle can usually be detected (Fig. 7.18).

A lesion at the L5-S1 disc space in which the sacral base has moved into a position of $-\theta X$ and a slight amount of $-Z$ translation, has been termed a sacral base posterior (56) (Fig. 7.19). In this situation, the disc space at L5-S1 is parallel or widened at the posterior. This is different from the usual slightly wedge-like configuration of the disc. Because of the posterior opening at the lumbosacral, the L4-L5 region will often become hyperextended ($-\theta X$) in a compensation reaction for the flexion of the lower motion segment (Fig. 7.19).

In the case of a herniation of the nucleus pulposus in either a posterolateral or central direction, the patient will often present with a hypolordotic posture of the entire lumbar spine. This flexion compensation is an effort to open the posterior aspect of the disc and decrease pressure on the nerve roots. There is usually an associated muscle spasm that guards and splints the injured area. The hypolordosis has sometimes been erroneously ascribed to the presence of the muscle spasm. This is probably not the case. The posterior muscle groups lie posterior to the center or apex of the normal lumbar lordosis. If contracture or spasm of the muscle groups did affect the posture, then they would tend to pull the two ends of the lordosis together, thereby producing a hyperlordotic configuration (18).

Static Compensation Reaction in the Coronal Plane

The antero-posterior radiograph is also of help in detecting compensation reactions. A posterolateral protrusion of the nucleus pulposus will usually produce a wedging malposition of the involved segment. Also, while not caused by the protrusion directly, a unilateral protrusion may affect one nerve root and thereby initiate an antalgic lean of the patient away from the side of involvement (8). This would occur in protrusions lateral to the nerve root. Herniations that are medial to the nerve root may produce an antalgic lean towards the side of leg pain (the side of nerve root involvement) (See Examination of the Acute Low Back).

Disc protrusions lateral to the nerve root tend to cause a rotatory scoliosis (spinous process deviation to the concavity of the curve) above the level of involvement. Protrusions medial to the nerve root tend to cause a simple scoliosis (spinous towards the convexity). These are extreme generalizations. Their usefulness in the clinical assessment of the patient is unclear. Accurate determination of the direction of protrusion, is achieved through CT or MR imaging (68).

On the A-P radiograph, the probable site of subluxation will often wedge off the horizontal and deviate away

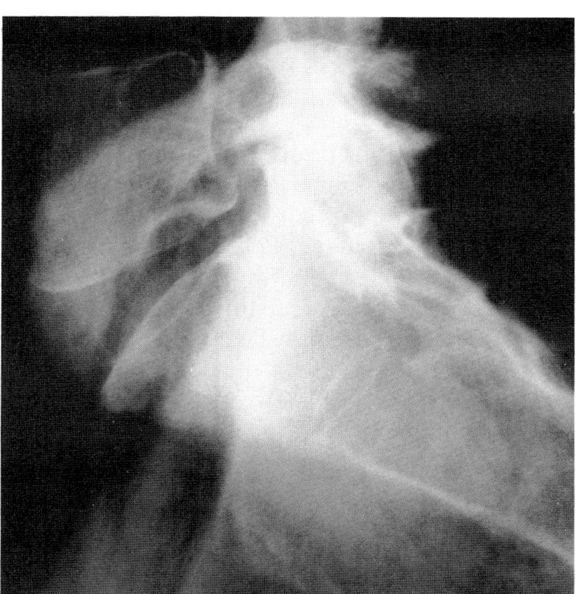

Figure 7.18. Retrolisthesis ($-Z$) and extension ($-\theta X$) positional dyskinesia of L5. There is an associated increased sacral base angle.

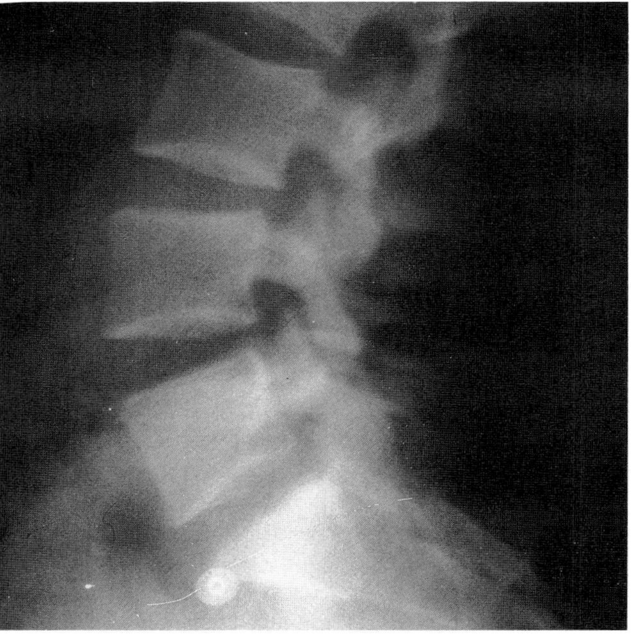

Figure 7.19. A base posterior sacrum with compensation in hyperextension of L4 ($-\theta X$).

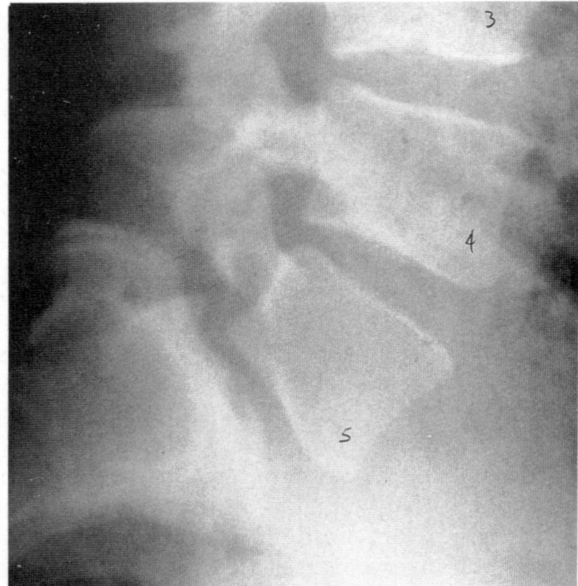

Figure 7.20. Spondylolisthesis of L5. Meyerding's grading of spondylolisthesis is based on the percentage of slip in comparison to the length of the end-plate of S1; 25% (Grade 1), 50% (Grade 2), 75% (Grade 3), 100% (Grade 4).

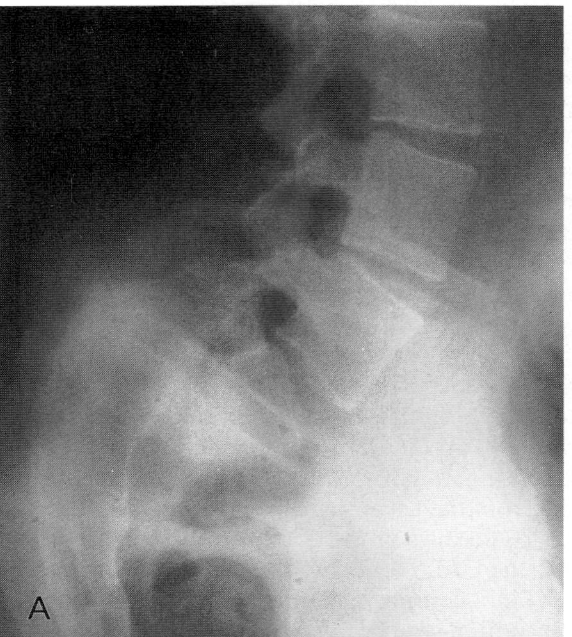

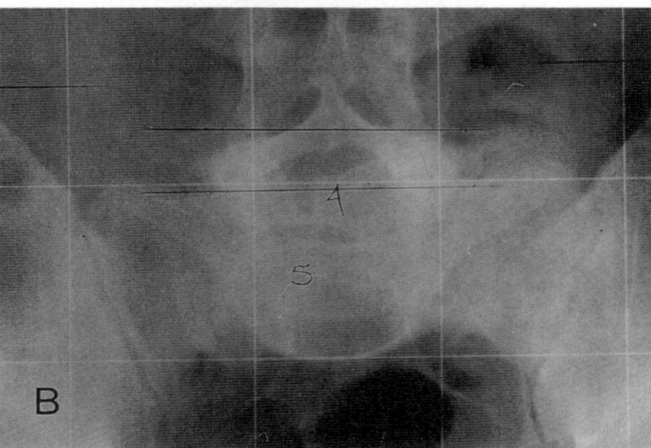

Figure 7.21. **A,** A Grade 4 spondylolisthesis. **B,** The inverted Napoleon hat sign, indicative of a Grade 4 spondylolisthesis.

from the center of gravity. The compensation however, will tend to wedge towards horizontal and back towards midline (See Chapter 5).

SPONDYLOLISTHESIS

Spondylolisthesis is defined as a slippage anterior of one vertebra on the segment below. This forward displacement can happen in any area of the spine, occurring most frequently at L5 (Fig. 7.20).

Spondylolysis is a lysis of the neural arch at the pars interarticularis. It often occurs in conjunction with spondylolisthesis.

Classification

There are five classifications of spondylolisthesis, depending on the etiology of the slippage (34). Type 1 is called isthmic and refers to either a stress fracture in the pars, or an elongation without separation. Lysis of the pars from fracture is the most common cause for anterior slippage. The stress fracture usually develops shortly after the child begins to learn to walk. There is no evidence that lysis of the pars is congenital, because autopsies of stillborns and fetuses have never shown the defect. There may be however, a genetic weakness in the pars, such as a thin cortex, which makes it susceptible to stress fracture (69).

Most patients with isthmic spondylolisthesis of L5 have a prominent spinous process at that level and a steep sacral base angle (70). The steep sacral base angle will place more anterior shear at the articulation possible leading to elongation or the development of a stress fracture. The prominent spinous process may also be implicated in the development of this disorder. Gracovetsky (71) (See Chapter 2) points out that a small spinous will be pulled posteriorward by the lumbodorsal fascia (LDF) during forward bending. This is a protective mechanism to resist the tremendous anterior shear that occurs at that level. A large spinous process will cause the opposite effect. Here, the LDF will exert an anterior shear force heightening the possibility of the development of a stress fracture at the pars.

Type 2 spondylolisthesis is termed congenital and refers to congenital malformations of the posterior elements. This condition is rare and may be manifested by aplasia of the articular facets (Fig. 7.21).

When the three-joint complex undergoes severe degenerative changes due to previous trauma, the supporting ligaments can be lax enough so as to allow forward slippage. In the case of an L4 degenerative spondylolisthesis, the main pathologic finding is marked erosion of the superior articular processes of L5 (55). The amount of forward slip is usually small. This scenario is called a degenerative spondylolisthesis or Type 3 (Fig. 7.22). If the degeneration occurs concomitantly with an elongation of the neural arch, the anterior slippage can be quite large.

Type 4 spondylolisthesis is characterized by elongation of the pedicles. This could be called an isthmic type of spondylolisthesis. Traction forces (+Z) cause elongation of the neural arch.

Type 5 spondylolisthesis is anterior movement of the vertebra caused by a destructive process in the neural arch. Tuberculosis, metastasis, and other diseases that compromise the structural integrity of the bone are included in this category.

A forward displacement of the vertebral body will lead to more nuclear pressure on the posterior end-plates. Through Heuter-Volkmann's Law (8), this increased pressure at the posterior will retard the growth of the epiphyseal plate, thereby creating a wedge-like appearance of the vertebral body on the lateral radiograph (See Fig. 7.20). This is a common finding in patients with spondylolisthesis.

Instability

In an experiment by Pearcy (72), it was shown that grade one and two spondylolistheses do not show increased mobility during flexion and extension stress radiography. These patients were in pain however, and the lack of signs of instability, could have been related to overall reduction of motion due to protective muscle spasm. Penning and Blickman (73) found no abnormal translation at the site of the spondylo, but did see increased motion one segment above. Instability of a joint with spondylolisthesis cannot be assumed.

An interesting report by Friberg (74), has shown that axial traction tends to reduce the slippage of spondylolisthesis by lessening the anterior shear component across the S1 superior end-plate (Fig. 7.23). Compression of the spine tended to increase the anterior slippage. In contrast, retrolisthesis increased during traction and decreased during compression (Fig. 7.24).

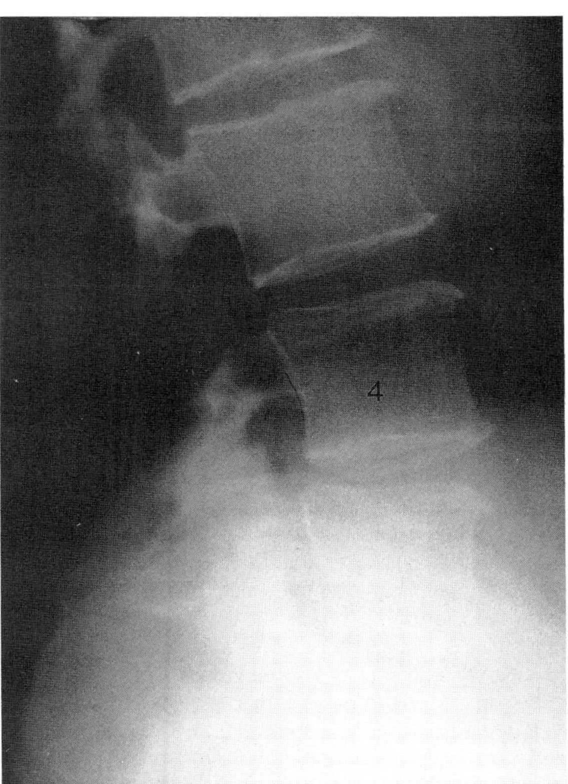

Figure 7.22. A degenerative spondylolisthesis of L4.

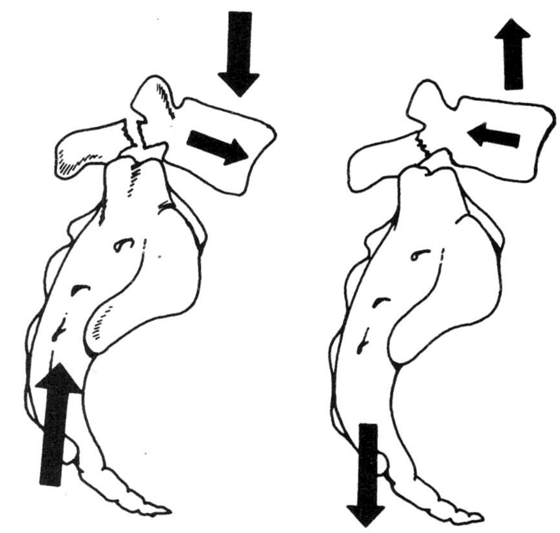

Figure 7.23. Traction reduces a spondylolisthesis, and compression increases the forward displacement.

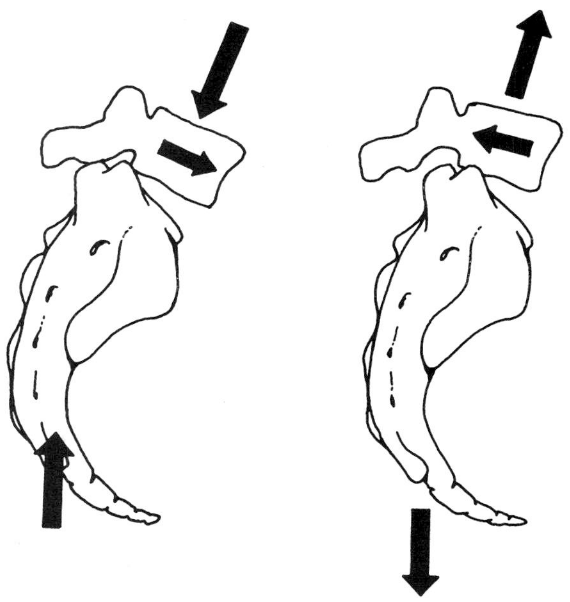

Figure 7.24. Traction will further displace a retrolisthesis, and compression tends to reduce it.

Management

Dysfunction at a joint with spondylolisthesis is just as common as in other areas without defects. Treatment however, is somewhat different from other lumbar levels.

The patient with a symptomatic spondylolisthesis will usually present with moderate to severe pain on extension of the lumbar spine. A hyperlordosis may be noted, as well as a prominent spinous process at the level of the defect. The lateral and oblique radiograph will confirm the clinical impression.

The sacrum will tend to be restricted in posterior to anterior motion (+Z translation) in relation to L5 during motion examination of a fixated L5-S1 spondylolisthesis. If instability or normal motion is present, then adjustments are contraindicated. Spondylolisthesis, by itself, is not a contraindication to prudent manipulation (75). The adjustment is designed to restore the restricted mobility at L5-S1 while using the S2 segment of the sacrum as the short lever arm. Improvement of the forward slippage rarely occurs.

In most cases, the adjustments are curtailed after symptomatic improvement, because this region of the spine affords less structural stability. If the dysfunction persists however, and affects other motion segments above, then corrective measures should be used.

For the acute patient, a lumbar support is often helpful. It should be worn for the first few days after trauma to provide support for healing to occur, and for reduction of symptomatology due to decreased stretching of the compromised soft and hard tissues.

LATERAL RECESS STENOSIS

The lateral recess is an area bordered laterally by the pedicle, posteriorly by the superior articular facet, and anteriorly by the posterolateral surface of the vertebral body and the adjacent intervertebral disc (76). The lateral recess can become narrowed and lead to entrapment of the nerve (Fig. 7.25). Degeneration is the primary etiology. Disc injury will lead to posterior displacement of the vertebra (retrolisthesis) which narrows the lateral recess. Disc displacement (e.g., annular bulge) can also narrow the recess. Soft tissue scarring in the area will further occlude the foramen (77).

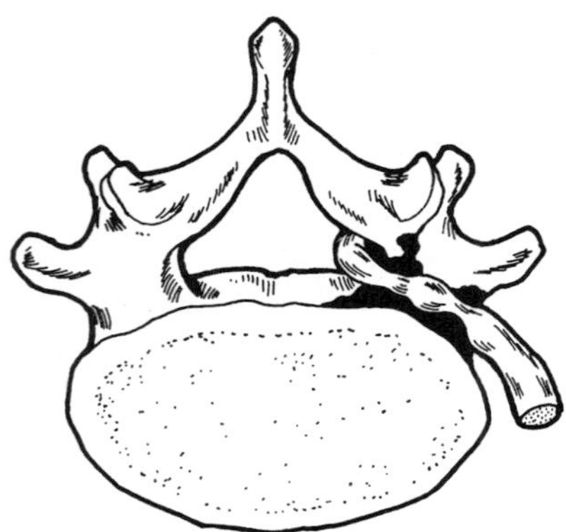

Figure 7.25. Caudal-cephalad view of lateral recess stenosis caused by bony proliferation. Modified from Porter RW, Hibbert C, Evans C. The natural history of root entrapment syndrome. Spine 1984;9:418–421.

The radiograph will usually show degeneration of the central joint with retrolisthesis of the superior segment. The CT scan can demonstrate the bony encroachment conclusively.

If the joint is unstable, symptomatology may only be detected during certain postures, such as hyperextension. Straight leg raising is usually only slightly limited. Back pain, though often present, is not necessary for the diagnosis. Referral pain patterns can occur in the buttock, trochanter, posterior thigh, calf, ankles, and toes (63). Signs of nerve root compression at the affected level will usually be present.

Kirkaldy-Willis (78) has outlined three tests helpful in making the diagnosis of dynamic lateral nerve entrapment (Fig. 7.26A-C). The entrapment can be dynamic or fixed, so different body positions must be tested. Persis-

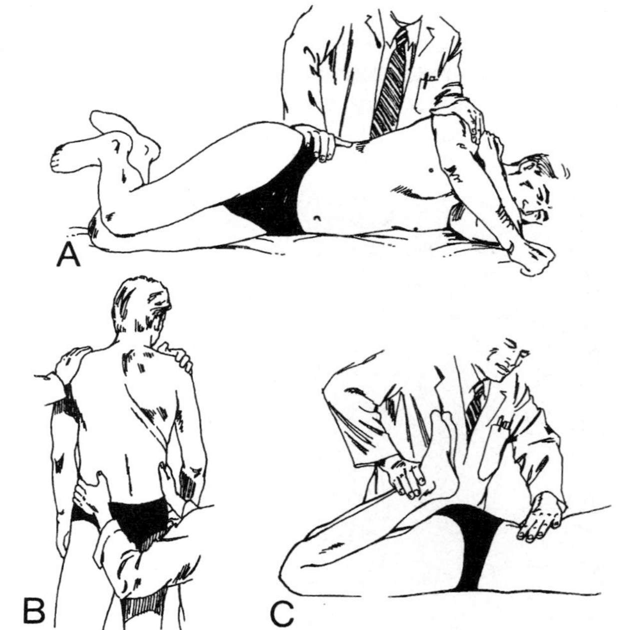

Figure 7.26. A, Patient lying in the lateral recumbent position on the examination table with the painful side down. The doctor then holds the upper body and pushes the hip away from them. This procedure can sometimes accentuate left sided pain. **B,** Patient standing erect. The doctor can hold the patient's pelvis while an assistant rotates the shoulders from one side to the other. This will sometimes cause leg pain. **C,** Patient prone on the examination table, the knees are flexed and compression is applied to the lumbar spine. This will cause hyperextension in the area and possibly accentuate symptomatology in some patients. Modified from Kirkaldy-Willis WH. The site and nature of the lesion. In: Kirkaldy-Willis WH, ed. Managing low back pain. New York: Churchill Livingstone, 1983:100.

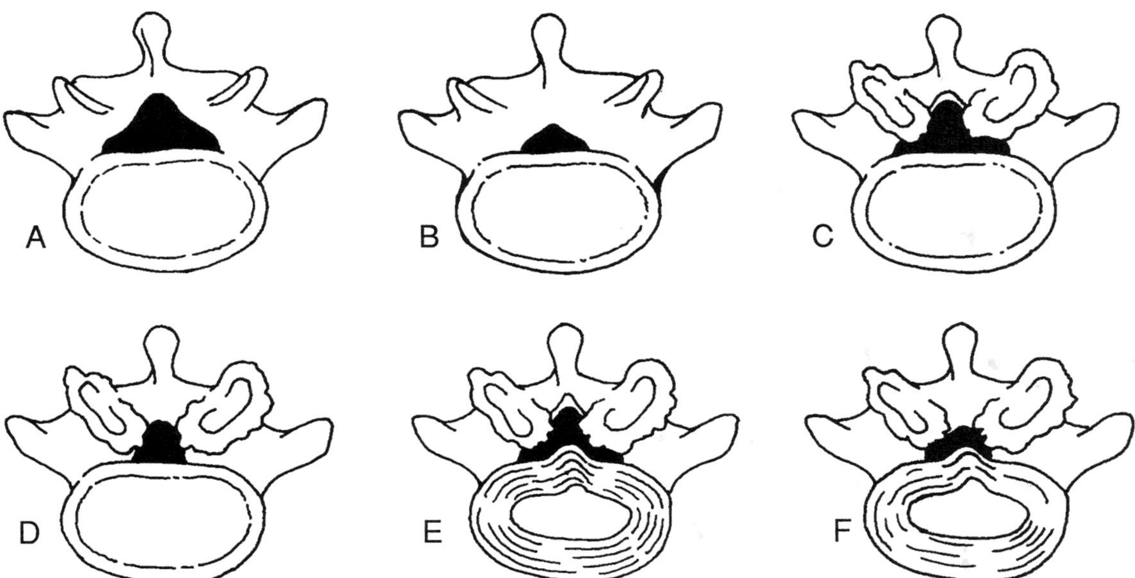

Figure 7.27. **A,** Normal spinal canal. **B,** A congenitally small canal. **C,** The effect of posterior joint degeneration on an otherwise normal canal. **D,** Posterior joint hypertrophy and a congenitally small canal. **E-F,** The added effect of a small disc herniation. Modified from Arnoldi CC, Brodsky AE, Cauchoix HV, et al. Lumbar spinal stenosis and nerve root entrapment syndromes. Clin Orthop 1976;115:5.

tent or fixed retrolisthesis leads to entrapment of a constant nature, because the joint is not periodically moving away from the nerve. Fixed lateral recess entrapment commonly occurs as a sequela to degeneration of the central and posterior joints.

The combination of loss of disc height, retrolisthesis, and hypertrophy of the posterior articulations will lead to severe narrowing of the recess. This situation, commonly seen in the geriatric patient due to the pronounced degeneration, holds the worse prognosis for conservative management. Chiropractic treatment in the preceding scenarios consists of moving the posteriorly displaced segment forward to open up the recess, and to reduce subluxation of the posterior joints (79). If instability is present at that level, then adjustments may be indicated at a fixated motion segment, usually below.

Narrowing of the recess can also be brought on by a protruding annulus in the area. An adjustment may have the effect of moving the annular material forward, away from the nerve, if the posterior displacement can be reduced. If there is inflammation in the area, adjusting the articulations may dissipate some of the inflammatory edema, thus decreasing nerve root compression.

There is some clinical research evidence that manipulation is effective for patients with lateral recess stenosis (80). Relatively few individuals will require surgical decompression of lateral recess stenosis (68).

CENTRAL CANAL STENOSIS

Central canal stenosis is caused by advanced structural changes and is most common in older patients. These individuals usually present a symptom pattern of altered sensation with pain in one or both legs. If compression is of a long duration, motor weakness may be present (78). Pressure on the cauda equina comes from a narrowed central canal, primarily due to enlarged posterior joints, posterior osteophytes of the vertebral body, and sometimes a small disc herniation (Fig. 7.27). Occasionally, signs of central stenosis can occur in the young if there is a congenitally small spinal canal. The presence of a central disc herniation in these cases, can lead to symptomatology characteristic of central stenosis (Fig. 7.27).

The back pain associated with central stenosis is usually not severe. Leg pain patterns can border on the bizarre. Patients may complain that their legs feel cold, or that they feel like they are made of rubber (78).

Restriction of lumbar movement depends primarily on the extent of degeneration in the joints. Nerve compression tests will usually be positive with multiple dermatomal levels involved. The straight leg raising test may only be moderately positive.

Neurogenic claudication (NC) can occur. The patient will report being able to walk only a short distance before resting because of accentuation of the leg pain. Neurogenic claudication can be differentiated from the vascular form (VC). If the patient can ride a stationary bicycle (lumbar spine in flexion) for several minutes without pain, this differentiates NC from VC. Vascular claudication will be provoked when greater circulatory demands are placed on the leg muscles (78).

The radiograph will usually show moderate to severe levels of degeneration, unless it is of a young patient with a congenitally small spinal canal. The CT scan is generally used to accurately evaluate the dimensions of the canal. A method described by Dailey and Buehler (81), for use on lateral lumbar radiographs compares well with CT scan measurements.

Treatment consists of adjustments to the fixated motion segment. If retrolisthesis is present, then this should be reduced. An obese patient will require dietary consultation or referral. If severe degenerative changes are present and the patient does not respond to conservative measures, then surgical consultation may be indicated. Advancing neurologic deficits also require neurosurgical consultation or referral. In a study on the natural history of central stenosis (82), it was found that most patients did not deteriorate (i.e., symptomatology) at two to three years follow-up. These authors also evaluated the effects of decompression for central stenosis. They found that 60% of the patients improved and 25% deteriorated. Neurogenic claudication was significantly reduced. In a group of untreated patients, 30% improved and 60% were unchanged. The operation did not prevent neurophysiologic deterioration.

ACUTE LOW BACK SYNDROME

The acute low back syndrome can be an extremely disabling condition. The patient is usually severely impaired with regards to movement, and may experience excruciating pain. The clinical presentation can be somewhat unnerving to the inexperienced practitioner. Chiropractic care can usually offer dramatic relief provided the doctor is sure of the diagnosis and confident in the application of treatment. Hesitance to take action is usually caused by uncertainty in the diagnosis and fear of further traumatizing the patient. If the doctor strives to do a thorough and clinically meaningful examination for all patient presentations, the acute patient can be easily accommodated. It is typical of individuals not well versed in the management of the acute low back patient, to treat by "avoiding the lesion." Here, the doctor will go to great lengths to achieve a proper diagnosis (e.g., CT, MRI, etc) of an L5-S1 disc herniation, and then do everything possible to avoid adjusting the patient at the involved level. Such avoidance may result in adjusting a fixated sacroiliac joint and/or the thoracolumbar junction, in hopes of providing some relief without addressing the acute spinal level. Attempting to adjust levels near the acute disc may actually cause a worsening of the patient's symptomatology. Only experience in managing patients with acute symptomatology will provide the necessary tools for clinical prowess. The information in this section will hopefully facilitate the appropriate management of such cases.

Acute vs. Chronic

Most acute presentations of the low back are an acute exacerbation of a chronic condition. The patient will usually relate in the history of several episodes of back pain over the preceding years. The fact that many of these conditions have chronic overlays will facilitate the examination. The radiograph may show early signs of disc degeneration at a motion segment, alerting the clinician to a possible level of involvement. Figure 7.28 and 7.29 illustrates the effect of acute injury in a patient with retrolisthesis of L5.

EXAMINATION

Acute symptomatology of the low back is generally caused by subluxations of the lower lumbar levels, and rarely from one or both sacroiliac articulations. The doctor must keep in mind however, that an unbiased examination of the entire spine is requisite, to avoid overlooking levels of involvement which could be contributory (e.g., upper cervical region). The subluxation should be accepted where it is found. The doctor must avoid leading the examination with a bias.

The patient will usually relate a particular traumatic event preceding the pain, such as lifting a heavy object while in a stooped, awkward position. The flexed, laterally bent and axially rotated position, is a common mechanism of lumbar disc injury. In addition to pain in the

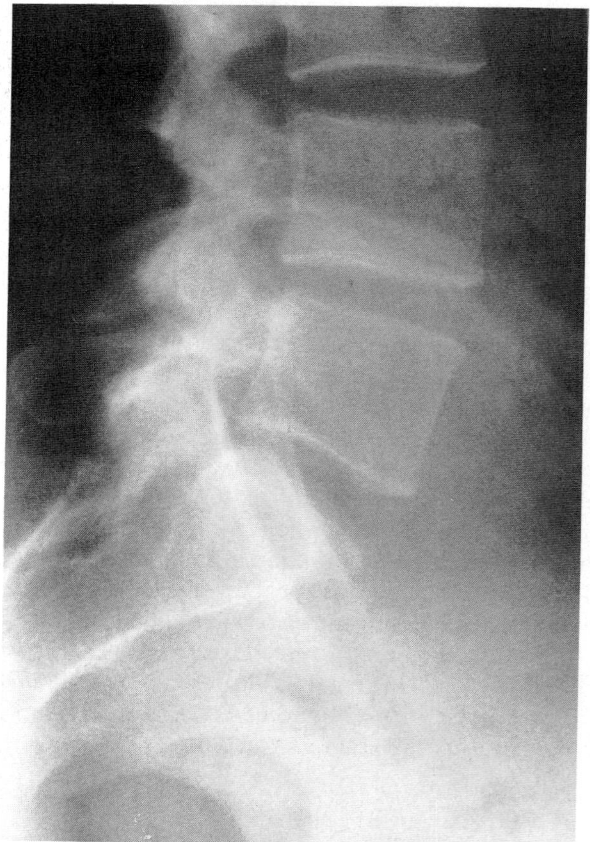

Figure 7.28. Radiograph demonstrating retrolisthesis at L5. The patient presented with chronic low back pain.

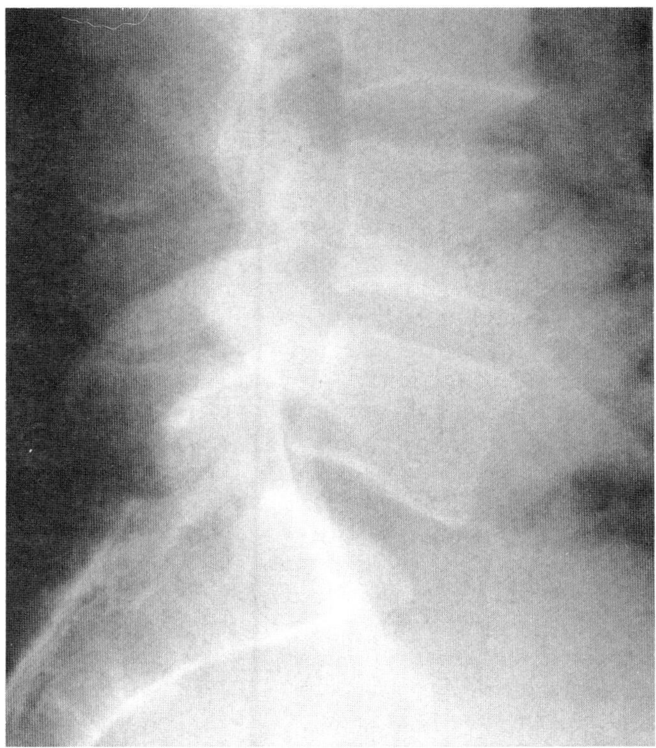

Figure 7.29. An exacerbation of the patient's condition one year later (See Fig. 7.28). Disc swelling has reduced the amount of retrolisthesis at L5.

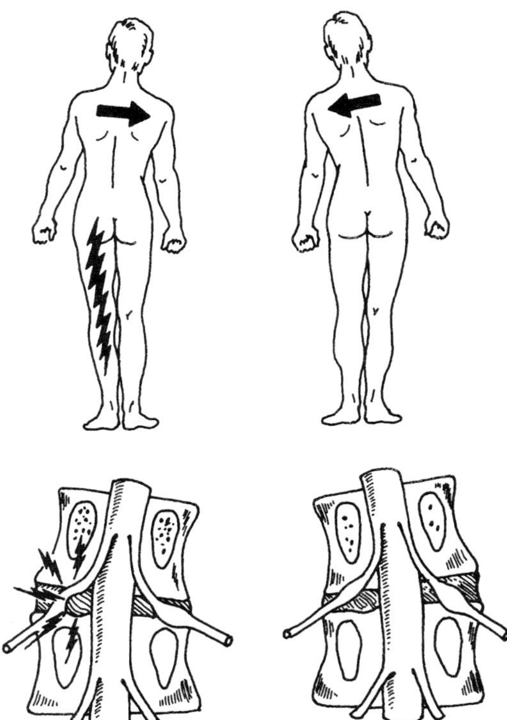

Figure 7.30. Characteristic antalgic lean of an individual with a medial (to the nerve root) disc protrusion.

lower back, the patient may also complain of radiation into one or both extremities.

Flattening of the lumbar lordosis is often present. This may be due to pelvic flexion in an attempt by the patient to reduce contraction of the erector spinae through activation of the lumbodorsal fascia (See Chapter 2). A reduced lumbar lordosis may slightly pull an annular bulge away from the nerve root as well as increase the vertical dimensions of the lateral recesses. The patient can also "draw-up" one or both legs to decrease nerve root tension. Bogduk (83) has speculated that the flattening could be due to spasm of the multifidus or erector spinae muscles. Most of the paraspinal muscles in acute low back injury are in a sustained contraction. If the flattening was due to erector spinae spasm, it would likely pull in the lordosis, not reduce it, because the main function of the erector spinae muscles is to extend the lumbar spine.

Ambulation will usually be difficult and the patient may require assistance. After a history that includes checking for signs of cauda equina syndrome[a] (a surgical emergency), the patient should be prepared for a physical and radiographic examination (See Chapters 4 and 5).

Porter and Miller (68) found no correlation between the side of antalgic list and the direction of disc protrusion in 100 patients attending a back pain clinic. Because the CT scan and operation are performed in positions different from upright stance, this lack of correlation may be suspect. MRI and CT are the most important instruments available to the chiropractor for determining the nature of the disc lesion. In the absence of these tests, clinical assessment of trunk list in relation to the side of sciatica appears to be helpful in the management of the patient. With a disc protrusion medial to the nerve root, the patient will generally lean towards the side of leg pain (Fig. 7.30). With a protrusion lateral to the nerve root, the patient will lean away from the side of leg pain (Fig. 7.31). If the protrusion is beneath the nerve root (subrhizal), the patient will typically present in a forward bent position. A broad based central herniation may cause a forward lean as well as bilateral symptomatology. In general, clinical observations suggest that the central, medial, and subrhizal disc protrusions are somewhat more difficult to resolve (i.e., requires more frequent and prolonged adjustive therapy), than protrusions lateral to the nerve root.

The physical examination will be modified somewhat when the patient is in severe pain. Effort should be made to use as few orthopedic tests as possible to obtain the desired information. Going overboard with ten or twenty tests, purely for documentation purposes, will simply put the patient through undue pain and distress. The adjustment will be more comfortable if the patient is less aggravated during the examination. The cough impulse and

[a]Cauda equina syndrome is defined as a dull pain in the upper sacral region with anesthesia or analgesia in the buttocks, genitalia, or thighs; accompanied by disturbed bowel and bladder function.

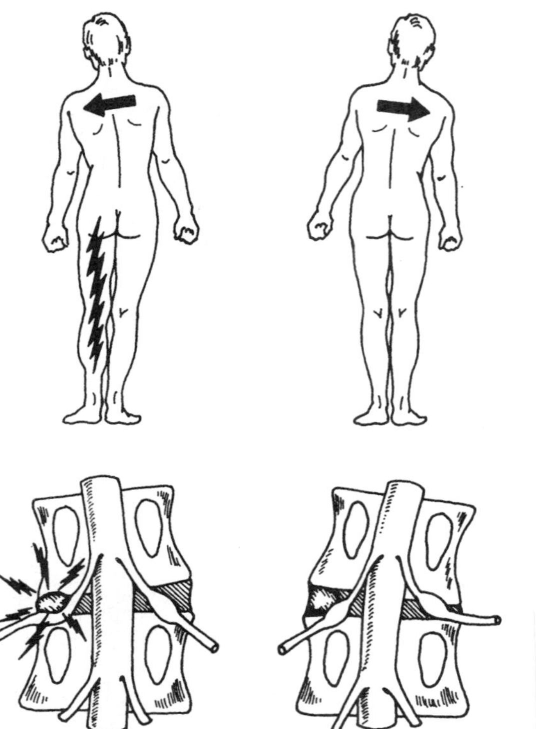

Figure 7.31. Antalgic lean associated with a lateral (to the nerve root) disc protrusion.

straight leg raise tests tend to be the most sensitive for patients with sciatica caused by lumbar disc herniation (84). Static examination procedures such as the history, static x-ray, static palpation and instrumentation, are the primary assessment measures for the acute patient during the initial examination.

Radiography

All efforts should be made to x-ray the patient in the upright position. This posture will place the injured tissues under stress and accentuate the appearance of any biomechanical improprieties. Porter and Miller (68) found that trunk list in patients with back pain was abolished when the patient was recumbent. This list may be important in determining if the protrusion is lateral or medial to the nerve root.

The lateral lumbar radiograph should be scrutinized first. Disc space alterations may be indicative of the level of involvement. Slight disc degeneration at a particular segment should be noted. The disc spaces should all have relative symmetry. An acutely swollen disc may increase the disc space height, but this can take up to three days to occur. If the patient presents immediately after the trauma, this finding may be absent.

George's line should be checked for the presence of retrolisthesis. In the acute patient, intervertebral swelling may lessen the amount of displacement that is detected (Fig. 7.32A).

A base posterior sacrum will show a relatively parallel disc space at L5-S1. If severe, the disc space can be opened at the back. In some patients, swelling of the posterior joint space, makes it more difficult to determine which short lever arm to use to affect the segment (See Fig. 7.29).

From the AP radiograph, several observations can be made. Distortions in the pelvis such as a rotated sacrum, will usually show obvious measurement findings with a concomitant axial rotation of the lumbar spine. Proper patient positioning is critical to identifying pelvic positional dyskinesia (See Chapter 6).

A high intercrestal line with the L5 vertebra deep-seated between the iliac crests will tend to protect the lumbosacral articulation. A relatively low intercrestal line, with absent or reduced iliolumbar ligaments, will tend to make the L5-S1 motion segment more vulnerable to injury (18). These are generalizations however.

An adjustment of a vertebra is usually specifically applied with respect to the segment below. A rare exception to the above, is an acute lumbar disc herniation at L4-L5 with L5 in a posterior position with respect to the sacrum. In this case, the L5 segment can be adjusted to the motion segment above (i.e., L4).

It is important to be aware that adjusting the motion segment with the herniated disc may be contraindicated, if the joint exhibits signs of hypermobility or instability. In general, more lesions at the L5-S1 motion segment will require adjusting (either an L5 or base posterior adjustment) than those at L4-L5 (L4 adjustment to L5 or L5 contact and set to L4). The incidence of disc herniation at both levels is roughly equal. An interesting study by Kortelainen et al. (84) attempted to correlate neurologic signs with the level of disc herniation. Four hundred three patients were studied. Fifty-six percent of the herniations occurred at L4-L5, however pain projection into the S1 distribution was most common. The traditional view point is that lesions at L4-L5 will tend to affect the L5 nerve root and that disc protrusions at L5-S1 will affect the S1 distribution. Multiple levels of involvement (e.g., L4-L5, L5-S1, SI joint) are likely to be found in patients with a chronic condition.

Release Phenomenon

Various clinicians (85,86) have described a phenomenon whereby the patient may experience pain along the distribution of a nerve once compression has been released (release phenomenon).

A faint tingling and numbness appear when a nerve is first compressed; then nothing is noted until the pressure on the nerve has been released. A painful paresthesia will then develop some time after the pressure on the nerve trunk has ceased (86). When adjusting patients with an acute low back syndrome, it is important to advise them that after the adjustment there may be a dull aching sensation along the distribution of the nerve. The pain is usually mild, and can be abated with cryotherapy if needed.

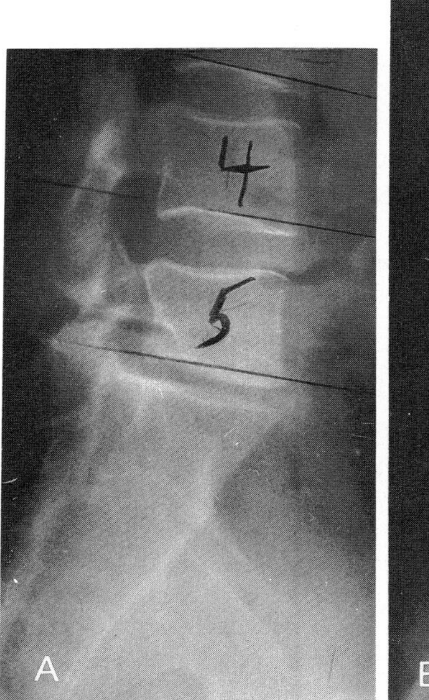

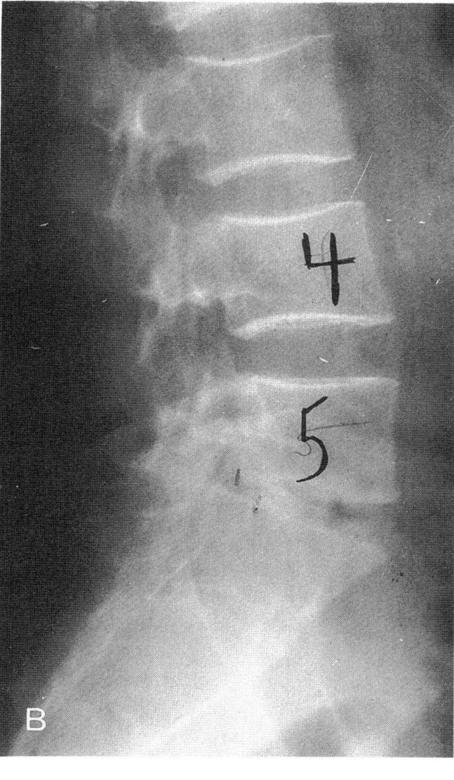

Figure 7.32. **A,** The swollen and flexed disc at L4-L5 tends to lessen the amount of retrolisthesis at L5. Notice the flattening of the lumbar lordosis. **B,** Two days later, the swelling is still apparent, but reduction of the flexion at L4 makes the retrolisthesis at L5 more noticeable.

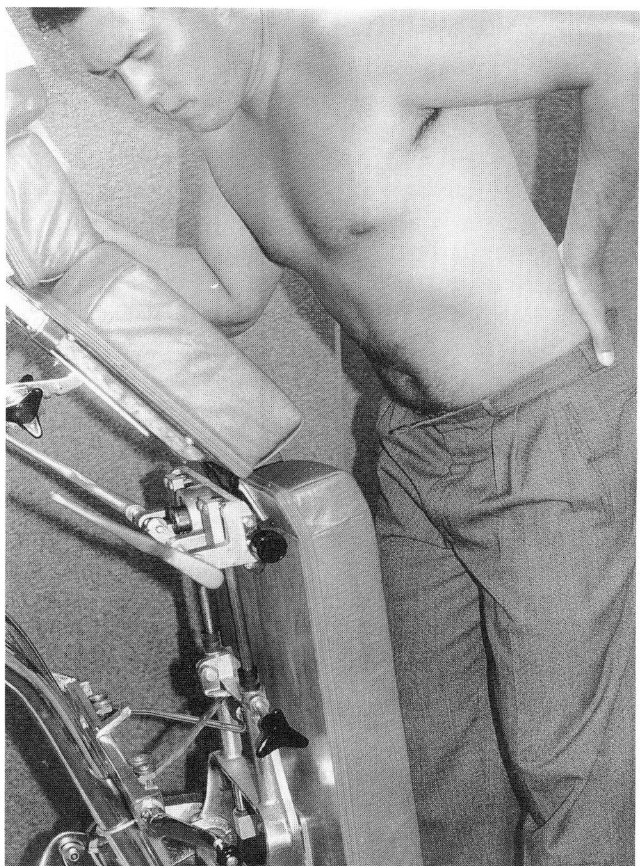

Figure 7.33. The hi-lo table can be positioned to accommodate the flexed posture of a patient with an acute disc injury.

Discussion of this issue with the patient before the pain occurs will increase the patient's confidence in the care he or she is receiving. The decision to decrease or increase the frequency of adjusting should be based on the findings of the low back rather than extremity symptomatology. Nonetheless, as the pain moves below the knee, it is usually a sign to decrease the frequency of adjusting.

The release phenomenon must always be differentiated from peripheralization of pain caused by increased nerve root compression. The patient whose low back pain is suddenly relieved after a long lever rotational manipulation, but who now suffers from intense sciatica, most likely has consequently developed a ruptured disc. Sharp pain in the lower extremity is rarely a good sign.

Prone Reduction

The patient with an acute disc injury will typically present in a flexed posture. To achieve a more normal position, the assistance of a mechanical table is often needed. The hi-lo table can be put in the upright position with the pelvic and abdominal sections raised, to conform to the flexion position of the patient (Fig. 7.33). The patient can then be placed against the vertically positioned table. The hi-lo table can then be gradually lowered to a horizontal position.

Cryotherapy may be applied in the prone position for 15–20 minutes to reduce superficial inflammation, and anesthetize the skin so that more comfort can be afforded the patient when contact is made over the posterior tis-

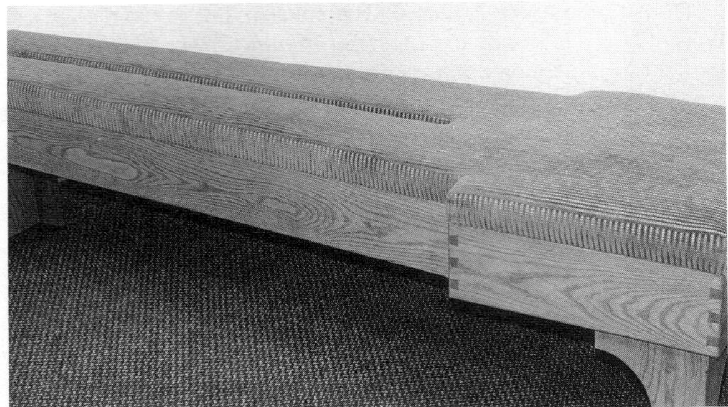

Figure 7.34. Slot table.

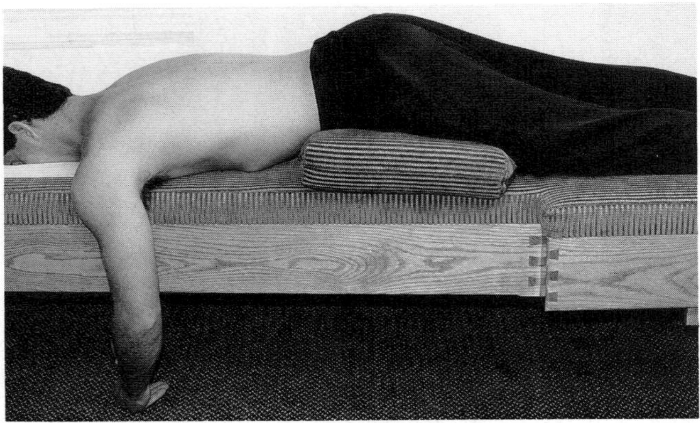

Figure 7.35. Patient positioning for a lumbar disc injury.

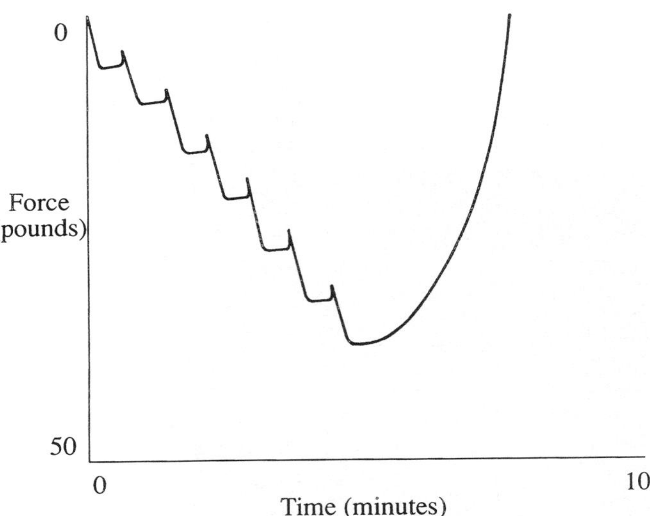

Figure 7.36. Mobilization or "pumping" procedure for a lumbar disc injury. A light pressure is applied to the involved segment (i.e., the segment that will eventually be adjusted). The pressure is held for a few seconds followed by progressively more force. Patient tolerance is continually monitored during the maneuver. The patient may not be able to tolerate force beyond what is initially applied. Peripheralization of symptomatology is a contraindication for the procedure.

sues. Gradually, the pelvic and abdominal sections are lowered until the flexion posture has been reduced as much as possible. This must be accomplished very gradually and to patient tolerance. It may take ten minutes or more to achieve a relatively flat position. The flexed posture can also be accommodated on the slot table (Figs. 7.34–7.35). The determined level of involvement can then be slightly translated forward in a "pumping action" (i.e., mobilization) to dissipate fluids in the area and encourage an anterior migration of bone and disc material. A slight pressure is first applied and then held for several seconds (85). From here, slightly more pressure is applied, then held (Fig. 7.36). The doctor should avoid bringing the joint to tension and then releasing it entirely before applying the next sequence. Patient tolerance will dictate how the procedure is applied. In some cases, the pressure may need to be completely released before another sequence of mobilization is begun. After 5–20 mobilization procedures are applied, the pressure should be carefully released.

Cryotherapy can be applied again while the patient is in the prone position. Although instant relief can sometimes occur, the patient's level of symptomatology usually will not immediately change after the treatment. Deterioration should not result however. If the leg pain becomes more severe or develops while the patient undergoes the procedure, then the mobilization should be ceased.

The doctor should always apply adjustments and mobilizations that tend to centralize the patient's symptoms. If leg pain is worsened with a particular therapy, then this contraindicates the procedure. An adjustment can be made with the patient in the prone position on either the knee-chest or hi-lo table (87), however, reduction in the side posture position is often more comfortable for the patient.

Side Posture Reduction

Mobilization of the motion segment can be accomplished in the side lying position, which is used if the patient cannot tolerate being placed prone. The patient will usually need to lie on the side that is most comfortable. The doctor should not attempt to move the patient into the correct position on the table. Rather, the patient can be allowed to use the doctor's body, to aid in movement. The patient's tolerance to pain is something only they know, the doctor should avoid testing it, beyond offering an arm for stabilization. Occasionally, lifting the legs from the floor to the table as the patient moves into the side posture position may be helpful. After the patient is placed in side posture, ask if the leg pain, if any, is worsening. Peripheralization of symptoms during a particular position, is a contraindication for that posture. If the protrusion is posterolateral (i.e., medial, lateral or beneath the nerve root), then the involved side should be placed "up" in the side posture position. If the bent leg also has nerve root tension signs, then positioning may be more difficult on this side. Occasionally the involved side may need to be placed towards the table. Care must be taken to modify the pretensioning procedure before the thrust. Tension should be developed by decreasing the lateral flexion component of the listing.

Before attempting a thrust into a patient, the area should be iced thoroughly so that there is little increase in symptomatology when attempting to locate the contact point of the involved segment. The spinous process contact is generally preferred, because this contact point will have a tendency to move the entire segment forward with a posterior to anterior (+Z) thrust. Thrusting onto a mamillary process will tend to "spin" the vertebra somewhat. After the thrust, it is especially important to hold pressure on the segment (Fig. 7.37). Backing off rapidly, or "recoiling," can be extremely painful for the patient in acute pain. The doctor will only get one attempt to make a reduction, so the first should count.

As when getting onto the table, the patient should help themselves up with only minimal assistance from the doctor. The doctor should carefully guide the legs off of the table while the patient pushes up with the arm (Fig. 7.38). Moving the legs off of the table first, will act as a counter weight for the upper body, thereby facilitating getting into a vertical position. Once seated on the table, the patient should be encouraged to stand as soon as possible, because disc pressure will increase while in the seated position. After the adjustment, the patient should be encouraged to walk as long as possible or until the pain begins to increase. The patient can remain recumbent after the treatment or may be encouraged to walk if possible. Sitting and forward bending should always be avoided because of the increase in disc pressure.

A patient with an acute lumbar disc lesion can be adjusted at six hour intervals although usually two adjustments per day are all that is required (84). A positive response is generally seen after only a few treatments. If improvement is not observed, then a reevaluation should be made.

Despite the localization and clear cut symptomatology, the entire musculoskeletal system should be examined. The presence of upper cervical subluxation especially, should not be overlooked as a complicating variable (85). Theoretically, neurologic tension in this area leads to abnormal paraspinal muscle hypertonicity, contributing to the patient's dysfunction.

A study by Tich'y et al. (88) showed a beneficial effect on symptomatology of sciatica patients when their posterior rib articulations from T5 through T7 received manipulative therapy. This again illustrates the importance of examining the entire spine in the patient with an apparently localized disorder such as an L5 disc herniation.

Walking should be encouraged as a form of therapy. Not only does this keep the individual from sitting, which would place more stress on the lumbar spine, but it is known that those individuals who walk more in their occupation have a lower incidence of lumbar disc degeneration (89). The walking might create movement in the area, without compromising the restraining elements, especially the ligaments. Swimming is another excellent therapy, which because of its antigravity medium, places very little stress on the lumbar spine, while causing movement at the various articulations.

The use of flexion distraction treatment as well as William's flexion exercises, is not advocated here. Our goal is to restore the lumbar lordosis, not reduce it. A study by Ponte et al. (90) found that extension exercises were superior to those involving flexion in decreasing low back pain and hastening the return to pain-free lumbar motion. Considering the fact that 90% of the damage that occurs

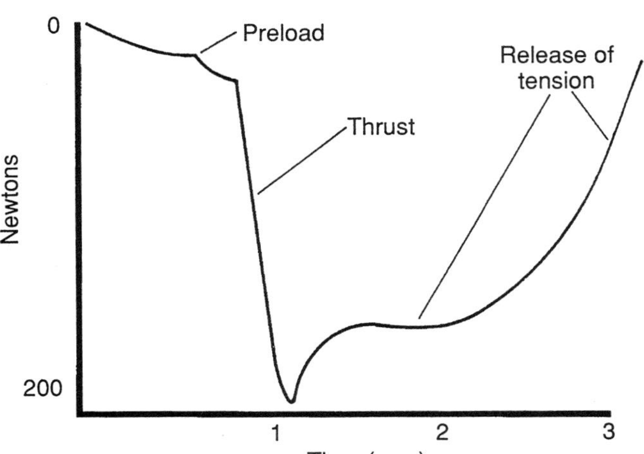

Figure 7.37. Set-hold characteristic of the adjustive thrust.

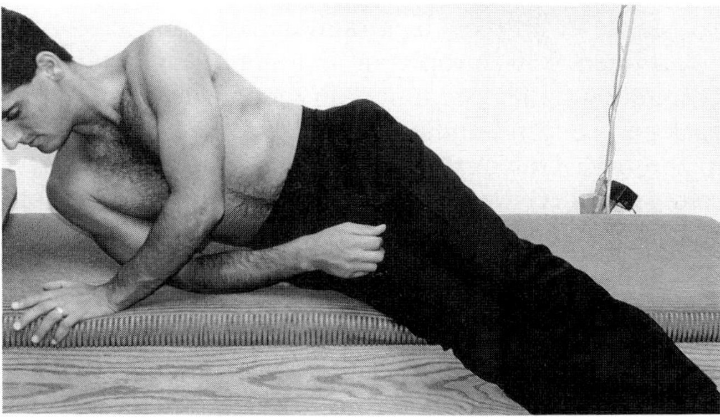
Figure 7.38. Getting off of the pelvic bench requires pushing up with the arm, while the legs provide the necessary counterbalance to the upper body.

in low back injury is posterior to the nucleus pulposus, flexion therapies would most likely stretch already torn and sprained ligamentous elements. Long-term use of flexion and traction procedures could lead to ligamentous laxity, muscular stretch and weakness, as well as intervertebral joint instability (87). Schnebel et al. (91) studied the effects of flexion and extension on changing nerve root compression in experimental disc herniation. The amount of compressive force and tension in the nerve root increased with flexion of the spine and decreased with extension. This would also agree with the work of Brieg (92) on spinal cord tension (See Chapter 2). It is acknowledged however, that there is some empirical evidence (38) that flexion distraction therapy, in conjunction with a multitude of other therapies, appears to provide some measure of symptomatic improvement for patients with low back pain.

The ruptured lumbar disc, with a free fragment compressing the nerve root, may require operation. Surgical or expert consultation is recommended for patients unresponsive to chiropractic care, those with progressive neurologic deficits, and patients with cauda equina syndrome.

White et al. (93), in a prospective controlled study on patients with herniated lumbar discs, found that those patients treated with fusion, had a significantly longer average time to return to work after surgery, versus a group of patients who only underwent laminectomy. Their conclusion was that fusions were not necessary and that simple laminectomy would suffice. It is well known that fusion patients will likely develop instability at levels above the fusion site at a later date (66).

CHRONIC LOW BACK PAIN

Waagen et al. (94) have presented a double blind clinical trial of the effects of adjustive therapy delivered by chiropractors on a group of chronic low back pain patients. The treatment group had significantly more pain relief compared to a control group as well as improvement in spinal mobility.

Meade et al. (95), in a randomized controlled trial, determined that chiropractic treatment was superior to hospital outpatient treatment in the management of low back pain. Seven hundred forty-one patients participated in the trial. Outcomes were primarily determined by a change in the Oswestry disability index. The authors concluded that for patients with low back pain in whom manipulation is not contraindicated, chiropractic almost certainly confers worthwhile long-term benefit, in comparison with hospital outpatient management. The benefit is more clearly seen in those with chronic or severe low back pain. The authors recommended that chiropractic care be included in the National Health Service of Britain based on the results of the study.

Facet Syndrome

Pain arising from the posterior joints of the lumbar spine appears to be quite common. Isolating two aspects of a three joint complex will often lead to ineffective management however. Facet injury likely does not occur in the absence of injury to the intervertebral disc (5,96). Nevertheless the "facet syndrome" has crept into the diagnostic jargon of physicians and therefore deserves some mention.

Perhaps as many as 80% of patients with chronic low back pain have some of their symptomatology arising from the posterior joints (97). Retrolisthesis and disc degeneration will lead to telescoping of the facet joints and the production of pain from nerve entrapment and stretched joint capsules (Fig. 7.39).

An increased sacral base angle or hyperlordosis can place additional compressive stress on the posterior joints (98). Pain is primarily due to stretching of the articular capsules, or bone to bone contact giving rise to periosteal pain. Hourigan and Bassett (98) have compiled the typical signs and symptoms of patients with lumbar facet syndrome (Table 7.2).

Because facet syndrome is often caused by facet overriding due to hyperextension and retrolisthesis of the segment, closed manipulative reduction is the treatment of

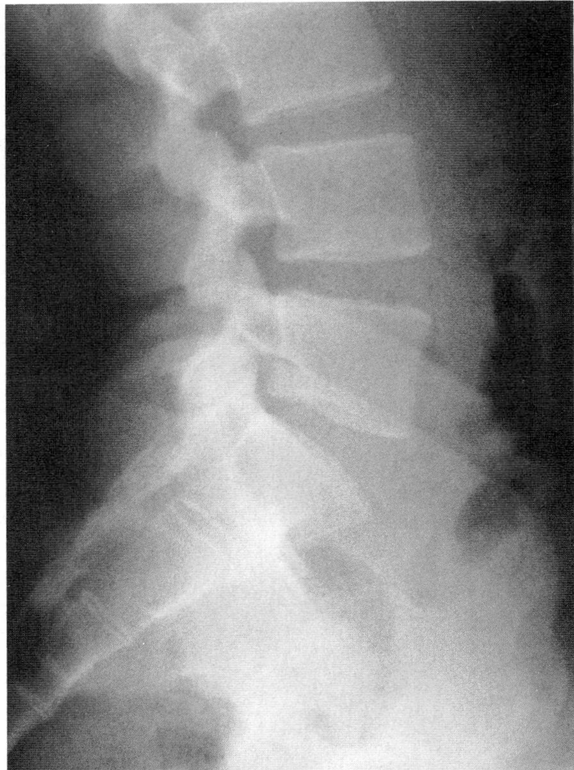

Figure 7.39. The retrolisthesis of L5 has a primary hyperextension ($-\theta X$) component. This is typical of patients who present with pain from the posterior joints.

Table 7.2.
The Classic Symptoms and Signs of Lumbar Facet Syndrome[a]

Classic Symptoms
1. Hip and buttock pain
2. Cramping leg pain, primarily above the knee
3. Low back stiffness, especially in the morning or with inactivity
4. Absence of paresthesias
Physical Signs
1. Local paralumbar tenderness
2. Pain on hyperextension of the lumbar spine
3. Absence of neurologic deficit
4. Absence of root tension signs
5. Hip, buttock, or back pain on straight leg raising

[a]Modified from Hourigan CL, Bassett JM. Facet syndrome: clinical signs, symptoms, diagnosis, and treatment. J Manipulative Physiol Ther 1989;12:294.

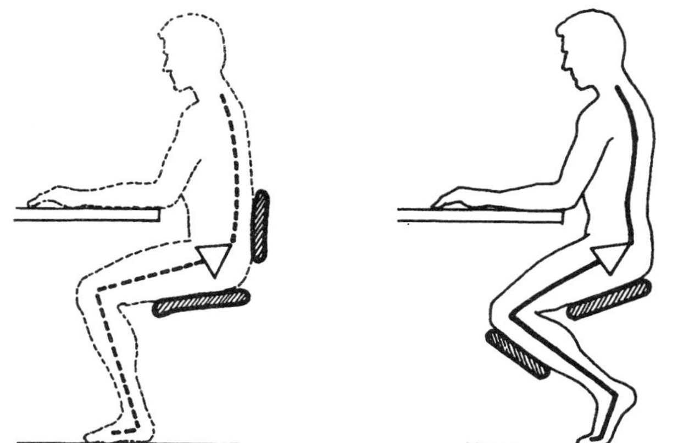

Figure 7.40. Postural changes of the lumbar lordosis from moving to the knee-support chair. Modified from Bendix A, Jensen CV, Bendix T. Posture, acceptability and energy consumption on a tiltable and a knee-support chair. Clinical Biomechanics 1988;3:70.

choice. Banks (99) has shown that reduction of the hyperextension component of the lesion is readily attainable with side posture manipulation. A statistically significant decrease in the average disc angle at the involved level was detected in his sample of 13 patients with clinical diagnoses of facet syndrome.

Plaugher et al. (23), in a retrospective, consecutive case analysis study, detected an average (mean) reduction in retrolisthesis of 34% in 49 patients. The technique employed, emphasized posterior to anterior forces (+Z) in the side posture position. Post radiologic evaluations were made after an average of eight treatments.

LUMBAR KYPHOSIS

Lumbar kyphosis can be caused by a variety of subluxation patterns. A common cause is severe axial rotation of the lumbar spine or pelvis. Sacral rotation, or a rotated fifth lumbar could be contributory. If the patient also has an ipsilateral degeneration of the acetabulum, then an ASIn subluxation of the ilium may be involved (85).

BILATERAL SCIATICA

Bilateral symptoms in any patient should be a cause for concern. Carcinoma and diabetic neuropathy must be ruled out. Mechanical causes of bilateral sciatica include a large centralized disc herniation or extreme degeneration of the motion segment (85).

LIFESTYLE AND ERGONOMIC FACTORS

Deyo and Bass (100) have studied the potential risk factors of smoking and obesity on low back pain. Generally, greater obesity leads to a higher incidence of low back pain, especially in those grossly overweight. Back pain prevalence tends to rise with increased levels of smoking.

Videman et al. (101) studied patient-handling skills of a group of nurses and compared this with the incidence of back injuries. They discovered that poor patient handling skills, low number of repetitions in a sit-up test, and high work-load scores were major risk factors for having a back injury. It was concluded that back injuries could be prevented by the teaching of patient-handling skills.

The biomechanics of lifting without injury (See Chapter 2) should be explained to the patient. For those individuals with lumbar disc injury who must sit for long periods, the use of a knee-support chair may decrease symptomatology by increasing the lumbar lordosis, thus reducing internal disc pressures (102) (Fig. 7.40)

REHABILITATION

Muscle

Mayer et al. (103) determined flexion and extension strength of the lumbar spine in pain-free and symptomatic patients. Low back pain patients had decreased strength for both flexion and extension motion, and greater variability. Extensor strength tended to be more affected than flexor strength. The discrepancies between symptomatic patients and controls was more noticeable in females. High speed drop-off ratios were also much lower in the symptomatic group. Their conclusion was that strength deficits are a major factor in the deconditioning syndrome associated with chronic low back pain.

While it is unlikely that reduced strength is what caused the injury initially, it behooves the practitioner to consider rehabilitative exercises as part of the overall management approach, especially if the patient must return to an ergonomic environment where large demands are going to be placed on the muscular system.

In a study of the effects of modern rehabilitation on chronic low back pain and disability, disappointing results were observed (104). The four week program consisted of three to five training sessions a day, six days a week. The training employed ergometer bicycling, tread-

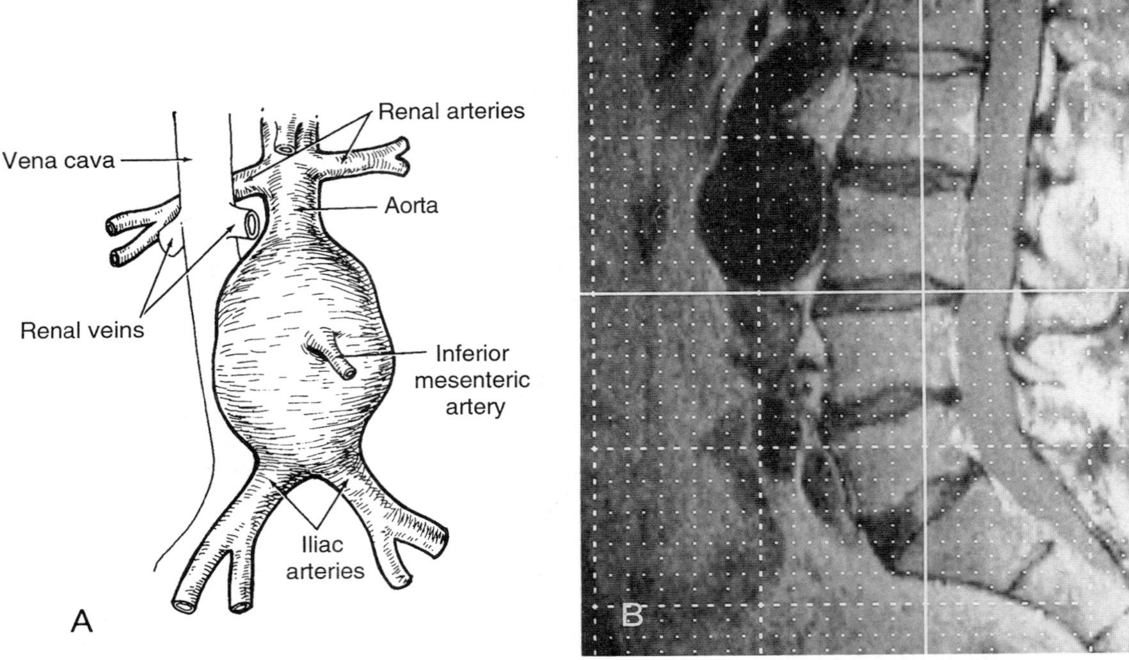

Figure 7.41. **A,** An aneurysm of the abdominal aorta. Modified from Stedman's medical dictionary. 25th ed. Baltimore: Williams & Wilkins, 1990:77. **B,** An aneurysm of the abdominal aorta.

mill running, group training with aerobics, swimming, paddling, skiing, hiking, and riding. This type of program has been previously shown to increase muscle power by 14% and aerobic capacity by 30% (105). At 18 months follow-up, only 15 of the 66 (23%) low back pain patients had returned to work. It is clear from this report that rehabilitation alone has little effect on a person returning to work. Perhaps if chiropractic care were combined with the program, a more positive result would have emerged. This question remains unanswered until further research is performed.

A clinical trial by Donchin et al. (106), showed that a calisthenics program increased lumbar flexion more than back school, in a group of chronic low back pain patients. The trial attempted to determine if the therapies had a significant effect on prevention of pain in 142 hospital employees reporting at least three annual episodes of the condition. After three months of treatment, pain was also significantly reduced in the calisthenics group.

Stankovic and Johnell (107) evaluated the effects of McKenzie (108) extension exercises in a prospective randomized clinical trial on patients with acute low back pain. Comparisons were made between extension exercises and maneuvers designed to improve the lumbar lordosis, and a "mini back school" that consisted only of back care education. In this study, McKenzie's treatment for acute low back pain was significantly better than patient education in a back school, with regard to return to work during the initial period, sick-leave during the initial episode, recurrences during the first year, pain, and spinal movement.

UNUSUAL CAUSES OF LOW BACK AND LEG PAIN

Aneurysm of the Abdominal Aorta

Vernon et al. (109) report on two patients with abdominal aortic aneurysms (AAA) that presented to chiropractors' offices with a chief compliant of low back pain (Fig. 7.41A-B). The first case had radiographic evidence of a pulsating mass in the lower abdomen consisting of slight erosion of the anterior vertebral body of L4 and a faint curvilinear calcification to the left of L4. The patient was subsequently referred for a diagnostic ultrasound examination that confirmed the clinical impression. No other physical findings were present in this patient which would have indicated the possibility of AAA. The second case was initially diagnosed as a herniated nucleus pulposus and was referred for CT examination. CT findings suggested the possibility of AAA which was later confirmed with diagnostic ultrasound.

An excellent review of AAA has been provided by Hopkins (110). In England, an AAA is found in 3% of the population over age 50. It causes death in 1.5% of these cases (110). The incidence appears to be increasing in the U.S. This is due, in large part, by the use of modern scanning techniques that can detect much smaller aneurysms. Aneurysms grow at the rate of about 4 to 5 mm a year.

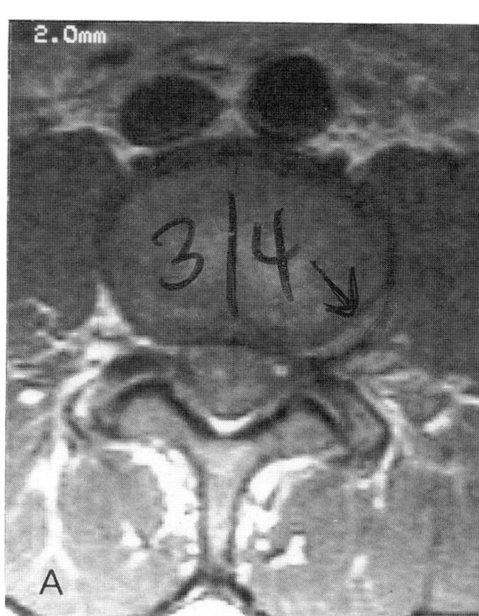

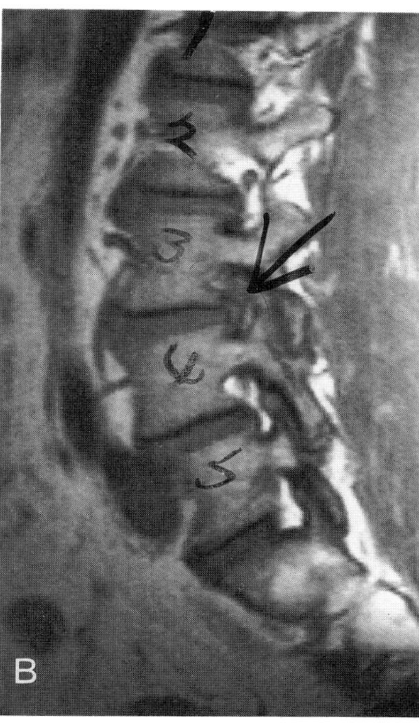

Figure 7.48. **A,** Axial MRI demonstrating annular protrusion. This posterolateral bulge is likely to affect the lateral bending characteristics of the motion segment. **B,** Disc protrusion at L3-L4.

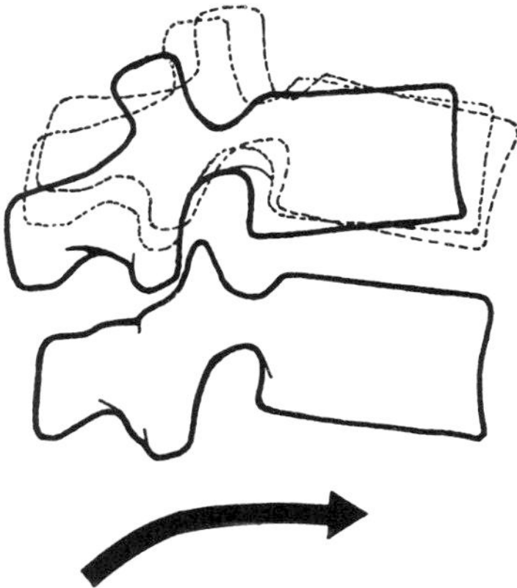

Figure 7.49. Primary pattern of thrust for adjustments of the lumbar spine

vic organs). Rather, the fifth lumbar is said to be posterior to the sacral base and adjusted from posterior to anterior. A cervical vertebra may be anterior to the segment below. The inferior segment, if subluxated, can then be adjusted to partially remedy the situation.

Severe ligamentous laxity precludes a good prognosis for reduction of positional dyskinesia. There is little scientific evidence that adjustments can affect the positional dyskinesia component of the subluxation complex (23, 67, 99, 120). Nevertheless, the listing is used to maximize the potential for repositioning to occur.

A three-dimensional listing system is a good communication tool (provided others understand it) that assists in the reproducibility of adjustments, both between adjustments of a series performed by one doctor, and adjustments administered by different chiropractors.

The pattern of thrust must take into account the center of mass of the vertebra and be directed through it anteriorward. In most instances, an arcing motion upward will be made at the beginning of the thrust. This flexes the segment to decrease any hyperextension of the segment. The vertebra is then driven straight forward, through the plane line of the disc or perpendicular to the lumbar lordosis (Fig. 7.49).

The spinous process contact is usually preferred to the mamillary, because of the more direct contact that can be made. The mamillary contact is usually less able to reduce the posteriority of the segment, which may be a major component of the listing. Intersegmental axial rotation is usually relatively minor in the lumbar spine, unless a coronally orientated facet joint is involved. Lateral flexion can be a major dysfunctional direction. This is chiefly corrected by "kinking" the segment into lateral flexion during positioning and preload or "tension." Further lateral flexion can be attained by introducing a screw motion or torque during the thrust. The posterior to anterior vector is followed by an inferiorward or caudal arcing motion or torque (Z axis) that attempts to laterally flex the motion segment further. The segment is then held in this position for 1–2 seconds, or longer if the doctor wishes to take full advantage of ligamentous, muscular, and tendinous creep. These viscoelastic structures respond most favorably to constant loads applied over a long period of time. If a nuclear fragment is being directed centrally, then "holding" the segment is thought to accentuate this effect.

In some acute situations, it may be difficult to hold a sustained pressure.

Careful attention should be made to protecting the surrounding normal or hypermobile segments in an effort to minimize any harm to these articulations. The doctor should try to create a fulcrum at the articulation to be adjusted by stressing the spine at the involved level through prepositioning.

The amount of force involved in an adjustment in the side posture position is on the order of 80–100 lbs (119). The force would be much less for pediatric or geriatric patients and any other situation where less force is desired. The amount of the thrust is always to patient tolerance and should be as comfortable as possible. The acute patient situation may be exacerbated somewhat during a thrust, but pain should rapidly subside after the maneuver. An increase in symptomatology is a contraindication for further manipulation until a reevaluation is made.

When the vertebra has subluxated posterior it is listed with the letter "P". This represents a $-Z$ translational vector and is corrected in the adjustment by thrusting in a posterior to anterior direction. Other letters of the listing include "R" or "L" for listing either spinous rotation to the right ($+\theta Y$) or left ($-\theta Y$).

If the vertebra is also tilted in the coronal plane (wedging) then this too is listed. When the spinous process of the vertebra ($\pm\theta Y$) has rotated to the higher side of the wedged disc, an "S" (superiority) ($\pm\theta Z$) is placed after the rotational component. If the spinous process has rotated to the inferior side of the wedge, then an "I" will follow the spinous rotation letter.

The contact point (mamillary or spinous) follows the listing as either an "m" or "sp." PLI and PRI listings are adjusted using a mamillary contact (the exception is L5). P, PL, PR, PRS and PLS listings are adjusted with a spinous process contact. If no wedging is present ($\pm\theta Z$), PL and PR may be adjusted with a mamillary contact, if the spinous process has rotated towards the concavity of a scoliosis (Fig. 7.50A-B).

The radiographs provided with the adjustment descriptions are not meant to represent the total examination, but rather a way to conceptualize the three-dimensional thrust. The radiograph is a two dimensional image of a three-dimensional patient. An artist's rendition of some listings, from the perspective of the doctor before the thrust, is provided. This will hopefully orient the doctor from two dimensions to three. The displacements illustrated are not meant to be anatomically correct, and may be exaggerated somewhat, to illustrate the vectors of the thrust. Keep in mind, that the pattern of thrust may vary during the adjustment.

Simply achieving an audible is not the sole indicator of a successful adjustment. An audible should occur however, unless there is marked edema in the area.

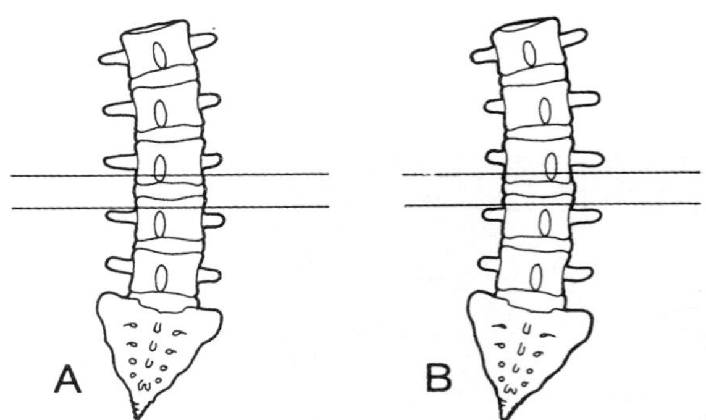

Figure 7.50. **A,** A mamillary contact is used if the spinous has rotated towards the concavity of a scoliosis. The thrust of an adjustment should never be towards the concavity of a curve. **B,** The spinous contact can be used for the adjustment because it has rotated toward the convexity of the scoliosis.

Because the adjustment is a highly coordinated event, the doctor should refrain from thinking "cerebrally" during the actual thrust. The doctor should only conceptualize the movement of the vertebra towards a more normal position. In this way the fixation component is necessarily addressed, without traumatizing the joint by moving it into the direction of injury.

Special Listings of L5

In most instances the wedging of the disc is corrected by pretensioning and thrusting from the opened side of the wedge towards the center. It is generally not preferred, to attempt to open the closed side by making a superiorward arcing motion during the thrust. This is due to the freely movable nature of the segment below. The exception to this, is the case of L5, because the sacrum and pelvis can remain relatively stable during an adjustment. If a lumbar scoliosis is present, then this supersedes the requirement for adjusting from the open towards the closed side of the wedge if the contact segment is L5 (56). Essentially, the wedging of L4-L5 is used to determine if there is a special listing for L5. When there is wedging of L4, then the opened side is placed up in the side posture position (Fig. 7.51A-C). Doing this, may mean that the L5 segment wedging is opposite to the L4 level. To decrease the lateral flexion component of the listing, the L5 segment is torqued superiorly with a cephalad arcing motion towards the end of the thrust. If no scoliosis or wedging is present at L4, then conventional or simple listings are used for L5.

ADJUSTMENT

Side Posture Position

The side posture position is generally the preferred position for adjusting the lumbar spine (See Chapter 6) (Fig. 7.52). The doctor should first place the pillow at the

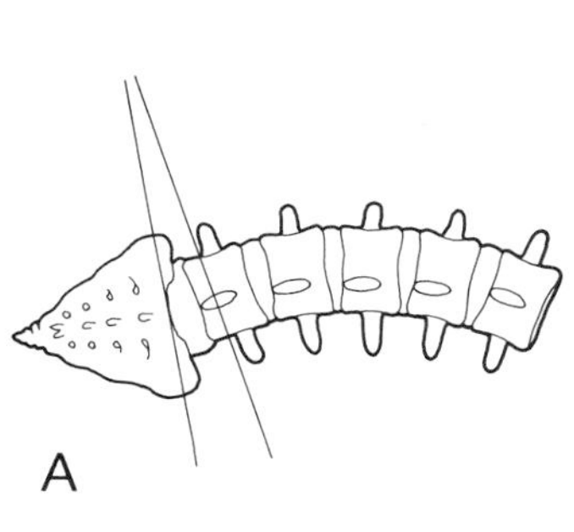

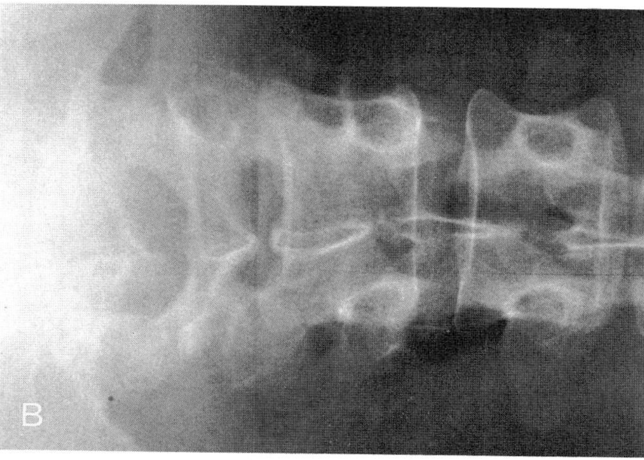

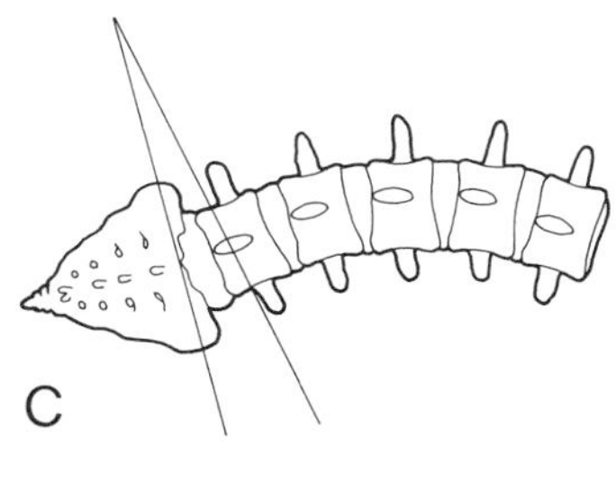

Figure 7.51. **A,** The spinous process of L5 has rotated toward the open side of the wedge. Contact is made on the left mamillary process of L5 (PRS-m). The figure is placed horizontally, to depict the listing while in the side posture position. **B,** The AP radiograph demonstrates a special listing of L5 (PRS-m). **C,** The spinous process of L5 has rotated toward the closed side of the wedge, which is the convexity of the scoliosis. The special listing is PLI-sp of L5.

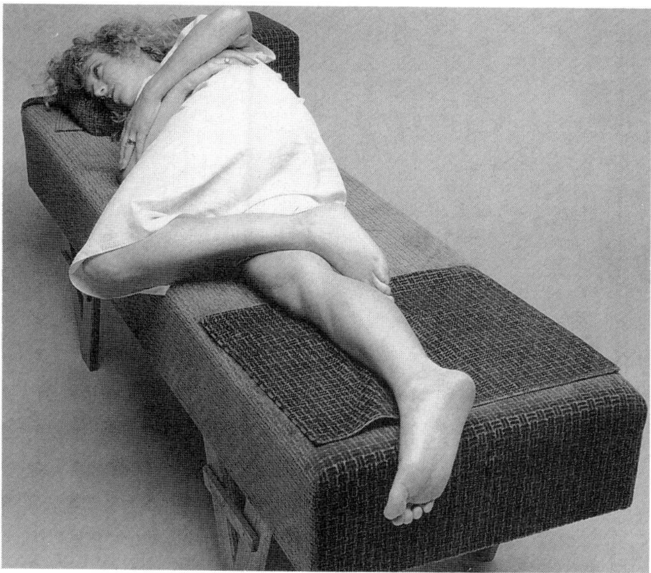

Figure 7.52. Side posture position.

appropriate end of the table. The patient is then instructed to sit in the center of the table and then to lie on either the right or left side. The inferior leg is kept straight, in line with the rest of the spinal column. The superior leg is bent, with the patient's foot tucked behind the popliteal fossa. The inferior foot should be allowed to roll forward when the patient is brought closer to the doctor. This can be accomplished by allowing the foot to hang off of the end of the table. The inferior shoulder should be pulled caudally.

The doctor then contacts the appropriate short lever arm by taking a tissue pull in the direction of correction (Fig. 7.53). When identifying the contact point, it is helpful to use the radiograph. The AP view can be used to determine the relationship of the spinous process to its mamillary process. The lateral view is of help in determining the shape of the spinous process in relation to others in the area. Wiggling the leg forwards and back should be avoided. Because L5 is the last freely movable vertebra, this method could theoretically be used to differentiate a movable L5 from an immovable S1. If L5 is fixated, as it should be if an adjustment is considered, there may or may not be movement at this level.

As can be seen in Figure 7.54 the patient is rolled over towards the doctor so that a posterior to anterior line of correction is easily attained. To be rolled forward this far, the patient needs to be prepositioned towards the center of the table. Different doctor and patient somatotypes prohibit broad generalizations for the side posture position. The key points to keep in mind are as follows:

1. The joint should be brought to tension by rolling the patient over with the contact on the spinous or mamillary process
2. As the patient is rolled forward the shoulder should be allowed to roll forward as well, in order that the thoracic spine is not excessively rotated.
3. The body drop should be into the pelvis, directly opposite the thrusting vector of the contact hand (e.g., pisiform).
4. The segment contacted is held for several seconds after the thrust.
5. If a patient lifts the inferior leg before the thrust, it shows absence of relaxation. So, instruct the patient to let the leg go. Similarly, if the patient attempts to arch the spine anteriorward while rolled forward, this would necessitate contracted erector spinae muscles. In some instances, the patient may need to be asked to flex the lumbar spine before the thrust. If this needed, it is important to not axially rotate the lumbar spine during the flexed posture because this is a vulnerable position for torsional injury.

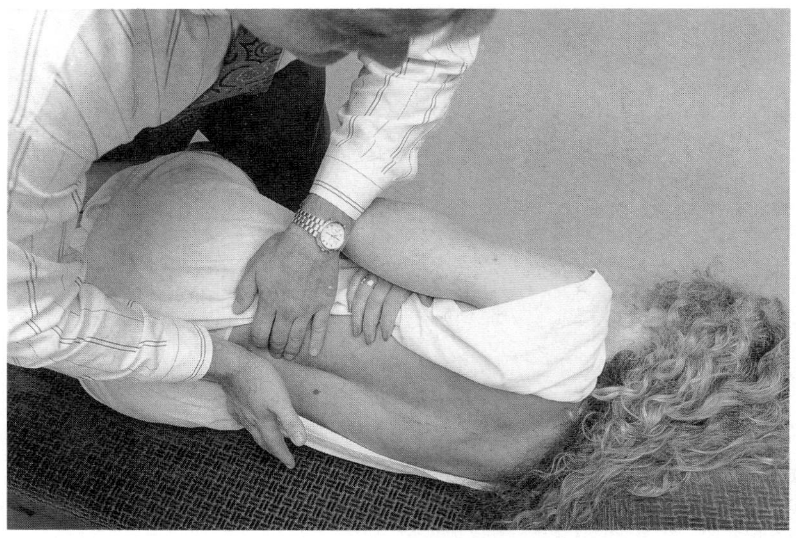

Figure 7.53. Placing the contact hand on the spinous process of L5 while taking a tissue pull with the stabilization hand. The tissue pull should be similar to the pattern of thrust.

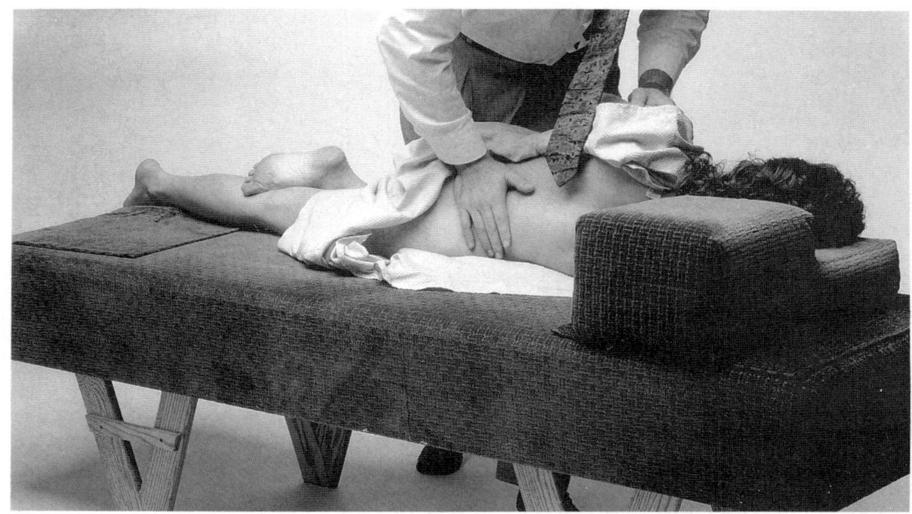

Figure 7.54. Set-up for a posterior L5 adjustment. Notice the lack of any twisting to the thoracic and lumbar spine. The patient is in a nearly prone position, which facilitates the posterior to anterior thrust without compromising the doctor's spine.

Name of technique: Gonstead

Name of technique procedure: Posterior L5 (−Z) side posture adjustment (Fig. 7.55A-B).

Indications: Retrolisthesis of L5 with decreased anteriorward translation during flexion.

Contraindications: All other listings, normal FSU, hypermobility, instability, destruction or fracture of the neural arch or spinous process, infection of the contact vertebra.

Patient position: Right or left side posture position.

Doctor's position: Standing at a 45° angle facing cephalad.

Contact point: Posterior, inferior border of the spinous process.

Supporting Hand: Contacts the anterolateral portion of the shoulder and axilla region with a slight cephalad distraction.

Pattern of thrust: A slight inferior to superior pattern followed with a marked posterior to anterior vector along the sacral base angle. It is important to keep in mind that the sacral base angle is reduced when the patient lies in the side posture position. It is further reduced when the patient's thigh is flexed just before the thrust.

Category by algorithm: Short lever specific contact procedure.

Name of technique: Gonstead

Name of technique procedure: Posterior, inferior L5 ($-Z, -\theta X$) side posture adjustment (Fig. 7.56A).

Indications: Retrolisthesis of L5 (7.56B) with decreased anteriorward translation and flexion during forward bending.

Contraindications: All other listings, normal FSU, hypermobility, instability, destruction or fracture of the neural arch or spinous process, infection of the contact vertebra.

Patient position: Right or left side posture position.

Doctor's position: Standing at a 45° angle facing cephalad.

Contact point: Posterior, inferior border of the spinous process.

Supporting Hand: Contacts the anterolateral portion of the shoulder and axilla region with a slight cephalad distraction.

Pattern of thrust: A moderate inferior to superior pattern followed with a posterior to anterior vector along the sacral base angle. It is important to keep in mind that the sacral base angle is reduced when the patient lies in the side posture position. It is

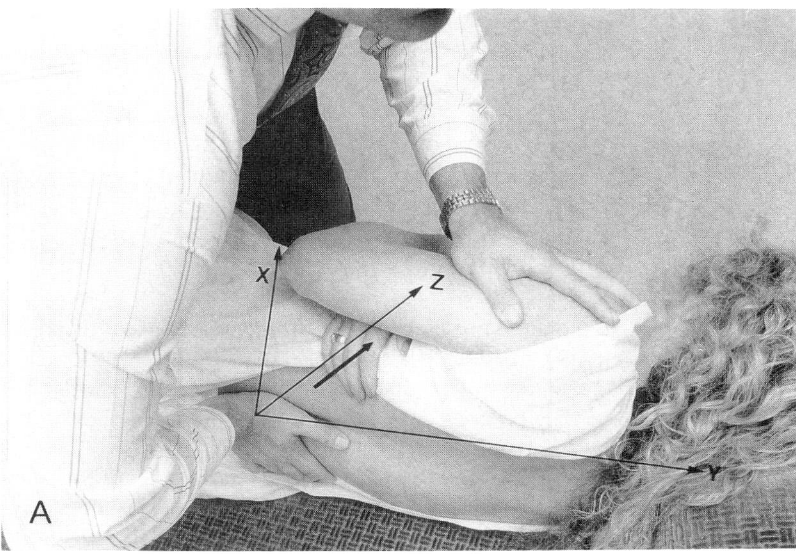

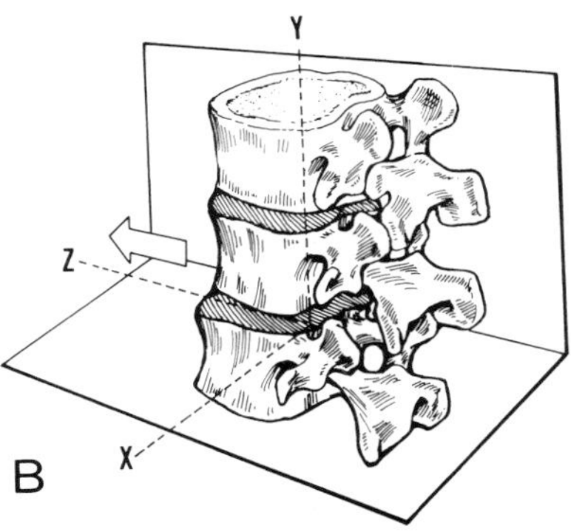

Figure 7.55. **A,** Pattern of thrust for a posterior L5. In this example, the patient is kept in a side posture position during the thrust. Doing so, necessitates that the doctor lean over the patient to maximize the posterior to anterior vector. **B,** Pattern of thrust for a posterior segment.

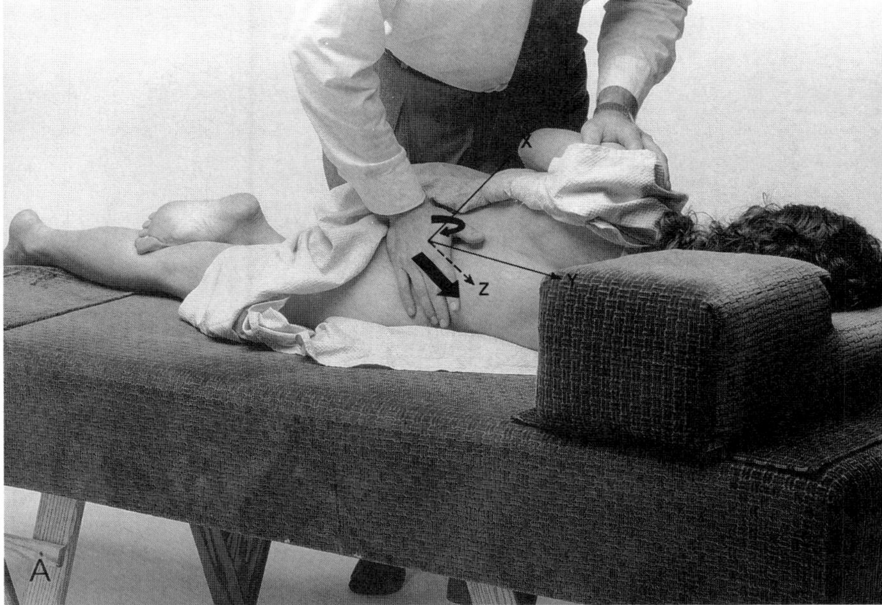

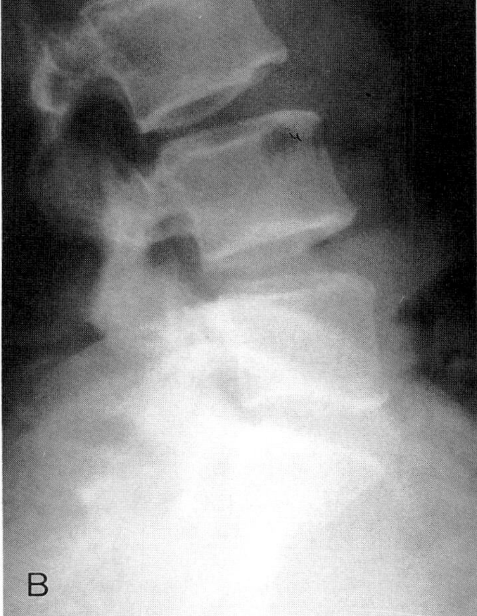

Figure 7.56. **A,** The pattern of thrust for a posterior and inferior (P-inf) ($-Z, -\theta X$) L5. **B,** Retrolisthesis of L5.

further reduced when the patient's thigh is flexed before the thrust.

Category by algorithm: Short lever specific contact procedure.

Name of technique: Gonstead

Name of technique procedure: PLS ($-$Z, $-\theta$Y, $+\theta$Z)L5 side posture adjustment (Fig. 7.57).

Indications: Retrolisthesis of L5 with decreased anteriorward translation and flexion during forward bending. Fixation dysfunction in right spinous rotation ($+\theta$Y) and left lateral flexion ($-\theta$Z).

Contraindications: All other listings, normal FSU, hypermobility, instability, destruction or fracture of the neural arch or spinous process infection of the contact vertebra.

Patient position: Right side posture position.

Doctor's position: Standing at a 45° angle facing cephalad.

Contact point: Posterior, inferior, left lateral border of the spinous process. The tissue pull for the lateral flexion positional dyskinesia should be from superior to inferior.

Supporting Hand: Contacts the anterolateral portion of the shoulder and axilla region with a slight cephalad distraction.

Pattern of thrust: Posterior to anterior vector along the sacral base angle. It is important to keep in mind that the sacral base angle is reduced when the patient lies in the side posture position. It is further reduced when the patient's thigh is flexed before the thrust. Lateral to medial ($+\theta$Y), with an inferiorward arcing motion ($-\theta$Z) toward the end of the thrust.

Category by algorithm: Short lever specific contact procedure.

Name of technique: Gonstead

Name of technique procedure: PRS-inf ($-$Z, $+\theta$Y, $-\theta$Z, $-\theta$X) L5 side posture adjustment (Fig. 7.58A-D).

Indications: Retrolisthesis of L5 with decreased anteriorward translation and flexion during forward bending. Fixation dysfunction in left spinous rotation ($-\theta$Y) and right lateral flexion ($+\theta$Z).

Contraindications: All other listings, normal FSU, hypermobility, instability, destruction or fracture of the neural arch or spinous process, infection of the contact vertebra.

Patient position: Left side posture position.

Doctor's position: Standing at a 45° angle facing cephalad.

Contact point: Posterior, inferior, right lateral border of the spinous process. The tissue pull for the lateral flexion positional dyskinesia should be from superior to inferior.

Supporting Hand: Contacts the anterolateral portion of the shoulder and axilla region with a slight cephalad distraction.

Pattern of thrust: Slightly inferior to superior and posterior to anterior along the sacral base angle. It is important to keep in mind that the sacral base angle is reduced when the patient lies in the side posture position. It is further reduced when the

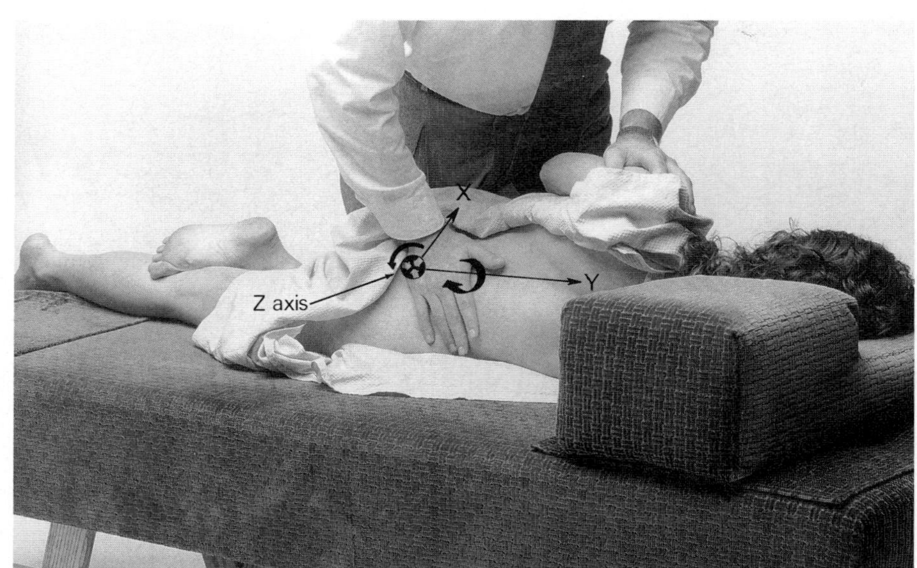

Figure 7.57. PLS L5 adjustment.

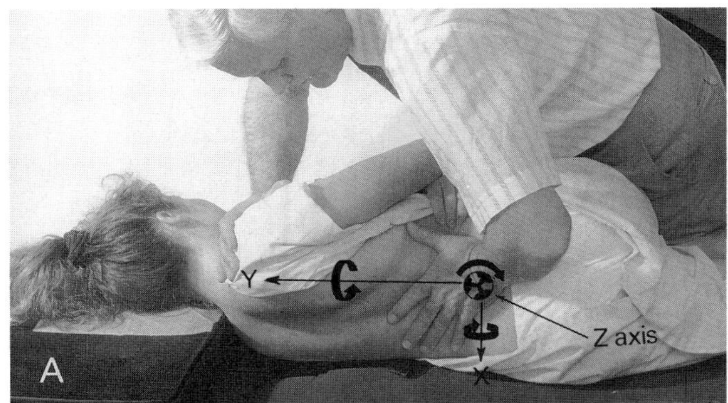

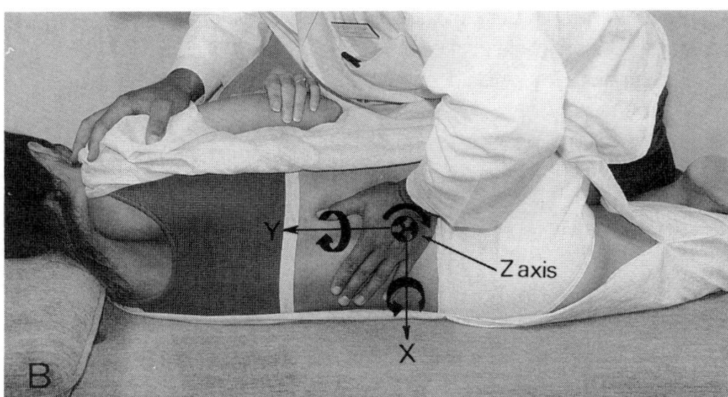

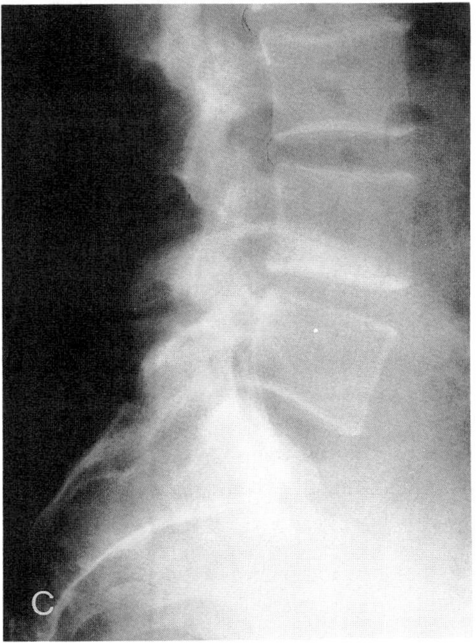

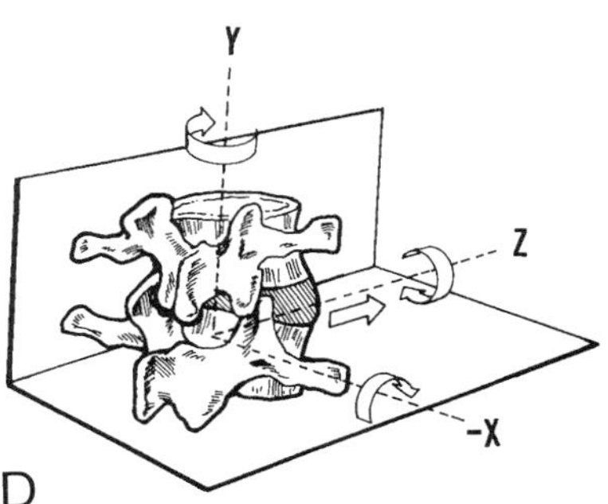

Figure 7.58. **A,** PRS-inf side posture adjustment. **B,** PRS-inf side posture adjustment. **C,** Retrolisthesis of L5. **D,** Pattern of thrust for a PRS-inf listing.

patient's thigh is flexed before the thrust. Lateral to medial ($-\theta Y$), with an inferiorward arcing motion ($+\theta Z$) toward the end of the thrust.

Category by algorithm: Short lever specific contact procedure.

Special listings of L5 can be adjusted in the side posture position (Fig. 7.59) using the Gonstead method. The torque, if applicable, will be superiorward.

Name of technique: Gonstead

Name of technique procedure: PRS-m L5 ($-Z$, $+\theta Y$, $-\theta Z$) side posture lumbar adjustment (Fig. 7.60).

Indications: Retrolisthesis of L5 with left lateral flexion positional dyskinesia and left body rotation. Left convex scoliosis with right lateral flexion of the L4-L5 motion segment necessitates using the left mamillary process as the contact point (special listing).

Contraindications: All other listings, normal FSU, hypermobility, instability, destruction or fracture of the neural arch or spinous process, infection of the contact vertebra.

Patient position: In the right side posture position.

Doctor's position: Standing at a 45° angle facing cephalad.

Contact point: Left mamillary process with the pisiform. The fingers should be oriented along the axis of the spine.

Supporting Hand: Contacts the anterolateral portion of the shoulder and axilla region with a slight cephalad distraction.

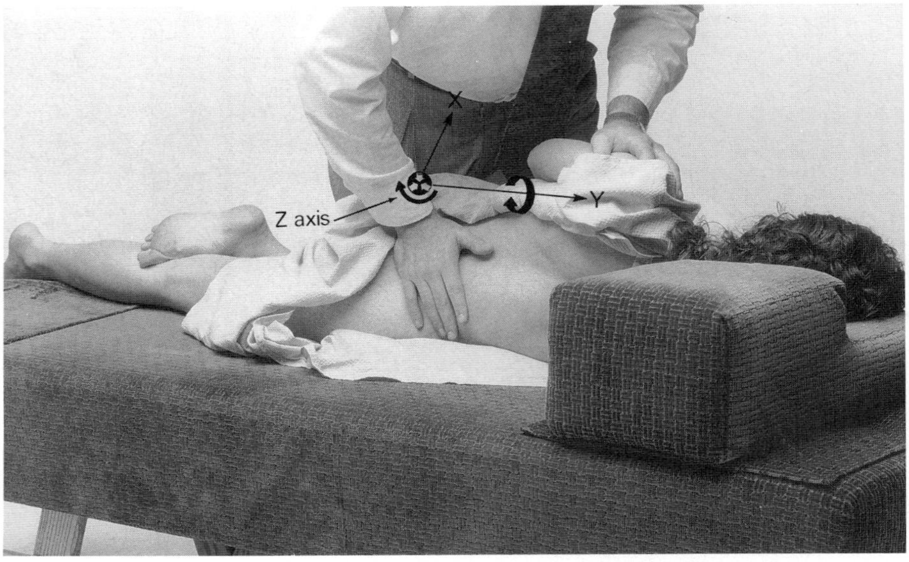

Figure 7.59. L5 PLI-sp special listing side posture adjustment. The contact point is the posterior, inferior and lateral aspect of the spinous process of L5 with the pisiform. The pattern of thrust is depicted.

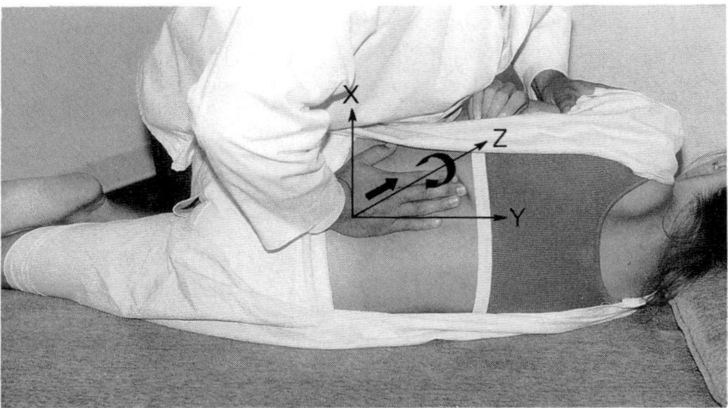

Figure 7.60. L5 PRS-m special listing side posture adjustment. Contact is made on the left mamillary process of L5. The pattern of thrust is depicted.

Pattern of thrust: Posterior to anterior ($+Z$) with a superiorward arcing motion ($+\theta Z$) toward the end of the thrust.

Category by algorithm: Short lever specific contact procedure.

Technique: Gonstead

Technique procedure: L4 PL ($-Z$, $-\theta Y$) side posture adjustment (Fig. 7.61A).

Indications: Retrolisthesis ($-Z$) of L4 (Fig. 7.61B) and left spinous rotation ($-\theta Y$). Fixation dysfunction in flexion and right spinous rotation ($+\theta Y$).

Contraindications: All other listings, normal FSU, hypermobility, instability, destruction or fracture of the neural arch of the contact vertebra, infection of the contact vertebra.

Patient position: On the right side.

Doctor's position: Standing at a 45° angle facing cephalad.

Contact point: Posterior, inferior and left lateral border of the spinous process of L4.

Supporting Hand: Contacts the anterolateral left shoulder and axilla region with a slight cephalad distraction.

Set Up: With the patient on the right side, the contact hand (R) is placed so that the pisiform is over L4, with the fingers pointing at approximately a 45° angle from the longitudinal axis of the spine. The patient is then rolled over towards the doctor with the pisiform contact thereby moving the L4-L5 articulation into the paraphysiologic elastic zone. The patient's left shoulder is allowed to roll forward minimizing axial rotation of the spine. The doctor stabilizes the patient's pelvis into the table.

Pattern of thrust: Posterior to anterior ($+Z$) through the L4-L5 disc plane with a slight lateral to medial ($+\theta Y$) vector of thrust.

Category by algorithm: Short lever specific contact procedure.

Name of technique: Gonstead

Name of technique procedure: PLS L3 ($-Z$, $-\theta Y$, $+\theta Z$) side posture lumbar adjustment (Fig. 7.62A).

Indications: Retrolisthesis of L3 (Fig. 7.62B) with right body rotation right lateral flexion positional dyskinesia (Fig. 7.62C).

Contraindications: All other listings, normal FSU, hypermobility, instability, destruction or fracture of the neural arch or spinous process, infection of the contact vertebra

Patient position: Right side posture position.

Doctor's position: Standing at a 45° angle facing cephalad.

Contact point: Posterior, inferior, left lateral border of the L3 spinous process with the pisiform of the doctor.

Supporting Hand: Contacts the anterolateral portion of the shoulder and axilla region with a slight cephalad distraction.

Pattern of thrust: Posterior to anterior (+Z), lateral to medial (+θY) with an inferiorward arcing motion (−θZ) towards the end of the thrust.

Category by algorithm: Short lever specific contact procedure.

Name of technique: Gonstead

Name of technique procedure: L3 PLI-m (−Z, −θY, −θZ) side posture adjustment with pisiform contact (Fig. 7.63).

Indications: Decreased anterior translation (+Z) motion of the segment, right lateral bending (+θZ) and left axial rotation (+θY). Retrolisthesis, lateral flexion malposition (−θZ) and left rotational (−θY) positional dyskinesia of L3.

Contraindications: All other listings, normal FSU, hypermobility, instability, destruction or fracture of the mamillary process or superior zygapophyseal joint of L3, infection of the contact vertebra.

Patient position: Left side posture position.

Doctor's position: Standing at a 45° angle facing cephalad.

Contact point: Right mamillary process with the left pisiform of the doctor. The AP radiograph should be used to determine the location of the mamillary process in relation to nearby structures. The fingers do not cross the spine.

Supporting Hand: Contacts the anterolateral right shoulder and axilla region with a slight cephalad distraction.

Set Up: The patient is rolled over towards the doctor with the pisiform contact, thereby moving the L3-L4 articulation from the neutral zone to the elastic zone (maximal preload or "tension").

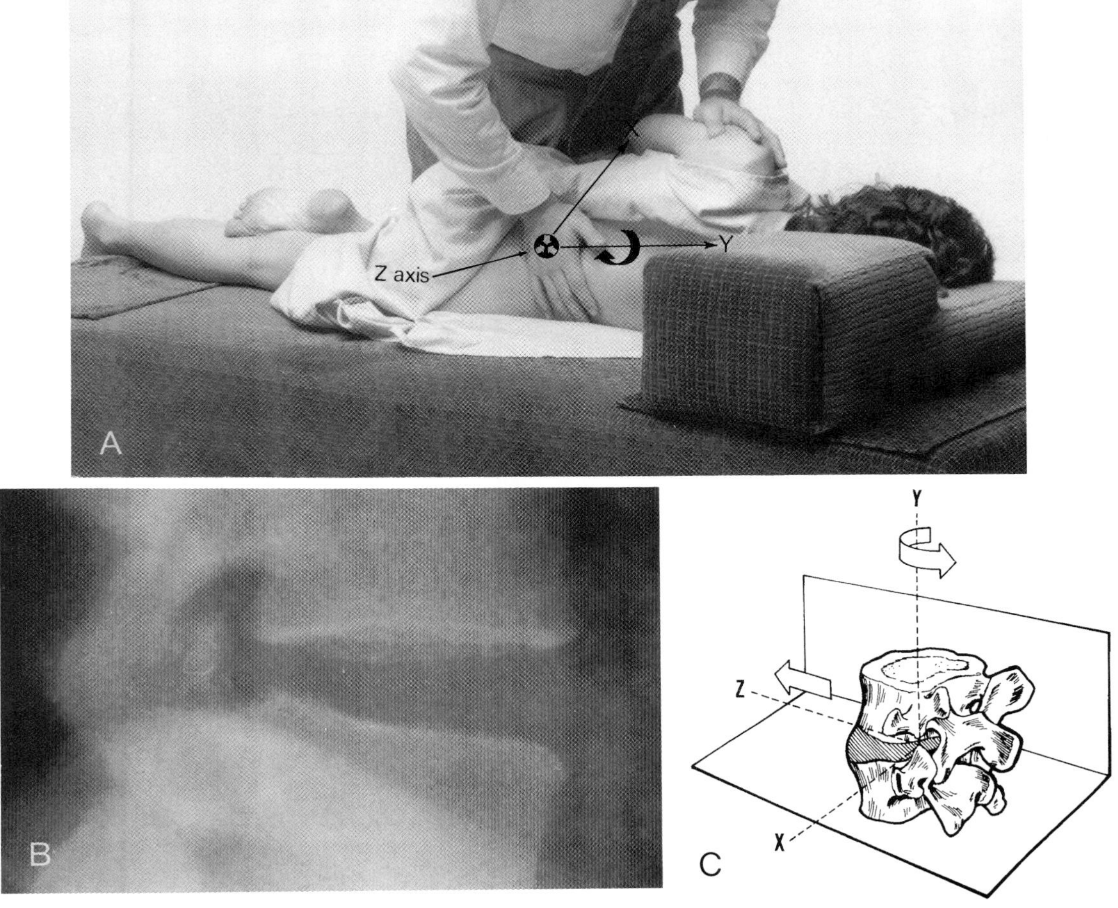

Figure 7.61. **A,** L4 PL side posture adjustment. **B,** Retrolisthesis of L4. **C,** Pattern of thrust for a PL L4.

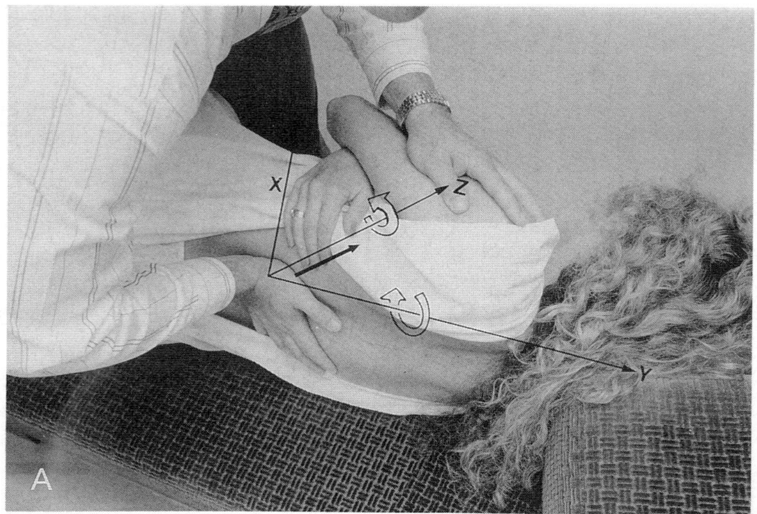

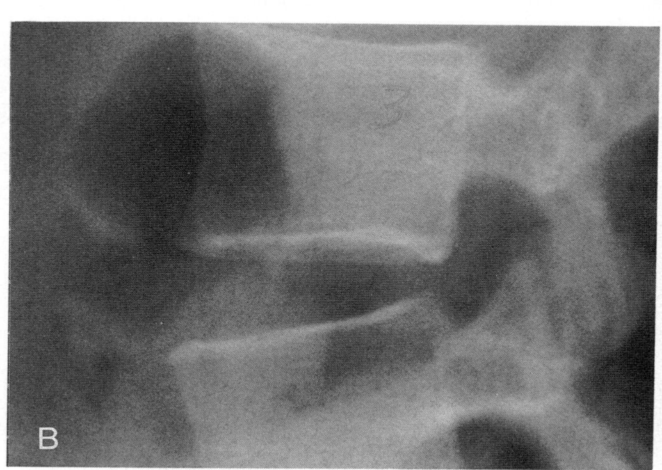

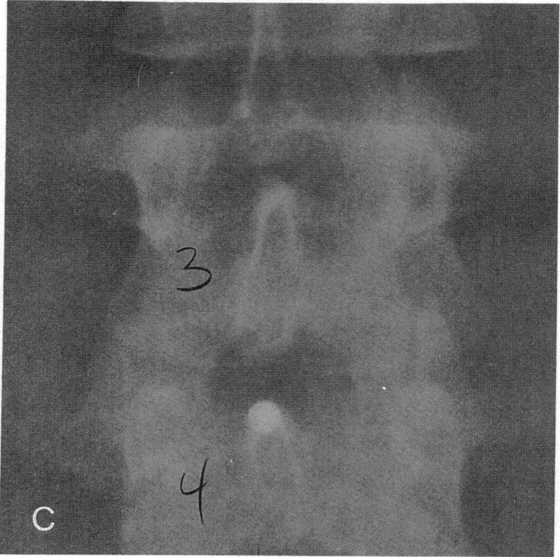

Figure 7.62. **A,** L3 PLS side posture adjustment. **B,** Retrolisthesis of L3. **C,** Left spinous rotation ($-\theta Y$) and slight wedging ($+\theta Z$) of L3.

The patient's shoulder is allowed to roll forward minimizing axial rotation of the spine. The doctor stabilizes the patient's pelvis into the table.

Pattern of thrust: Posterior to anterior ($+Z$) with an inferiorward arcing motion ($+\theta Z$) toward the end of the thrust.

Category by algorithm: Short lever specific contact procedure.

Name of technique: Gonstead

Name of technique procedure: L2 PRI-m ($-Z$, $+\theta Y$, $+\theta Z$) side posture adjustment with pisiform contact (Fig. 7.64).

Indications: Decreased anterior translation ($+Z$) motion of the segment, left lateral bending ($-\theta Z$) and right axial rotation ($-\theta Y$). Retrolisthesis, lateral flexion malposition ($+\theta Z$) and left rotational ($+\theta Y$) positional dyskinesia of L2.

Contraindications: All other listings, normal FSU, hypermobility, instability, destruction or fracture of the neural arch of L2, infection of the contact vertebra.

Patient position: Right side posture position.

Doctor's position: Standing at a 45° angle facing cephalad.

Contact point: Left mamillary process with the right pisiform of the doctor. The fingers do not cross the spine.

Supporting Hand: Contacts the anterolateral left shoulder and axilla region with a slight cephalad distraction.

Set Up: The patient is rolled over towards the doctor with the pisiform contact, thereby moving the L2-L3 articulation from the neutral zone to the elastic zone (maximal preload or "tension"). The patient's shoulder is allowed to roll forward minimizing axial rotation of the spine. The doctor stabilizes the patient's pelvis into the table.

Pattern of thrust: Posterior to anterior (+Z) (along the L2-L3 disc plane) with an inferiorward arcing motion ($-\theta$Z) toward the end of the thrust.

Category by algorithm: Short lever specific contact procedure.

Name of technique: Gonstead

Name of technique procedure: Base posterior side posture adjustment (Fig. 7.65A).

Indications: Retrolisthesis (−Z) of sacral base and/or $+\theta$X positional dyskinesia of L5-S1 (Fig. 7.65B). Decreased extension of the lumbosacral junction.

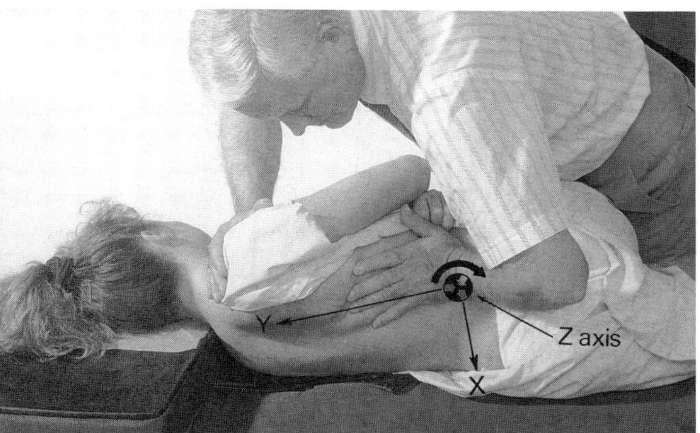

Figure 7.63. L3 PLI-m side posture adjustment.

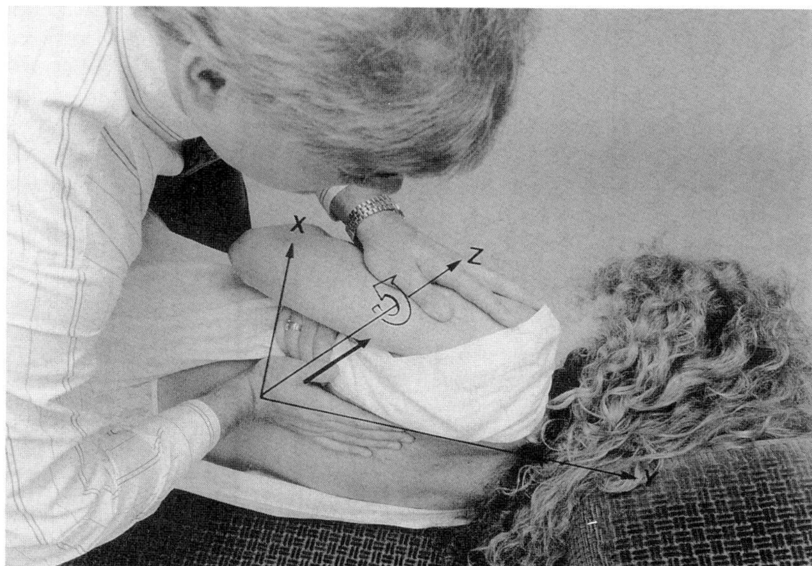

Figure 7.64. L2 PRI-m side posture adjustment.

Contraindications: All other listings, normal FSU, hypermobility, instability, destruction or fracture of the neural arch or S1 tubercle, infection of the contact vertebra.

Patient position: On either the right or left side depending on the doctor's or patient's preference. If a lumbar scoliosis is present, then the convexity of the curve should be placed up.

Doctor's position: Standing at a 45° angle facing cephalad.

Contact point: First sacral tubercle with a soft pisiform contact (i.e., left hand).

Supporting Hand: Contacts the anterolateral right shoulder and axilla region with a slight cephalad distraction.

Set Up: With the patient on the left side the contact hand (L) is placed so that the pisiform is over S1, with the fingers pointing at approximately a 45° angle from the longitudinal axis of the spine. The patient is then rolled over towards the doctor with the pisiform contact thereby moving the S1-L5 articulation into the paraphysiologic, elastic zone. The patient's right shoulder is allowed to roll forward minimizing axial rotation of the spine. The doctor stabilizes the patient's pelvis into the table.

Pattern of thrust: Posterior to anterior (+Z) through the lumbosacral articulation with a cephalad arcing motion ($+\theta$X) toward the end of the thrust.

Category by algorithm: Short lever specific contact procedure.

Name of technique: Gonstead

Name of technique procedure: Side posture L5 spondylolisthesis adjustment (Fig. 7.66A).

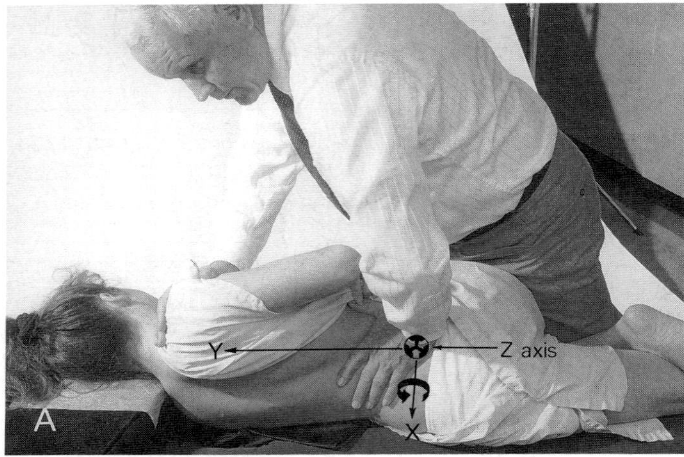

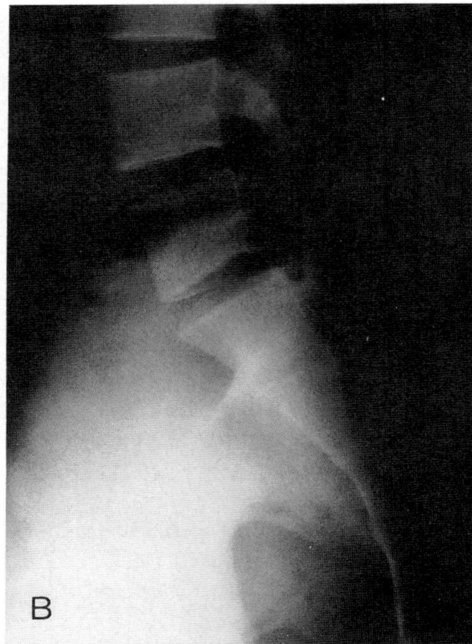

Figure 7.65. A, Base posterior side posture adjustment. **B,** A base posterior sacrum.

Figure 7.66. A, L5 spondylolisthesis side posture adjustment. Contact is made on the S2 tubercle. **B,** Spondylolisthesis of L5.

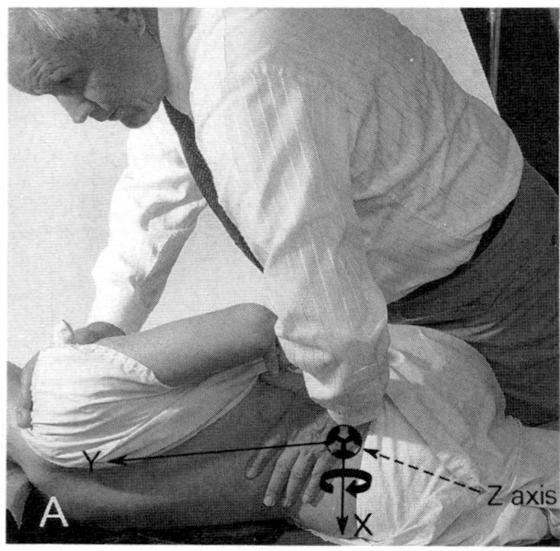

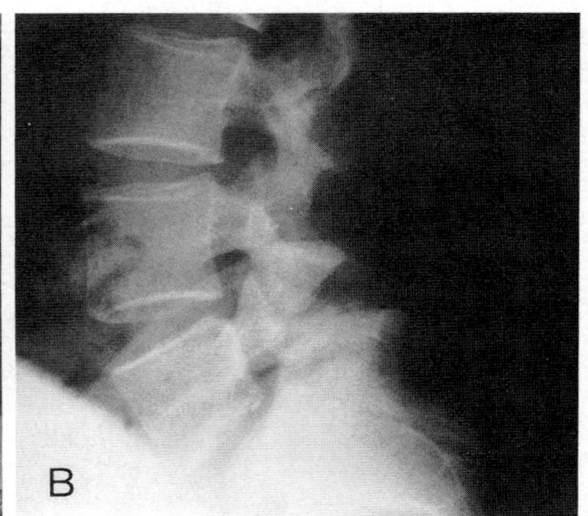

Indications: L5 spondylolisthesis (Fig. 7.66B) (Grade one or two) with decreased anterior translation of the sacral base during motion analysis. Grade three and four spondylolistheses are usually adjusted in the prone position.

Contraindications: All other listings, normal FSU, hypermobility, instability, destruction or fracture or infection of the sacrum.

Patient position: On either the right or left side depending on the doctor or patient preference. If a lumbar scoliosis is present, then the convexity of the curve should be placed up.

Doctor's position: Standing at a 45° angle facing cephalad.

Contact point: S2 tubercle with a pisiform contact.

Supporting Hand: Contacts the anterolateral portion of the shoulder and axilla region with a slight cephalad distraction.

Pattern of thrust: Posterior to anterior (+Z) followed by an inferiorward arcing motion ($-\theta X$).

Category by algorithm: Short lever specific contact procedure.

KNEE-CHEST TABLE

The knee-chest table was developed in the early 1900's to facilitate adjustments of the spinal column (121) (Fig. 7.67). Originally used with upper cervical technique, Gonstead modified both the table, and the thrusting action; a set-hold procedure (56). The table gets its name from the position the patient assumes when on the table (Fig. 7.68). The face and chest are supported by a head or chest piece and the lower trunk is left unsupported. The patient's knees rest on the base of the table. The chest piece or knee position can be adjusted so that the patient obtains a comfortable position with the spine relatively level from front to back. The segment being adjusted should be at the highest point on the spine, if possible.

General Indications

Patients beyond the first trimester of pregnancy may find it difficult to assume a prone position because of the protuberant abdomen (121). Because most thoracic adjustive procedures involve translatory thrusts along the Z axis (posterior to anterior), the pressure on the fetus may be harmful or cause anxiety in the patient. It is for these reasons that the table is especially suited for the gravid patient (See Chapter 14).

The knee-chest table provides a mechanical advantage to the doctor when adjusting the thoracic and lumbar spines. The knee-chest position lessens the amount of work by the doctor, which becomes critically important in the large or obese patient. In the typical side posture position for lumbar adjustments, the doctor must use coordination and strength to position the patient correctly and keeping them stable during and after the thrust. As much as possible, the patient should be asked to move into the appropriate position.

The advantage of the knee-chest table for adjustments of the thoracic spine and lumbar spine is accomplished through the torso being allowed to move freely in an anteriorward direction during the thrust. This is not so

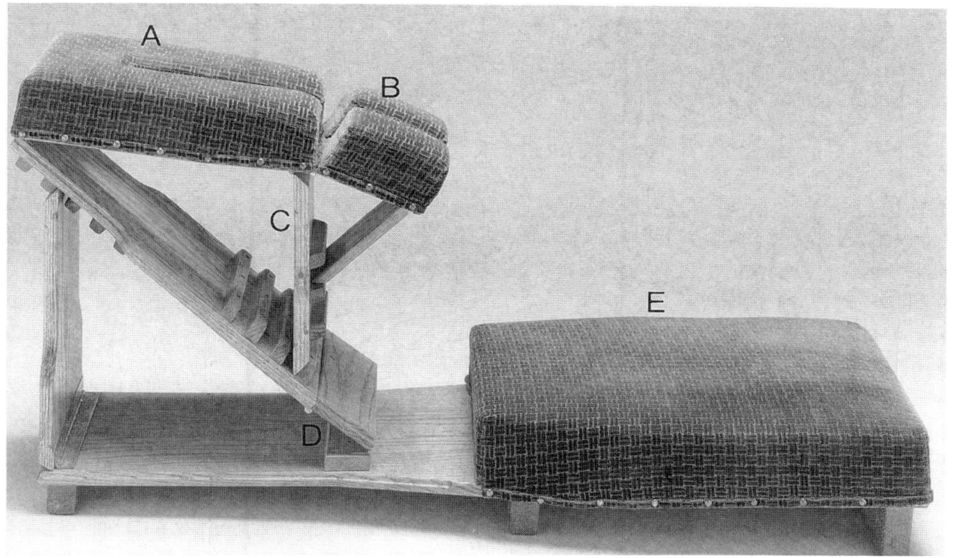

Figure 7.67. **A,** Knee-chest table. **A,** Face section. **B,** Chest piece. **C,** Adjustable pillar. **D,** Small adult-child adjustment portion. **E,** Knee section.

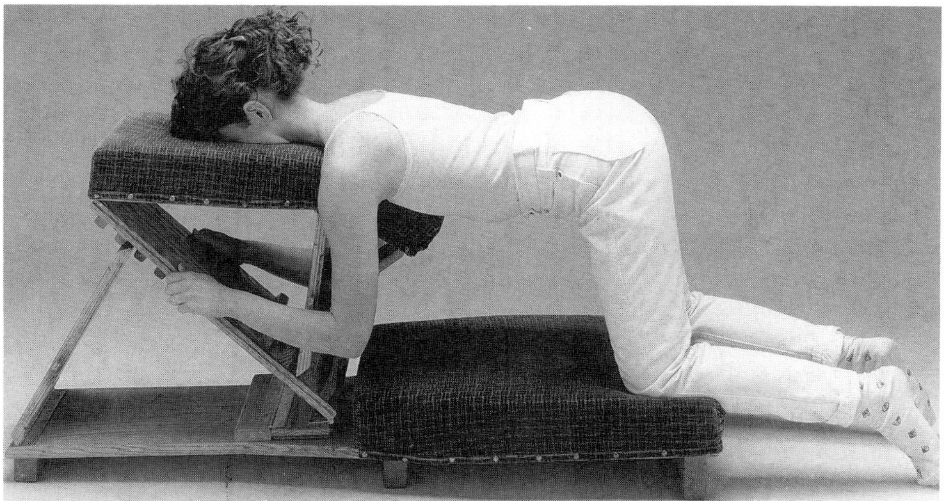

Figure 7.68. Patient position on the knee-chest table. The small adult configuration is presented.

when a normal flat table is used for the prone adjusting position. In the latter, the rib cage and torso provide increased stiffness to the anteriorward thrust, thereby necessitating a proportional increase in the amount of force. The magnitude of force is much less in nearly all knee-chest adjustments, compared to side posture. Because less force is needed to accomplish the adjustment, from the lack of resistance offered by the unrestrained torso, the table is well equipped to handle those patients sensitive to high force techniques, such as the geriatric with osteoporosis.

The table can be used for adjustments to all vertebral segments. The table is rarely used for adjustments to the sacroiliac articulations (See Chapter 6). Clinical experience has been that the more flexible and shallow the sagittal curvatures are, the more easily the patient is adjusted in the knee-chest position (85). Conversely, the hyperkyphotic patient may be more easily adjusted on a typical flat or contoured table with support for the torso.

Adjustive Thrust

Because the mechanical advantage of the doctor is increased when the patient is in the knee-chest position, great care must be taken when the actual thrust is given (121). The patient should be completely relaxed and not supporting the chest with the upper extremities. The doctor guides the patient towards maximal +Z "tension," allowing the abdominal and pelvic area to protrude towards the knee-piece. "Tension" can be described as a preload of the motion segment which brings the articulations to the end of their physiologic range of motion, before the paraphysiologic zone. In this position, the bodies of the lumbar vertebrae are separated at the anterior, allowing for eased +Z translational movement of the segment. The thoracic spine is translated anteriorly, similar to the lumbar spine, though less +Z translation is permissible because of the stiffness of the kyphosis to compression.

Preload is applied to the spine by contacting the appropriate short lever arm (spinous, mamillary, transverse, or the cervical lamina) and translating the joint involved along the +Z axis to the limit of its physiologic range. The transverse process of L5 can be used as a contact point if it is large. Care must be taken to translate the segment by taking into account the plane lines of the bodies of the vertebrae and the orientation of the articular facets. The arcing motion of the thrust through the center of mass of the vertebra is described in Figure 7.69. Directing the thrust normally to the spinal sagittal curves while minimizing vectors that create flexion or extension moments of the segment lessens the amount of longitudinal force encountered by the adjacent motion segments (121,122).

Once the joint has been brought to maximal preload, a high velocity and short amplitude thrust is administered. At the end of the thrust (i.e., at maximal translation), the segment is held for one to two seconds, followed by a gradual "backing off" of the pressure (Fig. 7.70). The toggle-recoil thrust is markedly different (See Chapter 2). The careful holding after the thrust reduces any "whiplash" effect the spine would otherwise undergo. Failure to use this specific type of thrusting action is perhaps the major misuse of the table (121). The thrust is given during maximal expiration, or between respirations, when the patient is completely relaxed.

Besides purely Z axis translatory movements, variation in contact points and the use of thrusting vectors that create motions in either the frontal (X-Y) or horizontal planes (X-Z), make the table useful for a variety of positional or dysfunctional configurations or movements of the segment (121).

Lumbar Adjustments

The chest support section should be positioned so that the patient's thoracic spine is level with, or slightly lower than, the lumbar spine (121). The knees are placed in a position such that the femurs are approximately 5 to 10° off vertical with the acute angle at the anterior. The doctor, facing the side of the patient, then places the most

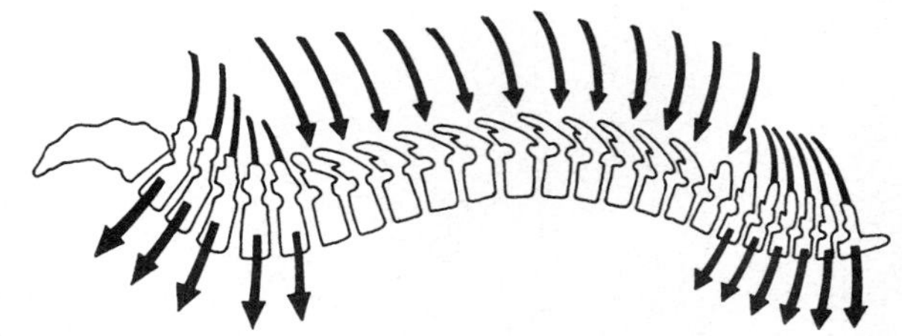

Figure 7.69. Major pattern of thrust for the spinal segments with the patient in the knee-chest position. Modified from Dr. Craig Ripley. Plaugher G, Lopes MA. The knee-chest table: indications and contraindications. Chiropractic Technique 1990;2: 164.

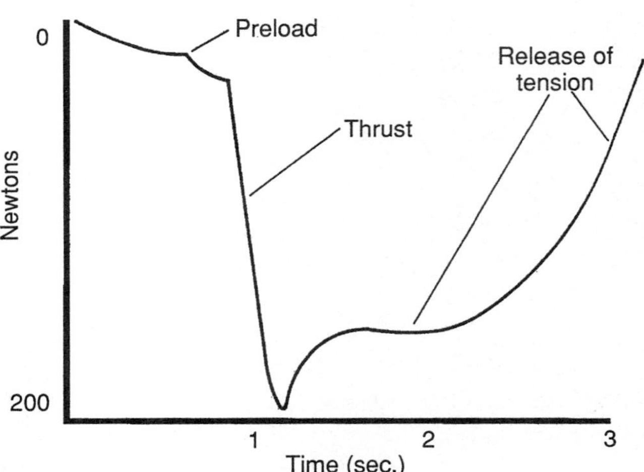

Figure 7.70. Set-hold adjustive force pattern.

30. Gordon SJ, Yang KH, Mayer PJ, et al. Mechanism of disc rupture: a preliminary report. Spine 1991;16:450–456.
31. Hutton WC. The forces acting on a lumbar intervertebral joint. J Manual Medicine 1990;5:66–67.
32. Klein JA, Hukins DWL. Relocation of the bending axis during flexion-extension of lumbar intervertebral discs and its implications for prolapse. Spine 1983;8:659–664.
33. Adams MA, Hutton WC. Prolapsed intervertebral disc: a hyperflexion injury. Spine 1982;7:184.
34. Cailliet R. Low back pain syndrome, 3rd ed. Philadelphia: FA Davis Co., 1981.
35. Farfan HF, Cossette JW, Robertson GH, Wells RV. The instantaneous center of rotation of the third lumbar intervertebral joint. J Biomech 1971;4:149.
36. Adams MA, Hutton WC. The relevance of torsion to the mechanical derangement of the lumbar spine. Spine 1981;6:241.
37. Kirkaldy-Willis WH. The site and nature of the lesion. In: Kirkaldy-Willis WH, ed. Managing low back pain. New York: Churchill Livingstone, 1983.
38. Cox JM. Low back pain syndrome, 4th ed. Baltimore: Williams & Wilkins, 1985.
39. Smith AD. Posterior displacement of the fifth lumbar vertebrae. J Bone Joint Surg 1934;16A:877–888.
40. Cailliet R. Neck and arm pain, 3rd. ed. Philadelphia: FA Davis Co., 1981.
41. Voutsinas SA, MacEwen GE. Sagittal profiles of the spine. Clin Orthop 1986;210:235–242.
42. Rydevik BL, Myers RR, Powell HC. Pressure increase in the dorsal root ganglion following mechanical compression: closed compartment syndrome in nerve roots. Spine 1989;14:574–576.
43. Mensor MC, Duvall G. Absence of motion at the fourth and fifth lumbar interspaces in patients with and without low-back pain. J Bone Joint Surg 1958;41A:1047–1054.
44. Rahlman J. The mechanism of intervertebral joint fixation. J Manipulative Physiol Ther 1987;10:177–187.
45. Akeson WH, Amiel D, Woo SL-Y. Immobility effects on synovial joints: the pathomechanics of joint contracture. Biorheology 1980;17:95–110.
46. Mellin G. Decreased joint and spinal mobility associated with low back pain in young adults. J Spinal Disorders 1990;3:238–243.
47. Stokes IAF, Counts DF, Frymoyer JW. Experimental instability in the rabbit lumbar spine. Spine 1989;14:68–72.
48. Pearcy M, Portek I, Shepherd J. The effect of low-back pain on lumbar spinal movements measured by three-dimensional x-ray analysis. Spine 1985;10:150–153.
49. Carrick FR. Treatment of pathomechanics of the lumbar spine by manipulation. J Manipulative Physiol Ther 1981;4:173–178.
50. Bronfort G, Jochumsen OH. The functional radiographic examination of patients with low-back pain: a study of different forms of variations. J Manipulative Physiol Ther 1984;7:89–97.
51. Speiser RM, Aragona RJ, Heffernan JP. The application of therapeutic exercises based upon lateral flexion roentgenography to restore biomechanical function in the lumbar spine. Chiro Res J 1990;1(4):7–16.
52. Paajanen H, Erkintalo M, Kuusela T, Dahlstrom S, Kormano M. Magnetic resonance study of disc degeneration in young low-back pain patients. Spine 1989;14:982–985.
53. Schiebler ML, Camerino VJ, Fallon MD, et al. In vivo and ex vivo magnetic resonance imaging evaluation of early disc degeneration with histopathologic correlation. Spine 1991;16:635–640.
54. Tertti M, Paajanen H, Laato M, et al. Disc degeneration in magnetic resonance imaging: a comparative biochemical, histologic, and radiologic study in cadaver spines. Spine 1991;16:629–634.
55. Kirkaldy-Willis WH, Wedge JH, Yong-Hing K, Reilly J. Pathology and pathogenesis of lumbar spondylosis and stenosis. Spine 1978;3:319–328.
56. Herbst RW. Gonstead chiropractic science and art. Chicago: Sci-Chi Publications, 1968.
57. Farfan HF, Gracovetsky S. The nature of instability. Spine 1984;9:714–719.
58. Dupuis PR, Yong-Hing K, Cassidy JD, Kirkaldy-Willis WH. Radiologic diagnosis of degenerative lumbar spinal instability. Spine 1985;10:262–276.
59. Hayes MA, Howard TC, Gruel CR, Kopta JA. Roentgenographic evaluation of lumbar spine flexion-extension in asymptomatic individuals. Spine 1989;14:327–331.
60. Kalebo P, Kadziolka R, Sward L. Compression-traction radiography of lumbar segmental instability. Spine 1990;15:351–355.
61. Weiler PJ, King GJ, Gertzbein SD. Analysis of sagittal plane instability of the lumbar spine in vivo. Spine 1990;15:1299–1306.
62. Goobar JE, Pate D, Resnick D, Sartoris DJ. Radiography of the hyperextended lumbar spine: an effective technique for the demonstration of discal vacuum phenomena. J Can Assoc Radiol 1987;38:271–74.
63. Kirkaldy–Willis WH. Managing low back pain. New York: Churchill Livingstone, 1983.
64. Hubka MJ. Another critical look at the subluxation hypothesis. Chiropractic Technique 1990;2:27–29.
65. Frymoyer JW, Selby DK. Segmental instability: rationale for treatment. Spine 1985;10:280–286.
66. Lehmann TR, Spratt KF, Tozzi JE, et al. Long-term follow-up of lower lumbar fusion patients. Spine 1987;12:97–104.
67. Lopes MA, Plaugher G, Ray S. Closed reduction of lumbar retrolisthesis: a report of two cases. Proceedings of the 1991 International Conference on Spinal Manipulation. Washington DC: Foundation for Chiropractic Education and Research, 1991:110–114.
68. Porter RW, Miller CG. Back pain and trunk list. Spine 1986; 11:596–600.
69. Cyron BM, Hutton WC. Variations in the amount and distribution of cortical bone across the partes interarticularis of L5. A predisposing factor in spondylolysis? Spine 1979;4:163–167.
70. During J, Goudfrooij H, Keessen W, Beeker THW, Crowe A. Toward standards for posture. Postural characteristics of the lower back system in normal and pathologic conditions. Spine 1985;10:83–87.
71. Gracovetsky S. The spinal engine. Wien: Springer-Verlag, 1988.
72. Pearcy M, Shepherd J. Is there instability in spondylolisthesis? Spine 1985;10:175–177.
73. Penning L, Blickman JR. Instability in lumbar spondylolisthesis: a radiologic study of several concepts. Am J Radiol 1980;134:293.
74. Friberg O. Lumbar instability: a dynamic approach by traction-compression radiography. Spine 1987;12:119–129.
75. Mierau D, Cassidy JD, McGregor M, Kirkaldy-Willis WH. A comparison of the effectiveness of spinal manipulative therapy for low back pain patients with and without spondylolisthesis. J Manipulative Physiol Ther 1987;10:49–55.
76. Ciric I, Mikhael MA, Tarkington JA, Vick NA. The lateral recess syndrome: a variant of spinal stenosis. J Neurosurg 1980;53:433–443.
77. Porter RW, Hibbert C, Evans C. The natural history of root entrapment syndrome. Spine 1984;9:418–421.
78. Kirkaldy-Willis WH. Managing low back pain. 2nd ed. New York: Churchill Livingstone, 1988.
79. Ben-Eliyahu DJ, Rutili MM, Przybysz JA. Lateral recess syndrome: diagnosis and chiropractic management. J Manipulative Physiol Ther 1983;6:25–31.
80. Mior SA, Cassidy JD. Lateral nerve root entrapment: pathological, clinical, and manipulative considerations. J Can Chiro Assoc 1982;26:13–20.
81. Dailey EJ, Buehler MT. Plain film assessment of spinal stenosis: method comparison with lumbar CT. J Manipulative Physiol Ther 1989;12:192–199.

82. Johnsson K-E, Uden A, Rosen I. The effect of decompression on the natural course of spinal stenosis: a comparison of surgically treated and untreated patients. Spine 1991;16:615–619.
83. Bogduk N. A reappraisal of the anatomy of the human lumbar erector spinae. J Anat 1980;131:525–540.
84. Kortelainen P, Puranen J, Koivisto E, Lahde S. Symptoms and signs of sciatica and their relation to the localization of the lumbar disc herniation. Spine 1985;10:88–92.
85. Lecture notes. Gonstead Seminar of Chiropractic. Mt. Horeb, WI, 1990.
86. Cyriax J. Textbook of orthopaedic medicine. Vol 2. 8th ed. London: Bailliere Tindall, 1974.
87. Barrale R, Diamond R, Filson RM, Wittmer M. Manipulative management of lumbar disc bulge. Chiropractic Technique 1989;1:79–87.
88. Tich'y J, Mojzisova L, Horak J. Sternocostal joints, low back pain and lumbar discopathy. Czechoslovakian Medicine 1988;11:205–216.
89. Evans W, Jobe W, Seibert C. A cross-sectional prevalence study of lumbar disc degeneration in a working population. Spine 1989;14:60–64.
90. Ponte DJ, Jensen GJ, Gent BE. A preliminary report on the use of the McKenzie protocol versus Williams protocol in the treatment of low back pain. J Orthop Sports Physical Ther 1984;Oct:130–139.
91. Schnebel BE, Watkins RG, Dillin W. The role of spinal flexion and extension in changing nerve root compression in disc herniations. Spine 1989;14:835–837.
92. Brieg A. Adverse mechanical tension in the central nervous system. Stockholm: Almqvist & Wiksell International, 1978.
93. White AH, Von Rogov P, Zucherman J, Heiden D. Lumbar laminectomy for herniated disc: a prospective controlled comparison with internal fixation fusion. Spine 1987;12:305–307.
94. Waagen GN, Haldeman S, Cook G, Lopez D, DeBoer KF. Short term trial of chiropractic adjustments for the relief of chronic low back pain. Manual Medicine 1986;2:63–67.
95. Meade TW, Dyer S, Browne W, Townsend J, Frank AO. Low back pain of mechanical origin: randomised comparison of chiropractic and hospital outpatient treatment. Br Med J 1990;300:1431–1437.
96. Butler D, Trafimow JH, Andersson GBJ, McNeil TW, Hockman MS. Discs degenerate before facets. Spine 1990;15:111–13.
97. Shealy CN. Facet denervation in the management of back and sciatic pain. Clin Orthop 1976;115:157–64.
98. Hourigan CL, Bassett JM. Facet syndrome: clinical signs, symptoms, diagnosis, and treatment. J Manipulative Physiol Ther 1989;12:293–297.
99. Banks SD. Lumbar facet syndrome: spinographic assessment of treatment by spinal manipulative therapy. J Manipulative Physiol Ther 1983;6:175–180.
100. Deyo RA, Bass JE. Lifestyle and low-back pain: The influence of smoking and obesity. Spine 1989;14:501–506.
101. Videman T, Rauhala H, Asp S, et al. Patient-handling skill, back injuries, and back pain: an intervention study in nursing. Spine 1989;14:148–156.
102. Bendix A, Jensen CV, Bendix T. Posture, acceptability and energy consumption on a tiltable and a knee-support chair. Clinical Biomechanics 1988;3:66–73.
103. Mayer TG, Smith SS, Keeley J, Mooney V. Quantification of lumbar function. Part 2: sagittal plane strength in chronic low-back pain patients. Spine 1985;10:765–772.
104. Oland G, Tveiten G. A trial of modern rehabilitation for chronic low-back pain and disability: vocational outcome and effect of pain modulation. Spine 1991;16:457–459.
105. Harstad H, Alvsaker K, Nessioy I. Effect of training and treatment at Rauland Rehabilitation Center. Tidsskr Nor Laegeforen 1989;109:212–215.
106. Donchin M, Woolf O, Kaplan L, Floman Y. Secondary prevention of low-back pain: a clinical trial. Spine 1990;15:1317–1320.
107. Stankovic R, Johnell O. Conservative treatment of acute low back pain. A prospective randomized trial: McKenzie method of treatment versus patient education in "mini back school." Spine 1990;15:120–123.
108. McKenzie RA. The lumbar spine: mechanical diagnosis and therapy. Waikanae, New Zealand: Spinal Publication, 1981.
109. Vernon LF, Peacock JR, Esposito AP. Abdominal aortic aneurysms presenting as low back pain: a report of two cases. J Manipulative Physiol Ther 1986;9:47–50.
110. Hopkins NFG. Abdominal aortic aneurysms. Br Med J 1987;294:790–91.
111. Wedge JH, Tchang S. Differential diagnosis of low back pain. In: Kirkaldy-Willis WH, ed. Managing low back pain. 2nd ed. New York: Churchill-Livingstone, 1988:229–243.
112. Keating JC. Interexaminer reliability of motion palpation of the lumbar spine: a review of quantitative literature. Am J Chiro Med 1989;2:107–110.
113. Pochaczevsky R, Wexler CE, Meyers PH, Epstein JA, Marc JA. Liquid crystal thermography of the spine and extremities. J Neurosurg 1982;56:386–395.
114. Pochaczevsky R. Thermography in posttraumatic pain. Am J Sports Med 1987;15:243–250.
115. Plaugher G. Skin temperature assessment for neuromusculoskeletal abnormalities of the spinal column: a review of the literature. J Manipulative Physiol Ther 1992;(July/Aug).
116. Plaugher G, Lopes MA, Melch PE, Cremata EE. The inter- and intraexaminer reliability of a paraspinal skin temperature differential instrument. J Manipulative Physiol Ther 1991;14:361–367.
117. Van Schaik JPJ, Verbiest H, Van Schaik FDJ. Isolated spinous process deviation a pitfall in the interpretation of AP radiographs of the lumbar spine. Spine 1989;14:970.
118. Gerow G. Osseous configurations of the axial skeleton: specific application to spatial relationships of vertebrae. J Manipulative Physiol Ther 1984;7:33–38.
119. Cremata EE, Plaugher G, Cox WA. Technique system application: the Gonstead approach. Chiropractic Tech 1991;3:19–25.
120. Leach RA. An evaluation of the effect of chiropractic manipulative therapy on hypolordosis of the cervical spine. J Manipulative Physiol Ther 1983;6:17–24.
121. Plaugher G, Lopes MA. The knee chest table: indications and contraindications. Chiropractic Technique 1990;2:163–167.
122. Lee M. Mechanics of spinal joint manipulation in the thoracic and lumbar spine: a theoretical study of posteroanterior force techniques. Clin Biomech 1989;4:249–251.
123. Haney PL, Mootz RD. A case report on nonresolving conservative care of low back pain and sciatic radicular syndrome. J Manipulative Physiol Ther 1985;8:109–114.
124. Grieve GP. Common vertebral joint problems. New York: Churchill Livingstone, 1981:91.
125. Mathews JA, Yates DAH. Reduction of lumbar disc prolapse by manipulation. Br Med J 1969;20:696–697.

8 Thoracic Spine

STEVEN S. TANAKA and GREGORY PLAUGHER

On Sept. 18, 1895, Harvey Lillard called upon me. He was so deaf for seventeen years that he could not hear the noises on the street. Mr. Lillard informed me that he was in a cramped position and felt something give in his back. I replaced the displaced 4th dorsal vertebra by one move, which restored his hearing fully.

DR. D.D. PALMER

The Science, Art, and Philosophy of Chiropractic

1910

The intricate complexity of the thoracic spine is best illustrated by considering its intimate connection with the rib cage, its proximity and neurologic connections with the viscera of the thorax and abdomen, and its influence on the cervical and lumbar spine. This interconnection makes possible a wide range of diverse interactions. Although widespread disability exists for cervical and lumbar spine disorders, the thoracic spine is conspicuously absent from the picture. If pain is not a major disability factor for the patient, wherein lies the putative morbidity? This question can best be answered by analyzing the mechanical traumas that do affect the region. From this perspective, one can appreciate how and where disease occurs.

Degenerative joint disease is relatively common in the thoracic spine. Circumferential tears of the annulus are an early occurrence in the degeneration process. At a later date, fissures develop, radiating from the nucleus outward, primarily at the posterolateral angles. Radial fissures occur most frequently in the thoracic spine (1).

Degenerative joint disease at the central joint leads to anterior disc thinning. This is possibly due to the increased compressive loads that are encountered here. Subchondral bone and end-plate sclerosis signify that normal disc nutrition has been interrupted. Stabilization processes, such as anterior osteophyte formation, occur later in the course of the disease. These anterior osteophytes can compress the sympathetic trunks, which are in close proximity (2).

For optimal health of the region, it is necessary to prevent or minimize degeneration. Normal joint movement is likely to limit the degenerative processes of the joint (3). Magnetic resonance imaging (MRI) is useful in identifying early changes in the disc (4). Whether or not chiropractic care can facilitate normal joint function early in the course of the disease largely determines the extent to which future morbidity can be influenced (See Chapter 13).

CLINICAL ANATOMY AND BIOMECHANICS

Osseous Structures

The thoracic spine is usually formed by 12 vertebrae (See Anomalies). The middle thoracics are considered the typical thoracic vertebrae. They have deeply imbricated spinous processes (Fig. 8.1A-B), coronally oriented facets (Fig. 8.2), hemifacets for the costovertebral articulations on the superior and inferior aspects of the lateral vertebral bodies, and vertebral bodies equal in anteroposterior and transverse diameters (5). There are also articular surfaces on the transverse processes that form the vertebral surface of the costotransverse joints.

The upper thoracic vertebrae, especially T1, are cervical-like, while the lower thoracic tend to resemble the lumbar spine. The thoraco-lumbar junction (i.e., T10-L1) has mortice-like zygapophyseal joints (6). This arrangement markedly restricts axial rotation and extension. When adjusting this area, it is important to not hyperextend the segment. Instead, the vertebra should be moved forward through the center of mass of the segment. Forces that cause extension or flexion of the motion segment will

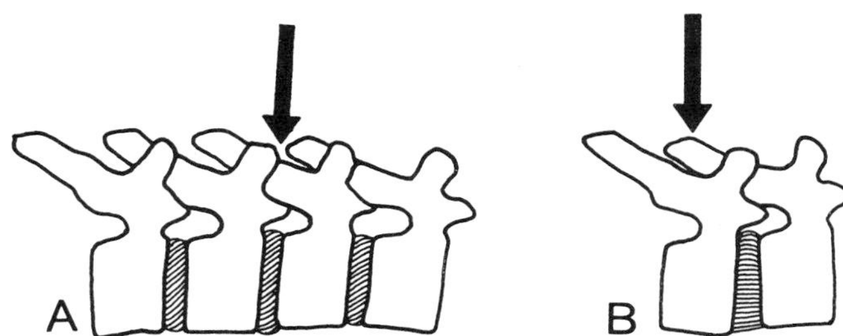

Figure 8.1. **A,** Imbrication of the middle thoracic vertebrae. If a spinous contact is used for the adjustment, the force should be directed just caudal to the superior vertebra. **B,** Inappropriate contact point. If the force is directed near the tip of the spinous, then hyperextension of the segment will occur. The subjacent vertebra may be moved as well.

create the most movement at adjacent levels (7). Figure 8.3 demonstrates the primary pattern of thrust for thoracic motion segments.

Ligamentous Structures

The thoracic spine has ligaments that are typical of the spine in general. The anterior longitudinal ligament tends to be narrower than in the cervical spine. The interspinous and capsular ligaments are also thinner and looser than in the cervical spine. The posterior longitudinal ligament is broad and uniform in the upper thoracic spine. In the lower thoracic spine it is denticulated, narrow over the vertebral bodies, and broad over the intervertebral disc (8).

The intervertebral disc has a much less developed nucleus in comparison with the cervical and lumbar spine (8). The disc's ability to swell is somewhat reduced in the thoracic spine (9). The disc is avascular, and its nutritional requirements rely on imbibition through the semipermeable end-plates from avascular buds between the spongiosa and the end-plates. Movement is required for this flow of nutrients, and the disc deteriorates with its loss (3). The thoracic disc height is smaller in relation to the vertebral body thickness, when compared to other regions of the spine. Support is also provided by the costovertebral and costotransverse ligaments. The end-plates of the normal disc are relatively parallel. A kyphosis is achieved through the wedge-like shape of the vertebral bodies (8).

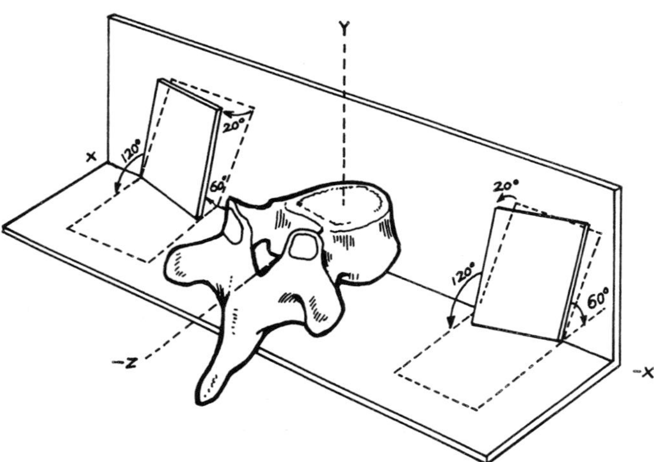

Figure 8.2. The orientation of the articular facets of a low thoracic (T9) vertebra.

Costovertebral Joint

The typical costovertebral joint is a pair of demifacets on adjacent vertebral bodies at the lateral margins, which articulate with the convex rib head in a synovial joint. There is capsular attachment to the annulus of the disc and the posterior longitudinal ligament. The intermediate interarticular ligament subdivides the joint and attaches the rib head to the facets. There are also ligaments attaching the rib head to the adjacent vertebral bodies (8,10) (Fig. 8.4).

Costotransverse Joint

The posterior tubercle of the rib neck articulates with a facet on the transverse process in a synovial joint. These joints are absent in the lower two or three ribs. The costovertebral and costotransverse joints allow rotation around an axis formed by the two articulations (10,11).

Clinical observations suggest that subluxation of the ribs is relatively rare, compared to the incidence of vertebral dysfunction (i.e., three-joint complex). Axial rotation of the motion segment can often create pain along the posterior rib margin. Intercostal neuritis is more likely due to irritation near the nerve root than entrapment elsewhere.

Subluxation of the rib at the anterior can occur when there is moderate rotation of the thoracic spine (e.g., scoliosis). These subluxations can be reduced from the anterior (See Chapter 16), but if the spine is not derotated, reoccurrence is likely. Traumatic blows to the thorax can also subluxate the anterior ribs. These injuries reduce quickly with an adjustment, provided that there is not severe ligamentous laxity and that the adjustment quickly follows the trauma. The rib usually fractures before severe trauma occurs at the costotransverse or costovertebral joints.

Figure 8.3. The primary pattern of thrust for the spine in the prone position.

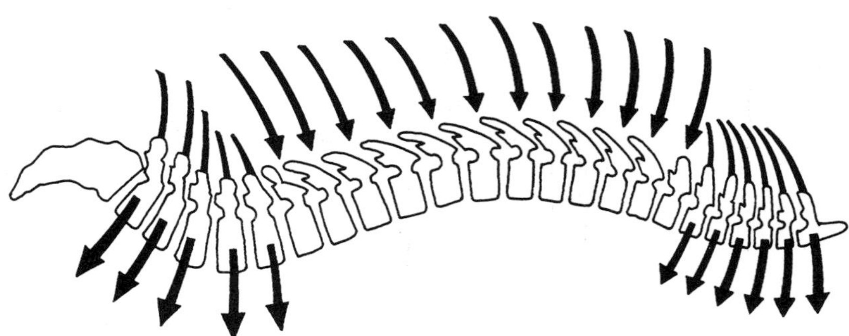

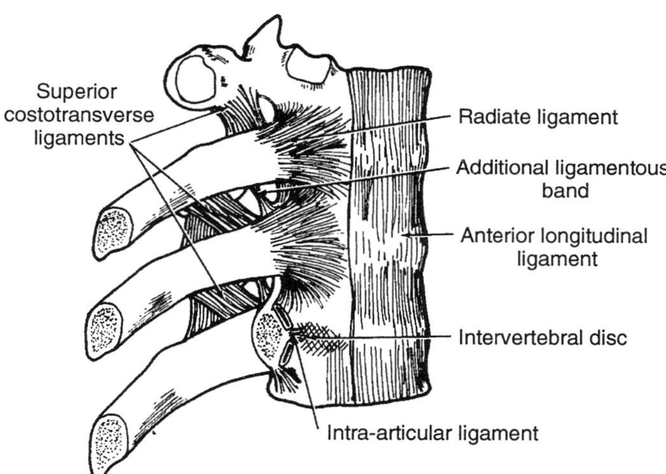

Figure 8.4. The right anterolateral aspect of the costovertebral articulations. At the lowest joint shown, most of the radiate ligament and the anterior portion of the head of the rib have been excised to demonstrate the two joint cavities and the intraarticular ligament between them. Modified from Williams PL, Warwick R. Gray's anatomy. 36th British ed. Philadelphia: W.B. Saunders Co., 1980:450.

Nervous System

SPINAL CORD

The cervical cord enlargement continues down to the T2 segmental level, and the lumbar cord enlargement is between the T9 and T12 segments (12). The epidural space between the spinal cord and the margins of the thoracic neural canal is relatively narrow (13). Dislocation, subluxation, and fracture into the spinal canal can cause cord injury. In the pediatric, gross cord and nerve root injury can occur with only relatively slight radiographic alterations (14–16)

Blood Supply. The cord is supplied by the anterior and posterior spinal arteries. The "Arteria Radicularis Magna" or "Artery of Adamowicz" is located in the lower thoracic spine and supplies the lower two-thirds of the spinal cord. The intercostal arteries send branches to the vertebral body and spinal muscles. Branches also enter through the intervertebral foramen and supply the posterior vertebral body, nerve root, dura mater, vertebral arch, and extradural contents of the canal (10). The narrowest part of the thoracic canal from T4 to T9 is also the area of poorest blood supply (3). Brieg (17) has shown how tension in the spinal cord will lead to decreased blood flow to the cord tissue. Hyperflexion of the spinal canal, or adhesions in the area may lead to tension in the meninges and spinal cord (17).

NERVE ROOTS

There are 12 pairs of thoracic nerve roots which course through the intervertebral foraminae formed by the same numerical vertebra and its subjacent neighbor. The nerve root divides into the anterior and posterior primary divisions, the sinuvertebral or recurrent meningeal nerve, and the white and gray communicating nerves that join the sympathetic trunk. The posterior primary division of the nerve root has medial and lateral branches. The medial branch innervates short medial back muscles and the skin of the back as far as the midscapular line. Lateral branches innervate the sacrospinalis muscles. The lateral branches of the lower six thoracic nerve roots send sensory branches to the skin of the lower lateral back, and the T12 lateral branches send fibers along the iliac crest descending to the skin of the front part of the gluteal region. Some filaments reach as low as the greater trochanter of the femur (8,12).

The anterior primary division of the nerve root becomes the intercostal nerve with the exception of T12 which becomes the subcostal nerve (8,12). Anterior branches of the anterior primary division supply the intercostal muscles, parietal pleura, and the skin over the anterior thorax and abdomen (12).

The major portion of the T1 nerve root and portions of T2 and T3 enter the brachial plexus (12). They have sensory branches that innervate the axillae and the medial side of the arm and forearm. Lesions in this area can cause symptoms characteristic of thoracic outlet syndrome.

The T12 nerve root enters the lumbar plexus and becomes the iliohypogastric nerve (12). A lateral branch innervates the upper lateral thigh and an anterior branch descends anteriorly to the symphysis pubis. Pain in either of these areas can result from nerve irritation at the spinal level. The lower three to four thoracic nerve roots send branches to the periphery of the diaphragm and the serratus posterior inferior muscle (12).

The recurrent meningeal or sinuvertebral nerve is formed by the ventral ramus and a root from the gray ramus communicans and reenters the intervertebral foramen to innervate the dura, epidural and posterior vertebral body vascular structures, posterior superficial layers of the annulus fibrosis, epidural fat and the posterior longitudinal ligament (18–20).

The gray communicans connects the sympathetic trunk to the ventral rami. Branches from it also innervate the lateral portion of the intervertebral disc (19,20).

SYMPATHETIC NERVOUS SYSTEM

Traditionally, preganglionic cell bodies from the lateral columns were thought to be confined to the thoracic and upper lumbar levels (8,12). Mitchell (21) however, has identified preganglionic sympathetic cell bodies at all levels of the spinal cord. Randall (22) has confirmed these observations at the lower lumbar levels. Richter and Woodruff (23) mapped the lumbar sympathetic dermatomes through operations (at all levels) on the various lumbar ganglia.

The preganglionic efferent fibers travel with the ventral root, and via the white communicating rami, enter the sympathetic chain ganglia that lie along the lateral vertebral bodies. On entering the chain ganglia, the fibers may synapse in the ganglia with ganglionic cells, pass superiorly or inferiorly along the sympathetic chain and synapse at other levels, or continue through the ganglia out to the intermediary sympathetic ganglia. The collateral or intermediary sympathetic ganglia include the celiac, superior mesenteric, and inferior mesenteric ganglia.

The greater and lesser splanchnic nerves arising from the lower seven thoracic sympathetic ganglia travel to the celiac and superior mesenteric ganglia, where they synapse. The postganglionic fibers go through the celiac plexus to the abdominal viscera. Lower thoracic sympathetic fibers may travel to the inferior mesenteric ganglion from which postganglion fibers pass through the hypogastric plexus to the lower abdominal and pelvic viscera (12) (See Chapter 13).

VERTEBRAL ANOMALIES

Vertebral anomalies are frequently found in the thoracic spine. There may be differences in number of vertebral segments (Fig. 8.5) and developmental anomalies of bone tissue. Malformed spinous processes are common. Using static palpation of these structures solely to identify vertebral rotation is questionable. Hemivertebrae are due to failure of one of the vertebral body ossification centers to grow. They can be seen with other anomalies, such as Klippel-Feil syndrome and meningocele. A solitary hemivertebra will cause a structural scoliosis (See Chapter 9). An anterior-posterior hemivertebra is rare and can cause a gibbus formation. It is associated with cretinism and achondroplasia. A "scrambled spine" is multiple hemivertebrae (24).

Nuclear impression or persistent notochord is an irregularity of the end-plates and causes a characteristic "Cupid's Bow" or double hump contour of the end-plates. Block vertebrae may occur in the thoracic spine. Klippel-Feil syndrome is defined as multiple block vertebrae. Sixty percent of these patients show the triad of a short webbed neck, low hairline, and diminished range of motion. Sprengel's deformity is a failure of the scapula to descend during gestation; 25 to 35% of Klippel-Feil patients will have Sprengel's deformity (25). Females are twice as likely to display it as males (24).

Schmorl's nodes are commonly seen in the thoracic spine. These are nuclear herniations through the end-plates. This condition may be due to an inherent weakening of the end-plate, trauma, or a pathologic process. The radiographic appearance is of a small protrusion into the vertebral body through the end-plate that has a surrounding rim of sclerosis. Sclerosis of the end-plate most likely interferes with the nutritional requirements of the disc (See Chapter 2).

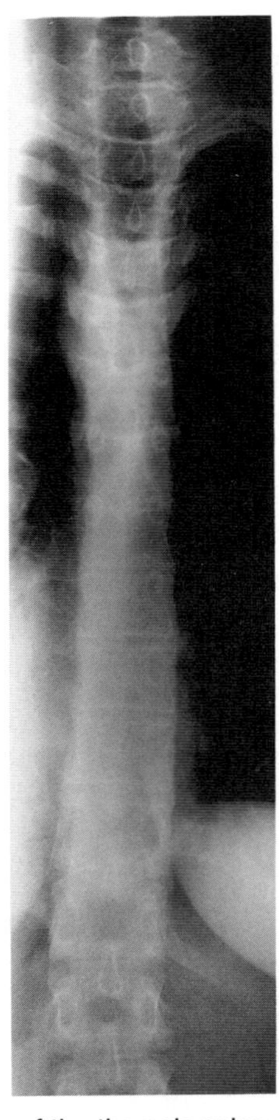

Figure 8.5. AP view of the thoracic spine. There are thirteen thoracic vertebrae.

Venous clefts or Clefts of Hahn appear radiographically as a lucent horizontal line through the vertebral body. These clefts are commonly seen in childhood and often persist into adulthood. This phenomenon represents the communication of the basivertebral vein and the anterior external plexus. They are common in the lower thoracic spine but are of unknown clinical significance (24).

Rib cage anomalies, such as bifurcated ribs, rib foramen, synostosis and accessory ribs, or the absence of ribs, can occur. Srb's Anomaly (24) is an involution of one or both first ribs caused by shortening and incomplete fusion of the first and second ribs. A bony plate is formed with absence of the intercostal space. A pseudoarthrosis may be present (24).

Most radiologists consider costochondral calcification to be a normal variant. Gonstead (26) hypothesized that costochondral calcification was a strong indicator of chemistry imbalance in the body especially when accompanied by calcification of the thyroid gland and a kyphotic cervical spine.

Rib Cage and Respiration

The biomechanics of the thoracic spine cannot be studied without including the rib cage. Inspiration is largely an active process, whereas exhalation is mostly passive. There is a slight amount of axial rotation around the axis formed by the costovertebral and costotransverse joints that allows elevation and depression of the ribs. In the lower thoracic spine, the elevation is accompanied by lateral or transverse expansion of the rib cage, whereas in the upper thoracic spine the elevation is accompanied by AP expansion. Because of the elevation and expansion of the rib cage, the costal cartilage is the element that absorbs the torque that occurs at the costosternal junction. This torque action is then released during exhalation thus reducing muscular effort (11).

The rib cage increases the moment of inertia of the thoracic spine, acts as a barrier to impacts, and increases the overall stiffness of the region due to the multiple ligamentous attachments (See Chapter 2).

Posture

The dorsally convex thoracic curve and the sacrum form the primary curves of the spinal column. The thoracic curve is present at birth and is formed predominately by the wedge-like configuration of the vertebral bodies. The disc spaces are relatively parallel. White and Panjabi (27) report that the common range for the thoracic curve is between 20 and 40°. The apex of the curve occurs at about the T6-T7 segmental levels (28). In the young, the thoracic curve tends to be less in females when compared with their male counterparts. The female curve does progress with age, however, so that during middle age the magnitudes are comparable for both sexes. Fon et al. (29) studied the range of the thoracic curve compared with chronologic age in 316 patients who were undergoing elective surgery or had a preemployment radiographic examination (Table 8.1 and Table 8.2). For the examination, the patient's arms were above the shoulders for the lateral view. This may have diminished the curve in some individuals. Since all of the sagittal curves are interdependent (30), it is important to not analyze the thoracic region in isolation (Fig. 8.6A-B)

Table 8.1.
Degree of Kyphosis in Males by Age[a]

Age (Years)	n	Mean	SD	Minimum	Maximum
2–9	26	20.88	7.85	5	40
10–19	28	25.11	8.16	8	39
20–29	37	26.27	8.12	13	48
30–39	26	29.04	7.93	13	49
40–49	20	29.75	6.93	17	44
50–59	10	33.00	6.46	25	45
60–69	9	34.67	5.12	25	62
70–79	3	40.67	7.57	32	66

[a]Modified from Fon GT, Pitt MJ, Thies AC. Thoracic kyphosis: range in normal subjects. Am J Roentgenol 1980;134:982.

Table 8.2.
Degree of Kyphosis in Females by Age[a]

Age (Years)	n	Mean	SD	Minimum	Maximum
2–9	23	23.87	6.67	8	36
10–19	22	26.00	7.43	11	41
20–29	24	26.83	7.98	7	40
30–39	26	28.42	8.63	10	42
40–49	32	32.66	6.72	21	50
50–59	17	40.71	9.88	22	53
60–69	7	44.86	7.80	34	54
70–79	6	41.67	9.00	30	56

[a]Modified from Fon GT, Pitt MJ, Thies AC. Thoracic kyphosis: range in normal subjects. Am J Roentgenol 1980;134:982.

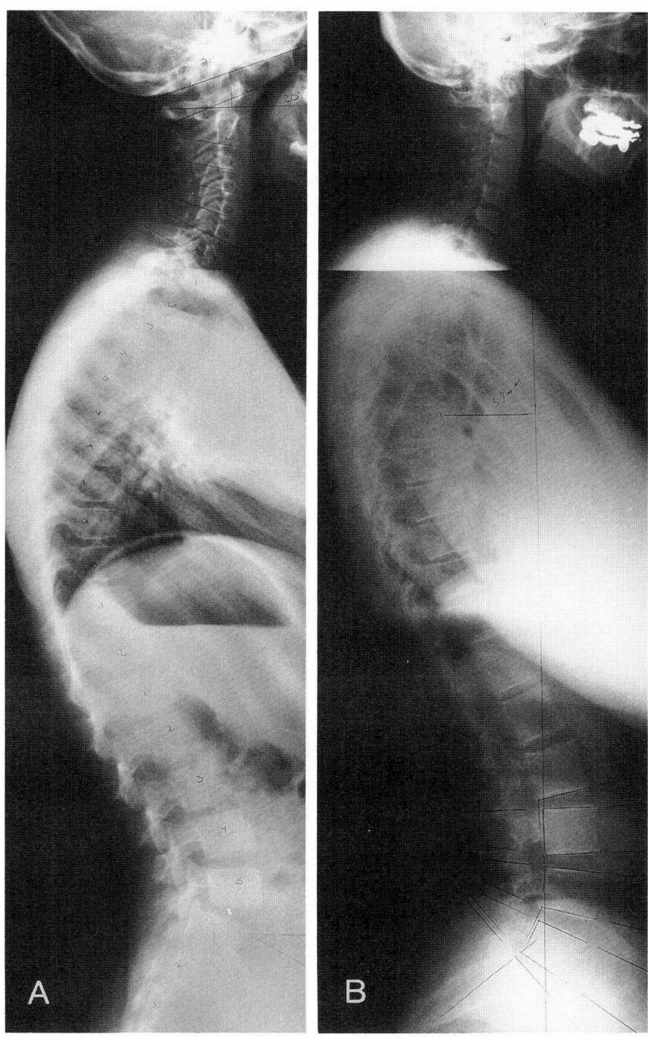

Figure 8.6. **A,** Sagittal perspective of the thoracic curve. Notice the hyperextension of the lumbar spine. **B,** Sagittal perspective of the thoracic curve. The apex of the curve is at approximately the T6-T7 segmental levels. This patient's lower thoracic vertebrae are very lumbar-like (i.e., square).

Table 8.3.
The Range of Motion (i.e., Elastic + Neutral Zones) of the Thoracic Spine During Lateral Bending and Y Axis Rotation[a]

Motion Segment	One Side Lateral Bending: Limits of Ranges (Degrees)	One Side Lateral Bending: Representative Angle (Degrees)	One Side Axial Rotation: Limits of Ranges (Degrees)	One Side Axial Rotation: Representative Angle (Degrees)
T1–T2	5	5	14	9
T2–T3	5–7	6	4–12	8
T3–T4	3–7	5	5–11	8
T4–T5	5–6	6	5–11	8
T5–T6	5–6	6	5–11	8
T6–T7	6	6	4–11	7
T7–T8	3–8	6	4–11	7
T8–T9	4–7	6	6–7	6
T9–T10	4–7	6	3–5	4
T10–T11	3–10	7	2–3	2
T11–T12	4–13	9	2–3	2
T12–L1	5–10	8	2–3	2

[a]Based on data from White AA, Panjabi MM. Clinical biomechanics of the spine. 2nd ed. Philadelphia: JB Lippincott, 1990:103.

Kinematics

With the exception of axial rotation, the ranges of motion of the thoracic spine are much less than other regions of the spinal column. There are also marked regional differences within the thoracic spine. The upper dorsal region behaves much like the lower cervical spine, and the T10–12 area has similarities to lumbar spine motion.

LATERAL FLEXION ($\pm\theta Z$)

The neutral zone (See Chapter 2) in lateral flexion is 2.2° (27). The neutral zone can increase with degeneration, after unfavorable surgery, with repetitious loading, and after trauma (27). The range of motion (neutral zone + elastic zone) is approximately 6° in the upper and middle thoracic spine, and 8° or so in the lower (27). Lateral flexion is limited by the ipsilateral facet joint and contralateral flava and intertransverse ligaments (11). The rib cage limits movement as well (Table 8.3).

ROTATION ($\pm\theta Y$)

The neutral zone in axial rotation is 1.2° (27) (Table 8.3). Rotation is limited primarily by the costosternal structures (11). The range of motion is approximately 2° in the lower thoracic area and 10° or so in the upper regions (27). The greatest amount of axial rotation and therefore, the greatest amount of stress, occurs in the middle thoracic area (31). During walking, the counterrotation of the shoulders to that of the pelvis may cause strain at the transition zone (i.e., T6-T8) and increase symptomatology in a patient with subluxation in the area.

FLEXION/EXTENSION ($\pm\theta X$)

The thoracic spine is more stiff when extended than when it is flexed (32,33). In general, there is less range of motion for extension. The neutral zone from the neutral position for flexion and extension is 1.5°. The upper thoracic total range of motion is approximately 4° at each motion segment. There are 6° at the middle thoracics and 12° at the lower segments (27).

Flexion is limited by the posterior ligaments, such as the interspinous, flava, capsular, and posterior longitudinal. Extension is limited by the spinous processes and the facet joints and, to an extent, by the anterior longitudinal ligament and anterior portion of the annulus (11).

THORACIC SUBLUXATION COMPLEX

Subluxations in other regions of the spine may and often do cause compensatory changes in the thoracic spine. Correction of these subluxations can reduce or eliminate the compensation reactions. It is important to only adjust those segments exhibiting fixation dysfunction. Stress radiographic methods are useful to detect this dysfunction as well as to reveal compensatory hypermobilities and normal segments.

Compensation Reaction

The direction a vertebra subluxates depends on the anatomy of the articulations (posterior and central joint orientations), the global postural mechanics (kyphosis), and the mechanism of injury. Some thoracic injuries occur with the spine in a flexed position. It follows, therefore, that if ligaments are damaged when the motion segment is flexing, then the vertebra will be in an extreme flexion position after the trauma (34,35). Treatment should be directed at this level and not at the compensation above.

For every subluxation, the motion segments above will usually compensate. It is less common for the compensation to occur below. One example may be the individual with a kyphotic cervical spine (primary) which leads to a flattened thoracic curve (secondary). In the cervical spine, extension malposition will be compensated for by flexion of the segments above. The range of motion for sagittal plane motion in the cervical region ($\pm\theta X$) is large (approx. 15°) for each individual motion segment; therefore, subluxations in the sagittal plane are easily compensated for. This is in sharp contrast to the thoracic spine, where range of motion in the sagittal plane is quite limited, especially extension from T1 to T6. This is also the most common site for thoracic "dishing" to occur (36). The hypothetical sequence of events for a typical thoracic (i.e., T7-T8) flexion injury occurs as follows:

1. Subluxation is produced due to hyperflexion injury with ligamentous (including disc) damage. There may be only slight radiographic (neutral lateral) alterations, unless there is swelling or degenerative joint disease, or marked flexion positional dyskinesia of the motion segment.
2. The T7-T8 functional spinal unit is sprained with T7 hyperflexed on the subjacent motion segment (Fig. 8.7).
3. The T6-T7 motion segment does not compensate by moving into extension because of its limited ability to do so.
4. Compensation occurs over multiple levels (e.g., 3–4) because of the limited range of motion in extension at individual motion segments from T1 to T6.
5. Because the flexion lesion at T7 directs the segments above towards the thoracic cavity, these segments will palpate or visualize as being relatively anterior or "dished."

The area of the dishing will usually be painful and edematous and be resilient to compressive palpation (+Z). The correction is made by adjusting a segment caudal to the compensation. The spinous contact is usually preferred in this regard.

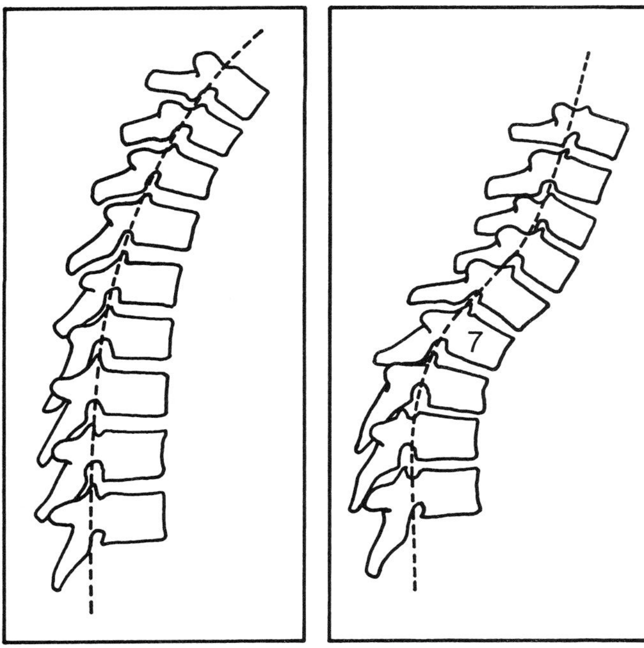

Figure 8.7. A hyperflexed T7 creates an anterior position of the thoracic curve above.

Strain and Sprain

Myotendinous strains or ligamentous sprains follow trauma to the thoracic spine. Sprains or strains occurring in the rib cage, cervical spine, or upper extremities may affect the biomechanics of the thoracic spine. Strains are exacerbated by resisted contraction. Sprains are exacerbated with passive motion of the injured joint. Subluxations are considered to have damaged (sprained) ligamentous elements. It is important to not direct the force of an adjustment into the direction of ligamentous injury.

Disc Disease

Intervertebral disc disorders such as herniation are not common in the thoracic spine. This region accounts for only 2% of the intervertebral disc herniations (13). The most probable explanation for this is the limited motion of the thoracic spine due to the rib cage. Herniations are more common in the lower thoracic spine (Fig. 8.8). Disc damage without herniation is relatively common. Radial fissures of the disc are often found in the thoracic spine (1). The true prevalence of thoracic disc herniation and related pathologies is likely to be determined with increased use of advanced imaging devices such as MRI (37).

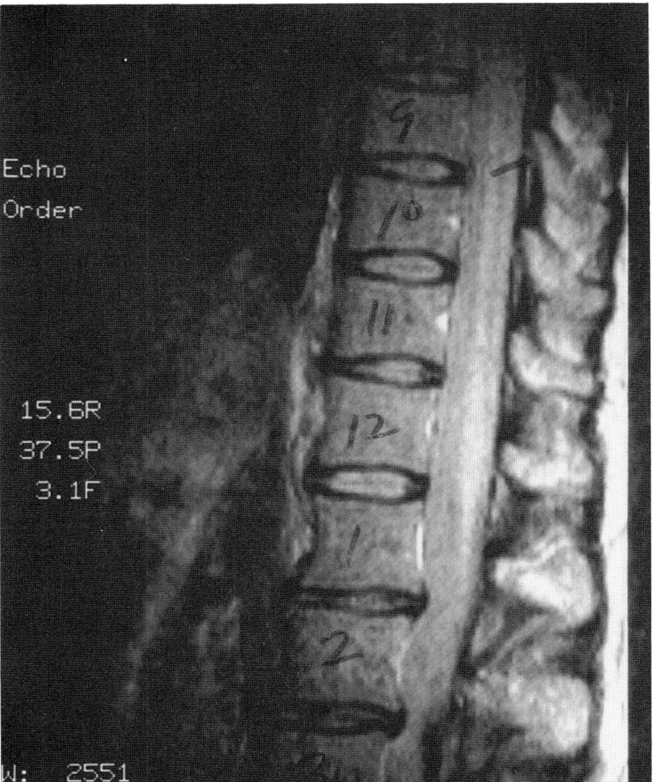

Figure 8.8. Herniation of the T9 intervertebral disc. A slight retrolisthesis is also detected at the affected level. There are annular protrusions at L1 and L2 with retrolisthesis of both segments.

Nerve root compromise from direct disc protrusion is uncommon in the thoracic spine because the intervertebral foramina are primarily level with the body rather than the disc. The limited movement of the thoracic spine also protects the neural elements by keeping their positions relatively constant (13). Because of the tremendous anterior compressive load at the central joint due to the kyphosis, protrusions of the disc tend to be posteriorward, affecting the cord rather than the nerve roots (13). Thoracic disc disease is usually associated with myelopathy.

A history of recent trauma may not be present because many patients with disc protrusions have a gradual onset of symptoms (38). Thoracic disc protrusion with myelopathy tends to produce lower extremity and lower GI tract disorders (13). Paraplegia is often present with lower thoracic disc herniation. Magnetic resonance imaging or computerized tomography scan should confirm the diagnosis.

Initially, the patient should receive conservative management. The area of involvement should be tested by preloading the joint (bring to tension). If neurologic signs or symptoms increase with the maneuver, the adjustment is less likely to be successful. As with all adjustments, the force should be as specifically directed as possible. If neurologic signs or bowel and bladder dysfunction increase, neurosurgical referral is warranted.

Thoracic Myelopathy

Thoracic myelopathy can be caused by disc disease as previously noted. Thoracic hyperkyphosis can also cause myelopathy by pressing the cord against the anterior canal wall. In extreme kyphosis, the dura mater may be stretched to the point of putting pressure on the posterior cord. Scoliosis rarely causes myelopathy, but traction in an attempt to straighten the spine may compromise the soft tissue within the cord. Halo-pelvic traction for kyphoscoliosis can compromise the brainstem (17). Thoracic myelopathy often manifests itself in lower extremity and lower gastrointestinal disorders (13).

Nerve Root Disorders

Nerve root compression or irritation can cause symptoms along the course of the involved spinal nerve. In the thoracic spine, radiculopathy commonly takes the form of intercostal pain. Brachial referral patterns can occur directly from thoracic subluxation or as a result of compensatory hypermobility in the cervical spine above. The lowest thoracic segments contribute to the cluneal nerve which can give rise to referral patterns along the iliac crests and lower back.

Herpes zoster or shingles is a disorder associated with the dorsal root ganglia. Nerve root irritation may make the peripheral nerve more susceptible to clinical infection with the herpes virus.

Horner's syndrome is often associated with upper thoracic subluxation (36). This syndrome usually follows acceleration/deceleration injuries of the neck which stretch the sympathetic chain.

Scheuermann's Disease

Scheuermann's disease is not an osteochondrosis. The mechanism causing the condition is unknown, although trauma arresting growth plate development is one of many theories (39). The disease affects the growth plate of the vertebral body, especially at the anterior.

The typical profile is a male, age 13 to 17. Presenting clinical features include pain, fatigue, and increased thoracic kyphosis (24).

The characteristic radiographic signs are decreased anterior vertebral body height, increased thoracic kyphosis, and Schmorl's nodes affecting at least three contiguous segments. There may also be limbus bones, decreased disc height, osteophytes, postural changes to the cervical and lumbar spine, and persistent venous channels (24).

Disc herniation, although rare, can occur with Scheuermann's disease. The involved segment is usually at the area with the greatest kyphotic angulation. Spastic paraparesis and sphincter dysfunction are common sequelae. These patients should initially be managed by chiropractors, provided the neurologic signs are stable and not deteriorating. When the condition is chronic, an adequate trial of care is necessary. The results of surgery for this disorder are mixed (40–43).

Degenerative Joint Disease

Degenerative joint disease is progressive and noninflammatory. The most likely causes are repetitive microtrauma or a macrotraumatic event. The most common radiographic features include osteophytes, sclerosis, and disc space narrowing (Fig. 8.9A-B). Anterior narrowing of the disc is relatively common and may lead to an increased kyphosis. Anterior osteophyte formation can compress the sympathetic trunk (2). Costovertebral and costotransverse arthrosis, which usually occurs in the lower thoracic area, may cause pain and simulate an upper gastrointestinal disorder (24). Osteophytes are not seen on the left side of the anterior vertebral body. This is thought to be due to pulsations of the descending aorta (24). Treatment is directed to the fixated segment(s). Prevention or diminishment of this sequential process lies in early intervention (See Chapter 14). Unfortunately, children rarely report long-lasting symptomatology which would otherwise alert the doctor or parent that a chiropractic examination is in order.

Interscapular Pain

Interscapular pain of nonvisceral or nonmetastatic cause has often been referred to as benign (44). Bourne (45) sug-

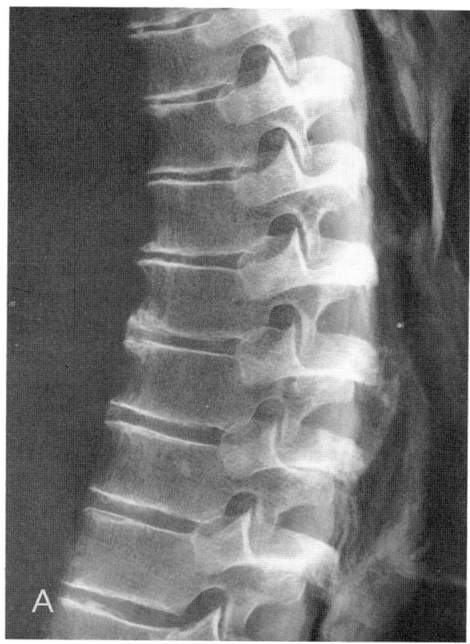

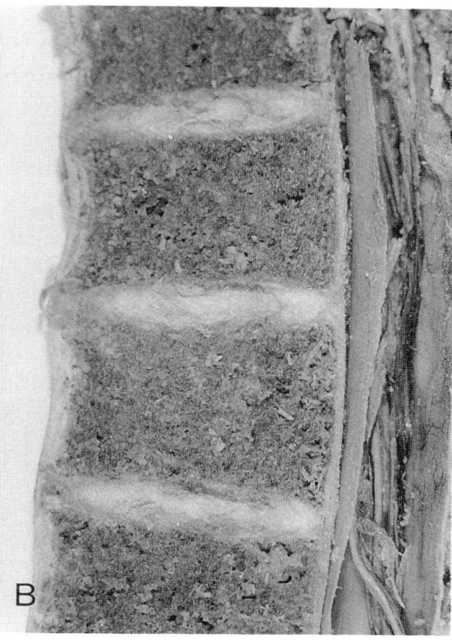

Figure 8.9. A, Radiograph of the cadaver specimen demonstrating subchondral sclerosis and anterior osteophyte formation. **B,** Cadaver specimen demonstrates a slight anterior disc protrusion and osteophyte formation.

gests that the term "benign" be discarded, because it has no other purpose than to reassure the patient that malignant disease has not been diagnosed. The patient does not consider the pain to be benign and is seeking relief for what can be severe and incapacitating symptoms. The pain is often described as dull, aching and continuous and is aggravated by coughing, sneezing, and deep breathing. A few patients may have hyperesthesia of radicular distribution (44). The pain may appear to be of rib origin to the novice clinician. Clinical observations and recent evidence (4) suggest that there is a primary spinal component. Bruckner et al. (4) found that 90% of patients with this disorder had intervertebral disc dehydration (determined with MRI) compared with only 13% of a control group. The finding of spinal tenderness was usually just above the level of disc pathology (4). The most tender area may be a hypermobile compensation. If multiple segments appear to be involved, at least initially, it may be wise to adjust the lowest tender level. Manipulating multiple segments in a nonspecific fashion will do little to help in determining the offending motion segment. Reliance on objective parameters such as skin temperature differentials and stress radiographic abnormalities is encouraged. Occupational factors, such as prolonged bending, are often related to chronic interscapular pain (46). If there is a "dishing" of the thoracic curve, it is wise to focus treatment just below the sectional deformity (35) (See Compensation Reaction).

Spinal Stenosis

Stenosis in the thoracic spine is not common, especially when compared with the cervical or lumbar regions. Narrowing of the thoracic spinal canal can be due to a variety of factors, such as trauma, disc herniation, hypertrophy of the posterior elements lining the canal, and tumor. The imaging system of choice for visualizing canal stenosis is MRI (47).

Rheumatoid Arthritis

Rheumatoid arthritis is not common in the thoracic spine. Corticosteroid treatments for patients with rheumatoid arthritis may result in iatrogenic disorders such as osteoporosis and compression fractures (24).

Viscerosomatic Disorders

Symptoms localized to the thoracic region can be referred from visceral organs. The pathways appear to be the sympathetic nervous system and appear to be associated with the embryologic neuromeres. Referring organs include the gallbladder, lungs, pancreas, heart, and kidneys.

If during the course of care, the patient responds poorly or if complaints continually return, there may be a viscerogenic referral pattern. In these cases, it is important to analyze for the subluxation based on objective criteria. If the signs of subluxation appear to not correspond with the magnitude or nature of the complaint, then further investigation or specialist consultation is warranted.

Somatovisceral Disorders

Musculoskeletal/neuromusculoskeletal disorders (e.g., subluxation) can cause symptoms similar to those caused by referral from malfunctioning visceral organs. Perhaps the most common of these is the angina-like symptoms due to thoracic spinal problems. This has been called pseudocardiac disease (48) or cervicoprecordial angina (49,50). The condition may cause chest pain and left shoulder and arm pain. Thoracoabdominal radiculopathy can occur and may be confused with primary visceral pathology (51). Marinacci and Courville (52) studied this phenomenon in a group of patients suspected of having gallbladder or intestinal disease. One-half of the patients were operated on before the diagnosis of nerve root irritation was considered. For the management of patients with primary spinal pathology and concomitant visceral symptomatology or pathology, the reader is referred to Chapter 13.

EXAMINATION

The analysis of the thoracic spine begins with a history (53). Other than general health information, queries should include smoking, alcohol use, trauma, osteoporosis or other metabolic disorders, and current or past visceral disorders. These might have an effect on the evaluation of the thoracic spine. The patient may relate a specific traumatic event to the onset of symptomatology. In other cases, a more insidious nature may prevail. This is especially true of interscapular pain. The patient must be gowned or unclothed for the examination. This includes follow-up examinations as well, because subtle signs of injury such as skin texture changes (54), edema and erythema would go undetected.

Inspection

Symmetry and skin quality are first observed. Sagittal and coronal curvatures are noted as are shoulder heights and scapular position. The most common evaluation in the thoracic spine is a scoliosis check. Scoliosis in a child must be studied for progression (See Chapter 9). Scoliosis is often associated with a loss of the normal thoracic curve. A kyphoscoliosis may develop in some individuals. An extremely kyphotic thoracic curve, especially if it has progressed to a marked gibbus deformity, must be evaluated for fracture or underlying pathology such as osteoporosis. "Dishing" of the thoracic spine may indicate loss or reversal of the normal thoracic curve, but often the thoracic curve is normal or near normal and the overlying musculature is atrophied. Imbrication of the spinous processes may give a "dished" appearance to the thoracic spine.

Altered scapular position may indicate muscle weakness. Shoulder symmetry should be observed because asymmetry can indicate injury, scoliosis, congenital malformations, or handedness. Aberrant shape of the chest (e.g., pectus excavatum) may indicate other underlying pathology or anomaly.

Surgical scars should be noted. Coloration and skin quality are observed, since neurotrophic changes or pathology may alter quality and color. Lipomas and moles are often found in the thoracic region. They may direct the doctor to a vertebral subluxation level, if associated with a dermatomal or pattern distribution. Café-au-lait spots must be investigated if large or numerous, as they may indicate neurofibromatosus or fibrous dysplasia.

Range of motion is measured, noting pain and restriction. Interruptions in smooth bending motions (inflexion points) indicate fixation dysfunction or anomaly (See Chapter 4). The radiograph may be used to make the differentiation. Pain on passive motion is suggestive of joint or ligamentous sprain. Pain during resisted isometric motion is indicative of muscle or tendinous strain.

Thorax expansion is studied by comparing girths on full exhalation and full inhalation. Measurements are taken at the nipple-line. In males, there should be a change of at least 1½ to 2½ inches; in females, 1 to 1½ inches. Lesser values may indicate ankylosing spondylitis and costotransverse or costovertebral articulation ankylosis or pulmonary dysfunction (55,56)

Instrumentation

A paraspinal skin temperature differential instrument (e.g., Nervoscope) can be used to scan the thoracic spine for temperature asymmetries. Plaugher et al. (57) found good reliability for the Nervoscope in the thoracic spine (i.e., T4-T8) both between examiners and during test-retest. This study used 19 relatively pain-free females as subjects. Because static radiologic findings are often equivocal in the thoracic spine, more weight is given to the findings of temperature analysis and palpation in this region. The glide speed for a Nervoscope should be approximately two inches per second (35) (See Chapter 4) and the instrument is moved in a caudal direction during the scan.

Static Palpation

The thoracic spine should be palpated for tenderness and edematous "pitting" in the interspinous area and over the transverse process (See Chapter 4). The lowest tender thoracic spinous is often the level of involvement (26). Tenderness can be elicited by applying pressure to the spinous tip, followed by continued pressure over the upward length of the process. Pain arising in any particular segment of the thoracic spine is much more precisely localized than is the case with the upper and lower regions of the spinal column. This is due to the lack of large numbers of intersegmental neurologic connections as seen in the cervical and lumbar spine (18).

Compensatory areas often have associated musculature alterations that are tight and rope-like. The area or site of subluxation, in contrast, is usually more edematous and flaccid on palpatory assessment.

Rubbing over the area of the subluxation often pro-

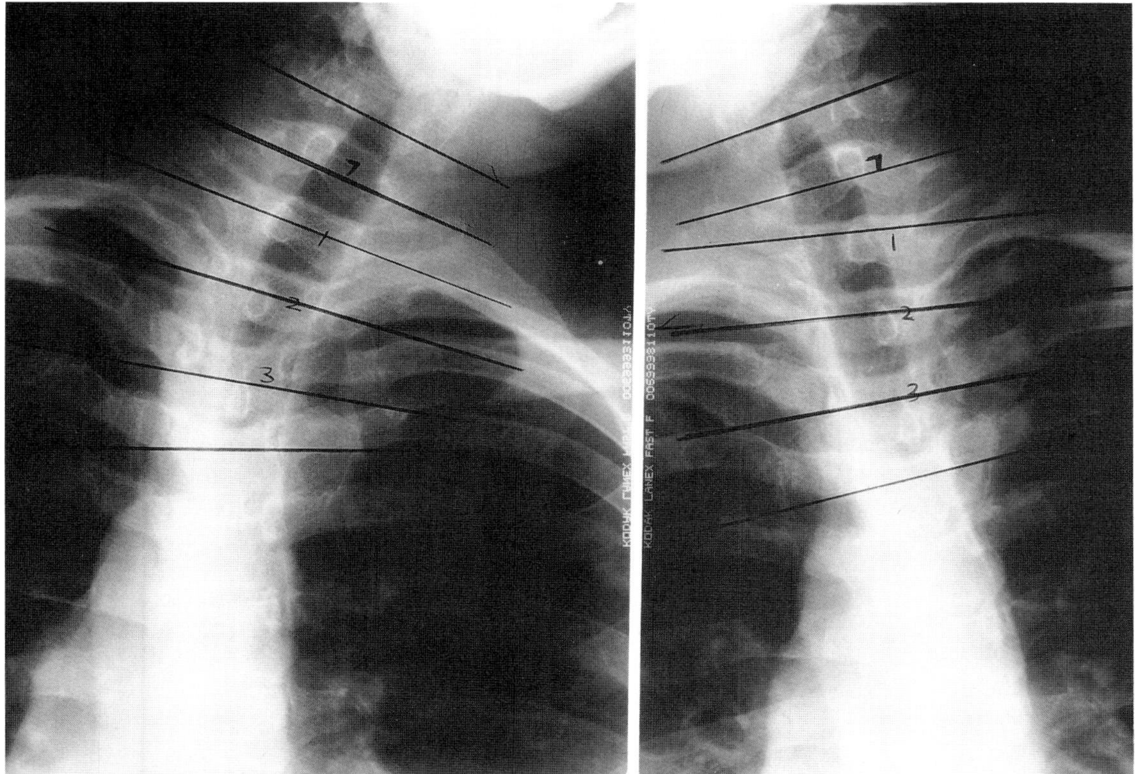

Figure 8.10. Right bending (*left panel*) demonstrates relatively normal lateral flexion. There is absence of the normal coupling pattern at T3. Left bending shows marked restriction at multiple levels. Notice the increased lateral bending at C7-T1 in compensation. This patient was initially adjusted at T3 (PRI-t) and later at T2 (PRI-t) and T1 (PLS).

duces a persistent hyperemia (red response). If hyperemia is asymmetrical or persists for an abnormally long period of time, then this may indicate underlying autonomic dysfunction in the area (58). Skin texture should be noted. Texture and color changes may indicate neurotrophic (e.g., trophedema) (See Chapter 3) or other pathologic changes.

Subdermal masses, such as lipomas or cysts, can be readily palpated. Palpation of the paravertebral musculature can detect spasm, tonic changes, etc.

Osseous anomalies, such as deviated spinous processes, may be visualized and palpated, as can vertebral landmarks, such as the typically prominent spinous processes of T1, T4, and T10. These will aid in vertebral count. The T9 spinous process is usually very small. The doctor should correlate the palpation examination with the AP neutral upright radiograph. Projectional distortion of the radiograph must always be accounted for (See Chapter 5). Active "trigger points" in the paravertebral myofascial tissues should be noted.

Motion Palpation

The main purpose of motion palpation is to detect fixation dysfunction. Unless a fracture is present (See Chapter 12), an adjustment is not given unless there is fixation of the motion segment. Hypermobilities, which appear to be due to direct injury, pathology, or as a compensatory reaction, are usually not distinguishable from normal segments, unless extreme. Stress radiography is useful in identifying hypermobile or normal motion segments (Fig. 8.10).

The doctor should motion palpate flexion and extension, lateral flexion, rotation and coupled extension, lateral flexion, and rotational movements. In flexion and extension, interspinous separation and approximation are detected. The upper thoracic spine is usually evaluated by extreme extension of the cervical spine or the patient elevating and crossing the arms and the examiner raising and lowering them while digitally evaluating the interspinous space closure and opening. Lateral flexion is palpated by pushing the spinous process opposite from the side of passive lateral flexion. Rotation and coupled movements are usually determined by applying digital pressure against the spinous or transverse processes (35,59).

Orthopaedic Tests

Adam's sign is a test to differentiate structural from functional scoliosis (See Chapter 9). If pain and restriction are present, this test should be followed by tests for intervertebral disc syndrome. Adam's test is performed standing, sitting, or kneeling. Lateral curvatures and rib cage asymmetries are noted in the upright position. The patient then flexes forward. If the curvature straightens, the scoliosis is considered functional. If it persists, it is structural.

Beevor's sign is a test for nerve root lesions. The patient lies supine with fingertips interlocked behind the head. The patient attempts to flex the head toward the feet. If the umbilicus moves cephalically, there may a T10-T12 nerve root lesion. If the umbilicus moves caudally, there may be a T7-T10 nerve root lesion (55). A positive test may occur in patients with poliomyelitis or meningiomyelocele.

The Soto-Hall test was originally developed for cervico-thoracic fractures. The patient is supine. The examiner places one hand under the occiput and the other stabilizes the chest. The examiner passively flexes the head toward the sternum. Localized pain may indicate osseous or ligamentous injury (55,56).

If firm spinous percussion or placing a tuning fork on the spinous results in an increase in pain, a fracture is suspected. Tuning fork examination is also used if a rib fracture is a possibility. Compression tests should accentuate the pain from a rib fracture.

Neurologic Tests

Muscle stretch or deep tendon reflexes are not typically evaluated for thoracic root levels, but lumbar reflexes should be tested as pathology in the thoracic spine may affect these (60). Dermatomal evaluation can be done with an open pin, cotton wisp for light touch, hot and cold objects for temperature, or tuning fork for vibratory sense.

Infrared or telethermography is useful in identifying sensory-autonomic alterations (61).

Plain Film Radiography

The 14″ x 36″ anteroposterior and lateral full spine radiograph usually provides an adequate view of the thoracic spine with the proper filtration and high speed (e.g., 1200) screens. The two exposure lateral film usually has its cut-off point at the T9-T11 levels (35). Great care must be taken during the exposures to ensure that all segments are visualized (See Chapter 5). The single exposure lateral full spine is preferred, although facility limitations pertaining to the necessary film focal distance precludes widespread usage. The upper thoracic region is frequently difficult to penetrate, and a spot view, such as a "swimmer's" projection or other imaging modalities, such as tomography, may be required if osseous pathology or fracture is suspected.

Positional dyskinesia of the thoracic spine is often difficult to visualize on the lateral film. Not typically detected is the obvious posterior inferior malposition seen in the cervical or lumbar spine. Because of the rib cage, the kyphosis and the orientation of the apophyseal joints, positional dyskinesia tends to be posterior and superiorward (i.e., hyperflexion) (35).

Global thoracic lateral flexion views are helpful in evaluating the subluxation. If lumbar lateral flexion is included, visualization of normal and abnormal motion is more complex. The T6 motion segment is considered the transition area between the coupled motion of spinous rotation to the concave side in the lower thoracic and the coupling of spinous rotation to the convex side in the upper thoracic spine (Fig. 8.11A-C) (See Chapter 2). When the thoracic spine is isolated, the spinous processes of the entire region should rotate to the convex side of bend (31,62).

The listing is derived primarily from the results of stress radiographic analysis and the neutral AP radiograph (Fig. 8.12A-B). Radiopaque markers can be used to help locate the dysfunctional motion segment (Fig. 8.13). The authors have provided several studies of the thoracic spine in lateral bending. This should provide the reader with an appreciation of the complex biomechanics of the region (Figs. 8.14–8.16). The examiner should note the presence of lateral flexion (or lack of) toward the side of bend. The spinous process should rotate toward the convexity of bend. The adjustment is designed to restore the main motion of lateral bending as well as coupled motions.

Visualization of rib fractures is often difficult, especially if there is recent injury. Expert consultation may be warranted in these cases.

Special Procedures

Certain suspected pathologies, or nonresponse, or deterioration after treatment may require additional investigation, such as visceral palpation, MRI, CT scan, thermography, laboratory tests, sonograms, somatic evoked potential tests, electromyelography, and nerve conduction velocity tests. Magnetic resonance imaging is best used for soft tissue evaluation, whereas computerized tomography is superior for osseous tissue analysis, such as canal size or bone pathology. These ancillary procedures are especially important if extraspinal or visceral disorders are suspected. In certain cases, the mental status may need to be evaluated for functional overlays. Referral to a clinical psychologist is warranted for these patients.

THORACIC ADJUSTMENT

The segmental contact points for adjusting the thoracic spine are the spinous process and the transverse process. Spinous contact on the imbricated segments (e.g., T5-T9) is the uppermost portion of the spinous, immediately subjacent to the next cephalic vertebra (See Figure 8.3). This contact is used to direct the thrust as close to the vertebral body as possible.

Patient position: The patient should be positioned on the knee-chest table so that the thoracic spine is slightly higher than the lumbar spine. There should be a slight incline on the chest support to allow for anterior expansion of the thoracic spine when the posterior to anterior (+Z) thrust is given. The knees should be placed so that the femurs are nearly perpendicular to the floor (See Chapter 7) to accommodate the anterior movement of the stomach.

Doctor's position: Standing on the right side of the patient.

Contact point: The posterior, inferior and right lateral border of the spinous process of T12 is contacted with the cephalad (right) pisiform.

Supporting hand: Placed over the contact hand.

Pattern of thrust: Posterior to anterior (+Z), with a quick arcing motion (+θX) at the beginning of the thrust. This is especially important at the thoraco-lumbar junction because extension of the segment will be painful for the patient. Lateral to medial (−θY), with an inferiorward arcing motion (+θZ) toward the end of the thrust.

Category by algorithm: Short lever specific contact procedure.

Name of technique: Gonstead

Name of technique procedure: PRI-t (−Z, +θY, +θZ) T9 Knee Chest Pisiform Contact Adjustment (Fig. 8.20).

Indications: Retrolisthesis of T9 with decreased +Z motion and decreased −θY and −θZ motion.

Contraindications: All other listings, normal FSU, hypermobility, instability, destruction or fracture of the neural arch or transverse process, infection of the contact vertebra.

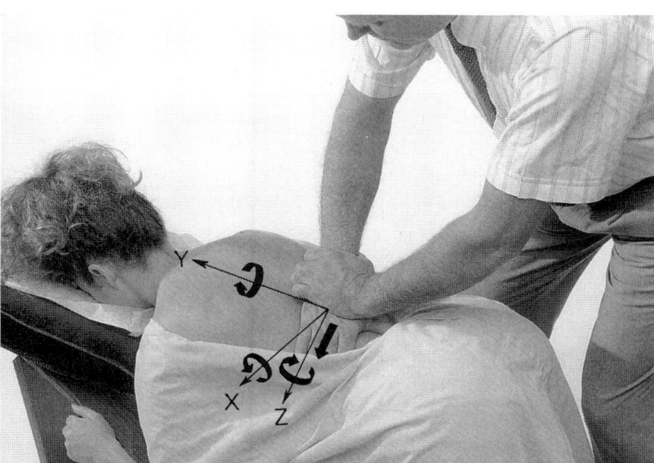

Figure 8.19. T12 PRS pisiform contact adjustment.

Patient position: The patient should be positioned on the knee-chest table so that the thoracic spine is slightly higher than the lumbar spine. There should be a slight incline on the chest support to allow for anterior expansion of the thoracic spine when the posterior to anterior (+Z) thrust is given. The knees should be placed so that the femurs are nearly perpendicular to the floor (See Chapter 7) to accommodate the anterior movement of the stomach.

Doctor's position: Standing on the side of spinous laterality (R) directly over T9 reaching across the spine to the transverse process being adjusted. The patient is further stabilized with the doctor's knees.

Contact point: Left transverse process of T9 with the right pisiform.

Supporting hand: The left pisiform is placed over the contact hand.

Pattern of thrust: Posterior to anterior (+Z), lateral to medial, with an inferiorward arcing motion toward the end of the thrust (−θZ).

Category by algorithm: Short lever specific contact procedure.

Name of technique: Gonstead

Name of technique procedure: PRI-t (−Z, +θY, +θZ) T8 Knee Chest Thumb-Pisiform Adjustment (Fig. 8.21).

Indications: Retrolisthesis of T8 with decreased +Z motion and decreased −θY and −θZ motion.

Contraindications: All other listings, normal FSU, hypermobility, instability, destruction or fracture of the neural arch or transverse process, infection of the contact vertebra.

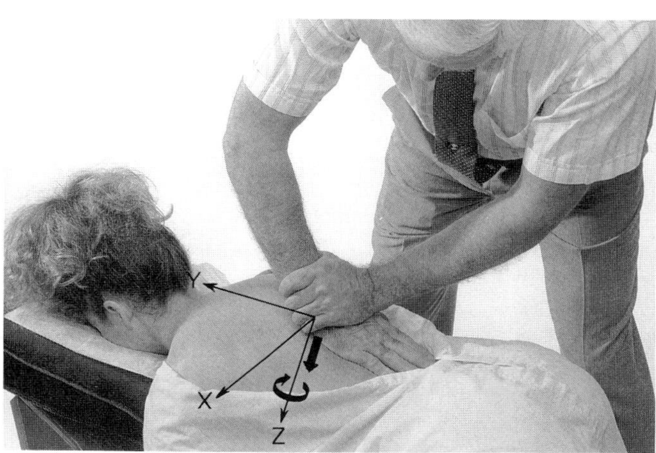

Figure 8.20. T9 PRI-t pisiform contact adjustment.

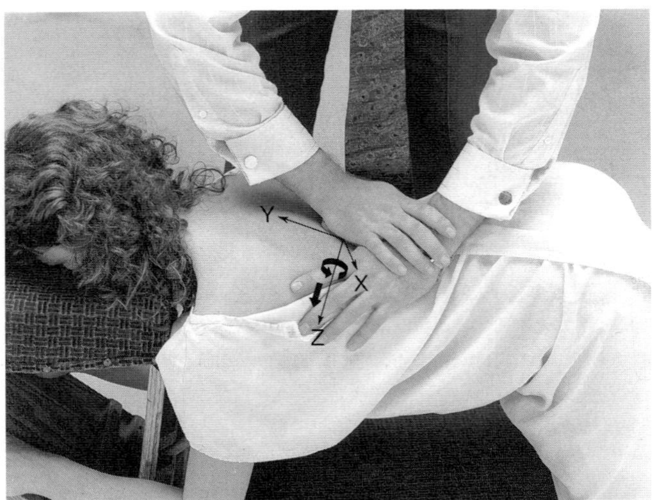

Figure 8.21. T8 PRI-t thumb-pisiform contact adjustment.

Patient position: The patient should be positioned on the knee-chest table so that the thoracic spine is slightly higher than the lumbar spine. There should be a slight incline on the chest support, to allow for anterior expansion of the thoracic spine when the posterior to anterior (+Z) thrust is given. The knees should be placed so that the femurs are nearly perpendicular to the floor (see Chapter 7) to accommodate the anterior movement of the stomach.

Doctor's position: Standing on the side of spinous laterality (R) directly over T8 reaching across the spine to the transverse process being adjusted.

Contact point: Left transverse process of T8 with the thumb.

Supporting hand: The right pisiform is placed over the thumb.

Pattern of thrust: Posterior to anterior (+Z), lateral to medial, with an inferiorward arcing motion toward the end of the thrust ($-\theta$Z).

Category by algorithm: Short lever specific contact procedure.

Name of technique: Gonstead

Name of technique procedure: PRS (−Z, $+\theta$Y, $-\theta$Z) T8 Knee Chest Pisiform Contact Adjustment (Fig. 8.22).

Indications: Retrolisthesis of T8 with decreased +Z, $-\theta$Y and $+\theta$Z motions.

Contraindications: All other listings, normal FSU, hypermobility, instability, destruction or fracture of the neural arch or spinous process, infection of the contact vertebra.

Patient position: The patient should be positioned on the knee-chest table so that the thoracic spine is slightly higher than the

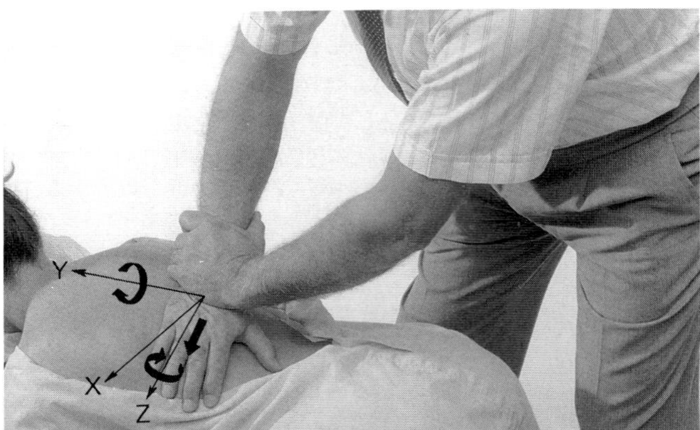

Figure 8.22. T8 PRS pisiform contact adjustment.

lumbar spine. There should be a slight incline on the chest support to allow for anterior expansion of the thoracic spine when the posterior to anterior (+Z) thrust is given. The knees should be placed so that the femurs are nearly perpendicular to the floor (see Chapter 7) to accommodate the anterior movement of the stomach.

Doctor's position: Standing on the right side of the patient.

Contact point: The posterior, inferior and right lateral border of the spinous process of T8 is contacted with the cephalad (right) pisiform.

Supporting hand: Placed over the contact hand.

Pattern of thrust: Posterior to anterior (+Z), with a quick arcing motion ($+\theta$X) at the beginning of the thrust. This is especially important at this level due to the imbrication of the spinous processes. Lateral to medial ($-\theta$Y), with an inferiorward arcing motion ($+\theta$Z) toward the end of the thrust.

Category by algorithm: Short lever specific contact procedure.

Name of technique: Gonstead

Name of technique procedure: P (−Z) T8 Knee Chest Double-thumb Contact Adjustment (Fig. 8.23).

Indications: Retrolisthesis of T8 with decreased +Z motion.

Contraindications: All other listings, normal FSU, hypermobility, instability, destruction or fracture of the neural arch or spinous process, infection of the contact vertebra.

Patient position: The patient should be positioned on the knee-chest table so that the thoracic spine is slightly higher than the lumbar spine. There should be a slight incline on the chest support to allow for anterior expansion of the thoracic spine when the posterior to anterior (+Z) thrust is given. The knees should be placed so that the femurs are nearly perpendicular to the floor (see Chapter 7) to accommodate the anterior movement of the stomach.

Doctor's position: Standing behind the patient.

Contact point: Spinous process of T8. The thumbs are placed on the lateral, posterior, inferior borders of the spinous process.

Supporting hand: Not applicable.

Pattern of thrust: Posterior to anterior (+Z), with a quick arcing motion (+θX) at the beginning of the thrust.

Category by algorithm: Short lever specific contact procedure.

Name of technique: Gonstead

Name of technique procedure: PRS (−Z, +θY, −θZ) T4 Knee Chest Pisiform Contact Adjustment (Fig. 8.24).

Indications: Retrolisthesis of T4 with decreased +Z, −θY and +θZ motions.

Contraindications: All other listings, normal FSU, hypermobility, instability, destruction or fracture of the neural arch or spinous process, infection of the contact vertebra.

Patient position: The patient should be positioned on the knee-chest table so that the thoracic spine is slightly higher than the lumbar spine. There should be a slight incline on the chest support to allow for anterior expansion of the thoracic spine when the posterior to anterior (+Z) thrust is given. The knees should be placed so that the femurs are nearly perpendicular to the floor (see Chapter 7) to accommodate the anterior movement of the stomach. The stabilization strap for the head may be used for this adjustment.

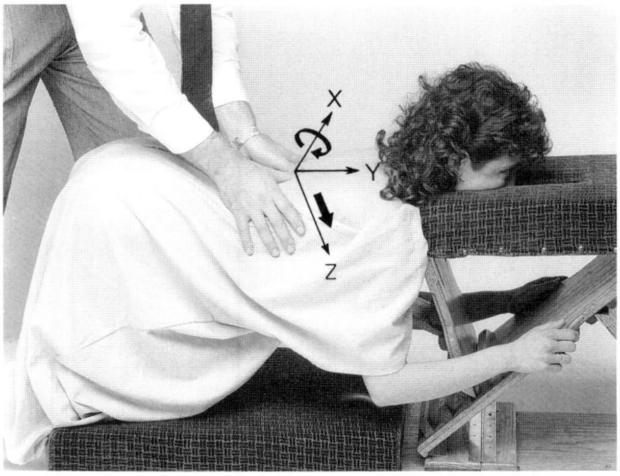

Figure 8.23. T8 P double-thumb contact adjustment.

Doctor's position: Standing on the right side of the patient.

Contact point: The posterior, and right lateral border of the spinous process of T4 is contacted with the cephalad (right) pisiform. The hand will cross the spine.

Supporting hand: Placed over the contact hand.

Pattern of thrust: Posterior to anterior (+Z), lateral to medial (−θY), with an inferiorward arcing motion (+θZ) toward the end of the thrust.

Category by algorithm: Short lever specific contact procedure.

Name of technique: Gonstead

Name of technique procedure: PLI-t (−Z, −θY, −θZ) T3 Knee Chest Pisiform Contact Adjustment (Fig. 8.25).

Indications: Retrolisthesis of T3 with decreased +Z motion and decreased +θY and +θZ motion.

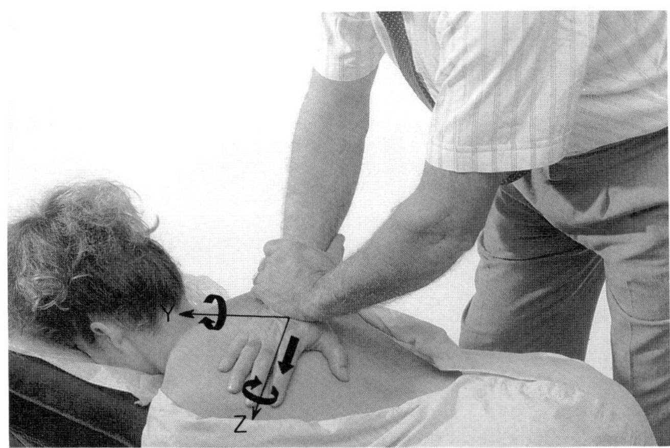

Figure 8.24. T4 PRS pisiform contact adjustment.

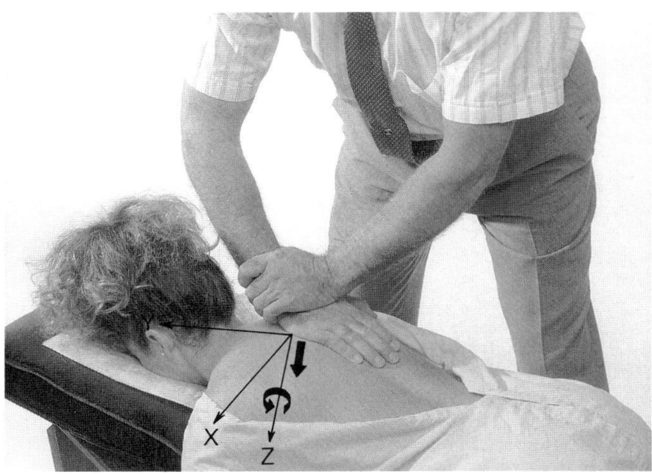

Figure 8.25. T3 PLI-t pisiform contact adjustment.

Contraindications: All other listings, normal FSU, hypermobility, instability, destruction or fracture of the neural arch or right transverse process, infection of the contact vertebra.

Patient position: Knee-chest position. The upper thoracic spine should be slightly higher than the rest of the spine.

Doctor's position: Facing the patient's right side, provided the patient is stable in this position.

Contact point: Right transverse process of T3 with a soft pisiform contact. The contact hand does not cross the spine.

Supporting hand: The left hand is placed on top of the right.

Pattern of thrust: Posterior anterior (+Z) with a clockwise torque (+θZ) toward the end of the thrust.

Category by algorithm: Short lever specific contact procedure.

Name of technique: Gonstead

Name of technique procedure: PRS (−Z, +θY, −θZ) T1 Knee Chest Pisiform Contact Adjustment (Fig. 8.26).

Indications: Retrolisthesis of T1 with decreased +Z, −θY and +θZ motions.

Contraindications: All other listings, normal FSU, hypermobility, instability, destruction or fracture of the neural arch or spinous process, infection of the contact vertebra.

Patient position: The patient should be positioned on the knee-chest table so that the thoracic spine is slightly higher than the lumbar spine. There should be a slight incline on the chest support to allow for anterior expansion of the thoracic spine when the posterior to anterior (+Z) thrust is given. The knees should be placed so that the femurs are nearly perpendicular to the floor (see Chapter 7) to accommodate the anterior movement of the stomach. The stabilization strap for the head should be used for this adjustment (not shown).

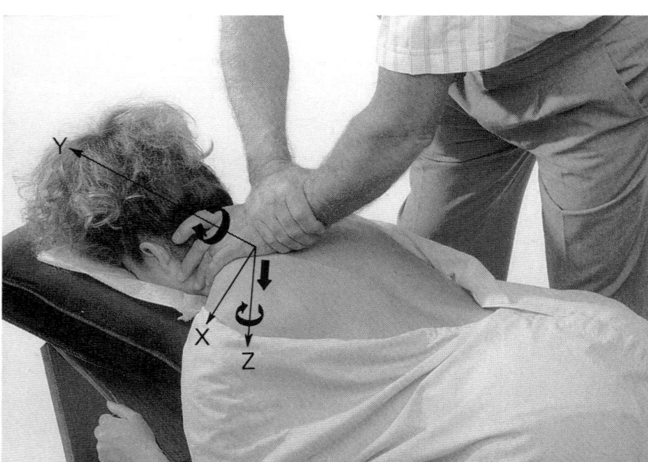

Figure 8.26. T1 PRS pisiform contact adjustment. The stabilization strap is not shown.

Doctor's position: Standing on the right side of the patient.

Contact point: The posterior, and right lateral border of the spinous process of T1 is contacted with the caudal (left) pisiform. The hand will cross the spine.

Supporting hand: Placed over the contact hand.

Pattern of thrust: Posterior to anterior (+Z), lateral to medial (−θY), with an inferiorward arcing motion (+θZ) toward the end of the thrust.

Category by algorithm: Short lever specific contact procedure.

Cervical Chair

The first two or three thoracics may be adjusted in a manner similar to the cervical spine. The wrist is kept fairly neutral as there is less of the radial flexion used in the thrust. The thrust tends to be more from the shoulder. The contact point with the distal end of the first finger is the inferior tip of the spinous process or the transverse process as determined by the listing.

Name of technique: Gonstead

Name of technique procedure: PRI-t (−Z, +θY, +θZ,) T2 Cervical Chair Adjustment (Fig. 8.27).

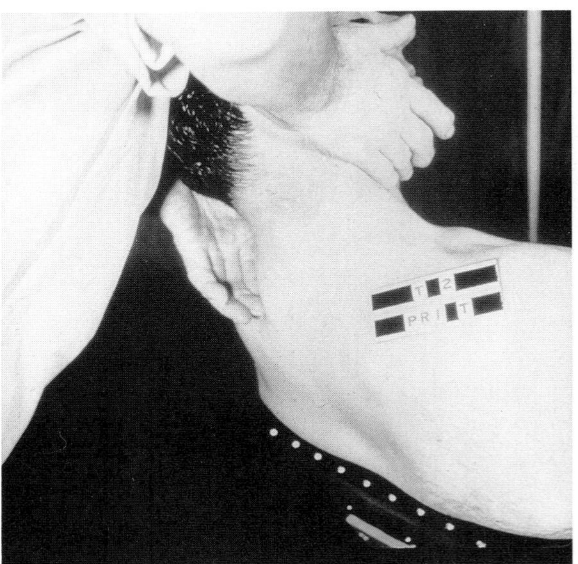

Figure 8.27. T2 PRI-t cervical chair adjustment.

Indications: Retrolisthesis of T2 with decreased +Z motion and decreased $-\theta$Y and $-\theta$Z motion.

Contraindications: All other listings, normal FSU, hypermobility, instability, destruction or fracture of the neural arch or left transverse process, infection of the contact vertebra.

Patient position: Seated in the cervical chair. The stabilization strap should be over the right shoulder unless the patient is of a heavier build.

Doctor's position: Standing behind the patient, favoring the left side.

Contact point: Palmar surface of the left distal phalanx of the index finger placed on the spinous lamina junction of T2 vertebra. The middle finger should be directly adjacent to the index finger to give the index finger stability. The contact hand (L) is stabilized by placing the thumb (not shown) on the ramus of the mandible or the sternocleidomastoid muscle (if the doctor's hand is too small). When the contact hand is properly placed, an arch is formed by the lateral position of the thumb and index finger.

Supporting hand: The right hand is placed so that the palmar surface supports the cervical spine. This will bring the thenar eminence on the sternocleidomastoid muscle and the thumb facing anterior and inferior at a 45° angle. The stabilization should attempt to restrict movement of the foundation for the adjustment (i.e., T3) and segments above the level of subluxation. The illustration shows the doctor stabilizing the head with his chest and stabilization of the middle and upper neck. No thrust, especially posteriorward, should be made with the supporting hand.

Pattern of thrust: Posterior to anterior through the plane line of the disc, slightly medialward, with an inferiorward arcing motion toward the end of the thrust.

Category by algorithm: Short lever specific contact procedure.

Name of technique: Gonstead

Name of technique procedure: PLS ($-$Z, $-\theta$Y, $+\theta$Z,) T2 Cervical Chair Adjustment (Fig. 8.28).

Indications: Retrolisthesis of T2 with decreased +Z motion and decreased $+\theta$Y and $-\theta$Z motion.

Contraindications: All other listings, normal FSU, hypermobility, instability, destruction or fracture of the neural arch or spinous process, infection of the contact vertebra.

Patient position: Seated in the cervical chair. The stabilization strap should be over the right shoulder unless the patient is of a heavier build.

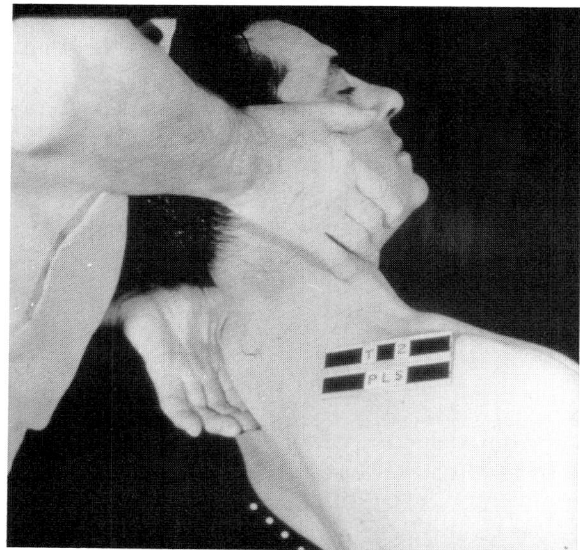

Figure 8.28. T2 PLS cervical chair adjustment.

Doctor's position: Standing behind the patient, favoring the left side.

Contact point: Palmar surface of the left distal phalanx of the index finger placed on the left posterior portion of the spinous process. The middle finger should be directly adjacent to the index finger to give the index finger stability. The contact hand (L) is stabilized by placing the thumb (not shown) on the ramus of the mandible or the sternocleidomastoid muscle (if the doctor's hand is too small). When the contact hand is properly placed, an arch is formed by the lateral position of the thumb and index finger.

Supporting hand: The right hand is placed so that the palmar surface supports the cervical spine. This will bring the thenar eminence on the sternocleidomastoid muscle and the thumb facing anterior and inferior at a 45° angle. The stabilization should attempt to restrict movement of the foundation for the adjustment (i.e., T3) and segments above the level of subluxation. The illustration shows the doctor stabilizing the head with his chest and stabilization of the middle and upper neck. No thrust, especially posteriorward, should be made with the supporting hand.

Pattern of thrust: Posterior to anterior (+Z) through the plane line of the disc, medialward ($+\theta$Y), with an inferiorward arcing motion ($-\theta$Z) toward the end of the thrust.

Category by algorithm: Short lever specific contact procedure.

Rib Adjustments

A rule of thumb for adjustments from the posterior is to adjust the upper half of the rib cage lateral to medial and superior to inferior; the lower half is adjusted somewhat medial to lateral and inferior to superior. The contact point is the rib just lateral to the spine, and a light, quick thrust is used. Occasionally, the contact is the anterior rib at the costochondral junction (See Chapter 16). Rib subluxations are typically found by palpation. An awareness of the condition of the ribs is important before adjusting one, and the rib should be adjusted only after reduction of spinal subluxations has failed to reduce the fixation or symptoms.

ADJUNCTIVE THERAPIES

Additional therapeutic procedures are used as necessary to aid in the reduction of the thoracic subluxation complex. In acute cases, ice may be used. It must be removed when the area feels numb (usually one half hour). Exercises, especially in extension, and postural maneuvers designed to restore normal patterns of motion, may be beneficial. These need to be individually designed to offer optimal biomechanical efficiency. Nutritional support may be necessary, especially in trauma cases requiring repair of damaged tissues. In certain cases of instability, especially in a patient engaged in physical activity that adversely affects the thoracic spine, a back support may be required.

In cases where physical activities exacerbate the thoracic spine subluxation complex, activity retraining to biomechanically efficient activity or even abandonment of the patient's particular occupation or recreational activities may be required. In some acute cases, short-term use of appropriate electrotherapeutic modalities can be beneficial for some patients who otherwise may be unresponsive to care.

In cases of nonresponse or worsening of the condition, referral to another chiropractor, such as one versed in a particular adjustive technique or specializing in internal disorders, neurology, radiology, or orthopaedics, or a medical specialist may be required, particularly in light of the intimate connection between the viscera and the thoracic spine.

REFERENCES

1. Eckert G, Decker A. Pathological studies of the intervertebral discs. J Bone Joint Surg 1947;29:447–454.
2. Nathan H. Osteophytes of the spine compressing the sympathetic trunk and splanchnic nerves in the thorax. Spine 1987;12:527–532.
3. Grieve GP. Common vertebral joint problems. New York: Churchill Livingstone, 1981.
4. Bruckner FE, Greco A, Leung AW. Benign thoracic pain syndrome: role of magnetic resonance imaging in the detection and localization of thoracic disc disease. J Roy Soc Med 1989;82:81–83.
5. Norkin C, Levangie P. Joint structure and function: a comprehensive analysis. Philadelphia: FA Davis Co., 1983.
6. Singer KP, Giles LGF. Manual therapy considerations at the thoracolumbar junction: an anatomical and functional perspective. J Manipulative Physiol Ther 1990;13:83–88.
7. Lee M. Mechanics of spinal joint manipulation in the thoracic and lumbar spine: a theoretical study of posteroanterior force techniques. Clin Biomech 1989;4:249–251.
8. Williams PL, Warwick R, eds. Gray's Anatomy. 36th British ed. Philadelphia: WB Saunders, 1980.
9. White AA. Analysis of the mechanics of the thoracic spine in man. Acta Orthopaedica Scand 1969(suppl):127.
10. Schafer RC. Clinical biomechanics: musculoskeletal actions and reactions. Baltimore: Williams & Wilkins, 1983.
11. Kapandji IA. The physiology of the joints. Vol. 3. The trunk and vertebral column. New York: Churchill Livingstone, 1974:128–166.
12. DeGroots J, Chusid JG. Correlative neuroanatomy. 20th ed. East Norwalk, CT: Appleton and Lange, 1988.
13. Krämer J. Intervertebral disk disease. New York: Thieme Medical Publishers, 1990:114–117.
14. Glasauer FE, Cares HL. Traumatic paraplegia in infancy. JAMA 1972;219:38–41.
15. Taylor AR. The mechanism of injury to the spinal cord in the neck without damage to the vertebral column. J Bone Joint Surg 1951;33B: 543–547.
16. Melzak J. Paraplegia among children. Lancet 1969;July 5:45–48.
17. Brieg A. Adverse mechanical tension in the central nervous system. Stockholm: Almqvist & Wiksell International, 1978.
18. Wyke B. The neurological basis of thoracic spinal pain. Rheum Phys Med 1970;10:356–367.
19. Bogduk N. The innervation of the lumbar spine. Spine 1983;8:286–293.
20. Bogduk N, Twomey LT. Clinical anatomy of the lumbar spine. New York: Churchill Livingstone, 1987:92–102.
21. Mitchell GAG. Anatomy of the autonomic nervous system. London: E and S Livingstone Ltd, 1955:116–118.
22. Randall WC, Cox JW, Alexander WF, Coldwater KB, Hertzman AB. Direct examination of the sympathetic outflows in man. J Appl Physiol 1955;7:688–698.
23. Richter CP, Woodruff BG. Lumbar sympathetic dermatomes in man determined by the electrical skin resistance method. J Neurophysiol 1945;8:323–338.
24. Yochum TR, Rowe LJ. Essentials of skeletal radiology. Baltimore: Williams & Wilkins, 1987.
25. Hensinger RN, MacEwen GD. Congenital anomalies of the spine. In: Rothman RH, Simeone FA. The spine. 2nd ed. Philadelphia: WB Saunders, 1982:220.
26. Lecture notes. Gonstead Seminar of Chiropractic. Mt. Horeb, WI:1990.
27. White AA, Panjabi MM. Clinical biomechanics of the spine. 2nd ed. Philadelphia: JB Lippincott, 1990.
28. Bernhardt M, Bridwell KH. Segmental analysis of the sagittal plane alignment of the normal thoracic and lumbar spines and thoracolumbar junction. Spine 1989;14:717–721.
29. Fon GT, Pitt MJ, Thies AC. Thoracic kyphosis: range in normal subjects. Am J Roentgenol 1980;134:979–983.
30. Voutsinas SA, MacEwen GD. Sagittal profiles of the spine. Clin Orthop 1986;210:235–242.
31. Gregersen GG. Lucas DB. An in vivo study of the axial rotation of the human thoracolumbar spine. J Bone Joint Surg 1967;49A:247–262.
32. Panjabi MM, Brand RA, White AA. Three-dimensional flexibility and stiffness properties of the human thoracic spine. J Biomech 1976;9:185–192
33. Panjabi MM, Brand RA, White AA. Mechanical properties of the human thoracic spine. J Bone Joint Surg 1976;58A:642–652.
34. Zachman ZJ, Bolles S, Bergmann TF, Traina AD. Understanding the anterior thoracic adjustment: (a concept of a sectional subluxation). Chiropractic Technique 1989;Jan/Feb:30–33.
35. Herbst RW. Gonstead chiropractic science and healing art. Mt. Horeb, WI: Sci-Chi Publications, 1968.

36. Fracheboud R, Kraus S, Choiniere B. A survey of anterior thoracic adjustments. Chiropractic 1988;1:89–92.
37. Ross JS, Perez-Reyes N, Masaryk TJ, Bohlman H, Modic MT. Thoracic disk herniation: MR imaging. Radiolology 1987;165:511–515.
38. Otani K, Yoshida M, Fujii E, Nakai S, Shibasaki K. Thoracic disc herniation: surgical treatment in 23 patients. Spine 1988;13:1262–1267.
39. Bradford DS, Moe JH, Winter RB. Scoliosis and kyphosis. In: Rothman RH, Simeone FA, eds. The spine. 2nd ed. Philadelphia: WB Saunders, 1982:398–401.
40. Yablon JS, Kasdon DL, Levine H. Thoracic cord compression in Scheuermann's disease. Spine 1988;13:896–898.
41. Roth M, Lambert H, Chiuchen K. Hernie disease thoracique double et malade de Scheuermann: Apropos d'un cas. Rev Med Suisse Romande 1965;85:296.
42. Muller R. Protrusion of thoracic intervertebral disc with compression of the spinal cord. Acta Med Scand 1951;139:99–104.
43. Bradford DS, Garcia A. Neurological complications in Scheuermann's disease. J Bone Joint Surg 1969;51A:567–572.
44. Bruckner FE, Allard SA, Moussa NA. Benign thoracic pain. J Roy Soc Med 1987;80:286–289.
45. Bourne IHJ. Benign thoracic pain. J Roy Soc Med 1988;81:123–124.
46. Watts RA. Benign thoracic pain. J Roy Soc Med 1987;80:660–661.
47. Gatterman B. Etiological considerations of thoracic spine stenosis. D.C. Tracts 1990;2(2):57–60.
48. Murphy DR. Myofascial pain and pseudocardiac disease. Dynamic Chiropractic May 10, 1991;9(10):8.
49. Myers GE. When angina is a pain in the neck. Medical World News 1977: April 18.
50. West HG. When angina is a pain in the neck. D.C. Tracts 1989;1(3):141–142.
51. Sellman MS, Mayer RF. Thoracoabdominal radiculopathy. Southern Med J 1988;81:199–201.
52. Marinacci AA, Courville CB. Radicular syndromes simulating intra-abdominal surgical conditions. Am Surg 1962;28:59–63.
53. Cremata EE, Plaugher G, Cox WA. Technique system application: the Gonstead approach. Chiropractic Technique 1991;3:19–25.
54. Gunn CC, Milbrandt WE. Early and subtle signs in low back sprain. Spine 1978;3:267–81.
55. Cipriano JJ. Photographic manual of regional orthopedic tests. Baltimore: Williams & Wilkins, 1985.
56. West HG. Physical and spinal examination procedures utilized in the practice of chiropractic. In: Haldeman S, ed. Modern developments in the principles and practice of chiropractic. New York: Appleton-Century-Crofts, 1980:269–296.
57. Plaugher G, Lopes MA, Melch PE, Cremata EE. The inter- and intraexaminer reliability of a paraspinal skin temperature differential instrument. J Manipulative Physiol Ther 1991;14:361–67.
58. Wright HM, Korr IM, Thomas PE. Local and regional variations in cutaneous vasomotor tone of the human trunk. Neural Transmission 1960;22:34–52.
59. Faye LJ. Motion palpation and chiropractic technique. Huntington Beach, CA: Motion Palpation Institute, 1990.
60. Magee DJ. Orthopedic physical assessment. Philadelphia: WB Saunders, 1987.
61. Plaugher G. Skin temperature assessment for neuromusculoskeletal abnormalities of the spinal column: a review of the literature. J Manipulative Physiol Ther 1992;(July/Aug).
62. Aragona RJ. Vol VII: Efficient clinical procedures for reducing thoracic biomechanical instability distortion coefficients of V.S.S. and V.S.C. Manchester, NH:1985:54–68.
63. Plaugher G, Lopes MA. The knee chest table: indications and contraindications. Chiropractic Technique 1990;2:163–167.

9 Scoliosis

GREGORY PLAUGHER with the assistance of MARK A. LOPES

Hippocrates first described the type of deformity whereby the spine deviates laterally; however, it was Galen (A.D. 131–201) who actually coined the term *scoliosis*. Galen also created the terms lordosis and kyphosis to describe postural deviations in the sagittal plane. Today, *scoliosis* is defined as being an appreciable lateral curvature of the spine in the coronal plane. Most authors consider a deviation greater than 10° (Cobb's method) to be a scoliosis, and a curve less than 10°, a convexity. This chapter will provide a literature review of scoliosis, especially scolioses afflicting the adolescent, classifications of curvatures, and, treatment and management strategies that may prove beneficial for this often crippling disorder.

BACK PAIN

Back pain associated with adolescent scoliosis appears not to have a higher incidence than the population of adolescents as a whole; however, adult scoliotic patients do seem to have a higher incidence of back pain (1). With age, many curvatures progress, albeit slowly, possibly explaining the higher incidence of back pain in adult scoliotics.

VISCERAL DISTURBANCES

It has been hypothesized that scoliosis is associated with visceral disturbances (2). The osteodegenerative changes that occur around the nerve roots in patients with scoliosis may affect visceral function through somatovisceral reflexes. Whether scoliotic individuals have higher incidences of visceral pathology has not yet been determined. Severe curvature, however, especially in the thoracic spine, has been associated with cardiac and pulmonary complications caused by compression of the lungs and vessels of the heart (3,4).

EARLY DEATH

Autopsy studies have revealed an interesting correlation between severe curvature and the average age of death. More severe curvature is related to earlier death. Moreover, the mean age of death (30–50 years) was especially correlative if the curves had started during adolescence (5–7).

In the long-term, patients with scoliosis show a marked increase in mortality, with the cause of death in 60% of cases being cardiopulmonary complications (8). Another long-term follow-up study (9) revealed similar results with a population of severe scoliotics. It is noted, however, that no radiographs were obtained during this study; therefore, the exact amount (degree) of curvature was not determined. It was concluded that the mortality rate of a patient with a severe scoliosis (>80°) is well over 100% when compared with the general population. Thoracogenic, congenital and neurogenic scoliosis were found to have a worse prognosis when compared with the idiopathic, rachitogenic or poliomyelitic types of scoliosis. Nachemson's study (9) revealed the cause of death in 80% of cases to be kyphoscoliotic cardiopathy with cor pulmonale.

COSMETIC DEFORMITY

Scoliosis is also an obvious cosmetic deformity that may have an effect on the personality of the individual. Specific psychological disorders or behaviors associated with scoliosis are not known. In one study (8) it was noted that 76% of the females involved in the investigation did not marry.

ETIOLOGY

There are many different causes for scoliosis. Most authors identify scoliosis as a multifactorial disorder involving mostly genetic and growth factors. It has been estimated that 80% of all scolioses have no singular identifiable cause (10). Idiopathic scoliosis is the major focus of this chapter.

Structural vs. Functional

Structural scolioses are those that remain in a curved position during forward bending. Nonstructural or functional scolioses are those curves that remit or improve during forward bending. Functional scolioses are commonly associated with leg length inequality. Lateral bending should improve a functional curve, whereas, in using the same movement, a structural curve will remain. There may be levels of the functional curve, however, which will exhibit some asymmetry of motion due to the beginning effects of ligamentous creep at the motion segment. Although the adolescent idiopathic scoliosis is commonly referred to as a structural curve, this may not be the case during the beginning stages of the disorder. A functional curve caused by a lateral flexion malposition of a spinal segment will, over time, undergo bone remodeling because of Heuter Volkmann's or Wolff's law, thereby creating a structural curve.

Classifications for Scoliosis

A review of the literature indicates that approximately 80% of scolioses have no known cause. The chiropractic community may find this number to be arguable. The chiropractic specialty revolves around subtle and large changes in the spinal column which may be associated with abnormal structure or function.

To learn more about biomechanical causes for scoliosis, case reports and case control studies of successes and failures in scoliotic patients need to be performed. Large populational studies could be performed with scoliosis patients, thereby allowing for a classification system that would be more reflective of the type of patient encountered in private chiropractic practice. Without this much needed research, chiropractic would surely follow the obtuse course of medicine whereby most cases have no known cause. A biomechanical approach, which emphasizes the subtle interactions between structure and function, needs to be used to direct treatment at the cause of the curvature rather than at the reaction to the dysfunctional motion segment.

The approximately 20% of cases that do have an identifiable cause, have varied etiologies. Winter has provided the majority of the categories for scoliosis classification (11). Additional categories that appear to be unique to the chiropractic profession have been included by the author:

Structural Scoliosis

- I. Idiopathic
  - A. Infantile (0–3 years)
    - 1. Resolving
    - 2. Progressive
  - B. Juvenile (3–10 years)
  - C. Adolescent (>10 years) (most common; 80% of all curves)
- II. Neuromuscular
  - A. Neuropathic
    - 1. Upper motor neuron lesion
      - a. Cerebral palsy
      - b. Spinocerebellar degeneration
        - i. Friedrich's disease
        - ii. Charcot-Marie-Tooth disease
        - iii. Roussy-Levy disease
      - c. Syringomyelia
      - d. Spinal cord tumor
      - e. Spinal cord trauma
    - 2. Lower motor neuron lesion
      - a. Poliomyelitis
      - b. Traumatic
      - c. Spinal muscular atrophy
        - i. Werdnig-Hoffman
        - ii. Kugelberg-Welander
      - d. Myelomeningocele (paralytic)
    - 3. Dysautonomia (Riley-Day)
  - B. Myopathic
    - 1. Arthrogryposis
    - 2. Muscular dystrophy
      - a. Duchenne (pseudohypertrophic)
      - b. Limb girdle
      - c. Facioscapulohumeral
    - 3. Fiber type disproportion
    - 4. Congenital hypotonia
    - 5. Myotonia dystrophica
- III. Congenital
  - A. Failure of formation
    - 1. Hemivertebrae (Fig. 9.1)
    - 2. Unilateral sacral inferiority (hemivertebra of S1)
  - B. Failure of segmentation
    - 1. Unilateral (unsegmented bar)
    - 2. Bilateral
    - 3. Mixed
- IV. Neurofibromatosis
- V. Mesenchymal disorders
  - A. Marfan's
  - B. Ehlers-Danlos
- VI. Rheumatoid disease
- VII. Trauma
  - A. Fracture
  - B. Surgical
    - 1. Postlaminectomy
    - 2. Postthoracoplasty
  - C. Irradiation

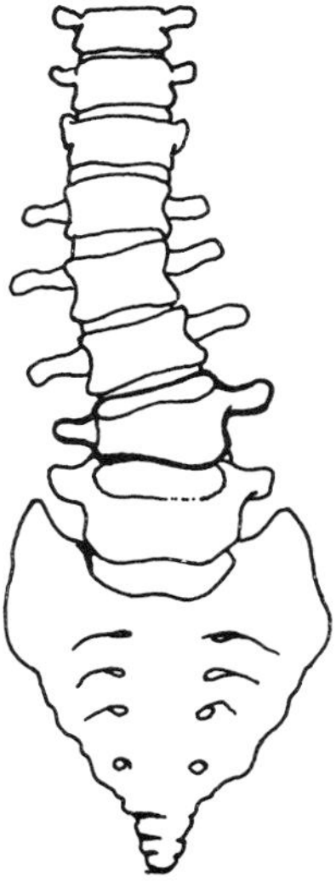

Figure 9.1. Biomechanical effect of a wedge vertebra. The patient has usually had years for adaptation to take place before the anomaly is discovered. Asymmetrical compression fracture can cause a wedge-like configuration of the vertebral body. In these instances, the demands in terms of adaptation are often greater than the ability of the spinal compensatory mechanism. The degenerated spine will have even less tolerance for this acute adaptational disturbance. There is often associated anterior/posterior plateau asymmetry that causes compensatory reactions in the sagittal plane as well.

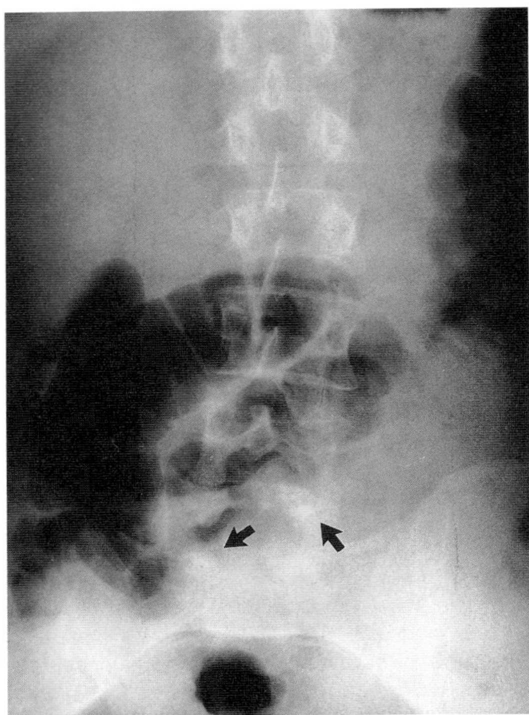

Figure 9.2. Spondylolisthesis with spondylolysis may at times present with other anomalies such as asymmetrical bony elements which cause scoliosis. Often, young scoliosis patients are monitored with only an AP radiograph. Without the lateral radiograph, important information may be missed. Two orthogonal radiographic exposures are mandatory for a minimal radiographic evaluation. Figure 9.2 is a radiograph of a patient with a lateral spinal deviation beginning at the level of a spondylolisthesis.

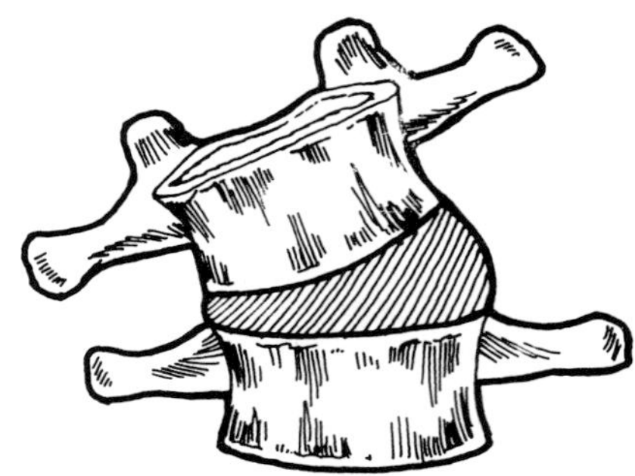

Figure 9.3. Lateral flexion (θZ) positional dyskinesia caused by disc lesions or other factors often will result in a compensatory lateral deviation above.

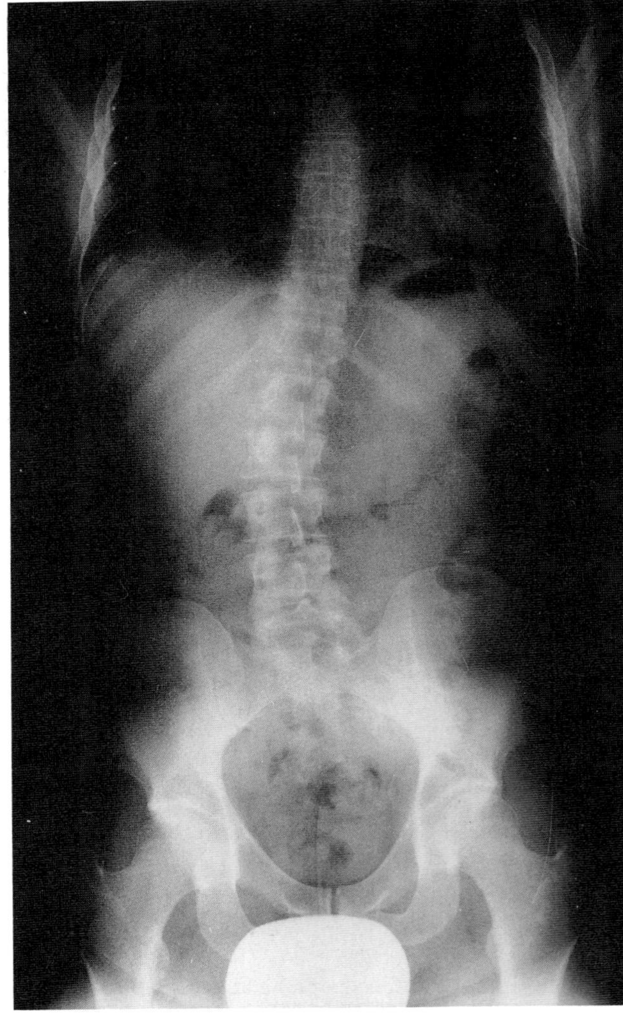

Figure 9.4. AP radiograph showing the effect of leg length inequality on the development of scoliosis.

VIII. Extraspinal contractures
  A. Postempyema
  B. Post burns
IX. Osteochondrodystrophies
  A. Diastrophic dwarfism
  B. Mucopolysaccharidoses (e.g., Morquio's syndrome)
  C. Spondyloepiphyseal dysplasia
  D. Multiple epiphyseal dysplasia
X. Infection of bone
  A. Acute
  B. Chronic
XI. Metabolic disorders
  A. Rickets
  B. Osteogenesis imperfecta
  C. Homocystinuria
XII. Related to lumbosacral joint
  A. Congenital anomalies of the lumbosacral region
    1. Unilateral sacral inferiority (See Congenital)
  B. Spondylolysis and spondylolisthesis (Fig. 9.2)
XIII. Tumors
  A. Vertebral column
    1. Osteoid osteoma
    2. Hystiocytosis X
  B. Spinal cord (see neuromuscular)

Nonstructural or Functional Scoliosis

I. Postural scoliosis
II. Hysterical scoliosis
III. Nerve root irritation
  A. Herniation of the intervertebral disc

B. Disc block subluxation (12) (Fig. 9.3)
C. Tumors
IV. Segmental (Fig. 9.3) and postural positional dyskinesia
V. Inflammatory (e.g., appendicitis)
VI. Related to leg length inequality (Fig. 9.4)
VII. Related to contractures about the hip

INFANTILE IDIOPATHIC SCOLIOSIS

Infantile scoliosis appears at birth or sometime before the age of three. Most (80–90%) remit spontaneously; therefore, no treatment is indicated. Those curves that do progress usually become quite severe and disabling. Infantile scoliosis is seen predominantly in the male and is usually left thoracic in nature. Mehta (13) has devised a rib angle differential measurement which appears to be helpful in distinguishing those curves that are likely to progress (14) (Fig. 9.5).

JUVENILE IDIOPATHIC SCOLIOSIS

Juvenile scoliosis is detected after the age of three and before puberty (Fig. 9.6A-D). Unfortunately, most of these curves are progressive in nature. If treatment is not directed in the early stages, severe deformity can result. Most curves begin before the age of ten and there is a preponderance in females (15).

Observation is very important in the juvenile group, because the great majority of these curves do progress. After initial examinations are performed, follow up radiographic examinations should be performed at approximately 4- to 6-month intervals. During the growth spurt, curve progression is greatest, making careful monitoring important. After the growth spurt, most curves have little progression. Many scolioses that started in the juvenile stage are discovered during adolescence. There are no sharp lines of differentiation between the varying age groups.

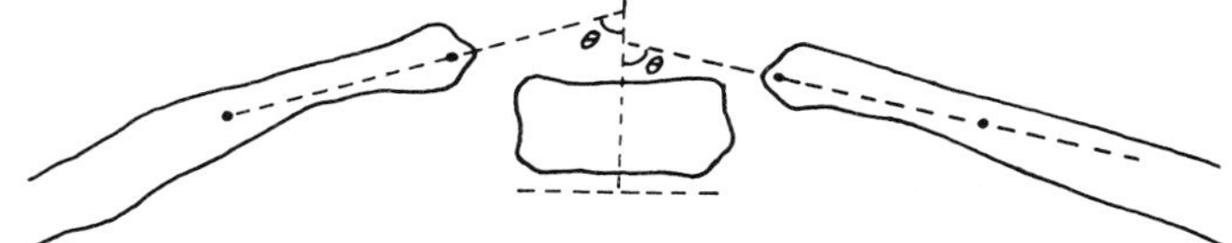

Figure 9.5. Shows the method of measurement for determining the rib-vertebra angles. If the difference between the right and left angles is >20°, then progression is likely for the infant. Kristmundsdottir and coworkers (14) found that if the rib-vertebra angle on the convex side (measured at the apex) is <68° then progression is also likely. From Mehta MH. The rib-vertebra angle in the early diagnosis between resolving and progressive infantile scoliosis. J Bone Joint Surg 1972;54B:230–243.

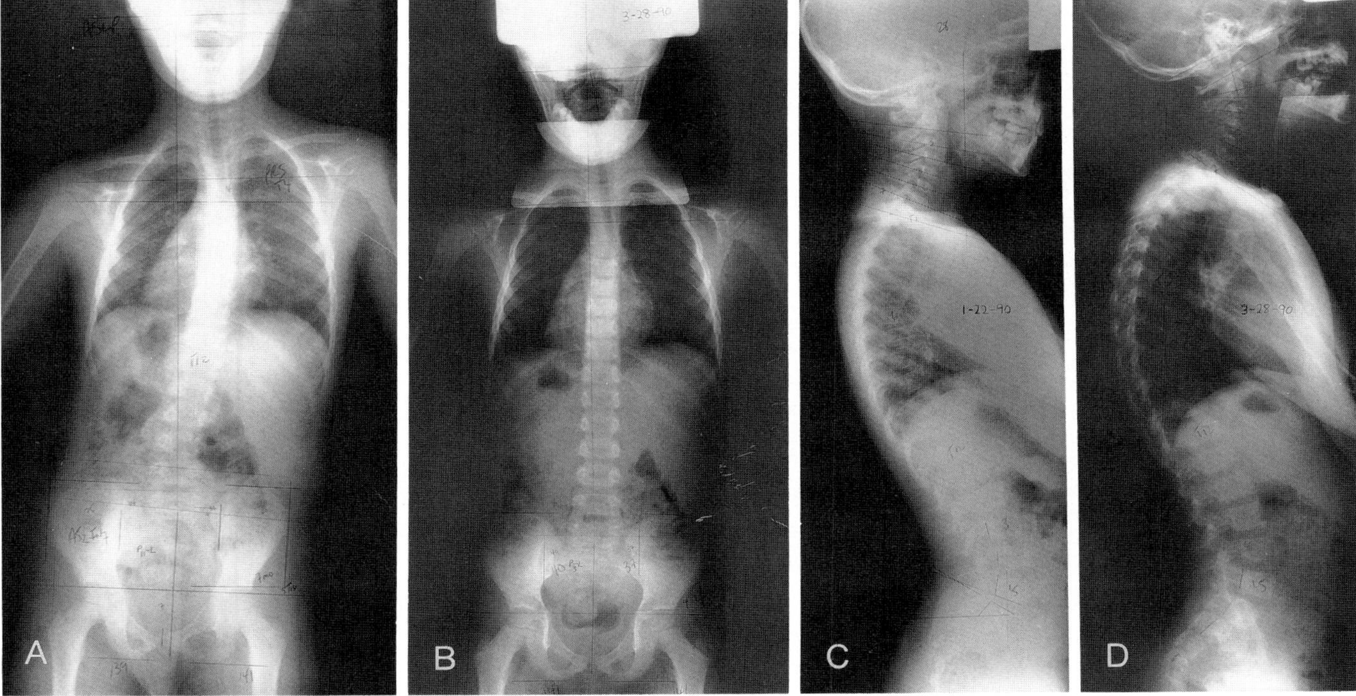

Figure 9.6. Juvenile scoliosis. This is an example of a nonantalgic rotational lesion (P-L, $+\theta Y$) of the sacrum causing a lateral deviation through the normal coupling mechanism of the spine. The left sacroiliac and T4-T5 articulations were adjusted. The comparative radiographs were taken after two months of chiropractic care (i.e., spinal adjustments). The AP radiographs demonstrate a marked reduction in the sacral rotation and lateral spinal deviation. The initial radiograph was taken on 1-22-90 (**A**) and the comparative one on 3-28-90 (**B**). **C,** Initial lateral radiograph. **D,** Posttreatment view.

ADOLESCENT IDIOPATHIC SCOLIOSIS

Most forms of scoliosis fall into the adolescent idiopathic type (Fig. 9.7A-B). The age range is from the onset of puberty to adulthood or skeletal maturity. The adolescent curve is usually discovered shortly after puberty. Curves greater than 20° tend to be more common in females, but the male to female ratio approaches 1:1 for curves less than 20°.

It is interesting to note that adolescent scoliosis patients are taller and heavier than their peers (16). The height change may be partially due to the thoracic hypokyphosis commonly observed.

Not all adolescent curves are progressive. This variation has been a problem in documenting the efficacy of a given treatment. It is rare, however, for the adolescent curvature to spontaneously improve as seen in the infantile types. Monitoring curve progression is especially important during the rapid skeletal development phase. It is complicated by the fact that onsets of puberty are quite varied from individual to individual. The time taken to reach skeletal maturation is also quite varied. For instance, individuals may take from two to five years to mature.

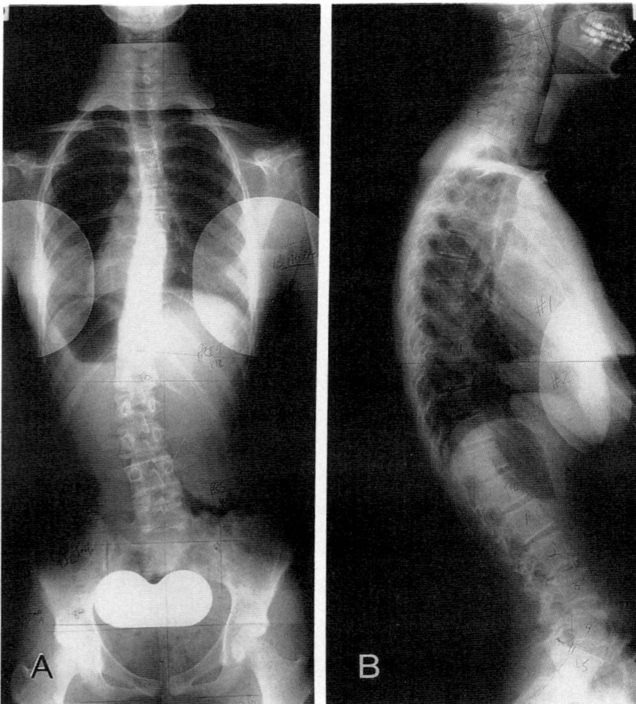

Figure 9.7. Adolescent scoliosis. **A,** This adolescent female has a number of anomalies, including spina bifida at L5 with sacralization and an anatomical short leg on the left. There are 4 lumbar and 13 thoracic vertebrae. A lateral flexion malposition ($-\theta Z$) is present at L4. Notice the placement of radiographic shielding for the breasts, gonads and thyroid. **B,** The lateral full spine shows abnormal posture in the sagittal plane. There is retrolisthesis of L4 on the sacralized L5 with hyperextension of the mid and upper lumbar vertebrae.

The average age of menarche is 12½ to 13½ in American girls, but approximately 1 to 2% of all females have not menstruated by the age of 16 (17). Males have an onset of puberty between the ages of 9½ and 13½. Growth usually ceases between the ages of 13 and 17. After the growth spurt, most curves (both male and female) have little progression.

Three-Dimensional Perspective

Most adolescent scoliotics present with not only a lateral deviation of the spinal column in the coronal plane, but also a flattening of the normal kyphosis, viewed from the sagittal plane. The normal kyphosis of the thoracic spine can be thought of as rotating toward one side or the other, thereby creating two dysfunctions simultaneously—scoliosis and hypokyphosis. It is integral to the examination when seeking biomechanical causes for scoliosis to look at the lateral radiograph for signs of dysfunction in the sagittal plane.

EXAMINATION

Those examinations that are specific to scoliosis are presented here. The spinal examination is presented in Chapters 4 and 5.

Posture

Postural analysis is essential to the examination and can be performed physically and radiographically. The analysis is performed in part to determine which curves are compensated. Compensation refers to the spine assuming a horizontal or level position in response to a postural dysfunction.

Anterior carriage of the head is a common finding in patients with scoliosis. This is commonly due to dysfunction in the lower spine rather than in the neck itself.

In the coronal plane, compensated curves with the rib cage centered over the pelvis have usually been present for the longest duration. Rib and shoulder girdle remodeling is usually extensive and these curves hold a poor prognosis for correction (Fig. 9.8). The well-compensated curve is also unlikely to progress. Adult scoliotics tend to have very well compensated curves. Uncompensated patterns occur more often in the juvenile or adolescent or in the acute patient with antalgia.

Radiography

The radiographic examination will give the most detailed information with regard to posture and compensation reaction. This examination usually entails a minimum of an AP and a lateral full spine radiograph.

The AP radiograph includes an evaluation for leg length inequality and associated pelvic posture. For a

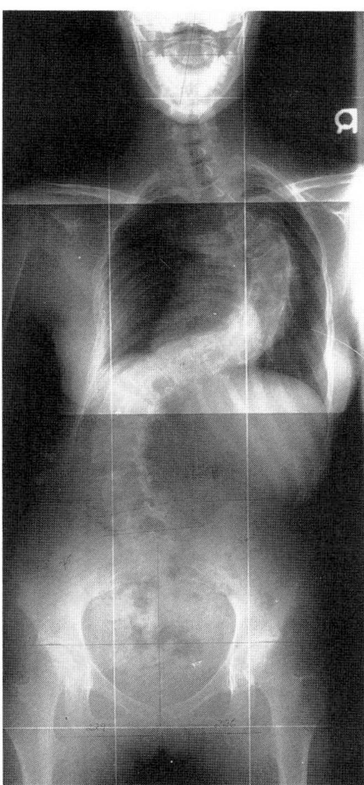

Figure 9.8. This 19-year-old female patient has a well-compensated 90° scoliosis. Lack of proper treatment during the child's growing years resulted in this situation. She presented for chiropractic evaluation with complaints of migraine headaches and dysmenorrhea. Treatment consisted of adjustments at L5-S1 and gentle mobilization at the apices of the double major curvature.

complete treatise on the evaluation of leg length and appropriate orthotic or lift therapy the reader is directed to Chapter 6.

The radiographic examination should include those views necessary to determine skeletal maturity. Skeletal maturity is determined through observation, radiologic analysis, and a careful history, which includes the age of menarche in the female. The iliac crest, visible on the AP full spine or on the AP pelvic radiograph, is best evaluated using the Risser method (18). The crest is divided into four quadrants, and the epiphyseal excursion grade is calculated by determining the extent of excursion (Fig. 9.9):

Grade 1 = 25% excursion
Grade 2 = 50% excursion
Grade 3 = 75% excursion
Grade 4 = 100% excursion
Grade 5 = Full excursion and complete fusion of the ilium to the epiphysis

The vertebral body epiphysis can also be of help in determining skeletal maturity because complete fusion of the epiphysis to the body occurs at the cessation of vertebral growth. The lateral film best visualizes the vertebral epiphysis.

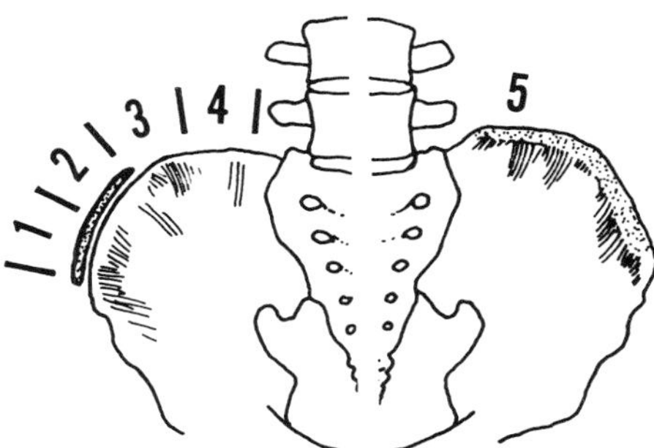

Figure 9.9. Risser's sign. A Risser sign of 2 or less indicates a high likelihood of curve progression. A Risser sign of 5 is depicted on the *right*.

TECHNOLOGY

Because breast tissue is highly sensitive to radiation, the AP radiograph should be performed with adequate shielding or, in the absence of shielding, in a posterior to anterior fashion. Thorough x-ray shielding is important during all radiographic examinations, and this is especially true in the young, because maturing bone marrow is a very radiosensitive tissue.

Eighty-four inches or greater film focal distance (FFD) should be used. This will result in less skin dose to the patient (19) and also decrease the extent of magnification distortion. Appropriate patient identifying information should be present on the film, including technologic factors for the radiograph. Film focal distance is especially important in order that future technicians can use similar technique. Keeping the FFD constant, although not affecting angular measurements on the film, will remove one variable should the amount of the scoliosis angle change due to improper patient positioning during the examination.

A supplemental radiograph of importance, is the sacral base tilt or Fergusen projection (Fig. 9.10). This view is taken posterior to anterior or anterior to posterior depending on facility limitations and is performed with gonadal shielding. Visualization of the L5-S1 disc space in the standing position is done with this view as well as determination of the presence of anomalies at the lumbosacral junction, especially unilateral sacral inferiority (20).

The Cobb's method of measurement is preferred for analysis of the curvature of scoliosis. A report by Goldberg indicated an average intraobserver disagreement of 1.9° (21). Figure 9.11A and B details the method of mensuration.

Lateral flexion x-rays should be performed to ascertain the flexibility of the curvature and to determine potential sites for spinal adjustment. These motion segments would exhibit fixation dysfunction in a particular plane of motion due to soft tissue effects. All attempts must be made to differentiate between fixation dysfunc-

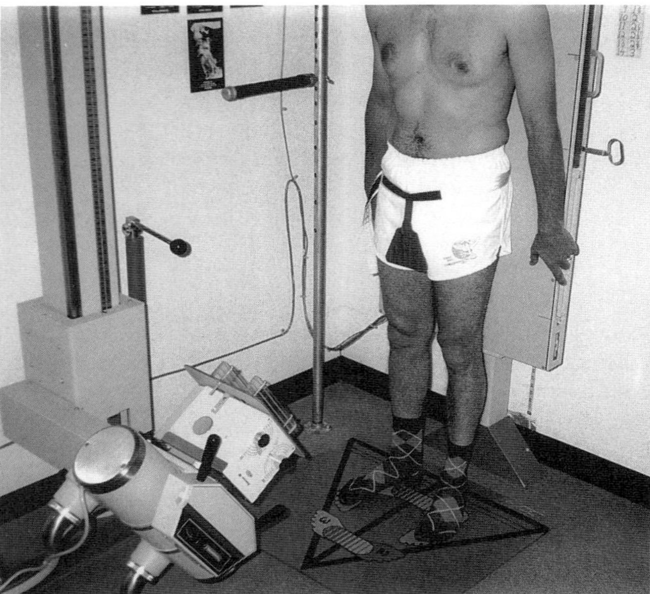

Figure 9.10. Patient positioning for the sacral base tilt-up radiograph. This positioning will demonstrate the L5-S1 disc space and disclose malformations such as wedged vertebrae or disc space asymmetries.

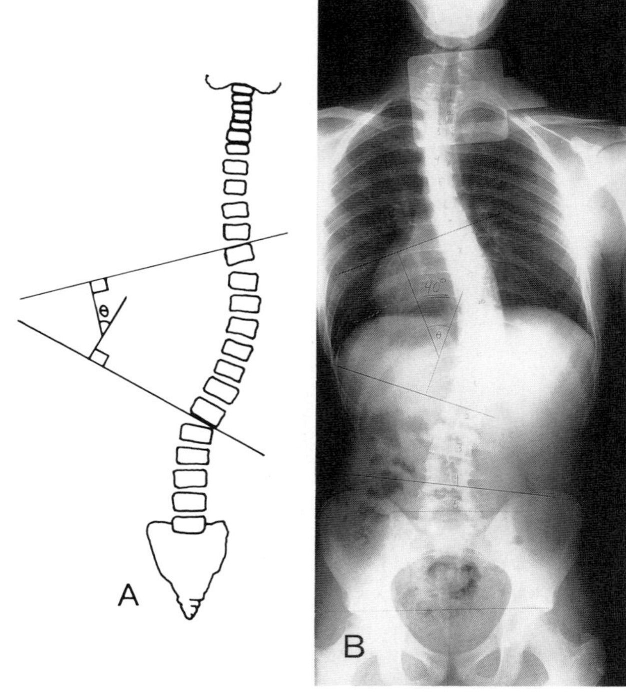

Figure 9.11. **A,** Cobb's scoliosis measurement is depicted. *Lines* are drawn representing the lateral tilt of the two most angulated vertebrae towards the concavity of the curve. From these lines, *perpendicular lines* are drawn which then intersect forming the angle θ. Comparative examinations must use the identical end-vertebrae for their analyses. As can be seen from the picture, slight changes in the angulation of one end-vertebra, would have a pronounced effect on the measured angle. **B,** This adolescent male has a Cobb's angle of 40°.

tion and motion restriction caused by anomalous changes in the vertebrae themselves.

Tomography, helpful in evaluating congenital problems, may also be indicated along with other advanced imaging such as computerized axial tomography (CT) or magnetic resonance imaging (MRI).

Physical Examination

In addition to the normal spinal examination, for the presence of vertebral lesions, the orthopaedic examination includes Adam's maneuver (Fig. 9.12). This test simply stresses the vertebral column making a functional curve remit and a structural one appear as a raised area lateral to the spine due to axial rotation of the vertebrae.

The clinician should also be watchful for the presence of café-au-lait spots which may indicate neurofibromatosis. A patch of hair over the lumbosacral region may indicate a diastematomyelia and abnormal scarring with extreme elasticity of the skin may be indicative of Ehlers-Danlos syndrome.

HANDEDNESS

In a report by Goldberg and Dowling (22), an attempt was made to determine correlation, if any, between the convex side of a scoliosis and the handedness of the individual. The sample of 254 females had curve patterns assessed in terms of the lower thoracic portion only. Of 228 right-handed children, 197 had a right convex curve. The 26 left-handed children had convexities to the left in 12 cases. The correlation between scoliosis configuration and handedness, although not occurring in every instance, was statistically significant.

CURVE PROGRESSION

The natural history of scoliosis must be considered before evaluating the effectiveness of a given treatment. A lateral curvature has been shown to do one of three things during the child's development:

1. Progress; the largest amount occurring during growth spurts.
2. Remain stationary.
   a. Adult curves; those with only a single scoliosis and those which are past skeletal maturity.
   b. Functional curves; especially those seen with leg length inequality which appear to have little tendency towards progression.
3. Spontaneously improve or remit commonly seen in infants and to a much lesser extent in adolescents.

Treatment, therefore, must be effective in altering the natural history of the disease before it can be of any value.

Although manipulation is not a contraindication for scoliosis patients and most likely has a positive effect on back pain, especially in the adult (10), spinal adjustments should be directed at eliminating the cause of the curvature. Though adjustments may be helpful in managing pain the patient is experiencing, a rapidly progressive scoliosis (>50°) in an adolescent or juvenile should be managed by both the chiropractor and an orthopaedist familiar with the disorder.

Slowing or stopping the advance of a progressive scoliosis is a positive clinical result. Improving or correcting progressive or stationary curves is another positive result. Intervention must be evaluated in light of the specific natural history of that patient's curve. Chiropractic care must be objectively evaluated, especially in those cases in which spontaneous improvement was likely regardless of the form of treatment.

Determining which curves will progress is somewhat difficult. Clarisse (23) found that curve progression past 30° was documented in 53% of the cases in which the patient's initial curves were in the range of between 10° to 29°. When evaluating curve progression in the pre-menstrual patients, 12% of lumbar curves progressed, as did 42% of single thoracic curves and 67% of double major curves.

Another study (24) involving 727 patients showed that curve progression was intimately associated with skeletal maturity (Risser sign), age of menarche and type of curvature (double, thoracolumbar, etc.) present. Progression greater than 10° in curves less than 19° and progression of 5° for curves between 20° and 29° was considered significant. Spontaneous remission occurred in about 11% of the cases. Menarche had occurred in 68% of the patients with a nonprogressive curve and in only 32% of the patients with progressive scoliosis. For curves less than 19° and also having a Risser sign of 2, 3 or 4, there was little progression (<2%). However, 68% of patients with 20 to 29° curvatures with a Risser sign of 0 or 1 were progressive. The magnitude, as well as the pattern of the curve, have effects on progression (Fig. 9.13).

The follow-up in a premenstrual patient with a double major curve needs to be quite aggressive because the majority of these curves do progress (Fig. 9.14A-B). The follow-up in adults with single curves less than 20° needs to be less frequent. Radiographic guidelines for comparative examinations after chiropractic treatment are undefined. If the curve has been determined to be progressive, then a comparative radiographic examination after 3 to 6 months is not unusual. If the physical examination findings are inconsistent with the radiologic picture, then reexamination is in order.

CHIROPRACTIC RESEARCH

Scientific evidence substantiating the uses of different therapies in the treatment of scoliosis is lacking. The Milwaukee brace, which for years was the mainstay of conservative management of idiopathic scoliosis, has never been adequately tested (25,26).

Similarly, chiropractors have claimed success with scoliotic individuals (20,27), but to date no clinical trials (controlled or otherwise) have been performed. Case reports, for which there are little technical difficulties in performing, are sorely missing (28). Controlled studies are difficult at times to perform, because withholding treatment in this often crippling disorder is unethical. Retrospective studies would be a beginning for our research endeavors in this area. One report (29) demonstrated no significant change in curvature after 9 adjustments in a series of 13 adult patients. Another study (30) showed significant reduction in lumbar scoliosis after a combination of manipulation and lift therapy. Others (31) have demonstrated the benefits of lift therapy in the adult with scoliosis.

Figure 9.12. Adam's test. Two rib humps (lumbar and thoracic) indicating structural asymmetry are shown.

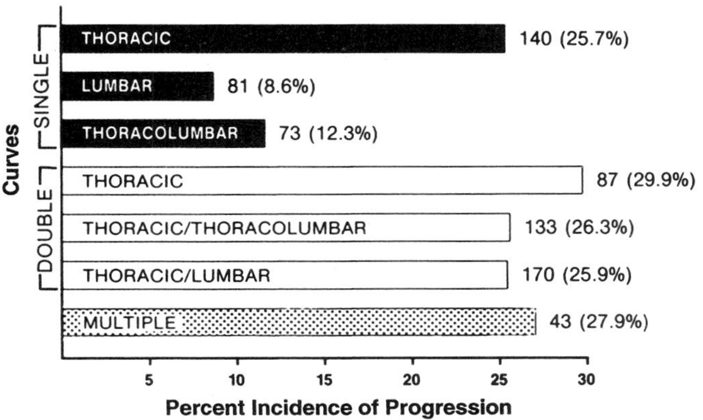

Figure 9.13. Incidence of scoliosis progression. Modified from Lonstein JE, Carlson JM. The prediction of curve progression in untreated idiopathic scoliosis during growth. J Bone Joint Surg 1984;66A:1061–1071.

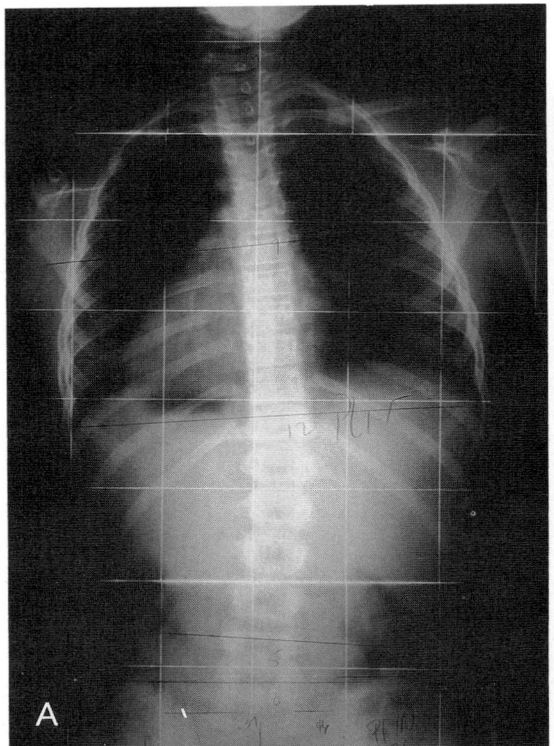

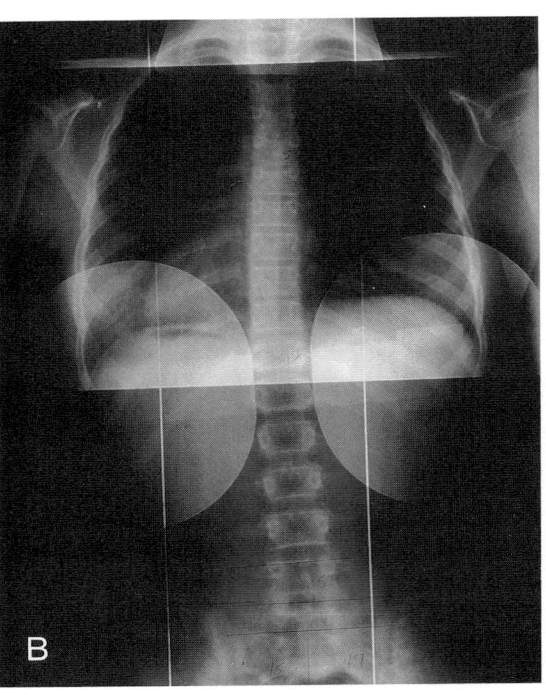

Figure 9.14. Spinal curvature in an adolescent. **A,** Pretreatment radiograph. **B,** Curvature that has reversed the direction of laterality after a series of spinal adjustments. This case demonstrates the need for comparative examination to evaluate the effectiveness or lack thereof of treatment.

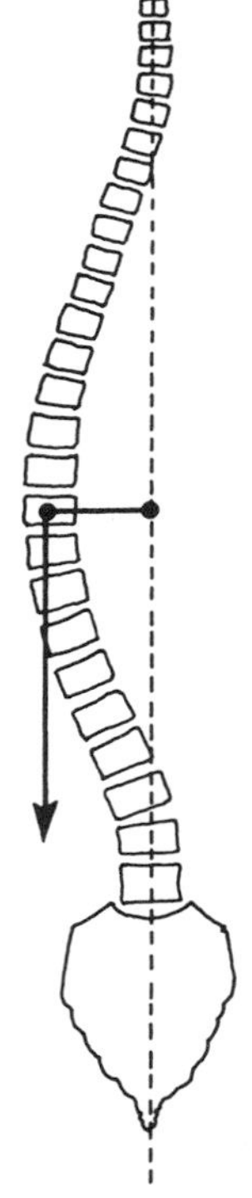

Figure 9.15. Lateral deviation creates asymmetrical loads on the motion segments, predisposing them to injury.

CHIROPRACTIC MANAGEMENT

The specific short lever arm adjustment is designed to restore function at a dysfunctional motion segment. Because scoliosis is a global postural problem, finding the causes of the curvature is difficult but important.

The most caudal portion of the curve may be the genesis of the scoliosis. Lateral flexion malpositions have been suggested (20,32) to be significant areas of involvement in the scoliotic patient. These malpositions could be due to disc, or disc and posterior joint trauma. The apex of the curvature is another likely site for dysfunction. The long lever arm (Fig. 9.15) at this area allows a large lateralward moment to be created on the spine because of the force of gravity. This stress is concentrated on the motion segment at the apex of the scoliosis.

If it is determined that the apex is freely movable, then adjustments are contraindicated. Mobile and hypermobile functional spinal units are contraindicated for any manipulative therapy. Intersegmental spinal mobility is best evaluated with stress plane film analysis or videofluoroscopy.

It is important to approach all adjustments from the convexity of the curve to reduce the likelihood of increasing the deviation. Generally, this is also probably the best approach for reducing the curvature.

Disturbances in the vestibular apparatus have been associated with scoliosis patients (33). Also, dysfunction in proprioception has been documented (34). Whether this is a cause of the scoliosis or simply an effect of the disease is presently unclear. Lewit (35) has hypothesized that mechanical dysfunction in the upper cervical spine may have an influence on the curve or its genesis. The doctor should examine all segments of the spinal column for signs (e.g., edema, tenderness, etc.) of a vertebral subluxation complex, because the etiology of the deformity may occur at any level (See Chapters 4 and 5) (Figs. 9.16–9.18.).

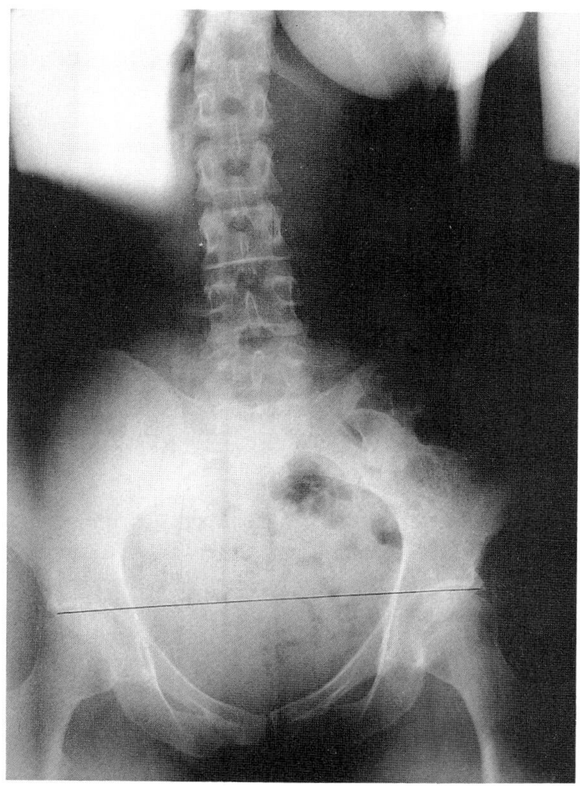

Figure 9.16. AP radiograph demonstrating a short leg in a 31-yr-old female patient.

Scoliosis and Exercise

Exercises have not been shown either to correct the curvature or halt curve progression in most scoliotics. This apparent ineffectiveness does not mean that exercise is not an important adjunct to overall spinal fitness.

After the initial phase of adjustments, general exercises such as swimming and walking and other nonspinal stressors may be implemented. This will prepare the patient for more stressful spinal maneuvers in the future and also improve cardiovascular function.

After a few weeks of general exercise,the patient can then progress to specific therapies designed to strengthen weak paraspinal musculature and stretch chronically contracted fascia and muscles. Nautilus trunk flexion and extension machines or similar designs are helpful in strengthening the torso musculature.

Asymmetric lateral flexion isotonic and isometric exercises to the side of convexity will help to stretch those tissues on the concavity of the curvature. In the case of compound curves this becomes more difficult. The patient must be careful in avoiding hypermobile motion segments with the stretch or exercise because this may accelerate creep at those levels.

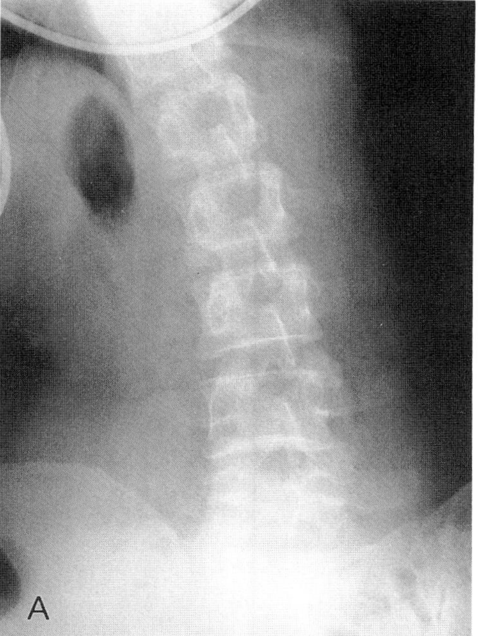

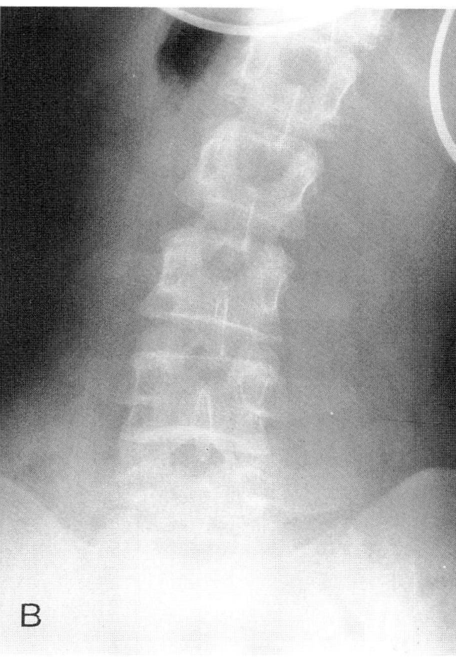

Figure 9.17. Stress x-rays of patient in Figure 9.16, indicate global postural coupling dysfunction during left lateral flexion (**A**) and fixation dysfunction at L5-S1 during right bending (**B**). The treatment for this patient included spinal adjustments (L5-S1), specific postural maneuvers to reverse the abnormal coupling pattern during left bending, and a heel lift.

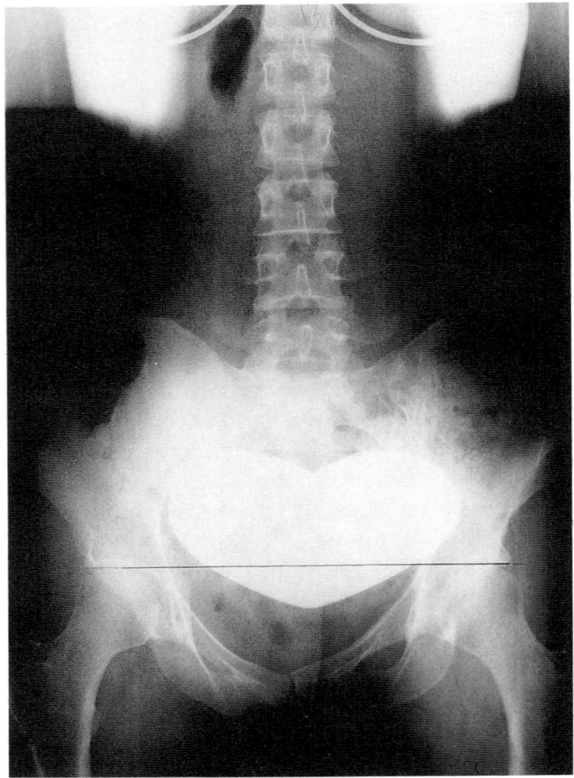

Figure 9.18. Comparative radiograph of patient in Figure 9.16. Patient is wearing a shoe lift.

Braces

Bracing for scoliosis is a controversial subject. Although some authors feel that it is an excellent therapy, others discount any supposed efficacy. Braces are seldom recommended for curves greater than 50° or less than 20°. One report (36) indicates that the Boston brace has little effect on curve magnitude. In a series of 107 patients, it was determined that scolioses with apices at T10-T12 showed slight improvement (i.e., 2°), whereas other areas remained unchanged. A preliminary study by Price et al (37) showed that nighttime brace therapy (Charleston) compares favorably to the results obtained from full time orthoses (i.e., Milwaukee).

One serious complication of brace therapy to which the physician should be aware is that of persistent vomiting associated with wearing the brace. The device may press the superior mesenteric artery against the duodenum. The brace should be removed immediately if vomiting occurs due to the risk of abdominal obstruction and death (38).

Compliance with orthoses such as the Milwaukee brace is quite low due to the cumbersome nature and unattractiveness of the device. Compliance rates are about 50% with most children.

Patient Compliance

Compliance with chiropractic care in the adolescent is made difficult because of the repetitive nature of treatment in the absence of symptomatology. Rehabilitative or reconstructive care entails multiple adjustments unlike a typical pediatric patient without a spinal curvature. Education for parents is essential so that they understand the need for prolonged and often expensive treatment.

Electrical Stimulation

Electrical muscle stimulation in the treatment of idiopathic scoliosis has gained popularity in recent years (28,39,40). Whether electrical muscle stimulation is a helpful adjunct to chiropractic adjustments, or has the ability to halt progression or, indeed, corrects lateral deviations of the spinal column has yet to be determined. Muscle stimulation's effectiveness is still largely unknown but appears to be equal to bracing in terms of slowing progression (39).

Studies differ on appropriate position for the electrodes. Some authors have used a position close to the midline of the spine, whereas others have advocated a more lateral approach (41,42). Sleep disturbance has been reported to be a problem in some patients. This is due to the sometimes irritating effects of the electrodes. Although sleep disturbance is a problem, it is manageable and compliance rates in patients using stimulation appear to be much higher than brace therapy (40). Unfortunately, the patient must sleep in the prone position with electrical stimulation, necessitating head rotation which places rotational stress on the cervical spine.

Electrical stimulation and its role in the chiropractor's practice has been summarized by Dutro and Keene (40). This summary emphasized that proper patient protocol including patient education is mandatory, in order for the therapy to have maximal results. It is suggested that the doctor work closely with the equipment manufacturer and an experienced clinician before integrating the therapy into practice.

TERMINOLOGY

The terminology committee of the Scoliosis Research Society has developed a glossary of terms which will be of use to the practitioner with an interest in scoliosis. These terms create a common language between health care disciplines and should be used when detailing reports about scoliotic individuals.

Glossary

Adolescent scoliosis. Spinal curvature presenting at or about the onset of puberty and before maturity.

Adult scoliosis. Spinal curvature existing after skeletal maturity.

Apical vertebra. The most axially rotated vertebra in a curve; the most deviated vertebra from the vertical axis of the patient.

Café-au-lait spots. Light brown irregular areas of skin pigmentation. If sufficient in number and having smooth margins, they are suggestive of neurofibromatosis.

Compensatory curve. A curve, which can be structural, above or below a major curve, that tends to maintain normal body balance by keeping the majority of the trunk over the midline.

Congenital scoliosis. Scoliosis due to congenital anomalous vertebral development.

Curve measurement. Cobb's method: select the upper and lower end vertebrae with the steepest inclination towards the concavity of the curve. Erect perpendiculars to lines drawn through the end-plates of the end vertebrae. If the end-plates are poorly visualized or anomalous, then draw a line which bisects the centers of the pedicles.

Double major scoliosis. A scoliosis with two structural curves.

End vertebra. 1. The most cephalad vertebra of a curve, whose superior surface tilts maximally towards the concavity of the curve. 2. The most caudal vertebra whose inferior surface tilts maximally towards the concavity of the curve.

Fractional curve. Compensatory curve that is incomplete because it returns to the erect. Its only horizontal vertebra is its caudad or cephalad one.

Full curve. A curve in which the only horizontal vertebra is at its apex.

Gibbus. A sharply angular kyphotic deformation.

Hyperkyphosis. A sagittal alignment of the thoracic spine in which there is more than the normal amount of kyphosis.

Hypokyphosis. A sagittal alignment of the thoracic spine in which there is less than the normal amount of kyphosis.

Hysterical scoliosis. A nonstructural deformity of the spine that develops as a manifestation of a conversion reaction.

Idiopathic scoliosis. A structural spinal curve for which there is no known cause.

Iliac epiphysis, iliac apophysis. The epiphysis along the wing of an ilium.

Inclinometer. An instrument used to measure the angle of thoracic inclination or rib hump.

Infantile scoliosis. Spinal curvature which is developing during the first three years of life.

Juvenile scoliosis. Spinal curvature which is developing between the skeletal age of three and the onset of puberty.

Kyphos. A change in alignment of a segment of the spine in the sagittal plane that increases the posterior convex angulation; an abnormally increased kyphosis.

Kyphoscoliosis. A spine with a scoliosis and a true hyperkyphosis. A rotatory deformity with only apparent kyphosis should not be described by this term.

Lordoscoliosis. A scoliosis associated with an abnormal anterior angulation in the sagittal plane.

Major curve. Term used to designate the largest structural curve.

Minor curve. Term used to describe the smallest curve. This curve is always more flexible than the major curve.

Nonstructural curve. A curve that has no structural component and that corrects or overcorrects on recumbent or standing lateral bending radiographs.

Pelvic obliquity. Deviation of the pelvis from the horizontal in the frontal plane. Fixed pelvic obliquities can be attributable to contractures either above or below the pelvis. Functional obliquity can be caused by leg length inequality.

Primary curve. The first or earliest of several curves to appear, if identifiable.

Rotational prominence. In the forward bending position, the thoracic prominence on one side is usually due to vertebra axial rotation causing rib prominence. In the lumbar spine, the prominence is usually due to axial rotation of the lumbar vertebrae.

Skeletal age, bone age. The age obtained by comparing an AP radiograph of the left hand and wrist with the standards of the Gruelich and Pyle Atlas.

Structural curve. A segment of the spine with a lateral curvature that lacks normal flexibility.

Vertebral ring apophysis. The most reliable index of vertebral immaturity, seen best in lateral radiographs or in the lumbar region in AP lateral bending roentgenograms.

REFERENCES

1. Kostiuk JP, Bentivoglio J. The incidence of low back pain in adult scoliosis. Spine 1981;6:268–273.
2. Ussher NT. Spinal curvatures: visceral disturbances in relation thereto. California West Med 1933;38:423.
3. Bergofsky EH, Turino GM, Fishman AP. Cardiorespiratory failure in kyphoscoliosis. Medicine 1959;38:263–317.
4. Fishman AP. Pulmonary aspects of scoliosis. In: Zorab PA, ed. Proceedings of a Symposium on Scoliosis. London: Vincent House, 1965:52.

5. Chapman EM, Dill BD, Graybiel A. The decrease in functional capacity of the lungs and heart resulting from deformities of the chest: pulmocardiac failure. Medicine 1939;18:167–202.
6. Rieder J. Die respirations und zirculationsstorungen bei kyphoscoliosis dorsalis. Diss. Berlin 1881 (citation from Sulser).
7. Sulser UJ. Zur klinik und pathologischen anatomie der kyphoscoliose mit besonder berucksichtigung der lebenserwartung. Cardiologia 1958;32:231.
8. Nilsonne U, Lundgren KD. Long term prognosis in idiopathic scoliosis. Acta Orthopaedica Scandinavica 1968;39:456–465.
9. Nachemson A. A long term follow-up study of non-treated scoliosis. Acta Orthopaedica Scandinavica 1968;39:466–476.
10. Nykoliation JW, Cassidy JD, Arthur BE, Wedge JH. An algorithm for the management of scoliosis. J Manipulative Physiol Ther 1986;9:1–14.
11. Winter RB. Classification and terminology. In: Moe JH, Bradford D, Lonstein J, Ogilvie J, Winter RB, eds. Moe's textbook of scoliosis and other spinal deformities. 2nd. ed. Philadelphia: WB Saunders Co, 1987.
12. Barge FH. Tortipelvis. Davenport: Bawden Bros. Inc., 1980:121.
13. Mehta MH. The rib-vertebrae angle in the early diagnosis between resolving and progressive infantile scoliosis. J Bone Joint Surg 1972;54B:230–243.
14. Kristmundsdottir F, Burwell RG, James JI. The rib-vertebra angles on the convexity and concavity of the spinal curve in infantile idiopathic scoliosis. Clin Orthop 1985;201:205–209.
15. Tolo VT, Gillespie R. The characteristics of juvenile idiopathic scoliosis and results of its treatment. J Bone Joint Surg 1978;60B:181–188.
16. Rogala EH, Drummond DS, Gurr J. Scoliosis: incidence and natural history, a prospective epidemiological study. J Bone Joint Surg 1978;60A:173–176.
17. Nelson WE. Nelson's textbook of pediatrics. Philadelphia: WB Saunders, 1979.
18. Aspegren DD. Scoliosis. In: Cox JM, ed. Low back pain. 5th ed. Baltimore: Williams & Wilkins, 1990:323.
19. Hildebrandt RW. Chiropractic spinography: a manual of technology and interpretation. 2nd ed. Baltimore: Williams & Wilkins, 1985.
20. Barge FH. "Idiopathic" Scoliosis. Davenport: Bawden Bros. Inc., 1986:17–129.
21. Goldberg MS, Poitras B, Mayo NE et. al. Observer variation in assessing spinal curvature and skeletal development in adolescent idiopathic scoliosis. Spine 1988;13:1371–1377.
22. Goldberg C, Dowling FE. Handedness and scoliosis convexity: a reappraisal. Spine 1990;15:61–64.
23. Clarisse P. Prognostic evolutif des scolioses idiopathiques mineures de 10 degrees to 29 degrees en periode de croissance. Doctoral Thesis: Univ. Claude Bernard, Lyon, 1974.
24. Lonstein JE, Carlson JM. The prediction of curve progression in untreated idiopathic scoliosis during growth. J Bone Joint Surg 1984;66A:1061–1071.
25. Miller JAA, Nachemson AL, Schultz AB. Effectiveness of braces in mild idiopathic scoliosis. Spine 1984;9:632–635.
26. Cochran T, Nachemson A. Long-term anatomic and functional changes in patients with adolescent idiopathic scoliosis treated with the Milwaukee brace. Spine 1985;10:127–133.
27. Cox JM, Aspegren DD. Scoliosis: diagnosis, detection and treatment. J Am Chiro Assoc 1986;23(1):45–52.
28. Aspegren DD, Cox JM. Correction of progressive idiopathic scoliosis utilizing neuromuscular stimulation and manipulation: a case report. J Manipulative Physiol Ther 1987;10:147–156.
29. Plaugher G, Cremata EE, Phillips RB. A retrospective consecutive case analysis of pre-treatment and comparative static radiological parameters following chiropractic adjustments. J Manipulative Physiol Ther 1990;13:498–506.
30. Possin DM, Mawhiney RB. The efficacy of chiropractic treatment in adult lumbar scoliosis. Chiropractic 1989;2:99–102.
31. Irvin RE. Reduction of lumbar scoliosis by use of a heel lift to level the sacral base. J Am Osteopath Assoc 1991;91:34–44.
32. Herbst RW. Gonstead chiropractic science and art. Mount Horeb, WI: Sci-Chi Publications, 1968.
33. Byrd JA. Equilibrium dysfunction and sensitivity to vibration in scoliosis. Clin Orthop 1988;229:114–119.
34. Barrack RL, Whitecloud TS, Burke SW, Cook SD, Harding AF. Proprioception in idiopathic scoliosis. Spine 1984;9:681–685.
35. Lewit K. Manipulative therapy in rehabilitation of the motor system. Boston: Butterworths, 1985.
36. Ylikoski M, Peltonen J, Poussa M. Biological factors and predictability of bracing in adolescent idiopathic scoliosis. J Pediatr Orthop 1989;9:680–683.
37. Price CT, Scott DS, Reed FE, Riddick MF. Nighttime bracing for adolescent idiopathic scoliosis with the Charleston bending brace: preliminary report. Spine 1990;15:1294–1301.
38. Turek SL. Orthopaedics, principles and their applications. 3rd. ed. Philadelphia: JB Lippincott 1977, 1425–1427.
39. Axelgaard J, Brown JC. Lateral electrical surface stimulation for the treatment of progressive idiopathic scoliosis. Spine 1983;8:242–260.
40. Dutro CL, Keene KJ. Electrical muscle stimulation in the treatment of progressive adolescent idiopathic scoliosis: a literature review. J Manipulative Physiol Ther 1985;8:257–260.
41. Bradford DS, Tanguy A, Vanselow J. Surface electrical stimulation in the treatment of idiopathic scoliosis: preliminary results in 30 patients. Spine 1983;8:757–764.
42. Schultz A, Haderspeck K, Takashima S. Correction of scoliosis by muscle stimulation: biomechanical analyses. Spine 1981;6:468–476.

10 Lower Cervical Spine

GREGORY PLAUGHER with the assistance of RICHARD W. DOBLE, JR. and MARK A. LOPES

Biomechanical considerations of the cervical spine are extremely important due to the common occurrence of acceleration/deceleration injuries in this region. This chapter covers the cervical spine from the C2 vertebra through the C7-T1 motion segment. The cervical spine has been divided into two sections because of the uniqueness of both the upper and lower regions.

CLINICAL ANATOMY AND BIOMECHANICS

Posture

The cervical lordosis is formed primarily by the wedge shape of the intervertebral discs (1,2) (Fig. 10.1). There are several anatomic factors that determine the degree of lordosis. Hyperplastic articular pillars (3), small facet angles (4), and short pedicles (4) are important structural features that can lead to a cervical hypolordosis. Patients with hypolordotic cervical spines are more likely to develop symptoms (i.e., pain) than those without straightening (5).

The lateral radiograph of the cervical spine is appropriate for assessing the degree of curvature. During the exposure, the patient's head should be held erect in what the patient considers to be normal upright posture. Slight flexion or extension of the head will have little effect on the cervical curve because this motion is confined primarily to the C0-C1 motion segment. Weir (6), however, found that lowering the chin one inch will create a postural hypolordosis in many patients. Patient positioning is especially critical if comparative radiography is performed (Fig. 10.2A-H). It is important that the doctor understands that the sagittal curves of the spinal column are all interdependent (7). Treatment directed at only the cervical spine will usually provide incomplete spinal care. Compensation reactions of the neck may even result from dysfunction of the lumbar spine or pelvis.

Besides specific adjustments, the doctor may wish to consider the incorporation of postural exercises as an additional therapeutic modality. These exercises usually consist of moving the head and neck into a lordotic configuration. The first step involves asking the patient to translate the head posteriorward along the Z axis. This maneuver counters the usual anterior carriage of the head which is present in patients with a kyphotic or hypolordotic cervical curve. The $-Z$ translation should be followed with hyperextension of the head and neck. This maneuver is contraindicated if it provokes symptomatology. Patients with posterior and inferior subluxations may have difficulty with performing this exercise.

The use of a cervical pillow also may facilitate return of the lordosis (5). Ergonomic factors have a strong influence on cervical mechanics and symptomatology. Often, the work environment will require the head and neck to remain in a forward bent position for long time periods. The neck extensors will be under higher muscular loads and may fatigue in the forward bent position (8). This factor alone can create tension at the origins and insertions of the posterior neck muscles (e.g., trapezius), which then may lead to trigger points and ultimately neck pain or referred syndromes such as headache.

Zygapophyseal Joints

The three-joint complex comprises the two zygapophyseal joints of the functional spinal unit and the central intervertebral disc articulation. In contrast with the lumbar spine, the facet joints provide a greater contribution to the overall stability of this region. An example of the

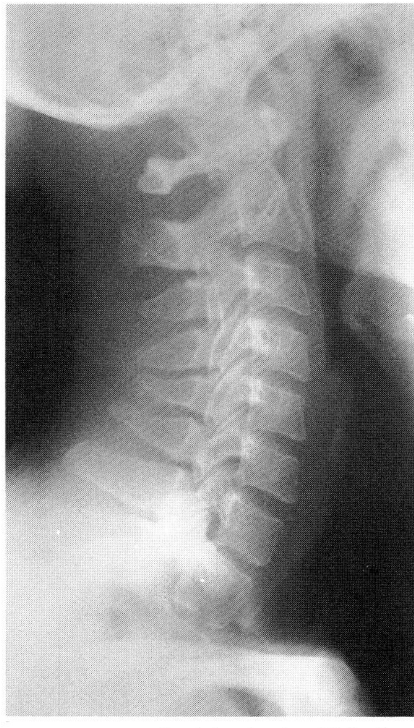

Figure 10.1. Normal cervical lordosis. This is a posttreatment radiograph.

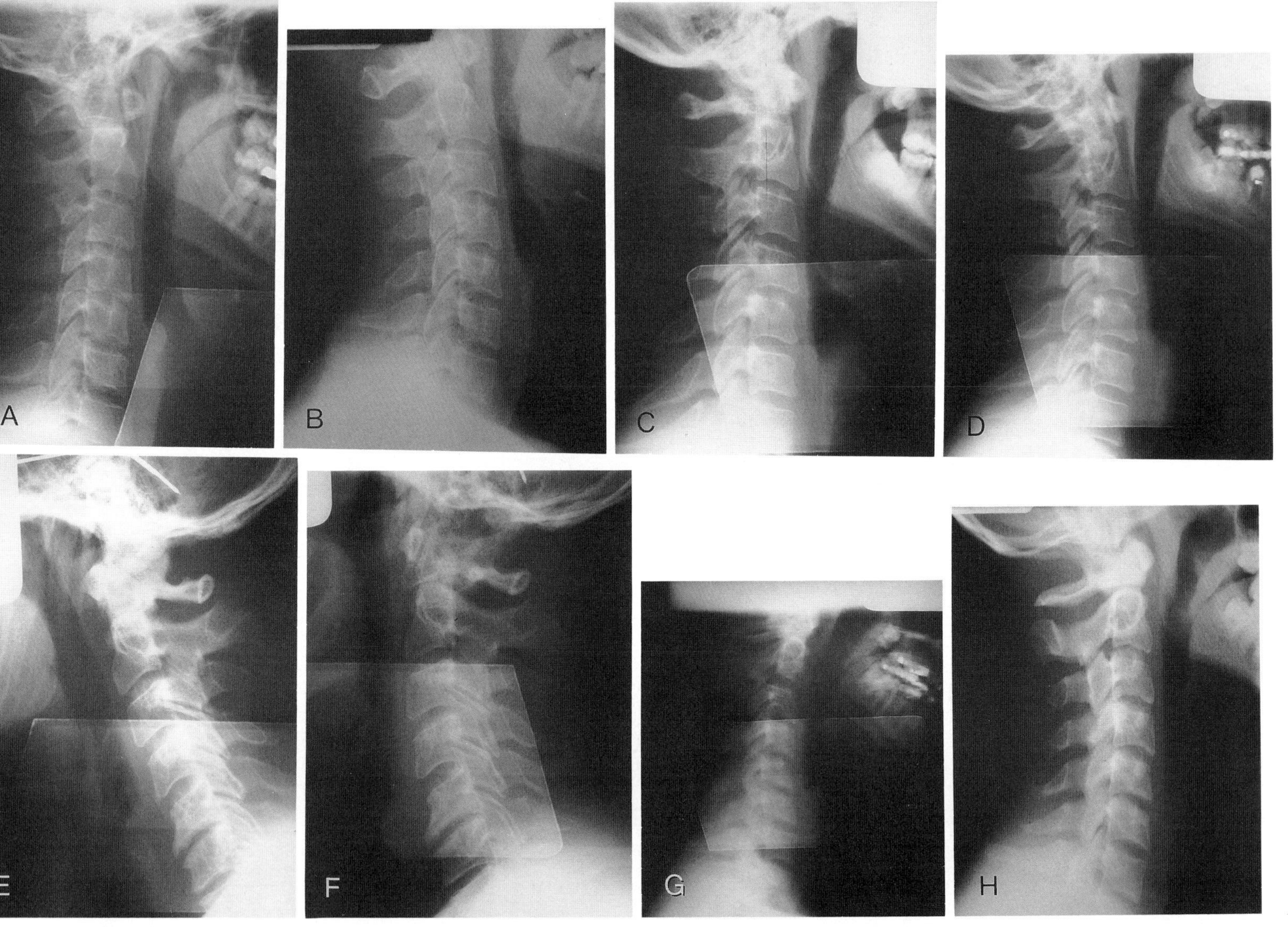

Figure 10.2. **A,** Pretreatment radiograph (11-27-90). **B,** Posttreatment radiograph of patient in **A** (1-23-91). **C,** Pretreatment radiograph (2-26-90). **D,** Posttreatment radiograph of patient in **C** (7-6-90). **E,** Pretreatment radiograph (5-23-90). **F,** Posttreatment radiograph of the patient in **E** (8-1-90). **G,** Pretreatment radiograph (7-13-90). **H,** Posttreatment radiograph of the patient in **G** (9-14-90).

importance of the facets may be found in the work of White and Panjabi (9), who showed that after disc resection of the cervical spine, the motion segment increased its motion in flexion and extension by 33%. In contrast, the motion increased by 140% after posterior element resection.

The capsular ligaments are less taut in the cervical region when compared with the thoracic or lumbar areas. This relative laxity is a reflection of the large ranges of motion permitted in this region.

Pattern of Motion

The *pattern of motion* can be defined as the path of movement of a vertebra while moving through its range of motion. The pattern of motion of a cervical motion segment is due to in large part to the orientation of the zygapophyseal joints. The facets are oriented at approximately a 45° angle to the horizontal (Fig. 10.3). This angle increases as one moves caudal. At C7-T1 the angle is approximately 60°. At the C2-C3 joint the angle is closer to 30°. The more horizontal the facet facings are, the more Z axis translation (anterior-posterior shear) is possible. The pattern of motion, therefore, is different at C2 compared with C7. The acuity of the arc of motion is increased in the lower cervical segments (Fig. 10.4) (See Chapter 2). Disc degeneration leads to flattening of the arc (9,10).

During flexion, the vertebra moves anterior and superior. With extension, the segment glides posterior and inferior (10). The pattern of motion illustrates biomechanical factors influencing adjustments applied to the lower cervical segments in the sagittal plane. When adjusting a subluxation involving an articulation fixed in extension, it is necessary to accentuate the component of "lift" of the spinous process ($+\theta X$) to move the segment toward a flexed position. The cervical adjustment has often been characterized as an "extension" adjustment. This type of adjustment is, in fact, a flexion adjustment,

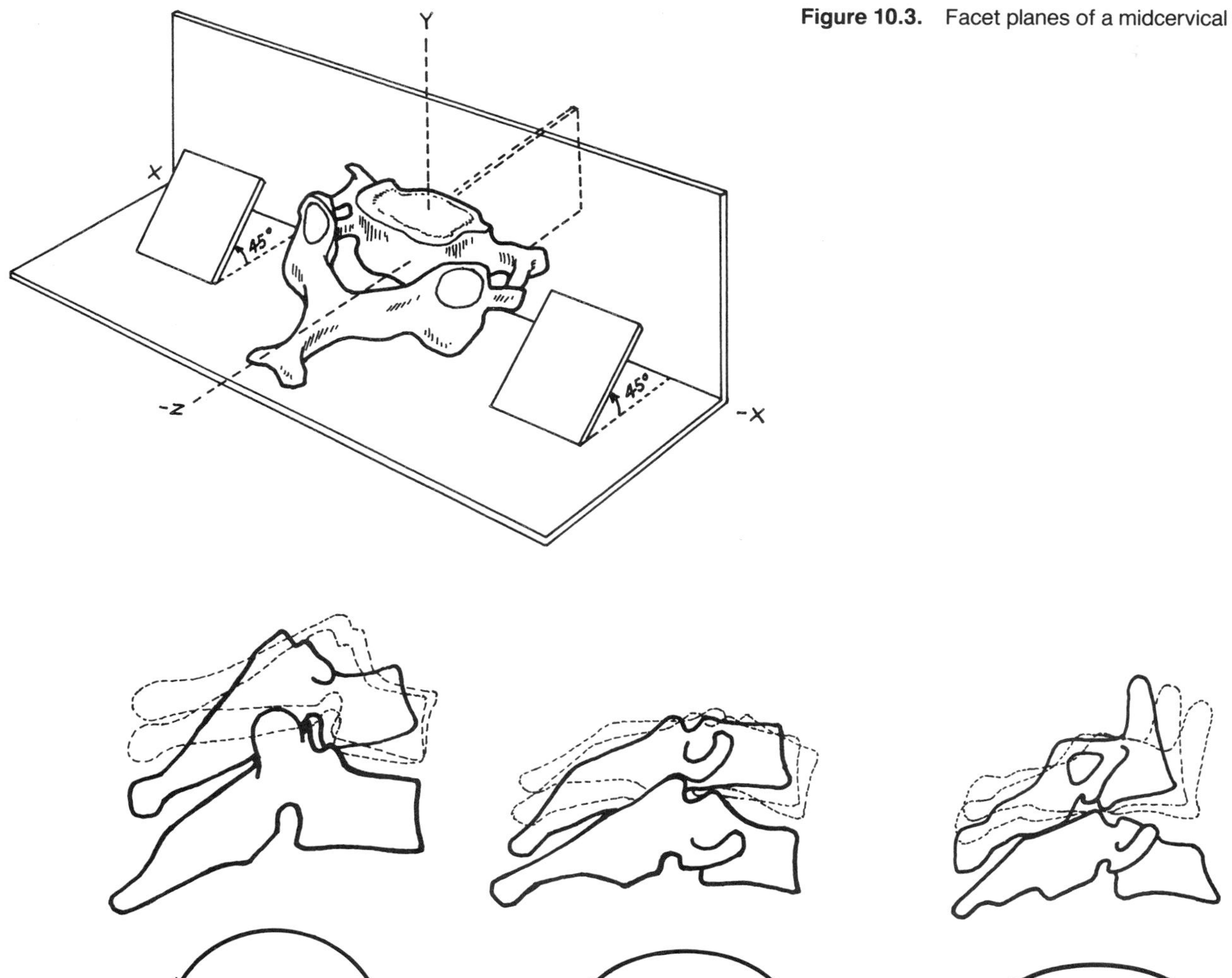

Figure 10.3. Facet planes of a midcervical vertebra.

Figure 10.4. Pattern of motion of C2, C4 and C7 during flexion/extension motion. Notice the increased arc at C7, which must be taken into account during an adjustment at this level.

with the primary vectors applied in the $+\theta X$ and $+Z$ directions.

When movements are analyzed with stress radiography, it is important to consider the intraregional differences of movement of the lower cervical spine. Normally coupled with $+\theta X$ motion during flexion is a very slight $+Z$ translation (See Chapter 5). This movement amounts to 1 or 2 mm when using a film focal distance of 72 inches. Similarly, a slight $-Z$ translation accompanies extension or $-\theta X$ motion. Normal translation varies from individual to individual. However, an isolated posteriorward translation of C5 during extension in the presence of surrounding motion segments displaying no translation may be considered abnormal.

The angle of the facet joints necessitates coupled axial rotation (Y axis) and slight flexion (X axis) during lateral bending. Because the facet joints resemble those of the thoracic spine at C7-T1 (coronal plane), very little coupled axial rotation is present. At the C2-C3 level there is normally 2° of axial rotation for every 3° of lateral flexion (9). This coupling gradually decreases as one moves caudally. At the C7-T1 articulation there is only 1 degree of axial rotation for 7.5° of lateral bend. It is important to know these regional variations to assess fixation dysfunction or hypermobility of the cervical spine accurately during lateral flexion stress radiography.

Intervertebral Disc

In contrast with the lumbar spine, where the intervertebral disc resists most of the compressive load, the cervical intervertebral discs form a tripod arrangement with the facet joints in resisting compressive loads. Approximately one-third of the compressive load is resisted by each zygapophyseal articulation and the central joint.

As a portion of vertebra height, the cervical disc is relatively tall, much like the lumbar disc and quite different from the thoracic disc. The nucleus pulposus comprises a large portion of the cross-sectional area (30–50%), therefore predisposing the total disc to swelling after trauma (9).

INNERVATION

The cervical disc can be an intrinsic source of pain. Branches of the vertebral and sinuvertebral nerves primarily innervate the outer one-third of the annulus fibrosis of the cervical discs (11).

Range of Motion

The *range of motion* is defined as the angular change between the two physiologic extremes of movement. Through a literature review, White and Panjabi (9) have established the intersegmental ranges of motion of the cervical motion segments. These values represent the total range of the motion segment. The analysis of flexion versus extension ranges would, therefore, have to take into account the neutral position from which the motions begin. Flexion-extension motion or rotation around the x axis, has the greatest angular range of the three possible degrees of freedom (See Chapter 2) concerned with rotations. The C5-C6 joint is the most mobile, having a total range of motion in the sagittal plane of 17°. The amount of intersegmental movement decreases to 9° at the C7-T1 and 8° at the C2-C3 motion segments. The representative angles for the total range of $\pm\theta X$ motion are as follows (9):

C2-C3: 8°
C3-C4: 13°
C4-C5: 12°
C5-C6: 17°
C6-C7: 16°
C7-T1: 9°

Lateral bending, or rotation around the Z axis is greatest at the cervical segments C3-C4 and C4-C5 with approximately 5.5° to each side. The representative angles to each side are as follows (9):

C2-C3: 5°
C3-C4: 5.5°
C4-C5: 5.5°
C5-C6: 4°
C6-C7: 3.5°
C7-T1: 2°

Rotation around the Y axis, or axial rotation, is greatest at the C4-C5 joint for cervical segments C2-C7. The representative angles for axial rotation in each direction are as follows (9):

C2-C3: 4.5°
C3-C4: 5.5°
C4-C5: 6°
C5-C6: 5°
C6-C7: 4.5°
C7-T1: 4°

Global range of motion of the cervical spine can be accurately assessed with simple goniometric methods (12). Cervical lateral flexion asymmetries have been studied by Nansel et al. (13). These asymmetries were found to be a relatively stable phenomenon and could be ameliorated with a single Gonstead-type lower cervical adjustment (14).

CERVICAL DISC DISEASE

Haley and Perry (15) studied disc injury in the cervical spine. In 53 of 99 cadavers, there was evidence of cervical disc protrusion. Twenty-seven had lumbar disc protrusions. It must be kept in mind, however, that a lumbar disc protrusion tends to be reduced when the lumbar spine has been unloaded, as in the recumbent position. Seven cases had protrusions in the thoracic spine. Two of

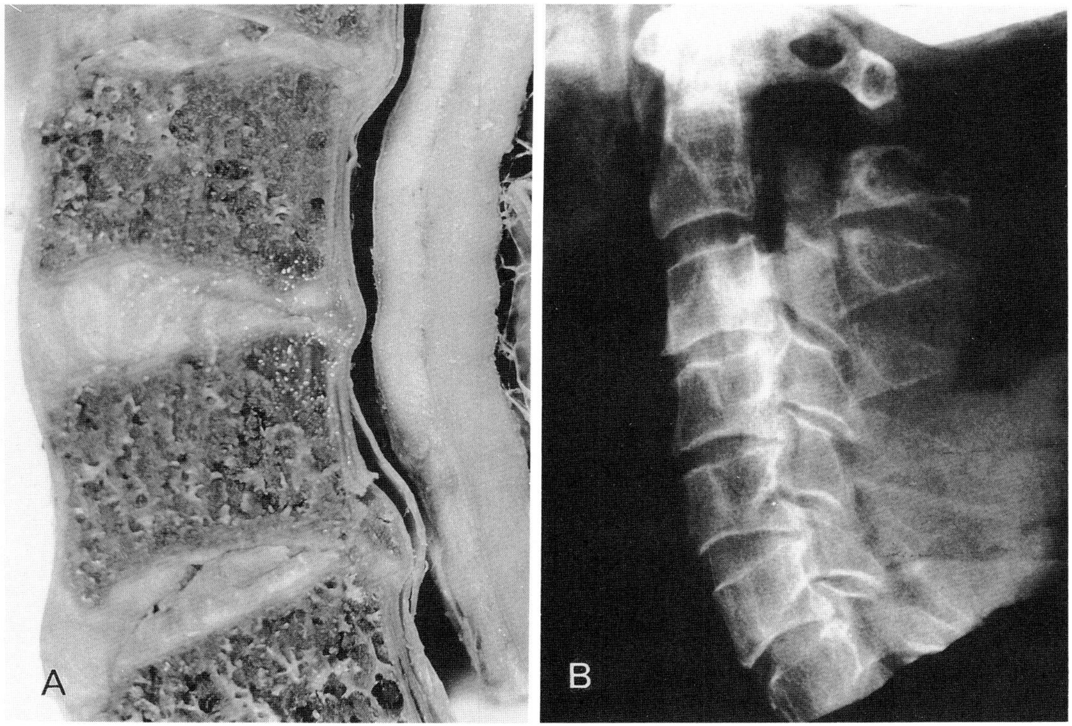

Figure 10.5. A, Cadaver specimen demonstrating multiple levels of disc protrusion and compression of the spinal cord. **B,** Radiograph of specimen in **A.**

these cases were associated with a marked thoracic scoliosis. Approximately 33% of cervical disc protrusions occur at C5 (15–17). Larger protrusions (4–6 mm) occur more frequently at C6. Most protrusions are central or posterolateral although lateral rupture and lateral protrusion form the most common combination. Although anterior migration of the nucleus does occur (15), it is more rare. The intervertebral foraminae of the cervical spine are elliptical and tightly enclose the neurovascular contents. Encroachment on the intervertebral foramen occurs frequently, especially when a disc protrusion is present. The prognosis of patients with disc protrusion is generally not good (15). Bony exostosis surrounding the disc material adds to the stenotic effect of the protrusion. Multiple levels (three to five) are often involved, which then can lead to spinal cord degeneration (15) (Fig. 10.5A-B). Ischemic degeneration of the cord and sensory portion of the nerve roots was the most common neurologic finding in the specimens studied with disc protrusion.

Management

The use of advanced imaging such as magnetic resonance to ascertain the extent of herniation more precisely makes conservative management of disc cases less difficult (Fig. 10.6A-D). MRI is also useful in differentially diagnosing other neurologic disorders such as tumors or multiple sclerosis (Fig. 10.7). Acute pain originating from disc protrusion or herniation most often presents itself as an acute aggravation of a preexisting condition. Protrusion or herniation is usually the result of cumulative and gradual disc degeneration (See Chapter 3). The condition often becomes clinically significant after a sudden movement or accident. Whether the patient relates a history of a gradual or sudden onset of pain, the acute cervical pain patient is often a challenging case. Disc derangement of a magnitude capable of producing severe pain is to be managed carefully. Chiropractic care, when indicated, must be administered to patient tolerance. The more experienced the clinician, the more likely the skill level of the practitioner will allow for a comfortable, early mobilization in the form of a spinal adjustment.

The symptomatic level(s) must be determined. The history and "hands-on" examination procedures are usually more useful than radiology in assessing the cause of the pain as well as determining patient tolerance to movement. Treatment by manual techniques in cases of mechanically induced acute neck pain depends mainly on patient tolerance. The decision as to whether or not mobilization is indicated depends on the doctor's ability to position the patient for treatment and apply the manual forces required to reduce the restriction of motion when present.

Hypermobile articulations are commonly encountered at the C4 to C6 spinal segments, which are also the most common sites of disc protrusion in the cervical spine. If the patient can move the neck enough to assess the ranges of motion of the cervical articulations, func-

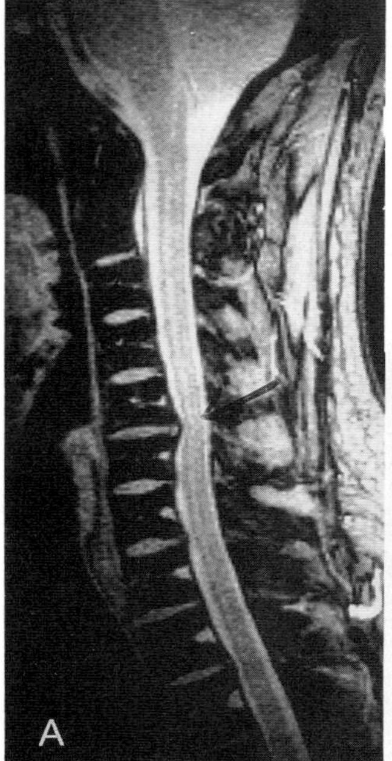

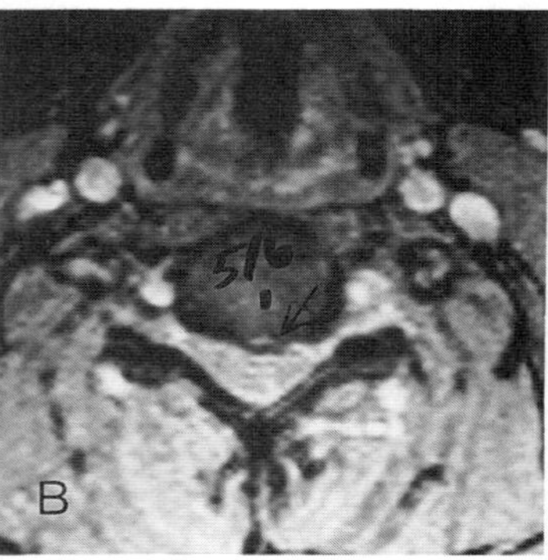

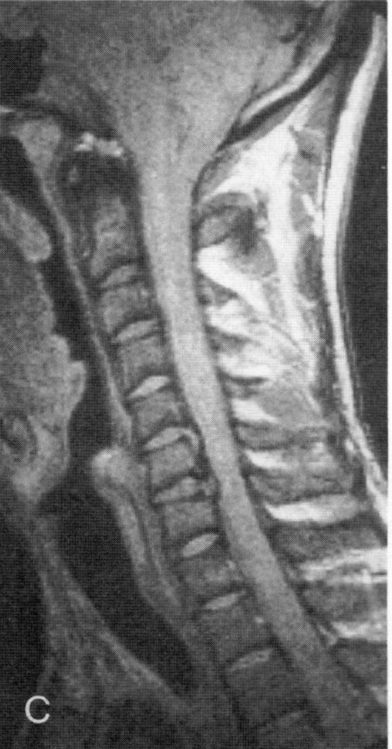

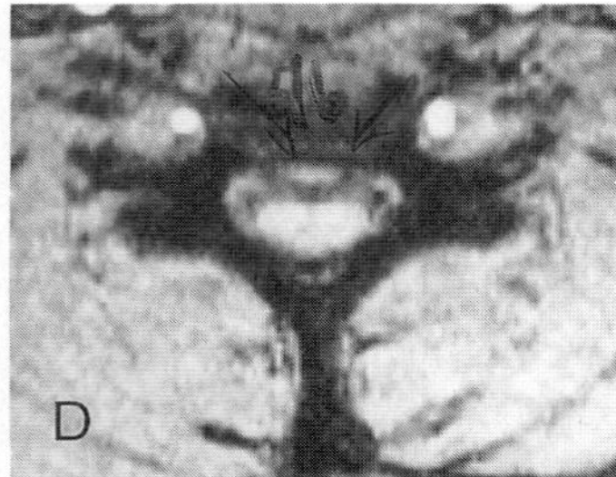

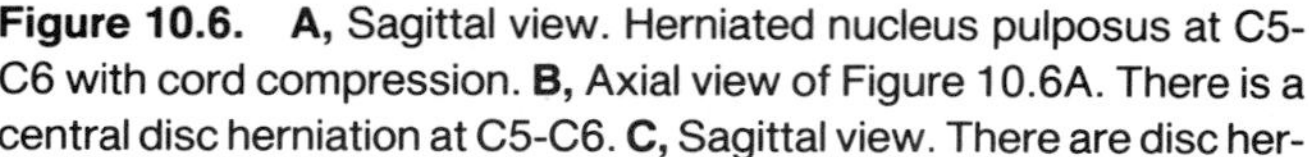

Figure 10.6. **A,** Sagittal view. Herniated nucleus pulposus at C5-C6 with cord compression. **B,** Axial view of Figure 10.6A. There is a central disc herniation at C5-C6. **C,** Sagittal view. There are disc herniations at C5-C6 and C6-C7 with subsequent cord compression. **D,** Axial view of **C**. There is a large broad based central herniation at the C5-C6 motion segment.

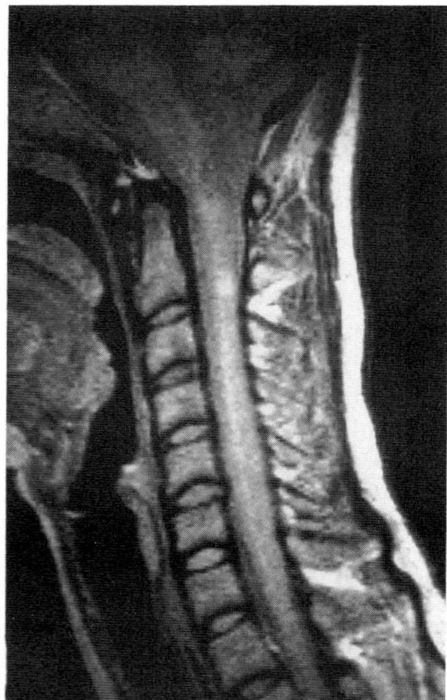

Figure 10.7. Image demonstrating white patchy areas in the superior portion of the spinal cord. These findings are characteristic of multiple sclerosis.

tional radiographs may be indicated. The patient is precisely adjusted at the fixated level like any other case (Fig. 10.8A-E). If the herniation occurs at a hypermobile and unstable motion segment, then attention should be focused at stabilization of those unstable levels. The patient's neurologic status is carefully monitored during the course of treatment. Important signs include muscle strength, reflexes and sensation (Fig. 10.9A-C). If, after following careful adjustive treatment, the patient does not respond favorably or deteriorates in their condition with progressive root or cord symptoms (e.g., spasticity, gait abnormalities, bladder incontinence), then neurosurgical referral is indicated (18).

Disc Degeneration

Narrowing and degeneration of the cervical discs occurs most often at the C5-C6 and C6-C7 disc spaces (19) (Fig. 10.10A-E). These findings correlate with the generally observed greatest range of motion in the sagittal plane at these levels. Most likely internal disc disruption leads to joint hypermobility and eventual disc resorption. The hypermobility may occur as a result of direct factors such as trauma to the joint as is often seen in acceleration/deceleration injuries. Compensation reaction to lower cervical immobility can also lead to gradual disc degeneration.

WHIPLASH INJURIES

Acceleration-deceleration injuries are commonly encountered in chiropractic practice. This subject is vast and diverse. For a more complete dissertation on these types of injuries, the authors advise seeking other sources (20).

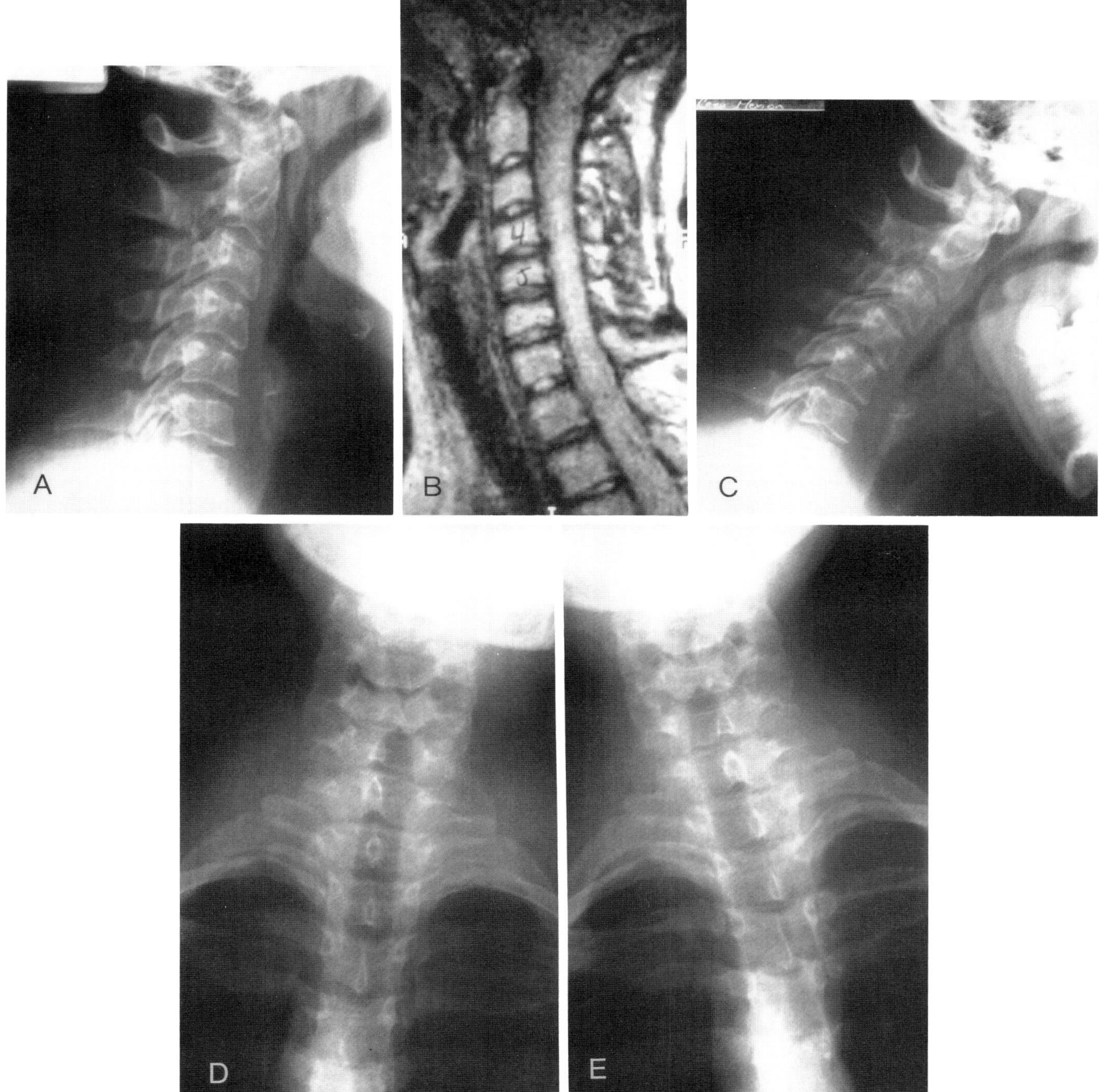

Figure 10.8. **A,** Flexion radiograph. Notice the decreased flexion at the C6 level. Much of the patient's limitation of movement is due to pain. There is a $-\theta X$ positional dyskinesia of C6. **B,** MRI demonstrating a disc protrusion at the C6-C7 level. **C,** Posttreatment (6 weeks) flexion radiograph demonstrating increased flexion movement. **D,** Pretreatment radiograph of right lateral bending. There is normal movement at C6-C7. **E,** Pretreatment radiograph of left lateral bending. Notice the decreased left lateral flexion ($-\theta Z$) at C6-C7.

If there is question as to the legitimacy of this disorder due to the often legal ramifications, the reader is referred to the review by Macnab (21). He poses the question as to why patients who have their head thrown backwards tend to become more "neurotic" than those who have it thrown forwards. Approximately 45% of patients still have symptoms two years or more after settlement of the legal dispute (21).

The patient suffering an acceleration-deceleration injury may present with a wide range of symptoms, the

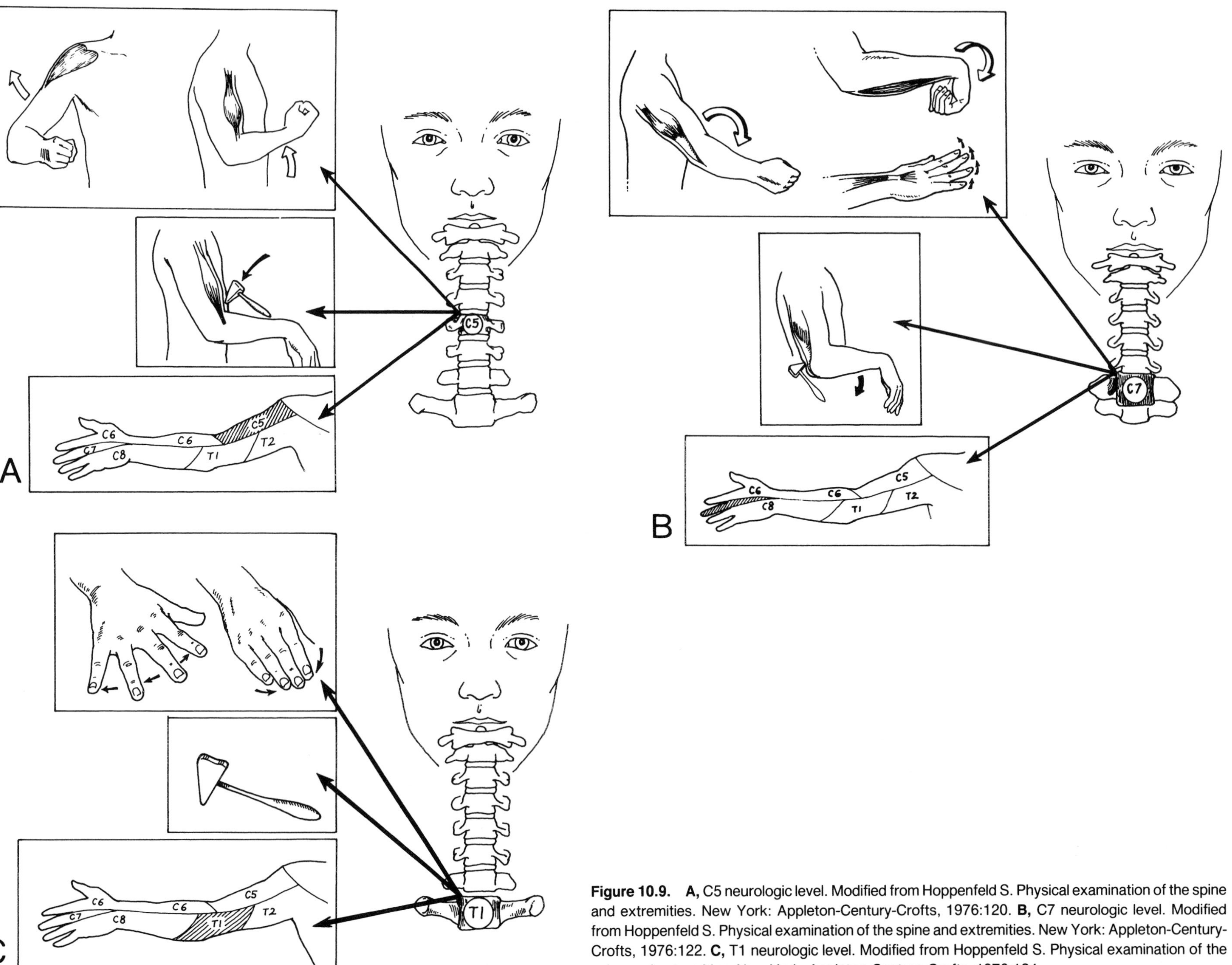

Figure 10.9. **A,** C5 neurologic level. Modified from Hoppenfeld S. Physical examination of the spine and extremities. New York: Appleton-Century-Crofts, 1976:120. **B,** C7 neurologic level. Modified from Hoppenfeld S. Physical examination of the spine and extremities. New York: Appleton-Century-Crofts, 1976:122. **C,** T1 neurologic level. Modified from Hoppenfeld S. Physical examination of the spine and extremities. New York: Appleton-Century-Crofts, 1976:124.

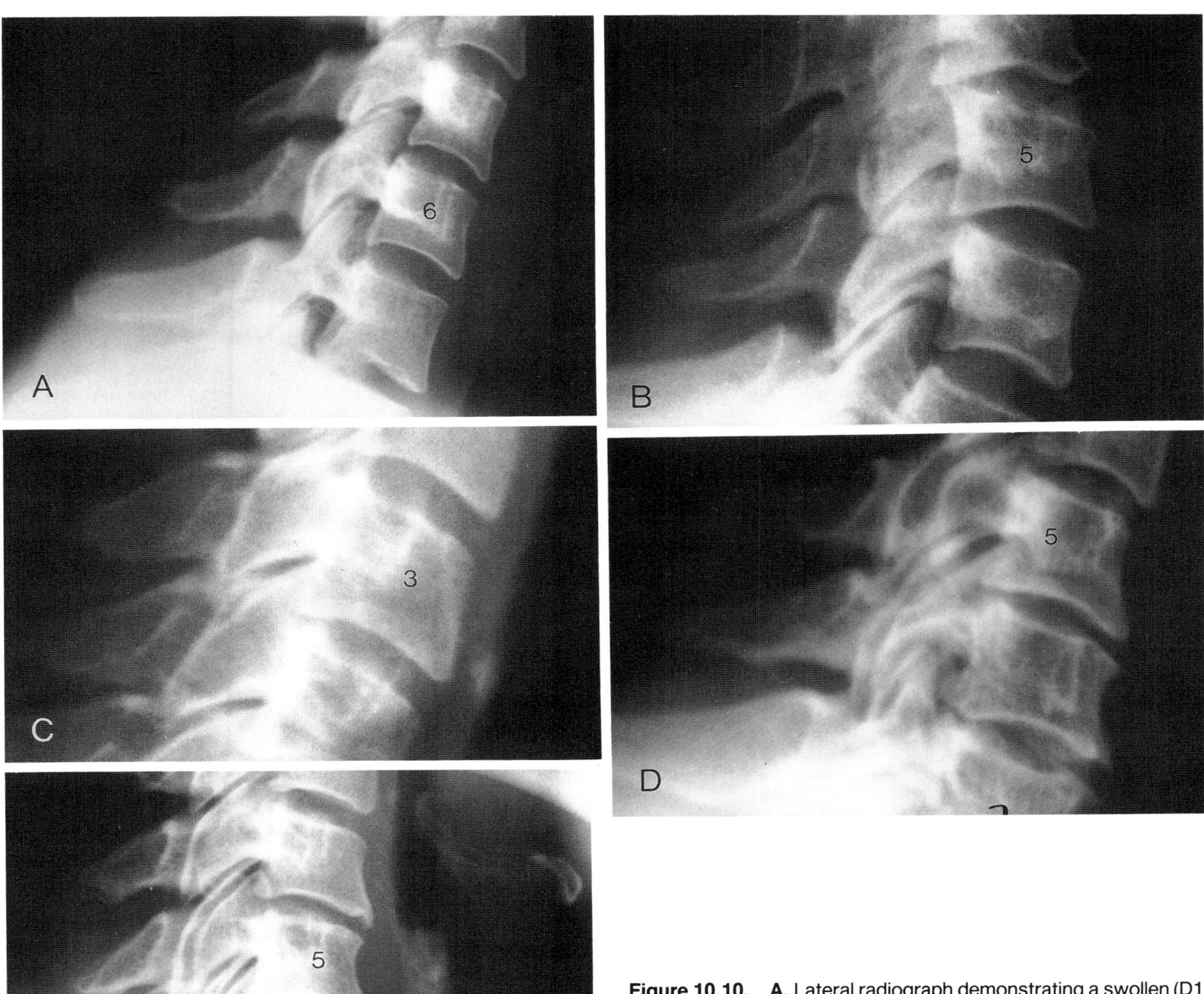

Figure 10.10. **A,** Lateral radiograph demonstrating a swollen (D1) disc at C6-C7. (See Chapter 2 for disc degeneration classification.) **B,** D2 disc at C5. Notice the hyperextension positional dyskinesia of C5. **C,** D3 disc at C3. There is a slight decrease in the anterior and posterior heights of the intervertebral disc. **D,** D4 disc at C5. There is a pronounced decrease in the anterior and posterior dimensions of the disc. **E,** D5 disc at C5. The disc is approximately one-third of its original height.

only constant one being neck pain. The total clinical picture may take several days or weeks to climax. Dizziness is a common symptom relating to whiplash type injuries. The onset is usually seven to ten days after the trauma (22). Low back pain is a common sequela of soft tissue injury of the cervical spine (23). It is important, therefore, that a full spinal assessment be performed for anyone involved in an apparently regionally specific injury such as cervical whiplash (Fig. 10.11).

Pathomechanics

After a vehicle collision from the rear, the lateral cervical radiograph will commonly show a patient with a reduced or completely reversed cervical lordotic curve. Extension malposition (Fig. 10.12) after hyperextension of the neck is usually the most detrimental positional dyskinesia, because the possibility of injury to the nerve roots in the lateral recess is more likely. The hyperextension posture

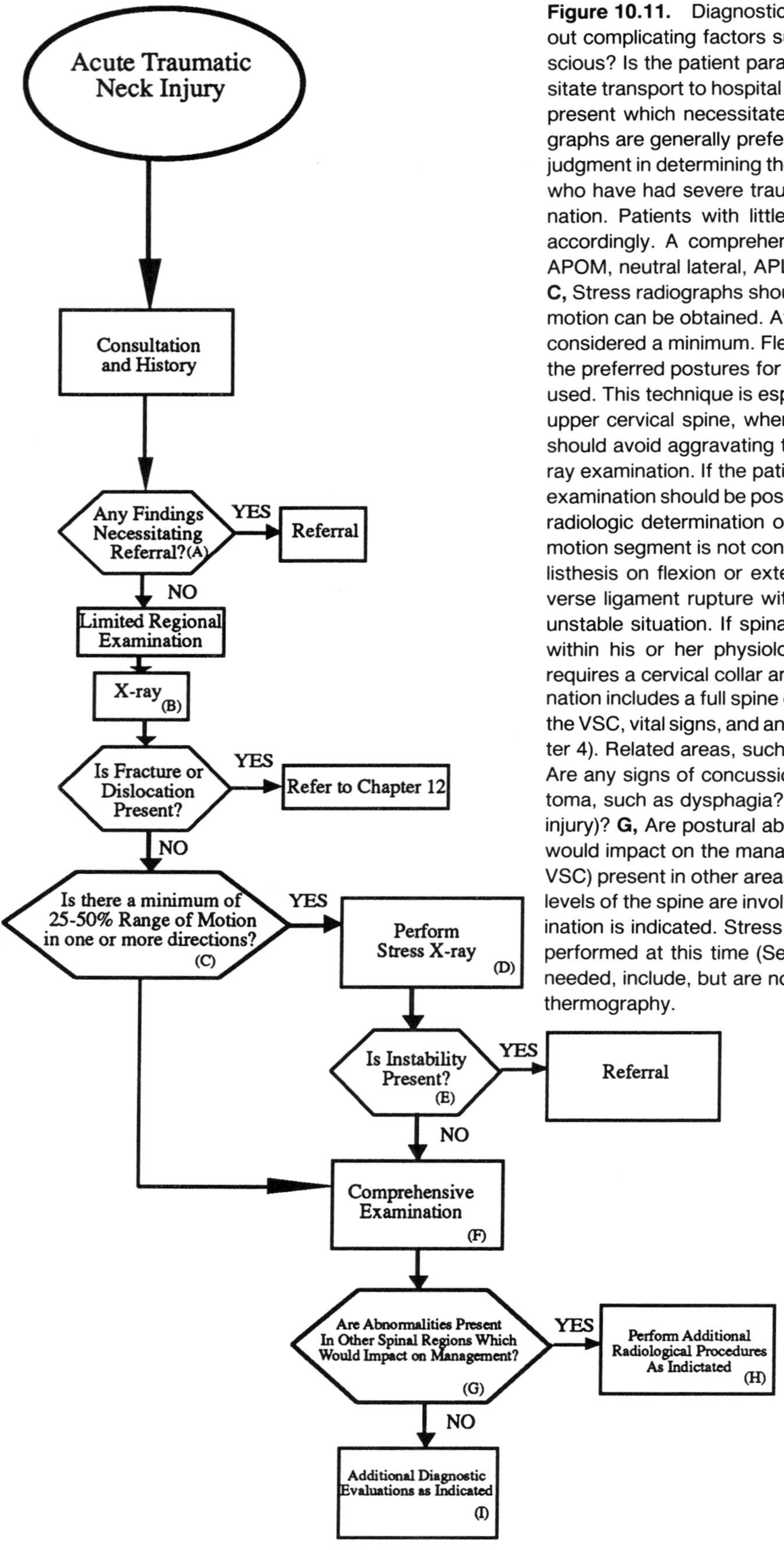

Figure 10.11. Diagnostic algorithm for an acute traumatic neck injury. **A,** Rule out complicating factors suggestive of severe head trauma. Is the patient conscious? Is the patient paraplegic or quadriplegic? Both of these findings necessitate transport to hospital for advanced imaging. Are any lesions (e.g., bleeding) present which necessitate referral to an emergency room. **B,** Sectional radiographs are generally preferred for ruling out fracture. The doctor must exercise judgment in determining the extent of the radiologic examination. Those patients who have had severe trauma should have a comprehensive neurologic examination. Patients with little likelihood of fracture or dislocation are evaluated accordingly. A comprehensive examination of the cervical spine includes an APOM, neutral lateral, APLC, right and left obliques, and AP pillar radiographs. **C,** Stress radiographs should only be performed for positions in which adequate motion can be obtained. At least 25% of motion in the plane under evaluation is considered a minimum. Flexion, extension, and right and left lateral bending are the preferred postures for evaluation. Cineradiographic procedures can also be used. This technique is especially helpful in diagnosing ligamentous injury of the upper cervical spine, where movements are more complex. **D,** The technician should avoid aggravating the patient's condition while performing the stress x-ray examination. If the patient's tolerance for the procedure is minimal, then the examination should be postponed. **E,** Is instability present? See Chapter 5 for the radiologic determination of instability of the cervical spine. Hypermobility at a motion segment is not considered an unstable situation. Severe antero-or retrolisthesis on flexion or extension may necessitate surgical stabilization. Transverse ligament rupture with anterior subluxation of the atlas is considered an unstable situation. If spinal cord compression occurs when the patient moves within his or her physiologic range, the patient is considered unstable and requires a cervical collar and referral. **F,** The comprehensive chiropractic examination includes a full spine evaluation for the presence of signs and symptoms of the VSC, vital signs, and an orthopedic and neurologic battery of tests (See Chapter 4). Related areas, such as the cranial nerves can be examined as indicated. Are any signs of concussion present? Any signs suggestive spinal cord hematoma, such as dysphagia? Is ear or nose bleeding present (suggestive of brain injury)? **G,** Are postural abnormalities present (e.g., leg length inequality) which would impact on the management of the patient? Are spinal abnormalities (i.e., VSC) present in other areas, such as the thoracic or lumbar spine? **H,** If multiple levels of the spine are involved, then an AP and lateral full spine radiologic examination is indicated. Stress radiographs of related areas, if needed, can also be performed at this time (See Chapter 5). **I,** Additional diagnostic evaluations, if needed, include, but are not limited to, MRI, CT, nerve conduction studies, and thermography.

tends to be more injurious because the loads are usually greater and the spinal cord and nerve roots are more susceptible to this type of loading (24). The hyperflexion injury from muscular reflexive contraction that usually follows the hyperextension is less forceful. The patient's head can also be thrown into hyperflexion by secondarily striking the vehicle in front. The most frequent and reproducible whiplash injuries are ruptures of the anterior longitudinal ligament and separation of the annulus fibrosis from the associated vertebrae. Experimental injuries can range from minor tears of the sternocleidomastoid to partial avulsion of the longus colli. If the longus colli muscle is torn, a retropharyngeal hematoma may develop. If the patient reports dysphagia, hematoma should be considered (See Chapter 5).

Clark et al. (25) have reported eleven significant radiologic signs of cervical spine trauma. In their review of 400 cases they categorized the significant findings as follows:

I. Abnormal soft tissues
   A. Widened retropharyngeal space
   B. Widened retrotracheal space
   C. Displacement of prevertebral fat stripe
II. Abnormal vertebral alignment
   A. Loss of lordosis
   B. Acute kyphotic angulation
   C. Torticollis
   D. Widened interspinous space
   E. Rotation of vertebral bodies
III. Abnormal joints
   A. Widened middle atlanto-axial joint
   B. Abnormal intervertebral disc
   C. Widening of the apophyseal joints

Macnab's (21) findings were that extension-acceleration injuries of the neck are more likely to produce soft tissue disruption than either lateral flexion or forward flexion traumas. If disc injury occurs, healing of the injured tissue is less likely to be complete. These early disc lesions do not routinely show changes on plain film radiography.

Concussion

It is known that electroencephalographic (EEG) alterations after whiplash injuries are common (9). These changes may be partly responsible for the wide ranging, bizarre clinical picture often reported by patients. These symptoms may be due to the stretch of the spinal cord and nerve roots and/or concussion of the brain.

Ommaya and Hirsch (26), using scaling techniques and extrapolating information from experiments on monkeys and chimpanzees, have concluded that head rotation (X axis) of 1800 Rad./sec^2 would result in a 50% probability of cerebral concussion. An angular acceleration of the head of 1800 Rad./sec^2 is reached when a car is hit from behind, producing a 5-g horizontal acceleration of the vehicle. (A "g" is equal to the amount of acceleration of gravitational force (9.8 m/sec^2).) Five g's of acceleration occurs when an automobile is accelerated to 18 kmh (11 mph) within 0.1 second. Severy (27), using anthropometric dummies and human volunteers at slow speeds, showed that a 13 kmh (8 mph) rear-end collision produces a 2-g acceleration of the vehicle and a 5-g acceleration of the head after a lapse of 0.25 second.

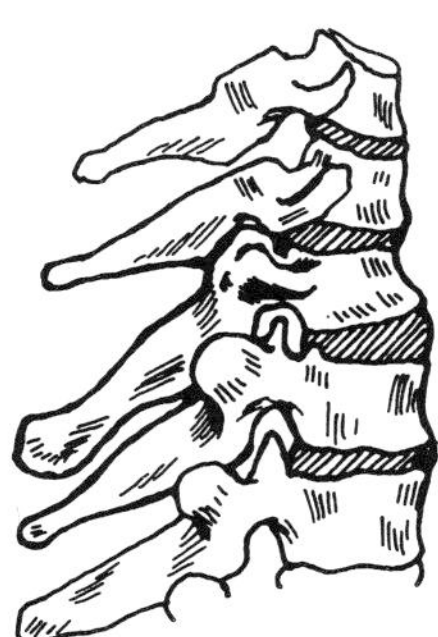

Figure 10.12. Extension ($-\theta X$) malposition of a cervical segment.

Seats

A stiffer seat produces less acceleration of the head than a soft one. The soft seat causes a delay before the vehicular speed reaches the back of the occupant. This delay results in a greater impact velocity between the seat and the occupant and, therefore, greater acceleration of the occupant after impact (9).

The use of headrests is important in lessening the severity of whiplash injuries. Placement is critical, however, because a low headrest will act as a fulcrum and accentuate the trauma. The headrest should be placed at the top-most portion of the head. Because of the "launching effect," the occupants will tend to rise slightly in the seat after a rear-end collision. Airbags will also lessen the severity of injuries caused by head-on collisions (28).

Treatment

The specific adjustment is the chiropractor's primary treatment modality. With the acute patient, this specificity cannot be emphasized enough. The stabilization of normal and hypermobile articulations is especially important because an abrupt stretch of a painful muscle spasm during an adjustment is likely to cause an exacerbation. Making contact on the involved vertebra can be eased if cryotherapy is applied over the contact point before the adjustment. The adjustment should be made with the patient in as much of a neutral position as possible. A rapid and low amplitude thrust followed by a careful "holding" with both hands is important. The doctor may only have one chance to make an adjustment, because unsuccessful attempts are likely to cause patient discomfort and lessen the patient's ability to relax for a future attempt.

TRACTION

The use of strong, intermittent traction can easily be challenged on the basis that it is irrational, counterproductive, nonphysiologic, and traumatic (29). It is astonishing that the claims for intermittent traction have gone so long uncontested. The passive stretch of already sprained ligamentous elements and reduction of the cervical lordosis are two of the more common arguments against cervical traction.

Mild, manual traction applied carefully, when indicated, may be accomplished with a specific segmental contact. A gradual force is applied at the level of subluxation. The supine position is preferred to lessen the load on the spine. The doctor should contact the patient similarly to the actual adjustment. A traction force is applied to the spine with the stabilization hand while a sustained pressure is applied with the segmental contact hand. Attention must be paid to patient tolerance. The segment should gradually "give-way" as creep deformation of the ligamentous elements occurs. The segmental pressure is applied in the direction of fixation dysfunction.

IMMOBILIZATION

The use of rigid or soft collars is usually not indicated in the management of whiplash-type injuries. If the patient is unable to hold the head in an upright position or if gross instability or fracture is present, then a cervical support will be required. Mealy et al. (30) compared immobilization (soft collar and bed rest) with early mobilization (Maitland technique) for patients who suffered whiplash injuries. In a randomized study, the results showed that at eight weeks after the accident, the degree of improvement seen in the actively treated group compared with the immobilized group was significantly greater for both cervical movement and the intensity of pain.

Prognosis

Greenfield and Ilfield (31) evaluated short-term prognostic factors in patients who sustained whiplash injuries from automobile accidents. The presence of interscapular and upper back pain appeared to correlate with a less favorable prognosis. Those patients who underwent a course of traction therapy also had a poorer prognosis.

The presence of neurologic signs in the upper extremities, such as paresthesia, or referred pain should reflect a relatively worse prognosis (32). Simple neurologic testing of dermatomes (See Chapter 4) can be performed or more objective testing methods may be used to aid assessment of these patients. Thermography is a useful modality for imaging these types of disorders (33). The presence of persistent thermographic abnormalities would also adversely affect the prognosis of the patient.

A poorer outcome is expected if there are preexisting degenerative changes (32). A hypolordotic or kyphotic cervical curve is more common in patients with persistent pain (34). Patients with restricted motion demonstrated on flexion/extension roentgenograms also tend to have a poorer prognosis for recovery (34).

STATIC RADIOGRAPHY

Plain film radiography in the neutral position is used essentially to rule out possible contraindications for manipulative therapy and as an aid in determining the site for treatment. The lateral projection is useful for determining which segments are in a hyperextended or flexed position. There appears to be a high correlation with extension malposition and the level of involvement (35) (Fig. 10.13A-B). This positional dyskinesia may be

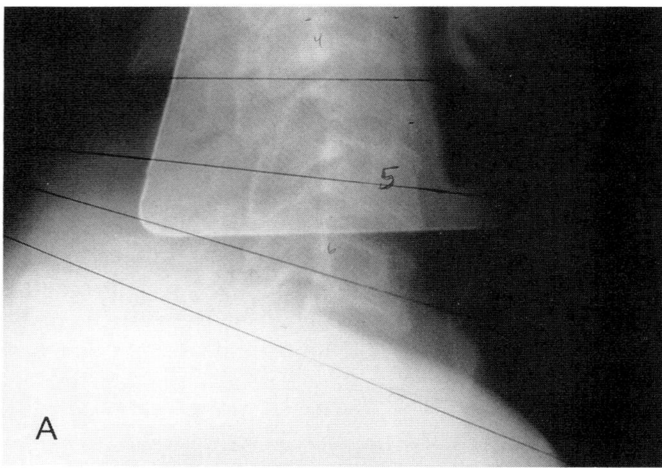

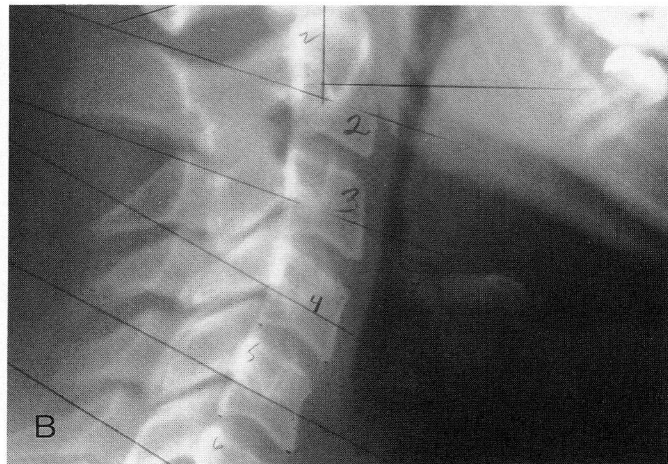

Figure 10.13. **A,** C5 extension malposition. **B,** C3 extension malposition.

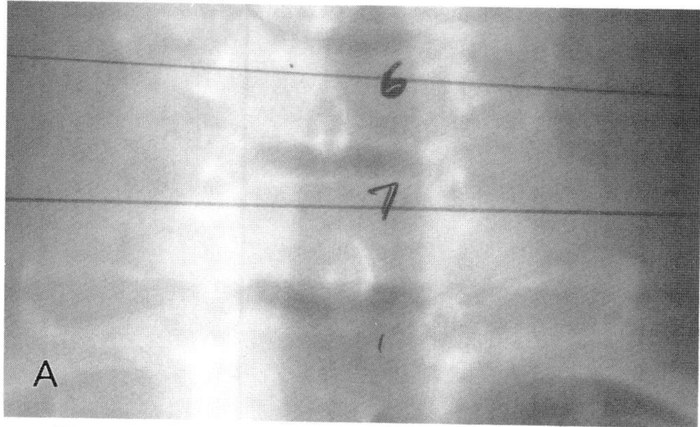

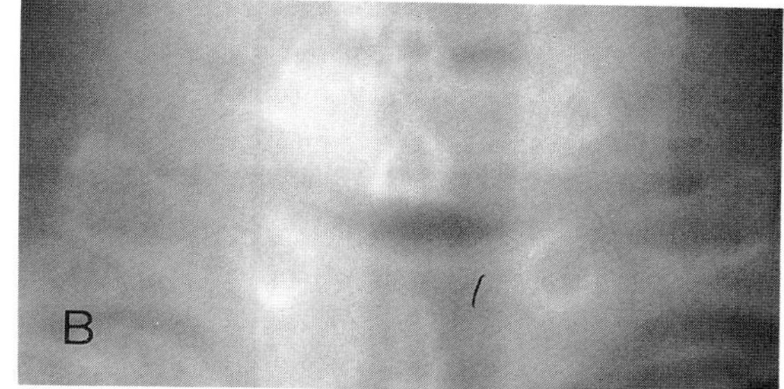

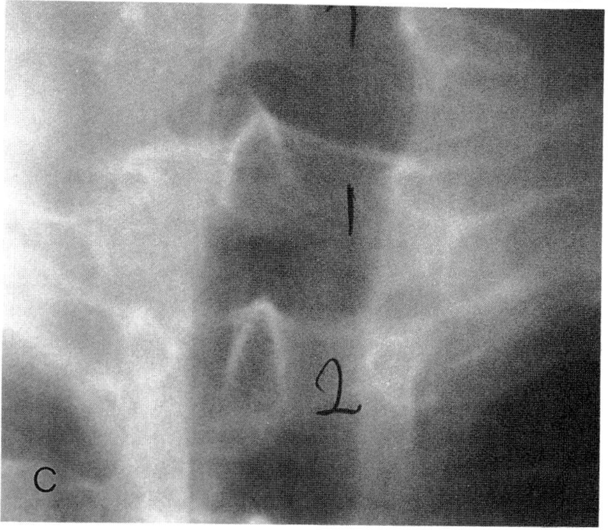

Figure 10.14. **A,** C6 PLS positional dyskinesia. **B,** C7 PLS positional dyskinesia. **C,** T1 PL positional dyskinesia. Notice the relative sizes of the pedicles at T1 compared with their equal dimensions at T2.

evaluated for relative mobility by taking a radiograph in the flexed position. If the vertebra moves anterior-superior during flexion, then an adjustment is usually contraindicated at that level. An exception to the above might be a segment that shows dysfunction in either lateral bending or rotation. In this case, the primary action of moving the vertebra anteriorward is deemphasized during the thrust and other movements are stressed.

The coronal plane radiograph is used to derive the rotational (Y axis) and lateral flexion components of the subluxation listing (Fig. 10.14A-C). If intersegmental motion palpation assessment of the joint appears to contraindicate the static listing, then radiographs taken at the extremes of lateral bending should be performed to obtain a more accurate diagnosis.

STRESS RADIOGRAPHY

Analysis of the spine in lateral bending as well as the extremes of flexion and extension is relatively common (Fig. 10.15–10.17). If more detailed information is necessary, the spine can be x-rayed in intermediate positions between the extremes of maximal flexion and extension (36). Dvorak et al. (37) found that analysis of the cervical spine in flexion/extension was more sensitive when passive movements were used. In their study of 59 adults, 19 hypermobile segments could be diagnosed during the active examination, whereas 31 hypermobile segments were found during the passive examination. It is important that the examiner wear a whole lead coat with long sleeves and lead gloves, as well as lead glasses during the passive radiologic assessment. Slight and marked restrictions in extension motion appear to be significant findings that indicate an abnormality of the joint (38). Paradoxical motion may be present as well. In this situation, the segment appears to flex when the neck is extended and vice versa. During flexion, excessive anterior glide or increased flexion indicates hypermobility secondary to ligamentous sprain or rupture. Fixation dysfunction is usually more easily detected in the flexed posture. The segment will remain in an extended position with head and neck flexion.

Cineradiography or videofluoroscopy of the cervical spine may be useful in identifying dysfunction that is not present on roentgenograms in the neutral or stressed positions (39–41). Videofluoroscopy appears to be able to detect midcervical (i.e., C4-C5) fixation dysfunction with a high degree of reliability (42). Videofluoroscopy has also been advocated for the evaluation of cervical spine instability (43).

COMPENSATION REACTIONS

Postural

The most common postural reaction to cervical trauma is a hypolordotic or kyphotic cervical curve. If an extension positional dyskinesia ($-Z$, $-\theta X$) is present, the vertebra above usually compensates by flexion. Hyperextension subluxations of the upper cervical spine (e.g., AS occiput or AS atlas) will usually result in a kyphotic deformation of the midcervical spine below.

Hyperkyphosis and compression fractures of the thoracic spine, as commonly occurs in patients with osteoporosis, may cause a compensatory hyperlordosis of the cervical spine. In general, hyperlordotic compensations of the cervical spine are less common than reversals of the cervical lordosis.

Dynamic

Dynamic reactions to vertebral injury include hypo- and hypermobility. Fixation dysfunction can be a result of direct injury (See Chapter 3) through adhesion formation or edema, or due to long-term effects of impaired postural movements. Hypermobility above the level of fixation dysfunction is quite common. The midcervical spine is a likely site for hypermobility to occur. The highest incidence of disc protrusion and degeneration in the cervical spine occurs in the midcervical area. Traction osteo-

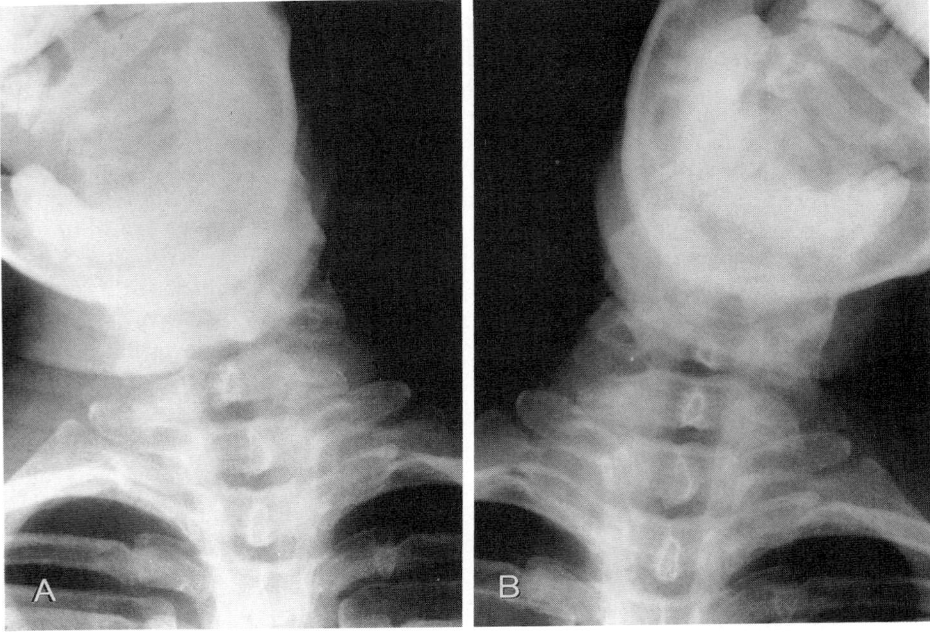

Figure 10.15. **A,** Left lateral bending. There is no coupling of the spinous process at C7 toward the convexity of bend. **B,** Right lateral bending. There is decreased lateral flexion (+θZ) at C7 and T1. Notice the compensatory hypermobility at C6.

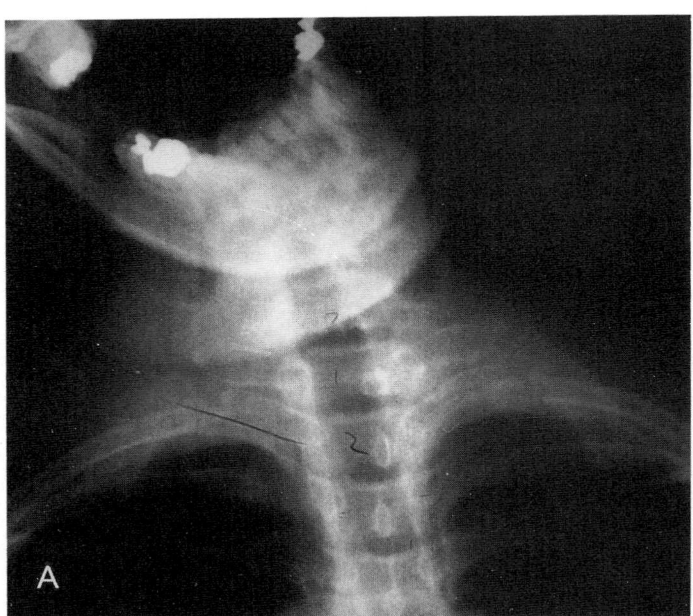

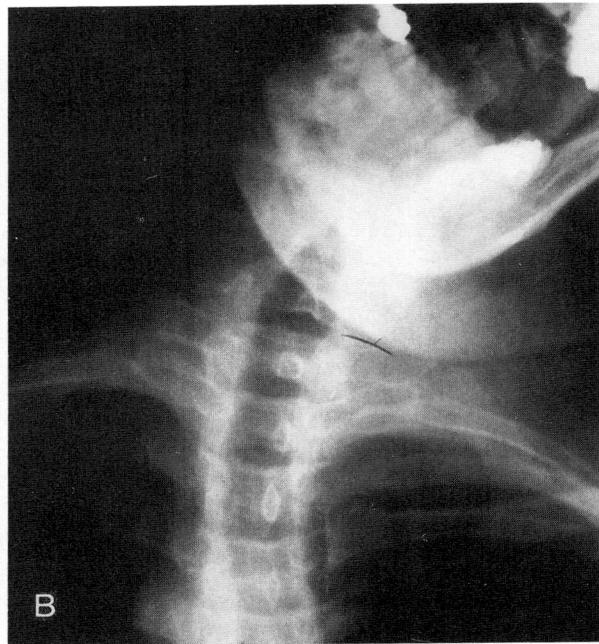

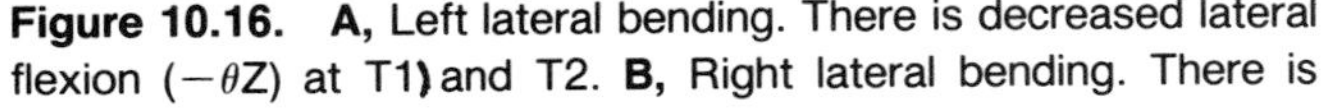

Figure 10.16. **A,** Left lateral bending. There is decreased lateral flexion (−θZ) at T1 and T2. **B,** Right lateral bending. There is decreased right lateral flexion (+θZ) and coupling motion (−θY) at C7. Notice the hypermobility at C6.

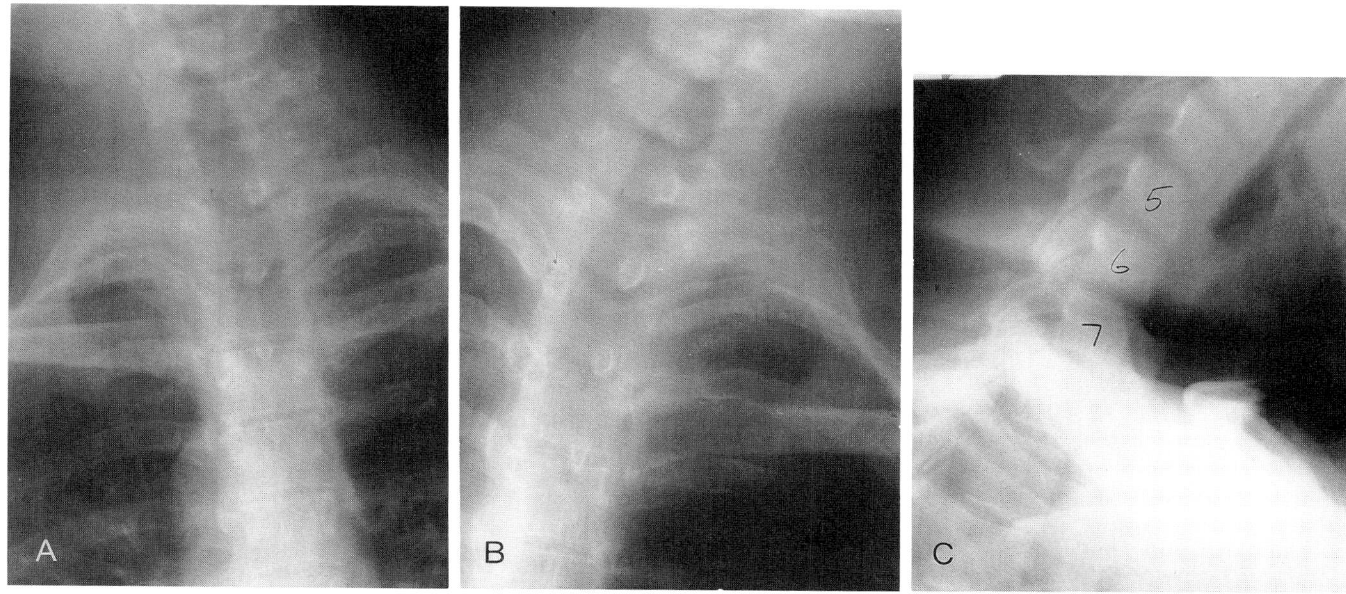

Figure 10.17. **A,** Left lateral bending. There is decreased lateral flexion ($-\theta Z$) at T1 through T3. **B,** Right lateral bending. There is decreased coupled motion ($-\theta Y$) at C7 through T4. There is severe lateral flexion ($+\theta Z$) dysfunction at C7. **C,** Flexion radiograph. There is decreased flexion ($+\theta X$) at C6 and C7. Notice the excessive anterior translatory ($+Z$) motion at C4.

phytes are an early sign of hypermobility/instability. Treatment (i.e., adjustments) should not be directed at these hypermobile (and often painful) areas. The fixated level is usually below the site of hypermobility. Stress radiography is an important tool for identifying levels of hyper- or hypomobility.

ACQUIRED TORTICOLLIS

Torticollis is defined as a twisting or tilting of the cervical spine. For a summary of pediatric torticollis, especially those encountered in the newborn, please consult Chapter 14. A variety of different therapies show little documented clinical efficacy (44). The older the patient or the more constant the symptoms, the worse the prognosis. The two major types of torticollis encountered in general practice are spasmodic and nonspasmodic.

Spasmodic Torticollis

Spasmodic torticollis is characterized by spasm of one or more cervical muscles. Commonly, the sternocleidomastoid is involved. The contracture of the muscles pulls the neck and head to one side. The spasms are usually caused by reflexive muscular contraction after irritation to the spinoaccessory nerve or upper cervical plexus. When the doctor attempts to passively straighten the head and neck, the patient will experience increased pain in the neck on the side of the lean. The pain is due to the forced stretching of a spasmed muscle. A subluxation of the upper cervical region, especially the C1-C2 motion segment, is a common cause of spasmodic torticollis. A spinal adjustment often brings immediate relief. Atlantoaxial rotatory fixation (See Chapter 11) may lead to spasmodic torticollis with spastic contracture of the sternocleidomastoid muscle. Stress radiography (e.g., flexion, lateral bending) may be performed to help determine the levels exhibiting fixation dysfunction. Acute pain and spasm makes motion palpation more difficult. The reliability of the information obtained is also uncertain.

Nonspasmodic Torticollis

Nonspasmodic torticollis is characterized by an antalgic lean away from a painful vertebral lesion. When passively moved towards a more vertical position, the patient will experience increased pain on the side of the neck being leaned away from. The etiology is often a subluxation of the lower cervical or upper thoracic area. Upper thoracic disc lesions are a common cause. A more caudal thoracic, such as a mid dorsal motion segment may be a contributing or primary factor. In the management of this condition, the lower segment, if two are involved, should be adjusted first, followed by the upper level during the adjustment session. Because of the substantial derangement of the intervertebral disc often encountered in nonspasmodic cases, the patient may require a more repetitive series of adjustments than with the spasmodic variety. Nonspasmodic conditions are usually a chronic problem presenting as an acute exacerbation. If the patient is prone to recurrent postural torticollis, ergonomic factors, such as sleep positions, must be evaluated (45).

Wood (46) has advocated not adjusting the spinal segment toward a central location (i.e., three-dimensionally toward center, opposite the components of the listing) in patients with torticollis. This "approach" is not advised by the authors, because moving the segment into the direction of ligamentous stretch is more likely to cause further injury.

THORACIC OUTLET SYNDROME

Thoracic outlet syndrome (TOS) refers to a group of disorders in which the neurovascular structures that run through the thoracic outlet are compromised by structures in and around it. It is helpful to further classify thoracic outlet syndrome based on etiology; scalenus anticus syndrome, costoclavicular syndrome, etc.

Symptoms of Thoracic Outlet Syndrome

The symptoms of TOS are associated with brachial plexopathy. The most common symptom is pain radiating down the medially aspect of the arm to the fifth digit. In many patients, headache may be the leading symptom of TOS (47). Other symptoms include the following:

1. A dull ache in the entire arm
2. Numbness and paresthesias in the arms
3. Grip weakness
4. Pain at night
5. Arm edema, rubor, coldness, cyanosis. Reynaud's phenomenon, and symptoms associated with vascular insufficiency.

Costoclavicular Syndrome

The costoclavicular area is the space between the first rib and the clavicle. Individuals with forward-drooping or rounded shoulders may develop symptoms when the clavicle is pressed down against the neurovascular bundle and the first rib. Postural exercises, as a supplement to spinal adjustive therapy, should provide relief for most patients. Less chronic postural dysfunctions will have a more favorable prognosis.

Scalenus Anticus Syndrome

The scalenes are often involved in TOS. This involvement can occur as a result of overdeveloped musculature such as may occur in bodybuilders or other athletes. There are often characteristic referred pain patterns due to trigger points in the scalenes. Pain may be referred from the lower part of the scalenus medius or scalenus posterior muscle to the anterior pectoral region about the nipple. The pain is aching and persistent.

The adjustive treatment of scalenus anticus syndrome should begin with determining if a subluxation is present in the cervical spine. Because the scalene muscles attach to the transverse processes of C2 through C6, nerve impingement may cause a reflex hypertonicity or spasm of the associated muscular elements. Trigger points in the scalene muscles may need to be addressed to break the pain-spasm-pain cycle.

Cervical Rib Syndrome

Cervical ribs occur in 0.5% of the population with 80% of these occurring bilaterally. Ten percent of patients with cervical ribs may have related symptomatology. Because the cervical rib has been present in the patient throughout life, the question must be asked as to why it is symptomatic now. It is most likely that the presence of a cervical rib will complicate the clinical picture rather than cause the disorder. Cervical ribs narrow the thoracic inlet and can compress the brachial plexus and the subclavian artery between it and the clavicle. This is most apparent when the arm is hyperabducted. A hasty decision to refer for surgery might prevent the patient from getting the best treatment. The patient with thoracic outlet syndrome who also has a cervical rib might present with neurovascular symptoms that are difficult to differentiate from costoclavicular, or scalenus anticus syndrome. Wright's and Adson's test may be positive. Subluxations of the lower cervical and upper thoracic spine should be ruled out. Other factors to consider are abnormal fibrous bands extending from the tip of an incomplete cervical rib to the first rib, an abnormally long transverse process of the C7 vertebra, an abnormal insertion of the scalene muscle(s) on to the first rib (48), or pseudoarthrosis of the clavicle and malunion of the clavicle with exuberant callus formation (49).

Vascular Thoracic Outlet Syndrome

Vascular TOS is rare (5–10% of all TOS) (49). Arterial dysfunction may be created by a long complete cervical rib which causes compression or kinking of the subclavian artery. This can lead to injury to the tunica intima and later aneurysm and mural thrombosis (49).

Venous TOS is even less common than the arterial variety (49). The subclavian vein lies outside the scalene triangle so the etiology has been perplexing. Factors to consider would be metastatic tumors (e.g., pancoast tumor).

Diagnostic Tests For Thoracic Outlet Syndrome

The diagnostic dilemma of TOS is differentiating it from C8-T1 radiculopathy (50). Foraminal compression tests, stress tests, electrodiagnostic studies and plain film radiography are useful tools for making the differentiation.

90° ABDUCTION EXTERNAL ROTATION TEST

The Abduction External Rotation (AER) Test is likely the most reliable test for assessing a narrow thoracic outlet (51,52). The arm is abducted to a right angle and externally rotated. The forearm should be flexed to 90° and the head turned to the opposite side of symptomatology. Pulse changes or increased symptomatology should be noted. If both the artery and the lower plexus are compressed, the patient will usually experience pain and paresthesia first in the ulnar distribution, followed by tingling into the entire hand (50). The early component is neurogenic and the late component is due to ischemia. Pure neurogenic TOS is suspected if paresthesia and pain persist without pulse diminution. If the patient's symptoms are not provoked with this maneuver, then they should be asked to open and close their fist slowly for three minutes. The test is diagnostic if crescendo fatigue, numbness, or aching pain develops in the hand and forearm. If the symptoms are relieved when the arm is dropped, the diagnosis is further strengthened (50).

EXAGGERATED MILITARY MANEUVER

This postural maneuver narrows the costoclavicular space by approximating the clavicle to the first rib (50). The patient is asked to brace the shoulders downward and backward forcefully while the chest is thrust forward. The chin should be slightly elevated.

ADSON'S AND WRIGHT'S TESTS

Patients with true neurogenic TOS may have a negative Adson test. Even if a positive finding is present, this test has no localizing value as to the exact site of compression (50). Many normal subjects show pulse obliteration with the Adson maneuver (51,53).

Wright's or the hyperabduction test may be positive in patients with TOS (50). This test compresses both the subcoracoid and the costoclavicular space, making localization of the site of entrapment more difficult.

SPINAL CANAL STENOSIS

The spinal canal can become stenotic due to congenital and acquired factors. Parke (54) has demonstrated that the spinal canal is funnel shaped and wider at the top. This configuration can be problematic if degenerative spondylophytic ridges narrow the dimensions of the canal (Fig. 10.18). There is an enlargement in the cervical spinal cord where the brachial plexus originates. This enlargement combined with a narrowed canal can lead to cord compression. Thus, the most common levels of involvement for cervical spondylotic myelopathy (CSM) are at the vertebral segments C4-C7 (55).

Degeneration of the motion segment occurs at the disc, the zygapophyseal joints, the vertebral body, and the surrounding ligaments. If the ligamentum flavum has been stretched or there is reduced disc space height, the ligament can infold into the posterior aspect of the canal. The ligament tends to thicken with repeated trauma. During extension movements, symptoms may be exaggerated due to compression from the ligamentum flavum. Flexion movements may also aggravate symptoms, because the spinal cord is stretched with this posture (See Chapter 2). The tension developed can lead to neural compromise. The cord can also become compressed against the posterior aspects of the disc and vertebral body (55).

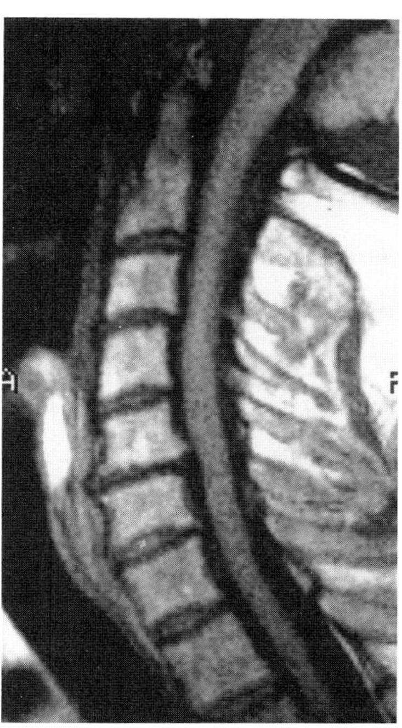

Figure 10.18. Sagittal view. Degenerative joint disease with spondylophyte formations encroaching on the thecal sac. There is moderate compression of the spinal cord at C5-C6 (See Figure 10.5).

ADJUSTMENT

Cervical Chair

The seated position is preferred for adjusting the cervical spine. In this position, the surrounding segments can be effectively stabilized and an inferior to superior pattern of thrust can be accomplished (35). Tension is developed usually through primarily lateral flexion movements. The doctor should avoid postures that compromise the vertebral arteries (i.e., rotation or rotation combined with extension) during the adjustment (See Chapter 11). The cervical chair has an adjustable back to accommodate most patients (Fig. 10.19). It is generally preferred to keep the seat-back in the most upright position.

The stabilization strap is used to prevent forward movement of the patient during the thrust. For right-sided contacts (e.g., PR, PLI-La) the strap is placed over the left shoulder and vice versa.

The patient should be seated in an upright position with hands on the lap and legs extended in front. The patient should not clench the hands or press against the

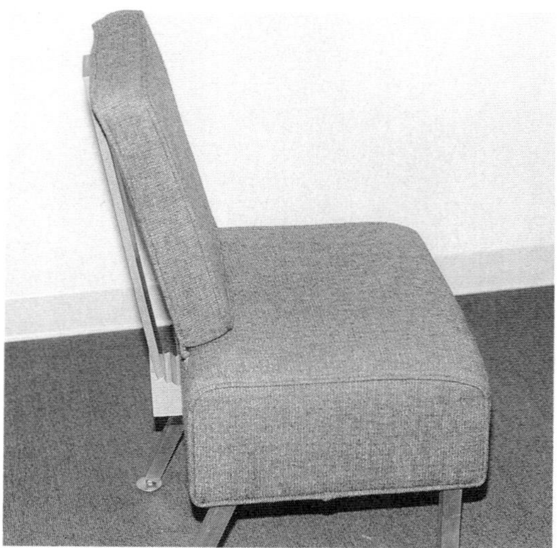

Figure 10.19. Cervical chair.

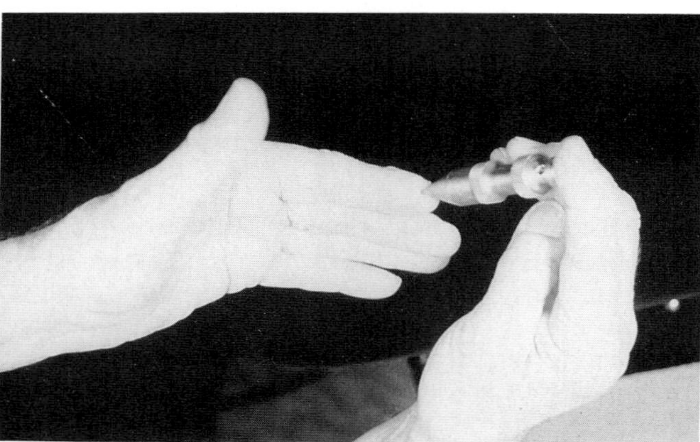

Figure 10.20. Doctor's contact point.

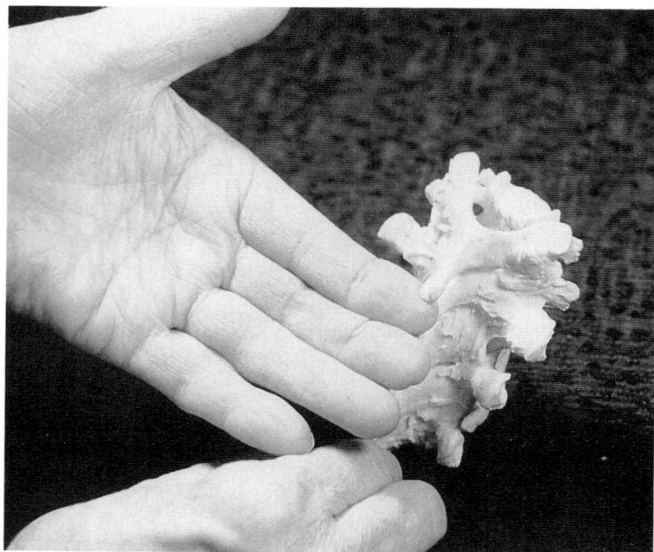

Figure 10.21. Contact point on the distal, inferior aspect of the spinous process.

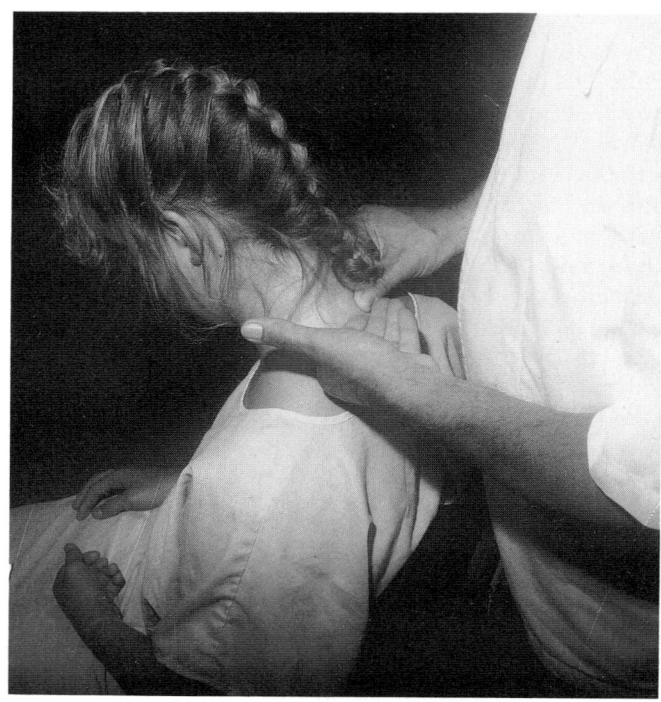

Figure 10.22. The tissue pull is made with the thumb of the stabilization hand in the line of correction.

floor with the soles of the feet. Both of these actions will create tension, thus making the adjustment more difficult.

The doctor's contact point for the adjustment is the distal, lateral and palmar aspect of the first digit (Fig. 10.20). The other fingers then back-up the first digit. If the listing demands a lamina contact (i.e., PRI-La or PLI-La), then the finger contacts the most medial portion of the lamina. For spinous listings (e.g., PR, PL, PLS, PRS, P, etc.), the doctor contacts the distal inferior border of the spinous process (Fig. 10.21). If the spinous is rotated to the left, then the doctor should slightly favor the left side and vice versa. A tissue pull is made with the stabilization hand in the line of correction. For example a PL listing would require a left to right and inferior to superior tissue pull (Fig. 10.22). The inferior to superior tissue pull is to accommodate the $+\theta X$ pattern of thrust of most lower cervical adjustments.

The thrust hand is stabilized by placing the thumb against the ramus of the mandible. Depending on the size of the doctor's hands and the size of the patient's neck, the thumb may be placed over or behind the ear. No pressure should be applied with the thumb during the thrust. It should simply move forward across the skin when the thrust is made from posterior to anterior. There should be a clear arch formed between the thumb and first finger (Fig. 10.23). This opening is sometimes referred to as a "rat hole." Maintenance of the arch appears to strengthen the hand for the thrust so that it remains rigid during the maneuver.

The palmar surface of the stabilization hand is placed over the cervical spine on the opposite side of the thrusting hand. The hand and fingers should stabilize the segments above and below the vertebra being adjusted (Fig. 10.24). No thrust is made with the stabilization hand. A slight inferiorward pressure can be applied by the fingers of the stabilization hand contacting the vertebra just beneath the segment being adjusted. This is done to stabilize the foundation that the vertebra is being "set-upon." The patient's head can rest against the doctor (Fig. 10.25), or can be maintained in the upright position solely with the doctor's hands. The set-up for the adjustment proceeds as follows:

1. The patient's head is flexed and a tissue pull is made in the line of correction.
2. The distal, lateral, palmar aspect of the first finger should contact the inferior and lateral border of the spinous or the medial portion of the lamina.
3. With the stabilization hand, the head is brought into an upright position and translated posteriorward.
4. The head is laterally flexed toward the side of contact (10–15°).
5. The stabilization hand covers the cervical segments from the opposite side.
6. The thrust is made with a very quick movement of the hand and forearm in the line of correction. No thrust is made with the stabilization hand.
7. The segment being contacted should be held for a moment after the thrust in order that the viscoelastic elements of the motion segment are maximally affected.

Name of technique: Gonstead

Name of technique procedure: P ($-Z$, $-\theta X$) C5 Cervical Chair Adjustment (Fig. 10.25).

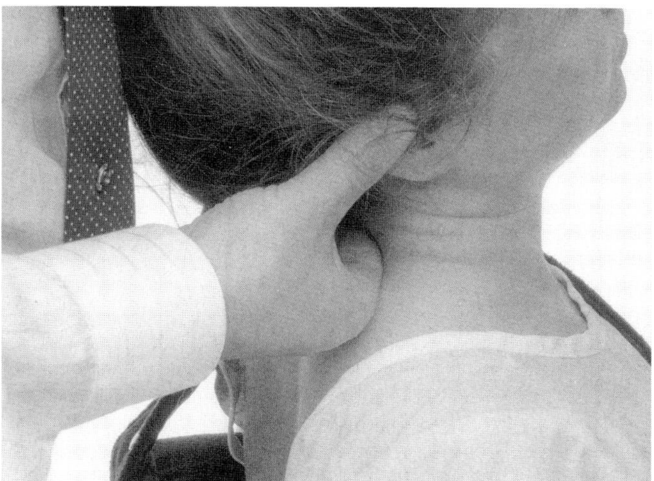

Figure 10.23. Maintenance of an arch between the thumb and first digit is critical to the performance of a cervical adjustment.

Indications: Retrolisthesis of C5 with decreased $+Z$ and $+\theta X$ motion.

Contraindications: All other listings, normal FSU, hypermobility, instability, destruction or fracture of the neural arch or spinous process, infection of the contact vertebra.

Patient position: Seated in the cervical chair as upright as possible with both lower extremities extended and the dorsal aspect of the patient's hands resting on the anterior thighs.

Doctor's position: Standing behind the patient and slightly to the right. The listing demonstrated could be adjusted with either the right or left hand.

Contact point: Palmar and lateral surface of the (R) distal phalanx of the index finger placed on the inferior lateral aspect of the C5 spinous process. The middle finger should be directly

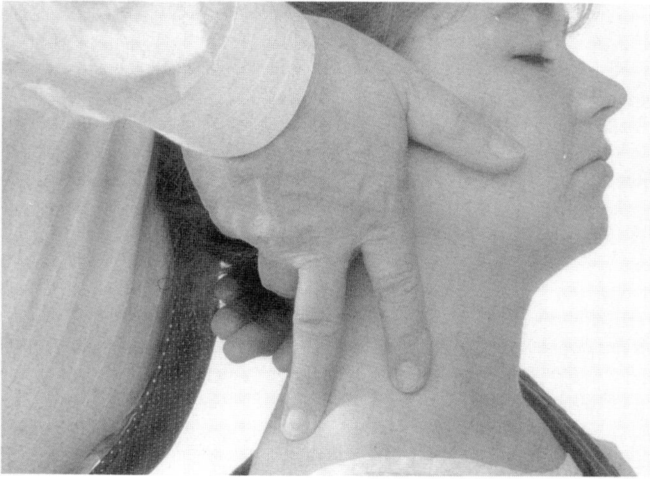

Figure 10.24. Stabilization hand for a T1 adjustment. Notice the line of drive for the thrusting hand along the plane line of the T1 disc.

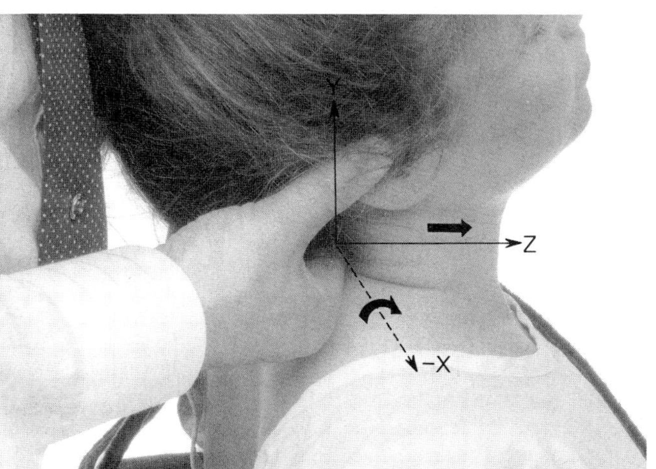

Figure 10.25. C5 P adjustment from the right side.

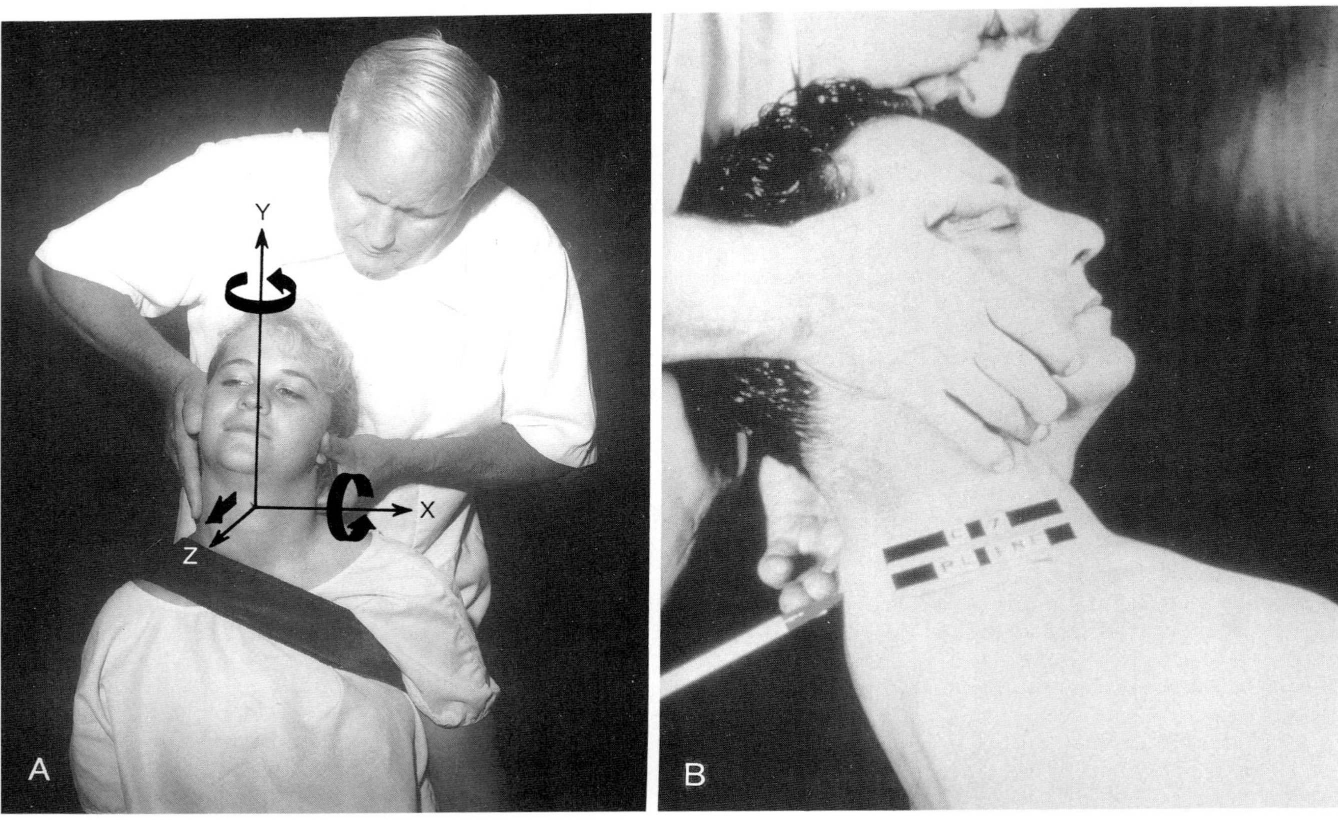

Figure 10.26. **A,** C7 PL adjustment. **B,** C7 PL adjustment.

adjacent to the index finger to give the index finger stability. The contact hand (R) is stabilized by placing the thumb on the ramus of the mandible, below the temporomandibular joint so that no pressure is applied to the head of the mandible. When the contact hand is properly placed, an arch is formed by the lateral portion of the thumb and index finger. Figure 10.25 demonstrates the thumb resting lightly over the patient's ear.

Supporting hand: The left hand is placed so that the palmar surface supports the lateral area of the cervical spine at the C5-C6 level. This will bring the thenar eminence below the ear and the thumb along the angle of the jaw.

Set Up: With the stabilization hand (L) on top of the patient's head, the head should be flexed slightly to separate the spinous processes. The palmar surface of the left distal phalanx of the index finger is then placed on the inferior aspect of the C5 spinous process. The thumb of the contact hand (R) should be placed on the ramus of the jaw facing anteriorward so that the arch is formed between the thumb and the index finger. The head is brought back into a more relaxed position by the stabilization hand, and it is placed along the posterior and lateral portion of the cervical spine. The chin is elevated slightly so that the posterior musculature is relaxed. The cervical spine is laterally flexed ($+\theta Z$) to the right approximately 10–15°. The slack is then reduced by applying a ($+Z$) pressure on the C5 spinous process with the (R) contact finger. The stabilization hand restricts head motion as the thrust is given. There is no pulling with the stabilization hand.

Pattern of thrust: An arcing motion through the vertebral body posterior to anterior ($+Z$) and inferior to superior ($+\theta X$) through the plane line of the intervertebral disc and facet articulations.

Category by algorithm: Short lever specific contact procedure.

Name of technique: Gonstead

Name of technique procedure: PL ($-Z, -\theta Y$) C7 Cervical Chair Adjustment (Fig. 10.26A-B).

Indications: Retrolisthesis of C7 with decreased $+Z$, $+\theta Y$ and $+\theta X$ motion.

Contraindications: All other listings, normal FSU, hypermobility, instability, destruction or fracture of the neural arch or spinous process, infection of the contact vertebra.

Patient position: Seated in the cervical chair as upright as possible with both lower extremities extended and the dorsal aspect of the patient's hands resting on their anterior thighs.

vial membrane. Posteriorly, each capsule is strengthened by an accessory ligament. The accessory ligament attaches to the axis at the base of the dens and to the lateral masses of the atlas. Anteriorly, these two bones are attached to each other by a continuation of the anterior longitudinal ligament (ALL). The ALL is attached at the lower portion of the anterior tubercle of atlas superiorly and to the front of the body of axis inferiorly. Posteriorly, the atlas and axis are joined together by a membrane that is attached to the lower portion of the posterior arch of atlas and to the upper edges of the laminae of the axis. This membrane is a continuation of the ligamentum flavum, and on its lateral extremity it is pierced by the second cervical nerve (13,14).

The anterior surface of the dens articulates with the posterior aspect of the anterior tubercle of atlas. This articulation is surrounded by a weak and loose fibrous capsule and is lined with a synovial membrane. Posteriorly, there is a bursa between the cartilage covered anterior surface of the transverse ligament of the atlas, and the posterior grooved portion of the dens of the axis.

The transverse ligament, the most important ligament of the C0-C1-C2 complex, is a strong thick band. It is a major portion of the cruciate ligament. The transverse ligament arches across the neural ring of the atlas and holds the dens in contact with the atlas. This ligament is broader in the middle and is attached to the atlas at two small tubercles on the medial border of the lateral masses of atlas. It divides the atlas into two unequal parts; the larger posterior portion surrounds the spinal cord and its associated membranes, whereas the smaller anterior portion contains the dens. The ligament is placed in such a way that if all other surrounding ligaments are cut, the transverse ligament, by itself, will be able to keep the axis in position. Patients with rheumatoid arthritis often have disruption of this ligament, which can lead to instability (15).

CRUCIATE LIGAMENT

The cruciate ligament was given its name because of its cross-like appearance (Fig. 11.3). It has three components:

1. Transverse ligament of atlas (Fig. 11.4);
2. Caudal crus—commences at the central portion of the transverse ligament, and runs inferiorward attaching at the center of the axis posterior body; and
3. Cranial crus—commencing at the central portion of the transverse ligament, running upward to the anterior margin of the foramen magnum.

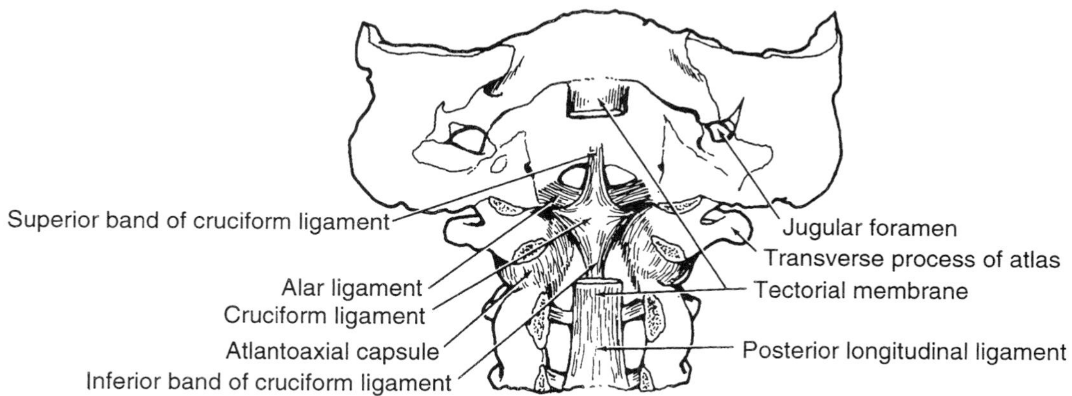

Figure 11.3. Posterior aspect of the upper cervical articulations after removal of the posterior portion of the occipital bone and the laminae of the subjacent vertebrae. Modified from Williams PL, Warwick R. Gray's anatomy. 36th British ed. Philadelphia: WB Saunders, 1980:449.

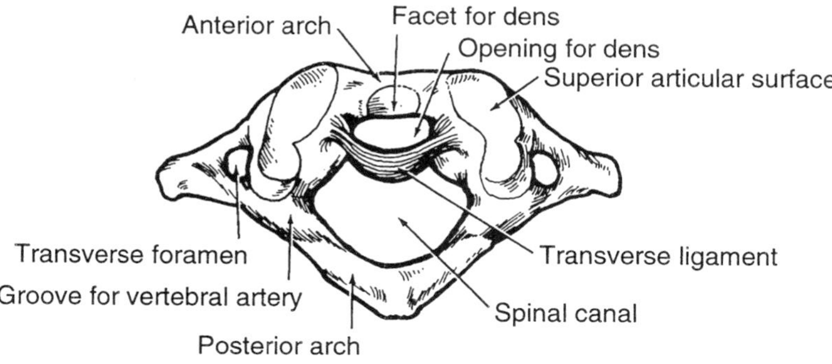

Figure 11.4. Atlas with transverse ligament. Modified from Williams PL, Warwick R. Gray's anatomy. 36th British ed. Philadelphia: WB Saunders, 1980:448.

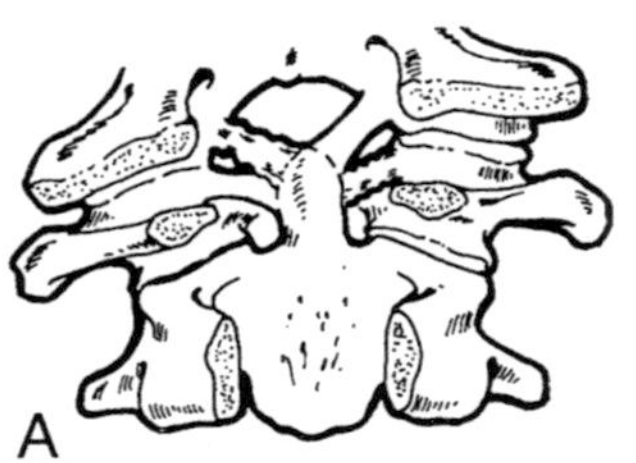

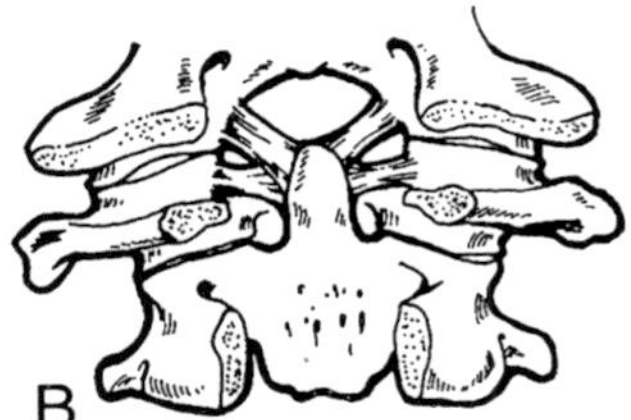

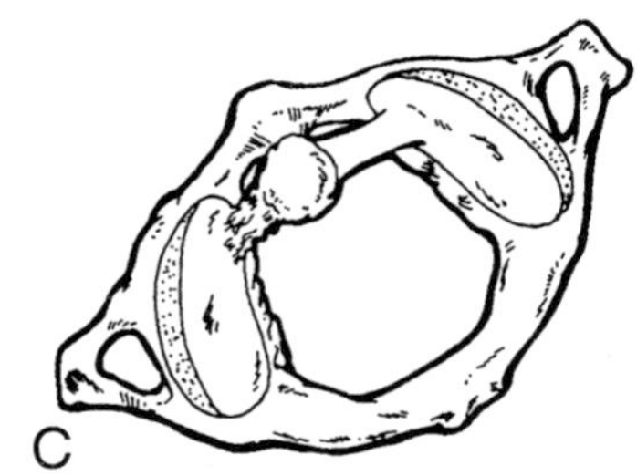

Figure 11.5. Alar ligaments. **A,** Left lateral bending. Notice the taut right upper and left lower ligaments. Modified from Jofe MH, White AA, Panjabi MM. Clinically relevant kinematics of the cervical spine. In: Sherk HH, Dunn EJ, Eismont FJ, et al., eds. The cervical spine. 2nd ed. Philadelphia: JB Lippincott, 1989:61. **B,** Neutral position. Modified from Jofe MH, White AA, Panjabi MM. Clinically relevant kinematics of the cervical spine. In: Sherk HH, Dunn EJ, Eismont FJ, et al., eds. The cervical spine. 2nd ed. Philadelphia: JB Lippincott, 1989:61. **C,** Left axial rotation ($+\theta$Y). Aerial view. Notice the taut right alar ligament. Modified from Jofe MH, White AA, Panjabi MM. Clinically relevant kinematics of the cervical spine. In: Sherk HH, Dunn EJ, Eismont FJ, et al., eds. The cervical spine. 2nd ed. Philadelphia: JB Lippincott, 1989:61.

The ligamentum nuchae attaches from the crest of the occiput to the posterior tubercle of atlas and the spinous process of the other cervical vertebrae. This ligament helps in stabilizing the skull on the cervical spine.

ALAR LIGAMENT

The alar ligaments, also termed the *check ligaments,* play a key role in controlling or checking rotation and lateral flexion at both the atlanto-axial, and occipito-atlantal joints (13,14). They are strong, round bands arising from the dens upward and lateralward, inserting into the medial borders of the condyles and atlas. In a study by Dvorak et al. (16), it was shown that severing of the alar ligament increased axial rotation at both the atlanto-axial and occipito-atlantal articulations. This increase in rotation was noted on the contralateral side of the ligament cut. The ligaments are placed on both sides of the dens symmetrically; one portion connects the dens to the atlas, and the other connects the dens to the occiput (Fig. 11.5A).

During left lateral flexion ($-\theta$Z), motion is controlled by the right upper portion connected to the occiput, and the left lower portion connected to the ring of atlas (11.5B). With left axial rotation ($+\theta$Y), the movement is checked by the right alar ligament (Fig. 11.5C).

Muscles

The upper cervical spine, which supports the cranium from above, and a group of freely movable vertebrae below, requires an organization of musculature able to execute motion and provide stability for the area. Some of the ligamentous structures are lax in this region. Support of the head on the neck is provided primarily by the upper cervical musculature (17). Joint motion is controlled by the facet planes and their associated ligamentous structures; however, it is the responsibility of the muscles to dictate patterns of motion in the upper cervical spine and to provide much of the stability (13,14). A study by Goel et al. (17) found that relatively small loads were needed to produce large amounts of rotation at the upper cervical complex. This finding supports the idea that the ligaments of the C0-C1-C2 complex are relatively lax.

Muscle tissue has abundant nerve supply. Joint dysfunction can cause the muscles to spasm or become hypertonic (18). The spasm/hypertonicity should resolve if treatment is focused on normalizing the joint dysfunction. The finding of trigger points and myofascitis is common in the upper cervical spine. These findings are often compensatory for disturbances below.

Flaccidity of the muscles will place more stress on the ligaments, possibly leading to ligament laxity and instability. Treatment protocols that focus solely on the muscles can lead to inappropriate management. Although muscles can be a source of pain, they should not be the only focus of a treatment paradigm. The use of trigger point therapy and transverse frictional massage would be indicated when fibrotic adhesions have developed in the area. Passive mobilization is encouraged after acute neck injuries (See Chapter 10).

Clinical observations suggest that individuals who have sustained soft tissue injuries respond quickly to treatment if they are well conditioned and have good muscle tone, provided all other variables are equal.

Once articular function has been restored, the use of exercises to help strengthen the associated muscular elements is strongly recommended. Posttraumatic muscle weakness, secondary to scar tissue or nerve damage, and joint weakness caused by creep of ligamentous structures may improve with specific exercises. The main purpose of these exercises is to stretch muscle and fascial elements that have been shortened and to contract muscles that have been in a chronic state of relaxation or hypotonicity. The patient should avoid movements that are in the direction of ligamentous sprain.

Patterns of Motion

FLEXION-EXTENSION $\pm\theta X$

Flexion at C0-C1-C2 is limited by a bursa that originates from the condyles and inserts into the dens of axis. It is referred to as the bursa apicus dentis. Extension at this joint is limited by the tectorial membrane which is a continuation of the posterior longitudinal ligament. Flexion-extension in this region is approximately 25° at the C0-C1 articulation and 20° at C1-C2 (13).

LATERAL FLEXION $\pm\theta Z$

The amount of lateral flexion allowed at both C0-C1 and C1-C2 is approximately 5° to either side (13). This motion is controlled by both components of the alar ligaments. During lateral flexion, there is a slight ipsilateral translation of the atlas ($\pm X$) to the side of the bend (viewed with stress radiography). Presence of this motion may contraindicate lateral to medial adjustive thrusts from the contralateral side.

ROTATION $\pm\theta Y$

Rotation in the upper cervical complex is approximately 40° at C1-C2, and 5° at C0-C1 (13). This movement is controlled or "checked" by the alar ligaments. For example, rotation to the right is controlled by the left alar ligament, and vice versa.

Neurology

Because of the anatomic relationship of the atlas and occiput with the brain stem, subluxation in this area may affect a variety of neural structures; cervical spinal cord, first and second cervical spinal nerves, superior cervical ganglion, and cranial nerves X, XI, XII. This region should not be overlooked as a potential cause of a variety of neurodysfunctional states. Experimental lesions in laboratory animals (3–6) have shown effects predominantly on the parasympathetic division of the autonomic nervous system. Clinical studies by Harris and Wagnon (19) demonstrated nonsympathetic effects on distal skin temperature when the patient was adjusted in the upper cervical spine. Gonstead (20) associated adjustments of the upper cervical spine (i.e., C0-C5) with effects primarily in the parasympathetic division.

It takes an average of 64° of rotation (Y axis) at the atlanto-axial articulation before the size of the neural canal is reduced to a diameter of 1 cm. The canal is 3 cm in width. One centimeter is taken up by the axis, 1 cm by the cord, and one-third is free space. An average of 63° of rotation is required to cause bilateral facet dislocation of the atlanto-axial articulation (21). Thus, direct cord compression due entirely to rotation of the bony elements appears unlikely. The models for dysfunction in the upper cervical region are very complex. Because of the proximity of the cervical sympathetic chain, the vagus, the various connective tissues and the cerebral spinal fluid, subluxation complexes are likely to have multiple neurologic effects.

When immobilization is present due to misalignment (positional dyskinesia), changes in the architecture of the connective tissue and the neuroreceptors occur (22). This contracture and constriction of the connective tissue will tighten the collagen matrix, thus putting more stress on the sensory receptors. As a result, slight movement will be perceived by the receptors as gross alterations in the joint. This abnormal sensory input can cause hyperactivity at the sensory receptor level feeding into the reflex pattern. This could be one reason changes in posture and nerve function have been observed after adjustments of the upper cervical spine.

Inflammation as a result of immobilization may cause hyperexcitability of nerves, particularly the dorsal root ganglia and spinal nerve roots. Inflammatory responses after trauma, disc herniation or end-plate fracture (Schmorl's node) may cause damage to the recurrent meningeal nerves, dorsal root ganglia, or spinal nerve roots (22).

Grostic (23) has proposed that the dentate ligament may be able to distort the cervical spinal cord from mechanical tensions in the area. The size and strength of the dentate ligaments indicate that they have a restraining function on the cord and restrict vertical movement. Combined with positional dyskinesia of the upper cervical region, the ligaments could traction different portions of the cord, thus leading to ischemia or direct mechanical irritation.

MECHANORECEPTORS

Mechanoreceptors within the upper cervical area play a key role in movement control and postural adaptations. They are divided into three types.

Type 1 mechanoreceptors are located in the stratum fibrosum of the capsules and ligaments. They are more dense in the proximal joints and are active both at rest and in movement. These receptors play an important role in positional sense, as they signal the angle of the joint throughout the range of motion (11,24,25).

Type 2 mechanoreceptors reside at the junction of the synovial joints and the fibrosum of the capsules. At the distal joints, they are high in density and are active at the beginning and termination of movement and adapt quickly to sudden movements. These receptors can also be found in the intraarticular and extraarticular fat pads.

Type 3 mechanoreceptors are located in the collateral ligaments. They adapt slowly and are active at the end of joint ranges.

There are also pain and proprioceptive fibers in the upper cervical area that communicate with the brain via a branch of the second cervical nerve or the greater occipital nerve.

Vertebral subluxation complex in the upper cervical region may influence posture via joint fixation and reflex compensatory mechanisms. In the past, it was hypothesized that such symptoms as vertigo, dizziness, and equilibrium disorders were either vascular or brainstem related. Recent literature indicates that mechanoreceptor injury can duplicate these symptom patterns.

Korr (18) states that the joint receptors in the capsules and ligaments send signals that inform the higher centers regarding joint angles, velocity, and direction of joint movement. Muscle spindle fibers are arranged in parallel, located within the muscle, and attached at both ends. These intrafusal fibers are innervated by gamma motor neurons that originate from the ventral horn and pass through the ventral root. The function of these fibers is to control contraction of the intrafusal fibers and through them, the sensitivity of the spindles. When a spindle fiber is slackened during muscle shortening, the spindle charge is reduced; and if a muscle is contracted, the discharge is increased. The term *gain* is used to explain the activity of the gamma fibers as their activity increases or decreases to maintain an average, even muscle tone. In the presence of a "lesion," the gain levels have been "stuck" on high settings (18). That is, the gamma discharge to the intrafusal fibers has been increased, which keeps the fibers in a shortened state and the spindles highly sensitive. The spindle will be continually discharging because of the influence of gravitational forces and postural reflexes in an effort to stretch the muscle back toward its resting length. However, because the CNS is ordering the muscle to resist, the more the stretch, the greater the resistance. Theoretically, manipulative procedures may be able to reset the spindle gain (18).

Vertebral Artery

Selecki (21) studied the effect of rotation on the vertebral arteries that exit from the foramina of the atlas and course their way down the cervical spine. He found that after 30° of rotation, the vertebral artery on the contralateral side was kinked and stretched. This phenomena occurred at the level of the foramen transverserii. At 45° of rotation the ipsilateral artery was also kinked. If both arteries are impinged, this may cause symptoms similar to stroke or TIA, such as nausea, vomiting, and visual disturbances. If only one vertebral artery is present, rotation to one side can cause vascular incompetence. Activities such as overhead work or stretching exercises of the neck may also produce circulatory symptomatology.

There have been several cases reported of Wallenberg's syndrome, as a result of rotational manipulations of the cervical spine (26–46). Stroke or stroke-like symptoms can occur in patients as a result of rotatory type manipulations, regardless if the patient has preexisting symptoms. Manipulative type procedures implicated in causing vascular accidents are not limited to the practice of chiropractic. Clearly, the need for rotary manipulations of the upper cervical spine is questionable, because a variety of alternate techniques are available without the associated morbidity (2,32).

The cervical adjustments advocated here involve a minimal amount of axial rotation (if any), which significantly reduces the possibility of causing vertebral artery injury. Different head positions will influence the extent of cerebral circulation. The position of the patient's head and neck before (i.e., set-up) and during an adjustment should maximize the patency of the vertebral arteries, i.e., avoidance of extension with rotation (Fig. 11.6).

UPPER CERVICAL DISORDERS

Vertigo

Vertigo as a result of upper cervical joint dysfunction has been generally accepted. In a study by Fitz-Ritson (47), 90.2% of a group of patients became symptom free after an average of 18 chiropractic treatments. Those patients that achieved the best results had suffered from acute upper cervical joint problems.

Vertigo seems to be present in large numbers of patients involved in whiplash-type injuries. Hinoki (48,49) reports that of his patients who were involved in whiplash injuries, 87% suffered from vertigo. The trauma that is introduced to the spine damages the proprioceptors of the muscles, joints, and tendons. Brunarski (50) states that the cervical proprioceptive input tends to overcompensate via somatosensory projection. Thus, cervicogenic vertigo is both a causative factor and an effect of autonomic dysfunction.

Atlanto-axial Rotary Fixation/Subluxation

Atlanto-axial rotatory fixation (AARF) is poorly understood, although it is well documented in the literature (51–55). This condition primarily occurs in children and is associated with torticollis. At times, it has been noted as a sequela to cervical infection, upper respiratory tract infection, or trauma. It is assumed that the disorder is caused by an increased laxity of the alar, capsular, and transverse ligaments. Children that have been diagnosed with this condition usually present with torticollis and decreased cervical range of motion. There may or may not be pain.

Altongy and Fielding (53) state that the reason most of these cases are delayed in diagnosis is because of the difficulty in obtaining a quality radiograph. This is due to the position of the patient's neck (rotation and lateral flexion).

Classic clinical features include the "cock robin" posi-

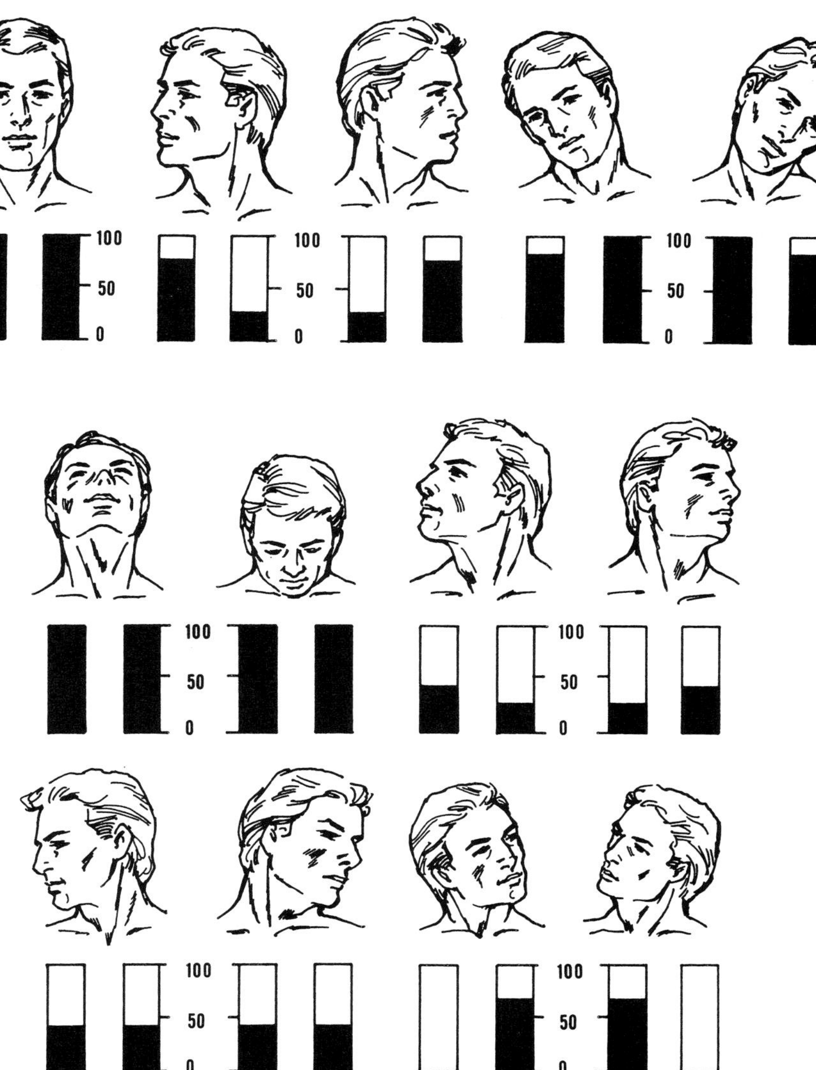

Figure 11.6. Influence of head and neck position on cerebral circulation: schematic depiction of obstruction of the vertebral artery. Adjustments of the upper cervical spine should use primarily lateral flexion and pure movements of flexion and extension to achieve tension. Modified from Junghanns H. Clinical implications of normal biomechanical stresses on spinal function. English language ed. Maryland: Aspen Publishers, Inc., 1990:25.

tion in which the head is laterally flexed to one side, rotated toward the opposite side, combined with slight flexion. Patients will usually have no neurologic signs; however, the greater occipital nerve may be irritated because it emerges between C1-C2 (54). Dvorak's maneuver (See Chapter 4) is usually positive, because 50% of the rotation of the cervical spine occurs at C1-C2. Motion palpation can also be used to compare the rotational and lateral flexion motions of the atlas on axis.

Radiographically, AARF can be diagnosed with the use of the antero-posterior open mouth, by checking for a persistently asymmetrical relationship of the articular masses of the atlas with the dens. Lateral bending radiographs are useful for determining the pattern of thrust for the adjustment. Cineradiography can be used if positioning is difficult. On rotation, the axis and the posterior arch of atlas move as one unit. Flexion/extension views assist in ruling out antero-posterior displacement. Lateral displacement of the dens in relation to atlas by more than 4 mm suggests AARF (54).

AARF is classified into two categories: type 1 and type 2. In type 1, anterior rotation fixation is present on one side of C1-C2 with no dislocation. This is seen in both adults and children. For type 2 , there is anterior dislocation of one lateral mass of C1 on C2 along with interlocking of the facets. This has been reported only in children and is associated with trauma. Orthopaedic treatment usually consists of halter traction for a period of two to three weeks during the acute stage. If progress is not satisfactory, surgery is performed (e.g., atlanto-axial, occipito-atlantal, or occipito-atlanto-axial arthrodesis).

Altongy (53) reports a case of a 9-year-old boy who presented with a 2-month history of neck pain and stiffness as a result of injuries sustained while break-dancing. Initial examination revealed decreased cervical spine range of motion with pain. No neurologic deficits were noted. Symptoms and physical findings were consistent with AARF. Radiographic findings confirmed AARF and the patient was admitted to the hospital. CT scan demonstrated a rotatory subluxation of the occiput on atlas,

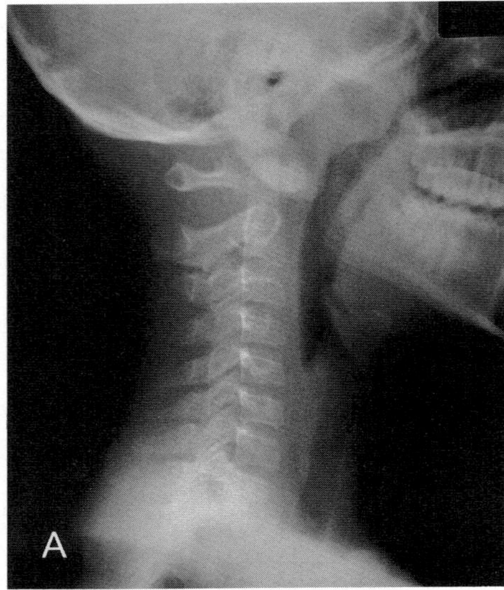

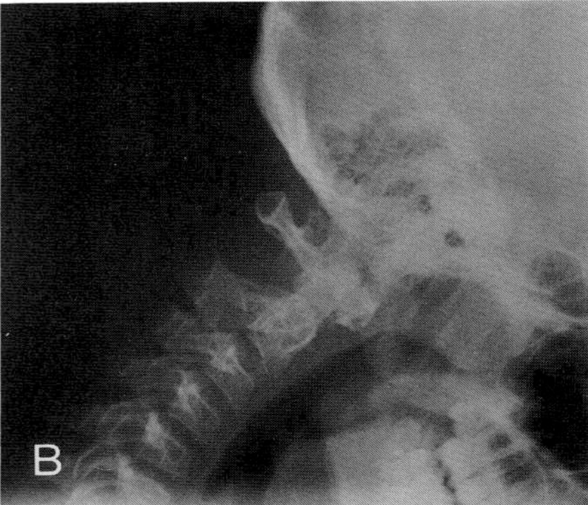

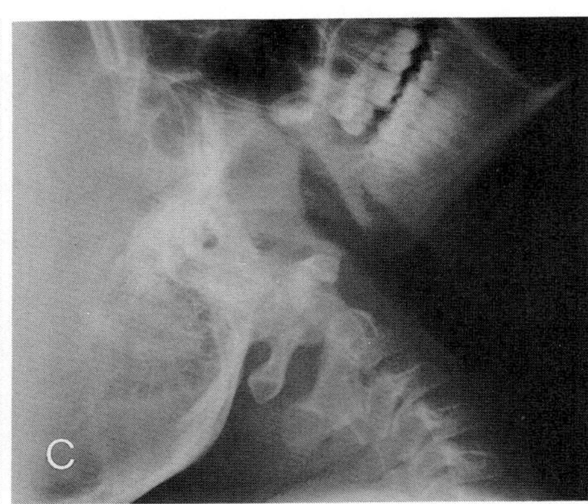

Figure 11.7. **A,** Neutral lateral radiograph demonstrating the "V" sign at the atlanto-dental interval. **B,** Flexion radiograph demonstrating further anterior translation of the atlas. The joint is clearly unstable. Adjustments at that level are contraindicated because there is no evidence of fixation dysfunction. **C,** Extension radiograph depicting posterior translation of the atlas.

and atlas on axis. Approximately 3½ weeks of traction ranging from 3.2 to 5.5 kilograms did not seem to resolve the problem. Post CT scan demonstrated some improvement of the subluxation but not complete reduction. At that point, a posterior atlanto-axial arthrodesis was performed during which "no gross malrotation could be appreciated through the exposure." A halo vest was applied and was worn for 6 weeks until fusion was solid. After 3 months, the brace was removed, and the child was able to rotate the head 45° bilaterally without pain. Thirty-six months after the operation, the patient had 70° of rotation bilaterally and no evidence of recurrence.

The chiropractic approach to AARF is much less drastic. The relative efficacy of any treatment remains unknown. When a patient presents with AARF, a complete examination of the upper cervical spine should be performed (See Chapters 4 and 5). Flexion-extension, standing AP and lateral views, and lateral bending radiographs. should be analyzed. If type 2 AARF has been ruled out, specific adjustments can be used to restore normal mechanical function by reducing the fixation dysfunction. Stretching exercises can be used to relax muscle hypertonicity. If after 2 to 3 weeks (i.e., several treatments), there has been no change in symptomatology, then a less conservative approach, such as halter traction, may be used. If surgery is performed (usually arthrodesis), adjustments at that level are contraindicated. The chiropractor can adjust above or below the fused areas, if indicated. A better understanding of AARF should open more avenues for treatment of this condition. Research in this area should be a high priority for the chiropractic profession.

Transverse Ligament Rupture

Bueller (56) describes anterior atlanto-axial subluxation (AAS) and various disorders that can arise as a result of this disturbance. The doctor must rule out the presence of AAS if certain objective and subjective signs such as headache, transient quadriplegia, neck weakness, or vertigo are present. Measurement of the atlanto-dental interval (ADI) (See Chapter 5) will help detect the amount of misalignment and spinal cord compromise. Standard lateral cervical views taken at 72 in. are analyzed to measure the ADI. Hinck and Hopkins (57) use the following formula to determine the normal ADI. They measure the inferior portion of the ADI and apply the following:

Male: 2.052-(0.0192 × age in years) ± 1.0 mm.
Female: 1.238-(0.0074 × age in years) ±0.9 mm.

They also state that the average normal measurement for children is 2.0 to 2.5 mm in extension, and 2.0 to 3.0 mm in flexion. If in adults a minute increase in the space is seen (4–5 mm), it is most likely caused by transverse ligament laxity.

The "V" sign (13), which often resembles a normal variant may be present in cases after significant trauma. This is indicative of a partial rupture or stretch of the transverse ligament (Fig. 11.7A-C). Fielding et al. (58) first reported this sign in 1974, interpreting it as a rupture of all the fibers of the transverse ligament except the lower fibers. This condition has not been proven to be clinically stable (13). Etiology of AAS can be classified into two categories:

1. Tearing or laxity caused by trauma.
2. Involvement of the dens as a result of trauma; erosions, resorptions, or congenital malformations.

Without bone damage, there are few cases in which the transverse ligament has ruptured and caused anterior displacement of the atlas on axis (59,60). The transverse ligament is quite strong and it is usually the odontoid that will break first during trauma. Instances in which rupture of the transverse ligament could be noted without dens fracture or other traumatic insult include:

1. Rheumatoid arthritis (61).
2. Yersinia arthritis (62).
3. Reiter's syndrome (63).
4. Down's syndrome (64); 10 to 20% of individuals with this genetic disease process show lack of or laxity of this ligament.
5. Ankylosing spondylitis (65).
6. Osseous metastasis, tuberculosis (65).
7. Psoriatic arthritis (66).

If severe AAS is suspected or evident, orthopaedic referral is necessary to determine the need for fusion. Lack of symptomatology still necessitates immediate referral, because fusion of the separation could prevent further potentially life-threatening injury.

Fracture

When a patient presents for examination and treatment after trauma, the upper cervical region should be scrutinized for the possibility of fracture or dislocation. Fractures or dislocations in this area can be neurologically or biomechanically unstable (See Chapter 12).

EXAMINATION (C1-C2)

The atlas is often in a compensatory position when analyzed in the coronal plane, due to the righting reflex. Because of this effect, it is necessary to rely on more than apparent radiographic findings to arrive at a differential diagnosis. Equally undesirable is to equate muscle bulging over the transverse process, or taut and tender muscle fibers, as pathognomonic of subluxation. A multiparameter examination is necessary. Examination of the upper cervical spine is generally performed with the patient in the seated position.

Static Palpation

Static palpation is used to detect edema or "bogginess" caused by tissue injury. This may be a result of direct trauma or autonomic nervous system effects. Static axial rotation of C1 can be palpated as an increased muscle/tissue bulging on the side of posterior rotation. Malformations and muscular asymmetries lessen the validity of this procedure.

Motion Palpation

Motion palpation involves examining the movement of atlas with respect to axis. It should not be relied on solely for the listing; however, motion palpation can be used to determine the presence of fixation dysfunction. The AS or AI component of the listing is best determined by analyzing the lateral radiograph, rather than relying on motion palpation.

ROTATION $\pm\theta Y$

Because the primary movement of C1-C2 is rotation (Y axis), fixation dysfunction can be readily determined. The doctor should rotate the patient's head from side to side. The atlas will rotate less on the side of fixation. Dvorak's maneuver (See Chapter 4) is used for determining upper cervical rotational fixation. As the patient's head is flexed and rotated, the upper cervical spine is isolated. By comparing motion bilaterally, the direction of fixation is determined.

LATERAL FLEXION $\pm\theta Z$

The doctor's segmental contact point is the transverse process of atlas between atlas and axis with either the thumb or the finger tips. If the doctor's hands cannot reach around the neck, the joint can be analyzed unilaterally. As the patient's head is bent from side to side, the motion of the segment is analyzed. The notion that the atlas compresses on the side of lateral flexion is questionable. The lateral mass of C1 most likely raises on the contralateral side of bend when C1 is laterally flexed on C2. The doctor, therefore, feels for the lack of motion on the contralateral side of fixation when the head is laterally flexed from side to side.

Instrumentation

Instrumentation (e.g., nervoscope) can also be used as part of the examination. During scanning, the instrument should be glided caudad to cephalad. The most common false-positive finding the doctor may encounter is due to suboccipital hair. Because of the close proximity of the articulations (i.e., C0-C2), it is difficult to determine which segmental level is involved when a true positive is present.

Inspection

Inspection is also used to derive the listing. If the atlas rotates anteriorly, there may be head tilt ipsilaterally. When the atlas rotates posterior (e.g., ASRP), there may be superficial muscle bulging on the side of posteriority. Lateral flexion malposition will also cause a slight head tilt, especially if the patient's eyes stay closed during the examination.

George's Test

George's test is performed to rule out vertebro-basilar artery insufficiency. It has historically been used to determine whether or not manipulation of the cervical spine is contraindicated. This test can, however, have a number of false positives that provide contradicting information; therefore, it should not be relied on exclusively to determine if an adjustment is contraindicated.

The test that is commonly used for detection of vertebral artery insufficiency (VBI) (67) is cervical rotation with extension. The patient's head should be put in maximal rotation and extension for a minimum of 10 seconds. The patient is asked if any unusual sensations such as nausea, or blinking lights are noticed. Vertebral artery occlusion may be reduced on the contralateral side of rotation; however, there can be occlusion of the ipsilateral artery with the presence of osteophytes. Patients are categorized as follows (67):

Type 1 patients show signs of vertigo, visual disturbances, motor/sensory symptoms.

Type 2 will have occasional dizziness, or mild transient symptoms.

Type 3 patients experience no symptoms that would be indicative of VBI.

Type 2 and 3 patients may be safely adjusted. Type 1 patients need not be classified as "non-adjustable." Ferezy (26) states that by normalizing the biomechanical function, the doctor may be preventing other ischemic attacks from arising. Of course, rotational type manipulations would be contraindicated.

Radiographic Analysis

When analyzing the radiograph, it is important not only to evaluate the specific segment in question but also the adjacent motion segments that may react in compensation to the involved level. Because the atlas rotates around the odontoid process of the axis, it is used as the point of reference.

First, the lateral cervical radiograph is used to help analyze the positional relationship between C1-C2. The odontoid process will be represented by a line that traverses it longitudinally. Two dots are placed, one in the center of the base of the odontoid and another so that it bisects the odontoid near its superior margin. The line drawn through these points is called the odontoid line (Fig. 11.8).

A line drawn perpendicular to the odontoid line is placed through the middle portion of the axis body, termed the *odontoid perpendicular line.*

The AP atlas plane line is drawn by placing two dots on the atlas, one in the center of the anterior tubercle, and the other in the center of the intersection of the posterior arch with the posterior tubercle. If the patient's head is tilted, so that one side of the arch no longer completely overlaps the other, the dot should be placed in the middle of the broadened image of the arch, or in the center of the space formed between the two sides of the posterior ring (2). When the atlas and axis have relatively normal alignment, the AP atlas plane line and the odontoid perpendicular line are parallel. Slight variances of this relationship, especially extension of the atlas on axis, are not

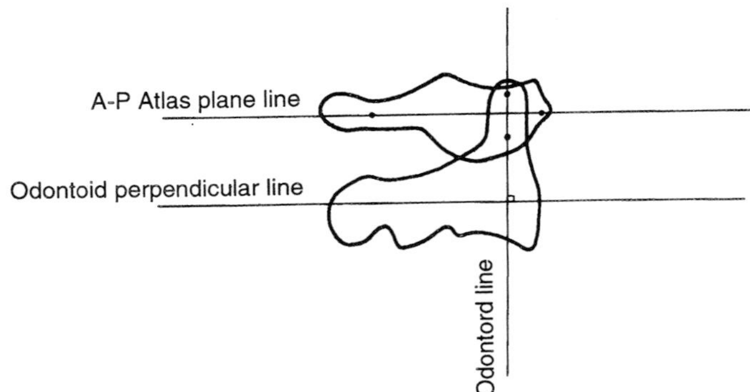

Figure 11.8. Relatively normal alignment between C1-C2. Modifed from Herbst RW. Gonstead chiropractic science and art. Mt. Horeb, WI: Sci-Chi Publications, 1968:119.

considered significant, unless accompanied by other clinical findings.

When viewing the atlas-axis relationship on the AP radiograph, optimal alignment will be depicted by lines that are parallel, providing there are no structural anomalies. The line that represents the plane of the axis is termed the "axis plane line." The plane of the atlas is represented by a line termed the "atlas plane line," which is drawn through like points on either side of the atlas, the most reliable of which are the transverse process-lateral mass junctions. These are the points where the superior and inferior borders of the transverse processes join the lateral masses. Because the superior borders of the transverse processes are often obscured by the overhanging occiput, the point where the inferior border joins the lateral mass is usually selected. When the atlas transverse plane line and the axis plane line appear parallel on the A-P radiograph, the atlas and axis are considered to be in relatively normal alignment.

ANTERIOR (+Z) POSITIONAL DYSKINESIA

Because the transverse ligament keeps the atlas close to axis, anteriorward displacement is rare, unless there is ligamentous rupture. It has been stated that the first letter in the listing is "A" because of the anterior slippage of the atlas on the axis (2). It is probably more accurate to state that the atlas rotates around the X axis, and while doing so it may slide anteriorward. If indeed, anteriority is present, and is a factor in the subluxation, it would be difficult to detect on the lateral radiograph unless the transverse ligament were torn or stretched. When contacting the atlas transverse process for an adjustment, the antero-lateral portion is used (Fig 11.9).

SUPERIORITY/INFERIORITY $\pm\theta X$

Superiority and inferiority ($\pm\theta X$) of the anterior tubercle can be detected radiographically. Hyperextension displacement is more common than hyperflexion positional dyskinesia. This misalignment ($-\theta X$) is best seen on the lateral radiograph. The AP atlas plane line and the odontoid perpendicular line will diverge anteriorly. The other possible direction of misalignment is inferiorward ($+\theta X$). Although uncommon, it should not be overlooked. This misalignment is also best detected with the lateral radiograph. The AP atlas plane line and the odontoid perpendicular line converge anteriorly with this positional dyskinesia.

If the line drawings on the lateral radiograph indicate that the misalignment is in a superior direction, the letter "S" is placed with the letter A, and if the lines indicate that the misalignment is in the inferior direction, the letter "I" is placed next to the letter A (Fig. 11.10A-B). At this point the listing of the atlas will either be AS or AI.

Another radiographic finding that should be checked for when analyzing the atlas is the space between the posterior portion of the anterior tubercle of atlas and the anterior portion of the dens. In the AS listing, an inverted "V" will be seen in that space. With the AI listing, there will be the appearance of a "V".

Whether the introduction of a torque ($\pm\theta X$) during the adjustment actually corrects the superiority or inferiority component remains to be seen.

LATERALITY $\pm\theta Z$ ($\pm X$)

It has been thought in the past that as the atlas subluxates, it shifts laterally. What likely happens, however, is that as it rotates around the z axis, it may move toward the convexity of lateral bend. The use of the AP radiograph appears to be the more reliable method to determine this displacement. Because of the superior lift of atlas on the side of lateral shift, a wedging of the axis plane line and the atlas transverse plane line will be evident. When the atlas misaligns laterally to the left, a diverging of these two lines occurs (Fig. 11.11) and the letter "L" is added to the listing. Possible listings include ASR, ASL.

ROTATION $\pm\theta Y$

Rotation is the fourth letter of the atlas listing, and may be determined by using the AP radiograph. The size of the

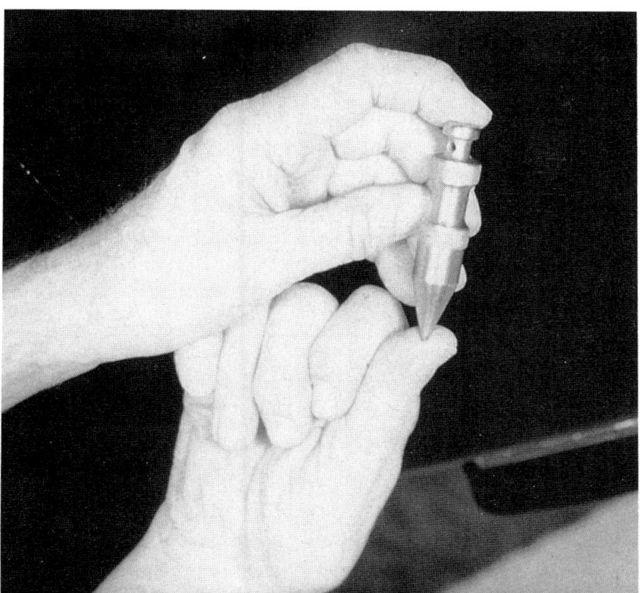

Figure 11.9. Contact point for adjusting the atlas.

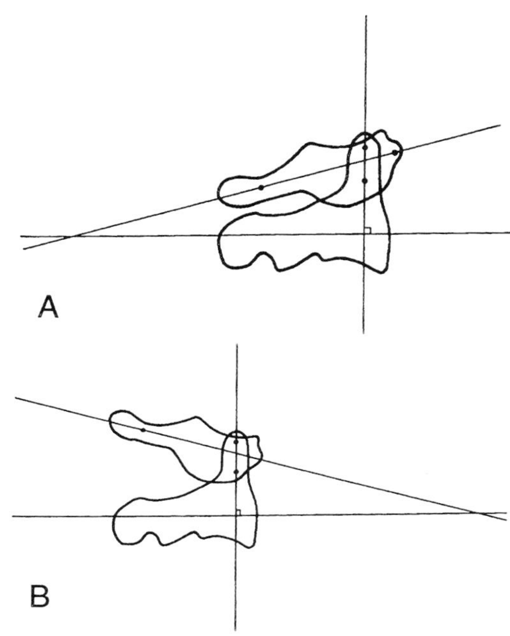

Figure 11.10. **A,** Diverging lines anteriorly indicating AS positional dyskinesia. Modifed from Herbst RW. Gonstead chiropractic science and art. Mt. Horeb, WI: Sci-Chi Publications, 1968:122. **B,** Converging lines anterior indicating AI positional dyskinesia of the atlas. Modifed from Herbst RW. Gonstead chiropractic science and art. Mt. Horeb, WI: Sci-Chi Publications, 1968:121.

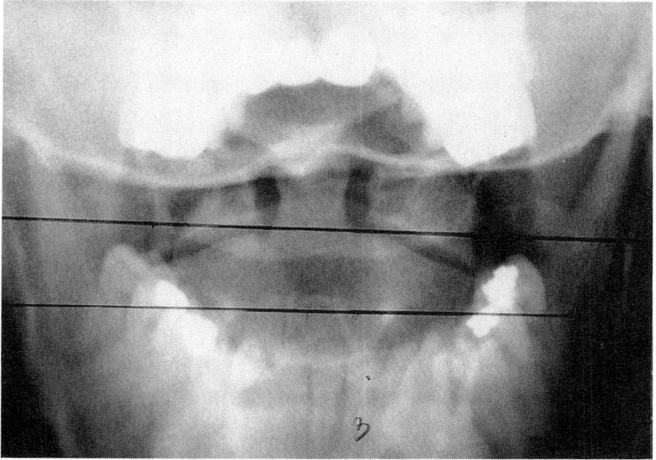

Figure 11.11. Radiograph demonstrating right lateral flexion positional dyskinesia (e.g., ASL).

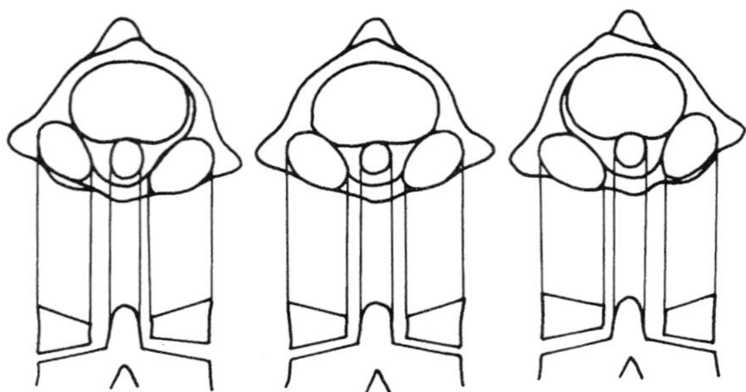

Figure 11.12. Shape of the lateral masses of C1 as it rotates. When the atlas rotates to the right, the distance between the dens and the right lateral mass of atlas increases. When it rotates to the left, there is an increase in the distance between the left lateral mass and the dens. Note that the lateral mass on the side of posterior rotation is smaller and vice versa. Modified from Shapiro R, Youngberg A, Rothman SLG. The differential diagnosis of traumatic lesions of the occipito-atlanto-axial segment. Radiol Clin North Am 1973;11:505.

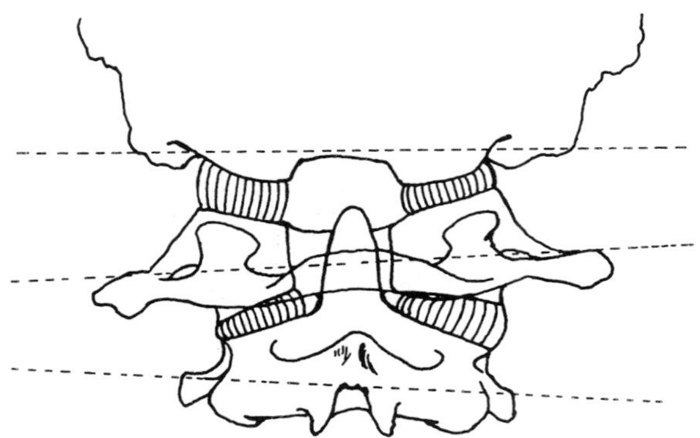

Figure 11.13. ASRA atlas. Notice the diverging lines on the right. The right lateral mass appears larger, indicating anterior rotation of the atlas on the right side ($+\theta Y$). The condyle has tipped up on the left in compensation. Modifed from Herbst RW. Gonstead chiropractic science and art. Mt. Horeb, WI: Sci-Chi Publications, 1968:123.

lateral mass on the side of laterality ($\pm\theta Z$) is analyzed. If the atlas has rotated anteriorly, the lateral mass will appear wider on that side. This is so, because as the atlas rotates, the obliquity of the lateral masses is altered in relation to the central ray (Fig. 11.12). If the rotational component is anteriority, the letter A is used (Fig. 11.13); and if it is posteriority the letter P is used (Fig. 11.14).

Another method of analyzing the radiograph for atlas rotation is by checking for the position of the occiput in relation to the atlas. When the atlas rotates anteriorly, the occiput may drop on that side. A line is drawn at the level of the occipital condyles, and it is compared with the AP atlas transverse line. On the side of atlas anteriority, the two lines may converge.

During examination of the AP radiograph, the

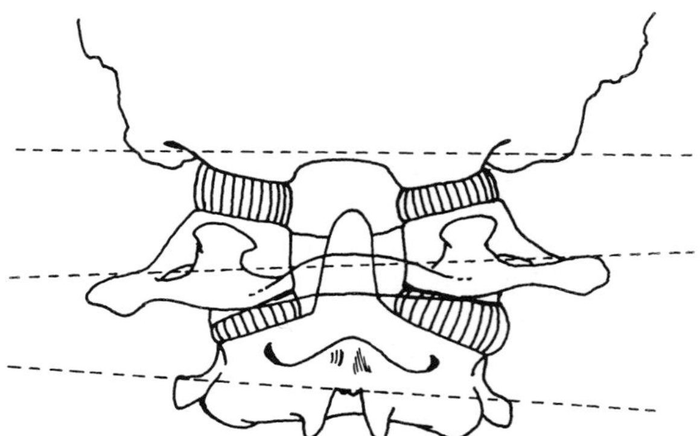

Figure 11.14. ASRP atlas. Notice diverging lines on the right ($-\theta Z$). The smaller lateral mass on the right indicates posterior rotation on the right side. The condyle has compensated on the left side by tilting superiorly ($+\theta Z$). Modifed from Herbst RW. Gonstead chiropractic science and art. Mt. Horeb, WI: Sci-Chi Publications, 1968:124.

indented concave surfaces of the lateral masses can be used to analyze for rotation. Because the upper medial surfaces of the lateral masses are concave and indented, they will appear as a radiolucency within the lateral mass. The side of anterior rotation will show a wider area of lucency, and posterior rotation will demonstrate a narrower area of radiolucency.

In Table 11.1 the majority of positional configurations that can occur are presented. Displacements in parenthesis will have equivocal or absent radiograph findings. The pattern of thrust is also provided.

ADJUSTMENT (C1-C2)

The seated upper cervical adjustment can be used to address multiple components of the atlas listing. AI atlas listings may be corrected in the prone or side lying position or adjusted in the cervical chair. The knee chest and hi-lo are considered alternate tables for adjusting AS listings. To reiterate, whether or not the torque ($\pm\theta X$) actually does correct the superiority of the subluxation remains to be seen. Its application does, however, appear to increase the acceleration and "smoothness" or fluidity of the adjustment.

Name of technique: Gonstead

Name of technique procedure: ASR ($+Z, -\theta X, -\theta Z, -X$) atlas adjustment (Fig. 11.15A).

Indications: Antero-superior translation ($-\theta X$), lateral flexion to the left ($-\theta Z$) (Fig. 11.15B). Flexion and right lateral flexion fixation dysfunction.

Table 11.1.
The Atlas Listings

Gonstead Listing	International	Pattern of Thrust
ASR	$(+Z), -\theta X, -\theta Z, (-X)$	Right to left, through the C1-C2 joint plane line, inferiorward arcing motion toward the end of the thrust.
ASRA	$(+Z), -\theta X, -\theta Z, -X, +\theta Y$	Right to left through the C1-C2 joint plane line, the head is rotated toward side of contact, an inferiorward arcing motion toward the end of thrust.
ASRP	$(+Z), -\theta X, -\theta Z, (-X), -\theta Y$	Right to left, through the C1-C2 joint plane line, the patient's head is rotated away from the side of contact, an inferiorward arcing motion toward end of thrust.
ASL	$(+Z), -\theta X, +\theta Z, (+X)$	Left to right, through the C1-C2 joint plane line, an inferiorward arcing motion toward the end of the thrust.
ASLA	$(+Z), -\theta X, +\theta Z, (+X), -\theta Y$	Left to right, through the C1-C2 joint plane line, the head is rotated toward the side of contact, an inferiorward arcing motion toward the end of the thrust.
AIR	$(+Z), +\theta X, -\theta Z, (-X)$	Right to left, through the C1-C2 joint plane line, a superiorward arcing motion toward the end of the thrust.
AIRA	$(+Z), +\theta X, -\theta Z, -X, +\theta Y$	Right to left, through the C1-C2 joint plane line, the head is rotated toward the side of contact, a superiorward arcing motion toward the end of the thrust.
AIRP	$(+Z), +\theta X, -\theta Z, (-X), -\theta Y$	Right to left, through the C1-C2 joint plane line, the head is rotated away from the side of contact, a superiorward arcing motion toward the end of the thrust.
AIL	$(+Z), +\theta X, +\theta Z, (+X)$	Left to right, through the C1-C2 joint plane line, a superiorward arcing motion toward the end of the thrust.
AILA	$(+Z), +\theta X, +\theta Z, (+X), -\theta Y$	Left to right, through the C1-C2 joint plane line, the head is rotated towards the side of contact, a superiorward arcing motion toward the end of the thrust.
ASLP	$(+Z), -\theta X, +\theta Z, (+X), +\theta Y$	Left to right, through C1-C2 joint plane line, the head is rotated away from the side of contact, an inferiorward arcing motion toward the end of the thrust.

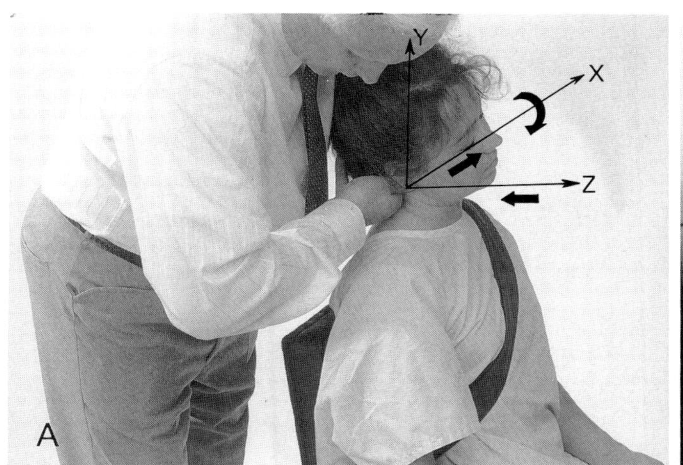

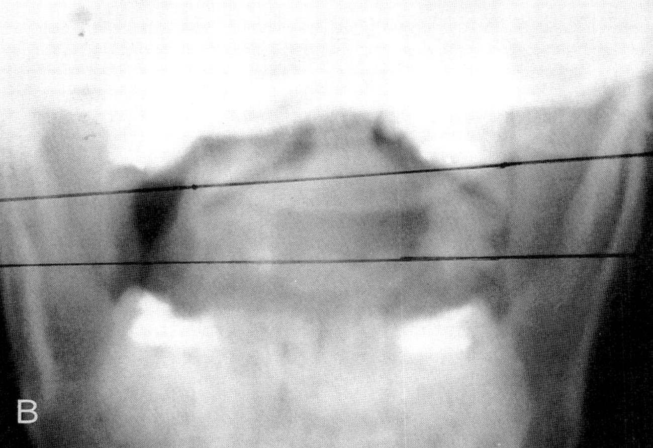

Figure 11.15. **A,** ASR atlas adjustment. **B,** Radiograph of an ASR atlas.

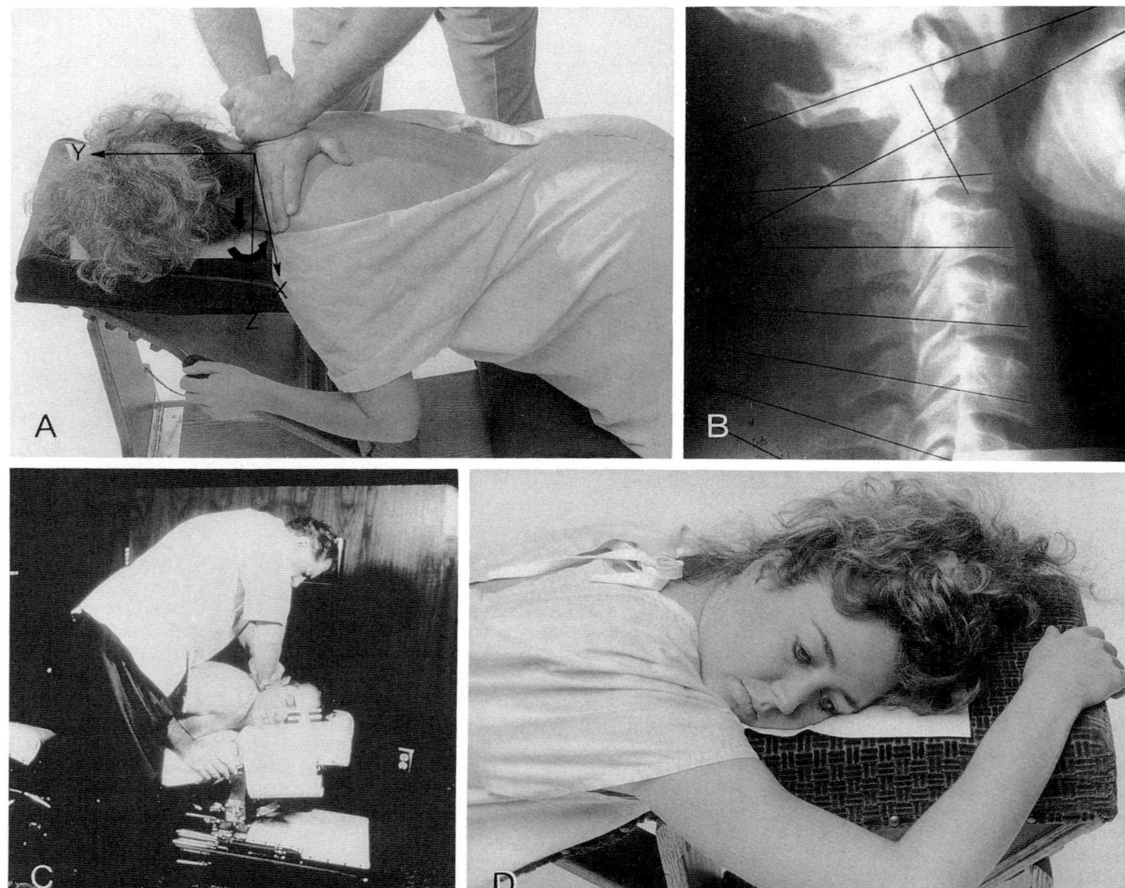

Figure 11.16. **A,** AIRA atlas adjustment. **B,** Radiograph of an AI atlas (lateral view). **C,** To avoid rotation in the cervical spine with the patient in the prone position, the torso is rotated to the side of head rotation to minimize excessive rotation of the cervical spine. **D,** Patient positioning on the knee-chest table for an AI atlas. The arm is raised to reduce tension in the cervical spine.

Contraindications: All other listings, normal FSU, hypermobility, instability, destruction of atlas, pathologic fracture of the neural arch, infection of the contact vertebra, transverse ligament rupture, C1-C2 arthrodesis.

Patient position: Seated in the cervical chair. The stabilization strap should be placed over the left shoulder.

Doctor's position: Standing behind the patient, favoring the right side.

Contact point: Tip of the right thumb. Segmentally, the anterolateral portion of the atlas transverse process.

Supporting hand: The left hand is used to stabilize the C2-C3 articulation on the opposite side (cupping the hand over the ear).

Pattern of thrust: Lateral to medial, through the C1-C2 joint plane line along with an inferiorward arcing motion toward the end of the thrust.

Category by algorithm: Short lever specific contact procedure.

Name of technique: Gonstead

Name of technique procedure: AIRA ($+Z, +\theta X, -\theta Z, -X, +\theta Y$) atlas adjustment, modified toggle (Fig. 11.16A).

Indications: Extension, right lateral flexion, and right anterior rotation fixation. Antero-inferior translation ($+\theta X, +Z$) (Fig. 11.16B), left lateral flexion ($-\theta Z$), and left axial rotation ($+\theta Y$) positional dyskinesia.

Contraindications: All other listings, normal FSU, hypermobility, instability, destruction of the atlas, or pathologic fracture of the neural arch, infection of the contact vertebra, transverse ligament rupture, C1-C2 arthrodesis, vertebral artery insufficiency.

Patient position: Prone on the knee-chest or hi-lo table (Fig. 11.16C), with the head rotated to the right. The right arm may be brought up by the head to help relax the paraspinal musculature (Fig. 11.16D).

Doctor's position: Facing perpendicular to the patient, with a slight angulation away from the patient to push anterior to posterior for correction of axial rotation.

Contact point: Soft pisiform of the inferior hand. Segmentally, the antero-lateral portion of the transverse process of atlas.

Supporting hand: The superior hand will wrap around the inferior hand (single hand contact).

Pattern of thrust: Lateral to medial, through the C1-C2 joint plane line, along with a superiorward ($-\theta X$) torque motion toward the end of the thrust.

Category by algorithm: Short lever specific contact procedure.

Name of technique: Gonstead

Name of technique procedure: ASRP ($+Z, -\theta X, -\theta Z, -X, -\theta Y$) atlas adjustment (Fig. 11.17).

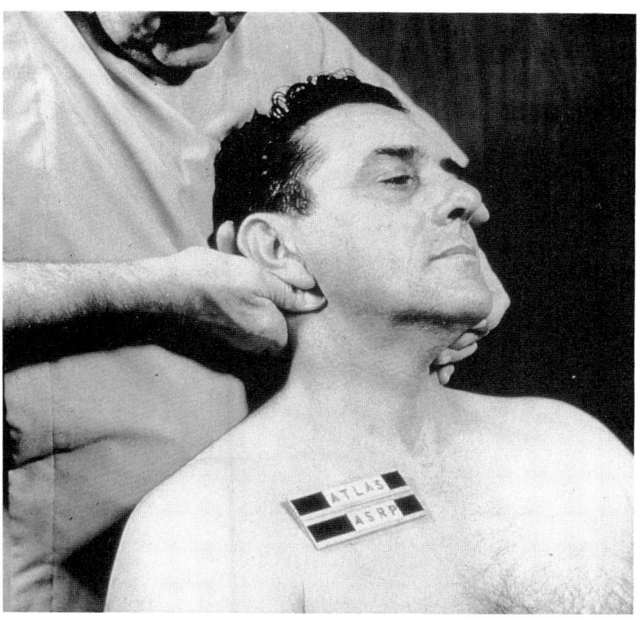

Figure 11.17. ASRP atlas adjustment.

Indications: Flexion, right lateral flexion, and left axial rotation fixation. Antero-superior ($+Z, -\theta X$) lateral flexion ($-\theta Z$), and right axial rotational ($-\theta Y$) positional dyskinesia.

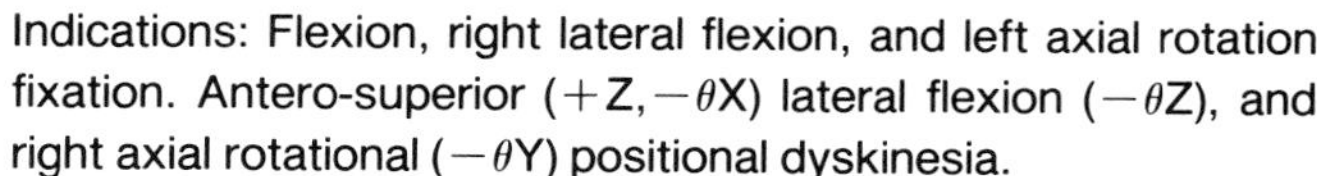

Contraindications: All other listings, normal FSU, hypermobility, instability, destruction of the atlas, or pathologic fracture of the neural arch, infection of the contact vertebra, transverse ligament rupture, C1-C2 arthrodesis.

Patient position: Seated in the cervical chair. The stabilization strap should be placed over the left shoulder. The head is rotated away from the side of contact proportional to the rotational (Y axis) component of the listing. If VBAI is present, there should be no axial rotation.

Doctor's position: Standing behind the patient, favoring the right side.

Contact point: Tip of the right thumb. Segmentally, the antero-lateral portion of atlas transverse process.

Supporting hand: The left hand is used to stabilize the C2-C3 articulation on the opposite side (cupping the hand over the ear).

Pattern of thrust: Lateral to medial, through the C1-C2 joint plane line, along with an inferiorward arcing motion at the end of the thrust.

Category by algorithm: Short lever specific contact procedure.

Name of technique: Gonstead

Name of technique procedure: ASL ($+Z, -\theta X, +\theta Z, +X$) atlas adjustment (Fig 11.18A).

Indications: Flexion fixation, left lateral flexion fixation. Antero-superior translation ($-\theta X$), right lateral flexion ($+\theta Z$) positional dyskinesia.

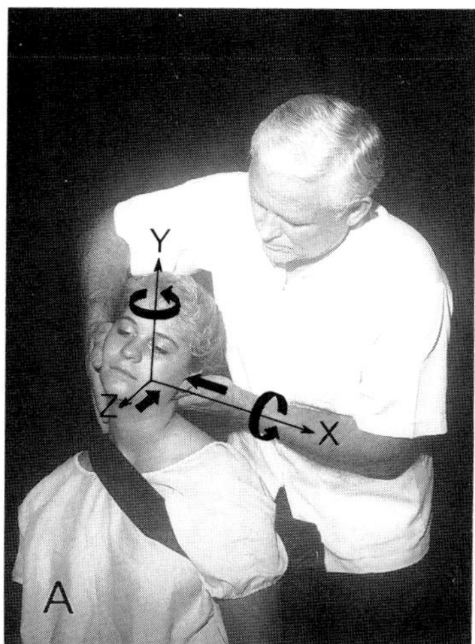

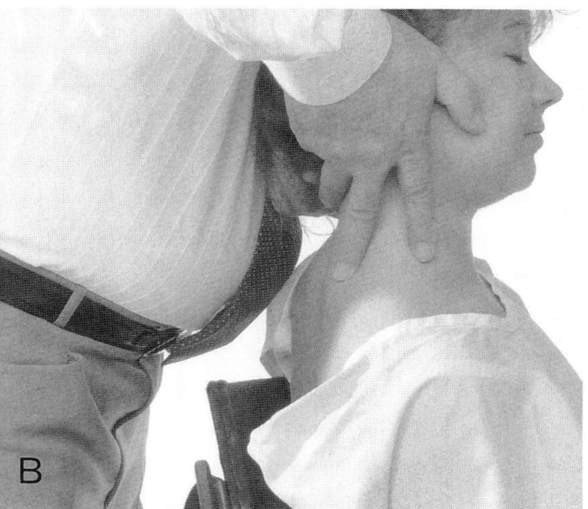

Figure 11.18. **A,** ASLA atlas adjustment. The head is turned toward the side of contact to correct the anterior rotation. **B,** Stabilization for the atlas adjustment.

Contraindications: All other listings, normal FSU, hypermobility, instability, destruction of the atlas, infection of the contact vertebra, transverse ligament rupture, C1-C2 arthrodesis.

Patient position: Seated in the cervical chair. The stabilization strap should be placed over the right shoulder.

Doctor's position: Standing behind the patient, favoring the left side.

Contact point: Tip of the left thumb. Segmentally, the antero-lateral portion of the left transverse process of the atlas.

Supporting hand: The right hand is used to stabilize the C2-C3 articulation on the opposite side (cupping the hand over the ear) (Fig. 11.18B).

Pattern of thrust: Lateral to medial, through the C1-C2 joint plane line, along with an inferiorward arcing motion toward the end of the thrust.

Category by algorithm: Short lever specific contact procedure.

EXAMINATION (C0-C1)

The condyle should be analyzed in relation to the atlas. Because of the close proximity of the C0-C1 and C1-C2 joints, it is easy to misinterpret the examination findings. Therefore, extra attention is advised when examining this area. As with C1-C2, all methods of examination discussed should be used (i.e., static palpation, motion palpation, instrumentation, and radiography).

Static Palpation

Static palpation at C0-C1 is used to detect edema and bogginess caused by tissue injury. Muscle and soft tissue bulging may also be palpated on the side of posterior rotation.

Motion Palpation

Motion palpation is primarily used to analyze flexion and extension motion. This is done by contacting the condyle with the fingertips while the patient's head is moved around the X axis. With a PS condyle fixation, extension will be limited.

Instrumentation

Instrumentation (e.g., Nervoscope) can be used in the same manner as when examining C1-C2. Suboccipital hair is likely to give spurious findings.

Inspection

Inspection is limited, but it can be used to derive the listing. The doctor may find a head tilt with associated positional dyskinesia of the occiput in lateral flexion.

Radiographic Analysis

The neutral upright posture of the occiput or foramen magnum should create maximal patency for the spinal canal. For this to occur, the foramen magnum line is relatively parallel to the AP atlas plane line (Fig. 11.19). Because of the difficulty in identifying landmarks for the foramen magnum line, a qualitative inspection of the region is generally performed. Both hyperextension and hyperflexion of the joint is considered abnormal. These findings must then be correlated with stress radiographic and clinical assessments.

AS ($-\theta X$), PS ($+\theta X$)

The condyles may move anterior and superior "AS" or posterior-superior "PS" in relation to the atlas. With anterior glide, the AP foramen line and the AP atlas line will converge posteriorly (Fig. 11.20A). The space between the posterior arch of atlas and the foramen magnum is reduced. With the PS misalignment, the two lines will converge anteriorly, and the space between the foramen magnum and the posterior arch of atlas is increased (Fig. 11.20B). Stress radiography, with the patient in maximum flexion and extension, can be used to determine if the positional dyskinesia noted on the neutral lateral radiograph is also fixated.

RS ($-\theta Z$), LS ($+\theta Z$)

Lateral flexion positional dyskinesia is determined with the AP radiograph. The transverse condyle line is used to determine the displacement. This line is drawn through like points on both sides of the condyles. The points that can be used are the mastoid notches (grooves on the mastoid process of the temporal bones). When like points have been determined and the lines have been drawn, optimal alignment in the coronal plane is assumed if the lines are parallel.

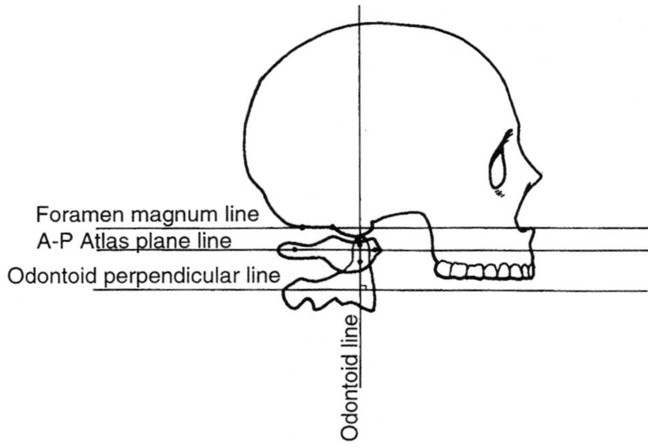

Figure 11.19. Relatively normal alignment of C0-C1. Modifed from Herbst RW. Gonstead chiropractic science and art. Mt. Horeb, WI: Sci-Chi Publications, 1968:133.

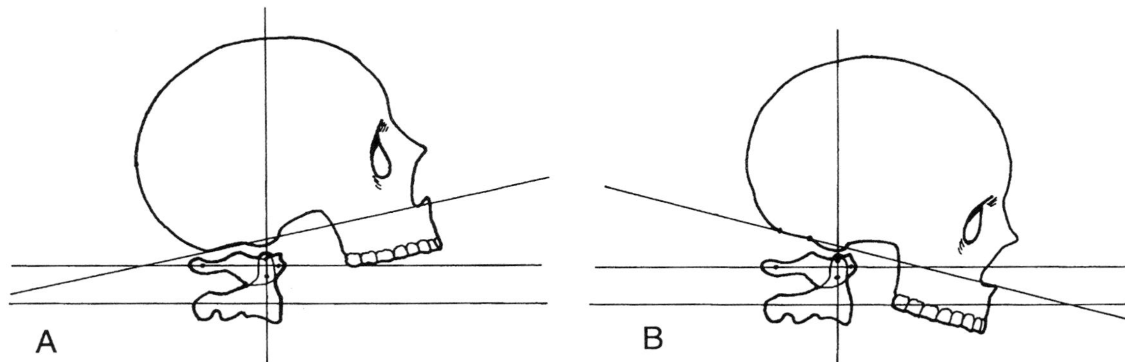

Figure 11.20. **A,** AS positional dyskinesia. **B,** PS positional dyskinesia.

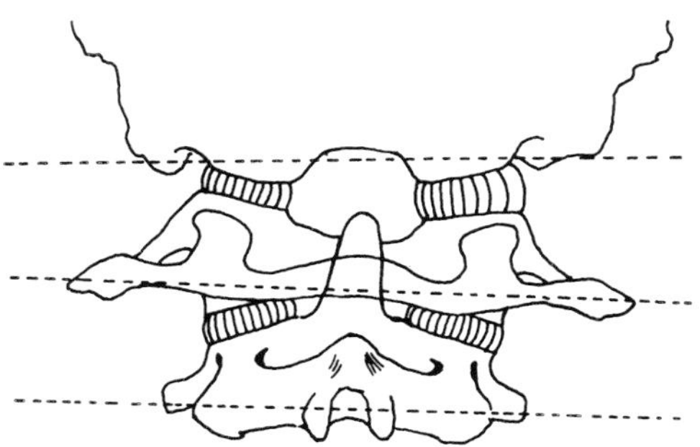

Figure 11.21. RSRA Condyle. Anterior view of condyle listing "AS" or "PS" cannot be determined from this view. Notice the diverging lines between C0-C1 on the right. The right lateral mass appears posterior on the right, indicating that the right condyle is rotated anterior. Modifed from Herbst RW. Gonstead chiropractic science and art. Mt. Horeb, WI: Sci-Chi Publications, 1968:138.

With misalignment, the atlas transverse plane line and the transverse condyle line will diverge. If lateral flexion is to the left, then a RS (right superior) listing is assigned.

AXIAL ROTATION (Y AXIS)

Rotation is indirectly analyzed from the radiograph. Because of the atlas' ability to compensate in axial rotation, its rotation is used to determine rotation at the condyle. If the lateral mass of the atlas is wider (anterior), on the side of the condyle involvement, the condyle is listed as posterior, and vice versa (Fig. 11.21).

ADJUSTMENT (C0-C1)

Condyle adjustments are performed in the seated position. Alternate moves can be performed either supine, or prone on the knee-chest or hi-lo table. The knee-chest PS condyle adjustment is considered the second option for patient positioning. Descriptions of the listing components and the patterns of thrust for their correction are presented in Table 11.2.

The doctor's contact point for a PS listing is the thenar pad (Fig. 11.22A-B). First, a superior glide is taken with the contact hand to displace excess occipital hair (Fig. 11.23A). The hand is then slid down as the proximal portion of the thenar pad hooks the supramastoid groove (Fig. 11.23B).

Name of technique: Gonstead

Name of technique procedure: PSRS ($+\theta$X, $-\theta$Z) condyle adjustment (Fig. 11.24).

Indications: Extension fixation, right lateral flexion fixation. Postero-superior glide ($+\theta$X, $-$Z), left lateral flexion ($-\theta$Z) positional dyskinesia.

Contraindications: All other listings, normal FSU, hypermobility, instability, destruction of the condyle, or pathologic/nonpathologic fracture of the condyle, infection of the contact bone, C0-C1 arthrodesis.

Patient position: The patient is seated in the cervical chair. The stabilization strap is placed over the left shoulder.

Doctor's position: Behind the patient, favoring the right side.

Contact point: Thenar pad of the right hand over the patient's right supramastoid groove.

Supporting hand: The left hand is used to stabilize the C1-C2 articulation on the opposite side.

Pattern of thrust: Lateral to medial, superior to inferior, posterior to anterior, through the C0-C1 joint plane line, with an inferiorward arcing motion toward the end of the thrust.

Category by algorithm: Short lever specific contact procedure.

Name of technique: Gonstead

Name of technique procedure: PSRSRP ($+\theta$X, $-\theta$Z, $-\theta$Y) condyle adjustment (Fig. 11.25).

Indications: Extension, right lateral flexion, and left rotational fixation. Postero-superior glide ($+\theta X, -Z$), right lateral flexion ($+X, -\theta Z$), and right axial rotation ($-\theta Y$) positional dyskinesia.

Contraindications: All other listings, normal FSU, hypermobility, instability, destruction of the condyle, or pathologic/nonpathologic fracture of the condyle, infection of the contact bone, and C0-C1 arthrodesis.

Patient position: The patient is seated. The stabilization strap is placed over the crown of the left shoulder. The head is turned away from the side of contact for correction of the rotational component.

Doctor's position: Behind the patient, favoring the right side.

Contact point: The thenar pad of the right hand over the patient's right supramastoid groove.

Table 11.2.
The Occipital Condyle Listings

Gonstead Listing	International	Pattern of Thrust
PSRS	$+\theta X, -\theta Z$	Posterior to anterior, superior to inferior, right to left, through the C0-C1 joint plane line, with an inferiorward arcing motion toward the end of the thrust.
PSRSRA	$+\theta X, -\theta Z, +\theta Y$	Posterior to anterior, superior to inferior, right to left, through the C0-C1 joint plane line, the head is prepositioned in right rotation.
PSRSRP	$+\theta X, -\theta Z, -\theta Y$	Posterior to anterior, superior to inferior, right to left, through the C0-C1 joint plane line, the head is prepositioned in left rotation.
PSLS	$+\theta X, +\theta Z$	Posterior to anterior, superior to inferior, left to right, through the C0-C1 joint plane line, with an inferiorward arcing motion toward the end of the thrust.
PSLSLA	$+\theta X, +\theta Z, -\theta Y$	Posterior to anterior, superior to inferior, left to right, through the C0-C1 joint plane line, the head is rotated toward the side of contact
PSLSLP	$+\theta X, +\theta Z, +\theta Y$	Posterior to anterior, superior to inferior, left to right, through the C0-C1 joint plane line, the head is prepositioned in right rotation.
AS	$-\theta X, +Z$	Anterior to posterior, superior to inferior, through the C0-C1 joint plane line.
ASRS	$-\theta X, -\theta Z$	Anterior to posterior, superior to inferior, right to left, through the C0-C1 joint plane line.
ASRSRA	$-\theta X, -\theta Z, +\theta Y$	Anterior to posterior, superior to inferior, right to left, through the C0-C1 joint plane line, the patient's head is prepositioned in right rotation.
ASRSRP	$-\theta X, -\theta Z, -\theta Y$	Anterior to posterior, superior to inferior, right to left, through the C0-C1 joint plane line, the patient's head is prepositioned in left rotation.

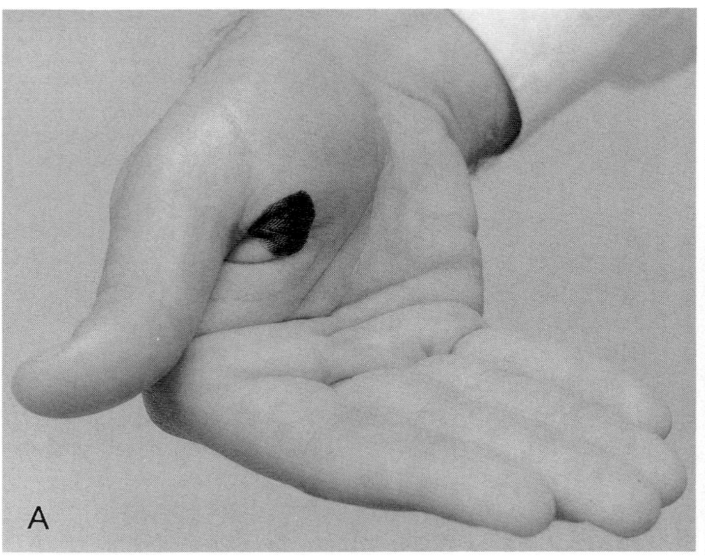

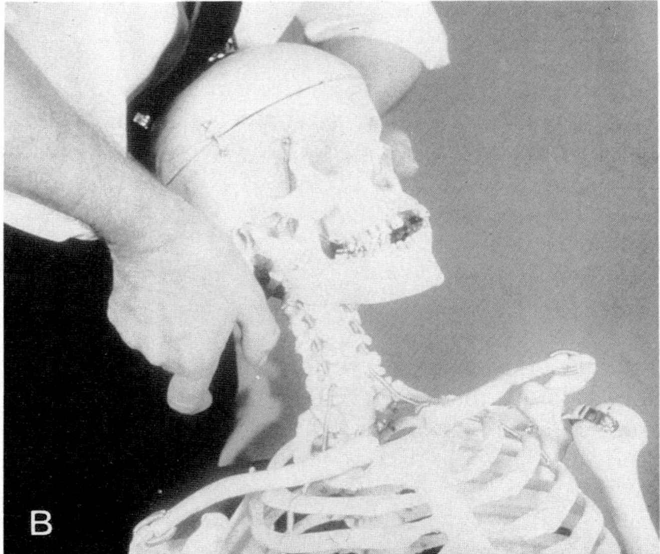

Figure 11.22. **A,** Thenar pad contact point for PS condyle adjustments. **B,** Contact for the PS condyle.

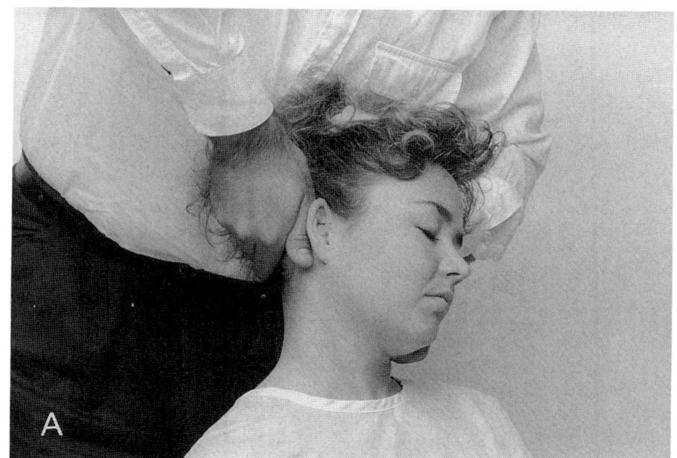

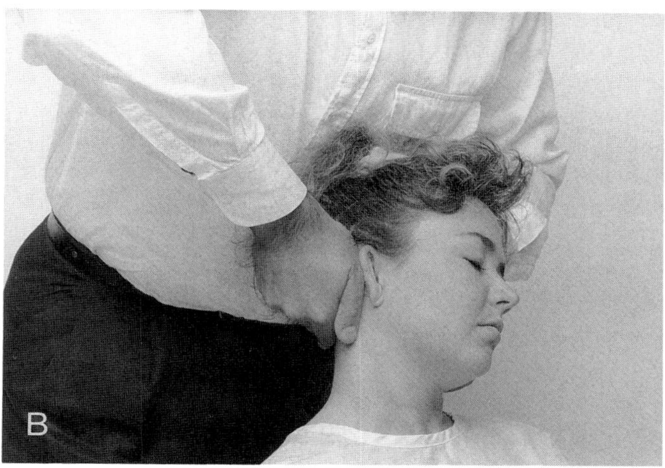

Figure 11.23. A, Getting set. The doctor slides the thenar pad superiorly past the supramastoid groove to move the hair out of the way. **B,** Sliding down to hook the supramastoid groove for the adjustment.

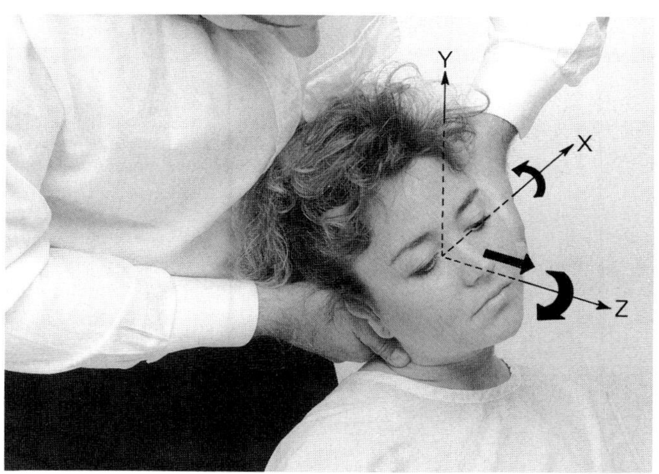

Figure 11.24. PSRS condyle adjustment.

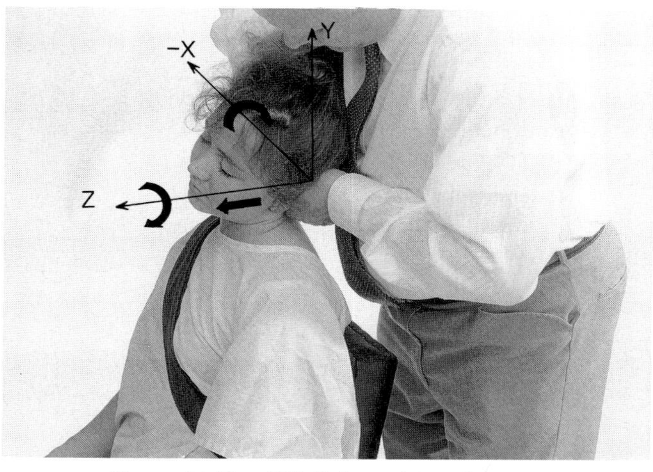

Figure 11.26. PSLSLA condyle adjustment.

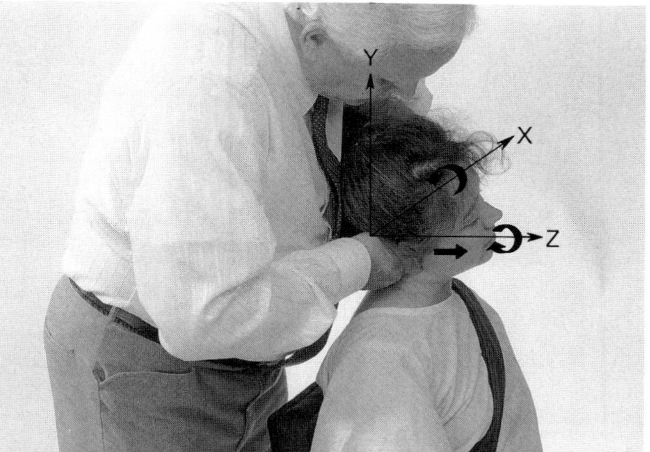

Figure 11.25. PSRSRP condyle adjustment.

Supporting hand: The left hand is used to stabilize the C1-C2 articulation on the opposite side.

Pattern of thrust: Lateral to medial, superior to inferior, posterior to anterior, through the C0-C1 joint plane line, along with an inferiorward arcing motion toward the end of the thrust.

Category by algorithm: Short lever specific contact procedure.

Name of technique: Gonstead

Name of technique procedure: PSLSLA ($+\theta X, +\theta Z, -\theta Y$) condyle adjustment (Fig. 11.26).

Indications: Extension, left lateral flexion, left anterior rotation fixation. Postero-superior glide ($+\theta X, -Z$), left lateral flexion ($+X, +\theta Z$), and left axial rotation ($-\theta Y$) positional dyskinesia.

Contraindications: All other listings, normal FSU, hypermobility, instability, destruction of the condyle, pathologic/nonpathologic fracture of the condyle, infection of the contact bone, C0-C1 arthrodesis.

Patient position: The patient is seated. The stabilization strap is placed over the right shoulder. The head is turned toward the side of contact for correction of the rotational component.

Doctor's position: Behind the patient, favoring the left side.

Contact point: Thenar pad of the left hand is placed over the patient's left supramastoid groove.

Supporting hand: The right hand will stabilize the C1-C2 articulation on the opposite side.

Pattern of thrust: Lateral to medial, superior to inferior, posterior to anterior, with an inferiorward arcing motion toward the end of the thrust, through the C0-C1 joint plane line.

Category by algorithm: Short lever specific contact procedure.

An alternate maneuver for adjusting the PS condyle can be performed in the knee-chest position (Fig. 11.27). If VBAI is present, then this position is contraindicated.

Name of technique: Gonstead

Name of technique procedure: AS ($-\theta X, +Z$) condyle adjustment (Fig. 11.28).

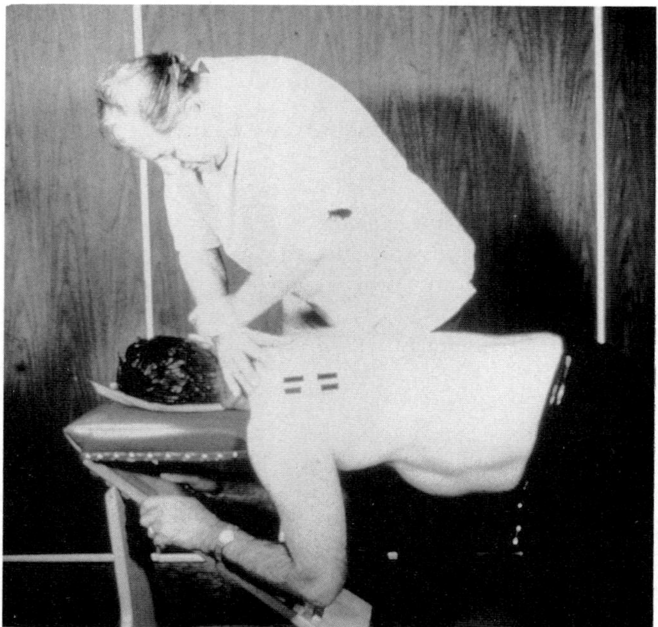

Figure 11.27. PSRS condyle adjustment on the knee-chest table.

Indications: Flexion fixation, antero-superior glide positional dyskinesia.

Contraindications: All other listings, normal FSU, hypermobility, instability, destruction of the cranium, infection of the contact bone, C0-C1 arthrodesis, fracture of the orbit.

Patient position: The patient is seated. The condyle block should be used to stabilize the lower cervical spine.

Doctor's position: Standing directly behind the patient.

Contact point: The hypothenar pad of either hand is placed over the glabella. Tissue pull is from superior to inferior.

Supporting hand: The other hand is used to stabilize, resting on top of the contact hand.

Pattern of thrust: Anterior to posterior, superior to inferior, in an inferiorward scooping motion through the C0-C1 joint plane line.

Category by algorithm: Short lever specific contact procedure.

Name of technique: Gonstead

Name of technique procedure: ASRS ($-\theta X, -\theta Z,$) condyle adjustment (Fig. 11.29).

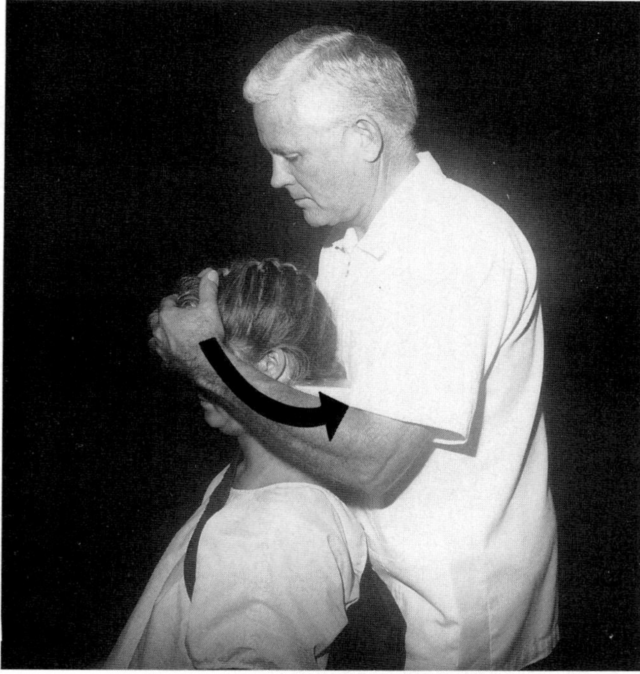

Figure 11.28. Lateral view of the AS condyle adjustment. Notice the "scooping motion" incorporated into the thrust.

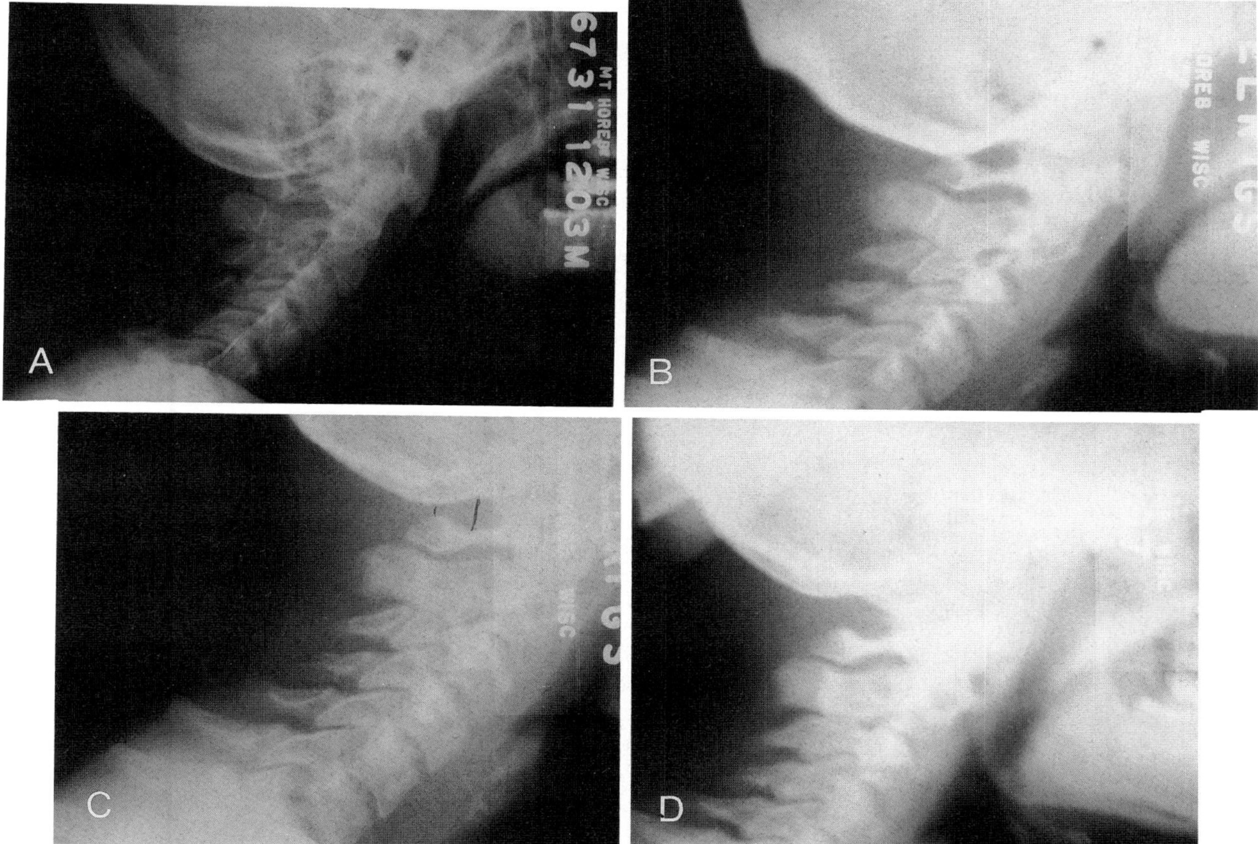

Figure 12.4. A, Anterosuperior occiput subluxation in a comatose patient. **B,** Posttreatment radiograph. **C,** Second posttreatment radiograph. **D,** Third posttreatment radiograph. The patient is now conscious.

reduction was performed on the anterosuperior condyle subluxation in the supine position (6). After the maneuver, a comparative radiograph in the lateral recumbent position was performed. This radiograph (Fig. 12.4B) demonstrates only minimal change in the osseous configuration of the C0-C1 motion segment. The patient continued to be unresponsive. The adjustment was repeated followed by another comparative radiograph. This radiograph (Fig. 12.4C) demonstrates a partial reduction in the displacement, however, the patient's condition remained unchanged. Encouraged by an apparently successful closed reduction, the adjustment was performed a third time. After the maneuver, the patient became conscious. Another comparative radiograph was performed (Fig. 12.4D) which demonstrates a marked reduction when compared with the initial displacement. Vital signs were obtained after the patient regained consciousness. The pulse rate was 58 and the blood pressure elevated to 90/60. The patient was observed for three days with no treatment. Adjustments were performed later at the L5-S1 motion segment to reduce retrolisthesis at that level. Adjustments were also administered to the thoracic spine. The patient was eventually able to ambulate with the aid of a walker.

Atlas Posterior Arch Fracture

A fracture at the junction of the posterior arch and lateral masses is the most common atlas fracture (3,7). A force exerted caudally ($-Y$) on the vertex of the head, as in a Jefferson fracture, but with a component of hyperextension ($-\theta X$) causes the posterior arch of the atlas to be forced between the posterior neural arch of the axis and the base of the occiput. This compressive force causes the posterior arch to move caudally while the lateral masses are held rigid, creating a fracture at the weakest point in the arch, the vertebral artery groove. The extension component of the mechanism of injury is further evidenced by the frequently accompanying hangman's fracture of C2 (also a hyperextension injury). A posterior arch fracture can best be visualized with a lateral radiograph. When the fracture is present, it should always be scrutinized closely for evidence of an accompanying hangman's fracture.

If no neurological signs are present, flexion and exten-

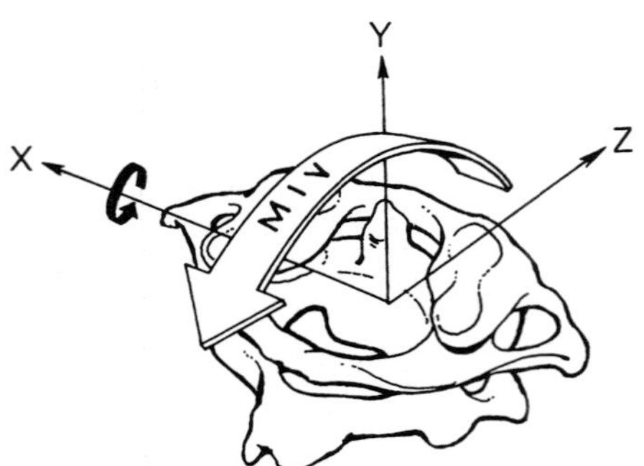

Figure 12.5. MIV for a hangman's fracture.

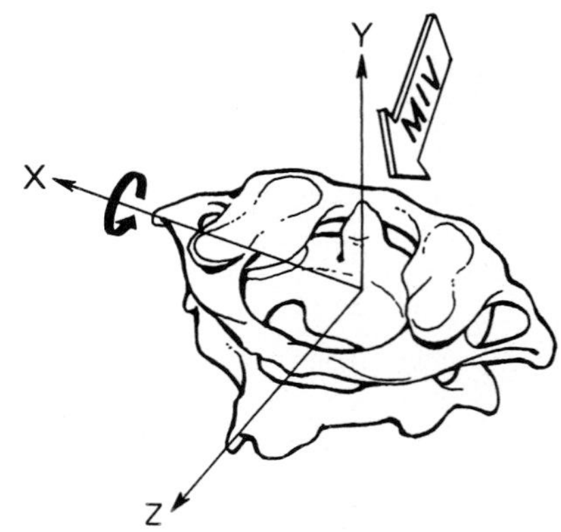

Figure 12.6. MIV for an odontoid fracture.

sion radiographs can further establish the fracture's stability status. Given that dynamic stress radiographs may recreate the mechanism of injury and further stress the damaged tissues, care should be taken with this procedure.

Like the Jefferson fracture, the posterior arch fracture is usually stable, but due to the presence of the delicate neurological structures and vertebral artery located in this area, extreme caution is advised (3,7).

Hangman's Fracture

The hangman's fracture, or traumatic spondylolisthesis of C2, is one of the most commonly occurring injuries of the cervical spine (7). The fracture is caused by forced hyperextension ($-\theta$X) (Fig. 12.5).

A rebound hyperextension action (7) following hyperflexion, from the head hitting the windshield or dashboard in rapid deceleration injuries (8), or hyperextension with compression, causes a separation at the pars interarticularis. The posterior arch of C2 remains in contact with C3 at the articular processes, but the body of C2 is displaced anteriorly, bringing with it the odontoid, atlas ring, and the skull. The lateral radiograph is the best view to evaluate the C2 anterolisthesis.

The hangman's fracture, is associated with anterior and middle column damage and although biomechanically unstable it is often times without neurological deficit because of the increased diameter of the spinal canal caused by the anterior slippage. Due to the location of delicate neurological structures, when nerve injury does occur, it can be devastating.

C2 Odontoid Fractures

Odontoid fractures have varied mechanisms of injury. Depending on the direction of force involved, each injury may have dramatically different neurological and mechanical manifestations.

Both +Z translational forces, as well as hyperflexion injuries, can lead to dens fractures by causing the atlas transverse ligament to forcibly sever the dens from its vertebral body. Negative Z forces, as well as hyperextension injuries, can create fractures through forces exerted by the posterior aspect of the anterior arch, posteriorly on the odontoid process (Fig. 12.6). The −Z and +Z translational injuries are usually caused by direct blows to the front or back of the head respectively.

The odontoid fracture can be visualized on the AP open mouth view as a jagged line through the dens, or on the lateral radiograph as an anterior or posterior displacement of the dens.

A dens fracture may be mistakenly interpreted on the AP open-mouth view due to the Mach effect (7). This is caused by a superimposition of the anterior and posterior arch of C1 appearing as a fracture line at the base of the odontoid. One helpful differentiating tool is that while the superimposition line is smooth and regular, the fracture line will be more jagged and irregular. Taking a lateral radiograph or altering the head position on the AP open mouth, should move the atlas ring enough to eliminate the superimposition. As with all suspected fractures, the doctor should exercise caution. If uncertainty exists, a flexion extension study should eliminate any remaining questions.

When determining if an odontoid fracture is present, the doctor must also rule out os odontoideum, a developmental nonunion of the dens to the body of C2. The gap between the dens and the body is much larger than occurs with most fractures and exhibits smooth sclerotic borders, as opposed to nonsclerotic jagged edges in the case of the fracture. The use of a bone scan and any preinjury x-rays should clarify the situation (7).

Three main types of odontoid fractures occur, as classified by Anderson and D'Alonzo (7). Type I is an avulsion of the top of the odontoid. It does not usually pose any neurological deficit or stability problems even with nonfused healing. Type II is the most frequently occurring and most likely not to reattach (7). As many as 38% heal with nonunion (3). It occurs at the junction of the dens and the vertebral body of C2.

Type III is a fracture occurring deeper into the C2 body (7). This fracture usually heals with no complications.

Odontoid fractures do not usually cause neurological compromise because of the extra canal space in this area of the spine. But since some fractures have an accompanying related anterior or posterior slippage, spinal canal encroachment (i.e., instability) can occur (3,7).

Rupture of the Atlas Transverse Ligament

Traumatic C1 transverse ligament rupture unrelated to preexisting ligament weakness is rare. As with most ligament-osseous relationships, the bone normally fails in trauma before the ligament tears. Certain conditions (7,8) predispose the ligament to rupturing; rheumatoid arthritis, psoriasis, ankylosing spondylitis, Reiter's syndrome, Down's syndrome, tonsillitis, pharyngitis and cervical adenitis. Any of these conditions, combined with a severe blow at the posterior of the skull in a +Z direction, can cause the ligament to rupture, with or without a corresponding odontoid fracture. In cases where the dens does not fracture (Fig. 12.7A), the cord is pinched between the posterior arch and the odontoid causing much more neurological involvement and damage than in instances where the odontoid also breaks (Fig. 12.7B). The latter allows the cord to snake around the insulting osseous structures.

The rupture is best visualized with the lateral radiograph. A finding of anterior slippage of the atlas on the axis is demonstrated with an increased atlanto-dental interval (ADI). The normal ADI is 3 mm in adults and 5 mm in children (See Chapter 5). This injury is unstable and often requires surgical stabilization (3).

CASE REPORT

This 36-yr-old female presented to hospital following cervical trauma. Initial radiographs taken there showed no transverse ligament disruption. She underwent a course of cervical traction of several days before electing to undergo chiropractic evaluation and treatment. Radiographs taken at this time demonstrated anterior displacement of C1 on C2, indicative of transverse ligament rupture. The patient complained of severe neck pain. The chiropractor adjusted C6 four times and then referred her to an orthopedist for surgical consultation. An arthrodesis at C1-C2 was performed subsequently (Fig. 12.8A-B). Approximately five months after surgery, she returned for chiropractic care with a complaint of severe headaches. Initially, the patient was adjusted at C2 and C5 four times. At later dates the patient was adjusted at T5, C6 and the sacrum. Cervical adjustments were performed in the seated position. The patient was eventually adjusted at C1, which then provided symptomatic relief for her headaches. This is an extremely interesting case study in which thrusts were applied at the level of an arthrodesis, which in most instances (See Chapter 11), would be considered a contraindication for direct adjustments at that level.

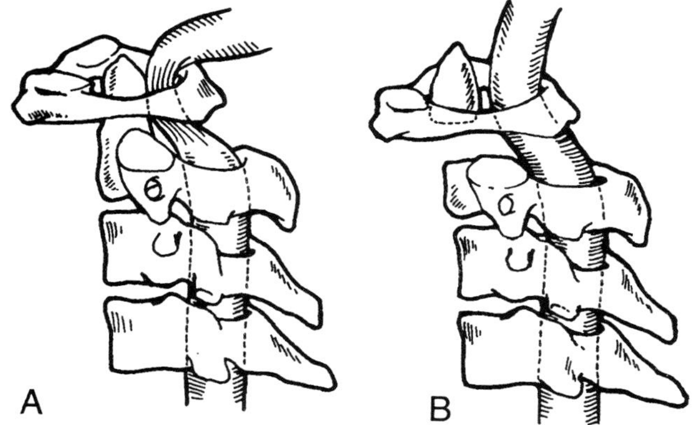

Figure 12.7. A, Effects on the spinal cord from a transverse ligament rupture. Modified from Yochum TR, Rowe LJ. Essentials of skeletal radiology. Baltimore: Williams & Wilkins, 1987:436. **B,** Effects on the spinal cord with a combined odontoid fracture. Modified from Yochum TR, Rowe LJ. Essentials of skeletal radiology. Baltimore: Williams & Wilkins, 1987:436.

Clay Shoveler's Fracture

A clay shoveler's fracture is an avulsion injury of the lower cervical or upper thoracic spinous processes. Due to their elongated spinous processes, C7 and C6 are the most frequently involved (3). The etiology is typically heavy lifting or forced flexion of the cervical spine, though direct trauma can also be a cause. The avulsion fracture is the result of extreme pulling from the muscles which are attached to the spinous processes, such as the upper trapezius or rhomboids.

The clay shoveler's fracture is best viewed on a lateral cervico-thoracic radiograph. The avulsed spinous process is usually displaced inferiorly and is often difficult to see due to the thick musculature at the cervico-thoracic area. Pre-patient filtration of the cervical spine is often helpful in producing a clearer radiograph (See Chapter 5).

The AP lower cervical radiograph often reveals two separated spinous processes on the same vertebra since the tip of the fractured spinous is visualized caudally to the base of the attached spinous of that vertebra.

Due to the non-neurologic proximity of the tip of the spinous process, the clay shoveler's fracture usually has no complications except when associated with other flexion injuries such as vertebral body compression or articular process misalignment. The spinous tip often does not reattach and will take on a smooth sclerotic edge as it heals (3,7,8).

Bilateral Interfacetal Dislocation

Bilateral interfacetal dislocation (BID) is caused by a severe hyperflexion injury to the cervical spine (Fig. 12.9). The mid cervical spine (C4-C7) is most commonly afflicted. Extreme hyperflexion brings the supporting soft

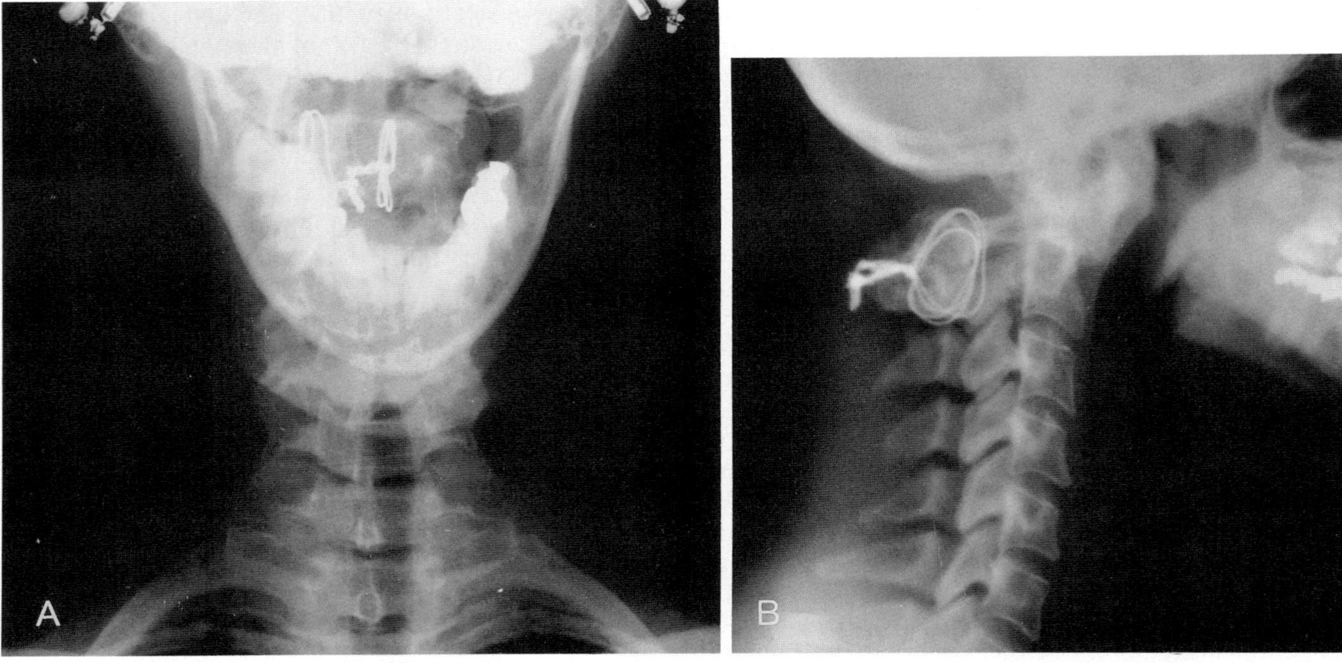

Figure 12.8. **A,** AP radiograph demonstrating a C1-C2 arthrodesis. **B,** Lateral radiograph demonstrating a C1-C2 arthrodesis. Notice the increase in the atlanto-dental interval.

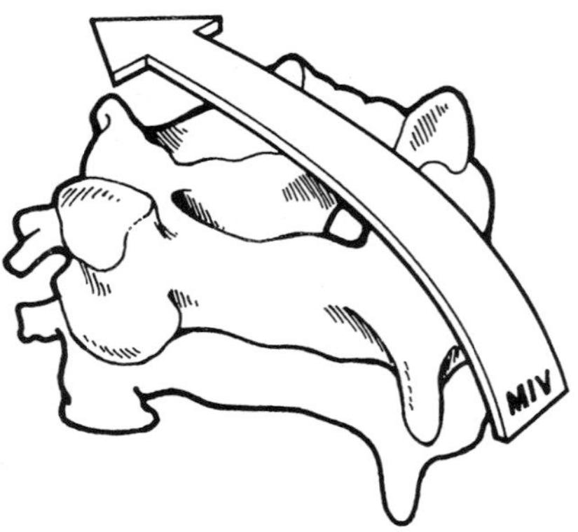

Figure 12.9. MIV for a bilateral interfacetal dislocation (BID). Modified from White AA, Panjabi MM. Clinical biomechanics of the spine. 2nd ed. Philadelphia: JB Lippincott, 1990:226.

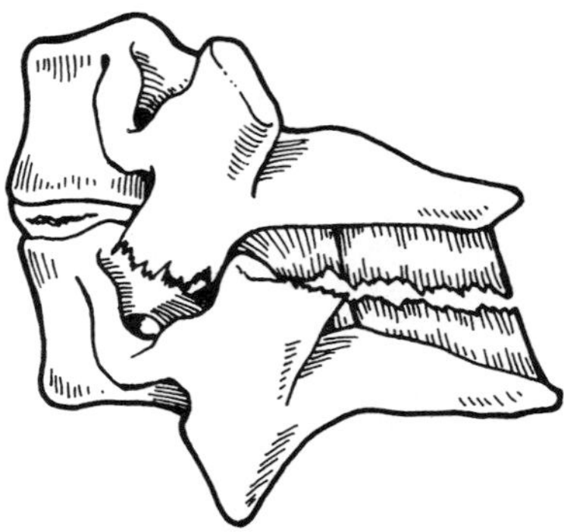

Figure 12.10. Ligamentous damage associated with the BID or unilateral facet dislocation. Modified from White AA, Panjabi MM. Clinical biomechanics of the spine. 2nd ed. Philadelphia: JB Lippincott, 1990:174.

tissues beyond their limits leading to ligamentous tearing (Fig. 12.10). This allows the inferior articular surfaces of the superior vertebra to ride up and over the superior articular surface of the vertebra below. In this particular situation, soft tissues fail before the bony structure. Affected soft tissues include the posterior longitudinal ligament, the midline ligaments, the annular fibers of the disc, the capsular ligaments, the apophyseal joints and occasionally the anterior longitudinal ligament.

After the injury, the superior vertebra usually comes to rest anterior to the vertebra below, with the inferior articulating processes resting in the intervertebral foramen. The body of the dislocated segment is usually anteriorly displaced a distance of at least ½ the AP vertebral body length of the vertebra below (7). Although rare, spontaneous repositioning can occur. In this scenario the neutral lateral cervical radiograph may not show bony misalignment, but the patient can have severe signs of cord injury. A radiograph taken in flexion will demonstrate the mechanical instability. As with all motion x-rays which reproduce the mechanism of injury, extreme care must be taken. Small chip fractures of the articular process may be found accompanying this dislocation (7). Since all three columns are involved, this injury is always considered unstable. Neurosurgical referral is indicated.

The so called "perched facet" (Fig. 12.11A-B) has

been proposed by White and Panjabi (3) to be a true dislocation. The injury can be uni or bilateral. Treatment is through controlled traction combined with muscle relaxation and sedation.

Unilateral Interfacetal Dislocation

The direction of injury in a unilateral interfacetal dislocation is flexion coupled with rotation (7). The dislocation occurs at only one zygapophyseal joint and leaves the injured inferior articular surface resting in the intervertebral foramen of the vertebra below.

The lateral view will give several indications of this condition. The body of the dislocated vertebra will be misaligned anteriorly on the body of the vertebra below, although usually not as far as in bilateral dislocations (See Case Report). There is also a disruption in the alignment of the facets which often exhibit a "bow tie" or "bat wing" appearance (8). Since unilateral dislocations are potentially unstable, protocol requires obtaining advanced imaging, such as MRI or CT, to determine the extent of injury.

CASE REPORT

This 19-yr-old male suffered an injury to the cervical spine while diving head first into a shallow portion of the ocean. The patient was driven to a hospital where clinical and computerized tomographic examinations of the cervical spine were performed. The CT scan clearly shows a displaced fracture of the vertebral body of C6 with a hairline fracture of the pedicle (Fig. 12.12A-E). The transverse process is also fractured. The patient's chief complaint was of moderate neck pain and numbness of the right upper arm and hand. The patient was placed in a Philadelphia collar and surgery was recommended. The patient then elected to travel out of state to seek chiropractic treatment. The patient presented to an outpatient facility with complaints of neck pain and numbness of the right arm and hand. This was twenty days after the initial trauma. Dynamometer evaluations revealed weakness of grip strength on the right side. Range of motion examination of the cervical spine demonstrated flexion limited to 80% of normal and extension limited to 60%. Right rotation of the cervical spine was limited to 50% of normal and left rotation was approximately 80% of normal. Radiologic examination disclosed the fracture dislocation of the C6 vertebra (Fig. 12.13A-B). Hyperextension of C7 on T1 was present. Intersegmental dysfunction was also present at the mid thoracic region (i.e., T5-T6) and at the lumbosacral junction. The patient was adjusted in the prone position on the hi-lo table using the spinous process of C7 as the contact point. A very light posterior to anterior and inferior to superior thrust was made in an attempt to reduce the hyperextension positional dyskinesia that was present at C7. The patient was treated sev-

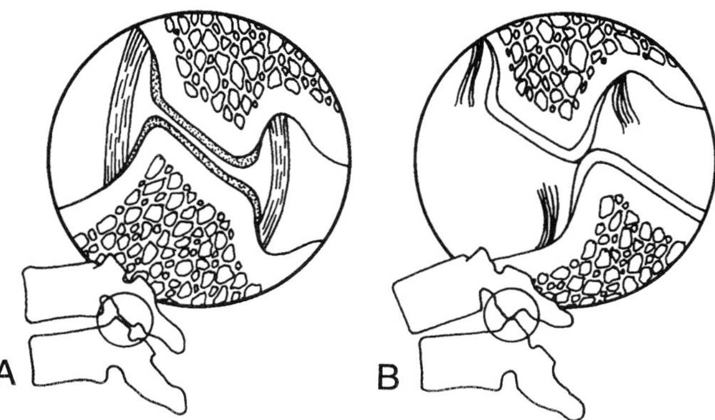

Figure 12.11. **A,** Normal anatomical relationship of the cervical spine. Modified from White AA, Panjabi MM. Clinical biomechanics of the spine. 2nd ed. Philadelphia: JB Lippincott, 1990:226. **B,** Perched facet is a true dislocation. It appears perched because the overlapped cartilage cannot be seen on the radiograph. Modified from White AA, Panjabi MM. Clinical biomechanics of the spine. 2nd ed. Philadelphia: JB Lippincott, 1990:226.

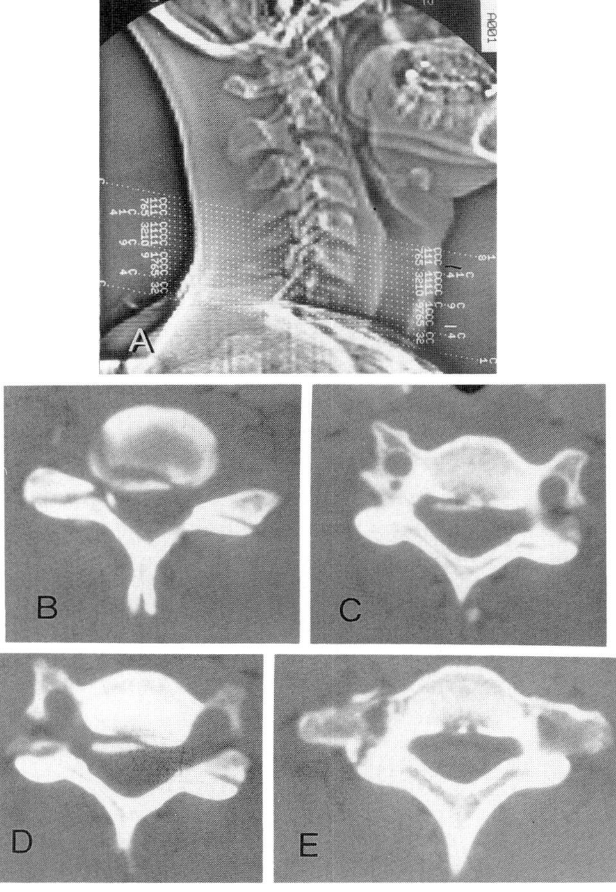

Figure 12.12. **A,** Scout view for the computed tomographic examination. **B,** Fracture displacement of the vertebral body. **C,** Hairline fracture of the pedicle. **D,** Fracture displacement into the spinal canal. **E,** Transverse process fracture.

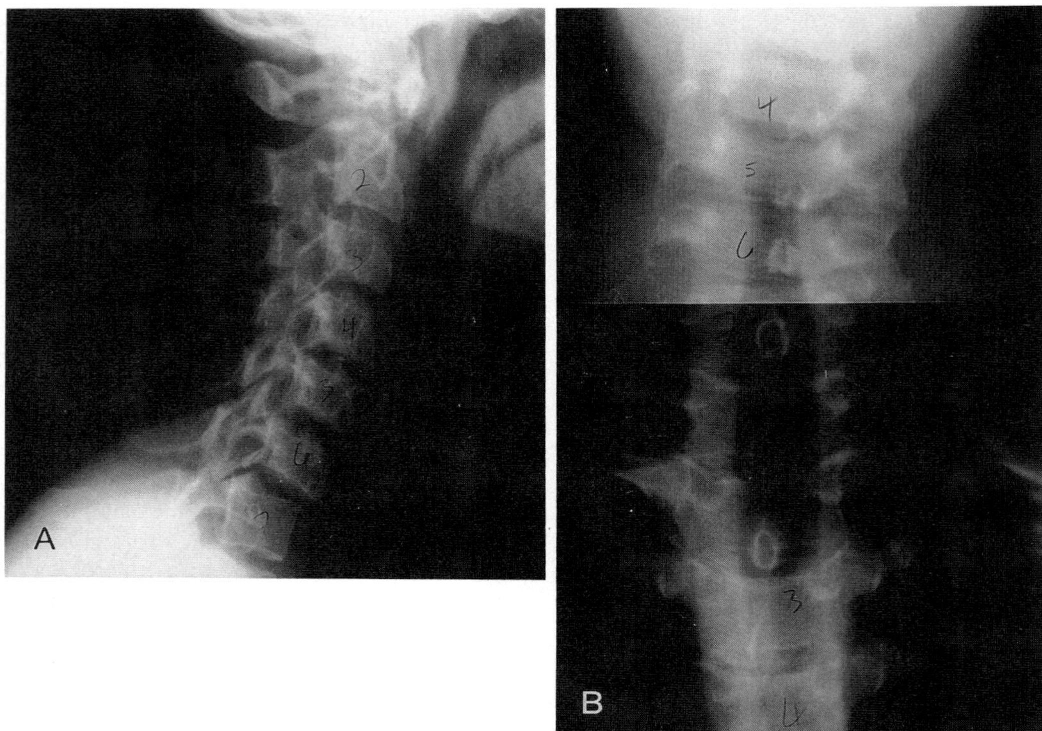

Figure 12.13. **A,** Lateral radiograph demonstrates the anterior dislocation at C6. **B,** AP radiograph demonstrates the rotated position of C6, characteristic of a unilateral facet dislocation.

eral times a month for two months and is currently seen on a periodic (maintenance) basis. He is completely asymptomatic and participates in sport activities (i.e., basketball, water-skiing).

LAMINA FRACTURES

Lamina fractures can be caused from forward flexion $(+\theta X)$ injury leading to avulsion of the lamina from the spinous process. Due to the strength of the ligamentous structures, the bone often fails before the ligament ruptures. The lamina fracture usually occurs in the mid cervical region. The lateral plain film radiograph is the best view to visualize this injury, which will appear as a radiolucent line through the lamina (7). Since the fracture is often difficult to detect with plain films, in some cases, a tomogram may be helpful in its identification. Lamina fractures can contraindicate spinal adjustments using the involved level as the contact vertebra (9).

Articular Pillar Fractures

Articular pillar fractures occur most commonly in the mid to lower cervical region, especially C6 (7). The most common mechanism of injury is hyperflexion with compression (7) coupled with lateral flexion (3,7,10). As the bony pillar fails and collapses, the body of the vertebra is often forced anteriorly.

This fracture may be seen on a lateral radiograph, but when suspected, it is best visualized with an articular pillar projection, taken in an AP direction with a caudal tube tilt of 20–30 degrees (7).

Vertebral Body Compression Type Fractures

WEDGE FRACTURES

The MIV for the wedge fracture is forced hyperflexion $(+\theta X)$ of the spine creating a compression on the anterior portion of the vertebral body. Most (⅔) wedge fractures occur at the fifth, sixth and seventh cervical segments (7). Supportive soft tissues are usually spared and no major ruptures occur to either the anterior longitudinal ligament, the disc structures, or the posterior ligamentous elements. Thus, the simple wedge compression fracture is a relatively stable injury.

The cervical wedge fracture is best seen on the lateral radiograph. The vertebral body is usually compressed anteriorly and the anterior vertebral body height measurement is generally at least 3 mm less than that of the posterior.

Prevertebral edema and hemorrhage can increase the retropharyngeal interspace (7). The measurement taken from the anterior margin of the vertebral bodies of the upper and mid cervical vertebra to the posterior aspect of the tracheal air shadow should not exceed 40% of the anterior to posterior measurement of C4. An increase in this measurement suggests anterior vertebral trauma (Fig. 12.14). The normally radiolucent fat stripe which runs within the prevertebral soft tissue may be locally displaced at the level of the trauma (8).

The wedge fracture often shows a disruption in the normal smooth and regular contour of the vertebral body at the point of cortex break. The best view for visualizing a compression fracture is the lateral radiograph. The AP view does not typically give a clear indication of the injury since no fracture line can be visualized. Once a fracture has been identified, the doctor should search for concomitant injuries. Nontraumatic compression fractures can occur with severe bone weakening diseases such as advanced osteoporosis or lytic metastasis.

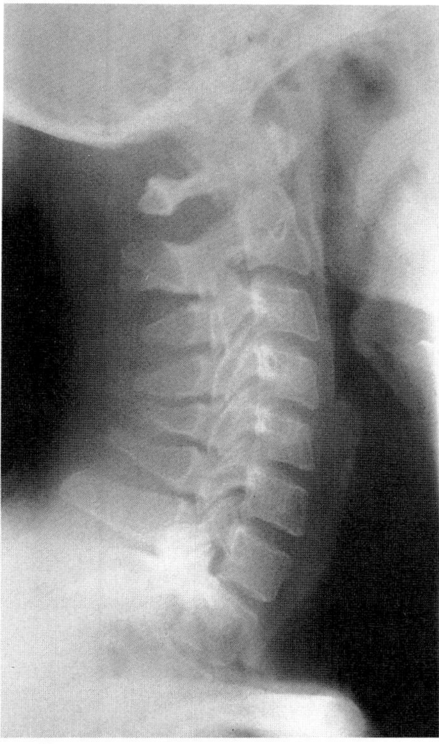

Figure 12.14. Cervical spine of a normal individual. Notice the tracheal air shadow.

Seizure attacks can lead to fracture of the cervical spine in rare cases. This accounts for approximately 2.5% of all hospitalized "non-traumatic" fractures of the spine (11). It is generally not contraindicated to use the fracture segment as a contact vertebra for an adjustment. If an adjustment is indicated, it can be performed in the prone or seated position using the spinous process as the short lever arm.

CASE REPORT

This patient suffered a diving injury (6–22–79) which compressed the C5 and C6 vertebral bodies (2). The patient immediately became quadriplegic. After treatment with halo traction the patient's condition improved and he regained control of the upper extremities but remained paraplegic. The patient subsequently underwent wire fixation arthrodesis from C4 to C6.

At the time of presentation to an outpatient chiropractic facility, the patient remained nonambulatory and paraplegic. This was approximately nine months after the accident. Physical and radiologic examinations were performed. The arthrodesis is visible on the lateral and anteroposterior radiographs (Fig. 12.15A-B).

The first thoracic vertebra was adjusted four times (PRI-t). The patient did not improve. The C7 vertebra was then adjusted (PL). The spinous process was contacted with the distal lateral tip of the index finger. All adjustments were made with the patient seated in the

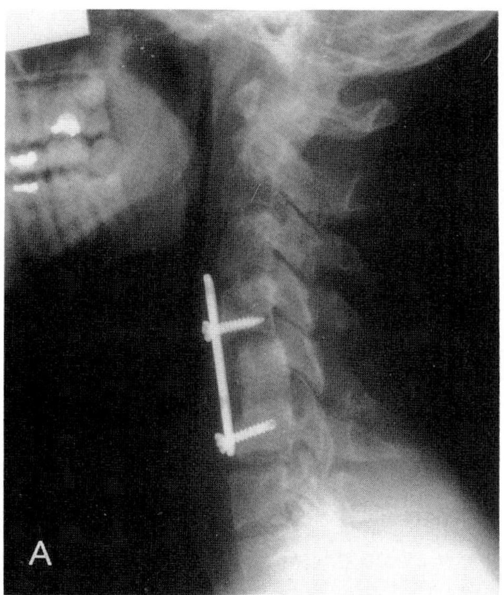

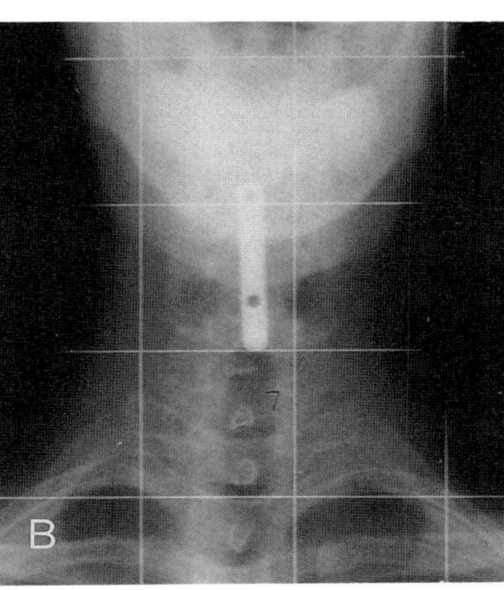

Figure 12.15. A, Anteroposterior radiograph of a C4-C7 arthrodesis. **B,** Lateral radiograph. Notice the retrolisthesis and hyperextension positional dyskinesia of C6.

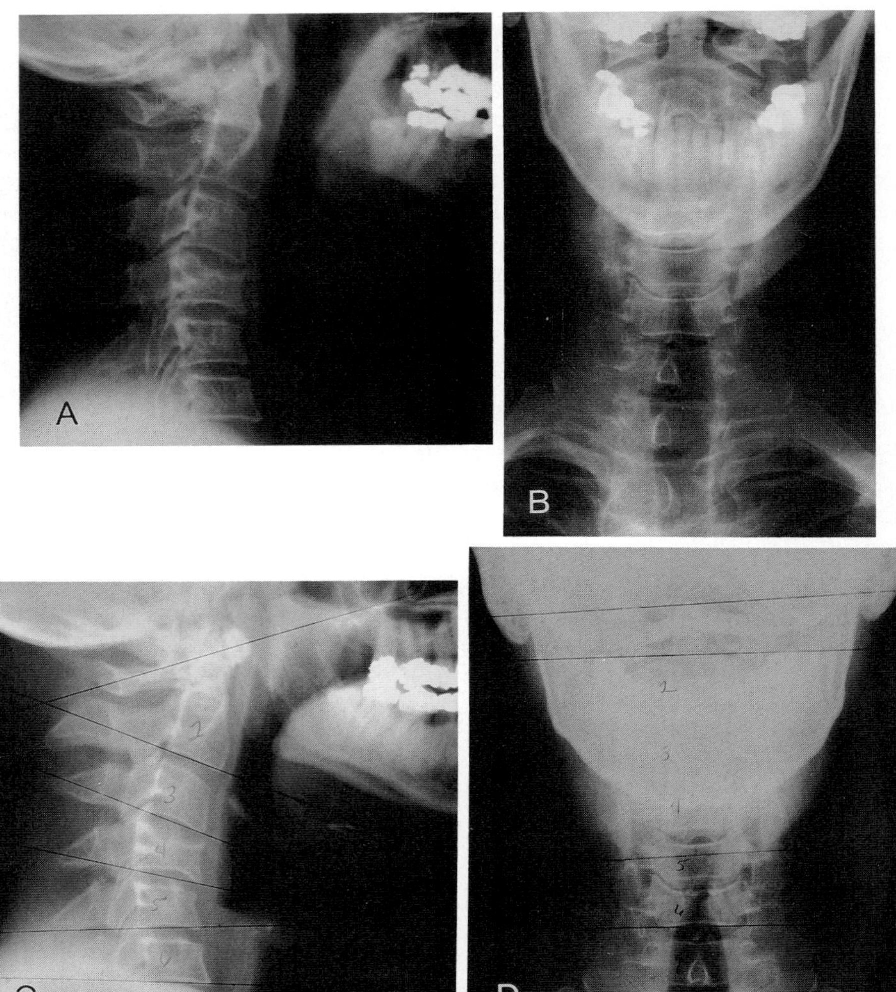

Figure 12.16. **A,** Pretreatment radiograph demonstrating a wedge fracture at C4. **B,** Pretreatment AP radiograph. **C,** Posttreatment radiograph. There is diminished $-\theta X$ positional dyskinesia at C0-C1 and no increase in the kyphotic deformity. **D,** Posttreatment radiograph. There appears to be a reduction in the rotational displacements of the lower cervical and upper thoracic vertebrae.

wheelchair. No objective or subjective improvements were detected after two treatments. The doctor then decided to adjust the C6-C7 motion segment (PL-inf) by contacting the C6 spinous process. Four treatments were administered monthly over the next six months. Range of motion improved and skin temperature asymmetries (12) diminished. The patient was then seen monthly for the next six months. During the course of chiropractic treatment, the patient also had extensive physical therapy (parallel bars, walker, Canadian crutches, etc.). He eventually was able to ambulate unaided.

CASE REPORT

This 35-yr-old patient presented for chiropractic evaluation approximately two years after an injury in which he sustained a compression fracture of C4 (Fig. 12.16A-D). The patient was hit in the back of the head with a tree limb which caused a hyperflexion injury of the cervical spine. He was treated with a halo apparatus and cervical traction. At the time of chiropractic evaluation the patient complained of left arm stiffness, inability to hold tools, muscular hypotonicity, tingling in both hands, burning sensations in the left leg and occasional clonus of the left foot.

The patient was adjusted at C6 in the cervical chair and at T6 and T8 in the prone position. Twenty-four treatments were rendered. The patient has been able to resume normal work including the use of tools. Full function of the upper extremities has been obtained and the left foot clonus has not reoccurred.

CASE REPORT

This 34-yr-old male presented for chiropractic evaluation approximately four months after sustaining a cervical spine compression trauma from diving into a pool. There was fragmentation of the disc into the spinal canal and the patient subsequently underwent arthrodesis at C6 and C7 (Fig. 12.17A-B). At the time of chiropractic assessment he complained of numbness and tingling in both arms and severe neck pain. Radicular symptomatology was exacerbated with less than five degrees of cervical motion. The patient also suffered from headaches. He underwent nine treatments where C4 was adjusted in the cervical chair and T5 in the prone position. All symptoms subsided after chiropractic treatment.

CASE REPORT

This 36-yr-old female patient presented for evaluation nine days after a motor vehicle accident, complaining of moderate to severe neck pain extending into the shoulders and arms, headache, thoracic pain, and low back pain descending into the right hip and leg, dizziness, insomnia, listlessness and constipation.

Radiographic examination revealed an avulsion fracture of the C2 spinous process and a compression fracture of the anterosuperior portion of the T1 vertebral body (Fig. 12.18A-D). The possibility of combined injuries should always be considered in the evaluation of the trauma patient. The patient has the right to have more than one thing wrong with them. Historical information, gathered from the patient, witnesses, police reports and other physicians relating to mechanism(s) of injury can often help in determining the extent of damage of the involved tissues.

A comprehensive examination (See Chapters 4 and 5) was performed. The patient was adjusted at C7 and C2. C7 was adjusted in the cervical chair three times per week for a period of approximately twelve weeks, at which time, her frequency of care was reduced to one visit per week for nine months. During this period, adjustments were alternated between C7 and C2. C2 was adjusted prone on the hi-lo table with a spinous contact. At one year follow-up, the patient reported reduced neck pain. The C2 spinous process separation has resolved (Fig. 12.18E-G). She continues to experience neck pain when under psychological stress.

Burst Fractures

The burst fracture is produced through a compressive (−Y) force to the head, leading to failure in a mid or lower cervical vertebra. The compressive force above pushes the nucleus through the end-plate, bursting the vertebral body at right angles to the MIV. There is a sandwich effect as the injured vertebra is squeezed between the two adjacent vertebrae.

Fragments are often driven posteriorward, damaging the posterior longitudinal ligament and compressing the anterior portion of the spinal cord. A classic anterior spinal syndrome may ensue, causing immediate and complete motor paralysis, and cutaneous sensory nerve loss of pain and temperature below the level of nerve damage. Bilateral vibration and position sense are often left unaffected (7,13).

The lateral radiograph demonstrates flattening of the comminuted vertebral body centrally. Anterior and posterior displacement of fragments can be visualized but do not necessarily give a clear indication of spinal stability (10).

The A-P radiograph often demonstrates a vertical fracture line in the body of the vertebra. This radiographic

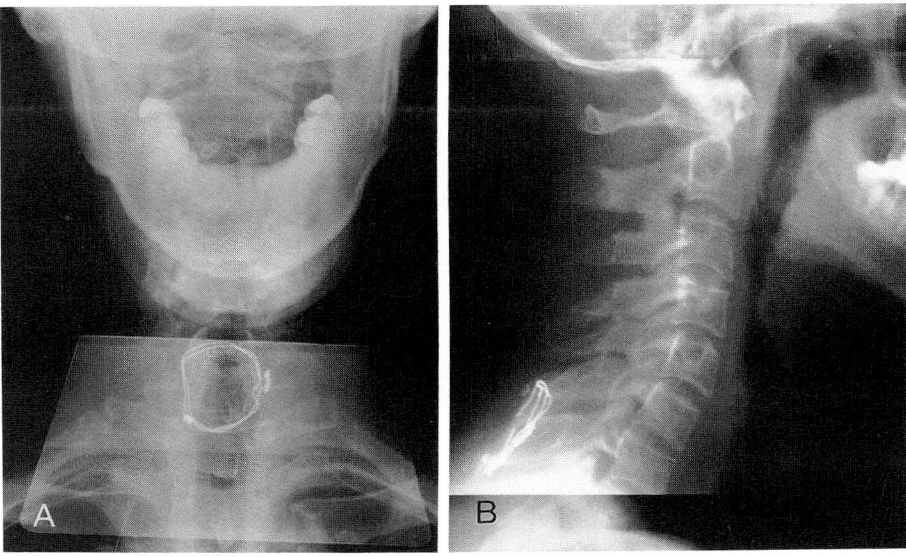

Figure 12.17. **A,** AP radiograph demonstrating the wire arthrodesis. **B,** Lateral radiograph demonstrates the C6-C7 arthrodesis. Notice the retrolisthesis at C4.

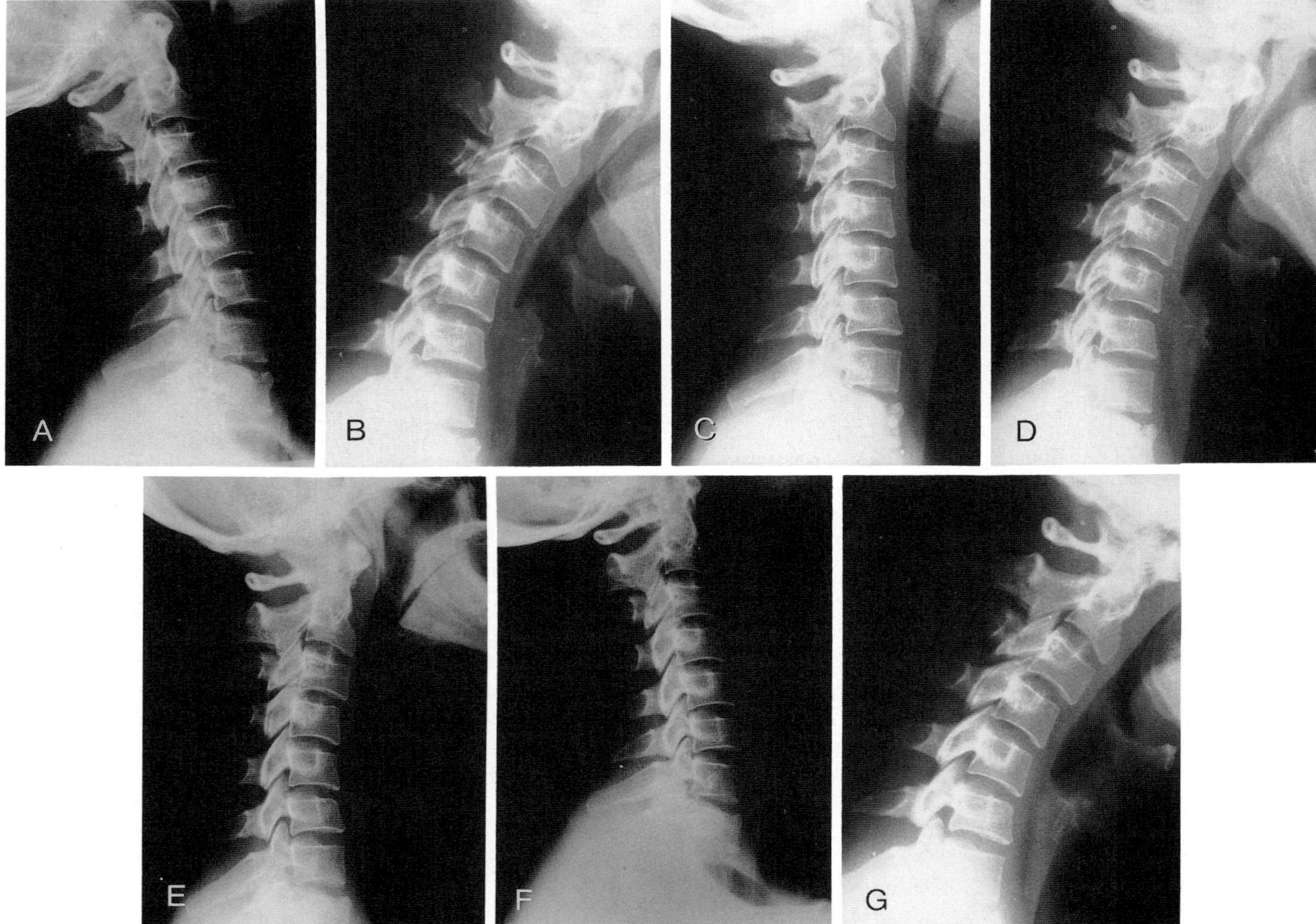

Figure 12.18. **A,** Extension radiograph (2–28–90). Notice the separation of the C2 spinous process and compression fracture of the anterosuperior margin of T1. **B,** Flexion radiograph (2–28–90). **C,** Neutral radiograph (4–2–90). **D,** Flexion radiograph (4–2–90). **E,** Neutral radiograph (5–10–91). **F,** Extension radiograph (5–10–91). **G,** Flexion radiograph (5–10–91).

sign is usually present in the burst fracture and absent in the simple compression fracture, making it useful as a differentiating factor (7).

The burst fracture is often missed, due to its tendency to reposition back to a more normal shape and position after the injury. This is due to the centering effect of the ligaments of the motion segment. This may leave the practitioner uncertain as to the level of neurologic deficit if the radiograph shows no alterations (3). The CT scan is the best method of determining the level of comminution and fracture (7). Due to the fact that the burst fracture involves the anterior and middle columns, it is always biomechanically and often neurologically unstable.

Lateral Bending Fractures

Forced lateral flexion ($\pm\theta Z$) of the cervical spine causes compression on the concavity of the curve and avulsive type forces on the convexity. The compressive forces, if severe enough, can cause vertebral body collapse on one side of an articular pillar. The fracture or dislocation can best be visualized with the AP radiograph (or with an AP pillar view) (3).

In severe cases, the transverse process on the convex side may fracture due to avulsion forces. The distal tip of the transverse process is forcibly pulled off by its attachment to strong ligaments and muscles. Due to its elongated processes, the C7 vertebra is the most common site of a transverse process fracture. The break is best visualized on an AP cervical view and will be differentiated from nonunion of the transverse process by the irregular edge in the fracture and the smooth sclerotic appearance of a nonunion process. Brachial plexus injury can occur on the convex side of bend, and worsens the prognosis. If the injury is isolated to the vertebral body, the segment is usually stable. When the posterior elements are also involved, or avulsion is present, the segment is considered unstable (3).

Teardrop Fractures

A teardrop fracture of the cervical spine may be caused by either a hyperextension ($-\theta X$) or hyperflexion ($+\theta X$) injury. The hyperextension type injury creates an avulsion of a triangular piece of bone from the anterior inferior aspect of the vertebral body. The damaging force is often severe enough to also rupture the anterior longitudinal ligament. The motion segment may be unstable if the anterior damage is combined with posterior compression. Along with anterior ligament avulsion damage, the posterior supportive laminar ligaments (i.e., ligamentum flavum) are usually compressed to such a degree that they are driven anteriorly into the spinal canal, causing posterior cord compression (7,8). This compression may cause central spinal cord syndrome which is characterized by loss of pain and temperature, but a sparing of sensation to touch (3).

Hyperflexion injuries can also cause teardrop type fractures as the anterior inferior aspect of one vertebra is compressively forced onto the anterior superior aspect of the vertebral body below. This may cause an often sizable chip of bone to break from the anterior inferior aspect of the vertebral body above. The posterior supportive ligaments can be torn, possibly allowing unilateral or bilateral facet dislocation to occur. There may also be associated acute anterior cervical cord syndrome (3,7). When ligamentous damage is present, the segment is considered biomechanically unstable.

FRACTURES OF THE THORACIC SPINE

Study of this area has long been neglected since fractures of the thoracic spine constitute only a small percentage of spinal fractures (14). Fractures occur less often in the thoracic area than in other parts of the spine given the protection offered by the rib cage, the orientation of the facet planes and the fact that considerable force is required. Due to the architecture of the thoracic vertebrae, the neural canal is smallest in this area, thereby subjecting its contents (the spinal cord and nerve roots) to damage when a vertebra is either fractured or subluxated. The main causes of thoracic fractures are auto accidents, falls from excessive heights, and direct blows to the area.

Unstable fractures result in loss of anterior vertebral body height and progressive kyphotic deformity (Gibbus) (Figs. 12.19–12.21), subluxation of the superior vertebra and disruption of the soft tissues, usually causing pain. Stable compression fractures may also present a similar symptomatology and if not treated properly, instability can ensue when anterior column height exceeds 50% due to progressive stress at the posterior elements.

As the cancellous bone collapses, there may or may not be a loss in compressive strength (3). The mechanical properties of spongy bone are depicted in Figure 12.22.

A less common type of injury is the burst-dislocation, combining elements of the burst fracture and fracture dis-

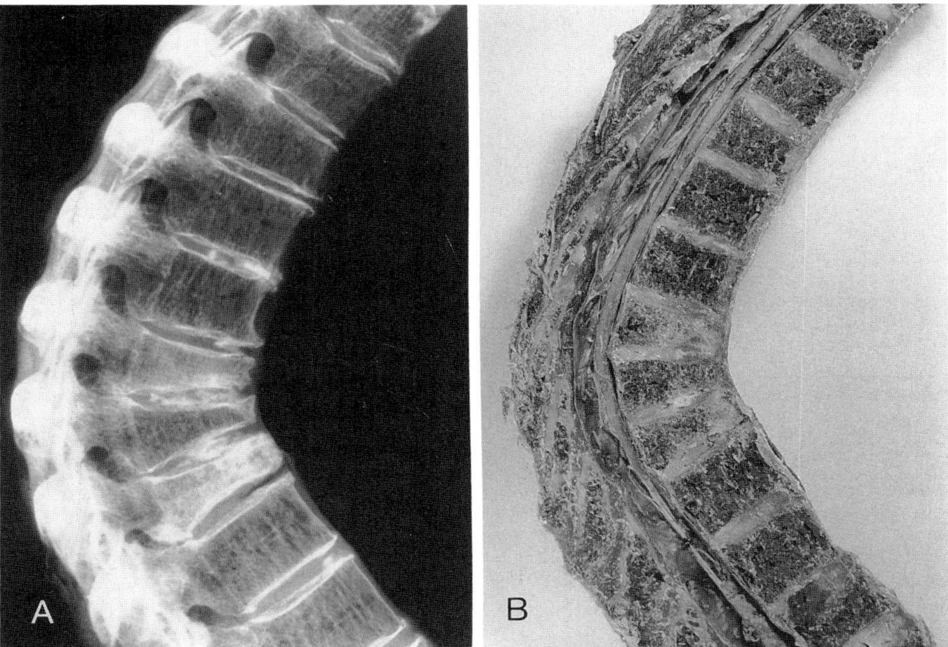

Figure 12.19. **A,** Radiograph of a cadaveric specimen demonstrating multiple compression fractures of the thoracic spine with a kyphotic or Gibbus deformity. **B,** Cadaver specimen.

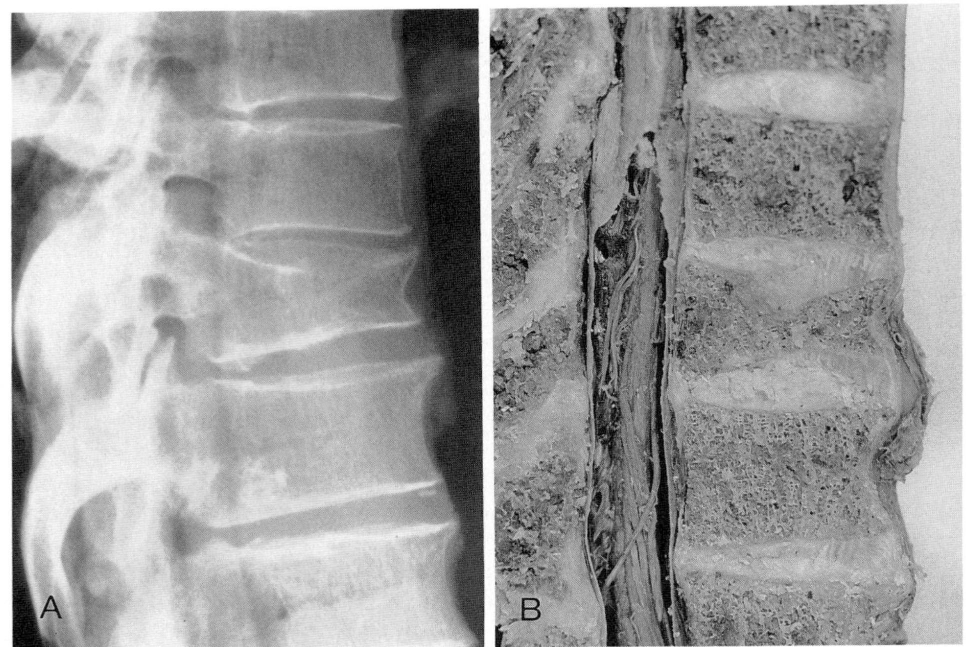

Figure 12.20. **A,** Radiograph of a cadaveric specimen demonstrating a compression fracture of a lower thoracic vertebra. **B,** Cadaver specimen.

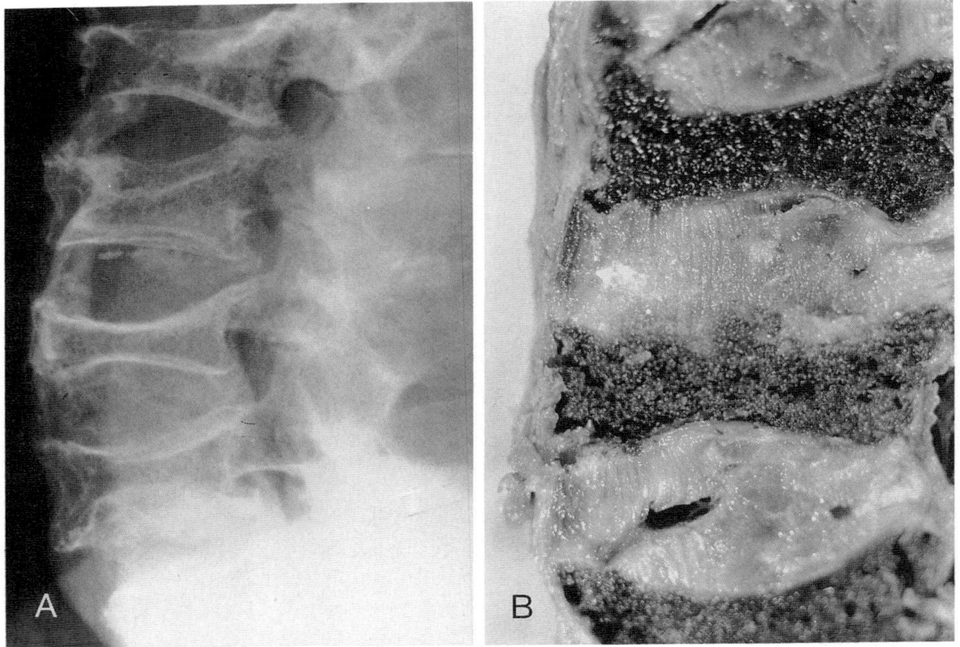

Figure 12.21. **A,** Radiograph demonstrating multiple compression fractures in a cadaveric specimen. **B,** Cadaver specimen.

location. In typical fracture-dislocations, the spinal cord is compromised with the superior fracture segment tethering the spinal cord contents across the relatively fixed inferior segment. In contrast, burst-dislocations shatter the inferior vertebral body and extensive posterior element fractures appear to add an element of decompression of the spinal canal at the time of injury. Without this decompression, a greater neurologic injury would be expected. Many unstable fractures of the thoracic spine occur from isolated direct blows.

CASE REPORT

This patient suffered an upper thoracic and left hand injury while involved in a high speed auto racing accident on 5–30–88. He remained in intensive care for two days. Injuries included a fractured ulna, median nerve damage, three fractured ribs, two fractured spinous processes, three fractured transverse processes, a brain concussion, and a compression fracture at T5 (Fig. 12.23). The attending orthopedic surgeons recommended Harrington rod surgery. The patient denied medical treatment and elected to undergo chiropractic evaluation and treatment for the spinal injuries. He was transported in a sling-type bed in a van and survived the 12 hour drive to a chiropractic care facility. After a thorough evaluation, treatment began. Since the patient was not ambulatory, several individuals had to logroll him so that the upper thoracic spine and neck remained in a neutral position when he was moved to the adjusting table. At first, treatments were rendered using the knee-chest table. After 1½ weeks the T5 segment was adjusted in the seated position. Four months after the accident, the patient, a chiropractor, was adjusting a limited number of patients. The patient was virtually pain-free approximately 18 months after the accident. He is regularly adjusted at two week intervals.

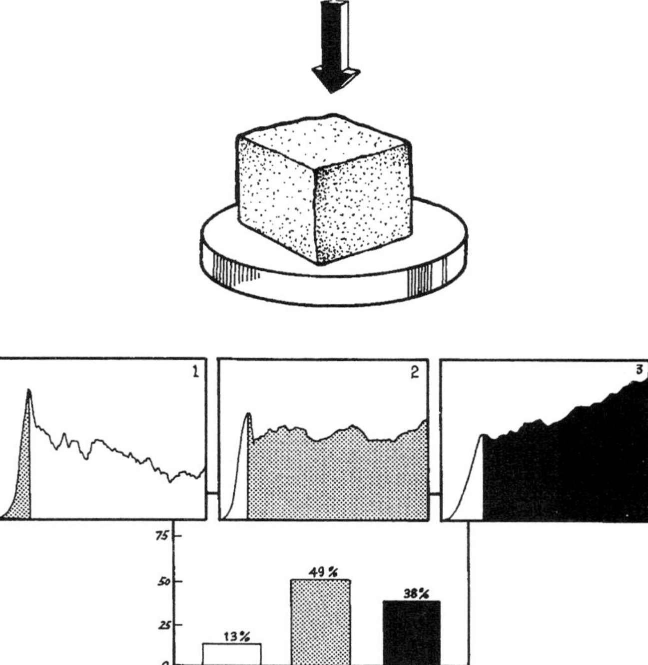

Figure 12.22. Cancellous bone failure patterns. There are three types of load-deformation curves presented. Type 1 demonstrates decreasing strength after the maximum load is reached. Type 2 maintains its strength and type 3, surprisingly, increases in strength after the failure point. The majority of the samples had type 2 curves. Modified from White AA, Panjabi MM. Clinical biomechanics of the spine. 2nd ed. Philadelphia: JB Lippincott, 1990:36.

CASE REPORT

This 10-yr-old female was involved in an automobile accident on 11–12–89. On 11–24–89 she presented for chiropractic evaluation and treatment with complaints of difficulty in breathing, interscapular and lower thoracic pain, and left anterior costal pain. The radiograph (Fig. 12.24) demonstrates compression fractures at T7 and T8. The patient was adjusted 12 times over a five month period at the sacrum (8X), T9 (4X), T4 (4X), C7 (1X) and C1 (3X). Two weeks after beginning chiropractic care, the patient reported no symptomatology.

CASE REPORT

This 85-yr-old male presented for chiropractic evaluation and treatment one week after thoracic spine trauma. He suffered a compression fracture of T8 (Fig. 12.25). Following a comprehensive assessment, the patient was adjusted. Over the course of several months the patient was adjusted at T9 (9X), T8 (1X), T12 (1X) and T10 (1X). Initially, a double thumb lamina contact was used. Breathing and thoracic pain improved. The patient continues to experience intermittent pain when lifting.

THORACOLUMBAR COMPRESSION FRACTURES

Most thoracic and lumbar fractures occur at the thoracolumbar junction. Approximately 60% are found between T12 and L2 and as many as 90% occur between T11 and L4 (1). The first lumbar is the most common level of involvement (1).

Several anatomical and functional factors contribute to the high incidence of fractures in this area: 1) the transition of facet orientation from thoracic coronal to lum-

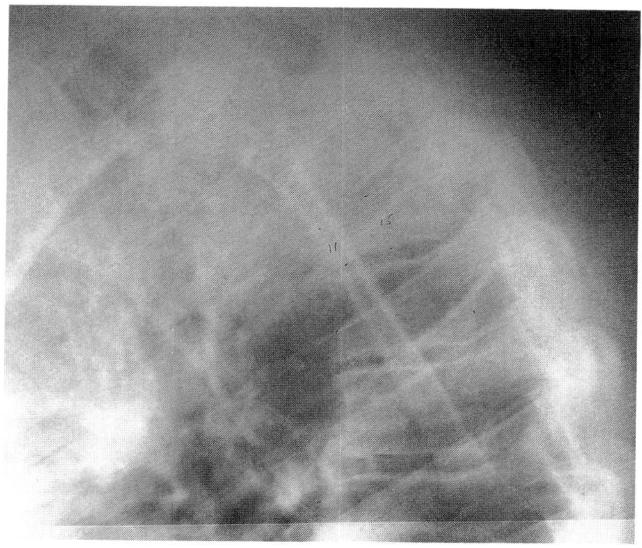

Figure 12.23. Compression fracture of T5.

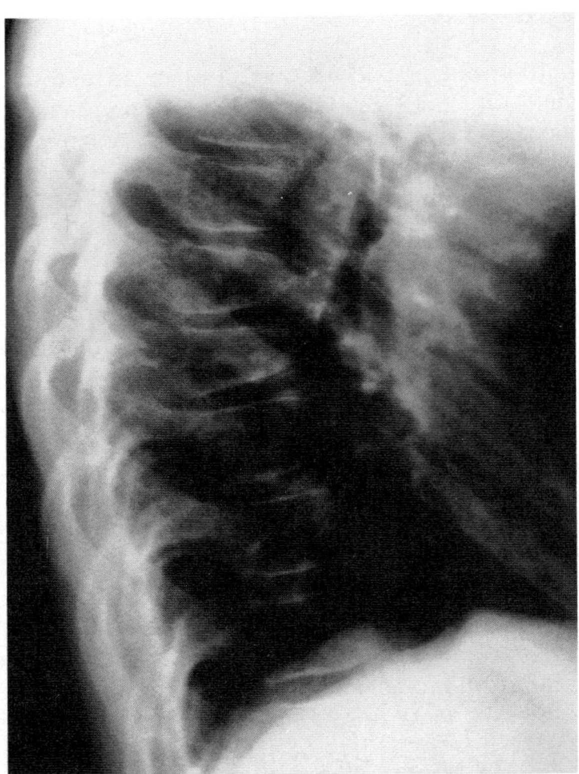

Figure 12.24. Radiograph demonstrating compression fractures of T7 and T8.

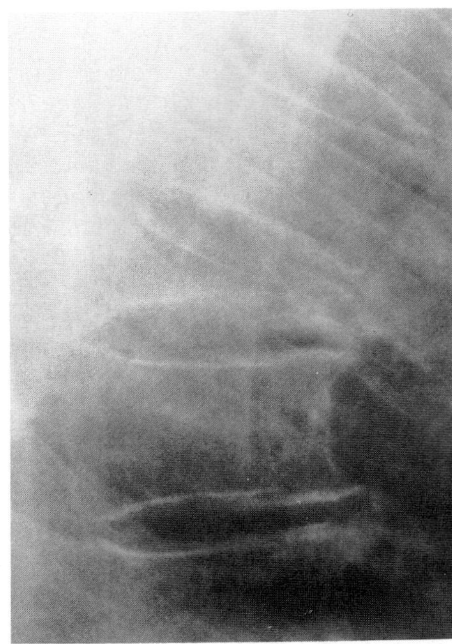

Figure 12.25. Radiograph demonstrating a compression fracture at T8.

bar sagittal, 2) the change from the thoracic kyphosis to the lumbar lordosis, 3) absence of thoracic costal stabilization in the lumbar spine, 4) increased range of lumbar motion compared to thoracic motion which is limited by costal attachments, and 5) the presence of mortise type joints which may increase susceptibility to fracture in this region by increasing the stiffness of the motion segment (3,15).

Compression or wedge fractures account for 48% of all fractures in the thoracic and lumbar spine (15,16). The MIV is hyperflexion with the center of rotation occurring at the center of the disc (15). Combined $+\theta X$ and $-Y$ forces on the anterior of the vertebral body cause failure. Since the posterior vertebral body elements, as well as the posterior ligamentous structures are usually unaffected, the typical thoracolumbar compression fracture is stable and exhibits minimal to moderate neurologic injury.

The compression fracture is best visualized on the lateral view, its primary radiographic finding being the wedge deformity, which is a decrease in anterior vertebral body height while the posterior body height remains unchanged. This leaves the vertebral body with a triangular shape. The "step defect" is another radiograph finding of the compression fracture (7). This finding can be seen on the lateral view as a sharp disruption in the anterior superior aspect of the vertebral body. As $-Y$ forces compress the anterior surface of the vertebral body, a piece of bone is forced anteriorly leaving a step in the normally smooth bony contour. In minor fractures with less than 30% loss of body height, the step defect may be the only radiographic finding.

A white line may also be seen in the superior section of the vertebral body running parallel to the vertebral endplate. This radiopaque line represents a recalcification healing of the fracture. As healing progresses past two months, this line decreases and eventually disappears (1,7). The healing process of recalcification also occurs in the step defect as time progresses. The step usually becomes smoother and less clearly delineated within two to three months (7). These two findings can help determine if the lesion is acute or healed, which can be very useful, especially in the geriatric patient, who may present with several fractures.

Forces that are predominantly $-Y$ in direction with little flexion ($+\theta X$), may lead to end-plate fractures (3). This fracture is often difficult to view on plain films but can be readily seen with tomography. End-plate fractures are the most common pathologic finding on lumbar dissection (17).

Although thoracolumbar compression fractures are not commonly associated with severe neurologic damage, some acute transient or chronic neurologic symptoms may occur. Abdominal ileus, or paralytic ileus is a loss of bowel function due to injury to the spine and irritation of the visceral (autonomic) nerve plexus and ganglia. This is usually transient and self resolving. Abdominal ileus is seen radiographically as excessive amounts of gas pockets in a slightly extended gastric lumen.

Clinical signs and symptoms can alert the practitioner to the possible existence of a thoracolumbar fracture, especially if there is a history of hyperflexion injury. The patient often complains of pain referred by the cluneal nerve to the iliac crests. Palpation of the paraspinal musculature, as well as spinous percussion with a hammer, should elicit pain. The presence of a gibbus formation is a strong indication of a compression fracture.

Computed tomography is usually not helpful in evaluating compression fractures since the axial view parallels the fracture line. Sagittal reconstruction is needed to identify the lesion. Greater than 50% loss of anterior vertebral body height is considered unstable due to the fact that it is often associated with posterior column ligamentous damage.

If the compressive forces (−Y) are of sufficient magnitude and there is less of a flexion bending moment, a burst fracture can occur (Fig. 12.26). With this injury, bony elements may be forced into the spinal canal causing cord compression.

CASE REPORT

This 57-year-old male presented to a chiropractic office with complaints after a lifting injury. The patient stated that he was lifting heavy pipes (approx. 100 lbs) when a sharp pain developed in the right lower portion of the back. After the injury, the patient was referred by his employer to a hospital where plain radiographs were performed. The patient was diagnosed as having a lumbar sprain and was prescribed muscle relaxant medication. The radiographs taken at this time (Fig. 12.27) clearly indicate a compression fracture at T12 which was not present on radiographs performed one year previously (Fig. 12.28). Clinically, thoracolumbar compression fractures may be missed, if a thorough examination is not performed. The patient then chose to seek chiropractic evaluation from the same physician who had successfully treated him for a cervical condition approximately one

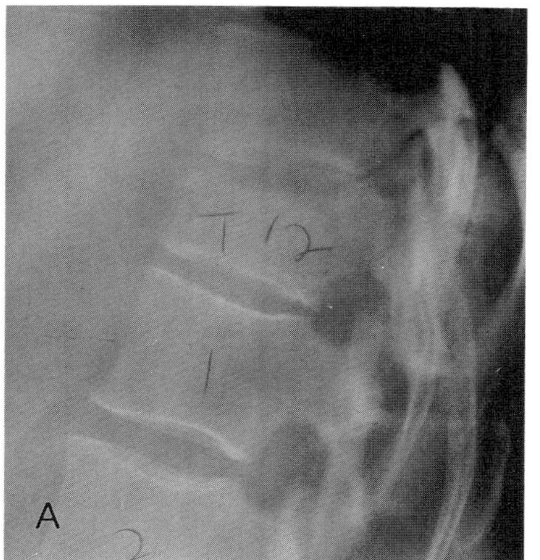

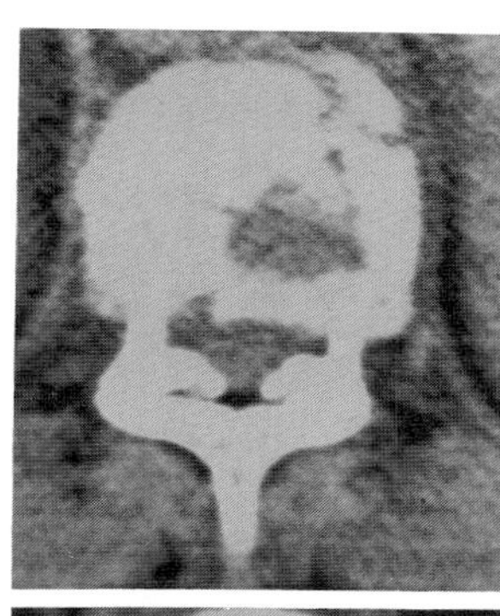

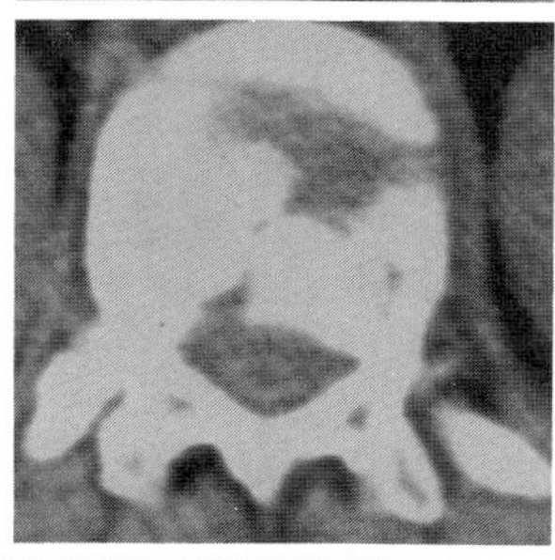

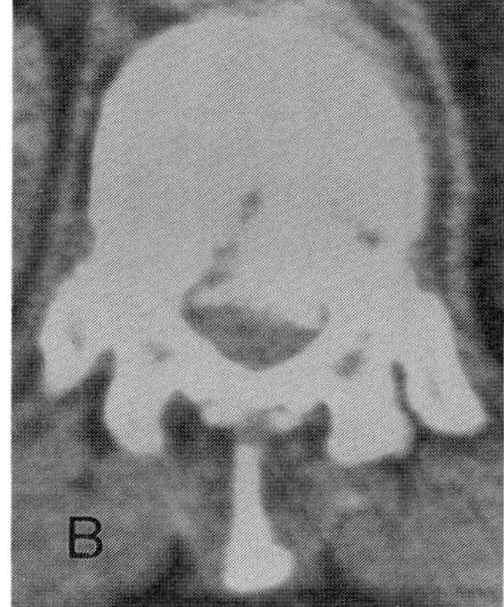

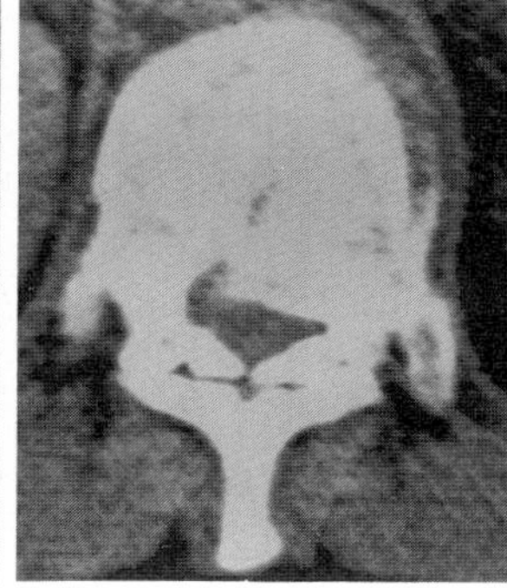

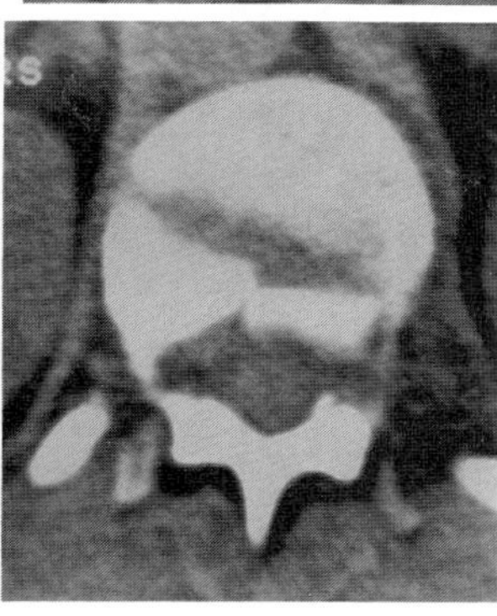

Figure 12.26. **A,** Burst fracture of T12. **B,** CT scan of patient in **A.**

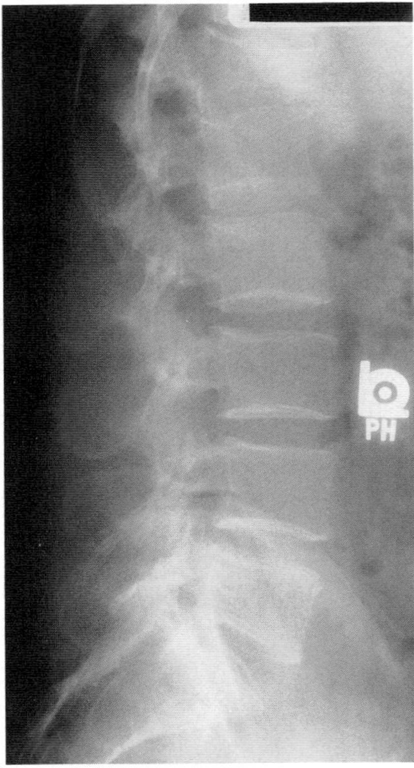

Figure 12.27. Compression fracture of T12. The films were reviewed in hospital.

year previous. Three days after the lifting injury the patient underwent examination. He presented with an antalgic forward lean. Anteroposterior and lateral full spine radiographs and clinical examinations were performed. A diagnosis was made of an acute compression fracture of T12 with associated neuritis and muscle spasm (Fig. 12.29). The patient was treated with an adjustment at the involved spinal level (T12). A double thenar contact was made on both transverse processes, very close to the spinous process. Because of the acute pain present on the spinous process, this contact point was avoided for the first few treatments. A hi-lo table was used for the adjustment and a very light pressure was made with attention to the patient's tolerance for the procedure. Over the next 10 days the patient was treated seven times. Gradually the force of the adjustment was increased and audible releases were heard after each treatment. The patient maintained employment during the treatment regimen and made moderate symptomatic improvement over the first week of care. Follow-up examinations were not obtained because the patient moved out of state.

ANTEROLATERAL COMPRESSION FRACTURES OF THE THORACOLUMBAR SPINE

Four patients involved in front-end collision auto accidents exhibited the same thoracolumbar wedge compres-

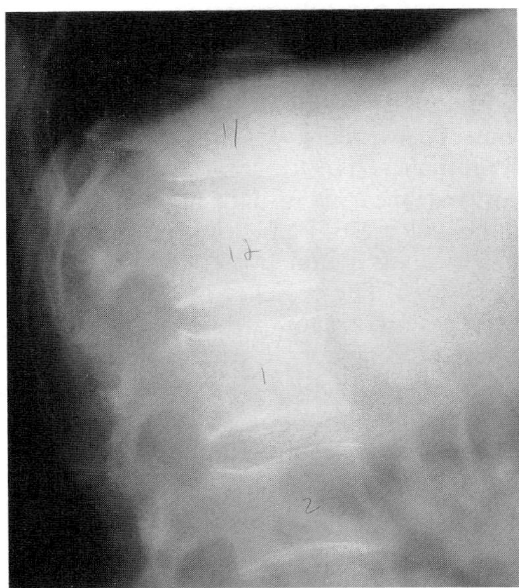

Figure 12.28. Radiograph of patient in Figure 12.27 one year before the lifting trauma.

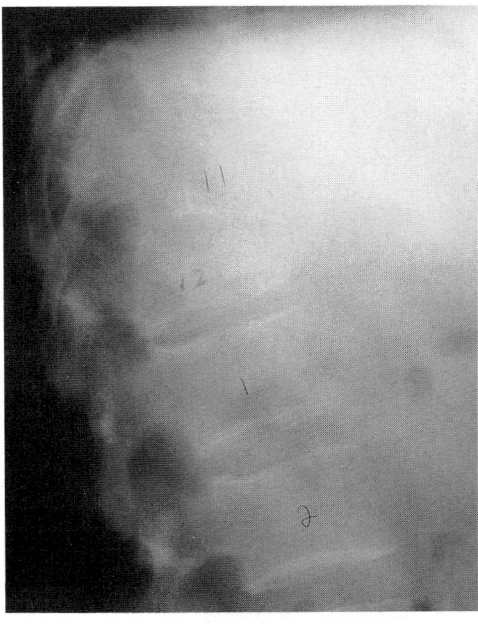

Figure 12.29. T12 compression fracture demonstrated on a full spine radiograph.

sion fracture accompanied by distraction trauma (18). All four were wearing a lap seat belt with shoulder harness and they sustained the wedge fracture in the anterior column on the side of the unrestrained shoulder, and the accompanying distraction injury occurred at the contralateral posterior column.

Biomechanical studies with cadavers using flexion-rotation about a shoulder harness exhibited the exact same fracture with distraction, leading to the conclusion that flexion-rotation is the mechanism of injury (18) (Fig. 12.30). Although none of the four patients in the study by Miniaci experienced any associated major injuries, due to the fact that both the anterior column and the contralateral posterior column were damaged, this injury must be considered unstable (18). In all four cases there was no neurologic deficit and all four fractures had healed at two years follow-up.

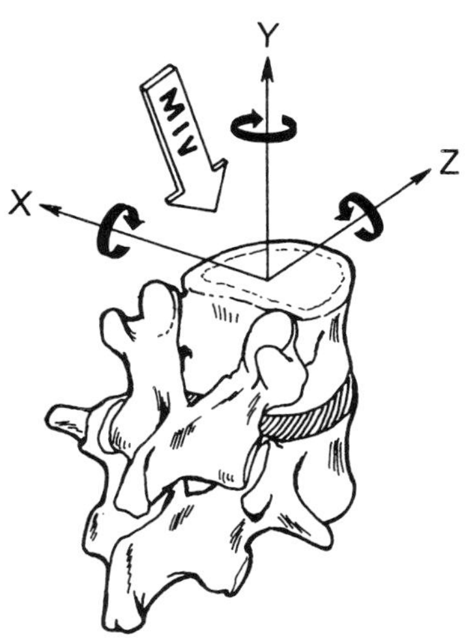

Figure 12.30. MIV for anterolateral compression fractures.

CASE REPORT

This patient suffered a compression fracture of the eleventh thoracic vertebra during a snowmobile accident (2) (Fig. 12.31A-B). No surgery was performed at this time. Upon presentation to an outpatient chiropractic facility, approximately three months after the initial trauma, the patient was paraplegic and confined to a wheelchair.

The right transverse process of T11 was contacted for the adjustment. The patient was prone for the maneuver (hi-lo table). The adjustment incorporated both $+Z$ and $+\theta Z$ patterns of thrust. During the course of treatment an L5 retrolisthesis was also adjusted. This maneuver was performed in the side posture position while avoiding axial rotation of the thoracolumbar junction. During this adjustment it was necessary to have an assistant stabilize the legs. The patient was periodically adjusted (1x/ month) over the next two years. During this time the patient underwent extensive physical therapy. He was eventually able to ambulate, although with some difficulty.

THORACOLUMBAR FRACTURE-DISLOCATIONS

Most fracture-dislocations of the lumbar spine occur at the thoracolumbar junction area (7). A forced hyperflex-

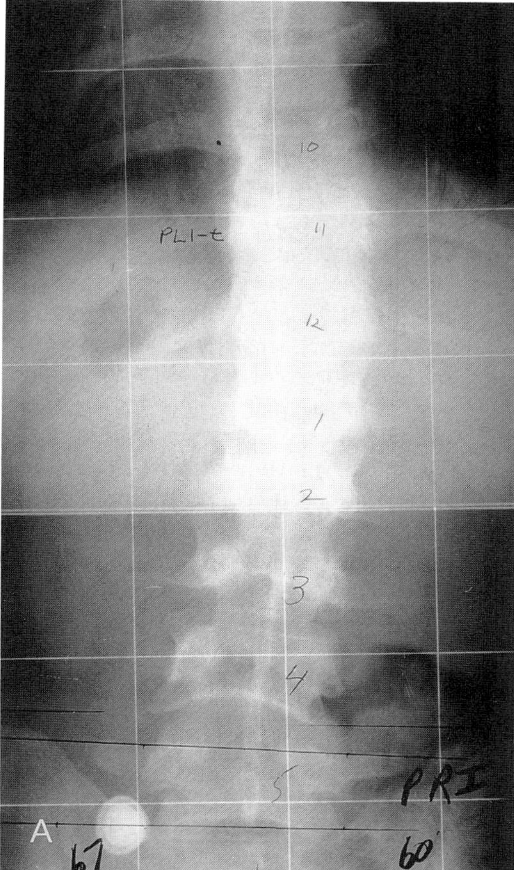

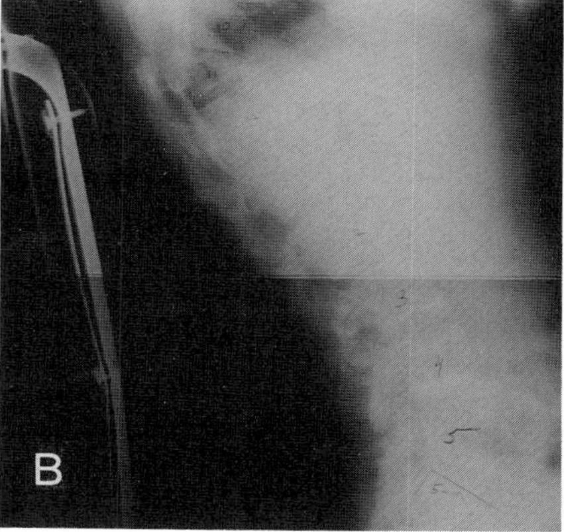

Figure 12.31. **A,** Anteroposterior radiograph of an anterolateral compression fracture of T11. **B,** Lateral radiograph of an anterolateral compression fracture of T11. The patient was seated in a wheelchair for the exposure.

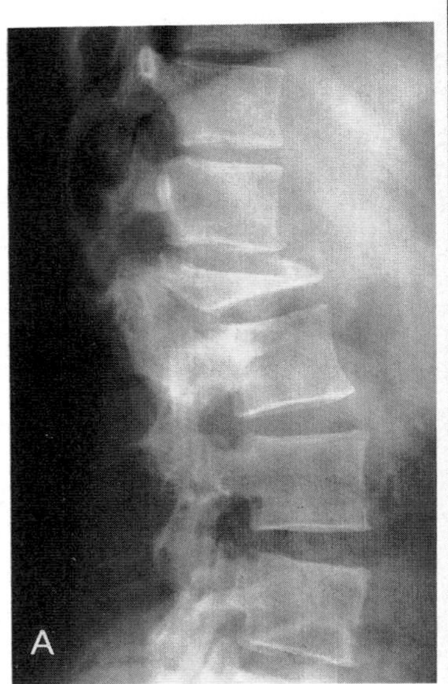

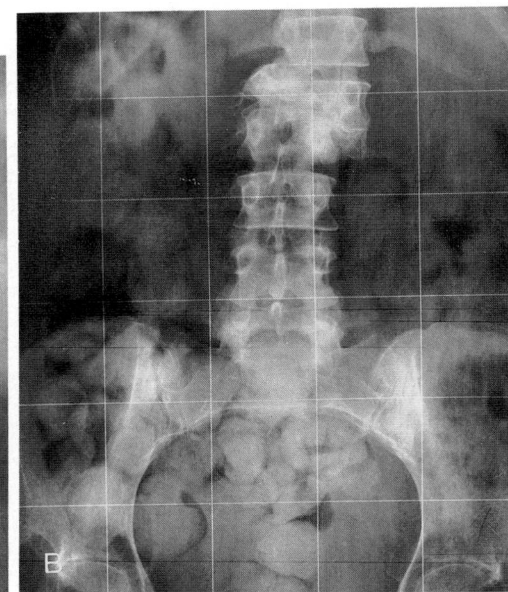

Figure 12.32. **A,** Lateral radiograph of a L1 fracture-dislocation. **B,** Anteroposterior radiograph of a L1 fracture-dislocation.

ion $+\theta X$ injury is usually the MIV, but forced rotation $\pm\theta Y$ and forced lateral flexion $\pm\theta Z$ are often associated (3). Due to the high strength of both bony and supportive soft tissues in the thoracic and lumbar spine, extreme multidirectional forces, from high speed auto accidents, high falls, or direct blows, are usually needed to produce the injury (3).

Anterior motion segment injuries include compression fractures, teardrop fractures and disc injuries. They are often coupled with posterior column distraction fractures, soft tissue tears, and dislocations. Middle column fracture and ligamentous injury can also occur.

Neurologic damage from compression of both the spinal cord and nerve roots may lead to permanent paralysis. These fracture dislocations can be well visualized on both AP and lateral radiographs. If there is a history of a hyperflexion injury which demonstrates vertebral body compression on the lateral view, the posterior bony elements should always be closely scrutinized to evaluate for fracture or dislocation which can complicate the treatment and final outcome of this injury. Since a fracture dislocation always involves damage to all three columns, the injury is considered unstable.

CASE REPORT

This 45-yr-old female suffered a fracture dislocation injury at L1 in October, 1977 (Fig. 12.32A-B). At the time of chiropractic evaluation (several months later), she had lower body paralysis and no bowel or bladder control. The patient was adjusted three times per week for three months, twice weekly for two months and once weekly for six months. After this, the patient was adjusted on an as needed basis for approximately one year. She was fitted with a back support (warm & form) after the first three months of care. The primary segment adjusted was L2 (hi-lo table), although C1, C6, T4, L5 and the right ilium were treated at various times. She regained bowel and bladder function after the fourth month of care. Her lower limb paralysis continues.

FRACTURES OF THE LUMBAR SPINE

Burst Fractures of the Fifth Lumbar Vertebra

There is an extremely low number of reported cases of burst fractures of the fifth lumbar vertebra. Court-Brown and Gertzbein (19) report a three case study of this fracture. In each of their examples there was a reduction in the original height of L5 by at least 60%. All three cases exhibited a loss of lordosis between L4 and the sacrum, and spinal compromise ranging from 70–85%. Two of the examples demonstrated posterior displacement of fracture fragments. One of the fractures was treated surgically with internal spinal instrumentation, and the other two were treated more conservatively with spinal bracing and bed rest. The surgical patient experienced complications of pseudarthrosis and persistent low back pain necessitating a second surgical procedure in which the instrumentation was removed. Despite two operations, only the surgical patient continued to suffer pain at two years follow-up. He also experienced the greatest loss of lordosis between L4 and the sacrum. Court-Brown and Gertzbein suggest conservative treatment of lumbar support and bed rest for many of these patients.

LAP SEAT BELT FRACTURES

The lap seat belt fracture, also called a Chance fracture, is a hyperflexion $(+\theta X)$ injury with the center of rotation anterior to the body of the vertebra (15) (Fig. 12.33). Since the center of rotation is anterior to that of a pure compression fracture, there is much greater tension put on the posterior bony elements. As the spinous processes separate to their physiologic limits, the bone often fails before the posterior ligamentous structures, creating longitudinal fractures through the spinous process, posterior arch, the pedicles and often into the posterior aspects of the vertebral body itself (Fig. 12.34). The anterior portion of the vertebral body may suffer mild compression type fractures as well. Although bone usually fails before the ligamentous structures, severe soft tissue injuries of the posterior ligaments, the posterior longitudinal ligament, and the disc itself are often associated with this injury due to the extreme tensile forces involved.

Standard plain film lateral radiographs may show fractures in the spinous, lamina, pedicles, and posterior portion of the vertebral body. Since there is often soft tissue injury as well as splaying of spinous processes, an abnormally increased posterior disc height is often visualized (7).

AP and lateral tomography can clearly demonstrate the fracture lines in a Chance fracture which are often poorly visualized in the axial view of CT. However, the reconstructed sagittal view of the CT scan can be quite helpful in visualizing and evaluating these horizontal fracture lines (15). The CT scan can also be useful in evaluating an associated burst fracture. In a group of Chance fractures described by Gertzbein (20), 70% had an accompanying vertebral body compression fracture. Fifteen percent had burst fractures and 15% had no vertebral body fracture. High force deceleration can cause the burst fracture due to increased $-Y$ forces, while low velocity can lead to the posterior distraction ($+\theta X$) injury. Because the center of rotation is more anterior, it causes posterior element soft tissue damage combined with posterior body fracture.

Flexion distraction type injuries are extremely uncommon in children due to their greater flexibility. However, with the use of lap seat belts, the major focus of flexion with posterior element distraction is placed on the lumbar vertebrae at the level of the seat belt. With the belt functioning like a fulcrum, the forced flexion is concentrated in one spinal area as opposed to being dissipated over a greater area, thereby increasing the likelihood of damage (21).

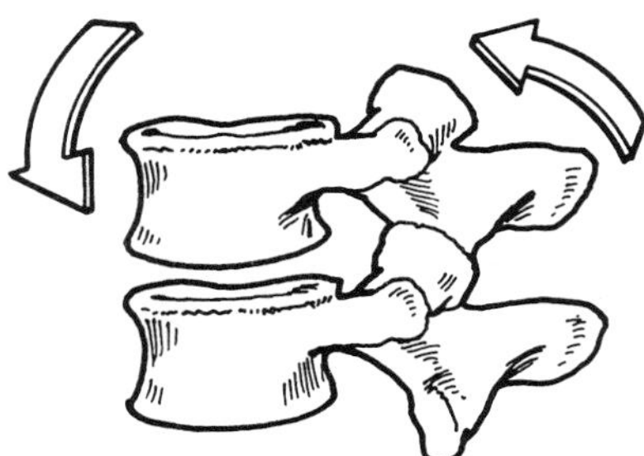

Figure 12.33. MIV for the Chance fracture. Modified from Kaye JJ, Nance EP. Thoracic and lumbar spine trauma. Radiol Clin North Am 1990;28:375.

Since the introduction of the lap seat belt, in the 1950s and 60s, the Chance fracture has occurred much more frequently (7). Approximately 50% of Chance fracture cases have associated intra-abdominal injuries (20).

The Chance fracture may or may not heal and return to being a stable motion segment. This is dependent on the tissues that are injured. A purely bony injury is most likely to heal. An injury with posterior supportive ligament or disc damage may never return to a stable situation. Regarding associated vertebral body fracture, the compression injury is much more likely to regain stability than the burst fracture (20). Neurologic deficit occurs in 15% of all Chance fracture cases and the upper lumbar spine, especially L1-L3, is the most frequent site of occurrence (7).

CASE REPORT

This 29-yr-old female presented on 3–21–88, one day after a motor vehicle accident. A full spine radiologic examination disclosed a traumatic spondylolisthesis at L4 (Fig. 12.35). The MIV for this injury is $+\theta X$ with the center of rotation anterior to the vertebral body.

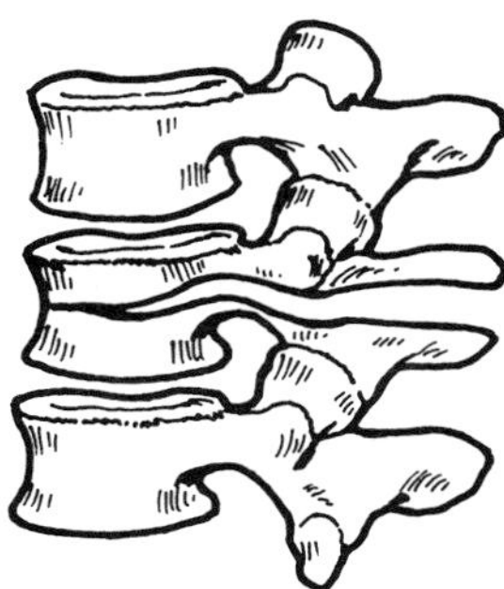

Figure 12.34. Involved bony elements of a Chance fracture. Modified from Kaye JJ, Nance EP. Thoracic and lumbar spine trauma. Radiol Clin North Am 1990;28:372.

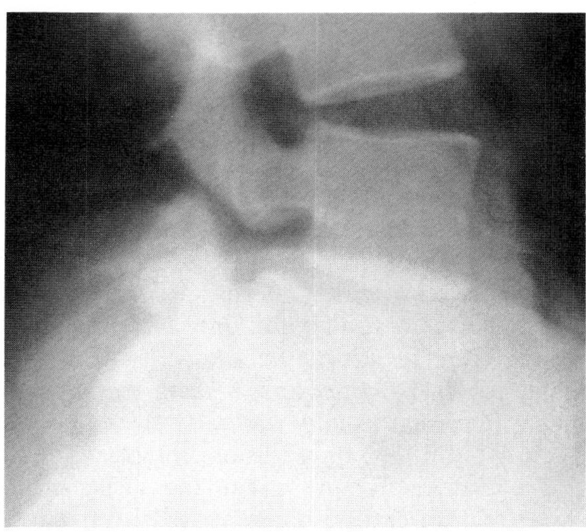

Figure 12.35. Traumatic spondylolisthesis of L4.

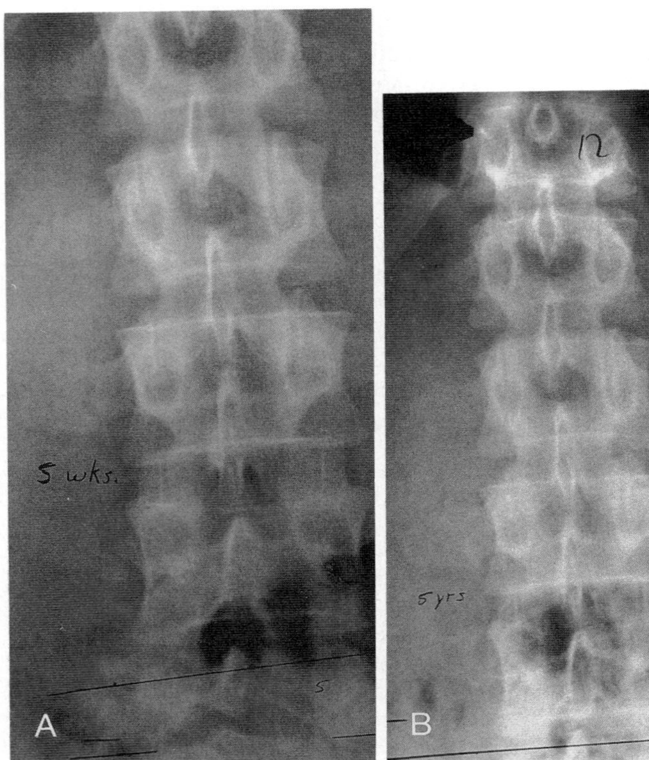

Figure 12.36. **A,** Transverse process fractures at L3 and L4 five weeks after the trauma. **B,** Radiograph (exposed 5 years later for other injuries) demonstrating bony union of the fractures at L3 and L4.

She was treated twenty-four times over a thirteen month course. Adjustments were performed at L5 (5X), sacrum (9X), the left ASIn (3X), T7 (5X), C7 (3X) and C2 (15X), in the prone, side posture, and cervical chair positions, without complication.

Initial symptoms included low back pain which radiated down the right leg, neck pain and headache. At one year follow-up, the patient reported no low back or leg pain. Psychological stress provoked occasional headaches. Since the injury, she has had two noncomplicated pregnancies.

TRANSVERSE PROCESS FRACTURES

Transverse process fractures of the lumbar spine usually occur from excessive lateral flexion coupled with a hyperextension injury. The break usually occurs at L2 and L3 and is the second most frequently occurring lumbar fracture (7). It is often found at more than one level. Fifth lumbar transverse fractures commonly accompany pelvic fractures, such as the vertical sacral type.

Radiographically, transverse fractures appear as radiolucent lines that usually run vertically or obliquely (Fig. 12.36A-B). When, on occasion, they traverse horizontally, a Chance fracture should be suspected. The transverse fracture can be differentiated from developmental nonunion by evidence of the fracture's jagged irregular border and fracture line. A urinalysis and kidney exam should be performed since renal damage may be found concurrently with transverse process fractures (7). Transverse process fractures are usually stable unless accompanied by other fractures or ligamentous damage.

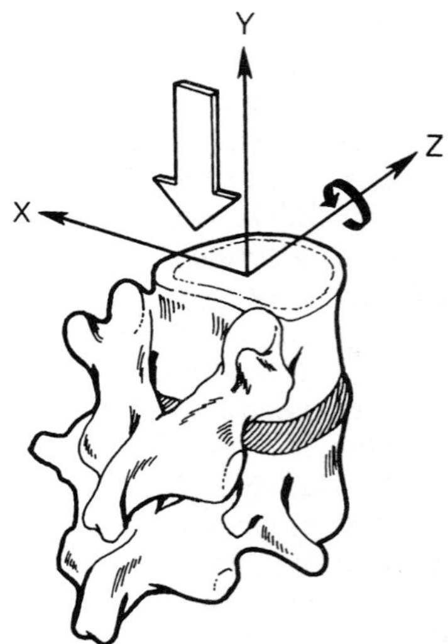

Figure 12.37. The MIV for a lateral wedge fracture.

LATERAL WEDGE FRACTURES

The lateral wedge fracture is very similar to the compression fracture but the $-Y$ force is directed lateral to the center, creating a $\pm\theta Z$ bending moment along with the $+\theta X$ injury vector (Fig. 12.37). The Z axis bending injury with vertebral body collapse to one side, can also create damage to the articular pillar and facet, the pedicle and lamina on the concavity of bend, as well as an avulsion fracture of the transverse process on the convexity (3).

Since the lateral wedge injury creates a greater amount of avulsion force to the soft tissue than does the simple anterior wedge fracture, the degree of permanent pain is also greater. Nicoll (22) states that in comparing the two injuries, there was total recovery in only 21% of lateral wedge fractures, while 40% of those with anterior wedge fractures completely recovered.

LUMBAR COMPRESSION FRACTURES

Lumbar compression fractures involve primarily a $-Y$ translational vector combined with flexion ($+\theta X$). Most of these injuries are stable since only the anterior column is involved. As with other compression fractures, they are best visualized with the lateral radiograph.

CASE REPORT

This male patient was asleep in the back seat, when the vehicle he was traveling in was involved in a head-on collision (2). Of the five passengers in the vehicle, he was the sole survivor. He sustained a compression fracture of the fourth lumbar vertebra (Fig. 12.38A-B). The patient had a course of medical treatment (medication) and physical therapy for his complaints at the time. He then presented for chiropractic evaluation with a complaint of severe low back pain and difficulty in ambulation, nearly six years following the initial trauma.

After examination, he was adjusted in the side posture position to reduce the retrolisthesis at L4 (PR-m). Two adjustments were given over the course of two days and one adjustment was administered four months later. The patient's lower back pain resolved and he subsequently became employed as an airline pilot.

CASE REPORT

This 18-yr-old female patient suffered a car accident in 1973 in which the third lumbar vertebra compressed (2) (Fig. 12.39A-B). She subsequently developed secondary

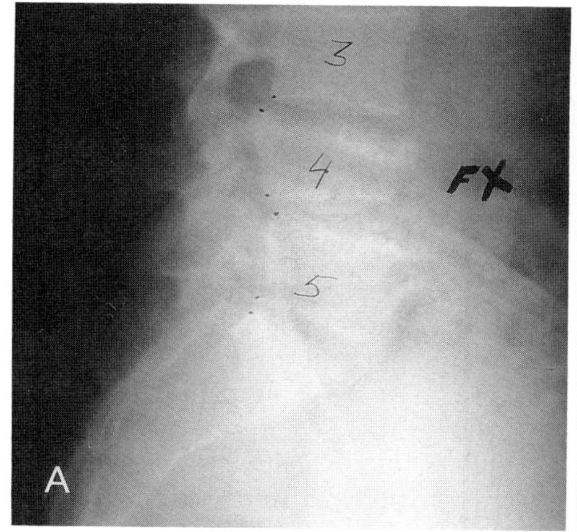

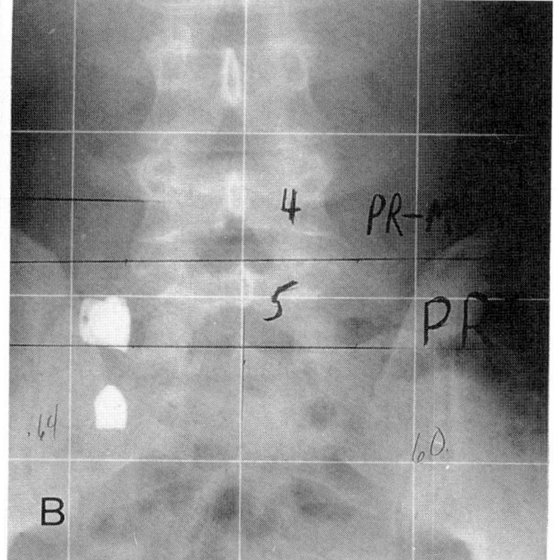

Figure 12.38. **A,** Lateral radiograph demonstrates a compression fracture at L4. Notice the retrolisthesis at the L4 level. **B,** Radiograph demonstrating the fracture at L4. Notice the widened interpedicular distance.

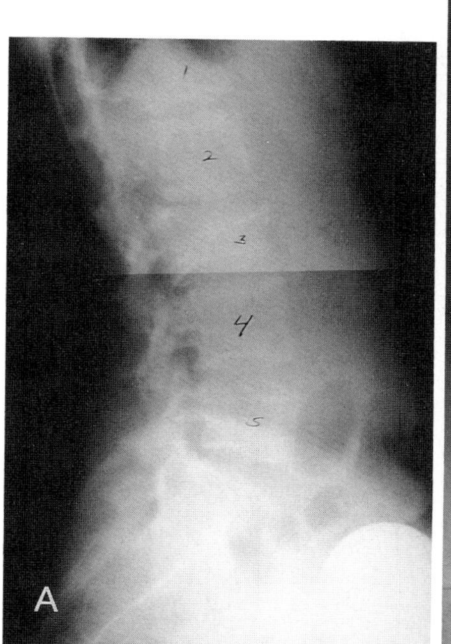

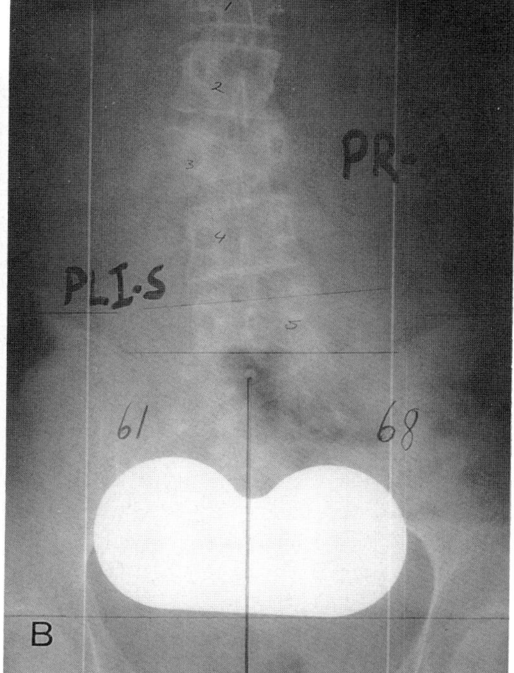

Figure 12.39. **A,** Lateral radiograph demonstrating a L3 compression fracture with retrolisthesis. **B,** AP radiograph depicting a wedge deformity at the fracture site.

amenorrhea. In 1984 she presented for chiropractic evaluation after a fall from a horse. Her symptoms consisted primarily of low back pain and secondary amenorrhea of eleven years duration. Adjustments of the L5, C7, and T3 vertebrae were performed nine times over the next eight months. The lumbar spine was adjusted in the side posture position by using a push move which emphasized reduction of the retrolisthesis. The seventh cervical was adjusted in the seated position and T3 was adjusted in the prone position. In February of 1985 she returned to the same clinic with a complaint of headaches. The third lumbar, T3 and C7 vertebrae were adjusted four times over the next month. The patient began menstruating during this time and became pregnant after three regular menses.

CASE REPORT

This 69-yr-old farmer fell from a roof on 11–28–89 and suffered a burst fracture of L3 and a compression fracture of L2 with cauda equina injury. Internal fixation was performed on 12–11–89. The patient presented for chiropractic evaluation on 4–29–91. Radiologic examination disclosed positional dyskinesia of the left ilium (PIIn) and L5 (PR-m). The internal fixation is demonstrated in Figure 12.40A-B. The patient received fourteen treatments. Initial symptoms of right foot numbness did not completely resolve. The patient reported improvement in bowel and bladder function (near normal). Intermittent rectal pain still occurs after riding farm equipment for long periods.

CASE REPORT

This patient suffered compression fractures of L5, L4, L3, and L2 while attempting to lift a water heater. He reported for chiropractic evaluation immediately after the injury. The preinjury radiograph of the lumbar spine is depicted in Figure 12.41A. The patient was adjusted using the knee-chest table for correction of retrolisthesis of the lumbar segments (Fig. 12.41B-F). He was advised to sleep on his side during the course of treatment.

LUMBAR NEURAL ARCH FRACTURE

Lumbar neural arch fractures occur posterior to the posterior longitudinal ligament (3). These fractures can be caused by hyperextension $-\theta X$ or from flexion $+\theta X$ coupled with axial rotation $\pm\theta Y$. Due to the sagittal position of lumbar facets, rotation is very limited. If they are forced beyond normal physiologic limits (less than 3 degrees at one segment), the facets will be damaged and the posterior elements such as the pars interarticularis or lamina will fracture (3).

Pars interarticularis fractures can also be caused by severe hyperextension. Although uncommon, when they

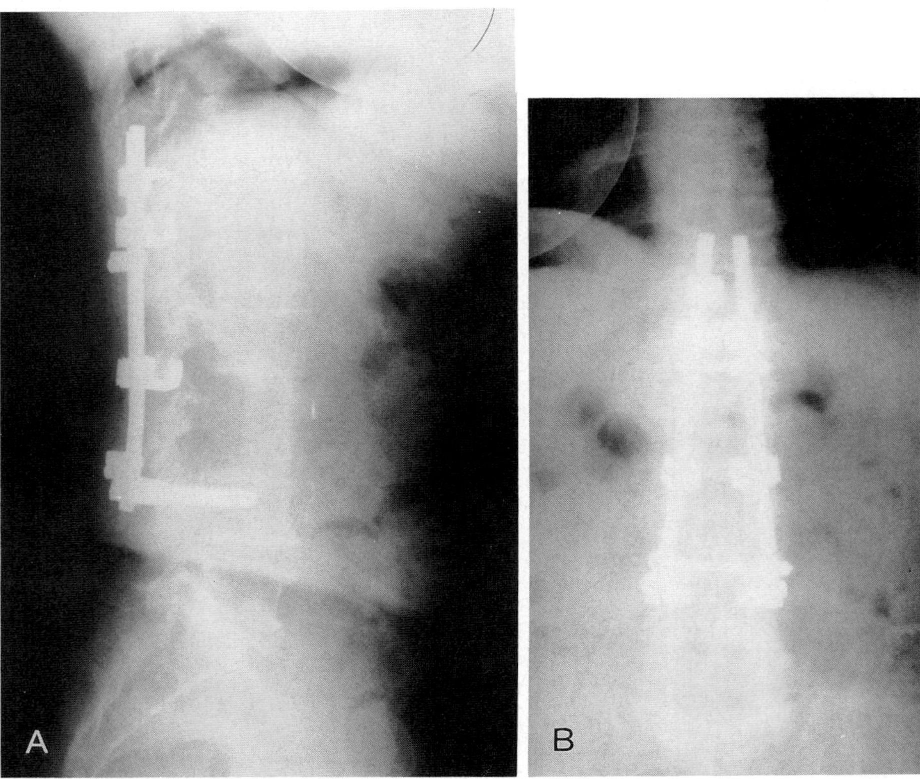

Figure 12.40. A, Lateral radiograph demonstrating the internal fixation. **B,** AP radiograph demonstrating the bilateral internal instrumentation.

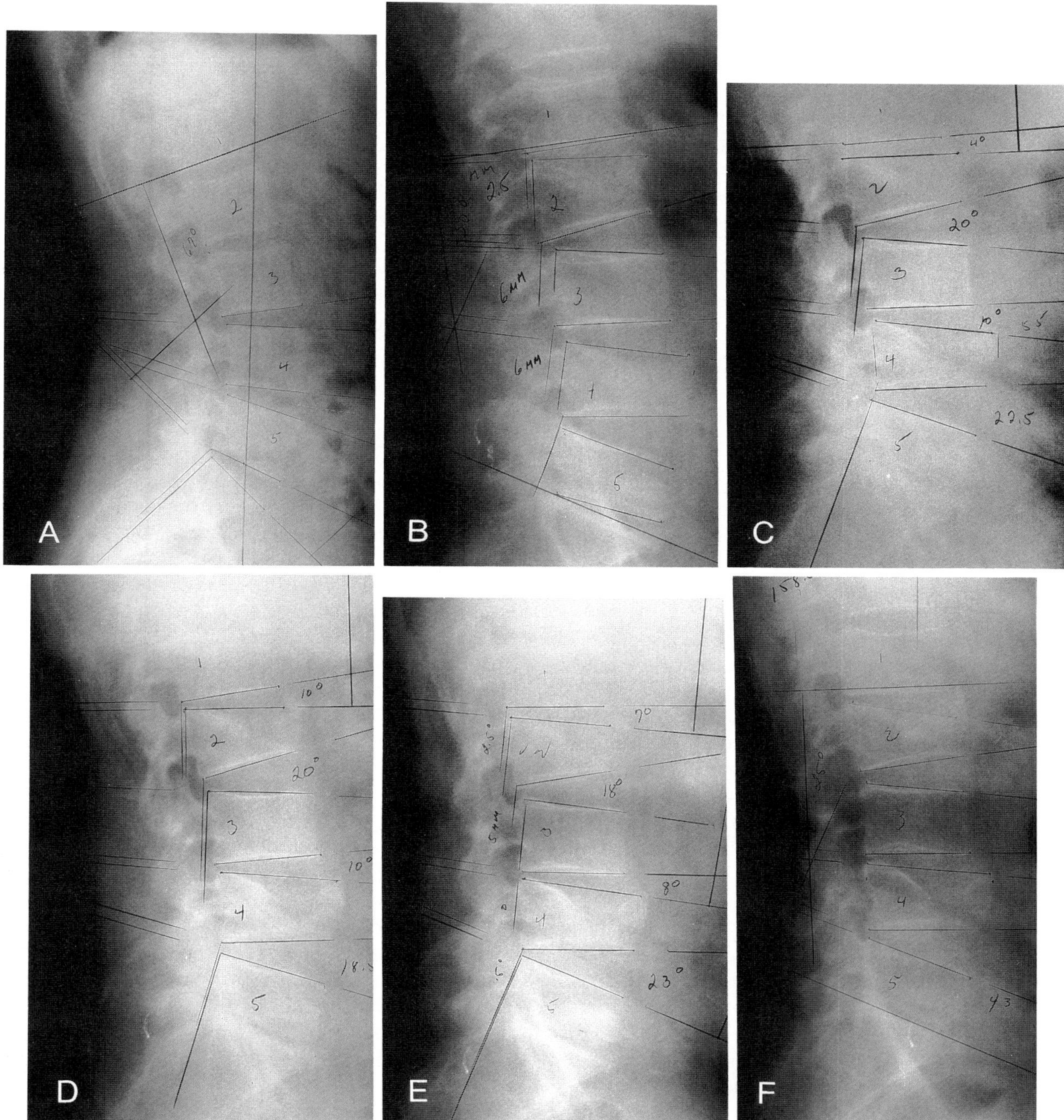

Figure 12.41. **A,** Preinjury radiograph (1–24–81). **B,** Pretreatment radiograph (1–31–85, posttrauma) demonstrating compression fractures at L5, L4, L3 (slight) and L2. Notice the retrolisthesis at L4, L3, L2 and L1. **C,** Posttreatment radiograph (2–21–85). Notice the reduction of retrolisthesis at L4. **D,** Posttreatment radiograph (3–7–85) in which retrolisthesis at L3 is reduced. **E,** Posttreatment radiograph (4–1–85). **F,** Posttreatment radiograph (10–2–85). Notice the reduction of retrolisthesis at L4, L3, L2 and L1 and preservation of the lumbar lordosis.

do occur, these fractures are usually at L4 or L5 and are most often unilateral. This acute traumatic fracture is not the same as the stress fracture associated with isthmic spondylolisthesis (7). The latter, which is usually bilateral, remains persistently displaced and does not typically undergo bony union (23). The unilateral acute pars interarticularis fracture often reunites (7).

PELVIC RING INJURIES

The pelvic ring is comprised of the sacrum and ischium in the posterior, the iliums laterally, and the pubic bones at the anterior. In cases of high force trauma with a magnitude great enough to cause a fracture, the pelvic ring usually breaks in more than one place. When a fracture is suspected or visualized on a radiograph, the entire pelvis should be scrutinized closely to rule out other fractures or dislocations in the sacroiliac joints or symphysis pubis.

Soft tissue injuries occur with pelvic injuries and can create an even more traumatic situation. Patients with pelvic injuries should be evaluated for the following complications: rupture of the diaphragm as evidenced by a chest x-ray, laceration or obstruction of the rectum, laceration or complete rupture of the urethra, bladder and ureters signaled by bruising in the perineum, retention of urine and fresh blood at the tip of the urethra, and laceration of the blood vessels causing hemorrhage. This is indicated by ecchymosis of the scrotum, inguinal area and buttocks (7). Acute injuries of the pelvic ring should undergo computed tomographic examination (24).

Classification

Many attempts at a logical and helpful classification of pelvic fractures have met with little success. Since most classifications are not based on mechanisms of injury, they provide the practitioner with little information regarding proper treatment protocols, accompanying soft tissue injury and prognosis.

Pennal and associates (25) developed a classification system that provides the necessary mechanistic perspective, hence aiding in treatment protocol and prognosis. Three common MIVs for pelvic fractures have been identified. They include lateral compressive (LC), anterior-posterior compressive (APC) and vertical shear (VS) forces. These mechanisms of injury are found alone or in combinations. The mechanisms are further classified according to severity (I–III), based in large part on radiographic findings (26).

LC

Lateral compressive forces (LC) cause the ipsilateral side of the pelvis to implode. This causes injury to both the anterior and posterior aspects of the pelvic ring. Anterior damage to the pubic ramus is pathognomonic of this injury and may be seen with or without symphysis pubis injury. One or both rami are fractured in a transverse direction. These fractures are best visualized with the inlet view and although the anterior component does not directly determine weight bearing capability, radiographic findings of injury here, are of help in determining mechanism(s) of injury, treatment protocol and prognosis.

LC-I

This is the most common and stable injury of the LC group. It is characterized by vertical sacral compaction (posterior injury) and a transverse rami fracture. The inlet view will often reveal a discontinuity of the sacral foraminae. The ipsilateral sacrotuberous and sacrospinous ligaments remain intact and are somewhat shortened in length.

LC-II

In this injury, a greater lateral force, or a more inferiorly directed lateral force than is associated with LC-I fractures, causes a vertical fracture of the iliac wing. A portion of the ilium usually remains in contact with the sacrum. The ipsilateral sacrotuberous and sacrospinous ligaments remain intact and although there is more movement in the direction of injury, the LC-II remains relatively stable.

LC-III

This crushing type of injury is caused when the patient is "sandwiched" between a fixed object and a contralateral compressive force. The fracture complex is characterized by an LC-I or LC-II fracture on the side of lateral force but is complicated by a contralateral "open book" injury. Here, the PSIS is forced medially and the ASIS moves laterally. This MIV forces open the anterior portion of the sacroiliac joint, damaging the sacrotuberous and sacrospinous ligaments and creating a failure in the anterior rami. This is by far the most unstable LC injury. There is gross mechanical instability and vascular damage on the open-book side of the pelvis.

APC

Anterior posterior compression (APC) injuries are produced by anteriorly or posteriorly directed forces which impact the ASIS, PSIS, ischial tuberosity and long axis of the femur (e.g., dashboard injury). The most characteristic radiographic findings are a separation of the pubic symphysis with or without a rami fracture. Separation of the pubic articulation beyond the average distance of 8 mm in nonpregnant adults and 10 mm in children (7) is considered indicative of trauma. Increasing magnitudes of injury are further classified (I–III).

APC-I

This is the least traumatic of the group with only mild pubic symphysis separation. There is gross sparing of the ligamentous structures (i.e., sacrotuberous, sacrospinous and sacroiliac ligaments), although plastic deformations are likely to occur. A slight widening of the SI joint may be visible on the radiograph.

CASE REPORT

This 25-yr-old female suffered a pelvic injury during an automobile accident in December of 1983 (Fig. 12.42A-B). The mechanism of injury was anterior to posterior,

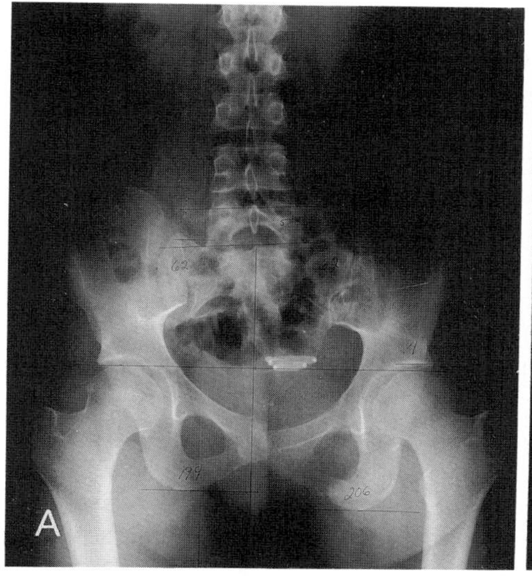
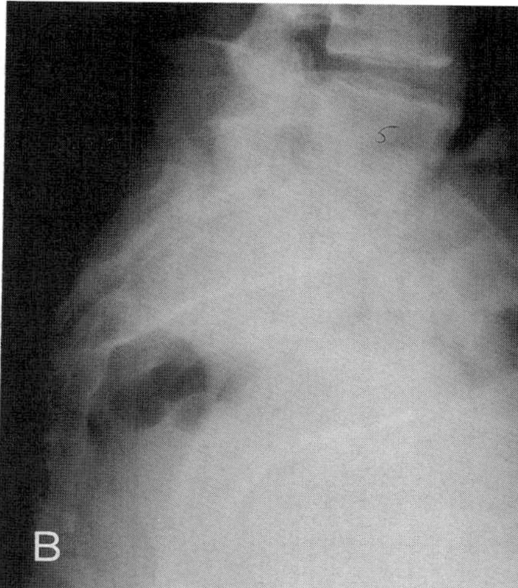
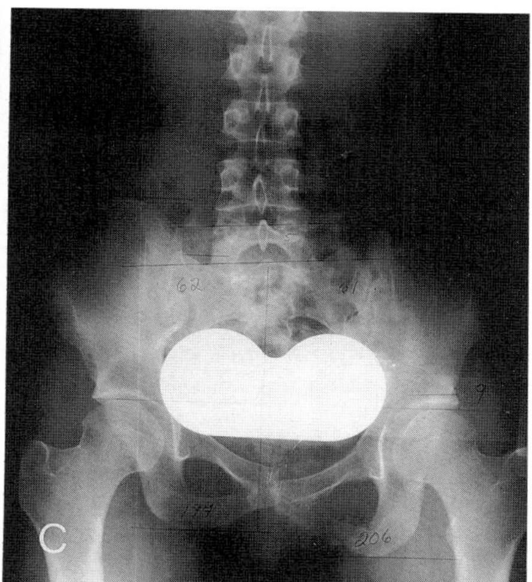

Figure 12.42. **A,** Pretreatment AP radiograph (5–7–84). Notice the separation of the symphysis pubis and widening of the left sacroiliac joint. The patient had difficulty bearing weight for this radiograph. **B,** Pretreatment lateral radiograph demonstrating a sacral fracture. **C,** Posttreatment radiograph (5–31–84) in which the patient is able to bear weight. Note that a 9-mm leg length inequality is now apparent.

due to the knees impacting the dashboard of the automobile. At the time of chiropractic evaluation the patient could not bear weight and used crutches to aid ambulation. The patient's medical doctor did not advise surgery and stated that she would require crutches for ambulation indefinitely. The patient was adjusted in the side posture position (left ASIn) three times over a three week period. After the first adjustment, the patient was able to ambulate unaided (Fig. 12.42C).

APC-II

This injury is characterized by damage to the anterior sacroiliac ligaments with widening of the joint space and symphysis pubis diastasis. The inlet view is used to diagnose the displacement. The sacrotuberous and sacrospinous ligaments are usually torn or there is an avulsion at their bony insertions on the ischial spine or sacral border. This class of injury may be seen bilaterally, depending on the specific injury contact and MIV. The pelvic ring is unstable in certain directions. Internal rotation of the ASIS will be excessively mobile and external rotation may be mobile if the fracture has spontaneously reduced. The severe force needed to create the open-book injury of an APC-II usually causes significant neural and vascular injury.

APC-III

APC-III injuries are the most unstable and severe of the pelvic fractures. A large force is needed to tear the anterior sacroiliac ligaments as seen in the APC-II. This injury causes further internal rotation of the PSIS to the point where the posterior sacroiliac ligaments are also compromised, leaving the hemipelvis totally disconnected from the sacrum. The injury is associated with the greatest amount of vascular damage, blood loss, and mortality.

VS

Vertical shear forces (VS) from above ($-Y$) and more commonly from below ($+Y$), cause the hemipelvis to separate at the symphysis pubis anteriorly and the SI joint, iliac wing or sacrum, posteriorly. This leaves the hemipelvis in a superior or inferiorly displaced position according to the direction of impact. The sacrospinous and sacrotuberous ligaments are usually severed. Common injury scenarios include landing on the feet from high falls and motor vehicle or cycling accidents. The $-Y$ displacements are often caused by crushing injuries from building and tunnel cave-ins. Due to the associated neurovascular damage, VS injuries can be life threatening. These fractures are best visualized with the AP or outlet views.

CM

Combined mechanical (CM) groups of injuries are due to obliquely directed forces or from multiple impacts from varying directions. After separating the components of the MIV, the practitioner must determine appropriate treatment for the soft tissue injuries and arrive at a prognosis.

AVULSION FRACTURES OF THE ILIUM

Avulsion fractures of the ilium involve separation of a fragment from the bone. They are common in young athletes who have yet to experience fusion of the involved growth center. Sprinters, long jumpers, gymnasts, hurdlers and cheerleaders are particularly prone to the fractures, due to the frequent and stressful flexing motion required (7).

There are two types of avulsion fractures of the ilium, anteroinferior iliac spine (AIIS) and anterosuperior iliac spine (ASIS). The former is avulsion by the sartorius muscle and can be ameliorated with hip flexion. The latter is avulsion by the rectus femoris muscle. Hip flexion usually causes great pain (7).

SACRAL CLASSIFICATION

Denis et al. (27) have devised a new classification for sacral fractures. Three zones are identified according to the level, location, and direction of the sacral fracture. Zone I involves the region of the ala, the area of the sacrum lateral to the foramina line. These alar fractures may include lateral compression fractures which cause minimal displacements, or open-book fractures where the displacement is severe. Neurologic damage is rare in a zone one injury except when the L5 root or the sciatic nerve is compromised.

Zone 2 fractures must include one or more foramina. Neurologic involvement is more frequently seen in fractures of this area. Sciatica is the most common complication, with bowel and bladder dysfunction occurring rarely.

Zone III fractures involve the region of the central sacral canal and are most often associated with neurologic deficits. Bowel, bladder, and sexual functions are most frequently compromised by Zone III fractures. Computed tomography scans are essential in evaluating the nature and extent of fractures of the pelvic ring (27).

Sacral Fractures

Fractures in the sacrum occur in one of two ways, either horizontally or vertically. Horizontal sacral fractures are usually a result of a fall on the buttocks from great heights, as in suicide attempts. This fracture is sometimes referred to as the "suicidal jumper's" fracture. This is the most common type of sacral fracture and usually affects the third and fourth sacral tubercle toward the end of the sacroiliac joint.

Horizontal fractures are best visualized on the lateral radiograph although they may be difficult to detect if air or fecal matter blocks the fracture site. A displacement or angling forward of the lower segment of the sacrum is often seen. This is the best radiographic indication of the injury. All horizontal fractures are considered zone three, since they pass through this zone.

Vertical sacral fractures can be visualized on an AP radiograph. The fracture lines generally run the entire length of the sacrum. As sacral fractures do not usually occur in isolation, the doctor should search carefully for associated fractures or dislocations of the pelvic ring or symphysis pubis (7).

LUMBOPELVIC FRACTURES

Generally, a combination of both anterior and posterior fractures constitute a pelvic ring injury (24). The anterior component could manifest as a pubic ramus fracture or pubic symphysis dislocation. The posterior lesion most frequently involves a fracture of the sacrum. These sacral fractures range from minimal compression fractures that remain stable to displaced fractures that may be extremely unstable. The first and second sacral foramina are the areas most commonly involved in pelvic ring fractures. The boundaries of the fracture include the articular process of the sacroiliac joint as a proximal landmark, through the free border of the sacrum as the distal landmark.

The lumbosacral junction is not jeopardized if the fracture boundary is lateral to the articular process of the sacroiliac joint. However, if the fracture is medial to the articular process of the sacrum, the lumbosacral junction will be damaged.

In a study of pelvic ring fractures and lumbosacral injuries, in which there was only partial posterior instability, Isler (24) found it very difficult to evaluate using routine radiologic examination. The author suggests that computerized tomography would considerably increase the number of diagnosed lumbosacral fractures. While unstable fractures can be easily diagnosed by conventional radiographs of the pelvis, computerized tomography provides detailed information concerning the range of soft and hard tissue injury. Since a locked L5/SI facet joint dislocation prevents the reduction of a displaced sacral fracture, it is particularly important to properly visualize and diagnose lumbosacral injuries. Also, lumbosacral pain that remains chronic after pelvic ring injuries have healed can be traced to degeneration of the lumbar sacral facet joints due to trauma from the original injury. It is estimated that 6% of the population in this study had a lumbosacral lesion in conjunction with the pelvic ring injury.

There are three major types of lumbosacral injuries associated with pelvic ring injuries: 1) articular lumbosacral injuries which may manifest as joint subluxation, fractures, dislocations, and complete locked dislocations; 2) extra-articular fractures where the lumbosacral posterior articulation remains intact, but there is a fracture either at the base of the L5 laminar pillar junction, or at the base of the L5 or S1 articular pillar; 3) complex injuries with multiple fractures of L5.

CHIROPRACTIC TREATMENT PROTOCOLS

Although the evaluation and treatment protocol for spinal fractures and dislocations is necessarily vague and extremely case dependent, certain basic practice guidelines must be followed to ensure the patient receives the most appropriate care (e.g., medical, chiropractic). A comprehensive investigation including a careful history, physical examination, plain film and any necessary advanced imaging examination, should be undertaken to arrive at an accurate assessment of the patient's condition. The clinician must then make certain clinical judgments based on this information. Many factors influence the clinician's decisions, including past experience with similar cases and knowledge of the clinical biomechanics and associated soft tissue injuries. The risks of the procedure should always be discussed with the patient and informed consent obtained. Extreme care should be taken in determining whether a patient is a candidate for chiropractic care. A cautious approach is advised since little data on clinical outcomes have been reported with closed reduction methods. Denying appropriate surgical treatment is not in the patient's best interest (28).

Whereas fixation dysfunction is the primary biomechanical factor for deciding the locus of an adjustment in nonfracture cases, misalignment of the segment or fracture displacement are the determining variables for fracture patients.

Examination

The patient must first be evaluated to determine if there are any abnormal vital signs which would necessitate immediate emergency room referral. This is true for the initial presentation as well as anytime during the course of care. If the vital signs are determined to be stable, then an evaluation is necessary to determine neurologic stability. Any neurologic instability (e.g., cauda equina) requires emergency room referral. Deterioration in neurologic status at anytime necessitates reevaluation and/or expert consultation and possible referral.

Classification

Patients may present at anytime during the course of recovery. The doctor should be familiar with acute, subacute and chronic presentations to manage the case effectively.

ACUTE

Emphasis should be on determining vital signs and indications for emergency room referral. Acute injuries require a comprehensive assessment to determine the patient's condition accurately. In many cases, advanced imaging such as MRI or CT and electrodiagnostic evaluation will be beneficial. All neurologically unstable patients require further evaluation and possibly referral. The patient will require stabilization when transport is made to the emergency room. Although there are reported cases of successful management of acute patients (2) no clear protocols have appeared in the literature.

SUBACUTE

The major determination should be to determine the stability of the vital signs, and the vascular and neurologic systems. The examination must be comprehensive (i.e., plain films (neutral and dynamic), and CT or MRI, if necessary). As in all cases of spinal fractures and dislocations, care must be case specific. Unstable injuries will often require surgical referral.

CHRONIC

These patients will usually have stable vital signs. Determination should be made if the fracture is biomechanically or neurologically unstable. If earlier plain films are available, then these should be obtained to compare with the most recent evaluations. This assessment is often helpful to determine if a progressive biomechanical instability is present.

PREVENTION

Since spinal fractures and dislocations are often devastating to an individual and costly to society, all efforts must be made to not only effectively treat them but to maximize efforts to prevent their occurrence and minimize their damaging effects. It has been estimated that the approximate cost to society for each new cervical spine injury with spinal cord involvement is $400,000 (10). There are approximately 10,000 new cases of spinal cord injury each year in the U.S. The total cost to society, therefore, is approximately $4 billion annually (10).

Spinal injuries may occur from so many different (unusual) situations (i.e., freak falls, being struck by falling objects and other accidents), that their prevention may be difficult or impossible to affect, but efforts can be made to minimize the frequency and damage of some more commonly occurring causes of spinal fractures and dislocations.

Public education aimed at both the prevention and emergency care of spinal injury victims can reduce the incidence of mortality and morbidity. Early instruction of the importance of spinal hygiene promotes increased spinal awareness and if properly applied, will increase both spinal strength and the ability of the spine to adapt under extreme loading conditions. The sagittal curves, symmetrical weight-bearing, normal mobility and proper postural positioning (29), increase the ability of the spine to yield, within normal physiologic boundaries, under high stresses and therefore limit residual effects.

During an impact injury, the body's position will determine the type and extent of tissue damage. In most instances, the anatomical position provides the highest degree of protection.

Motor vehicle accidents have greatly increased the occurrence and severity of many types of spinal fractures. Before the use of seat belts, unrestrained movements in the vehicle were common. Lap seat belts are responsible for reducing the instances of mortality in auto accidents which might otherwise occur from collisions with the dashboard, windshield, or other part of the interior (18). Lap seat belts provide some degree of body restraint, however, since this restraint is focused at one region of the body, a wide range of other injuries may occur (See Lap Seat Belt Fractures). These injuries include acceleration/deceleration injuries of the head and neck, head impacts with the steering wheel or dashboard or Chance fractures.

In an effort to decrease head impact, whiplash, Chance fractures and other spinal flexion injuries, shoulder harness restraints have been developed. These provide further support for the torso, but they can cause other injuries as a result of the forces pushing against the restraint. While one shoulder is restrained on impact, the other is thrown forward. In what is known as the "roll-out phenomenon," the upper trunk, neck and head "roll-out" from behind the restraint causing severe axial rotational stresses (18). To avoid damage from the roll-out phenomenon, a double shoulder harness seatbelt is currently in use in race cars. This type of restraint should be a standard feature in conventional automobiles.

The development of the air bag is one effort to decrease the bodily damage caused by automobile collisions. There are also other devices which can further decrease the likelihood of spinal injuries.

The properly positioned headrest decreases hyperextension injuries to the cervical spine. Headrests that are too short, provide a fulcrum for the cervical spine to hyperextend over, thus increasing injury to the soft and hard tissues (3).

Seats that provide support, while not reversing the lumbar lordosis nor exaggerating pressures onto the lumbar spine, help to keep the spine at its maximal strength position. This increases stability and decreases spinal injuries (3). Unfortunately the head and neck remain unprotected from many impacts, especially those from the side or front. Since these safety innovations are effective in reducing spinal injuries during motor vehicle accidents, it is imperative that manufacturers incorporate them and continue to develop new safety devices. It is equally critical that consumer education be advanced to increase utilization.

Many spinal fractures occur during athletics and recreation. Contact sports such as football and hockey create enough body impact for spinal injuries to occur. Proper protective gear must be used to minimize severe injuries. In football, the use of neck rolls, college style shoulder pads, and face masks that extend to or below the chin, can limit the amount of cervical motion and therefore decrease hyperflexion, extension and lateral flexion injuries. However, many athletes attempt to increase their mobility and thus opt for one or two bar masks, no neck rolls or less padding. As participants in contact sports become younger and younger, it is critical that they be maximally protected. This is especially important, since the young usually have increased spinal flexibility, thus risking injury to the spinal cord and nerve roots.

Diving, snowmobile riding, bicycling, horseback riding, skiing and other sports where high speeds or physical inertia is a factor, increase the potential for spinal fractures. The risks should be evaluated before participation is considered.

Only slight variations in postural position can dramatically affect stability and the occurrence, degree and type of fracture which occurs. Since biomechanical abnormalities will decrease spinal strength and increase the chance of injury, all competitive athletes, especially those in scholastic settings, should be properly screened for potential instability syndromes by professionals who specialize in spinal biomechanics.

Continued development of safety technology, accident prevention and educational programs, along with advances in the management of spinal fractures and dislocations when they do occur, should provide promising options for reducing the devastation caused by these injuries. The philosophical and political chasm between chiropractic and medicine has been ongoing. Cooperation between these two branches of the health care delivery system, in the area of spinal trauma, may greatly benefit society and ultimately the patients they both serve.

References

1. Winterstein JF. Diagnosis and management of stable thoracolumbar compression fractures. J Clin Chiro 1979;3(2):43–54.
2. Plaugher G, Cox DB, Thibodeau P. Chiropractic management of spinal fractures: a report of six cases. Proceedings 1991 International Conference on Spinal Manipulation, Washington DC, 1991:67–71.
3. White AA, Panjabi MM. Clinical biomechanics of the spine. Philadelphia: JB Lippincott, 1978.
4. Denis F. The three column spine and its significance in the classification of acute thoracolumbar spinal injuries. Spine 1983;8:817–831.
5. Denis F. Spinal instability as defined by the three-column spine concept in acute spinal trauma. Clin Orthop 1984;189:65–76.
6. Herbst RW. Gonstead chiropractic science and art. Mt. Horeb WI: Sci-Chi Publications, 1968.
7. Yochum TR, Rowe LJ. Essentials of skeletal radiology. Baltimore: Williams & Wilkins, 1987.
8. Gerlock AJ, Kirchner SG, Heller RM, Kaye JJ. The cervical spine in trauma. Philadelphia: WB Saunders Co., 1978.
9. Lecture notes. Gonstead Seminar of Chiropractic. Mt. Horeb, WI, 1990.
10. Panjabi MM, Duranceau JS, Oxland TR, Bowen CE. Multidirectional instabilities of traumatic cervical spine injuries in a porcine model. Spine 1989;14:111–115.
11. Vernay D, Dubost JJ, Dordain G, Sauvezie B. Seizures and compression fracture. Neurology 1990;40:725–726.
12. Plaugher G, Lopes MA, Melch PE, Cremata EE. The inter- and

intraexaminer reliability of a paraspinal skin temperature differential instrument. J Manipulative Physiol Ther 1991;14:361–367.

13. Chusid JG. Correlative neuroanatomy and functional neurology. 17th ed. Los Altos, CA: Lange Medical Publications, 1979.
14. Hanley EN, Eskay ML. Thoracic spine fractures. Orthopedics 1989;12:689–695.
15. Kaye JJ, Nance EP. Thoracic and lumbar spine trauma. Orthopedics 1990;28:361–377.
16. Singer KP, Willen J, Brerhahl PD, Day RE. Radiologic study of the influence of zygapophyseal joint orientation on spinal injuries at the thoracolumbar junction. Surg Radiol Anat 1989;11:233–239.
17. Farfan HF. Symptomatology in terms of the pathomechanics of low-back pain and sciatica. In: Haldeman S, ed. Modern developments in the principles and practice of chiropractic. East Norwalk, CT: Appleton & Lange, 1980:173.
18. Miniaci A, McLaren AC. Anterolateral compression fracture of the thoracolumbar spine. Clin Orthop 1989;240:153–156.
19. Court-Brown CM, Gertzbein SD. The management of burst fractures of the fifth lumbar vertebra. Spine 1987;12:308–312.
20. Gertzbein SD, Court-Brown CM. Flexion-distraction injuries of the lumbar spine. Clin Orthop 1988;227:52–59.
21. Moskowitz A. Lumbar seatbelt injury in a child: case report. J Trauma 1989;29:1279–1282.
22. Nicoll EA. Fractures of the dorso lumbar spine. J Bone Joint Surg 1949;31B:376.
23. Hadley LA. Anatomico-roentgenographic studies of the spine. 5th ed. Springfield, Illinois: Charles C Thomas, 1981.
24. Isler B. Lumbosacral lesions associated with pelvic ring injuries. J Orthop Trauma 1990;4:1–6.
25. Pennal GF, Tile M, Waddell JP, Garside H. Pelvic disruption: assessment and classification. Clin Orthop 1980;151:12–21.
26. Burgess AR, Tile M. Fractures of the pelvis. In: Rockwood CA, Green DP, Bucholz RW, eds. Fractures in adults. Philadelphia: JB Lippincott, 1991:1399–1479.
27. Denis F, Davis S, Comfort T. Sacral fractures: an important problem. Clin Orthop 1988;227:67–81.
28. Nykoliation JW, Cassidy JD, Dupuis P, Yong-Hing K, Crnec M. Missed cervical spine fracture-dislocations prior to manipulation: a review of three cases. J Can Chiro Assoc 1986;30:69–75.
29. Helleur C, Gracovetsky S, Farfan H. Tolerance of the human cervical spine to high acceleration: a modelling approach. Aviat Space Environ Med 1984;55:903–909.

13 Spinal Management for the Patient with a Visceral Concomitant

GREGORY PLAUGHER with the assistance of MARK A. LOPES, JAMES E. KONLANDE, RICHARD W. DOBLE, JR., and EDWARD E. CREMATA

Statistics on the percentage of visceral disorders (Type O) managed by chiropractors indicate a decline in the number of patients presenting to clinics with these complaints. In 1979, the number of patients presenting with a Type O disorder was 14%. For 1989 this number had declined to approximately 8% (1). Should this trend continue, by 1995 there will be few patients with these disorders being treated by chiropractors. This trend may be a result of a declining emphasis on visceral management by many chiropractic colleges. Recently, however, material on visceral disorders related to the spine has surfaced in the literature (2,3). If the chiropractic approach to low back pain had been abandoned early on due to the lack of research data, we would have never known its superiority to other conservative measures (4).

For the confident practitioner familiar with the management of visceral disorders, each case represents a chance to become reacquainted with the neuroanatomy and neurophysiology of the particular disease. The tasks of determining the primary levels of involvement, of adjusting them in a specific manner, and of monitoring the patient during resolution of the dysfunction become daily occurrences. The practitioner—with little clinical experience or one without a systematic approach—will find patient management to be an awkward exercise. Confidence is replaced with uncertainty and treatment becomes referral. For those who wish to take on this aspect of chiropractic practice, both challenges and rewards are plentiful.

CLINICAL OBSERVATIONS

Gonstead's empirical work with numerous patients during 55 years in practice are the foundation of our approach to a given condition. (Doctors who followed Gonstead's career found that he treated personally between 150 and 200 patients six and a half days per week. Gonstead worked at least 18 hours a day, usually not going to bed on the same day that he awoke. An 8-hour shift was considered half a Norwegian workday. The reception area at the Gonstead Clinic in Mt. Horeb, Wisconsin has seating for 106 patients (5).) Many have attempted to manage clinical conditions by using a theoretical approach. A treatment strategy that seems reasonable from an anatomic or physiologic standpoint may not necessarily produce favorable patient outcomes. Improvement is more likely if treatment and management are based on clinical experience or observation rather than theoretical protocols. Ultimately, the best approach will be through the accumulation of data from controlled clinical trials and descriptive case reports. Clinical trials provide more information for the practitioner, because they reveal useful or useless treatment for well-defined circumstances. The case report is important because it provides detailed information about how the patient was treated and monitored. The physiologic mechanisms involved in visceral disorders and how they may be remedied through chiropractic treatment will likely evolve as more basic science information becomes available.

HEALTH CARE TEAM

There are many disorders for which chiropractic treatment alone is not adequate. In these instances, the doctor should know with which health care professional to cooperate. If a spinal subluxation exists, then chiropractic care is indicated, provided no contraindications to treatment are present.

PROBLEM SOLVING

For each disorder there may be a variety of spinal levels which are related. The management approach should be systematic, insofar as the most likely related areas of spinal involvement are adjusted first. Adequate time for the healing process of the particular disorder is mandatory before determining the success or failure of the prescribed treatment. For example, a patient who has accumulated 40 years of dysfunction and degeneration may take years to heal or may not completely recover at all. In these situations, the practitioner must be patient and must realize his or her limitations with respect to the management of spinal related conditions. This perspective towards visceral management can only be gained through extensive personal clinical experience, and/or by learning from others with such experience. Publication of these clinical observations in scientific journals would ease the dissemination of this information.

Specificity is critical, because the results of an adjustment are diagnostic. If an unfavorable response is obtained after an adequate trial at a particular level, alternative levels are addressed. Limiting the number of areas initially adjusted at one time allows for a step-by-step approach to problem solving. If a reasonable clinical trial of adjustments at the specified levels has not resulted in a favorable outcome, additional diagnostic work-up is indicated. The general management of a patient with a visceral concomitant is presented in Figure 13.1.

CHRONIC SYSTEMIC DISORDERS

Gonstead (6) hypothesized that many chronic multifactorial diseases (e.g., cancer, migraine headache, osteoporosis, etc.) were related to imbalances of biochemistry from long-term glandular or organ dysfunction (e.g., thyroid, adrenal, ovary, liver, kidney, etc.). These chronic conditions usually did not respond until the organ or glandular function had been nearly restored. A minimum of 90 days might be needed to begin to see improvement in the patient's signs and symptoms. In the early stages of visceral involvement, symptomatic relief may occur within a few weeks. In chronic disorders, postadjustment improvement in the signs and symptoms of visceral dysfunction may suggest a strong spinal component. Local spinal improvement will likely occur before visceral changes in long-standing conditions. Care must be taken to avoid overadjusting these patients.

NEUROVISCERAL ASSOCIATION

The basic principle of chiropractic encompasses the primary role of the nervous system in the maintenance of homeostasis (health). Homeostasis depends on optimal communication between the brain and the rest of the organism (7). Nervous system dysfunction may result from a variety of stressors (e.g., genetic, psychological, environmental, mechanical). Optimizing neurospinal relationships helps the organism to cope with psychological or environmental stressors. In experiments with laboratory animals, it was found that those who underwent a course of manipulation had significantly less stress in response to cold when compared with controls (8–10).

The primary focus of chiropractic care is based on the premise that nervous system dysfunction from vertebral subluxation will interfere with the brain's regulation of physiology (11). Aberrant somatovisceral reflexes may be caused by spinal dysfunction (12–18). The mechanisms by which the nervous system becomes impaired through changes in the spinal column are diverse (See Chapter 3).

The approach to the management of the patient with a visceral concomitant presented here primarily involves normalization of parasympathetic and sympathetic function. Abnormal autonomic nervous system activity may be inhibitory or facilitative; however, the relationship between the two divisions is not a simple "balancing act." The etiology of a particular disease may be associated primarily with one division or the other. Beal (19), in his comprehensive literature review, found that spinal regions were often associated with different organic disturbances. Most of the clinical studies cited correlated well with the anatomic outflows of the autonomic nervous system. Vertebral dysfunction between T1 and L3 affected primarily the sympathetic nervous system. Disorders of the sacroiliac region affected the parasympathetic division, as did the upper cervical region.

Harris and Wagnon (20), in their study on the effects of adjustments on autonomic tone (i.e., distal skin temperature), found that different spinal regions had either a sympathetic or nonsympathetic effect. Actual parasympathetic stimulations were not theorized in this study because distal skin temperature is controlled entirely by sympathetic nerve endings. They correlated adjustments to the cervical region (C1-C7) and lower lumbar (i.e., L4-L5, L5-S1) as having a non-sympathetic effect. Adjustments to spinal segments T1 to L3 produced sympathetic effects.

Gonstead (6) observed that adjustments of occiput through C5, unfused sacral segments, and the sacroiliac joints (sometimes L5) had primarily a parasympathetic effect, whereas subluxations from C6 through L4 or L5 were associated with sympathetic disturbances.

Sympathetic preganglionic cell bodies are traditionally thought to be confined to the thoracic and upper lumbar levels (T1-L3) (7). Our review of the literature has indicated that preganglionic sympathetic cell bodies have been identified at all levels of the spinal cord (21–23). Additional research on the effects of chiropractic adjustments on the autonomic nervous system should be a high priority for the chiropractic profession.

Literature

We have reviewed somatovisceral relationships from a variety of sources (e.g., chiropractic, osteopathic, medical). Terminology for the spinal lesion is quite diverse. The following represents a partial list of descriptors found in the literature to describe the mechanical joint derangement of the spinal column:

1. Subluxation
2. Osteopathic lesion
3. Dysarthria
4. Somatic dysfunction
5. Vertebral subluxation complex
6. Vertebral subluxation syndrome
7. Bony lesion

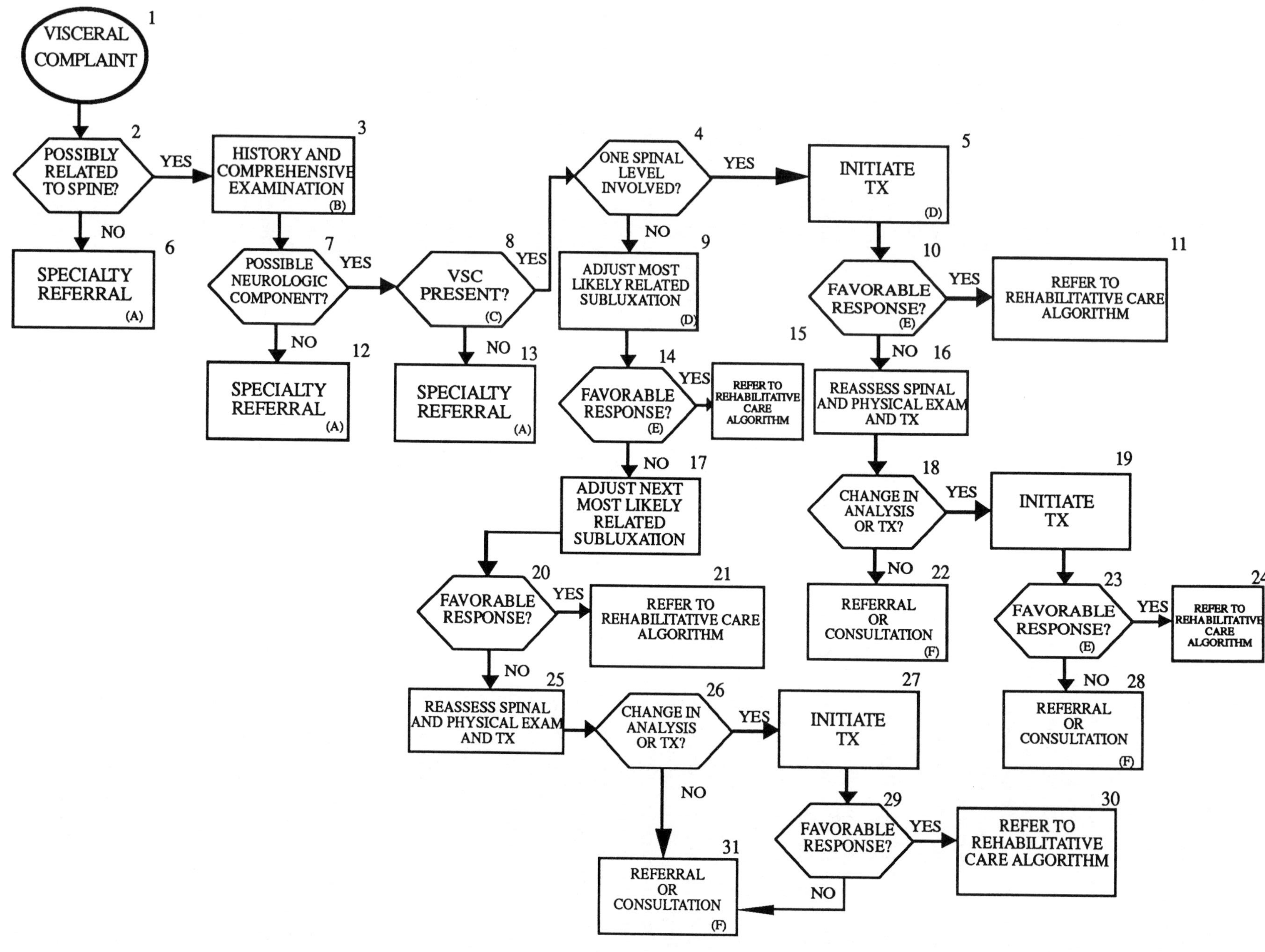
1 VISCERAL COMPLAINT
2 POSSIBLY RELATED TO SPINE?
YES
NO
6 SPECIALTY REFERRAL (A)
3 HISTORY AND COMPREHENSIVE EXAMINATION (B)
7 POSSIBLE NEUROLOGIC COMPONENT?
YES
NO
12 SPECIALTY REFERRAL (A)
8 VSC PRESENT? (C)
YES
NO
13 SPECIALTY REFERRAL (A)
4 ONE SPINAL LEVEL INVOLVED?
YES
NO
5 INITIATE TX (D)
9 ADJUST MOST LIKELY RELATED SUBLUXATION (D)
10 FAVORABLE RESPONSE? (E)
YES
NO
11 REFER TO REHABILITATIVE CARE ALGORITHM
14 FAVORABLE RESPONSE? (E)
YES
NO
15 REFER TO REHABILITATIVE CARE ALGORITHM
16 REASSESS SPINAL AND PHYSICAL EXAM AND TX
17 ADJUST NEXT MOST LIKELY RELATED SUBLUXATION
18 CHANGE IN ANALYSIS OR TX?
YES
NO
19 INITIATE TX
20 FAVORABLE RESPONSE?
YES
NO
21 REFER TO REHABILITATIVE CARE ALGORITHM
22 REFERRAL OR CONSULTATION (F)
23 FAVORABLE RESPONSE? (E)
YES
NO
24 REFER TO REHABILITATIVE CARE ALGORITHM
25 REASSESS SPINAL AND PHYSICAL EXAM AND TX
26 CHANGE IN ANALYSIS OR TX?
YES
NO
27 INITIATE TX
28 REFERRAL OR CONSULTATION (F)
29 FAVORABLE RESPONSE?
YES
NO
30 REFER TO REHABILITATIVE CARE ALGORITHM
31 REFERRAL OR CONSULTATION (F)

When citing reference material, the authors' lexicon may be used. The terms vertebral subluxation complex (VSC) and subluxation will be used most often, because they are germane to the chiropractic profession.

Nutritional Considerations

Integral to the management of visceral and other disorders is the implementation of nutritional supplementation to support the healing of tissues affected by the vertebral subluxation complex. Nutritional imbalances affect tissue responses to neural stimuli.

Recent research has revealed that modification of apparently normal diets might produce significant alterations in nutritional, neurologic, endocrine, and behavioral linkages (24). For example, diets that are deficient in the amino acid tryptophan, low in carbohydrates and or high in proteins and fats, tend to produce low levels of both tryptophan and the neurotransmitter serotonin in the brain (25). Low activity of serotonergic neurons is believed to result in a subnormal secretion of the pituitary hormone prolactin and less control of libido. It appears that prolactin reduces the sensitivity of the CNS centers controlling libido in both males and females. Therefore, elevated prolactin will have a dampening effect on both sexual and reproductive functions (26,27). This effect is counteracted by the elevated androgen secretion that occurs in adolescent males and in females who have high androgen secretion from adrenal cortical tissue. The latter effect would be enhanced by low activity of serotonergic neurons and high activity of dopaminergic neurons, because both conditions result in subnormal prolactin secretion (26). Diets related to obesity and the effects of weight gain on the various organ systems are also important to consider in overall patient management.

One might wonder why so much attention has been paid to scientific dietary concerns when it is apparent that the human race has survived for a very long time without the benefits of nutritional science. Numerous anthropologic and epidemiologic studies have shown that human survival apparently depended on the successful adaptation to a wide variety of environments and that those who lacked this physiologic characteristic did not survive. For example, each race appears to have numerous individuals who possess "thrifty genes." This term denotes those who possess the hormonal and other related characteristics that allow them to gain weight rapidly during periods when food is abundant, and the ability to withstand scarcity by drawing on the materials present in their body tissues.

A leading example of these factors at work is the Pima Indians who live in the area between Phoenix Arizona

Figure 13.1. Algorithm for the chiropractic management of a patient with a visceral concomitant. **A,** Specialty referral. This includes, emergency room, and primary contact physicians. If the patient is nonambulatory, then appropriate transportation (e.g., ambulance) should be arranged. The chiropractor should work closely with the referral physician because they were the primary contact provider. Many advanced testing equipment (e.g., MRI, CT, bone scan etc.) are available to the primary contact physician to determine which specialty referral is indicated. **B,** General intake history and comprehensive examination. This includes vital signs and tests of peripheral neurologic function; sensory, motor, reflex, and tests of autonomic function; skin temperature, red response, physical signs of denervation supersensitivity. Is the patient with the concomitant disorder manageable on an outpatient basis? Unstable patients require immediate referral or transportation to a hospital. Contraindications to manual force short lever arm techniques include fracture of the neural arch, infection, and severe osteolytic activity of the contact vertebra. General contraindications include adjustment protocols which would exacerbate the visceral concomitant. For example, a vertebrobasilar artery incident is likely to be worsened with the administration of subsequent manipulations. **C,** VSC Present? See Chapter 3 for the parameters related to the vertebral subluxation complex. If the visceral concomitant is probably not related (segmentally) to the VSC then specialty referral is indicated. For example, a patient may have a T4 subluxation but present with cauda equina syndrome. This scenario would dictate immediate referral (neurosurgeon or orthopedic surgeon). **D,** Adjust most likely related subluxation. The subluxation most likely related to the visceral concomitant would be a primary (See Chapter 3) subluxation, which is segmentally associated with the involved viscera. **E,** Favorable response. There are a number responses which could happen with a patient under chiropractic care. The first involves a reduction in the objective findings of subluxation followed by a resolution of the visceral complaint. This would clearly be the most favorable outcome. Another scenario may show clear reduction in the spinal dysfunction without a concomitant immediate reduction in the visceral disorder. Clinical judgment must dictate the appropriate course in this case. Often, the patient may require sufficient time for healing to occur in order for the resolution of symptomatology to take place. The doctor must weigh the patient's ability to recover with the possibility that additional therapies (e.g., nutritional) are needed or concurrent care with another specialty is indicated. The general well-being of the patient usually dictates their ability to recover. The geriatric with a chronic visceral disorder or someone under extreme psychological stress, will likely take more time to respond than someone with an acute adaptational disturbance. The possibility may exist that reduction of the subluxation related to the presenting visceral complaint may cause a compensation reaction in other portions of the spine. For example, the patient might have a T7 subluxation and stomach pain. Following a course of adjustments to T7, there may be compensation in the lower cervical spine (given preexisting subluxation in the area) which then causes vertebrogenic headache. The doctor may then choose to adjust these other areas, possibly in combination with the initially adjusted region. **F,** Referral or consultation. Another chiropractic opinion is often warranted when some confusion exists as to the appropriate level of involvement, or appropriate treatment (e.g., adjustment, diet therapy, etc.). Specialists (e.g., internist) with expertise in the disorder being managed are often helpful in patient management, especially when some degree of uncertainty in the diagnosis exists.

Table 13.1.
Estimated Total Deaths and Percentage of Total Deaths for the 10 Leading Causes of Death: United States, 1987

Rank	Cause of Death	Number	Percent
1	Heart disease[a]	759,400	35.7
2	Cancers[a]	476,700	22.4
3	Strokes[a]	148,700	7.0
4	Unintentional injuries[b]	92,500	4.4
5	Chronic obstructive lung diseases	78,000	3.7
6	Pneumonia and influenza	68,600	3.2
7	Diabetes mellitus[a]	37,800	1.8
8	Suicide[b]	29,600	1.4
9	Chronic liver disease and cirrhosis[b]	26,000	1.2
10	Atherosclerosis[a]	23,100	1.1

[a]Causes of death in which diet plays a part.
[b]Causes of death in which excessive alcohol consumption plays a part.

and East Central Sonora, Mexico. More than half of the Pimas suffer from adult onset diabetes, and they have over ten times the death rate from diabetic complications as Caucasian Americans (28). When the Pimas return to the use of their traditional diet they lose their excess body weight and most of their adult onset (Type II) diabetic characteristics. Researchers who induced nondiabetic Caucasians in Australia to adopt the Pima diet noted a significant reduction in physiologic risk factors such as the abnormal secretion of insulin in response to dietary sugar. It cannot be assumed, however, that every patient has similar physiologic traits. Therefore, the successful application of nutritional principles to the prevention of degenerative diseases requires that health practitioners identify those individuals most at risk. The urgent necessity for this screening of patients is shown by the fact that five of the ten leading causes of death in the U.S. are thought to be nutritionally related (See Table 13.1).

The gruesome statistics presented in Table 13.1 have led to a consensus by a panel of leading nutritional researchers from universities, medical centers and private industry that certain general recommendations on dietary modifications would benefit most Americans. This advice was compiled by the Nutritional Policy Board of the U.S. Department of Health and Human Services and published in the Surgeon General's Report on Nutrition and Health in 1988 (29). A brief summary of their recommendations is given in Table 13.2.

The identification of patients with needs for nutritional modifications are most urgent. This identification depends on a thorough screening with proper diagnostic methods. These methods include patient and family histories, physical examinations, dietary assessments, laboratory tests of blood and urine samples, and radiologic examinations.

Very few patients can carry out modifications of their diets without some very explicit descriptions of appropriate food and beverage selection. Examples of corrective dietary plans used by the U.S. Veterans Administration have been provided (See Appendix) (30).

Table 13.2.
Diet Recommendations

Issues for Most People:

- *Fats and cholesterol:* Reduce consumption of fat (especially saturated fat) and cholesterol. Choose foods relatively low in these substances, such as vegetables, fruits, whole grain foods, fish, poultry, lean meats, and low-fat dairy products. Use food preparation methods that add little or no fat.
- *Energy and weight control:* Achieve and maintain a desirable body weight. To do so, choose a dietary pattern in which energy (caloric) intake is consistent with energy expenditure. To reduce energy intake, limit consumption of foods relatively high in calories, fats, and sugars, and minimize alcohol consumption. Increase energy expenditure through regular and sustained physical activity.
- *Complex carbohydrates and fiber:* Increase consumption of whole grain foods and cereal products, vegetables (including dried beans and peas), and fruits.
- *Sodium:* Reduce intake of sodium by choosing foods relatively low in sodium and limiting the amount of salt added in food preparation and at the table.
- *Alcohol:* To reduce the risk for chronic disease, take alcohol only in moderation (no more than two drinks a day), if at all. Avoid drinking any alcohol before or while driving, operating machinery, taking medications, or engaging in any other activity requiring judgment. Avoid drinking alcohol while pregnant.

Other Issues for Some People:

- *Sugars:* Those who are particularly vulnerable to dental caries (cavities), especially children, should limit their consumption and frequency of use of foods high in sugars.
- *Calcium:* Adolescent girls and adult women should increase consumption of foods high in calcium, including low-fat dairy products.
- *Iron:* Children, adolescents, and women of childbearing age should be sure to consume foods that are good sources of iron, such as lean meats, fish, certain beans, and iron-enriched cereals and whole grain products. This issue is of special concern for low-income families.

HEADACHE

One of the most common complaints treated by a chiropractor is headache. It is estimated that between 50 and 100 million Americans suffer from chronic headaches each year. Headache sufferers cost businesses more than 50 billion dollars annually in lost labor. Each year 155 million workdays are lost due to headaches (31).

A thorough history is necessary to ascertain etiologic factors. The subjective findings are one of the most important clues in determining associated spinal levels of involvement. The headache may be described as sharp, dull, throbbing, stabbing, band-like, vise-like, or thumping. Temporal characteristics (e.g., morning, evening, postexercise, postprandial, etc.) should be determined. Headaches occurring later in the day and aggravated by stress may indicate muscular tension involvement. Those that are present on awakening may be associated with imbalances of body chemistry (e.g., hypothyroidism) (6), a strained sleeping position, or previous alcohol ingestion.

Associated symptoms with the headache can provide information as to the etiology. Patients with headaches associated with hypothyroidism will also have symptoms of that disorder; weight gain, intolerance to cold, persistent cough, etc. An aura or visual scotoma before a unilateral headache is commonly associated with classical migraine. Bilateral tinnitus is suggestive of a hypertensive etiology. A fever with neck pain on forced flexion may indicate an infection, such as spinal meningitis.

A common cause of headache is ingestion of alcohol which irritates the brain directly and lack of (or too much) sleep. More than one type of headache may be present with a given patient, making management more challenging. We present some of the more common headaches encountered in practice which may be ameliorated with chiropractic treatment. Some types of headaches have multifactorial etiologies. A reduction in symptomatology in these cases may not immediately follow improvement in the related biomechanical dysfunction.

Tension or Stress Headaches

Sustained contraction of the neck and shoulder muscles is a common cause of extracranial headache and is termed muscle tension or muscle contraction headache (MCH). This kind of headache is often initiated or exacerbated by stress and relieved by rest, analgesics, and movements that relax neck musculature. MCH is commonly described as a dull, pulling, ache manifesting itself in the region of the upper cervical musculature. The MCH commonly travels from the suboccipital area to the frontal region. The intensity is usually mild to moderate. The timing is towards the end of the day, although it is not uncommon for a MCH to last more than one day.

An anterior carriage of the cranium leads to sustained muscular contraction to keep the head upright (32) (Figure 13.2). Subluxations that cause or contribute to reduction or reversal of the cervical lordosis are often involved.

Spinal lesions contributing to MCH can range from the mid dorsal spine to the lower cervical region. Close attention should be directed to the cervicothoracic junction (C6 to T3) (33). Subluxations in the pelvic region, such as an ASIn ilium or a severely rotated sacrum may at times lead to compensatory hypolordosis of the spinal curvatures and should be considered in the overall management. All of the sagittal curves are interdependent. Adjusting a midthoracic subluxation in combination with a lower cervical or upper thoracic subluxation, is often indicated.

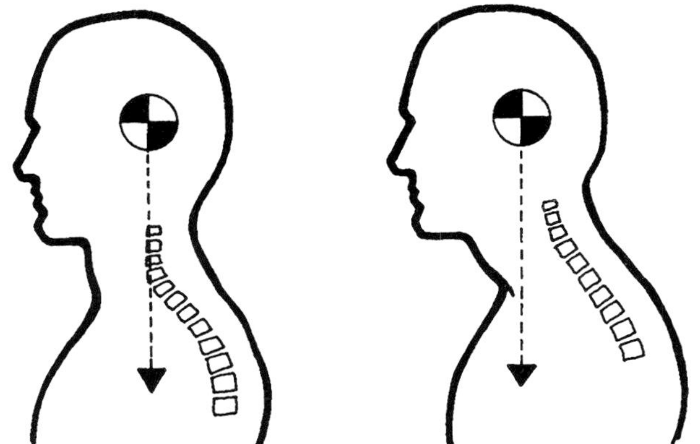

Figure 13.2. Anterior carriage of the head will move the center of mass forward, creating a lever for the acceleration of gravity to act on. This will necessitate compensatory contraction of the posterior neck musculature, to counterbalance the weight of the head.

Suboccipital Headache

Suboccipital headache is described as a focal area of pain in the suboccipital region which may be caused by irritation of the cervical nerves (34). Sustained muscular contraction from loss of the normal cervical lordosis appears to be a common denominator. Cervicothoracic subluxations (C6-T3) should be ruled out. Hypermobility of the upper cervical articulations in compensation for fixation dysfunction below may also be an important etiology. Occasionally, an upper cervical subluxation is involved (6). It is often difficult to differentiate between a suboccipital and muscle contraction headache.

Vascular Headaches

These headaches are characterized by a throbbing, pulsating pain, usually behind one eye, and sometimes accompanied with unilateral frontal radiation. The pain is rarely severe; however, sleep disturbance may occur. This type of headache is not relieved by analgesics. Overingestion of analgesics is common as patients receive little relief from them. Nausea and vomiting often results from such overingestion and should not be confused with a somatovisceral disorder. The patient often complains that "nothing seems to help." Vascular headaches include migraine (classical and common), and headaches with a hypertensive etiology.

CLASSICAL MIGRAINE

The migraine headache is a disorder characterized by recurrent attacks of headache with variable intensity, frequency, and duration. Migraines are commonly associated with nausea, vomiting, and anorexia and are often accompanied by neurologic and mood disturbances (35).

Classical migraine headache is the type that is preceded or accompanied by transient focal neurologic phenomena; visual aura of scintillating scotomas, fortification spectra, sensory disturbances such as paresthesia, and/or motor disturbances. It is commonly thought of as a central nervous system disturbance. There is also evidence that muscle contraction (tension or stress) headache can eventually lead to migraine (36). The various, sometimes arbitrary, classifications of headache appear to mingle as one studies the subject in detail (37). Vernon (38) has reviewed the literature on headaches that appear to have their origin in the cervical spine. Cervical spine causes of migraine and other types of headaches have been largely ignored by mainstream medical management. He presents two headache patients who responded favorably to chiropractic manipulation.

Classical migraine affects 10 to 30% of all migraine sufferers (37). Wight (35) showed a success rate of 75% in migraine patients treated with chiropractic methods. Parker et al. (39) demonstrated a 47% success rate in patients treated with manipulation (seven chiropractic treatments over a 2-month period) after a 2-year follow-up. Subluxations of the cervicothoracic junction (C6 to T4) and the thoracolumbar area (T12-L3) (6,33) may be associated with migraine headache.

Please see the dietary modification guidelines at the end of this section for adjunctive considerations for the rare patient who is unresponsive to adjustive treatment alone.

COMMON MIGRAINE

In contrast to the classical variant, common migraine headaches do not display sharply defined neurologic disturbances. They might only present with nausea in conjunction with the headache. The various symptomatology is more reflective of a peripheral nervous system disturbance. As in classical migraine, the cervicothoracic junction and the thoracolumbar region should be ruled out for subluxation complexes. In some individuals prone to migraine, adjustments of the upper cervical region may provoke an attack (6). There are instances in which cervical subluxations can cause various headache syndromes (38).

Dietary Considerations. Patients whose headaches are triggered by certain vasoactive dietary substances may wish to eliminate those foods from their diets during the early phases of chiropractic treatment. Approximately one-third of migraine headache sufferers will benefit from dietary modifications (40). The following is a list of foods to be avoided that was compiled by Theisler (31) for use in the management of the headache patient:

1. Ripened cheeses: Cheddar, Emmaantaler, Swiss, Gruyere, Parmesan, Stilton, Brie, provolone, Romano, and Camembert. *Cheese allowed:* American, cottage, cream, Velveeta, ricotta, and farmer.
2. Chocolate, cocoa, white chocolate, licorice.
3. Nuts, especially peanuts, peanut butter, pumpkin, sesame, and sunflower seeds.
4. Avocados, papaya, red plums, fresh pineapple, raisins, canned figs, banana (limit to one-half banana per day).
5. Milk, eggs, sour cream, yogurt, butter milk, and all dairy products.
6. Hot fresh breads, raised coffee cakes, and donuts.
7. Corn, tomatoes, olives, pickles, sauerkraut, onions (except for seasoning).
8. Broad beans, lima beans, navy beans, pea pods, pinto beans, soy beans, and snow peas.
9. Aged or cured meats: hot dogs, ham, bacon, bologna, chicken liver, pork; fermented sausage: salami, pepperoni.
10. Soy sauce, yeast, yeast extract, brewers yeast, Accent seasoned salt (monosodium glutamate), meat tenderizer.
11. Citrus fruits: oranges, grapefruit, lemons, limes (limit to one half cup serving per day).
12. Passion fruits: kiwi, strawberries, mango.
13. Foods containing large amounts of monosodium glutamate (e.g., Chinese).
14. Salted and dried fish, herring, snails.
15. Vinegar (except white vinegar).
16. Pizza.
17. Wheat products.
18. Anything fermented, pickled, or marinated.
19. All alcoholic beverages. If you must drink, do not exceed more than two normal sized drinks. Suggested drinks: Haute Sauterne, Riesling, Seagram's VO, Cutty Sark, vodka.
20. Shellfish.
21. Fasting.

HYPERTENSIVE HEADACHE

Hypertensive headache is characterized as a mild to moderate, generalized, throbbing pain of the occipital or vertex region of the head. The pain can be unilateral, and there may be an associated muscle contraction headache (37). Dizziness is often present, especially during motion of the head and neck.

Generally, the blood pressure must be elevated to above 200/120 mm Hg to cause this type of headache (37). The pain is alleviated by rest and antihypertensive drugs and aggravated by chemicals that increase blood pressure, such as caffeine or nicotine. Refer to the section on hypertension for appropriate chiropractic management.

Cluster Headache

Cluster headaches usually begin to appear in patients in their late teens or early twenties. They occur more commonly in males and are rare beyond the age of 40 (41). The pain comes in clusters, recurring as often as two or three times a day with intervals of asymptomatic times that last two or three weeks before the pain begins again. There may be associated unilateral tearing. The headache is constant and severe (knife-like) and lasts 30 to 45 minutes. There is no associated nausea or vomiting as in migrainous type headaches. Cluster headaches are correlated with HLA antigens, low serotonin levels in the brain, and there seem to be trigeminal nerve interactions as well (42). Because of possible trigeminal nerve involvement, spinal subluxations of the upper cervical region should be ruled out.

Chemistry Headache

The chemistry headache is a deep and generalized headache that is often alleviated by exercise. The intensity can vary from mild to severe. It is commonly seen after a change in activity level or extended sleep (e.g., patient awakens with it on a Saturday morning after sleeping in) (6). Spinal lesions should be ruled out from C6 to T4 (33), but all levels need to analyzed for the presence of a VSC.

Digestive Headache

Digestive headaches generally present after eating. Postprandial hypoglycemia should be ruled out. If the pain occurs within an hour of eating, the upper cervical region, especially C1-C2, could be contributory. Headaches that begin one-and-a-half to two hours after eating may be caused by dysfunction in regions with sympathetic outflows to the alimentary tract (T4-L3) (6).

Sinus Headache

The sinus headache is associated with inflammation, congestion, or infection of the sinuses. This generally mild pain may become quite severe during weather changes that affect humidity or barometric pressure (33). The headache is described as dull or gnawing and is located directly over the frontal or maxillary sinuses. They often begin in the morning and worsen as the day goes on. The upper cervical region (C0-C5), especially atlas or axis (6) should be checked for subluxation. A deviated nasal septum may be contributory (See Chapter 15) as well as drug use (e.g., cocaine).

Headaches of Temporomandibular Origin

Headache caused by temporomandibular joint (TMJ) dysfunction is usually described as a steady, dull pain radiating from the TMJ posteriorly to the temporal area (33). There may also be radiation towards the nasal region (6). It is caused by mechanical irritation of the nerves innervating and surrounding the temporomandibular joint. The pain can range from mild to severe depending on the extent of articular dysfunction. The headache is aggravated with movement of the joint. Refer to Chapter 15 for the management of TMJ dysfunction.

Post Whiplash Headache

Headaches are one of the most common sequelae of acceleration/deceleration injuries of the head and neck. These chronic, recurrent headaches can manifest themselves usually minutes and sometimes days after the initial trauma. The patient does not present with persistent focal neurologic signs as in migraine. The headache can be caused by cerebral concussion and/or irritation of the cervical nerves. Posttraumatic headache is often accompanied by symptoms of dizziness, difficulty in concentration, nervousness, personality changes, and insomnia (43). Appropriate spinal management of the spinal injury usually resolves the complaint (See Chapter 10).

Headache and Vertebral Basilar Artery Insufficiency

One of the most important headaches the chiropractor must consider is that associated with vertebral basilar artery insufficiency (VBAI). This must be considered in the differential diagnosis of head pain especially when the onset is sudden and intense. Additional rotational manipulations appear to accentuate the trauma, if they compromise previously damaged vascular structures. All adjustive procedures of the cervical spine must be carefully performed. Attention should be given to placement of the cervical spine in a neutral position during the adjustment. The extremes of extension, flexion, lateral bending and especially axial rotation will compromise the vertebral arteries.

Although the occurrence of basilar artery ischemia after manipulation is rare (about 1 death in 181 million manipulations) (44,45), there are many techniques that avoid the dangerous axial rotation and extension movements which usually precipitate the event. Symptoms associated with VBAI include, headache, nausea, vomiting, nystagmus, vertigo, suboccipital tenderness, and "drop attacks" (instantaneous and temporary quadriplegia on rotation and extension of the neck) (11).

Eyestrain Headache

Eyestrain headaches are typically precipitated with reading. Described as a mild to moderate ache that often becomes sharp, the pain may radiate from the orbit to the occiput and is commonly bilateral. Optometric consultation is indicated if the symptoms persist after chiropractic treatment.

GYNECOLOGIC DISORDERS

Research in the area of female disorders is plentiful although exact etiologies for many processes (e.g., dysmenorrhea) are unknown. Because of the paucity of clinical trials, many patients suffer from mismanagement by health professionals. This may be due to a reflection of the widespread belief that many of these disorders are benign and do not require a comprehensive management strategy. The patient suffering from any of the conditions which follow will think that the condition is anything but benign. The approach of the chiropractor is that painful menses is not normal despite its widespread occurrence. Successful treatment of these disorders has been reported by many chiropractors (46,47). It is important to differentiate a purely mechanical etiology from one that is hormonal (6).

Mechanical Etiology

Pelvic obliquity or torsion and its related ligamentous (e.g., broad) distortions may result in tipping of the uterus. This mechanical alteration can interfere with the normal flow of menstruation or lead to difficulties in childbirth.

Chiropractic care is aimed at the reduction of any subluxations in areas that cause pelvic torsion or alterations of the normal lumbar lordosis and sacral base angle. The mechanical effects of this treatment are thought to result from changes in the angle of contraction of the related muscle groups or via normalization of muscle tone through neurologic mechanisms.

Endocrinologic Etiology

The widespread allopathic use of oral contraceptives to modulate the menstrual cycle illustrates the importance of controlling hormonal levels in managing patients with female related disorders. Dysfunction of the ovaries, thyroid and adrenal glands may be vertebrogenic (See Endocrinologic Disorders). Hypothyroidism (48,49) and adrenal dysfunction (49) may be related to ovarian dysfunction.

The sympathetic fibers arising from the tenth and eleventh thoracic spinal cord segments innervate the ovaries and fallopian tubes. The parasympathetic supply is from the hypogastric plexus (vagus). Autonomic control is primarily vasomotor. Clinical management of these disorders may extend beyond the local anatomic innervation of the ovaries.

The symptoms associated with hormonal imbalances are more diverse and complex than those related to mechanical etiologies. These symptoms may range from premenstrual syndrome to amenorrhea.

The focus of chiropractic care is on normalizing endocrine function through autonomic nervous system effects by correcting vertebral subluxations related to specific end organs or tissues. A favorable response to treatment may be delayed from 60 to 90 days in these patients because of the time required in healing of glandular tissue (6).

DYSMENORRHEA

Primary or functional dysmenorrhea is cyclic pain associated with menses during ovulatory cycles but without demonstratable lesions (e.g., endometriosis) affecting the reproductive cycle. Its etiology is thought to result from uterine contractions and ischemia, the passage of tissue through the cervix, a narrow cervical os, or malposition of the uterus. Signs and symptoms include low abdominal pain (cramping, dull ache often with radiation to the low back or legs), endometrial casts or clots, urinary frequency, nausea, diarrhea, pelvic soreness, and headache.

Secondary dysmenorrhea is pain with menses caused by demonstratable pathology. Endometriosis, chronic pelvic inflammatory disease, adhesions, fibroids and polyps have all been implicated as possible etiologies.

The specific location and timing of cramping or pain assists in the differentiation of a mechanical from a hormonal etiology. Pain related to a mechanical problem is usually located in the lower anterior pelvis and coincides with the onset of menses. The pain may intensify after the start of flow. This structural dysfunction may be attributed to a loss of the normal lumbar lordosis. Subluxations that can reduce the lumbar curve include an ASIn ilium, rotated sacrum and severely rotated lumbar vertebrae. Other subluxations (e.g., PIEx ilium, Base Posterior Sacrum) may also be contributory.

Dysmenorrhea from hormonal dysfunction will generally present as abdominal pain and cramping beginning a few days before the onset of menstruation. Because of the generalized hormonal imbalance, other related symptoms may also be present (e.g., premenstrual syndrome). The primary levels of involvement are usually the upper lumbar spine (e.g., L1-L2) but can range from T12 to L5. The mechanisms involved are unclear but compensatory hypermobility in the lower thoracic spine may be a possible mechanism for initiation of nervous system dysfunction. In premenstrual syndrome, hypothyroidism may be a concomitant, therefore, the cervico-thoracic junction (C6-T3) should not be overlooked (6).

AMENORRHEA

Amenorrhea occurs physiologically before menarche, during pregnancy and early lactation, and after the menopause. Primary amenorrhea is defined as a delayed onset of menarche (age 18 years). The cessation of menses due to nonpathologic causes in a previously menstruating woman is termed secondary amenorrhea. Oligomenorrhea is characterized by infrequent menstruation in which the interval between cycles can range from 40 to 90 days (49).

Amenorrhea results from a disturbance in the production of estrogen and progesterone by the ovaries. Vertebrogenic amenorrhea is usually related to spinal dysfunction in the lower thoracic area to the lower lumbar region. The upper lumbar region (e.g., L1-L2) appears to be a common site for dysfunction in these patients (6).

Some cases of this disorder result from elevations in prolactin secretion. Stress, vigorous and frequent physical activity and tumors of the secreting cells of the pituitary can elevate blood concentrations of prolactin. High levels of serum prolactin inhibit the secretion and actions of the pituitary gonadotropins follicle-stimulating hormone (FSH) and luteinizing hormone (LH). The amenorrhea test panel for patients is serum levels of prolactin, FSH, and LH.

FIBROCYSTIC DISEASE

Fibrocystic disorders are the most common disease of the female breast (49). Hormonal imbalances are considered to be a fundamental etiology. An increase in estrogen and a decrease in progesterone levels are often detected. This could be the reason why there tends to be a lower incidence with oral contraceptive use. Gynecologic consultation is indicated because these patients are more likely to develop carcinoma of the breast. The dominant variant of fibrocystic disease that is associated with an increase risk of breast carcinoma is ductal and lobar epithelial hyperplasia. The cysts may become more noticeable with approaching menses. Chiropractic examination and treatment of patients with fibrocystic breasts should include all indicated spinal levels with concentration primarily on the upper lumber spine (6).

MENOPAUSE

Menopause normally occurs without side-effects. Hot flashes may be associated with ovarian/hormone dysfunction. The upper lumbars and the lower thoracic region should be examined closely because subluxations in these regions may be related (6).

MISCARRIAGE

Miscarriage can be caused by a variety of structural (e.g., uterus) or physiologic (e.g., hormonal) etiologies. Normal function of the nervous system is of paramount importance in sustaining a pregnancy. Miscarriages that occur early on in the pregnancy usually are related to hormonal dysfunction. The upper lumbar spine, therefore, should be checked closely. Hypomobility in the upper lumbar spine may cause compensatory hypermobility in the lower thoracic area, thus possibly eliciting aberrant somatovisceral reflexes. Late pregnancy abortion may be associated with a tipped uterus. The pelvic region and subluxations that can cause reduction of the normal lumbar lordosis (e.g., ASIn, rotated sacrum) may be related (6).

INFERTILITY

In the infertile female with normal ovulation, an examination of the spinal column is in order. Subluxations that influence the lumbar lordosis or affect ovarian hormone function should be ruled out. It is estimated that approximately 40% of infertility etiologies involve the male (50). Consultation with a specialist is indicated. Many drugs, such as corticosteroids, can affect fertility in the male.

HEART DISEASE

Diseases of the cardiovascular system are the most common causes of death for developed nations. Nutritional (e.g., cholesterol) and environmental (e.g., smoking) risk factors are commonly associated with these disorders. The contribution of the chiropractic profession in preventing and managing cardiovascular dysfunction is largely unexplored.

The efferent sympathetic preganglionic nerve fibers to the heart arise from the thoracic levels T1-T5. The upper segments supply the ascending aorta, pulmonary trunk and ventricles. The lower segments innervate the atria (7). The parasympathetic fibers to the heart are derived from cells near the nucleus ambiguous and the dorsal nucleus of the vagus. These nerves run in the cardiac branches of the vagus and synapse in the cardiac plexus and in the walls of the atria (7). The parasympathetic nerves slow the rate of the heart and cause constriction of the coronary arteries. Adjustments to the upper cervical region should be avoided in a patient with myocardial infarction or coronary artery spasm.

Sympathetic stimulation raises the heart rate and causes vasodilation. Nerve terminals storing norepinephrine are found in the sinoatrial and atrioventricular nodes, the atrial and ventricular myocardium, and the Perkinje system.

The heart apparently manufactures much of the norepinephrine that it needs and in this way can be thought of as an endocrine gland as well. Tissue concentrations of norepinephrine are reported to be lower during heart failure (51). Prolonged electrical stimulation of the norepinephrine discharging cardiac sympathetic nerves has been shown to elicit electrocardiographic signs of hypoxic myocardial damage and subendocardial hemorrhages and necrosis (52).

The parasympathetic nervous system also has a role in optimal cardiac function. Hall (53) showed that damage to the myocardium and coronary artery could be produced through daily administration of acetylcholine in experimental unanesthesized dogs. Continual stimulation of the vagus also has been linked to microscopic changes in the heart, including early hyaline degeneration of the myocardium (54).

Angina pectoris and myocardial infarction have both been associated with coronary thrombosis. There are reports, however, of patients with diagnosed angina pectoris or myocardial infarction who have normal coronary arteries as demonstrated with coronary arteriograms (55–59). This incidence may be as high as 30% of patients who are referred for cardiac catheterization (60). Rogers (61) cites two cases in which coronary artery spasm led to the patient's symptomatology and hypothesizes that there is a role for manipulative therapy, through normalization of autonomic function, in the management of coronary artery spasm in the absence of demonstrable thrombosis. Angina from dysfunction of the cervical spine (e.g., disc lesion) may be a more common occurrence than previously thought (62,63). Many of these patients will respond to nitroglycerin therapy, however, thus adding more confusion to the picture. Other reports (64–68) have described an association between mechanical lesions in the spine and angina pectoris. Burns (69) reports normalization of heart function after correction of lesions of the third thoracic vertebra in laboratory animals. She cites previous literature (70) indicating pathologic cardiac effects following the production of spinal lesions in laboratory animals. A report by Rogers (71) showed that spinal manipulative therapy was capable of normalizing the autonomic nervous system tone and being of benefit in nine patients with congestive heart failure.

In a study of 150 patients with heart disease, Koch (72) found that 92% of organic cardiac cases showed radiographic and palpatory evidence of soft tissue aberrations in the area of T2-T6. Many of the patients reported symptoms of musculoskeletal dysfunction just preceding and sometimes months before the initial cardiac distress. It is interesting to note that many presentations of myocardial infarction (MI) occur after primarily nondemanding activities, such as lawn mowing, washing, ironing, and not general body or leg activity, which would place the most demand on the cardiovascular system (73). There is a high incidence of heart disease among manual laborers. Upper extremity tasks do put a higher stress on the cervico-thoracic junction possibly explaining the occurrence. More research is needed in this area to clearly define the role of spinal manipulation in the management of heart disease.

Manipulative therapy has been shown (74) to normalize vasomotor tone through autonomic reflexes. Figar (75), using pre- and postplethysmyography, has shown that normalization of distal skin temperature occurs after cervical manipulation. Harris and Wagnon (20) have documented changes in distal skin temperature that corresponded to autonomic outflows after chiropractic adjustments.

Results of a blinded study by Beal (76) to test the occurrence of somatic dysfunction in patients with cardiovascular disease indicated a peak incidence of spinal lesions at the T2-T3 level. When the palpatory findings in the thoracic region were of a high magnitude, they were commonly associated with somatic dysfunction in the cervical spine as well. In an attempt to identify a link between palpatory findings (warm temperature, ropiness, increased density, edema, etc.) with the anatomic locus of acute myocardial infarction, Rosero (77) correlated anterior wall myocardial infarction and palpatory clues of increased warmth and resistance to mobility of the segments in question.

Nicholas (78,79) reports on a blinded, randomized investigation of somatic dysfunction in patients with myocardial infarction. Qualitative palpatory findings (increased firmness, warmth, ropiness, edema, heavy musculature) were significantly associated with the upper thoracic segments T1-T4. One of the authors' conclusions was that the palpatory examination is important in identifying those patients with a myocardial infarction and is of help in predicting those cases that may develop an MI. A double blind study by Cox (80) correlated palpable musculoskeletal findings with coronary artery disease. They found a peak incidence at the the fourth thoracic segment. Musculoskeletal examination was concluded as being a helpful supplement but not a substitute for standard methods in the diagnosis of coronary artery disease. Further investigation in this area is clearly indicated due to the high morbidity and mortality associated with heart disease.

Osteophytes of the spine which compress the sympathetic trunk may be a source of autonomic disturbance in some individuals (81). The incidence of osteophytic lipping of the thoracic spine and coronary heart disease has been investigated by Cox (82). Ninety-two patients underwent a blinded review of lateral radiographs. The results indicated that 43% of patients with significant coronary stenosis had thoracic osteophytes. A control group was found to have an incidence rate of only 15%. It was concluded that the presence of thoracic osteophytes was a good predictor (85%) (See Chapter 4) of coronary atherosclerosis but was not sensitive.

Lewit (83) states that restricted mobility of the upper thoracic spine is a possible risk factor in organic heart disease. He suggests that there is a role for manipulative treatment, especially in the case of paroxysmal tachycardia, but gives no data on results of treatment. Freedman (84) reports on a patient with diagnosed premature ventricular contractions, which normalized after chiropractic adjustments. Miller (85) reports an investigation in which subjective improvement in patients with chronic obstructive pulmonary disease was noted after manipulative treatment.

Bradycardia and Tachycardia

Bradycardia can be caused by excessive parasympathetic activity. Gonstead (6) hypothesized that this was due to a subluxation in the sympathetic region (T1-T4) which caused a relative parasympathetic override. On a rare occasion, the upper cervical region may be a factor. Tachycardia was most often correlated with upper cervical subluxation (6).

HYPERTENSION

Approximately 90% of hypertensive cases have an unknown etiology (86). This type of hypertension is termed essential or primary. Secondary hypertension (10% of cases) is due to renal (e.g., pheochromocytoma), endocrine (e.g., pituitary tumor), and other mechanisms. A diagnosis of hypertension is not made, generally, unless the elevated pressure is present on at least two separate occasions. The classifications of hypertension are as follows (87):

Diastolic:

BP<85	BP=85–89	BP=90–104	BP=105–114	BP>115
Normal	High-normal	Mild	Moderate	Severe

Systolic:

BP<140	BP=140–159		BP=160–199	BP>200
Normal	Borderline		Systolic Hypertension	

HYPERTENSION

The hypothalamic and medullary regions of the brain control blood pressure. From these centers, parasympathetic and sympathetic influences exert regulatory control over the major effecter organs; the heart, kidneys, and peripheral vascular components (88). The sympathetic nervous system (SNS) controls the increase of cardiac output by vasoconstriction of the peripheral vasculature to divert more blood to muscle and nervous tissue. The overall effect is an increase in the systemic blood pressure. The parasympathetic nervous system decreases blood pressure and cardiac output and increases the activity of the digestive system. Both systems are continually firing at a baseline rate, thus providing an equalizing vasomotor tone (88).

A review by Crawford et al. (88) identified the upper cervical region (C0-C2), the upper thoracics (T1-T6), and the lower thoracics (T11-T12), as potential sites for somatic dysfunction in patients with hypertensive disease. Gonstead (6) classified management of high blood pressure into three categories; diastolic, systolic, and mixed.

General Considerations

It is important to understand when referral to a medical specialty (e.g., internist) is indicated for patients with hypertensive disease. If the patient is younger, with only mild hypertension, there is less of an indication for immediate referral. The older patient, especially one without hypertensive medication, should be observed carefully. If positive results are not seen in a few treatments then referral is suggested. The long-term effects of chronic hypertensive disease can be severe. The kidneys are especially vulnerable. Proteinuria from kidney malfunction is easily detected with urinalysis.

A sudden increase in blood pressure can be dangerous. In this patient, the vessel walls have less time to compensate for the disease and an immediate referral for pharmacologic assistance is indicated. The patient should be managed with chiropractic after initial reduction of the pressure with hypertensive medication. Patients who experience a sudden increase in blood pressure should be examined for the presence of an upper cervical subluxation (6). Adjustments in this area should be of a specific nonrotary nature (See Chapter 11).

Monitoring the blood pressure is critical to patient management. It should be measured before and after each adjustment. The patient who is on hypertensive medication may experience low blood pressure after the treatment because of the combined effects of the medication and the adjustment. The chiropractor should work in conjunction with a medical specialist, so that the medication can be diminished should the patient respond to treatment. A rapid drop in pressure in a patient with chronic hypertensive disease may indicate myocardial infarction. Immediate referral to a hospital emergency room is mandated in this situation.

Dietary and lifestyle changes for the hypertensive patients should be considered in their overall management. Excellent sources are available for this information (89).

DIASTOLIC HYPERTENSION

Gonstead (6) found that patients suffering from diastolic hypertension had subluxations of the upper cervical region (C0-C5), especially atlas-axis. A low blood pressure during the morning which gradually elevates towards the end of the day was also related to this area of the spinal column.

SYSTOLIC HYPERTENSION

Gonstead (6) observed subluxations in systolic hypertensive patients primarily at the cervicothoracic junction (C7-T3) and the thoracolumbar areas (T10-L2). The splanchnic nerves terminate to form the renal plexus which influences blood volume and flow pressures through the kidneys (88). In a study using laboratory animals, Sato and Swenson (90) concluded that sympathetic stimulation of the lower thoracic segments resulted in a lowering of blood pressure. The influence of the autonomic nervous system on adrenal and renal function is thought to be the mechanism involved in many patients with hypertension (89).

MIXED HYPERTENSION

Those patients who have both a high systolic and diastolic blood pressure are more challenging in terms of management. Usually the lower thoracics are involved (T10-T12). If an upper cervical subluxation is present, it should be monitored only initially. Thoracic subluxations should be reduced (about a month) before moving to the upper cervical region (6). In some instances, the upper cervical area will need to be corrected. Those percentages and characteristics of patients who fall into this category is presently unknown. Close monitoring of the blood pressure after each adjustment will help in determining which levels are likely involved.

HYPOTENSION

Hypotension, or low blood pressure, may present in a variety of ways. One common presentation of the disorder is the orthostatic variant. Orthostatic hypotension is the abrupt decrease in blood pressure manifested on assuming an erect position. These individuals usually maintain a relatively normal blood pressure accompanied by sudden orthostatic decreases. Autonomic (primarily sympathetic) nervous system mechanisms normally compensate for the pooling of blood in the veins that results from arising to the erect position. The baroreceptors of the aortic and carotid sinus areas initiate reflexes resulting in sympathetic discharge. The sympathetic stimulation produces increased vasomotor tone and cardiac output and the restoration of blood pressure. The symptoms of orthostatic hypotension are usually mild and include lightheadedness and mental blurring but may even produce syncope and generalized seizures. These symptoms are transient and directly related to the change in posture to an erect position.

Orthostatic hypotension commonly results from the interference of the above autonomic nervous system reflexes by drugs such as antihypertensive medication, monoamine oxidase inhibitors used in mental and nervous disorders, barbiturates, and alcohol. Reductions in intravascular volume from hemorrhage, vomiting, diarrhea, and sweating may lead to dehydration and orthostatic hypotension. Various neuropathic diseases have also been associated with this disorder.

An individual who maintains a relatively low blood pressure at all times may experience symptoms related to orthostatic hypotension as well as generalized fatigue, low resistance to illness, and low tolerances to stress. These concomitant symptoms may result from associated disorders that may be causing the low blood pressure. Hypotensive individuals are commonly overlooked by physicians unfamiliar with the disorder or written off as subclinical or normal variants. The astute clinician, aware of the possible causes and management of hypotension, may provide much needed aid to these patients.

The successful management of these patients requires correction of the cause of the hypotension. The most common causes of ongoing hypotension are hypothyroidism, adrenocortical insufficiency, and anemia. Mild and easily overlooked manifestations of these conditions may contribute to low blood pressure. The assessment of the underlying cause(s) of hypotension includes a differential diagnosis of the above three disorders. A complete history, physical examination, and blood laboratory panel is requisite to accurately assess the possible causes of hypotension. Findings within the normal ranges for blood values may not completely rule out the possibility of abnormal internal function. Normal blood values are relatively wide ranges, and it is not unusual for patients to manifest symptoms and signs of a disorder in the presence of "normal" blood values. Laboratory results are subject to error and may need repeating to ensure accuracy.

Anemia

The history may reveal the most likely cause of hypotension and thereby direct the chiropractor to streamline the differential assessment and design a treatment trial that is practical for the patient. A past history of anemia is a strong clue to the probable cause of a presenting case of hypotension. The heart rate may help to differentiate between anemia and hypothyroid or hypoadrenia. With hypotension, one may expect an elevated heart rate if anemia is associated. Hypothyroid patients, however, will usually have a decreased heart rate. Blood laboratory analysis should confirm or refute an anemic condition causing the hypotension. Disorders that cause decreased red cell production or increased red cell destruction must be differentially assessed. Subclinical manifestations of anemia may be managed chiropractically and may be related to nutritional factors such as dietary lack of essential vitamins and iron, or malabsorption due to chronic gastrointestinal disorders. If Vitamin B12 deficiency is suspected, either due to dietary deficiency or malabsorption, a clinical trial of sublingual B12 may be indicated. If malabsorption is suspected, chiropractic assessment for a VSC and a possible somatovisceral relationship is indicated. The middle thoracic to upper lumbar areas are the most likely related areas of involvement; however, no area of the spine should be overlooked.

Adrenocortical Insufficiency

A pre- and poststress blood pressure test may reveal adrenal involvement. Take the blood pressure, and then have the patient hop on one leg 20 times and then the other leg 20 times. Take the blood pressure again. If the systolic pressure does not elevate by at least 20 points, adrenal insufficiency or hypofunction should be suspected. In the absence of the need for medical referral (neoplasm, inflammatory necrosis of the adrenal cortex, etc.), the patient should be managed chiropractically with consultation as to the possibility of stress reduction (a potential cause of adrenal insufficiency) and management of the related spinal areas, principally from T8 to T12. Nutritional support should also be considered (See Hypoadrenalism).

Hypothyroidism

A low functioning thyroid may be a more common cause of hypotension than is traditionally believed. The hypotension may be the result of bradycardia secondary to hypothyroid function (See Hypothyroidism). Concomitant findings associated with hypothyroidism include lethargy, weight gain, intolerance to cold, and dryness of the skin.

RESPIRATORY DISEASE

Infection

Manipulative therapy in the treatment of upper respiratory infections in children has been investigated by Purse

(91). In 4,500 cases of infection, there were 780 instances of complications ranging from simple conjunctivitis and acute otitis media to acute bronchitis and bronchial pneumonia. Upper cervical spinal motion restrictions were associated with acute otitis media. If spinal motion could be maintained or reestablished, complications rarely developed. The results of this study indicated manipulative therapy to be a superior treatment to antimicrobial therapy and that pharmacologic therapy is not indicated unless complications develop.

Other reports by osteopaths (92,93) have advocated a manipulative approach for the treatment of pneumonia. Treatments included mobilization of the cervical and thoracic spine as well as soft tissue manipulation of the paraspinal tissues. In addition, the thoracic pump, a manipulative maneuver designed to increase lymph flow in the region, is thought to be of help (94). In this treatment, the physician applies a pressure over the caudal or cephalad portion of the rib cage in an effort to increase the amount of tidal volume (95). Some authors have advocated an approach that emphasizes specific manipulation at fixated spinal levels and not manipulation applied in some general fashion (96).

Kline (97), in an investigation of combination treatments for respiratory infections, concluded that manipulative therapy in combination with antimicrobial agents was superior to manipulation alone. This study involved 252 patients and included conditions such as pneumonia, tracheobronchitis, tonsillitis, influenza, nasopharyngitis and general upper respiratory infections.

Somatic dysfunction associated with pulmonary disease appears to have a predilection for the segments T1 to T7 and in the upper cervical spine especially at the C2/C3 articulation (98). A report by Beal and Morlock (99) indicated a peak incidence of somatic dysfunction between the T2 and T7 motion segments. Nicholas (100) reports an incidence at T5 bilaterally in 60% of patients with respiratory dysfunction. Fifty percent of the patients demonstrated lower cervical involvement (C4-C7). A review of the literature by Beal (19) has indicated that somatic dysfunction in patients with lung disease occurs primarily at vertebral segments T3 to T5.

Asthma

The lungs are innervated by the pulmonary plexuses. The plexuses are formed by branches from the vagus and efferent sympathetic nerves that arise from the thoracic segments T2 to T5. The efferent vagal fibers are secretomotor to the mucous bronchial glands, and are vasodilator and bronchioconstrictive. When the efferent sympathetic fibers are activated, bronchodilation and vasoconstriction occurs.

There appear to be distinct autonomic abnormalities in asthma. Prolonged sympathetic stimulation in laboratory animals has been shown to decrease lung compliance by 38% (101). This occurs in the absence of gross pulmonary congestion and edema. Excessive mucous secretion and bronchial mucosal edema found in asthma patients are further evidence that asthma and autonomic abnormalities exist (102). A recent publication attributes the development of bronchial asthma to the blocking of β-adrenergic receptor(s) by an antibody (103).

A report by Murphy and Wilson (104) investigated the results of osteopathic adjustments to the fourth and fifth dorsal vertebrae in 20 cases of asthmatics. Seventy-five percent of the cases obtained some relief. A pilot study on the effectiveness of chiropractic treatment on asthma had inconclusive results (105). Controlled or comparison treatment clinical trials are needed.

For the chiropractic management of this condition, it is helpful to classify the asthma as either mucoid (wet) or nonmucoid (dry). Excessive mucous production often follows an acute respiratory infection that may provoke an acute asthmatic attack. The patient will have a "wet" sound during ventilation. There is some literature indicating that parasympathetic nervous system dysfunction will lead to this clinical picture. Clinical observations have associated the upper cervical portion of the spinal column (C0-C5) and asthma which is characterized by excessive mucous secretion (6). Less commonly involved are spinal lesions of the sacroiliac articulations. In the child it is important to consider displacements of unfused sacral segments (e.g., retrolisthesis of S2) as they may be contributory (6). Inhalation of steam may be of help in loosening mucous build-up.

The nonmucoid asthmatic will not have excessive mucous production. The airways will have a "dry" sound during the attack. This is also the type that afflicts the majority of adults who are afflicted with asthma. It has been hypothesized that because of sympathetic depression there is a parasympathetic over-ride which causes bronchoconstriction. During the acute episode the lower thoracic region should be suspected as an area of spinal dysfunction which may be contributory. The dry asthmatic type may have spinal lesions in the lower thoracic (T7-T12) and the cervical thoracic junction (C7-T3) (6). Evidence that adjustments to this area cause increased sympathetic nervous system activity is supported by basic neurologic data by Jindal and Kaur (106). They concluded that bronchodilation was chiefly controlled by the sympathetic nervous system.

During the first 6 weeks of treatment, lesions in the nonsympathetic portions of the spinal column (upper cervical, sacroiliac) should not be adjusted when managing a patient with a dry asthmatic condition (6). Because of hyperventilation, dehydration should be considered as a potential complication after an attack. The patient should avoid refined carbohydrates and fats in the diet (107). Vitamin supplementation including vitamins A, C, E and

B-complex should be encouraged (6). Vitamins C and E plus supplemental bioflavinoids have been found to help inhibit histamine release from mast cells that have been stimulated by various antigens (108).

General Respiratory Dysfunction

Side pain during inspiration may be the result of intercostal neuritis or muscle spasm. A subluxation of the midthoracic region should be suspected (6). Rib subluxations can be considered but tend to be less common than vertebral lesions (6). Dysfunction of the alimentary canal (e.g., hiatal hernia, hyperacidity, gastritis, etc.) may interfere with respiratory function.

Pertussis

Whooping cough is an acute, highly bacterial, contagious, disease characterized by a paroxysmal or spasmodic cough that usually ends in a prolonged, high-pitched, crowing inspiration (the whoop). The disease is serious in children under the age of two with mortality being 1 to 2% before the age of one year (49). It is rarely serious in older children and adults, but the elderly should be closely monitored because the disease can be troublesome in someone with a compromised immune system. Hospitalization is generally recommended for seriously ill infants. Chiropractic care should be provided at the bedside in these instances. Oxygen should be given if cyanosis develops. Monitoring of the nutritional state of the infant is important because preexisting or developing malnutrition can adversely affect the outcome.

The experience of many osteopathic physicians has indicated that those individuals who receive manipulative treatment fare far better than those who do not (109–114). In a comparative clinical investigation between an antibiotic treatment and osteopathic manipulation, Kurschner (115) found superior results in the manipulation group. The ninety-five subjects in the study had their outcomes evaluated by recording the average daily coughing spasms over the course of 12 days. Soft tissue manipulation was performed in the cervical, upper dorsal and middorsal regions. Forceful vertebral adjustments were carried out at those motion segments exhibiting motion restriction. Deviation of the hyoid bone and dysfunction of the articulations of the first and second ribs at the sternal attachments has been hypothesized to influence the course of whooping cough (109).

GASTROINTESTINAL DISEASE

Stomach

The autonomic innervation for the stomach is via the vagus and segmental sympathetics (T6-T10). Osteopathic researchers (115,116) have correlated somatic dysfunction in the upper cervical region (e.g., C1-C2) and in the middorsal region (T5-T10) in patients with disorders of the stomach (e.g., gastritis). Beal (19), in his review of the literature, found similar levels of involvement. Wiles (117) demonstrated motility changes in the stomach after upper cervical manipulations. DeBoer and colleagues (118) showed changes in gastrointestinal myoelectric activity (inhibition) in conscious rabbits after spinal manipulation. Dramatic effects were seen when T6 was stimulated. Similar manipulations at T1, T12 and L3 showed progressively smaller effects.

Gonstead (6) divided gastric disorders into two general types: those affected by the middorsal area (T4-T10) and those caused by upper cervical (e.g., atlas) lesions. Gastritis that was present between meals (empty stomach) and within one-half hour postprandial was generally related to dysfunction of the upper cervical region, especially atlas-axis. Pain 1½ to 2 hours postprandial was correlated with spinal lesions in the midthoracic region (T4-T10). Peptic ulcers were found to be generally related to upper cervical dysfunction (e.g., atlas-axis) and duodenal ulcers to dysfunction of the sympathetic efferents (T4-T10) (6).

Diarrhea

Nonspecific diarrhea (e.g., not due to food poisoning) is often caused by upper cervical subluxations, especially C1-C2 (6). Occasionally, the upper lumbars may be involved. One to two treatments should reveal some improvement in the condition. Dehydration is an important complication. If the skin shows signs of dehydration intravenous rehydration may be needed. Some patients have chronic diarrhea that results from achlorhydria and/or food sensitivities. In these cases folate supplementation may be needed to counteract the deficiency that results from long-standing diarrhea. Diarrhea is common in the child when removed from breast feeding.

Ulcerative Colitis

Ulcerative colitis is a disease of unknown origin. It is characterized by bloody diarrhea. In 10% of patients, a progressive initial attack may become fatal (49). Hemorrhage is the most common local complication. After a differential diagnosis that includes potential bacterial causes, mild cases of ulcerative colitis can be managed by the chiropractor. More severe cases may necessitate medical collaboration. The upper cervical region (C0-C5) should be examined closely and subluxations, if any, reduced as indicated. Jordan et al. (119) describe a case report of a patient who developed a C1-C2 subluxation in association with inflammatory bowel disease (Crohn's). Corticosteroid treatment in patients with severe manifestations is often advocated, however, the long-term side-effects for this form of therapy should be considered by the patient and doctor. Avoidance of sugar and other refined carbohydrates coupled with supplementation of essential minerals and glycosaminoglycans (for healing of tissue) may be helpful (108).

Constipation

Constipation is defined as infrequent or difficult passage of feces. Mechanical bowel obstruction should be considered in patients with acute constipation, particularly in infants. Diet is important in the management of patients with constipation without identifiable organic causes (e.g., diverticulitis). Bulking agents such as bran and psyllium may be helpful. Dietary supplementation of folate and lactobacilli may also be helpful in the overall management (108). The portions of the spinal column most often detected in patients with chronic constipation involve the upper dorsals (T3-T5), the lower thoracics (T8-T12), and the upper lumbars (L1-L4). Occasionally, the upper cervical region (i.e., C1-C2) may be involved (6).

ENDOCRINOLOGIC DISORDERS

Hyperglycemia

Diabetes mellitus is a disorder of carbohydrate metabolism resulting from a variable interaction of hereditary and environmental factors and characterized by abnormal insulin secretion or utilization. This leads to inappropriately elevated blood glucose levels that may manifest in accelerated nonspecific atherosclerosis and other metabolic and vascular disorders such as blindness, kidney disease and neuropathy. Clinical manifestations include polyuria, polydipsia, fatigue, weight loss, and glycosuria.

The nerve supply to the pancreas is derived from the celiac plexus which has preganglionic fibers arising from the vertebral segments T6-T10 (7). Little is known about the afferent supply to the pancreas. The right vagus supplies the pancreas with parasympathetic innervation (120). The nerve fibers are vasomotor (sympathetic) and parenchymal (parasympathetic and sympathetic). Some fibers make synaptic contact with acinar cells before innervating the islets. This suggests a close association between the exocrine and endocrine functions of the pancreas.

Historically, work in the area of carbohydrate metabolism and spinal lesions was carried out by Deason in 1911 (121). Bandeen (122), in 1926, found a specific area of the spine to treat in diabetes through uncontrolled clinical observations. The areas outlined ranged from the tenth dorsal through the first lumbar. They advocated procedures that would improve the mobility in this region. Other osteopathic clinicians found lesions of the lower thoracic region (T5-T10) in patients with pancreatic disorders (123–125). Gonstead (6), through his clinical observations found an association with spinal lesions of the T9-T10 and T10-T11 motion segments and diabetes mellitus.

Hypoglycemia

Blood glucose disturbances characterized by a hypoglycemic state have been detected in patients with subluxation of the upper cervical region, especially C1-C2 (6). This area of the spine is thought to influence the function of the pancreas through vagal interactions. The avoidance of alcohol and refined carbohydrates should be encouraged in the hypoglycemic patient. The mainstay of corrective diets has been a moderately high protein intake (to promote gluconeogenesis). Also, a high fiber intake appears to reduce the rapid insulin secretion that occurs in response to dietary carbohydrates (108).

Hypothyroidism

Although it has been speculated that hypothyroidism (in the advanced stage of the adult it is referred to as myxedema) is the result of an autoimmune disorder (49), the cause is basically unknown. The disease is characterized by weakness, lethargy, decreased sweating, intolerance to cold, enlargement of the tongue, and nonpitting edema of the subcutaneous tissues (126). Disturbances of the menstrual cycle in females and migraine headache may also be related to lowered thyroid function (6,48).

The nerves to the thyroid gland are derived from the superior, middle, and inferior cervical ganglia of the sympathetic chain (7). The ganglions receive their nerve supply from the upper thoracic segmental levels.

Marked reduction in thyroid hormone levels can be determined from blood panels measuring T3, T4. Increased thyroid stimulating hormone (TSH) production would also be present in the primary hypothyroid patient because the pituitary gland will attempt to compensate by secreting more TSH. Low TSH levels in a patient may be indicative of secondary hypothyroidism from pituitary insufficiency. Pain syndromes may be related to hypothyroidism. The theory behind this suggestion is that noxious signals from painful inflamed tissues (e.g., trigger points) are transmitted to the CNS where the secretion of ACTH from the pituitary is stimulated. This, in turn, leads to an elevated secretion of cortisol, which has been shown to reduce the intracellular conversion of T4 to T3, the latter having three to five times the metabolic activity of the former. The standard laboratory tests for serum levels of Free T4 and Free T3 do not indicate whether the intracellular thyroid hormone activity is proportionate or similar to the serum levels.

The use of a basal temperature test has been proposed as a more sensitive test in evaluating thyroid function because lowered body temperature may be indicative of low thyroid or metabolic activity (48). This is best measured at the axilla, and the normal value (morning, before arising) should be between 97.8 and 98.2 degrees. Infection (e.g., sinus infection) may raise the basal temperature, and other dysfunctional states (e.g., pituitary or adrenal gland insufficiency, starvation) may produce a false low reading. Differential diagnosis of the various causes is critical to appropriate management. The basal temperature test should be supplemented with the appropriate blood panel and clinical correlation. The sensitivity and specificity of the basal temperature test have yet to be determined.

Spinal dysfunction at the cervicothoracic junction (C6-T3) has been observed in patients with hypothyroidism (6). Foods high in goitrogens should be avoided. These include cabbage, turnips, rapeseeds, mustard seeds, groundnuts, cassava, and soybeans. They are natural inhibitors to the thyroid, and their effect is inactivated with cooking (89).

Hyperthyroidism

Hyperthyroidism (e.g., Graves' disease) is a disease of unknown origin. It is thought to be caused by antibodies (thyroid stimulating immunoglobulins) that act on TSH receptors to produce inappropriate overstimulation. The most frequent symptoms of hyperthyroidism are nervousness and hyperactivity, increased sweating, hypersensitivity to heat, palpitations, fatigue, increased appetite, weight loss, tachycardia, insomnia, weakness, and frequent bowel movements (occasionally diarrhea) (49). Subluxation of the upper cervical region (C0-C5) may be contributory to the disease process (6).

Hypoadrenalism (Addison's Disease)

Hypoadrenalism etiology is related to progressive destruction of the adrenal cortex from chronic infectious diseases (e.g., tuberculosis, histoplasmosis, cryptococcosis). Some cases of hypoadrenalcorticolism result from the autoimmune destruction of the adrenal cortex with the adrenal medulla left intact. In 70% of patients, the etiology is an idiopathic atrophy of the adrenal gland (49).

The suprarenal plexus is formed by branches from the celiac ganglion, celiac plexus, and the greater splanchnic nerve. It has a larger autonomic supply than any other organ relative to its size (7). The parasympathetic supply is from the vagus and the sympathetics arise from spinal cord levels T8 to L2 (19); therefore, subluxations in these areas should be ruled out (6). Large amounts of Vitamin C are found in the adrenal gland. It is therefore suggested that a supplement be considered in the patient's management. Because smoking increases the body's need for Vitamin C, it should be discouraged. Supplementation with liberal amounts of the B-complex vitamins may be helpful for the patient. These vitamins function as coenzymes for metabolic reactions, compensating for the increased metabolism (89).

Symptoms of hypoglycemia may occur in patients with hypoadrenalism. They should be advised to have food around in case of an attack and to eat small protein-rich meals throughout the day. A meal at bedtime might be useful for preventing early morning hypoglycemia (89).

Other cases of adrenal cortical insufficiency might be the result of the adrenogenital syndrome. In this disorder, certain enzyme deficiencies cause hormonal synthesis to be shunted away from major hormone production (cortisol and aldosterone) to increased production of androgens and some estrogens. The latter hormones do not exert negative feedback on the pituitary secretion of ACTH. This hormone tends to be elevated due to the lack of sufficient serum cortisol exerting a negative feedback. Therefore, the adrenal cortical activity is stimulated greatly, but the amounts of cortisol and aldosterone secretions are subnormal and the secretion of adrenal androgens are elevated. Female patients will tend to have very obvious signs of masculization, but the condition is difficult to detect in males.

Hyperadrenalism

Hyperfunction of the adrenal cortex can result from increased pituitary secretion of ACTH. Excessive production of androgens will result in adrenal virilism and hypersecretion of glucocorticoids produces Cushing's syndrome. Gonstead (6) has hypothesized that subluxations of the upper cervical region (C0-C5) could result in a relative sympathetic override causing hyperadrenalism. The pituitary's influence on adrenal function is well known. Burns (127) has shown how lesions of the upper cervical region can create dysfunction (e.g., edema) of the pituitary gland in laboratory animals.

ARTHRITIS RELATED DISORDERS

Gout

Gonstead (6) found somatic reflections in patients with gout at segmental spinal levels with innervation to the kidneys (T10-L2). He also advised drinking unsweetened cherry juice (not from concentrate) as an adjunct to the diet. The patient should avoid foods high in purine content (89) (See Table 13.3), alcohol, and foods rich in fructose (108).

CANCER

Relatively little is known about the proposed influence of neuromechanical lesions of the spinal column and the promotion of cancer. The sympathetic nervous system (SNS) is concerned with the initiation of the immune or inflammatory response. The chain of reactions that follows leads to cell-mediated, homograft immunity (128). The pathogenesis of cancer has been considered to be related to alteration of the immune system. Paralyzation of the SNS through physical, viral or chemical agents

Table 13.3.
High Purine Content Foods

Anchovies	Heart	Mussels
Bouillon	Herring	Partridge
Brains	Kidney	Roe
Broth	Liver	Sardines
Consommé	Mackerel	Scallops
Goose	Meat Extracts	Sweatbreads
Gravy	Mincemeat	Yeast (Bakers, Brewers)

could promote the evolution of spontaneous, induced or transplanted tumor (129).

Lesions of the SNS have previously been shown to increase the incidence (130,131), induction (132), and, take and growth (133), of a tumor. The participation of the autonomic nervous system in the mechanisms of chemical hepatocarcinogenesis has been well described by Gurkalo and Zabezhinski (134). Pharmacologic activation of the sympathetic nervous system by means of peripheral alpha-adrenoreceptor stimulation and through blocking of beta-adrenoreceptors and cholinoceptors stimulates proliferative activity and hence hepatocarcinogenesis. In contrast, the inhibition of alpha-adrenoreceptor function and stimulation of beta-adrenoreceptors and cholinoreceptors have an anticarcinogenic effect.

Gonstead hypothesized that many cancers, in the absence of obvious carcinogens (e.g., nicotine), were due to generalized inhibition of the sympathetic nervous system. Hypothyroidism was also apparently related. The spinal management of a patient with cancer should have special attention directed at the upper thoracic spine (C6-T3) and other areas that have effects on the sympathetic outflows. This is considered only in the absence of any contraindications to manipulation (e.g., lytic metastasis of the neural arch). Until such time as there is documented therapeutic proof of a positive effect of spinal adjustments on the course of any form of cancer, it is best to explain to the patient that your management is concerned only with reduction of neuromechanical lesions (i.e., subluxation) of the spinal column. Development or aggravation of a preexisting cancer might be prevented or inhibited by a low sugar, low fat, high fiber diet, supplemented with beta-carotene and vitamins A, C and E (108).

Leukemia

The spleen receives sympathetic innervation from spinal levels T7-T10. Its functions include phagocytosis, cytopoiesis, erythrocyte storage, and the initiation of immune responses. Laboratory animals with mechanical lesions of the ninth thoracic vertebra show a spleen larger in size than normal. Blood counts of these animals have a larger proportion of immature granular cells when compared with controls. Blood counts were made for 90 human subjects with ninth thoracic lesions but with no pathognomonic symptoms. Each case demonstrated increased leukocyte count with a greater proportion of granular myelocytes and immature granular cells. In another study, blood counts were performed on 63 patients with splenomedullary leukemia. In each patient, a lesion of the ninth thoracic vertebra was the most marked structural abnormality, other than the enlarged spleen (135). The blinding procedures in this investigation, if any, are unknown. In eight of the patients, the spleen returned to its normal size after correction of the vertebral lesion, and the patients made a complete recovery. The disease in these patients apparently had been in an early stage. About 20% of patients with chronic granulocytic leukemia will survive longer than 5 years and 2 % will survive longer than 10 years (49); therefore, 8 cases from the 63 presented represent an almost insignificant percentage (i.e., 13%) of recovery. It is nonetheless quite interesting, and more aggressive clinical research (cohort study or controlled clinical trials) should be pursued in this area.

NEUROLOGIC DISORDERS

Epilepsy

Epilepsy is a chronic disorder characterized by paroxysmal brain dysfunction due to excessive neuronal discharge (136). The cause for most seizures remains unknown. For those patients who show a high voltage spike on electroencephalography, this may be indicative of an intracranial lesion, usually in the temporal or frontal lobe. Plain radiographs of the skull may provide useful information, particularly in the adult. Computerized tomography (CT) and magnetic resonance imaging (MRI) are important diagnostic aids because approximately 20% of late onset epileptics have operable tumors such as meningiomas. Neurologic consultation is important in the differential diagnosis of epilepsy.

Ancillary tests should include serology for syphilis, electrocardiography to exclude heart block, and blood sugar tests. Hypoglycemia is a potential cause of epilepsy. This can be due to an islet cell tumor or caused by functional disorders of the spine (See Hypoglycemia). Gonstead observed that petit mal seizures were often related to the upper cervical region (6).

Most seizures rarely end with complications. A brief period of cyanosis usually occurs during the tonic phase due to paralyzation of the respiratory muscles. The patient then begins respiration during the clonic phase of contraction. During the clonic phase, the tongue can be bitten and there may be foaming of the mouth.

The condition "status epilepticus" is present when repeated seizures occur without any intervening period of consciousness. Emergency room referral is mandatory. Unless the convulsions are stopped, coma deepens, and death occurs. Status epilepticus can be precipitated by the sudden withdrawal of anticonvulsant medication, especially barbiturates. The seizures may occur several days after the withdrawal of the drugs (137). Headache is a common sequel to seizure, and patients will usually sleep for several hours after an attack.

TEMPORAL RELATIONSHIP

Nocturnal attacks are most likely to occur shortly after going to sleep or between 4 and 5 a.m. The most common time for a diurnal attack is soon after awakening (137). The seizure that occurs within one hour of awakening may be related to subluxation complexes in the upper lumbar spine and thoracic region (6). Gonstead observed that, generally, seizures during the day were associated with upper cervical subluxations, and those that occurred at night, with lesions in the sympathetic nervous system (6).

MANAGEMENT

In the child with epilepsy, an AS condyle should be ruled out because this subluxation can cause severe neurologic dysfunction (See Chapter 11). One to four adjustments should be sufficient for subluxation reduction depending on the chronicity. If there is a regular frequency to the seizure, the upper cervical spine should be suspected (6). Often times seizures will occur just before menstruation in the female. The upper lumbar and lower thoracic spine should be checked in these individuals, because there may be an association between ovarian function (i.e., hormone levels) and the seizure.

If the seizure occurs during the spinal examination this may be helpful in isolating a specific subluxation. Pressure should be applied to the subluxation in the appropriate line of correction or pattern of thrust. If the symptoms abate, then this line of correction should be duplicated during the adjustment (6).

Multiple Sclerosis

Multiple sclerosis (MS) is a disease of unknown origin. Medical treatment of multiple sclerosis usually involves ACTH and corticosteroids, neither of which have shown conclusively that they alter symptomatology during the acute phase or reduce the relapse rate in the chronic patient.

The diagnosis of MS is difficult. The onset is extremely variable and the disease may suddenly develop in otherwise healthy young adults (137). The two major factors in the diagnosis of MS are:

1. Signs and symptoms of disseminated disease
2. A tendency to relapse and remit

The initial symptoms of the disease are usually motor weakness, numbness or paresthesia, and ataxia of gait. Visual symptoms may also occur, such as blurring and diplopia.

The chiropractic management begins first with a proper diagnosis. Special studies such as MRI and CT scanning are helpful when the disease has advanced. Cerebrospinal fluid analysis should be performed because there may be an increase in mononuclear cells and total protein content. Neurologic consultation is recommended due to the need for comprehensive neuropsychological testing.

Many patients report a history of physical trauma at the spinal region which eventually becomes symptomatic (37). Any irritant to the nervous system (e.g., subluxation) could predispose an area to myelin sheath degeneration. Chiropractic treatment may make portions of the nervous system less vulnerable to other alleged mechanisms of MS such as autoimmune interactions or a slow acting virus. A history of a fall on to the buttocks may be reported by some patients necessitating a comprehensive examination of the lower spine, especially the sacroiliac joints and coccygeal region. Subluxation complexes of the upper cervical region (C0-C5) are often present in patients with multiple sclerosis (6). If the individual has a hypolordotic or kyphotic cervical curve, this will place adverse mechanical tension on the spinal cord (See Chapter 2). Efforts to restore the normal lordosis should be implemented. Due to the many remissions characteristic of the natural history of the disease, it is difficult to determine the usefulness of any particular therapy. A low fat diet supplemented with essential fatty acids should be encouraged because this appears to retard the disease process and reduce the incidence of new attacks (138). Heavy metal toxicity has been suggested by some to be related to the development of MS.

Bell's Palsy

Bell's palsy is defined as idiopathic unilateral facial paralysis of sudden onset. It is thought that the mechanism involved is edema of the seventh cranial nerve due to an immune or viral disease. This results in compression and ischemia in the facial nerve as it travels its course through the temporal bone. Other neurologic symptoms are usually not present. If other neurologic signs begin or there is an insidious onset which becomes progressively worse with time, this may indicate a central nervous system lesion such as tumor (139,140).

This disorder is more commonly associated with diabetics and pregnancy. Pain behind the ear usually precedes the facial weakness and complete paralysis may ensue within hours. Other conditions that can produce facial palsy include tumors, herpes zoster infection of the geniculate ganglion, Lyme disease, AIDS, and sarcoidosis. The upper cervical region (C0-C5) should be examined closely. The temporomandibular joint (TMJ) should also be checked because a small proportion of patients may also have dysfunction at this site (6).

Trigeminal Neuralgia

Trigeminal neuralgia, or tic douloureux, is a facial pain syndrome of unknown etiology that usually develops in middle or old age. The reason for the age relationship is unclear. The tic is from a sharp lightning-like pain of the superior mandibular or maxillary branch of the trigeminal nerve.

In many instances the trigeminal nerve is in close relation to vascular structures and compression of the nerve is thought to be the cause of the disorder, but this is yet to be proven. Sensory stimulation, such as the wind blowing on the face, touch, or cold, at "trigger zones" may precipitate an attack. These trigger zones can be very unpredictable. Flexion of the head appears to also precipitate an attack in some patients (141). The anxiety of not knowing what may trigger an attack can lead to severe depression or even suicide.

The upper cervical region is commonly involved in these patients (142). Temporomandibular dysfunction may also be present and should be addressed. The chiropractic management can be difficult at times. For example, it is important to not overadjust an area of involvement. The temperature pattern of a paraspinal thermography instrument should be watched closely. A pattern (e.g., 20-point differential to the right at C1) should be established before commencing adjustive treatment. Only when the pattern is present should an adjustment be performed. An instrumentation reading towards the opposite side on a given day would contraindicate an adjustment (6).

Polio

Approximately 400,000 new cases of polio occur in subtropical and tropical regions each year (143). In most cases the virus enters the oral cavity and causes mild symptoms of fever and gastrointestinal upset lasting a few days. It is frequently not diagnosed (144). A small percentage of patients will have symptoms of central nervous system invasion, such as muscle pain, neck stiffness, headache, high fever and paralysis. The degree of recovery depends on the the number of motor neurons affected. No sensory loss occurs (143). The fever may go as high as 104 to 106 degrees. It should not be artificially lowered and usually resolves after three to four days (6). The use of moist heat over the neck and afflicted muscles is often therapeutic (49). The upper cervical portion of the spinal column should be inspected for the presence of subluxation (6). Virtually any region of the spine may be involved, making management more difficult.

Psoriasis

Psoriasis is a fairly common chronic disease affecting 2 to 4% of the white population and far fewer blacks (49). It is characterized by dry scaling silvery papules and plaques that recur in various sizes on the skin due to accelerated epidermal growth. Many patients present with severe itching. This condition is considered by many to be incurable.

Seven to fifteen percent of people with psoriasis have arthritis associated with it. This arthritis is most common in the small articulations especially the distal interphalangeal joints in the hands, small joints of the feet, sacroiliac joints and the spine. Sixty to seventy-five percent of patients with psoriasis have HLA-B27 in the blood (49).

Spinal lesions in individuals with psoriasis have been found to vary from C7 to L1 (6). The patient should be advised to maintain a balanced diet with limited amounts of red meat and the avoidance of acidic foods. A report by Bittiner et al. (145) has indicated a positive effect after fish oil supplementation. The use of stimulants (e.g., caffeine) should be avoided (6). Exposure to sunlight and treatment with ultraviolet light have sometimes been found to be useful. The skin should be well lubricated after the UV application.

OPHTHALMIC DISORDERS

The eyes and the optic tracts can be considered extensions of the brain. These structures are subject to the same vasomotor reactions as those which affect the rest of the brain and the meninges (146). Retinal examination gives important information concerning the circulation through the brain itself. The nutrition of the eye depends on normal blood flow, which is subject to the vasoconstrictor activities of the nerve centers in the upper thoracic cord segments. The innervation is ipsilateral; the left sympathetic chain affects the blood flow of the left brain and the left eye. Dysfunction of the sympathetic nervous system through lesions of the upper thoracic motion segments may create circulatory disturbances leading to vision disorders.

The fifth and seventh cranial nerves may be affected by lesions of the occiput (146). The edema associated with the inflammatory response can exert pressure on the connective tissues at the base of the skull, the nerves, and their ganglia. Becka (147) has provided a review of the autonomic innervation of the eye. He states, "Cord segment irritation could result in stimulation of the sympathetic preganglionic fibers with resultant hypersympathicotonia, which could alter the balance of the system and result in ocular dysfunction." He and Wilson (148) cite a role for manipulative treatment of the spine in the treatment of amblyopia.

Visual recovery after chiropractic intervention has

been described in a case report by Gilman and Bergstrand (149). The 75-year-old patient made a full recovery after adjustments to the upper cervical region (i.e., atlas).

Briggs and Boone (150) demonstrated direct effects on pupillary diameter following upper cervical adjustments. A parasympathetic response was obtained following atlas adjustments; however, when segments C2 through C5 were adjusted, both parasympathetic and sympathetic responses were observed. The small sample of subjects precludes any definitive statement on whether a parasympathetic or sympathetic response will be seen after adjustments of the cervical spine.

In an experiment using laboratory animals, Burns (151) determined that manually created subluxations of the second thoracic vertebra exerted an immediate influence on the pupillary reactions of the eyes. These changes reversed after reduction of the lesions. Somatic dysfunction of the upper cervical region (C0-C3) and the upper thoracics (T1-T3) should be ruled out in anyone with functional disorders of the eye (151). Indirectly, lesions of the lower thoracic (e.g., T9) vertebrae may influence vision through the development of cataracts from diseases such as diabetes mellitus (146).

Direct manipulation of the eyelids, lacrimal apparatus, cornea, etc. has been advocated by Ruddy (152) in the treatment of many eye disorders (e.g., hordeolum, blepharitis, etc.). Experience has been that the major vertebral lesion should be sought out and reduced. Multiple areas should not be adjusted as this appears to not influence the patient in as optimal a manner (6,146).

OTOVESTIBULAR DISORDERS

Since the first adjustment in 1895 (153), an empirical basis for chiropractic treatment of otologic disorders has been present. The role of the sympathetic nervous system in disorders such as tinnitus, unilateral or bilateral functional hypoacouosis and vertigo is well known. Reflex stimulation of the sympathetic system and purely vascular (compression of the vertebral artery) factors have been implicated in the etiology of these disorders. Terret (154), in his review of the literature advises that patients with symptoms of tinnitus should be given a trial of spinal manipulative therapy, especially in light of the fact that most medical therapies for this disorder are entirely based on empirical evidence. One of the cases he reviews had symptoms of vertigo, tinnitus, and unilateral deafness. The patient finally responded to manipulative treatment when the T4-T5 motion segment was adjusted (similar to Harvey Lillard in 1895).

Management

In a noncontrolled study by Zerillo and Lynch (155), improvement in hearing was noted in 19 of the 59 patients (32%) who received chiropractic treatment. Vertigo remissed in 64% of the patients (n=80) and decreased in the remainder.

A study by Fitz-Ritson (156) of 235 patients with cervicogenic vertigo found that 90% were symptom-free after eighteen treatments. The patients that responded best tended to have primarily upper cervical joint problems (subluxations).

Gonstead (6) found that the upper cervical region, especially C1-C2, were involved in patients with vertigo. Tilting the head towards the involved side will usually accentuate the problem and may help in identifying the lesion. Positive results are generally seen after a few adjustments. Purse (91), in a large series of cases, found that patients with acute otitis media generally had concomitant upper cervical motion restrictions.

RENAL DISEASE

The sympathetic innervation of the kidney arises from segmental spinal levels T10-T12 (19). The vagus nerve supplies the parasympathetic innervation. The main function of the autonomics is vasomotor.

Several osteopathic clinicians and researchers (157–163) have found a correlation between renal disease (e.g., nephritis, failure) and somatic dysfunction of the thoracolumbar junction (T9-L3). Gonstead (6) associated subluxation complexes of primarily the T9-T10 and T10-T11 motion segments in patients with renal failure.

MALE REPRODUCTIVE DISORDERS

Impotence

A careful physical examination is important because neurologic and vascular disorders (e.g., diabetes mellitus), can be the etiology in 20% of cases (49,50). Many patients simply have an exaggerated sympathetic nerve activity accompanied by a depressed parasympathetic activity. The latter must be adequate for the male to have an erection.

Eighty percent of secondary impotencies are caused by psychic factors. Referral to a marriage counselor or clinical psychologist may be indicated if the patient does not respond to reassurance and education about the dysfunction.

Stresses or other circumstances that cause elevated secretion of prolactin (such as the destruction of the prolactin inhibitory dopaminergic nerves in Parkinson's disease) can produce impotence through desensitization of testosterone receptors in the brain.

Urinary bladder and sexual dysfunction and their relation to disorders of the low back have been investigated by Suarez et al. (164). In their series of 97 consecutive male patients they noted that visceral complaints were often associated with disorders such as lumbar disc herniation, spinal stenosis, and segmental instability.

Falk (165) has presented three patients with bowel and bladder dysfunction secondary to lumbar spine disorders. In each case the dysfunction appeared to improve after chiropractic treatment.

References

1. ACA Department of Statistics Completes 1989 Survey. J Am Chiro Assoc 1990;27:80.
2. Lawrence DJ, ed. Fundamentals of chiropractic diagnosis and management. Baltimore: Williams & Wilkins, 1990.
3. Gatterman MI. Chiropractic management of spine related disorders. Baltimore: Williams & Wilkins, 1990.
4. Meade TW, Dyer S, Browne W, Townsend J, Frank AO. Low back pain of mechanical origin: randomized comparison of chiropractic and hospital outpatient treatment. Br Med J 1990;300:1431–1437.
5. Goble ME. The master's touch: A history of C.S. Gonstead and his legacy. Gonstead Clinical Studies Society, MT Horeb, WI, 1990.
6. Audiotape, videotape, and written notes from the Gonstead Seminar of Chiropractic 1964–1991, Mt. Horeb WI.
7. Williams PL, Warwick R, eds. Grays Anatomy. 36th British ed. Philadelphia: W.B. Saunders Co., 1980.
8. Greenspan J, Melchior J. The effect of osteopathic manipulative treatment on the resistance of rats to stressful situations. J Am Osteopath Assoc 1966;65:1205–9.
9. Brdlik OB, Melchior JB. Manipulation of albino rats: an effect on reaction to cold stress. J Am Osteopath Assoc 1972;72:105.
10. Melchior JB, Brdlik OB. Manipulation of albino rats: an effect on reaction to cold. Am J Osteopath Assoc 1974;73:443–445.
11. Leach RA. The chiropractic theories: a synopsis of scientific research. 2nd ed. Baltimore: Williams & Wilkins, 1986.
12. Denslow JS, Korr IM, Krems AD. Quantitative studies of chronic facilitation in human motoneuron pools. Am J Physiology 1947;150:229–238.
13. Korr IM, Goldstein MJ. Dermatomal autonomic activity in relation to segmental motor reflex threshold. Fed Proc 1948;7:67.
14. Korr IM, Thomas PE, Wright HM. Patterns of electrical skin resistance in man. J Neural Transmission 1958;17:77–96.
15. Wright HM, Korr IM, Thomas PE. Local and regional variations in cutaneous vasomotor tone of the human trunk. J Neural Transmission 1960;22:34–52.
16. Wright HM, Korr IM. Neural and spinal components of disease: progress in the application of thermography. J Am Osteopath Assoc 1965;64:918–921.
17. Korr IM. Sustained sympathicotonia as a factor in disease. In: Korr IM, ed. The neurobiologic mechanisms in manipulative therapy. New York: Plenum Publishing Corp, 1978:229–268.
18. Korr IM. The spinal cord as organizer of disease processes: the peripheral autonomic nervous system. J Am Osteopath Assoc 1979;79:82–90.
19. Beal MC. Viscerosomatic reflexes: a review. J Am Osteopath Assoc 1985;85:786–801.
20. Harris W, Wagnon RJ. The effects of chiropractic adjustments on distal skin temperature. J Manipulative Physiol Ther 1987;10:57–60.
21. Mitchell GAG. Anatomy of the autonomic nervous system. London: E and S Livingstone Ltd, 1955:116–118.
22. Randall WC, Cox JW, Alexander WF, Coldwater KB, Hertzman AB. Direct examination of the sympathetic outflows in man. J Appl Physiol 1955;7:688–698.
23. Richter CP, Woodruff BG. Lumbar sympathetic dermatomes in man determined by the electrical skin resistance method. J Neurophysiol 1945;8:323–338.
24. Wurtman RJ, Wurtman JJ, eds. Nutrition and the brain, vol. 3 New York: Raven Press, 1979:V-VI.
25. Growden JH. Neurotransmitter precursors in the diet: Their use in the treatment of brain diseases. In: Wurtman RJ, Wurtman JJ, eds. Nutrition and the brain, vol. 3. New York: Raven Press, 1979.
26. Forsling ML, Grossman A. Neuroendocrinology: a clinical text. Philadelphia: Charles Press, 1986:82.
27. Widman FK. Clinical interpretation of laboratory tests. 9th ed. Philadelphia: F.A. Davis Co., 1983.
28. Willoughby J. Primal prescription. Eating Well 1991;1:52–59.
29. U.S. Department of Health and Human Services, Public Health Service. The Surgeon General's Report on Nutrition and Health. BH (PHS) Publication No. 88–50210, 1988.
30. U.S. Veterans Administration Nutritional Care Services. Diet Manual. Long Beach, CA: Veterans Administration Medical Center, 1987.
31. Theisler CW. Seminars in Chiropractic: Chronic headache pain. Baltimore: Williams & Wilkins, 1990:2.
32. Formisano R, Buzzi MG, Cerbo R, et al. Idiopathic headaches: a neurophysiological and computerized electromyographic study. Headache 1988;28:426–429.
33. Cremata EE. Chiropractic management of cephalgia. Dig Chiro Econ 1984;May/June:34–36.
34. Saadah HA, Taylor FB. Sustained headache syndrome associated with tender occipital nerve zones. Headache 1987;27:201–205.
35. Wight SJ. Migraine: a statistical analysis of chiropractic treatment. J Am Chiro Assoc 1978;12:63–67.
36. Takeshima T, Takao Y, Takahashi K. Pupillary sympathetic hypofunction and asymmetry in muscle contraction headache and migraine. Cephalgia 1987;7:257–262.
37. Balduc HA. Neurological system. In: Lawrence DJ, ed. Fundamentals of chiropractic diagnosis and management. Baltimore: Williams & Wilkins, 1990:112–113.
38. Vernon H. Spinal manipulation and headaches of cervical origin: a review of literature and presentation of cases. J Manual Medicine 1991;6:73–79.
39. Parker GB, Pryor DS, Tupling H. Why does migraine improve during a clinical trial? Further results from a trial of cervical manipulation for migraine. Aust NZ J Med 1980;10:192–198.
40. Mansfield LE, Vaughan TR, Waller SF, Haverly RW, Ting S. Food allergy and adult migraine: double blind and mediator confirmation of an allergic etiology. Annals Allergy 1985;55:126–129.
41. Bracker M, Rothrock JF. Cluster headache among athletes: a case conference. The Physician and Sportsmedicine 1989;17:147–151, 154, 158.
42. Fanciullacci M, Fusco BM, Alessandri M, Campagnolo V, Sicuteri F. Unilateral impairment of pupillary response to trigeminal nerve stimulation in cluster headache. Pain 1989;36:185–191.
43. Scherokman B, Massey W. Post-traumatic headaches. Neuro Clinic 1983;1:457–463.
44. Terret AGJ. Vascular accidents from cervical spine manipulation: report on 107 cases. J Aust Chiro Assoc 1987;17:15–24.
45. Terret AGJ. Letter to the editor. Chiropractic Technique 1990;2:201–202.
46. Browning JE. Pelvic pain and organic dysfunction in a patient with low back pain: response to distractive manipulation: a case presentation. J Manipulative Physiol Ther 1987;10:116.
47. Browning JE. Mechanically induced pelvic pain and organic dysfunction in a patient without low back pain. J Manipulative Physiol Ther 1990;13:406–411.
48. Barnes BO. Hypothyroidism: the unsuspected illness. New York: Harper & Row, 1976.
49. Berkow R, Fletcher AJ, eds. The Merck Manual, 15th ed. New Jersey: Merck & Co, Inc., 1987.
50. Petersdorf RG, Adams RD, Braunwald E, Isselbacher KJ, Martin JB, Wilson JD, eds. Harrison's principles of internal medicine, 10th ed. New York: McGraw-Hill Inc., 1983.
51. Braunwald E. The sympathetic nervous system in heart failure. Hosp Practice 1970;5:31.
52. Raab W. Nonvascular metabolic myocardial vulnerability factor

in coronary artery disease: fundamentals of pathogenesis, treatment and prevention. Am Heart J 1963;66:685–706.
53. Hall GE. An experimental production of coronary thrombosis and myocardial failure. J Can Med Assoc 1936;34:9–15.
54. Manning GW. Vagus stimulation in the production of myocardial damage. J Can Med Assoc 1937;37:314–318.
55. Ehrlich JC, Shinohara Y. Low incidence of coronary thrombosis in myocardial infarction: a study of serial block technique. Arch Pathol 1964;78:432–445.
56. Kemp HG, Elliott WC, Gorlin R. The anginal syndrome with normal coronary arteriography. Trans Assoc Am Physicians 1967;80:59–70.
57. Likoff W . Paradox of normal selective arteriograms in patients considered to have unmistakable coronary artery disease. N Engl J Med 1967;276:1063–1066.
58. Proudfit WL, Shirey EK, Sones FM. Selective cine coronary arteriography: correlation with clinical findings in 1,000 patients. Circulation 1966;33:901–910.
59. Marchandise B, Bourassa MG, Chaitman BR, Lesperance J. Angiographic evaluation of the nature of normal coronary arteries and mild coronary atherosclerosis. Am J Cardiol 1978;41:216–220.
60. Ockene IS, Shay MYJ, Alpert JS, Weiner BH, Dalen JE. Unexplained chest pain in patients with normal coronary arteriograms: a follow-up study of functional status. N Engl J Med 1980;303:1249–1252.
61. Rogers JT, Rogers JC. The role of osteopathic manipulative therapy in the treatment of coronary heart disease. J Am Osteopath Assoc 1976;76:71–81.
62. Brodsky A. Cervical angina: a correlative study with emphasis on the use of coronary arteriography. Spine 1985;10:699–709.
63. Matoba T, Ohkita Y, Chiba M, Toshima H. Noninvasive assessment of the autonomic nervous tone in angina pectoris: an application of digital plethysmyography with auditory stimuli. Angiology 1983;Feb:127–135.
64. Appleyard EC. Angina pectoris with special reference to its mechanical causes. J Am Osteopath Assoc 1938;37:245–247.
65. Hall LR. Angina pectoris with special reference to its mechanical causes. J Am Osteopath Assoc 1938;37:181–183.
66. Becker AD. Manipulative osteopathy in cardiac therapy. J Am Osteopath Assoc 1939;38:317–319.
67. Becker AD. Osteopathy's contribution to the treatment of cardiac disease. J Am Osteopath Assoc 1942;42:1–2.
68. Burns L, Treat L. Incidence of certain etiologic factors in cardiac disorders. J Am Osteopath Assoc 1953;52:369–372.
69. Burns L. Preliminary report of cardiac changes following correction of third thoracic lesions. J Am Osteopath Assoc 1942;42:3–8.
70. Burns L. Review of cardiac pathology in certain laboratory animals. J Am Osteopath Assoc 1945;45:115–116.
71. Rogers F, Glassman J, Kavieff R. Effects of osteopathic manipulative treatment on autonomic nervous system function in patients with congestive heart failure. J Am Osteopath Assoc 1986;86:605.
72. Koch RS. A somatic component in heart disease. J Am Osteopath Assoc 1961;60:735–740.
73. Goldberger E. Heart disease: its diagnosis and treatment. 2nd Ed. Philadelphia: Lea & Febiger, 1955.
74. Marcus AJ, Kernis ID. The effects of osteopathic manipulative techniques upon bloodflow using the electrical impedance plethysmograph. J Am Osteopath Assoc 1969;68:1047–1051.
75. Figar S, Krausove L. A plethysmographic study of effects of chiropractic treatment in vertebrogenic syndromes. Acta Univ Carol [Med] Praha 1965;21.
76. Beal MC. Palpatory testing for somatic dysfunction in patients with cardiovascular disease. J Am Osteopath Assoc 1983;82:822–831.
77. Rosero HO. Correlation of palpatory observations with anatomic locus of acute myocardial infarction. J Am Osteopath Assoc 1987;87:118–122.
78. Nicholas AS, DeBias DA, Ehrenfeuchter W, et al. A somatic component to myocardial infarction. Br Med J 1985;291:13–17.
79. Nicholas AS . A somatic component to myocardial infarction. J Am Osteopath Assoc 1987;87:123–129.
80. Cox JM, Gorbis S, Dick LM, Rogers JC, Rogers FJ. Palpable musculoskeletal findings in coronary artery disease: results of a double blind study. J Am Osteopath Assoc 1983;82:832–836.
81. Nathan H. Osteophytes of the spine compressing the sympathetic trunk and splanchnic nerves in the thorax. Spine 1987;12:527–532.
82. Cox JM, Rogers FJ. Incidence of osteophytic lipping of the thoracic spine in coronary heart disease-results of a pilot study. J Am Osteopath Assoc 1983;82:837–38.
83. Lewit K. Manipulative therapy in rehabilitation of the locomotor system. London: Butterworth and Co, 1985.
84. Freedman LJ. The beneficial effects of spinal adjustments on premature ventricular contractions: a case study. Research Forum 1985;Autumn:13–16.
85. Miller WD. Treatment of visceral disorders by manipulative therapy. In: Goldstein M, ed. The research status of spinal manipulative therapy. NINCDS Monograph No. 15, 1975:295–301.
86. Robbins SL, Cotran RS. Pathological basis of disease. 2nd ed. Philadelphia: W.B. Saunders, 1979: 1164.
87. Wickes DJ. Cardiovascular disorders in ambulatory patients. In: Lawrence DJ, ed. Fundamentals of chiropractic diagnosis and management. Baltimore: Williams & Wilkins 1990:221–264.
88. Crawford JP, Hickson GS, Wiles MR. The management of hypertensive disease: a review of spinal manipulation and the efficacy of conservative therapeusis. J Manipulative Physiol Ther 1986;9:27–31.
89. Krause MV, Mahan LK. Food, nutrition and diet therapy. Philadelphia: W.B. Saunders Co., 1984.
90. Sato A, Swenson R. Sympathetic nervous system response to mechanical stress of the spinal column in rats. J Manipulative Physiol Ther 1984;7:141–147.
91. Purse FM. Manipulative therapy of upper respiratory infections in children. J Am Osteopath Assoc 1966;65:964–972.
92. Horton ER. Osteopathic manipulative treatment in pneumonia. J Am Osteopath Assoc 1940;39:511–513.
93. Litton HE. Manipulative treatment of pneumonia. J Am Osteopath Assoc 1942;41:228–230.
94. Allen T. Use of thoracic pump in treatment of lower respiratory tract disease. J Am Osteopath Assoc 1967;67:408–411.
95. Facto LL. The osteopathic treatment for lobar pneumonia. J Am Osteopath Assoc 1947;46:385–392.
96. Hoag JM. Musculoskeletal involvement in chronic lung disease. J Am Osteopath Assoc 1972;71:698–706.
97. Kline CA. Osteopathic manipulative therapy, antibiotics and supportive therapy in respiratory infections in children: a comparative study. J Am Osteopath Assoc 1965;65:278–281.
98. Long FA. Study of the segmental incidence of certain spinal changes in various disorders. Osteopath Dig 1940;6:11.
99. Beal MC, Morlock JW. Somatic dysfunction associated with pulmonary disease. J Am Osteopath Assoc 1984;84:179–183.
100. Nicholas NS. Correlation of somatic dysfunction with visceral disease. J Am Osteopath Assoc 1975;75:425–428.
101. Droste PL, Beckman DL. Pulmonary effects of prolonged sympathetic stimulation. Proc Soc Exp Biol Med 1974;146:352.
102. Kaliner M, Shelhamer JH, Davis PB etal. Autonomic nervous system abnormalities and asthma. Ann Internal Med 1982;96:349–357.
103. Granner DK. Characteristics of hormone systems. In: Murray RK, Granner DK, Mayes PA, Rodwell VW, eds. Harper's biochemistry. 22nd ed. Norwalk: Appleton & Lange, 1990:465.

104. Murphy WP, Wilson PT. A study of the value of osteopathic adjustment of the fourth and fifth thoracic vertebrae in a series of twenty cases of asthmatic bronchitis. Boston Med Surg J 1925;192:440–442.
105. Jamison JR, Leskovec K, Lepore S, Hannan P. Asthma in a chiropractic clinic: a pilot study. J Aust Chiro Assoc 1986;16:137–143.
106. Jindal SK, Kauer SJ. Relative bronchodilatory responsiveness attributable to sympathetic and parasympathetic activity in bronchial asthma. Respiration 1989;56:1–2.
107. Cessna RM. The asthmatic patient. Nutritional Perspectives 1990;Oct:12–13.
108. Werbach MR. Nutritional influences on illness. Tarzana, CA: Third Line Press, 1987:24–25.
109. Heist ED. Whooping cough. J Am Osteopath Assoc 1925;25:94.
110. Andrews EC. Superiority of osteopathy in treatment of whooping cough. J Am Osteopath Assoc 1930;30:155.
111. Wagner LC. Pertussis—its diagnosis and treatment. J Am Osteopath Assoc 1933;32:478.
112. Cunningham EJ. Acute diseases of childhood. J Am Osteopath Assoc 1948;47:495–497.
113. Wagner LC. Recent advances in acute diseases of childhood. J Am Osteopath Assoc 1949;48:462–464.
114. Rosman D. Role of osteopathic lesion in acute infectious diseases. J Am Osteopath Assoc 1952;52:169–172.
115. Kurschner OM. A comparative clinical investigation of chloramphenicol and osteopathic manipulative therapy of whooping cough. J Am Osteopath Assoc 1958;57:559–561
116. Mattern AV. Gastro-duodenal ulcer and its non-surgical treatment. J Am Osteopath Assoc 1934;33:188–191.
117. Wiles M. Observations on the effects of upper cervical manipulation on the electrogastrogram. J Manipulative Physiol Ther 1980;3:226–228.
118. DeBoer KF, Schutz M, McKnight ME. Acute effects of spinal manipulation on gastrointestinal myoelectric activity in conscious rabbits. Manual Medicine 1988;3:85–94.
119. Jordan JM, Obeid LM, Allen NB. Isolated atlantoaxial subluxation as the presenting manifestation of inflammatory bowel disease. Am J Med 1986;80:517.
120. Rinaman L, Miselis RR. The organization of vagal innervation of rat pancreas using cholera toxin-horseradish peroxidase conjugate. J Auton Nerv Syst 1987;21(2-3):109–125.
121. Deason J. Relation of spinal lesions to carbohydrate metabolism. J Am Osteopath Assoc 1911;10:469–475.
122. Bandeen SG. Specific areas of the spine to treat in diabetes. J Am Osteopath Assoc 1926;Feb.
123. Magoun HI. Osteopathic diagnosis and therapy for the general practitioner. J Am Osteopath Assoc 1948;48:169–172.
124. Gutensohn MT. Diagnosis of pancreatitis. J Am Osteopath Assoc 1955;54:375–377.
125. Wilson PT. A case of diabetic acidosis. In. Academy of Applied Osteopathy 1942 Year Book. American Academy of Osteopathy, Newark, Ohio, 1942.
126. Chusid JG. Correlative neuroanatomy and functional neurology. 19th ed. Los Altos, CA: Lange Medical Publishers, 1985:413.
127. Burns L. Similar effects of different lesions. J Am Osteopath Assoc 1946;45:545–547.
128. Stein-Werblowsky R. The sympathetic nervous system and cancer. Experimental Neurol 1974;42:97–100.
129. Stein M, Schiavi RC, Camerino M. Influence of brain and behavior on the immune system. Science 1976;191:435.
130. Coujard R, Chevreau J. Cancers de types divers provoques par lesion du sympathique. C.R. Acad Sci 1957;244:2434.
131. Coujard R, Heitz F. Production de tumeurs malignes consecutives a des lesions des fibres sympathiques du nerf sciatique chez le cobaye. C.R. Acad Sci 1957;244:409.
132. Champy C. Lesions neuro-sympathiques precedant la cancerisation dans l'attaque de l'organisme par les substances cancerigenes. C.R. Acad Sci 1959;248:3665.
133. Inouye T. Neuropathologische Versuche ueber die Organaffinitact der boesartigen Geschwuelste. Arch Jap Chir 1959;28:1580.
134. Gurkalo VK, Zabezhinski MA. On participation of the autonomic nervous system in the mechanisms of chemical carcinogenesis. Neoplasma 1982;29:301–307.
135. Burns L. Certain boney lesions which affect blood. J Am Osteopath Assoc 1931;30:359–361.
136. Stedman's medical dictionary. 25th ed. Baltimore: Williams & Wilkins, 1990.
137. Bannister R. Brain's clinical neurology. 6th ed. London: Oxford University Press, 1985.
138. Swank RL. Multiple sclerosis; twenty years on a low fat diet. Arch Neurol 1970;23:460–474.
139. May M, Hughes GB. Facial nerve disorders: update 1987. Am J Otology 1987;8:167–180.
140. Palmieri NF. Idiopathic facial paralysis: mechanism, diagnosis, and conservative chiropractic management. Chiropractic Technique 1990;2:182–187.
141. Brieg A. Adverse mechanical tension in the central nervous system. Stockholm: Almqvist & Wiksell International, 1978.
142. Wilson PT. Tic douloureux. J Am Osteopath Assoc 1942;41:395–396.
143. Raymond CA. Worldwide assault on poliomyelitis gathering support, garnering results. JAMA 1986;255:1541–6.
144. Westbrook MT. Clients' evaluations of chiropractic treatment for post polio syndrome. J Austral Chiro Assoc 1990;20:143–151.
145. Bittiner SB, Tucker WFG, Cartwright I, Bleehen SS. A double-blind, randomised, placebo-controlled trial of fish oil in psoriasis. Lancet 1988;1:378–380.
146. Burns L. Eyes and vertebral lesions. J Am Osteopath Assoc 1941;40:487–489.
147. Becka EA. Autonomic innervation of the eye. J Am Osteopath Assoc 1966;66:161–165.
148. Wilson EE. Evaluation of osteopathic therapy in amblyopia. In: Collected papers by members of the osteopathic college of ophthalmology and otolaryngology. 1965;4:5–8.
149. Gilman G, Bergstrand J. Visual recovery following chiropractic intervention. Chiropractic 1990;6:61–63.
150. Briggs L, Boone WR. Effects of a chiropractic adjustment on changes in pupillary diameter: a model for evaluating somatovisceral response. J Manipulative Physiol Ther 1988;11:181–189.
151. Burns L. Study of certain structures concerned in pupillary reactions following second thoracic lesions. J Am Osteopath Assoc 1937;36:409–410.
152. Ruddy TJ. Osteopathic manipulation in eye, ear, nose and throat disease. J Am Osteopath Assoc 1942;41:447–452.
153. Palmer DD. The science, art and philosophy of chiropractic. Portland: Portland Printing House Company, 1910.
154. Terret AGJ. Tinnitus, the cervical spine, and spinal manipulative therapy. Chiropractic Technique 1989;1:41–45.
155. Zerillo G, Lynch M. Importance of chiropractic in oto-vestibular pathology. Chiropractic Interprofessional Research. Mazzarelli JP, ed. Torino: Edizioni Minerva Medica, 1982.
156. Fitz-Ritson D. Assessment of cervicogenic vertigo. J Manipulative Physiol Ther 1991;14:193–198.
157. Conn RW. Osteopathic principles supporting manipulative treatment in nephritis. J Am Osteopath Assoc 1941;40:494–496.
158. Ellis SA. Osteopathic and surgical diagnosis of the abdomen. J Am Osteopath Assoc 1907;6:406–411.
159. Gibson JW. The significance of spinal reflexes due to visceral disturbance. Western Osteopath 1925;20:11–12.
160. Magoun HI. Diagnosis in acute conditions. J Am Osteopath Assoc 1928;28:105–106.

161. Nelson CR. Symposium: urologic manifestations of man's constitutional inadequacies. Structural diagnosis and treatment. J Am Osteopath Assoc 1954;53:255–257.
162. Smith FH. Osteopathic treatment of organic kidney lesions. J Am Osteopath Assoc 1912;11:848–852.
163. Strachan WF. Manipulative treatment of kidney disease. J Am Osteopath Assoc 1933;33:176–177.
164. Suarez GM, Larocca H, Baum NH. Sexual and bladder dysfunction in patients with lumbar pain syndromes (abstract). J Urol 1986;135(4):264.
165. Falk JW. Bowel and bladder dysfunction secondary to lumbar dysfunctional syndrome. Chiropractic Technique 1990;2:45–48.

Appendix 13A. Increased Fiber Diet

Description

This is a regular diet with the substitution of whole grain breads and cereals, and increased amounts of fruits and vegetables. The diet contains approximately 8–9 grams of crude fiber in contrast to 3–4 grams in the regular diet.

Indications for Use

The aims of this diet are to:

1. Increase the weight and volume of residue reaching the large intestine.
2. Increase gut motility and normalize transit time.
3. Decrease intraluminal colonic pressure.

For many patients with chronic constipation and some with diverticular disease and irritable bowel syndrome, this diet may promote more regular bowel habits and partial relief of symptoms.

This diet is contraindicated when changes due to inflammation have caused stenosis or narrowing of the intestinal lumen.

Nutritional Adequacy

The diet provides at least the proportions of nutrients provided by the regular diet. However, absorption of calcium, iron, zinc and possibly other trace minerals may be compromised by this diet.

Dietary Guide

Food Group	Foods Included	Foods Excluded
Beverages	All	None
Breads	All. Include 3 or more servings daily of whole grain products.	None
Cereals	All. Include 1 serving of bran cereal daily.	None
Desserts	All. Suggestions include desserts with coconut, nuts, raisins, dates, seeds, or fresh fruit with skin.	None
Eggs	All	None
Fats	All	None
Fruits and Juices	All. Include at least 2 servings of fruit daily, preferably fresh fruit with skin.	None
Meats	All	None
Potatoes and Alternatives	All	None
Soups	All	None
Sweets	All	None
Vegetables	All. Include at least 4 servings daily, 2 raw.	None

Appendix 13B. Fat Restricted Diet

Description

This diet limits the quantity of dietary fat to approximately 50 grams per day.

Indications For Use

The physician may choose this diet for a variety of conditions. Some examples include pancreatitis, multiple sclerosis, gallbladder disease, and type I hyperlipoproteinemia. The diet may be used in other disease states in which a disturbance in the digestion or absorption of fat occurs.

Nutritional Adequacy

This diet meets the Recommended Daily Dietary Allowances with the exception of the iron requirement for women.

Kilocalories = 1700
Carbohydrate = 217 gm
Protein = 76 gm
Fat = 47 gm

Dietary Guide

Food Group	Foods Included	Foods Excluded
Beverages	All except those in other food groups.	See other groups.
Breads	Regular bread, rolls crackers except as noted.	Biscuits, pancakes waffles, muffins, sweet rolls, doughnuts. Other rich breads and rolls.
Cereals	All cooked or ready-to-eat cereals except as noted.	Dry cereals containing coconut or coconut oil.
Cheese	Dry curd or low-fat cottage cheese. Low-fat processed	Cheeses made from whole milk, cream cheese, spreads.

	cheese. Natural cheese made from skim milk: mozzarella, hoop, farmer, sapsago, ricotta, etc.	
Desserts	Sherbet, gelatin, ices, pudding made with non-fat milk, Angel food or sponge cakes, jelly roll.	Other desserts rich in fat: pastry, cake, cookies, ice cream, ice milk, custard, mousse. Desserts made with whipped topping, chocolate, nuts.
Eggs	Any style, limit to one per day.	Excessive fat or whole milk in preparation.
Fats	Limited quantity of butter, margarine, oil, mayonnaise, sour cream, regular salad dressing.	Other fats unless approved by the doctor or dietitian.
Fruits and Juices	All except as noted.	Avocado, coconut.
Meat and Substitutes	Limited quantity of lean beef, lamb, pork, ham, veal, chicken turkey. Liver. Lean luncheon meats such as chicken, turkey, ham, roast beef. All fish and shellfish.	Fatty meats, skin of poultry. Fried meats, poultry, fish. Sausage, bacon, frankfurters, bologna, salami. Duck and goose. Fish canned in oil.
Milk	Fluid, evaporated, or powdered non-fat milk. Non-fat yogurt, buttermilk.	Whole or low-fat milk, half and half, cream.
Potatoes and Alternatives	Plain white or sweet potatoes, rice, pasta, dried beans, and peas.	Fried potatoes, potato or corn chips. Dishes made with whole milk or added fat. Refried beans, pork and beans.
Soups	Bouillon, fat-free broth, fat-free vegetable soup. Cream soup made with non-fat milk.	All others.
Sweets	Plain sugar, jam, jelly, honey, syrup. Plain sugar candy.	Candies made with fat, chocolate, coconut.
Vegetables	All except as noted.	Vegetables prepared with added fat, cream or cheese sauces. Olives.
Miscellaneous	Spices and herbs of all kinds. Condiments except as previously noted. Spray-on vegetable coating for cookware.	Nuts, peanut butter. Rich gravies and sauces.

Appendix 13C. Low Cholesterol Diet

Description

Cholesterol from dietary sources is reduced to 300 mg. or less. Foods containing polyunsaturated fat are increased and foods containing saturated fat are limited so that the P/S ratio will be between 1.5 and 2.0.

Indications for Use

For patients with hypercholesterolemia (Type IIa).

Nutritional Adequacy

This diet meets the Recommended Daily Dietary Allowances with the exception of the iron requirement for women.

Kilocalories = 1800
Carbohydrate = 235 gm
Protein = 81 gm
Fat = 62 gm
Cholesterol = 170 mg

Dietary Guide

Food Group	Foods Included	Foods Excluded
Beverages	All except those noted in other food groups.	None.
Breads	All regular breads, rolls, crackers except as noted. Baked goods, pancakes, waffles, French toast containing no whole milk or egg yolk and made with allowed fat.	Egg or cheese bread, commercial sweet rolls, buttery rolls. Flavored crackers and snack foods made with saturated fat.
Cereals	All cooked or ready-to-eat cereals except as noted.	Cereals containing coconut or coconut oil.
Cheese	Low-fat cottage cheese, low-fat processed cheese. Natural cheeses made from skim milk: mozzarella, hoop, farmer's, Sapsago, ricotta, etc.	Cheeses made from whole milk. Cream cheese, cheese spreads.

Desserts	Sherbet, gelatin, ices. Puddings made with non-fat milk. Baked desserts made with skim milk and allowed fats.	Regular commercial baked desserts, custard, ice cream, ice milk. Desserts containing egg yolks, whole milk, saturated fat, chocolate, coconut.
Eggs	Any style egg or egg substitute. Limit egg yolks to 2–3 per week.	None.
Fats	Polyunsaturated oils and margarine. Oil-based salad dressings. Mayonnaise and mayonnaise type dressings. Use 1 tsp. for each ounce of meat consumed.	Butter, lard, suet, salt pork, meat drippings, gravy, cream, hydrogenated vegetable shortening, palm oil, coconut oil. Salad dressings containing cheese, cream, sour cream.
Fruits and Juices	All.	Large amounts of avocado.
Meat and Substitute	Limit quantity to 6 ounces per day. Use lean beef, lamb, pork, ham only four times per week. May use veal, chicken, turkey, fish, shellfish (except as noted) at other meals. Lean cold cuts such as chicken, turkey, ham, roast beef. "Natural style" peanut butter preferred- 2 tablespoons may substitute for 1 ounce of meat.	Fatty meats. Sausage, bacon, hot dogs, salami, bologna, organ meats, Goose, duck. Poultry skin. Shrimp. Meats in rich sauces or gravies. Hydrogenated peanut butter.
Milk	Fluid, evaporated or powdered, non-fat milk, non-fat yogurt, buttermilk, fluid non-dairy creamer such as Mocha Mix.	Whole or low-fat milk. Cream, powdered non-dairy creamer.
Potatoes and Substitutes	White and sweet potatoes, rice, pasta, dried beans.	Dishes made with whole milk, egg yolk, cheeses or fats not allowed. Potato chips made with saturated fat. Refried beans, pork and beans. Egg noodles.
Soup	Bouillon, fat-free broth, fat-free vegetable soup, cream soup made with non-fat milk.	All others.
Sweets	Plain sugar and sugar candies. Jam, jelly, honey, syrup.	All other candy.
Vegetables	All raw and cooked vegetables prepared with allowed fat. All vegetable juices.	Vegetables prepared with cream, butter, cheese sauces or saturated fats.
Miscellaneous	Spices and herbs of all kinds. Condiments except as previously noted. Small quantities of nuts except as noted. Cocoa powder. Spray-on vegetable coating for cookware.	Cashew and macadamia nuts.

14 Chiropractic Approaches to Pregnancy and Pediatric Care

CLAUDIA ANRIG HOWE

As the twig is bent, the tree inclines.

VIRGIL (19–70 BC)

The factors that cause a vertebral subluxation complex in children warrant our exploration and investigation. When does the first subluxation occur? Does the possibility of preventing or eliminating the impact of vertebral subluxation exist? These questions and hypotheses should be posed by Doctors of Chiropractic and the supporting research community. This chapter discusses the role of chiropractic care in children. Because many spinal abnormalities can be due to in-utero factors, the care of the pregnant patient is also presented.

In the mature spine, skeletal structure primarily dictates function, particularly joint movement. For the developing spine, the functional demands drive the formation of bones and joints. Hippocrates noted that individual constraint caused physical alterations, because they altered normal function (1,2). A constraint position held over a sufficient period of time can influence the outcome of physical form (1,2). These physical alterations can then lead to abnormal function.

DEVELOPMENTAL AND INJURY MECHANISMS

The morphogenesis of bone, cartilage, ligament, and muscle are influenced by biomechanical forces. The human fetus will develop seven times more quickly than the infant. Because of this rapid growth, the fetus is most sensitive to biomechanical forces that lead to constraining pressures and molding (2,3). There are two factors that can alter morphogenesis: intrinsic and extrinsic. Intrinsic hormonal and biomechanical mechanisms can influence the genetically predetermined shape of bone. The physical properties that contribute to internal resistance and deformation of bone are fatigue strength, elasticity, energy absorbing capacity, and density (2). The bone elasticity is subjected to the forces of shearing, compression, bending, torsion, and stretching (2). Other factors such as nutrition can also affect the growth of bone.

Suppression of longitudinal growth also may occur from excessive compression forces that are placed on the perpendicular growth plates (2). Unequal compression loading and stretching of a growth plate can alter deposition of bone thus leading to asymmetry of the osseous elements.

An abnormal position occurs when the fetus does not move into the vertex position at the 7th month. In-utero constraint is the most common cause of extrinsic deformation. Approximately 2% of babies are born with deformities because of extrinsic factors (1–3). The growth plate is also susceptible to torsional forces that may cause rotational alterations (2,4). Extrinsic forces that influence the musculoskeletal systems include: gravity (abnormal weight bearing affecting the force on bone), strong muscles producing tensile loading, and dynamic stressors (2). The forces of shearing, stretching, compression, torsion, and bending are all extrinsic factors which can alter the growth and shape of the musculoskeletal system.

In-Utero Constraint

Various causes of in-utero constraint include: primigravida (i.e., excessive abdominal wall strength); small mother; uterine malformation; and fibromata (2). Four positions of the fetus that can cause biomechanical compromise to the spine are: breech, face, brow, and transverse presentations.

The last trimester of gestation, when the growth of the fetus fills the uterine cavity, is the most likely time for constraint to occur. This fact is supported by evidence of therapeutically aborted fetuses of 20 weeks or less revealing no observable deformations (1).

Abnormal positions of the mother's uterus from alterations in ligament attachments could lead to asymmetrical forces on the fetus. These abnormal ligamentous changes can result from abnormal position or movements of the lumbar spine and pelvis. Changes in the position of the lumbar spine and pelvis may also play a role in the development of in-utero constraint.

Breech or cephalic presentations occur in approximately 4% of all pregnancies and account for 32% of extrinsic deformations of the fetus (1). There are three forms of breech: frank, complete, and footling (Fig. 14.1). In approximately 70% of breech presentations, the fetal

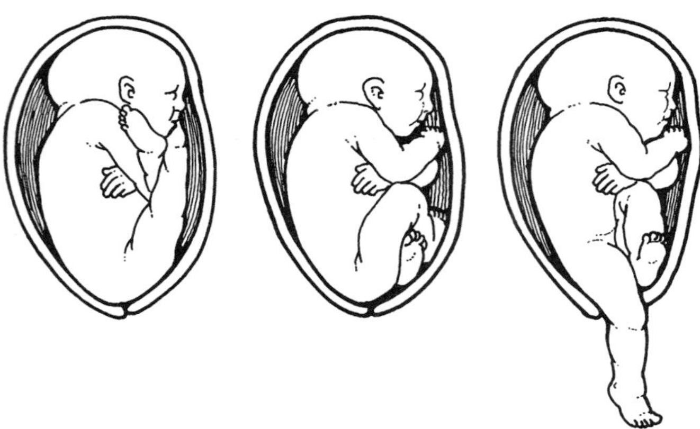

Figure 14.1. Three forms of breech presentation: frank, complete, footling. Modified from Graham JM. Smith's recognizable patterns of human deformation. 2nd ed. Philadelphia: WB Saunders, 1988:86.

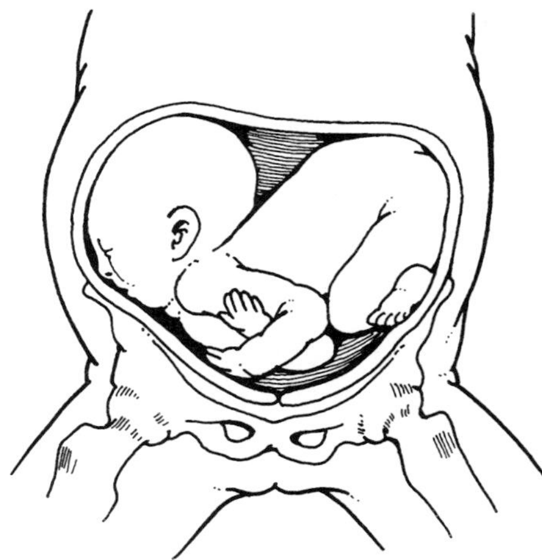

Figure 14.3. Transverse lie presentation. Modified from Graham JM. Smith's recognizable patterns of human deformation. 2nd ed. Philadelphia: WB Saunders, 1988:95.

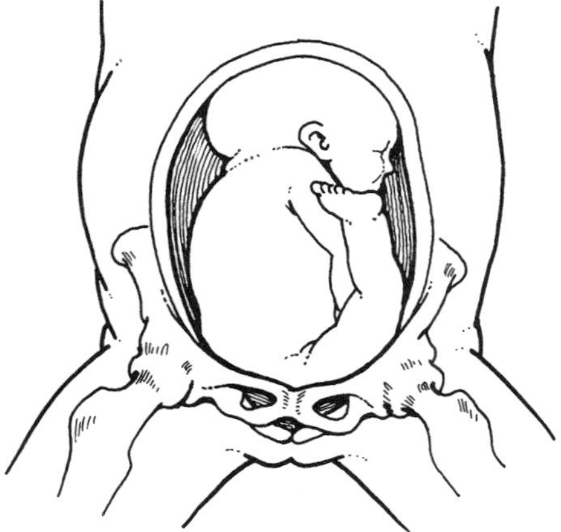

Figure 14.2. Breech presentation. Notice the position of the legs. Modified from Graham JM. Smith's recognizable patterns of human deformation. 2nd ed. Philadelphia: WB Saunders, 1988:86.

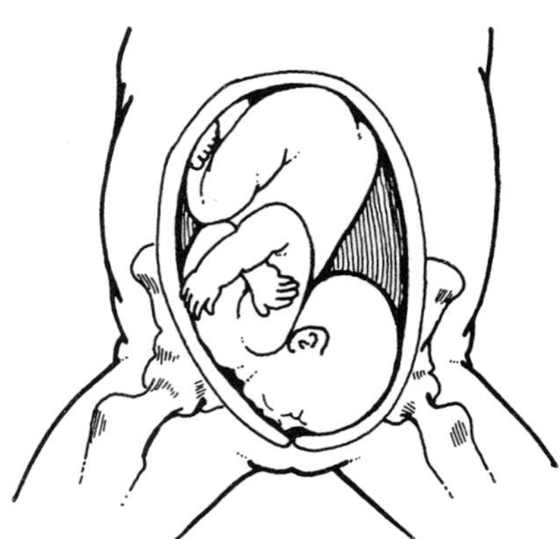

Figure 14.4. Face presentation. Modified from Graham JM. Smith's recognizable patterns of human deformation. 2nd ed. Philadelphia: WB Saunders, 1988:96.

movement is restricted by abnormal positioning of the legs (Fig. 14.2). The fetal position with legs extended in front of the fetus' abdomen is considered the cause of the fetus "catching" itself in the (breech) cephalic presentation.

Dunn (3) reviewed 6,000 cases of breech babies and found that 42% had postural scoliosis and that 20 to 25% had such deformities as torticollis, mandibular asymmetry and talipes equinovarus. Approximately 50% of breech infants will have hip dislocation (3).

The breech position places the head and cervical spine into a hyperextended position. The breech position pushes the cranium posterior and can either hyperextend or hyperflex the cervical spine—depending on the position of the chin (1,2). Breech positioning also can compromise the cervical, thoracic, lumbo-sacral and pelvic regions (2). Birth complications often arise because of the breech position.

Transverse lie positioning is seen in 1 of every 300 to 600 deliveries and is more common in multiparous females (1). Pressure against the lateral border of the uterus causes posterior displacement of the head and hyperextension or hyperflexion of the upper cervical spine (Fig. 14.3). The anterior compression of the cranium may force the occiput into a posterior superior (PS) subluxation. Transverse lie can lead to other postural deformities such as scoliosis (1); therefore, the entire spinal column should be examined after delivery.

Face presentation occurs approximately in 1 out of every 500 births. Brow presentation (Fig. 14.4) is even less common (1). Here, the face is compressed and the head and neck are forced into hyperextension. Both face and brow presentation have the potential of causing upper cervical subluxation, such as an anterior superior (AS) occiput.

Currently, two procedures that are used to treat the

breech fetus are: external manipulation (with associated high risk for complication) and cesarean surgery which can also lead to complications (1). Smith hopes that the future will hold new alternatives to the prevention and resolution of the breech presentation.

An alternative to the previously described approaches has been developed by Webster (5) (See In-Utero Constraint Turning Technique).

Chiropractic pre-natal care may be the first opportunity to reduce morphogenic changes from extrinsic factors. This may prevent or reduce the development of the vertebral subluxation complex and other associated biomechanical alterations.

Birth Trauma

The birth process can be another potential source of trauma to the spine which may lead to neuropathophysiologic effects. The cause of trauma in most instances is due to a forceful tractioning of the spine while in a hyperextended position. Longitudinal traction with rotation and flexion, or excessive lateral bending, also can cause injury (Fig. 14.5) (1,3,5–9). Towbin (9) found that mechanical injury from delivery procedures could produce cord compression and vertebral subluxation. These abnormalities may escape detection with standard radiographic methods because of the elastic properties of the pediatric spine.

Cesarian, forceps, (Fig.14.6) and suction or vacuum extraction (Fig.14.7) deliveries also can cause trauma to

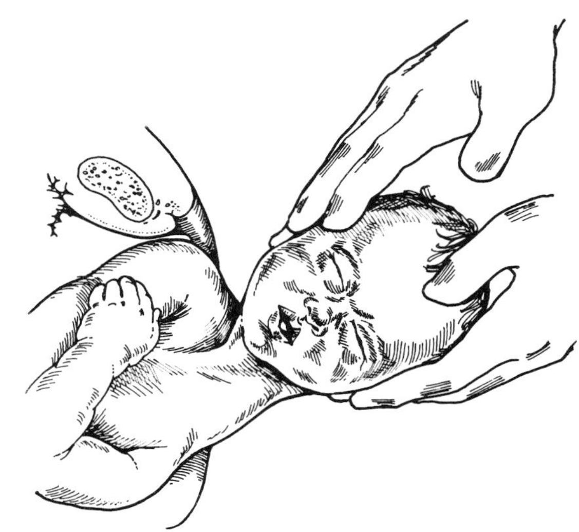

Figure 14.5. Delivery of the newborn. Upward traction on the head is used to deliver a posterior shoulder over the perineum. Modifed from Willson JR, Beecham CT, Forman I, Carrington ER, eds. Obstetrics and gynecology. St. Louis: CV Mosby, 1958:336.

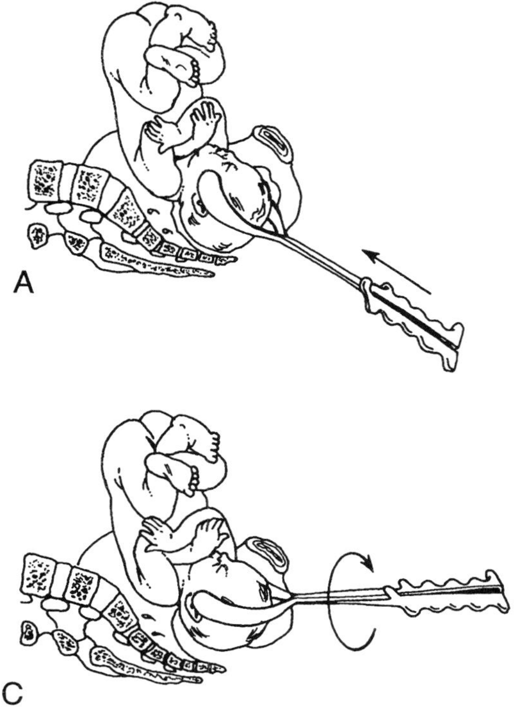

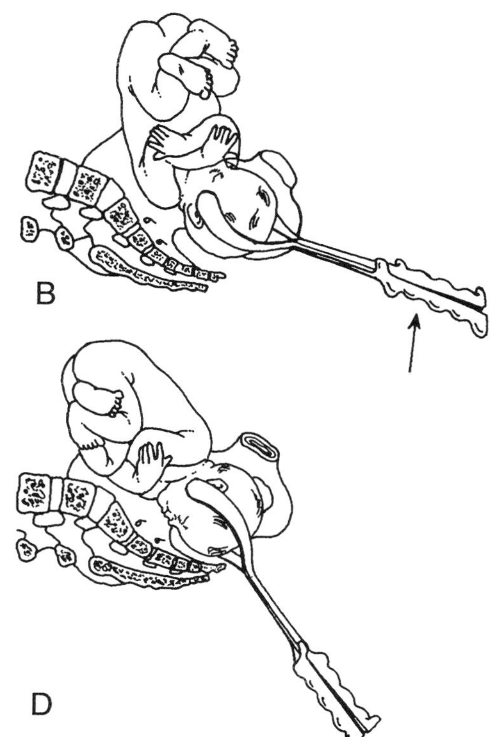

Figure 14.6. Forceps rotation of the head in occiput posterior presentation. **A,** The head is elevated in the axis of the birth canal. **B,** The handles are elevated. **C,** Rotation to the right. **D,** Rotation is completed. Modified from Pernoll ML, Benson RC. Current obstetric and gynecologic diagnosis and treatment. 6th ed. Norwalk, CT: Appleton & Lange, 1987:492.

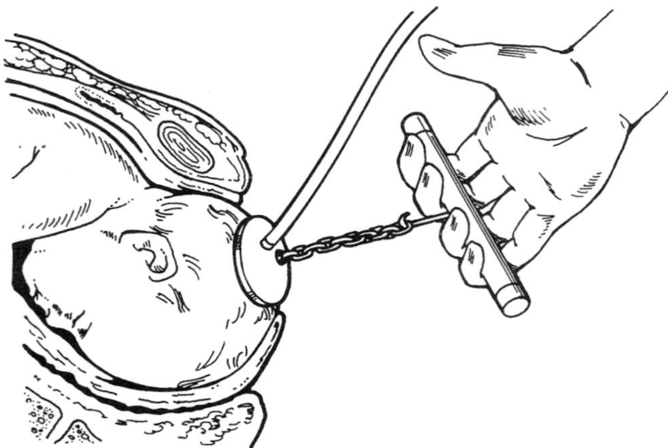

Figure 14.7. Bird's modification of Malmstrom's vacuum extractor method. Modified from Pernoll ML, Benson RC. Current obstetric and gynecologic diagnosis and treatment. 6th ed. Norwalk: Appleton & Lange, 1987:496.

the cervical and thoracic spine. The hand dominance of the obstetrician may lead to specific (left or right sided) cervical rotatory trauma. Approximately 70% of the general population have right handed dominance (10).

The complications of a vaginally delivered breech fetus, include both spinal and neurologic trauma (7). The delivery techniques are known to cause brachial plexus and cervico-thoracic nerve root damage (e.g., Erb's Palsy and Klumpe's paralysis) and potential upper spinal cord transectional lesion in severe cases. Approximately 24% of cerebral palsy cases could be caused by or attributed to delivery techniques for the breech fetus (1).

Gutmann's review of 1,000 infants (11) suggested that birth trauma often affected the atlanto-occipital joint resulting in blockage or vertebral subluxation. These abnormalities could alter peripheral nerve or brain stem function. Gutmann further speculates that abnormal nerve function may lead to lowered resistance and thus predisposition to disease.

Sudden Infant Death Syndrome (SIDS) appears to be related in some instances to birth trauma. Any process, whether genetic, biochemical, biomechanical or traumatic, which alters normal development and function of the respiratory control centers may cause this syndrome (12).

Post Natal Development of Spinal Asymmetry

The spine is composed of cartilaginous material up to the age of six. It is, therefore, readily susceptible to morphogenic alterations during this period (1,2,13,14). The average length of the spine (excluding the sacrum) of the newborn is approximately 20 cm. Within the first two years of life the length of the spine will grow to approximately 45 cm (13).

At birth, the infant's vertebrae consist of the centrum and the two halves of the neural arch. Uniting all parts is hyaline cartilage. A cartilaginous spine does not contraindicate carefully applied specific adjustments. Posterior synchondrosis (uniting of the vertebral arches) normally occurs first. The closure begins at C1 during the first year, and the process is completed by approximately the eighth year at the lumbar spine. Neurocentral synchondrosis (centrum ossification) is completed at approximately the third through the fifth year in the lumbar spine and by the fifth through the eighth year in the cervical spine. The sacrum and ilia do not completely ossify until the third decade of life.

Bone development is influenced by nerve and circulatory factors that control chemical and cytologic function (14). The shaping of bone and the joint surfaces depends on whole body motion. Motion restriction will lead to developmental asymmetries. Because the transitional areas (e.g., C0-C1, L5-S1) of the spine are more susceptible to biomechanical stresses, these regions are often affected more when asymmetrical loads or abnormal movements are encountered (14,15) (See Chapter 2).

For example, the infant or toddler learning to master the muscular coordination for standing or walking will have numerous falls to the sitting position. Pure symmetry and balanced movements unfortunately do not exist for the infant, toddler, pre-adolescent, or adolescent as they progress through their developmental stages. Micro and macro trauma, unilateral activities and sports, as well as postural and repetitive habits, are all considered a part of the normal childhood (6,13,14–17).

Jirout (17) has investigated the relationship of left-right hand dominance on the structure of the spine. In a radiographic study limited to the upper torso, 94% of the 600 human subjects demonstrated left-right positional asymmetries. The more prevalent right-handed dominance caused significant muscular imbalance, sufficient to shift the occiput and spinous processes of the involved vertebrae toward the right side. Another study of 100 subjects (17) confirmed right-handed dominance with right compensatory shift of the occiput and cervical region. In this report, left-handed exercises were given to right-hand dominant subjects. This resulted in a temporary shift of the spine to the left side.

The influence of hand dominance on idiopathic scoliosis has been studied by Goldberg and Dowling (18). Left-handed dominance was associated with a left convex scoliosis in the lower thoracic region. Right-handed individuals tended to develop right convex curves (See Chapter 9).

In a large radiographic study it was concluded that the atlas vertebra was asymmetrical in 99% of the cases. The report by Anderson (10) on 156 archaeological crania (comprised of Californian, Peruvian and Egyptian specimens), basioccipital angulation occurred in nearly 60% of the cases. He further states that right-handed dominance could influence the cervical spine with persistent tension at the left-sided musculature, thus resulting in structural deviation.

The influence of intrinsic (e.g., genetic) and extrinsic factors on the developing spine is well documented. The role of chiropractic care in ameliorating or preventing developmental spinal abnormalities is not well understood and merits further research.

Childhood Injuries

MOTOR VEHICLE INJURIES

In the United States the leading cause of death under the age of 25 is accidents (6). The leading cause of accidental deaths from the ages of 1 to 25 years is automobile related. Younger children tend to have more severe injuries. The head, neck, and facial region are the most frequently injured areas, although the whole body is also at risk (19,20). Two factors that increase the chance of injuries to younger children are the lack of or improper use of car restraints (e.g., car seats, seatbelts), and the presence of a larger head in relation to the upper torso. Underdeveloped cervical musculature may also contribute to increased forces sustained during impact. Glauser and Cares (19,20) discovered that during a collision, a child in a lap belt will elongate, jack-knife, and strike the back of the seat or dashboard.

The unrestrained child is most likely to receive the severest injury and die during an automobile accident. In a collision of 30 mph, it has been estimated that an unrestrained infant weighing 8 kg will accelerate and create the force of 350 kg. This is equal to the force generated by a fall from a third floor (6).

When hyperextension and hyperflexion trauma occurs, spinal traction, and cord compression or impingement can occur. Injuries from motor vehicle accidents are similar to those seen during birth trauma. Spinal cord injuries commonly occur at the lower cervical and upper thoracic region. The susceptibility of the spinal cord is increased in the midcervical region because of the enlargement for the brachial plexus at this area (19–21).

Melzak (21), Glauser (19), and Taylor (20) studied children involved in automobile accidents that resulted in traumatic paralysis. With rare exception, the radiographic evaluation revealed no fracture or dislocation; however, extensive spinal cord damage was present, resulting in the paralysis.

Although seatbelts and seat restraints can undoubtedly reduce the severity of injuries to children involved in motor vehicle accidents, they cannot completely eliminate traumatic acceleration/deceleration forces from impacting the child (6,19,20,22,23).

Vertebral subluxation with its associated components can occur from automobile accidents. The initial radiographic findings may only show slight alterations, however.

OTHER INJURIES

The home is the primary site for 2- to 3-year-old children to receive injuries. For 5- to 18-year-old children, school is the most frequent place for accidents to occur (6). Physical education, sports (See Chapter 2), and unorganized activities play a role in the occurrence of these injuries.

Bicycles are another childhood source of trauma. Over 50,000 children a year are treated for severe head trauma resulting from not wearing helmets while riding (24).

Playground equipment is responsible for 118,000 injuries a year to children. The majority of these accidents will be falls, 50% of which result in head and neck trauma (6).

Sudden hyperflexion or hyperextension of the neck, or vertical compression of the head or buttocks from falls, can cause either spine or spinal cord injury (16). Activities that are commonly associated with falls are skateboarding, roller-skating, horseback riding, surfing, water slides, or diving into shallow water.

Physically abused infants can sustain injuries to the spinal cord due to violent shaking of the head (16,22,23). An infant also can potentially fall from a high place (e.g., couch, bed) if left unattended. This could occur during routine diaper changing. In a study conducted by the National Safety Council, of 536 infants (25), 255 (47.5%) were discovered to have fallen head first from a high place (e.g., dressing table, bed) during their first year of life. Percy (26) reports that falls from a high place are not uncommon with young children and may cause rotational subluxation of the atlas and soft tissue damage of the cervical spine.

Maigne (25) reports that head and cervical trauma could create irritation to the cervical sympathetic fibers and may cause a variety of dysfunctional states: vasomotor and secretional problems; headaches; auditory, vestibular and visual problems; pharyngolaryngeal; and psychic disturbances. He reports positive results with these disorders when cervical adjustments are performed.

Goldthwait and Coe (25) theorized that faulty body mechanisms could alter the development of bone, eventually leading to adult functional disorders. Hinwood and Hinwood (25) report on a study of children under the age of eight. Although all subjects were considered "healthy" by conventional methods, nearly 40% had evidence of spinal subluxation.

Implications of Pediatric Vertebral Subluxation Complex

Lewit (15) discusses the possible ramifications of blockage (vertebral subluxation complex) if left uncorrected in the child. The consequences of vertebral subluxation may appear insignificant, with the exception of occasional transitory pain. If the vertebral subluxation is left uncorrected, compensatory reactions would develop at adjacent motion segments, further masking the effects of the original lesion. Long-term biomechanical strain deprives the disc tissue of needed nutrition, eventually leading to internal reabsorption and degeneration. Degenerative changes at the vertebra include traction osteophytes and spondylophytic ridges. Both hypomobile and hypermobile segments will undergo degeneration.

Heilig (14) points out that the longer the period of osseous development during which asymmetrical forces are acting, the greater the frequency, duration, and extent of spinal damage. If abnormal spinal function could be recognized and ameliorated early on, the greater the opportunity for normal developmental patterns to be established (14). Heilig implores his colleagues to consider osteopathic care for children because developmental changes can be most easily effected at an early age.

If accidents are the leading cause of death and severe injuries to children in the United States, one could postulate that such injuries, even those of lesser magnitude, are a potential cause of vertebral subluxation(s).

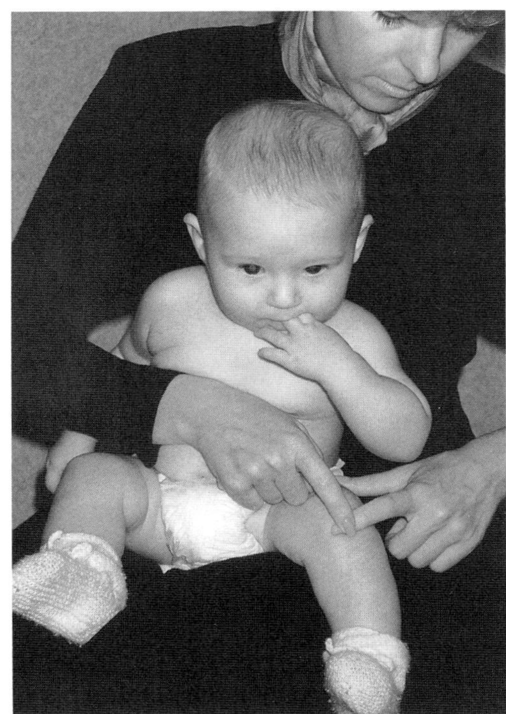

Figure 14.8. Elicitation of the patellar reflex.

NEUROLOGIC EXAMINATION OF THE NEONATE AND INFANT

The neurologic examination is a series of tests that assist the chiropractor in assessing the subcortical function of the newborn (0–4 months) or infant (4–12 months).

The newborn and infant examination can sometimes be challenging because of the lack of verbal communication. The examination presented here is considered supplementary to the usual neurologic spinal examination for adults and should be performed when indicated. Neurologic reflexes are used to evaluate the brainstem and spinal cord function.

Most newborn reflexes are present at birth or shortly thereafter. There are a few reflexes, however, that will manifest themselves from the 6th week up to the 24th month. If a reflex is absent, it may reflect general depression of motor function at a central or peripheral level. If asymmetry should occur in a reflex, this can indicate a central or peripheral focal motor lesion. For the normally maturing infant, the newborn reflexes will be replaced later by voluntary motor function. If a present finding persists beyond the normal age of disappearance, this may indicate a central motor lesion or a generalized developmental lag.

Note that although a doctor may expect a normal newborn/infant reflex, a recently fed or sleepy baby may manifest a depressed or brisk response.

Deep tendon reflexes (e.g., triceps, biceps, brachioradialis, patellar, and achilles) may be similarly elicited in the infant as in the adult. Rather than using a reflex hammer, the examiner should use a finger to tap directly the striking point or nailbed of the doctor (Fig. 14.8). The spinal reflex mechanisms (deep tendon reflexes and plantar response) may vary in response because of the lack of corticospinal pathway development in the infant. It is recommended that the doctor avoid labeling an abnormal reflex initially. Rather, the infant should be retested before concluding that there is indeed an abnormality.

A normal response of a deep tendon reflex is a brisk jerk. A cerebral disorder may be present if spontaneous clonus occurs with the feet, legs, and arms. Infants manifesting absence of reflexes also may suggest a neuromuscular disorder is present. The tricep reflex will not be present until after the 6th month.

Many authorities suggest that Babinski's sign is not a reliable test before the second year of life. The examiner may elicit a positive sign of extension of the toes or a negative sign of toe flexion.

The cranial nerves also can be tested in the newborn and infant. The same procedures for the adult are adapted to the infant. Two cranial nerve tests that are more difficult to assess in the infant are Cranial Nerve II (optic) and Cranial Nerve VII (vestibulocochlear), specifically the acoustic portion.

Infant Reflexes

ROOTING

The examiner strokes with a finger the cheek of the newborn unilaterally. Begin slightly above the mandible and glide toward the mouth. The normal response of the infant will be to move toward the stimulus. The response of the mouth is called "rooting." This test should be performed bilaterally (Fig. 14.9). This reflex, which is present after birth, will disappear during the waking hours after the 3rd to 4th month. The rooting reflex can usually be elicited during sleep in infants up to the 7th month. Absence of this reflex, particularly before the 4th month, indicates a severe generalized, central nervous system disorder.

SUCKING

The examiner inserts the first phalange of a clean finger into the newborn's mouth. The normal response should be a hearty "sucking" onto the finger (Fig. 14.10). This reflex is present after birth and continues to the 3rd or 4th month. Absence of this reflex may indicate a severe, generalized central nervous system disorder.

BLINK

The examiner shines a bright penlight into the newborn/infant's eyes. The newborn/infant with a normal response will blink the eyes tightly shut (Fig. 14.11). This reflex should be present from birth through the first year of life. Absence of this response may indicate blindness.

ACOUSTIC BLINK

This reflex is sometimes referred to as the cochleopalpebral test. The examiner claps the hands very close to the newborn/infant's ears. The normal response should be a bilateral eye blink to the loud noise (Fig. 14.12). This reflex is present from birth and has a variable time for disappearance. Absence of this response may indicate decreased or loss of hearing.

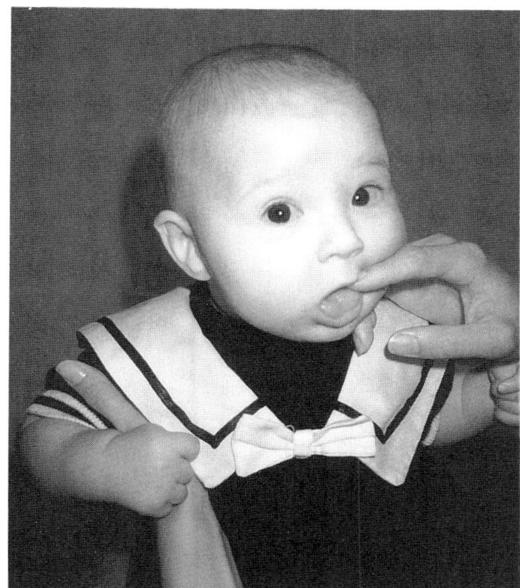

Figure 14.9. The newborn will "root" towards the side of the stimuli as a normal response. This test should be performed bilaterally.

MORO

This test is commonly called the "startle" reflex. The examiner creates a loud abrupt noise or change in the newborn's head position. The initial phase of Moro's response is a symmetric abduction and extension of the arms accompanied by extension of the trunk. The second phase includes adduction of the arms. The legs will be active, although to a lesser extent than the arms. This response is present from birth through approximately the 3rd month. If this response persists beyond this period, it

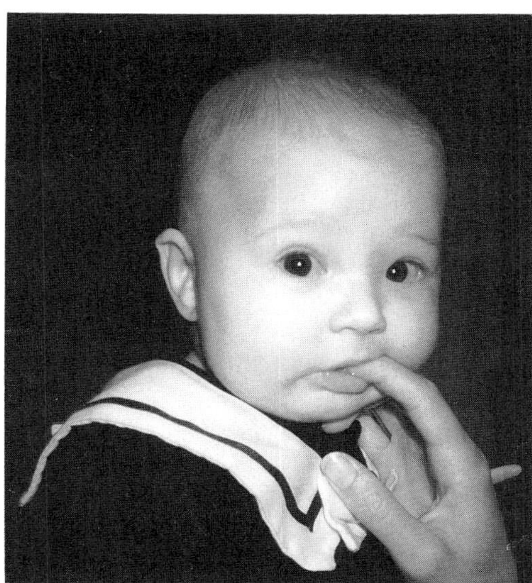

Figure 14.10. Sucking reflex. A normal response for this reflex is a hearty "sucking" onto the phalange.

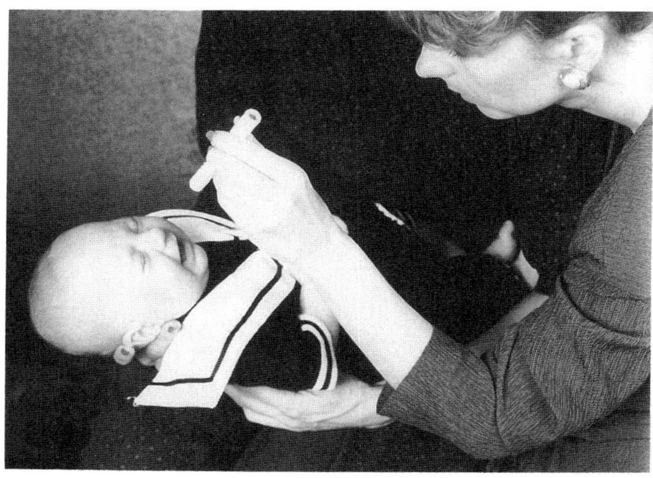

Figure 14.11. Blink reflex.

may indicate a neurologic disturbance (Fig. 14.13A-B). If asymmetry occurs in the upper extremity, this may suggest hemiparesis or injury to the brachial plexus. Asymmetry in the lower extremity may indicate lower spinal injury or congenital hip dislocation.

GALANT'S

This test is also known as the trunk incurvation test. While holding the newborn in a horizontal prone position, the examiner will stroke unilaterally the paraspinal musculature. The newborn should normally respond by arching the back and turning the head slightly to the ipsilateral side of the stroking stimulation. This test should be performed on both sides (Fig. 14.14). The response is present from birth to 2 months. Absence of the reflex may indicate a transverse spinal cord lesion.

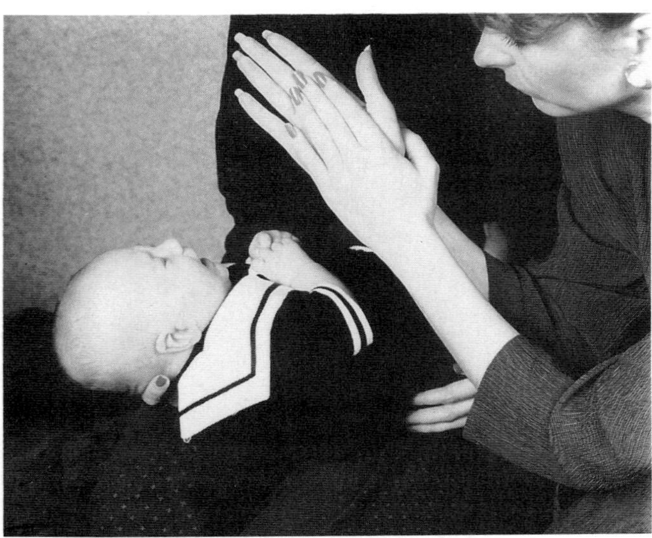

Figure 14.12. Acoustic blink reflex.

TONIC NECK

This test is also known as the "ATNR" (asymmetric tonic neck reflex). The examiner places a hand on the crown of the newborn/infant's head and rotates it to one side. The normal response is the extension of the arm and leg on the side of head rotation, and arm and leg flexion on the opposite side. This position is called the fencing posture. The test should be performed bilaterally (Fig. 14.15). This reflex is present by the 2nd week through the 6th month. It should be noted that this reflex in a normal newborn/infant should not always be present when the test is repeated. Findings that are abnormal and implicate major cerebral damage are a persistent present finding during each test under 6 months of age or a present finding beyond the 6th month.

NECK RIGHTING

The examiner rotates the head of the supine infant to one side. The normal response is for the trunk to rotate toward the side of head rotation (Fig. 14.16). This reflex is present from the 4th through the 6th month and disappears entirely at approximately 6 months.

PARACHUTE

The examiner holds the infant in the prone position while supporting the abdomen. Mimicking a rapid fall, allow the infant to drop a short, controlled distance. The normal response is for the infant to extend their arms, hands and fingers outward (Fig. 14.17). This reflex is present from the 9th month on.

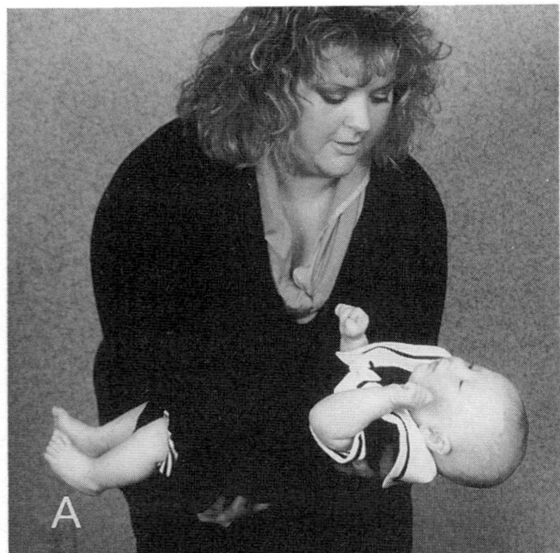

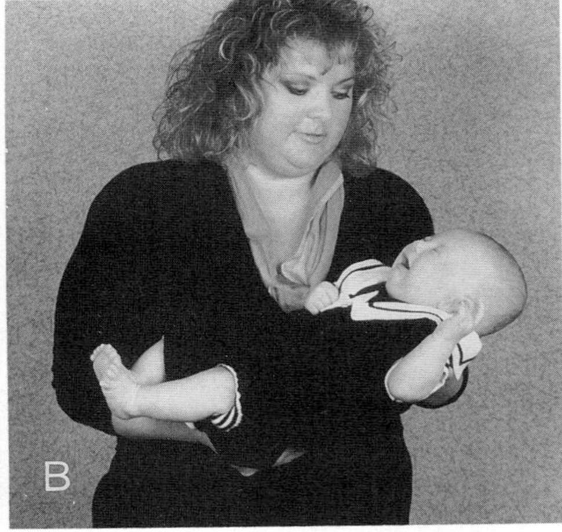

Figure 14.13. A, Moro's reflex. Phase one of Moro's reflex is a symmetric abduction and extension of the arms accompanied by extension of the trunk. **B,** Phase two of Moro's reflex includes adduction of the arms. The legs will be active in both phases with less noticeable participation.

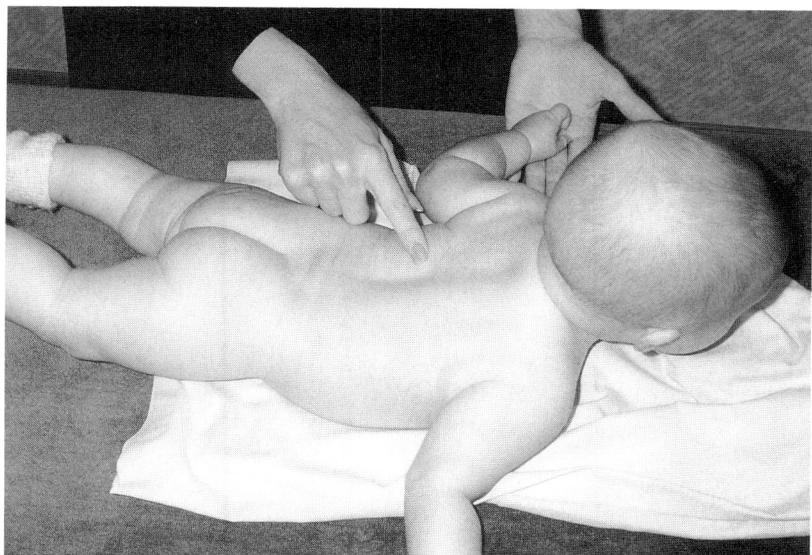

Figure 14.14. Galant's reflex.

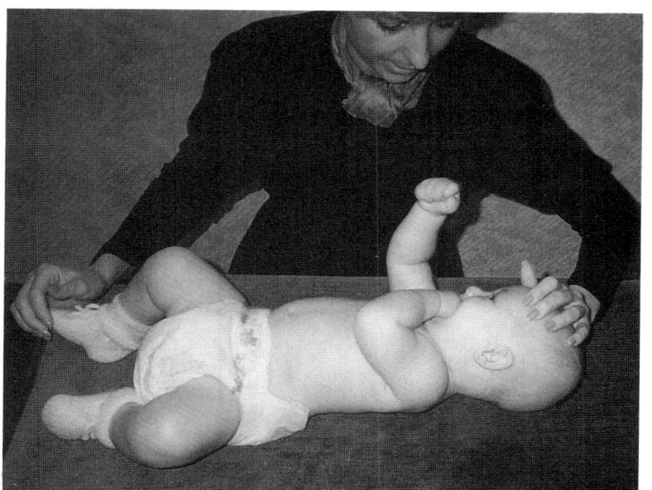

Figure 14.15. Tonic neck reflex.

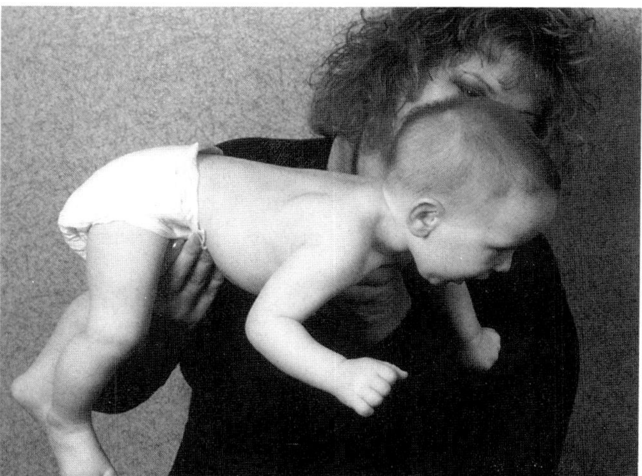

Figure 14.17. Parachute reflex.

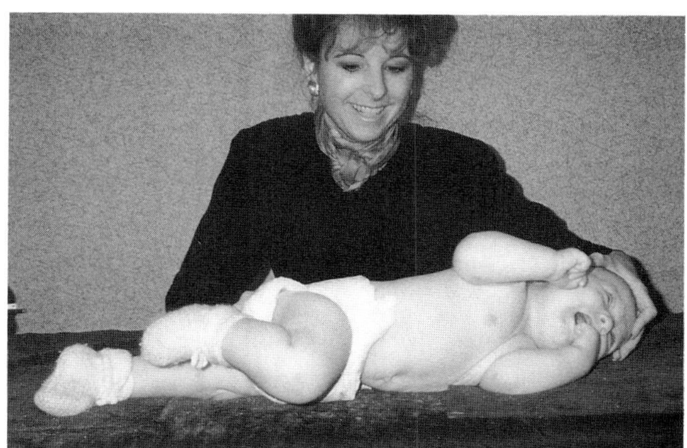

Figure 14.16. Neck righting reflex. The end stage of movement is presented (See text).

PLACING

Being careful not to displace the shoulder joints, the examiner supports the newborn from under the axillae. While touching the dorsum of the foot on a table top, the normal response will be flexion of the leg (Fig. 14.18A), followed by leg extension (Fig. 14.18B). This reflex is detected from birth to about the 6th week. Absence of this reflex may indicate paresis due to breech delivery or other factors.

STEPPING

The examiner carefully lifts the newborn from under the axillae and touches both soles of the feet on a flat surface. The normal response is the action of walking (Fig. 14.19). This reflex is present from birth to the 6th week. The

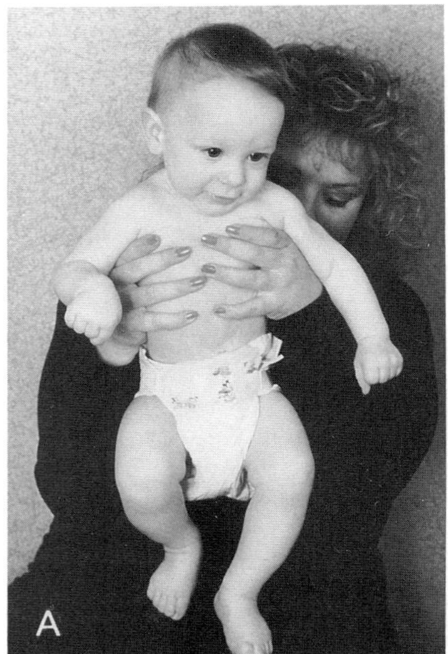

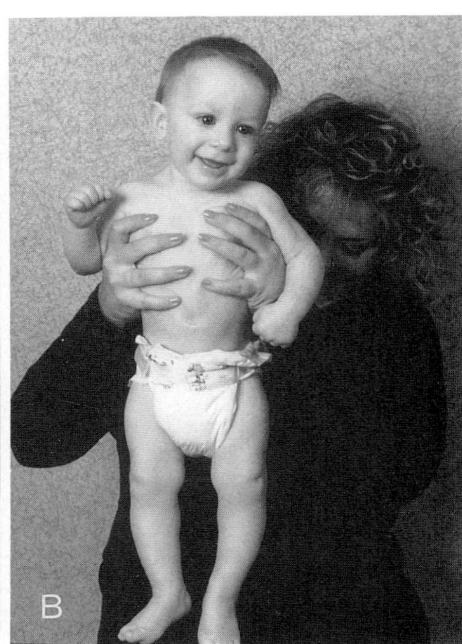

Figure 14.18. **A,** Placing reflex. **B,** End stage of the placing reflex. Notice leg extension.

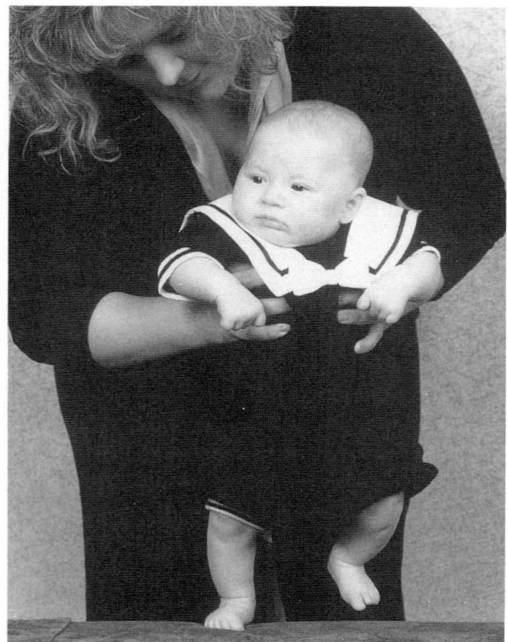

Figure 14.19. Stepping reflex.

absence of this reflex has the same indication as the placing reflex.

VERTICAL SUSPENSION

While lifting the newborn carefully under the axillae, the examiner will then quickly raise the child higher in the air. The normal response will be for the infant to flex both hips and knees (Fig. 14.20). This reflex is present from birth to approximately the 4th month. Absence of this reflex with fixed leg extensions, or adduction (scissoring effect), could indicate spastic paraplegia or diplegia.

PALMAR GRASP

The examiner places a finger in the palm of the newborn/infant from the ulnar side. The normal response will be a grasping action (Fig. 14.21).

DIGITAL RESPONSE

The examiner lightly strokes the ulnar side of the hand and fifth digit. The normal response is extension of the thumb and fingers (Fig. 14.22). Both the Palmar Grasp and Digital Response are present at birth and are normally not obtainable by the 6th month. If the grasp reflex persists beyond the 6th month, this may suggest cerebral dysfunction. A normal response for the newborn is to have the fist closed during the 1st month of life. If the newborn continues to keep the fist persistently closed beyond the 2nd month, this may indicate central nervous system dysfunction.

ABDOMINAL

The newborn/infant is placed in a supine position. The examiner, with a finger, performs a light but brisk stroke across the abdomen. To test T8 to T10, the stroke is performed in the right and left upper quadrants. The right and left lower quadrants will test T10 to T12 function. The stroke begins in the lateral superior corner of each quadrant and ends in the opposite medial inferior corner. A normal finding is abdominal muscle contraction and deviation of the umbilicus on the side of the stimulus.

This test will appear during the first 6 months of life. Absence of the reflex suggests either central motor lesion or a lesion of the spinal cord segment that was stimulated.

ANAL

The undiapered newborn/infant is placed in a prone position. With an object, lightly stroke the perianal region. A normal finding is contracture of the external anal sphincter. This reflex is usually present at birth and assesses function of the lower sacral segments.

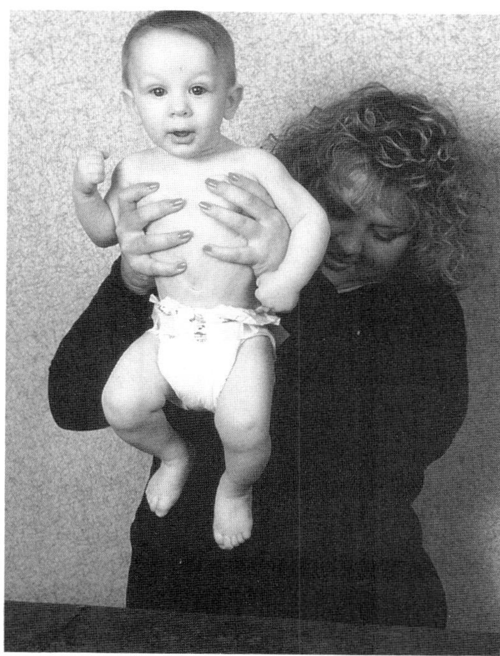

Figure 14.20. Vertical suspension reflex.

MOTOR FUNCTION ASSESSMENT

The process of general observation includes reviewing motor function in the newborn/infant. A normal activity level of the newborn/infant is symmetrical movement of the limbs. Motor function can be tested by taking each major joint through a range of motion. A finding of spasticity or flaccidity would indicate abnormal function. A gripping action of the newborn is a normal response unless it is continually present after the 2nd month, which indicates central motor lesion.

Diffuse cerebral dysfunction may reveal itself as generalized diminished muscle tone. A sign of a hypotonic state is abduction of the hips or a "frog leg" appearance. The arms may also be abducted in this state. Increased muscle tone (hypertonia) will cause adduction of the hips and create a lower limb scissoring effect.

ORTHOPAEDIC EXAMINATION

The orthopaedic examination, although not mandatory or necessary to detect the presence of a vertebral subluxation complex, may prove useful to differentiate other physical disorders. There are a restricted number of orthopaedic tests available for examining the newborn/infant.

The preadolescent and adolescent can be examined as adults. Chapter 4 should be referred to for the indicated orthopaedic tests. The Adam's maneuver, which is

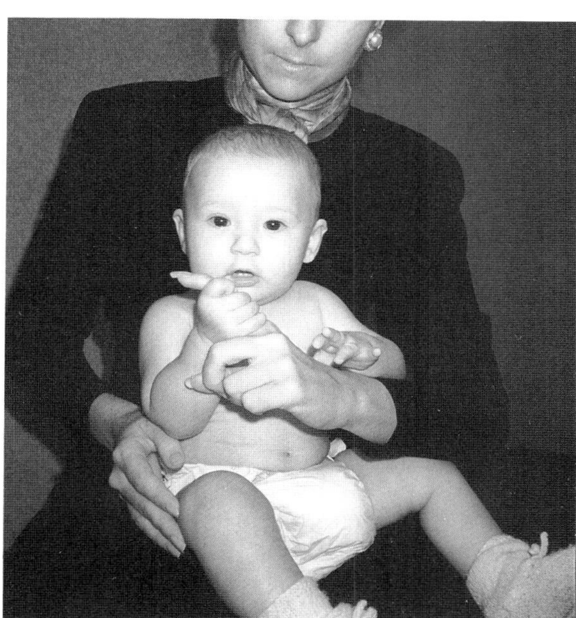

Figure 14.21. Palmar grasp reflex.

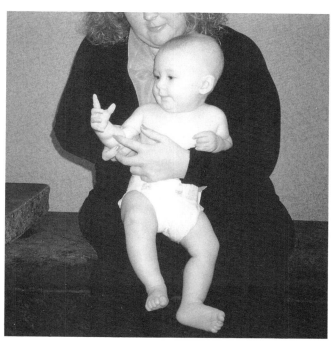

Figure 14.22. Digital response reflex.

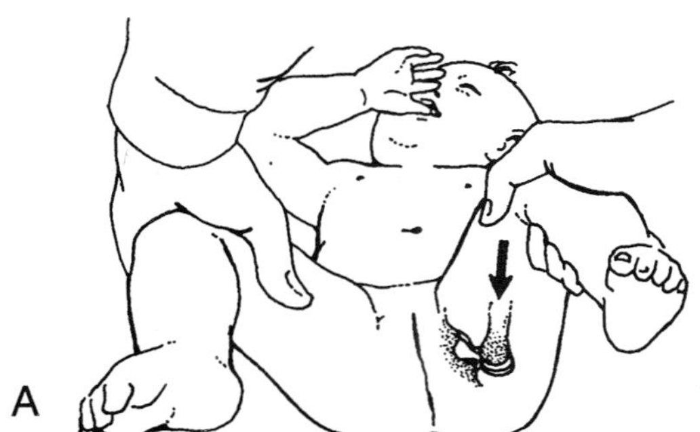

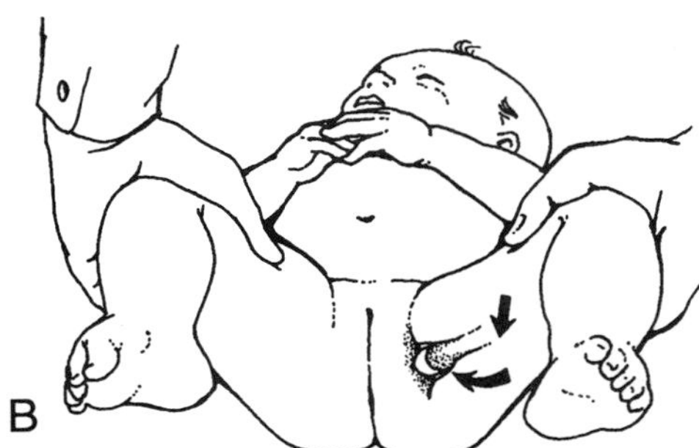

Figure 14.23. Technique for the Ortolani maneuver for hip dislocation. **A,** Downward pressure further dislocates the hip. **B,** Medialward rotation of the hip will force the femoral lead over the rim of the acetabulum, leading to a "clunk." Modified from Graham JM. Smith's recognizable patterns of human deformation. 2nd ed. Philadelphia: WB Saunders, 1988:25.

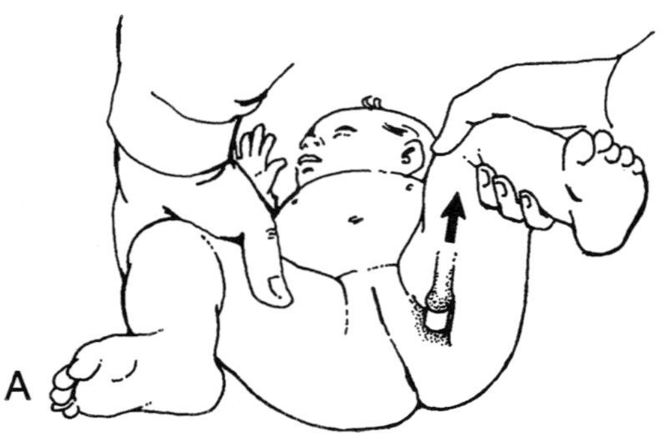

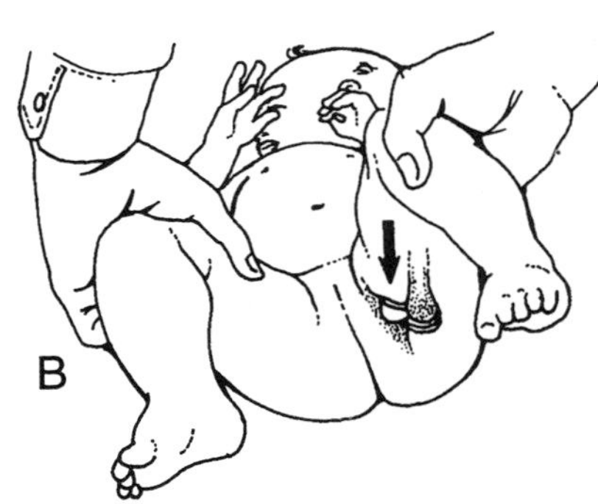

Figure 14.24. **A,** Barlow's sign is performed by strongly pulling on the femur causing distraction of the femur head. Modified from Graham JM. Smith's recognizable patterns of human deformation. 2nd ed. Philadelphia: WB Saunders, 1988:24. **B,** Passage of the femur head over the rim yields a "clunk." Modified from Graham JM. Smith's recognizable patterns of human deformation. 2nd ed. Philadelphia: WB Saunders, 1988:24.

explained and illustrated in Chapter 9, is useful to reveal the presence of a structural scoliosis.

Shortly after birth, the hip joint should be examined for possible congenital hip dislocation. Ortolani's and Barlow's signs are used to rule out displacement or subluxation of the femur head from its normal relationship with the acetabulum. The incidence of congenital hip dislocation is one to two for every 1,000 births (27). There are two classifications of hip dislocation: idiopathic (more common) and teratogenic. Idiopathic congenital dislocation of the hip has several poorly understood etiologies. In-utero constraint positioning, particularly the breech presentation, appears to be related (1,27). Approximately 50% of breech births (3.5% of all births) will manifest hip dislocation (1). Family history of the disorder also appears to be involved.

Females have a greater tendency for dislocation of the hip. Unilateral dislocation is found twice as often as bilateral dislocation. There is also a greater prevalence of primipara infants manifesting this disorder. Little is known about the teratogenic etiologies. They tend to be more severe and are thought to be related to a germ plasma defect.

ORTOLANI'S SIGN

Ortolani's sign is performed with the newborn in a supine position. The doctor places the length of the middle finger over the greater trochanters. The thumbs are then placed at the medial aspect of the inner thigh on the lesser trochanters. The doctor should first flex the newborn's knees to the chest, and then abduct the legs to 90°. A positive sign is elicited during the abduction phase. The femur will create a palpable "clunk" as it relocates out of the acetabulum over the posterior margin (Fig. 14.23A-B) of the hip. A positive finding indicates instability or dislocation.

BARLOW'S SIGN

Barlow's sign is performed on the supine infant. Hand placement is the same as described in Ortolani's sign. The doctor first pulls on the leg, distracting the femur, followed by a medialward push of the upper thigh (Fig. 14.24A-B). A noticeable "clunk" must be present in order for the test to be positive.

Both of the preceding tests should be performed bilaterally. A click or high pitch sound does not indicate a positive sign. An AP and "frogleg" radiograph will confirm the dislocation. For single hip dislocation, an In ilium may be involved (See Chapter 6). Bilateral dislocation may be related to a base posterior sacrum (See Chapter 7).

KERNIG'S TEST

Kernig's test is performed with the child in a supine position. The doctor lifts the child's leg and flexes it at the hip and the knee. The leg should then be straightened or extended from this position. Resistance because of pain is considered a positive sign. Both legs should be tested.

BRUDZINSKI'S TEST

Brudzinski's test is performed with the child in a supine position. After placing the hands on the child's head, the doctor then flexes the neck to the chest. A positive test is indicated when resistance, pain, or hip and knee flexion occurs.

Kernig's and Brudzinski's tests can both be performed if meningeal inflammation is suspected from infection (meningitis), or by blood, as seen with subarachnoid hemorrhage. Any positive findings should warrant further examinations.

SKIN TEMPERATURE INSTRUMENTATION

Hand-held paraspinal temperature differential instruments (e.g., Nervoscope) (See Chapter 4) can be a helpful component of the pediatric examination (28). The size of the newborn, infant or child will determine the setting of the width of the instrument's probes and the patient position for performing the analysis.

The adjustable probes of the instrument must be narrowed to adapt to a newborn or infant's spine, particularly in the cervical region. The newborn can be held against the chest of the parent. A prone position, across the lap of the parent or doctor or on the adjusting table, is an alternative to the upright position (Fig.14.25).

The newborn or infant's elastic skin may make the examination more difficult to perform and to obtain an accurate reading. If this is the case, a "dotting" procedure can be used (29). This replaces the normal gliding method. By lifting the probes from the skin, the paraspinal muscles can be "dotted" with the thermocouples every few millimeters.

Figure 14.26 demonstrates the toddler's ability to cooperate during the analysis. Many toddlers may find this examination ticklish and respond by squirming. A slower glide, while holding the abdomen or shoulder with the free hand, can prevent undesired movement.

PALPATION AND OBSERVATION

The newborn or infant is best palpated while placed against the chest of the parent (Fig. 14.27) or prone across the lap (Fig. 14.28). A posterior to anterior reduction in joint movement is frequently discovered at the involved motion segment.

Atlas subluxations will show reduction in axial rotation. Axial rotation dysfunction at other segments appears to occur less often, unless there has been a specific rotational trauma. Traumatic rotational lesions can occur in the cervical region if extreme rotation occurs during the birth process (7–9,22).

When palpating the cervical spine of the newborn, the

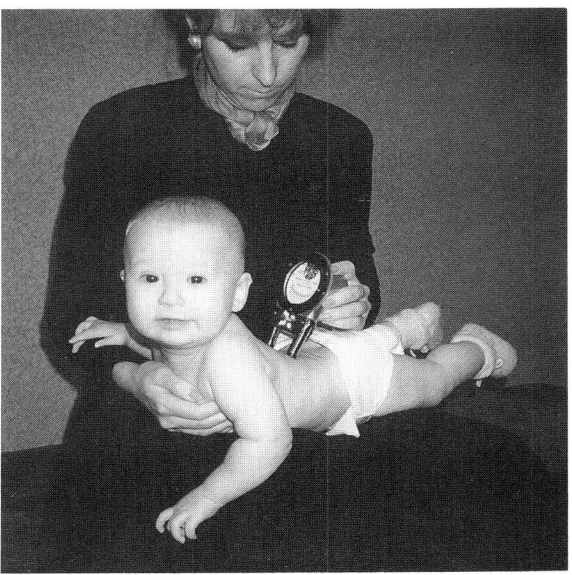

Figure 14.25. Skin temperature analysis of the infant.

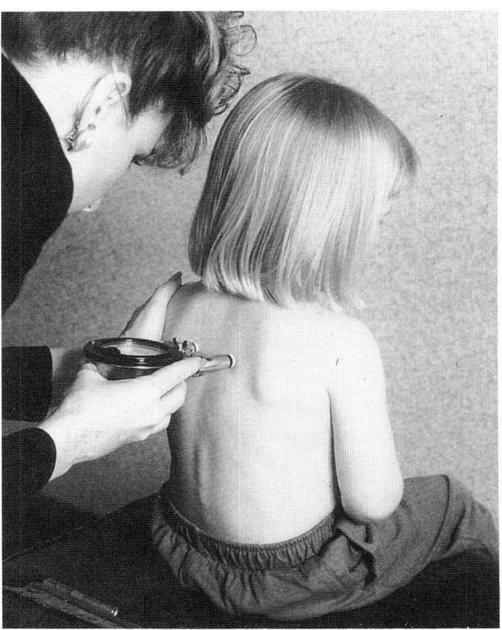

Figure 14.26. Skin temperature analysis in the upright position.

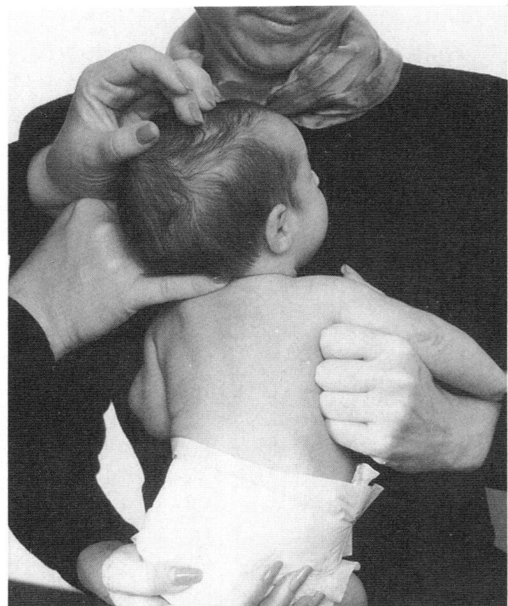

Figure 14.27. Newborn palpation can be performed against the chest of the parent.

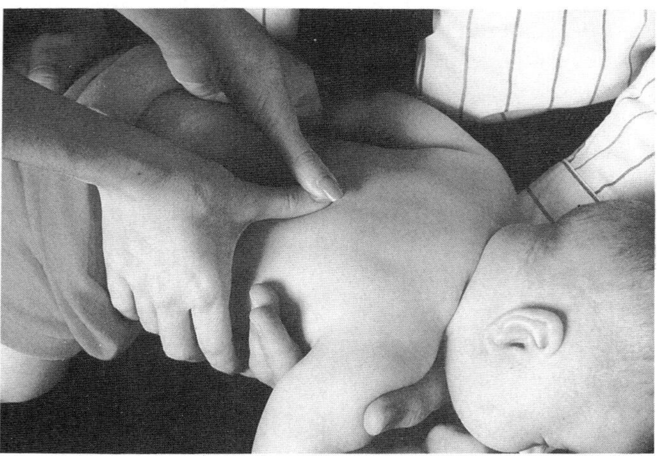

Figure 14.28. The doctor can palpate for posterior to anterior reduction in joint movement with the newborn/infant prone across the lap.

doctor's index finger, or the thumb and index finger can be used. For the thoracic and lumbar spine, a single or double digit, or thumb can be used to palpate (Fig. 14.29).

The palpation of the sacrum and ilium is performed in the prone position. Placing the distal end of the thumb or index pad on the sacral tubercles, the patient's legs should be raised and lowered bilaterally while creating a posterior-anterior motion (Fig. 14.30). The sacral segments most easily palpated for fixation dysfunction are S1 to S3. Posteriority of a sacral segment can be verified with a lateral radiograph.

The sacroiliac joint can be palpated by placing the thumb or finger on the superior medial aspect of the PSIS

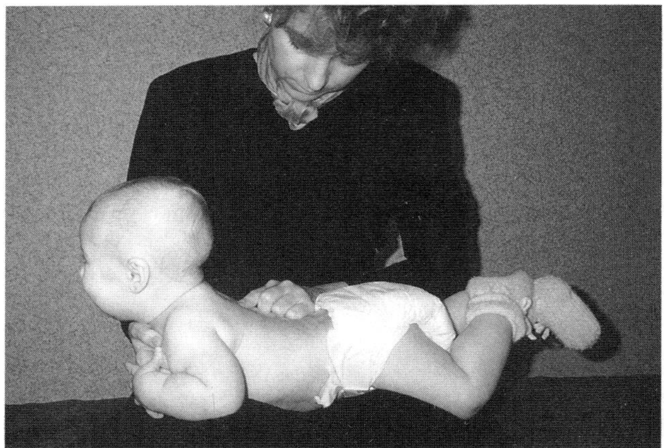

Figure 14.29. Palpation of the infant.

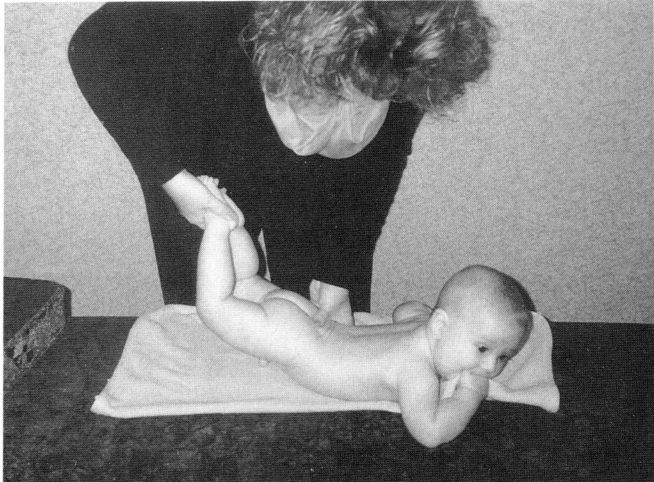

Figure 14.30. Motion palpation of the sacrum.

of the prone infant. The leg on the involved side should be first raised and then lowered (Fig. 14.31). The PI ilium can reveal edema at the superior portion of the joint as well as restriction in movement.

For palpation of the AS ilium, the thumb is placed on the inferior and medial aspect of the PSIS and the leg on the involved side is raised and lowered. Edema and joint restriction are usually present at the inferior portion of the joint of the subluxation. To confirm ilium findings, the doctor should place the undiapered baby in a prone position and observe the gluteal fold (Fig. 14.32). The PI ilium will have an increased gluteal fold, when compared to an AS subluxation.

The In or Ex ilium is difficult to palpate and is more easily determined through observation. In the prone position the undiapered infant with an Ex ilium will have a shorter ilia width, whereas the In ilium reveals a larger width.

Another way to determine the presence of an In or Ex ilium is to lift the infant in the air and observe the position of the legs and feet. The Ex ilium will cause internal rotation of the foot and the In ilium an external rotation. This observation can also be performed with the patient in a supine position.

A prone leg check also can be used to assist in evaluating ilium listings (Fig. 14.33). A short leg is observed with a PI ilium, and a long leg with an AS listing. Because of unequalized growth rate of the lower limbs of children, the leg check should not carry as much weight in the evaluation.

The toddler or adolescent can be palpated as an adult (Figs. 14.34 and 14.35). Observing the gait and stance of the toddler will assist the practitioner in determining the nature of the subluxation. Bilateral toe-in or "pigeon toe" syndrome may indicate a sacrum base posterior. This observation can be confirmed by a lateral lumbosacral radiograph (See Chapter 7). The Ex or In ilium will cause internal or external rotation of the foot in the standing position. This finding can be confirmed with the anterior-

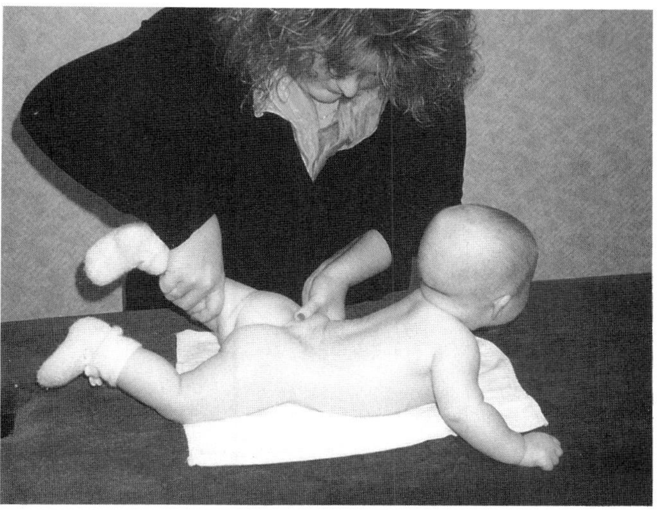

Figure 14.31. Motion palpation of the sacroiliac articulation.

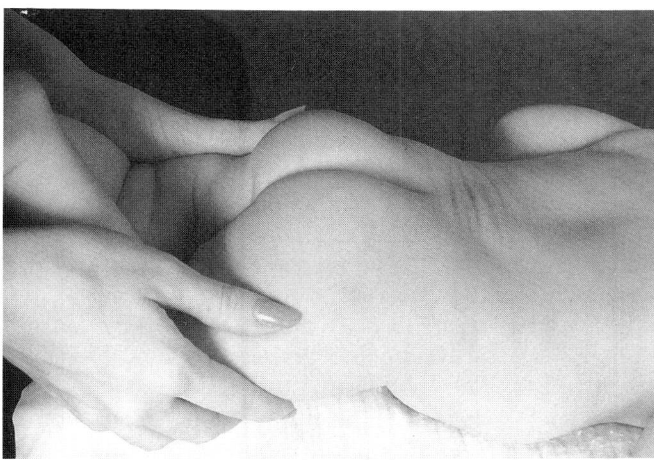

Figure 14.32. Observation of gluteal fold symmetry.

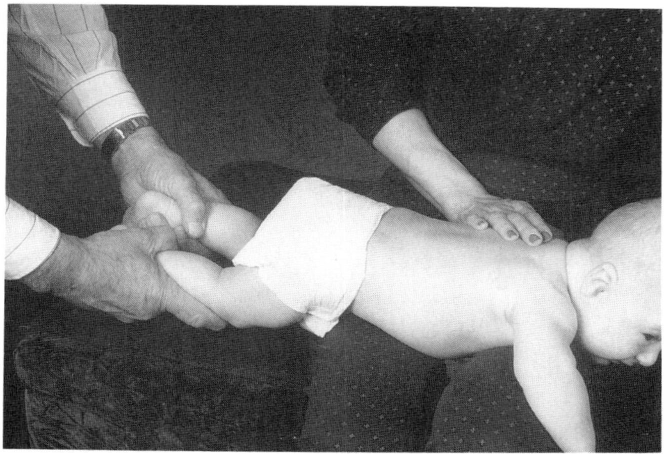

Figure 14.33. Prone leg check.

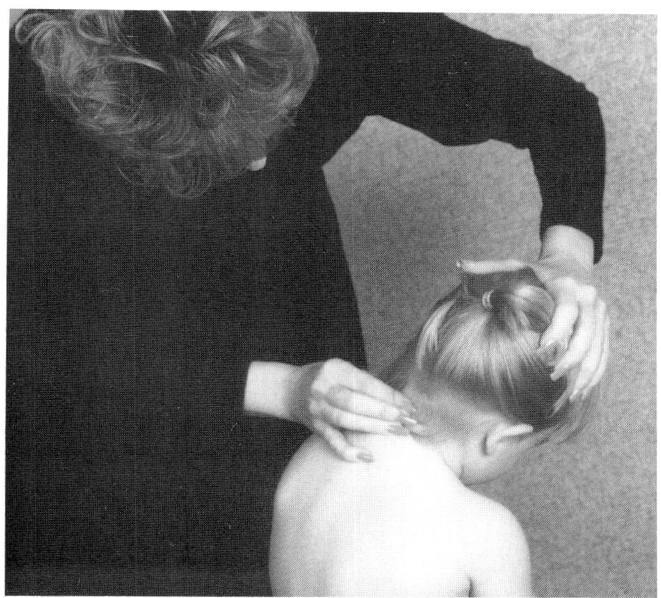

Figure 14.34. Palpation of the cervical spine in the child.

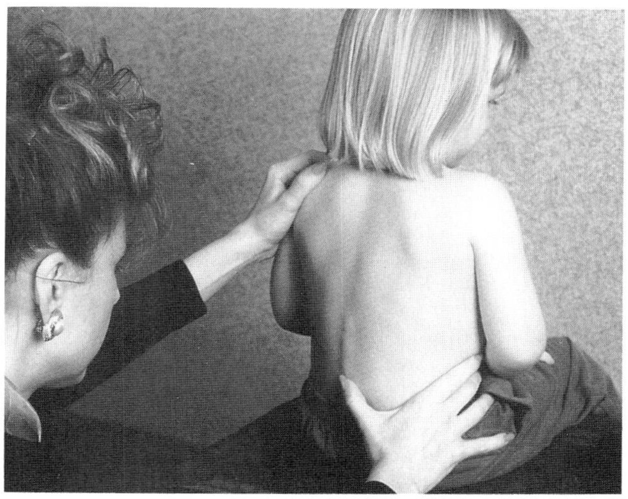

Figure 14.35. Palpation of the lumbar spine in the child.

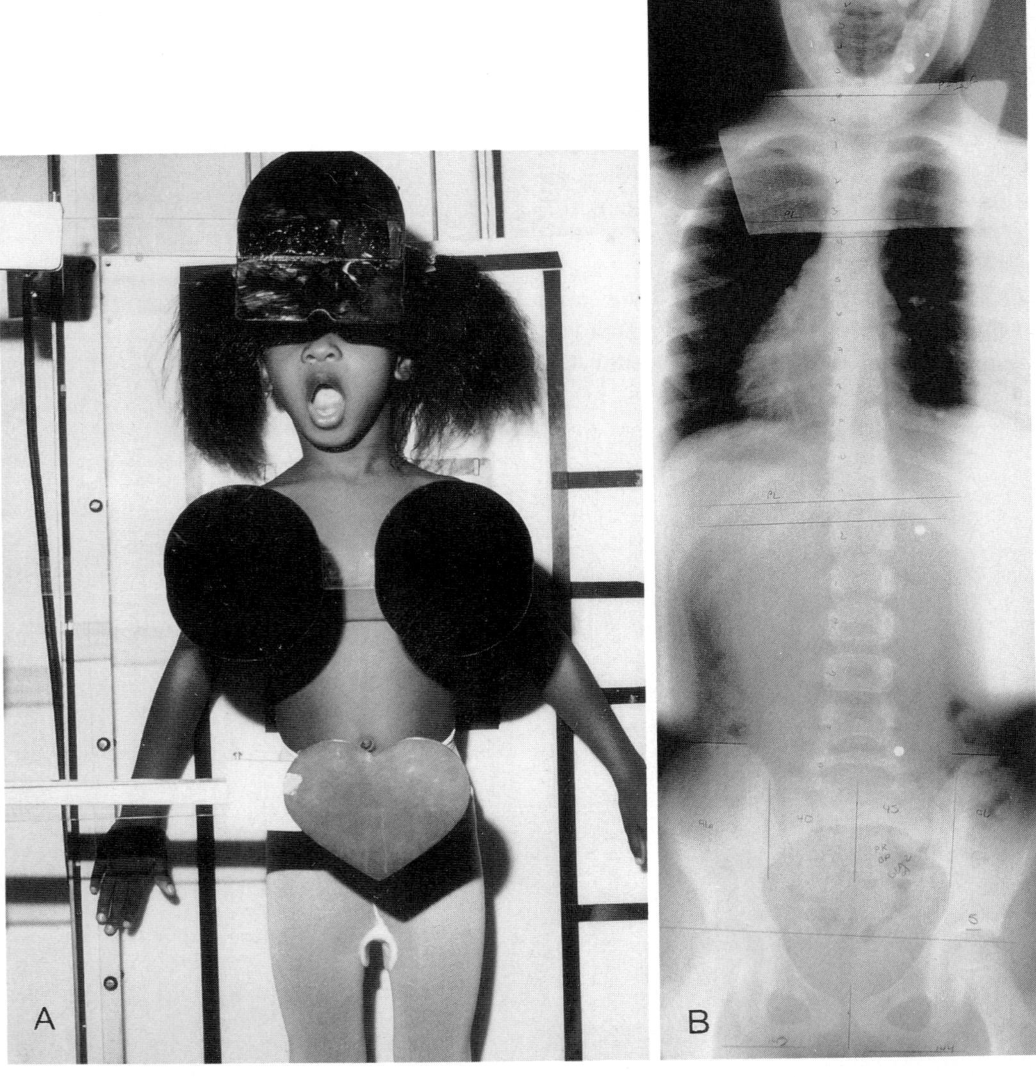

Figure 14.36. **A,** Prepatient filtration for the child. **B,** The radiograph demonstrates brain, breast, and thyroid prepatient filtration in this patient with a short right leg. The radiopaque markers are locations of skin temperature asymmetries.

posterior radiograph. Postural distortions detectable by physical or radiologic examination are discussed in Chapters 4 and 5.

PLAIN FILM RADIOGRAPHY

Chiropractic care may be more effective if it prevents the vertebral subluxation complex from developing permanent vertebral or soft tissue asymmetry. The pediatric spine is particularly vulnerable as the cartilage makes its transition to bone. During the formative years, abnormal vertebral remodeling and deformity may occur (10,13,14,17,30). Clinical research and observation suggest that biomechanical compromise can occur in utero (constraint positions) (1–3), or as a result of birth trauma (7–9,22,31). Later, micro and macro trauma will occur in the child throughout spinal development.

The issue of radiographing children has been a topic of discussion within the profession for many years. Questions such as, at what age and which circumstances would indicate the necessity to x-ray, are very important considerations (32). Radiographic procedures for any child should include every safety precaution to reduce exposure to ionizing radiation. Shielding for the reproductive organs, as well as the brain, eyes, breast, thyroid gland, and bone marrow should be provided (Fig. 14.36A-B). If the child is small enough, the use of a 14 × 17 film size should replace the standard 14 × 36, if a full spine radiograph is needed. As always, strict collimation to exclude the skull and femur bones from exposure should always be used.

Rare earth intensifying screens with a minimal 400 screen-film combination speed is recommended to reduce exposure time. Higher combinations such as 800 or 1200 speed are available and should be considered. A high kilovoltage technique (e.g., 90–100 kvp) and a long film focal distance (e.g., 84 inches) should be used to further reduce exposure (See Chapter 5). High frequency x-ray generators (e.g., Universal, G.E.) are preferred to decrease patient radiation dose.

A consideration in deciding when to radiograph a child is the child's ability to hold the stance for the film.

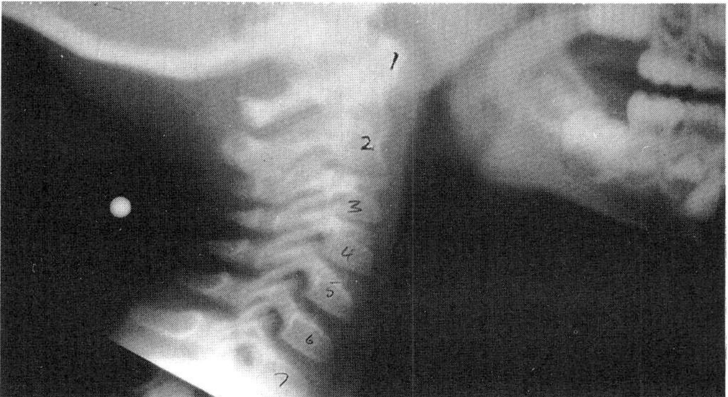

Figure 14.37. Radiograph depicting hyperextension positional dyskinesia of C3 in a four-yr-old. Notice the metallic marker, which was placed at the level of the skin temperature differential.

Positioning instructions should be adapted so that the child can understand the procedure. Patience in setting up the film can reduce the need for retakes. For the occasional, more difficult child to radiograph (e.g., cerebral palsy patient or the infant), the parents can assist. Lead shielding (e.g., apron, gloves) should be provided. The assistance of an outside radiologic facility may be necessary in some circumstances. If the doctor or parent chooses not to have a child radiographed, it is recommended that a x-ray waiver be signed by the parent or legal guardian.

Vertebral subluxation complexes can develop at a very early age (Fig. 14.37). Anomalies, spinal trauma, and acquired lesions such as spondylolisthesis are important in the evaluation of the patient (16,31,33–35) (Fig. 14.38A-B). Authorities within the radiologic community state that with the proper radiologic procedures, the usefulness of the information can assist in developing a more complete understanding of the pediatric spine. Spinal radiographs also are beneficial when specific thrust techniques are used.

SPECIAL CONSIDERATIONS

The pediatric patient has special requirements. The ability of the doctor to adapt procedures to the child is important in providing effective care.

The child's age, height, and weight are considerations. The newborn and infant will normally be most comfortable and cooperative if in physical contact with a parent during the evaluation and adjustment. The toddler's behavior may be the major factor in determining potential cooperation while on the cervical chair, pelvic bench,

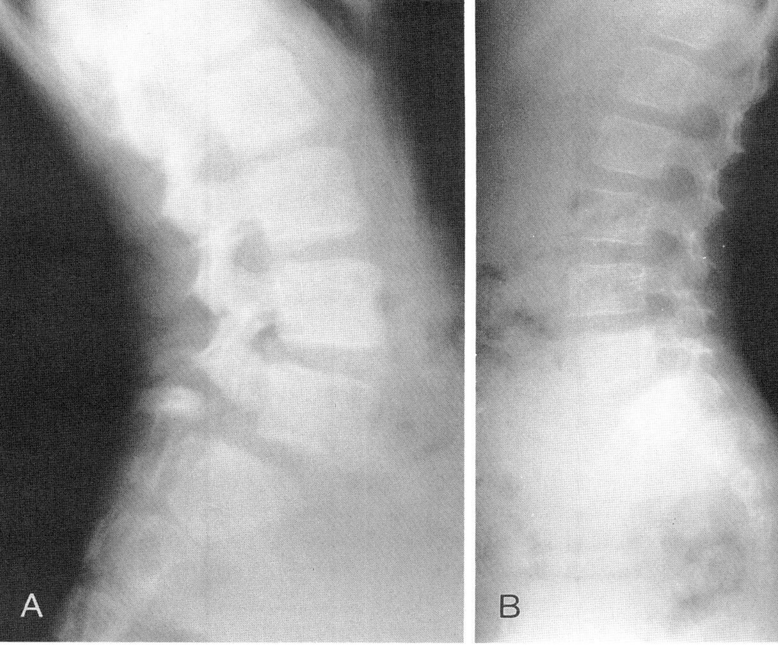

Figure 14.38. **A,** Spondylolisthesis of L5 in a ten-yr-old. **B,** Spondylolisthesis of L5 in a six-yr-old.

knee chest, or hi-lo table. Placement of the pediatric patient for the adjustment can vary from the adult. Where the child can receive the most comfortable and effective adjustment can only be determined on an individual basis.

The doctor's contact point for adjustments has traditionally been the pisiform and the broader aspects of the hand. The smaller size of the newborn, infant, and toddler will require the use of the distal ends of the fingers to ensure specificity. The age of the child will also determine the disc plane line before the thrust. The cervical curve, which is relatively flat at birth, begins to form the lordotic arch that becomes permanent, between the 3rd and 9th month of life (30). At approximately the 12th month, upright posture will complete the permanent lumbar curve. The thoracic and sacral curves are present at birth and remain so throughout the individual's lifetime.

The doctor's unfamiliarity with the pediatric spine, coupled with a general lack of gross morphologic changes of the motion segment, has often led to approaching the adjusting process in a generally unspecific fashion. Because many structural changes may take years to evidence neuropathophysiologic disorders such as symptoms, careless adjustments may have been considered relatively benign. The approach advocated here is to adjust only those articulations that are subluxated and require intervention. The haphazard introduction of a force directed into a dysfunctional motion segment, or thrusting into a normal or hypermobile articulation, should be avoided.

There are many potential sources of trauma (e.g., birth process, falls, automobile injuries) which can cause damage to the spine, spinal cord, and its supportive components (6–9,16,19,21–24,35,36). These physical traumas to children may result in stillbirth, SIDS, paralysis, functional disorders, and even death. If spinal trauma has been established to occur with children, it would behoove the chiropractor to learn from those mechanisms of injury. To repeat known mechanisms of injury to the pediatric spine with inappropriate adjustments, would obviously not benefit the child.

The pediatric patient placement and the adjustment should always prevent or minimize the following forces to the pediatric spine: traction ($+Y$), extension ($-\theta X$), rotation ($\pm\theta Y$), flexion ($+\theta X$) and lateral flexion ($-\theta Z$ or $+\theta Z$). The closer to the neutral position the spine can be maintained during patient placement and during the adjustive thrust, the less the likelihood of causing spinal injury.

In general, the most effective vector of thrust for the pediatric spine is from posterior to anterior ($+Z$) (Personal communication, Dr. Jan Jirout), excluding C1 laterality and rotation.

The depth of thrust can only be determined by the doctor. The amount of thrust should always be enough to accomplish the purpose of eliminating the vertebral subluxation. If the patient is relaxed and comfortable during the procedure, the amount of force is much less than in the adult. The foremost consideration by the doctor providing any pediatric care should always be the comfort of the child. A quick acceleration is generally required for the adjustment.

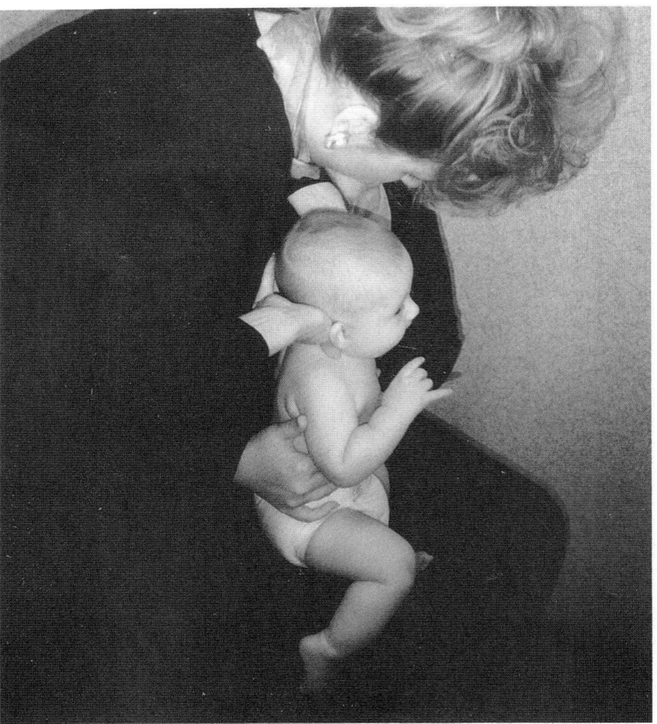

Figure 14.39. PS occiput adjustment with a thenar contact.

UPPER CERVICAL SPINE

Occipito-atlantal

The PS ($+\theta X$) occiput listing can be adjusted in two positions for the newborn or infant. The first is shown with the parent in Figure 14.39. The contact point is behind the infant's ear, slightly above the mastoid process, with the thenar of the doctor's hand. The thumb can replace the thenar eminence as the doctor's contact point (Fig. 14.40). To assist in stabilization, the parent should support the chest and back of the infant as demonstrated.

In positioning for a PS-RS ($+\theta X$, $-\theta Z$), the doctor can place the infant between the legs and apply a gentle pressure with the thighs. The chest of the doctor also can be used to stabilize the infant. The stabilization hand is placed on the opposite mastoid process. The fingers of that hand wrap around the posterior aspect of the cervical spine. This will protect the upper and midcervical regions from undesired movements during the thrust.

The toddler and doctor in Figure 14.41 display the proper set-up for stance, contact, and stabilization hand positioning for a PS-RS-RP ($+\theta X$, $-\theta Z$, $-\theta Y$), with the head rotated away slightly from contact hand, and a PS-LS-LA ($+\theta X$, $+\theta Z$, $-\theta Y$), with the head rotated slightly toward the contact hand (Fig. 14.42) (See Chapter 11).

The AS ($-\theta X$) condyle is an uncommon subluxation. This positional dyskinesia can cause severe neurologic disturbances. Micro or macro trauma is usually the cause of the AS condyle misalignment. In-utero constraint of the fetus may be one factor in the development of the AS condyle. The face or brow presentation is typically described as a compression of the head and cervical spine into an extended position. This presentation is found in one out of every 500 births and contributes to a malady of disorders (1–3). From a biomechanical standpoint, hyperextension of the cervical spine compounded by facial compression could create a posterior occipito-atlanto-axial vertebral subluxation as well.

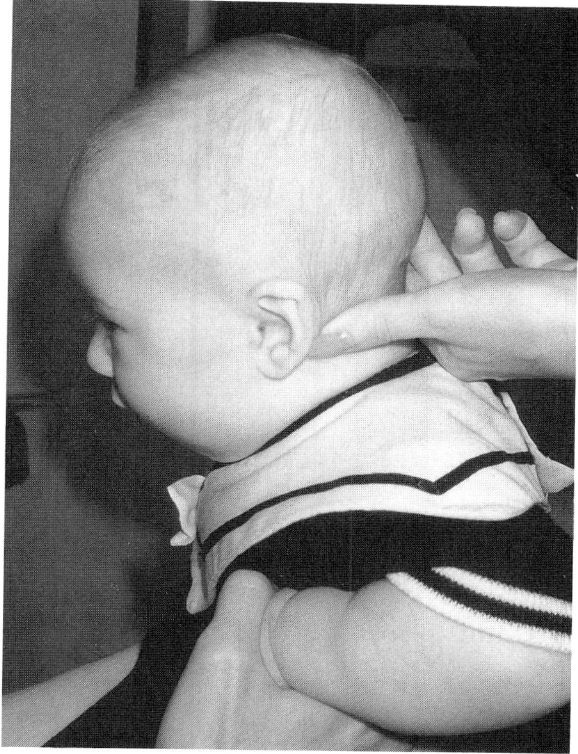

Figure 14.40. Thumb contact for PS occiput adjustment.

A newborn or infant with an AS condyle will display on postural examination a cervical hyperlordosis with a raised chin. The infant and toddler will manifest the hyperlordosis of the cervical spine. Over years of adaptation, however, compensation reactions of the midcervical spine can develop a kyphotic posture in the adult. The lateral radiograph will confirm the clinical impression. A lateral radiograph taken with the neck in flexion will demonstrate a lack of separation of the occiput from the posterior arch of the atlas (Fig. 14.43A-B). During motion palpation, the doctor should apply an anterior to posterior, superior to inferior, gliding motion. The AS condyle will cause restriction in joint play and muscular tenderness will be elicited at the posterior occipito-atlantal junction. The side of laterality and rotation can be confirmed with an APOM radiograph for both the AS and PS condyle subluxations.

Using a properly sized condyle block is important when adjusting a newborn or infant with an AS condyle. The block acts as a stabilizer for the cervical spine, thus protecting it from injury (See Chapter 11). The newborn or infant should be placed in a supine position with the condyle block supporting the cervical spine from C1 to

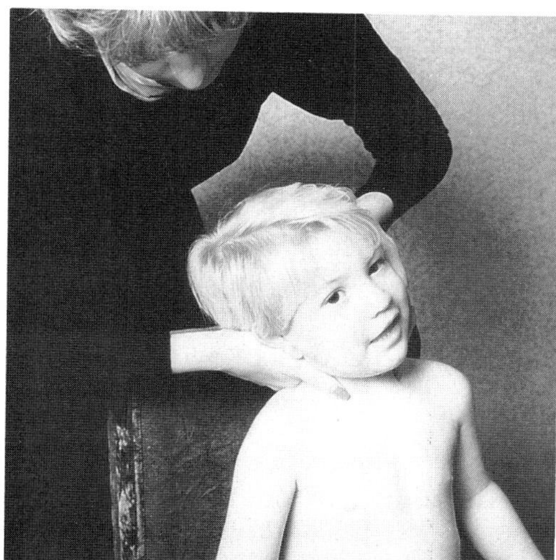

Figure 14.41. PS-RS-RP ($+\theta X, -\theta Z, -\theta Y$) adjustment with the toddler's head rotated accordingly away from the contact hand to correct axial rotation.

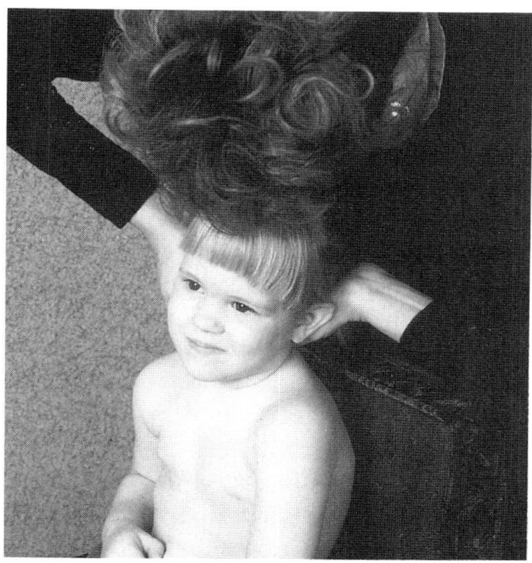

Figure 14.42. The toddler's head is rotated slightly toward the contact hand for axial rotation correction as depicted in this PS-LS-LA ($+\theta X, +\theta Z, -\theta Y$) listing.

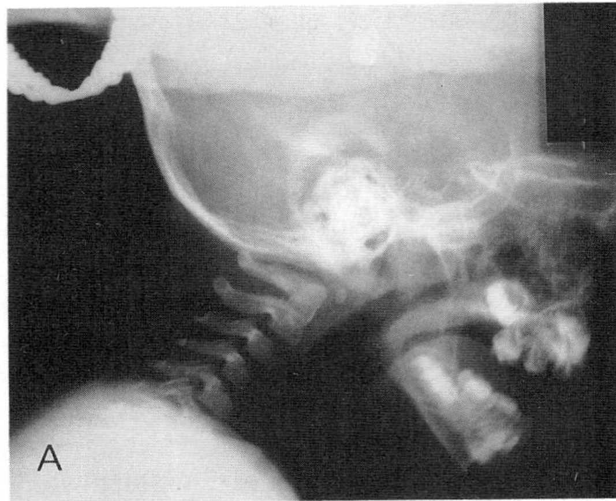

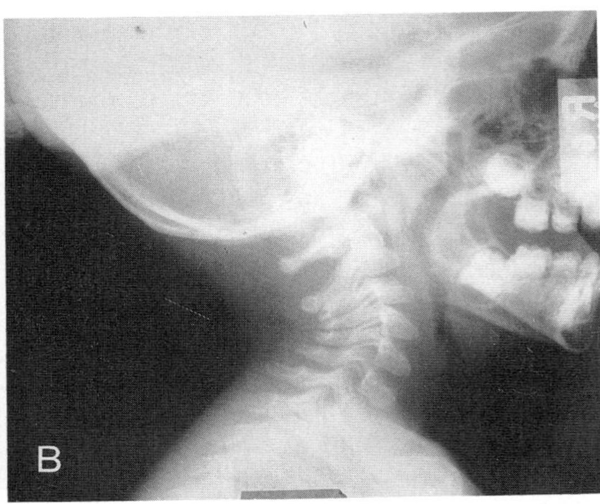

Figure 14.43. **A,** AS ($-\theta X$) subluxation. Cervical flexion discloses lack of separation of the occiput from the posterior arch of atlas. **B,** Posttreatment radiograph in the neutral position demonstrates more normal alignment.

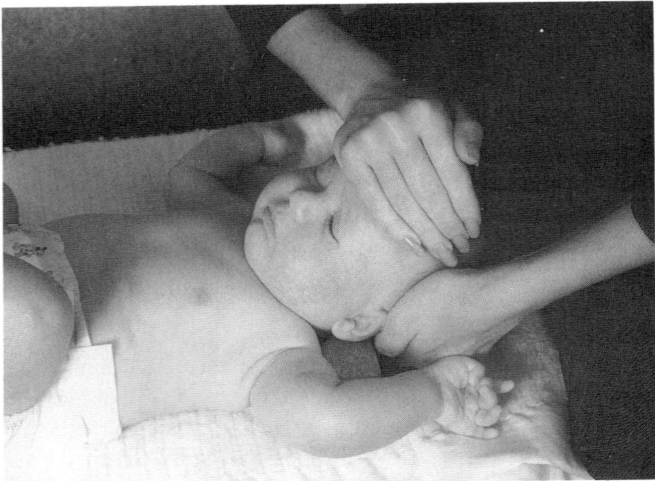

Figure 14.44. On the side of occiput laterality the doctor will squat or sit on a bench, contacting the glabella of the frontal bone on the side of laterality of the listing. The opposite hand will cup the posterior occiput and slightly lift to separate the occipito-atlantal joint as seen with this AS-LS listing. Notice the condyle block positioning.

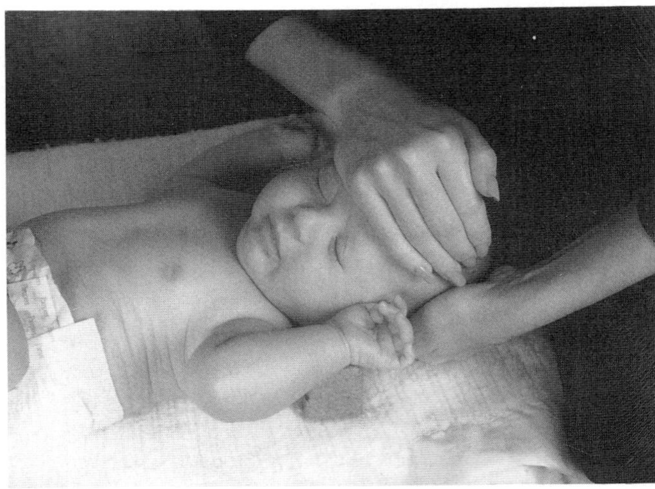

Figure 14.45. Slightly rotating the newborn's head away from the contact hand will correct axial rotation in an AS-LS-LP listing.

C7. To correct condyle laterality, (LS or RS listing), the doctor will stand or squat on the side of the lateral contact point. The flat palm of the contact hand is then placed on the glabella of the frontal bone. The opposite hand will cup the posterior occiput and create a slight lifting effect to separate the occipito-atlantal joint. In Figure 14.44 an AS-LS ($-\theta X$, $+\theta Z$) adjustment is demonstrated. The thrust is an arcing motion from anterior to posterior, and slightly superior to inferior ($+\theta X$). To correct the rotational component of anteriority or posteriority, the infant's head is pre-positioned in slight rotation before the thrust. For anteriority, the head should be turned slightly toward the contact hand. In Figure 14.45, turning the head away from the contact hand will correct the posterior rotation of the AS-LS-LP ($-\theta X$, $+\theta Z$, $+\theta Y$) listing.

If no laterality or rotation exists, an alternate approach can be used for correction of the AS component. The same supine position and condyle block placement is followed. However, the doctor will stand, squat or sit behind the center of the infant's head. Both thenar eminences are then placed on the glabella. The doctor's fingers will reach behind and contact the posterior occiput for the lift. The thrust is anterior to posterior ($-Z$) with a slight superior to inferior arc ($+\theta X$). Figure 14.46 demonstrates the AS condyle adjustment.

The toddler and adolescent set-up is performed in the cervical chair. The doctor will drop down the back of the chair to accommodate the height of the child and the condyle block placement. Once the proper condyle block size is chosen, it is placed on the posterior cervical spine (C1 to C7) with the abdomen of the doctor holding it in place (Fig. 14.47). In the cervical chair set-up, the flat palm of the hand will contact the glabella and supraorbital margin on the side of condyle laterality (AS-LS or AS-RS). The stabilization hand will be placed on the opposite supra orbital margin with the fingers overlapped or interlinked. The doctor should keep their elbows close to the patient's head. Tension pre-load is created by slightly flexing the chin downward. Figure 14.48 illustrates the set-up for the AS condyle adjustment. An AS-RS ($-\theta X$, $-\theta Z$) condyle is shown in Figure 14.49. To assist in stabilizing the patient set-up without the back of the chair, the knee of the doctor can be drawn up onto the cervical chair. Figure 14.50 depicts an AS-RS-RA adjustment, whereas Figure 14.51 illustrates an AS-RS-RP ($-\theta X$, $-\theta Z$, $-\theta Y$) correction. The rotational component of anteriority or posteriority is corrected when the doctor pre-positions the head before the thrust.

Atlanto-axial Region

The anterolateral tip of the transverse process is contacted for the AS portion of the atlas listing. To correct laterality of the atlas (ASL or ASR), the doctor contacts the involved side. The patient placement may vary depending on the comfort and cooperation of the patient. Figure 14.52 shows the parent holding the newborn for an ASL ($-\theta X$, $+\theta Z$) listing. Unnecessary head rotation should be avoided for correction of an ASL or ASR listing. The doctor also can position the infant sitting between the legs, while applying a slight thigh pressure to reduce infant movement (Fig. 14.53 illustrates an ASR listing). Protection of the cervical spine with the stabilization hand is important.

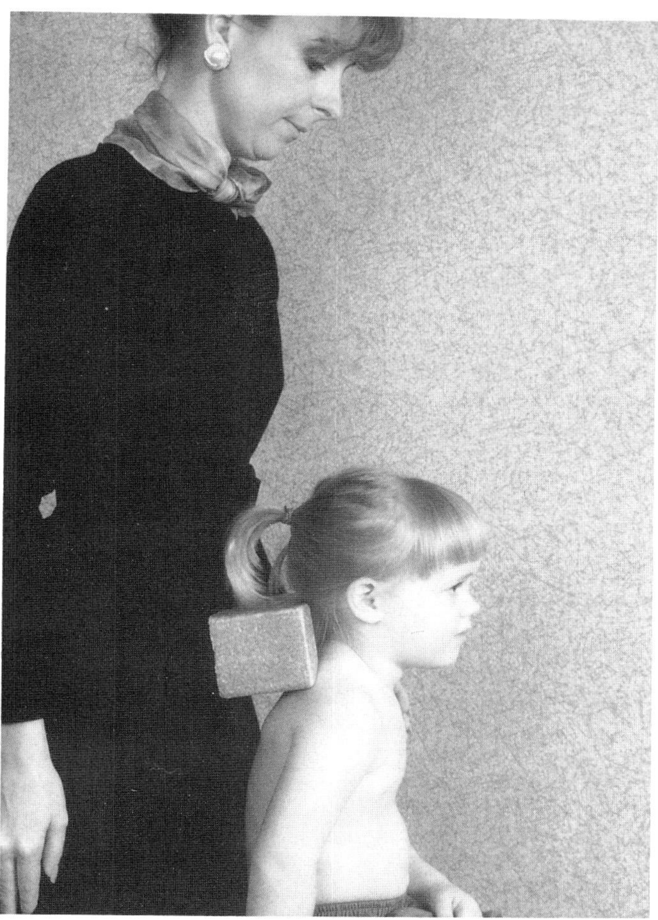

Figure 14.47. The back of the chair is dropped to accommodate the height of the toddler or adolescent. The doctor will hold with their abdomen the proper condyle block size for the posterior cervical (C1 to C7) spine.

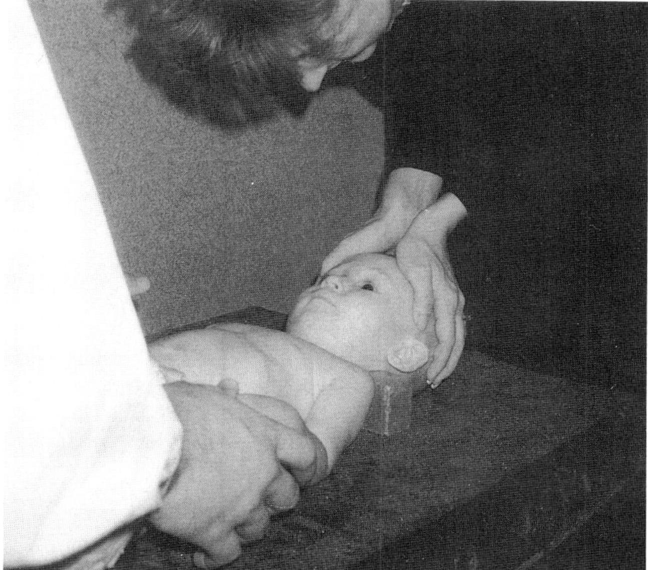

Figure 14.46. The AS condyle without laterality or rotation can be corrected by contacting the glabella with both thenar eminences. The doctor will stand, squat or sit behind and center to the infant's head.

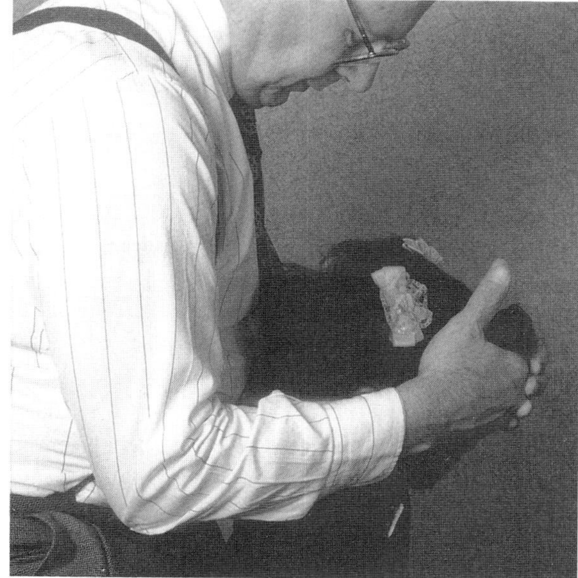

Figure 14.48. The child's chin will be slightly flexed to create pre-load tension for the AS condyle adjustment.

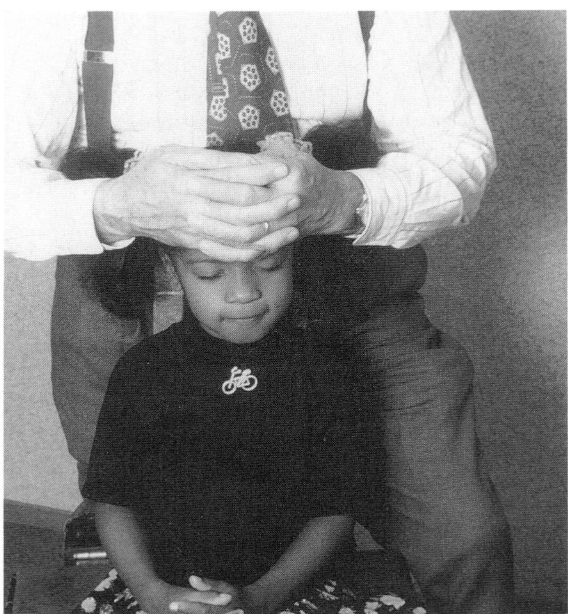

Figure 14.49. The flat palm of the hand will contact the glabella and supraorbital margin on the side of condyle laterality. The stabilization hand will be placed on the opposite supraorbital margin with the fingers interlinked. The doctor's elbows should be kept close to the patient's head as seen in the AS-RS set-up.

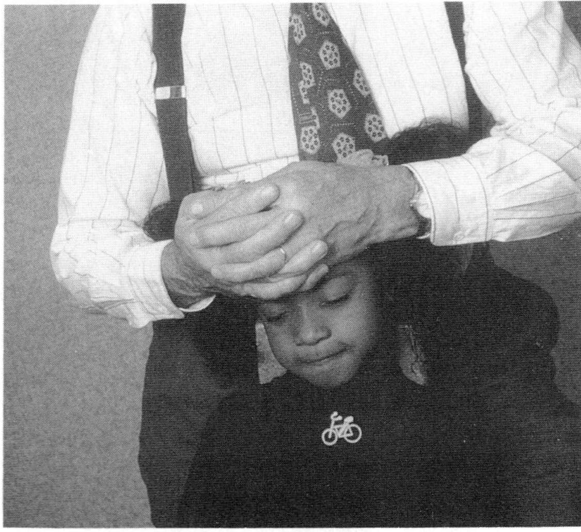

Figure 14.50. To assist in stabilization, the knee of the doctor can be drawn up onto the cervical chair to support the patient set-up. Rotating the child's head toward the contact hand will correct axial rotation as seen in this AS-RS-RA set-up.

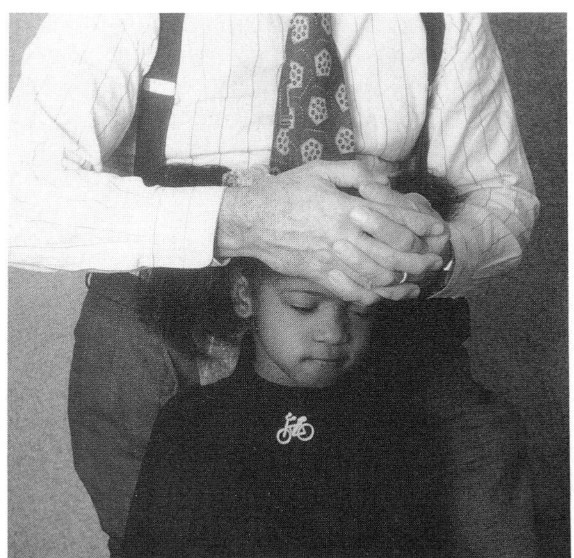

Figure 14.51. Rotating the child's head away from the contact hand is depicted in this AS-RS-RP set-up.

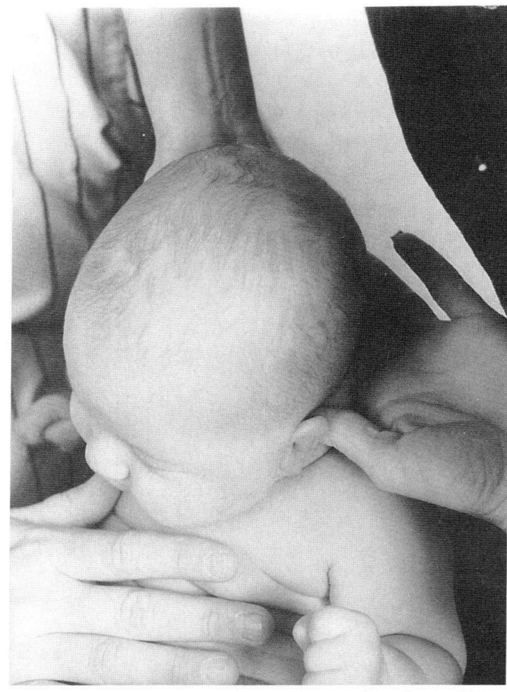

Figure 14.52. The parent can stabilize the newborn as the doctor contacts the anterior-lateral tip of the transverse process of the atlas for the AS portion of the listing. To correct laterality of the atlas, the doctor contacts the involved side as shown with this ASL set-up.

In the sitting position, the amount of head rotation before applying the thrust is in direct proportion to the degree of atlas rotation. For an anterior listing (ASLA, ASRA), the head is rotated toward the side of the contact hand. Posterior rotation (ASLP, ASRP) is corrected by turning the head away from the side of the contact hand. As seen in Figure 14.54, slight rotation is used to correct the rotational component of the ASLA ($-\theta X$, $+\theta Z$, $-\theta Y$) listing. With more atlas rotation, Figure 14.55 shows the appropriate set-up for an ASRA ($-\theta X$, $-\theta Z$, $+\theta Y$) adjustment.

A third alternative for adjusting the atlas is to lie the

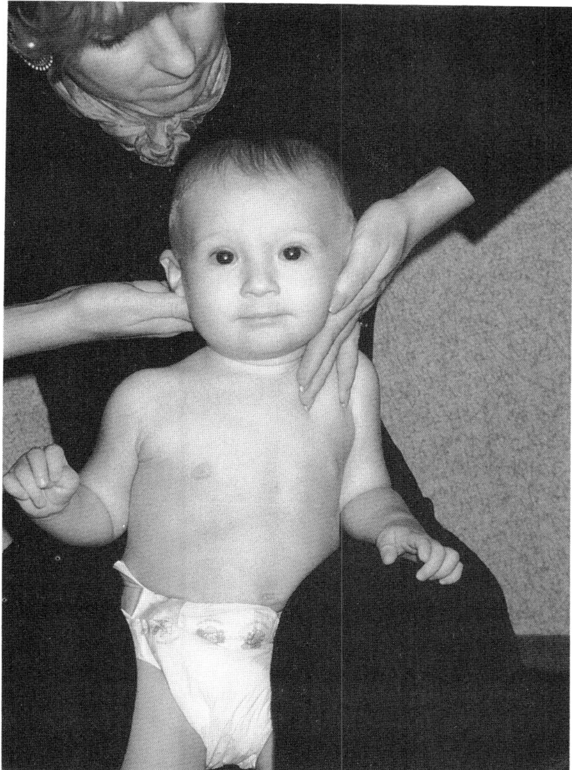

Figure 14.53. This ASR set-up shows the infant placement between the doctor's legs with slight thigh pressure. The stabilization hand will protect the cervical spine from unnecessary motion during the thrust.

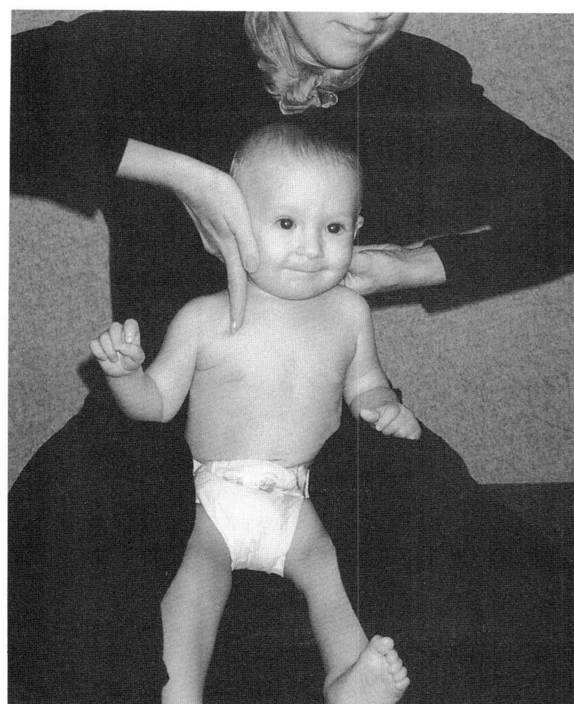

Figure 14.54. The ASLA listing will have head rotation toward the contact hand.

newborn or infant in a side posture position with the head in a neutral plane. The thumb, thumb-index, or the distal end of the index finger, can be used for adjusting the atlas. Figure 14.56 demonstrates a distal index finger on top of the thumb pad for an ASR ($-\theta X$, $-\theta Z$) listing in the side

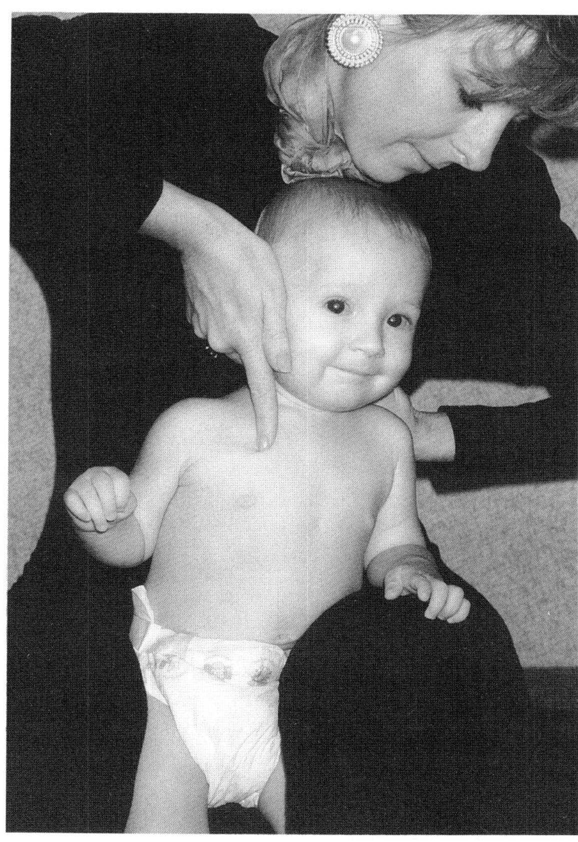

Figure 14.55. To correct more axial rotation, the doctor will rotate proportionally the newborn's head as seen with this ASLA set-up.

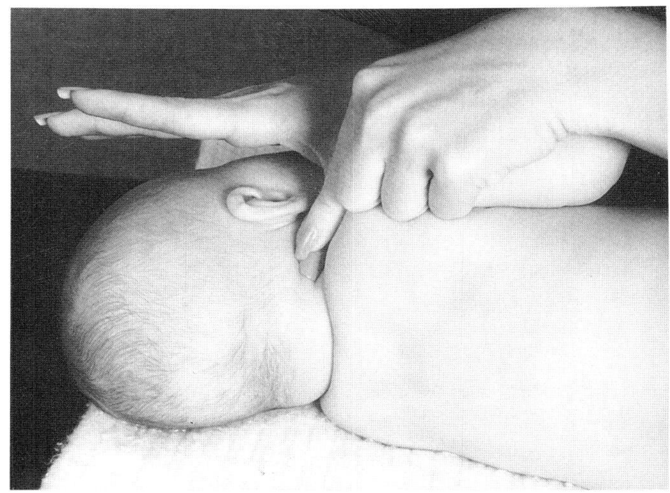

Figure 14.56. Side posture position with the head in the neutral plane for an ASR adjustment.

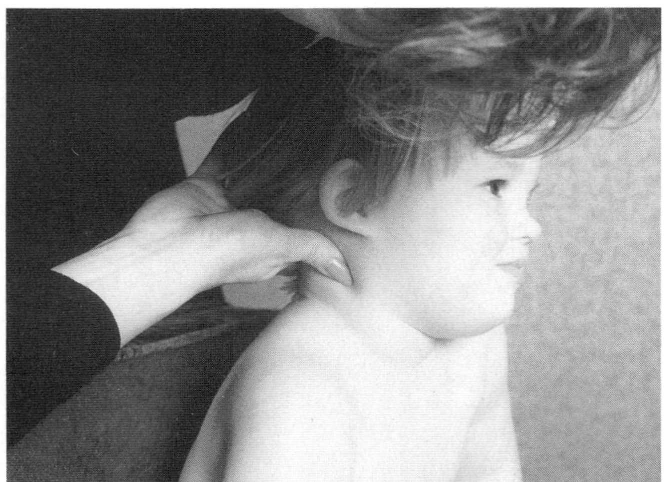

Figure 14.57. To prepare for a toddler atlas set-up, the head is first laterally flexed away from the side of contact. The doctor will contact the anterolateral tip of the atlas transverse process with the distal end of thumb.

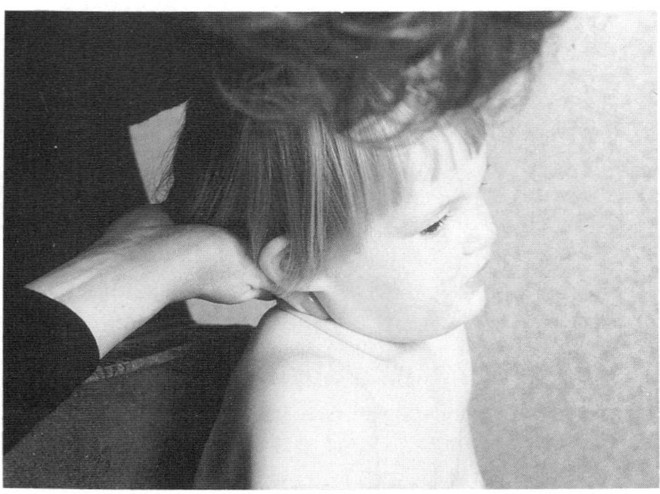

Figure 14.58. The cervical spine is then laterally flexed toward the thumb after the atlas is contacted.

posture position. The thrust is a set and hold (See Chapter 2). The adjustment should not be performed as a toggle-recoil. Because the purpose of the thrust is to correct atlas superiority and laterality, it is advised that a rotated atlas (e.g., ASLA, ASLP, ASRA, ASRP) not be adjusted in the side posture position. The thrust vector for correction of rotation is more difficult to achieve in this position.

With the toddler, set-up procedures are similar to the adult patient. To prepare for the atlas set-up, the head is first laterally flexed away from the side of the contact hand as seen in Figure 14.57.

After contacting the anterior lateral tip of the transverse process of the atlas with the distal end of the thumb, the cervical spine is laterally flexed toward the thumb (Fig. 14. 58). The contact wrist should remain relatively

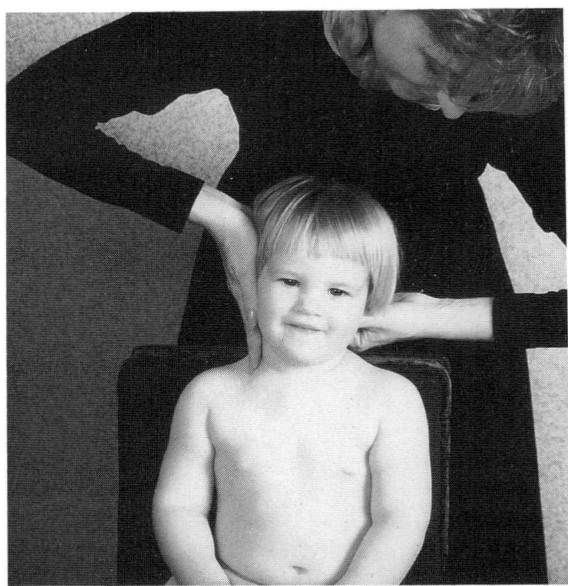

Figure 14.59. This ASR set-up illustrates the relatively flat wrist of the contact hand and proper stabilization hand positioning and doctor stance.

flat. Figure 14.59 illustrates the proper doctor stance, contact, and stabilization hand positioning for an ASR listing. The stabilization hand is an important consideration. The doctor should gently place a hand on the opposite side of contact on the lateral aspect of the cervical spine. The purpose of the stabilization hand is to avoid compromising the other motion segments during the adjustment. During the thrust, the stabilization hand should never produce any counterforce. Figure 14.60 depicts an ASLP ($-\theta X$, $+\theta Z$, $+\theta Y$) adjustment.

LOWER CERVICAL SPINE (C2-C7)

The set-ups for the cervical region (C2 to C7) for the newborn or infant have many variations. After performing a spinal analysis, the contact finger and patient placement must be chosen. The primary vector for correction of the subluxation is from posterior to anterior ($+Z$).

If a straight posterior subluxation is present, the distal end of the index finger can be placed on the spinous process with the patient in a prone position (Fig 14.61). The infant also can be placed in a prone position on the parent's lap while using the parent's hand for stabilization. Figure 14.62 shows the distal end of the fifth phalange with the stabilization fifth phalange placed on top for a posterior second cervical listing. The side posture position can be used with the index finger making contact on the spinous process for adjustments of a posteriorly ($-Z$) displaced cervical segment (Fig. 14.63).

A sitting position set-up can be accomplished with the assistance of the parent. The parent should support the chest and back of the infant. Figure 14.64 demonstrates a posterior midcervical set-up, using a spinous process contact. Again, the stabilization hand should not provide a counterforce. The PL or PR listing adds a lateral to medial vector to the posterior to anterior vector for correction.

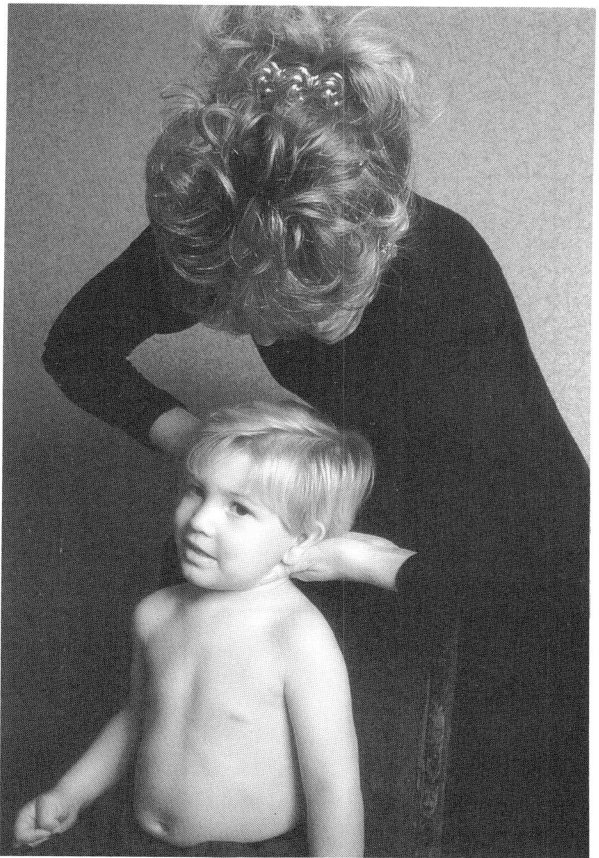

Figure 14.60. Rotating the head of the toddler away from the contact hand will pre-position for correction of axial rotation of the ASLP listing.

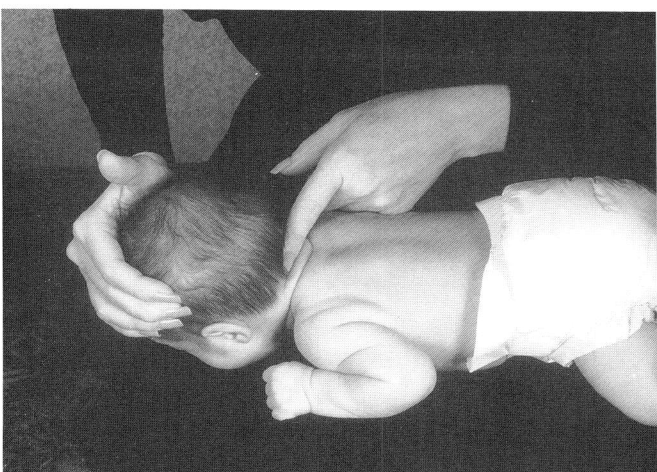

Figure 14.61. Posterior cervical adjustment with an index finger contact.

The third component of the listing [lateral flexion dyskinesia ($\pm\theta Z$)] is corrected by an inferiorward arcing motion or torque added at the end of the thrust. The pediatric spine is very flexible, and special attention must be made to avoid excessive lateral flexion or hyperextension of the cervical region. The reader is referred to Chapters 10 and 11 for additional information.

The toddler can be adjusted in the cervical chair. To raise the height of the toddler in the chair, the pelvic bench pillow can be placed underneath the patient. Figure 14.65 depicts a PR ($-Z$, $+\theta Y$) set-up on the fourth cervical vertebra. Figure 14.66 demonstrates a sixth cervical PL ($-Z$, $-\theta Y$) adjustment. Notice the placement of the stabilization hand in a seventh cervical PR set-up (Fig. 14.67).

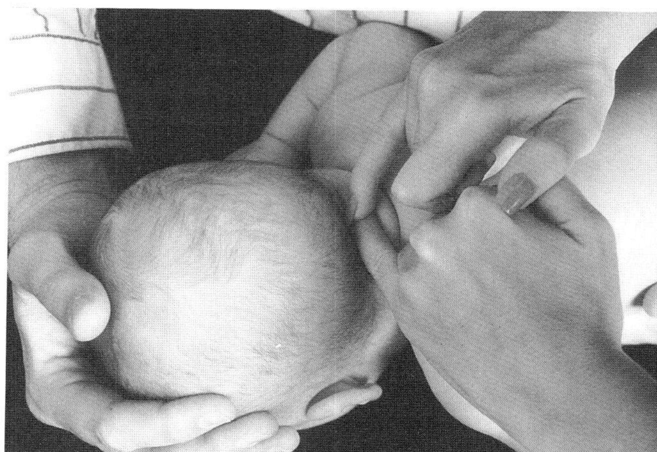

Figure 14.62. The infant can be placed prone on the lap of the parent, while they further assist by stabilizing the infant's head with their hand. This set-up depicts the distal end of the fifth phalange with the stabilization fifth phalange placed on top for a posterior second cervical listing.

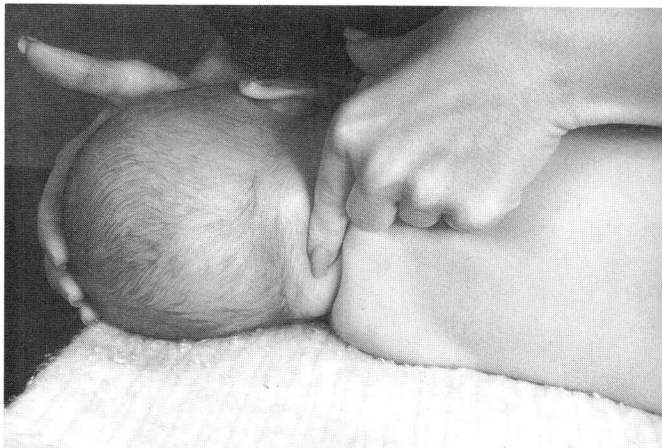

Figure 14.63. The side posture position with the distal end of the index finger contacting the spinous process of a posterior fourth cervical. The doctor's opposite hand should stabilize the crown of the infant's head.

The right-handed set-up would be used for a PR ($-Z$, $+\theta Y$), or PRS ($-Z$, $+\theta Y$, $-\theta Z$) listing on the spinous process or a PLI-la ($-Z$, $-\theta Y$, $-\theta Z$) listing, using the lamina as the contact point. Pre- and posttreatment radiographs are shown in Figure 14.68A-B.

The upper thoracic region also can be adjusted in the sitting position. Figure 14.69 illustrates a toddler in a cervical chair third thoracic set-up. Depending on the listing, the doctor can contact the spinous process or transverse process with the distal end of the index finger. The upper thoracic region will require a more superior to inferior pattern of thrust.

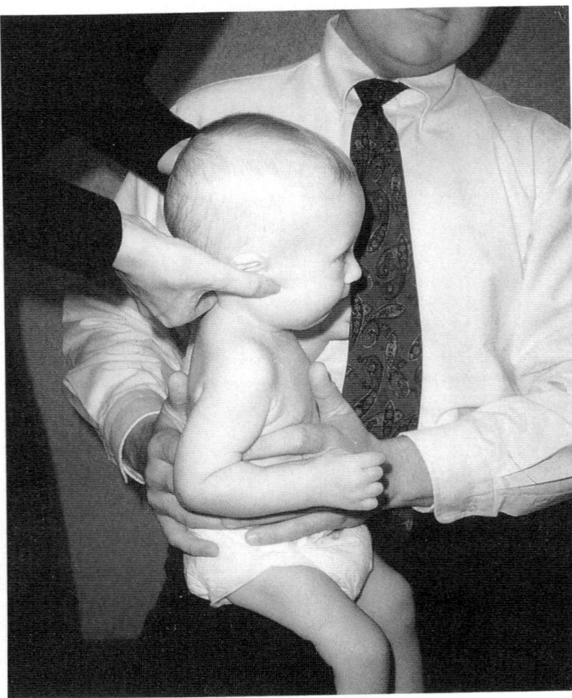

Figure 14.64. With the assistance of the parent holding the infant's stomach and back, a sitting position is shown for this posterior mid cervical adjustment.

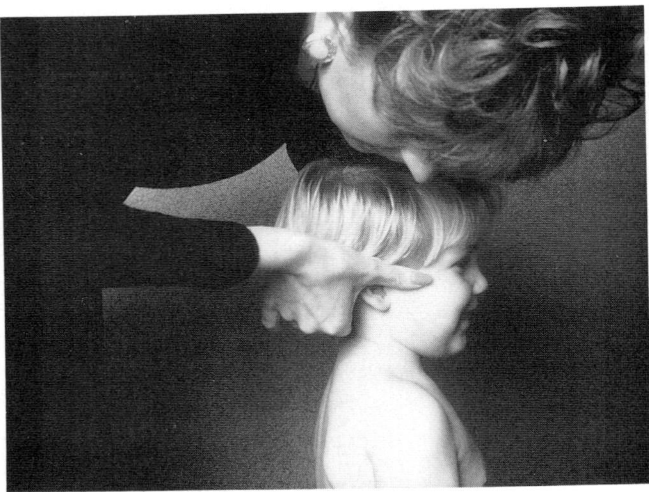

Figure 14.65. The toddler's height is raised in the chair before the set-up by placing the pelvic bench pillow underneath. The back of the cervical chair has been lowered for illustration purposes only for this PR fourth cervical adjustment.

THORACIC SPINE

Correction of thoracic subluxations is accomplished primarily using adjustments in the posterior to anterior ($+Z$) direction. Rotational displacements (e.g., $-Z$, $-\theta Y$/PL or $-Z$, $+\theta Y$/PR) can occur as well and are

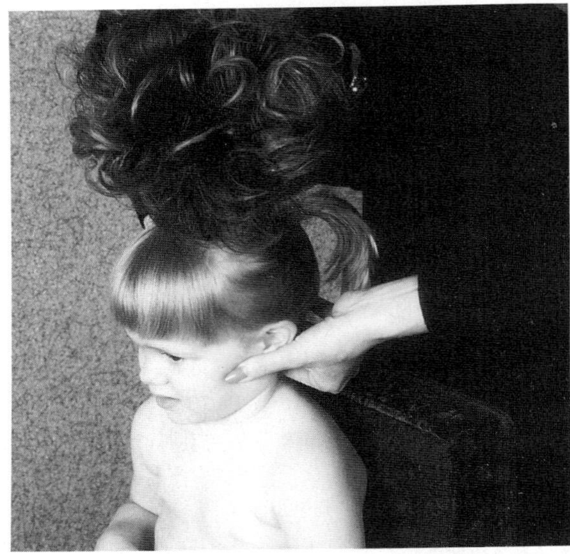

Figure 14.66. PL ($-Z, -\theta X, -\theta Y$) C6 adjustment.

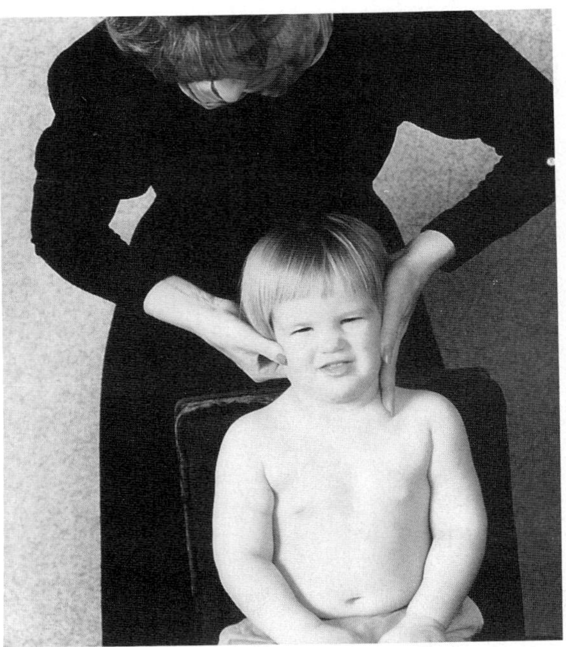

Figure 14.67. PR ($-Z, -\theta X, +\theta Y$) C7 adjustment. Notice the stabilization hand.

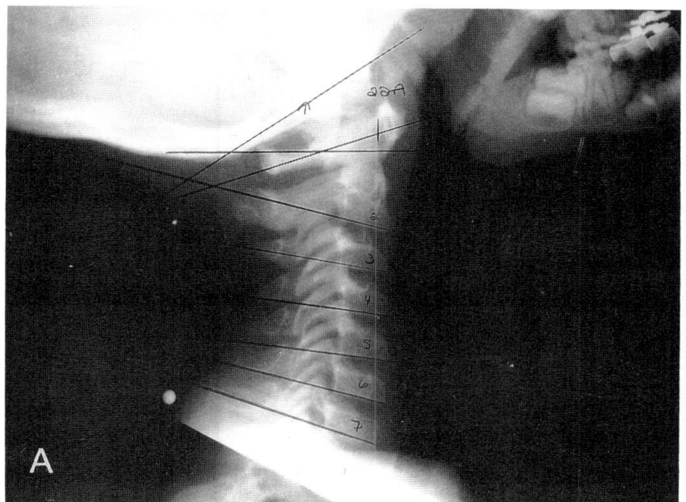

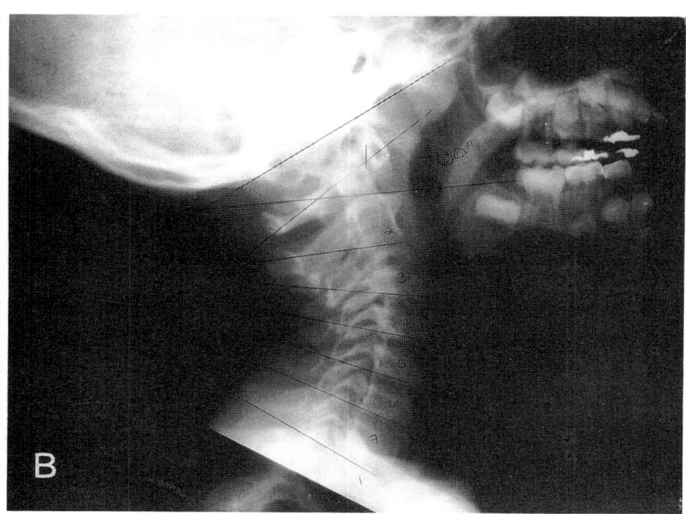

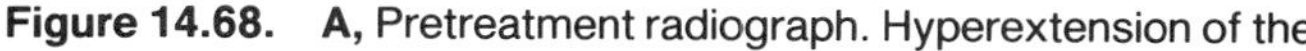

Figure 14.68. **A,** Pretreatment radiograph. Hyperextension of the head was the child's normal position. **B,** Posttreatment radiograph.

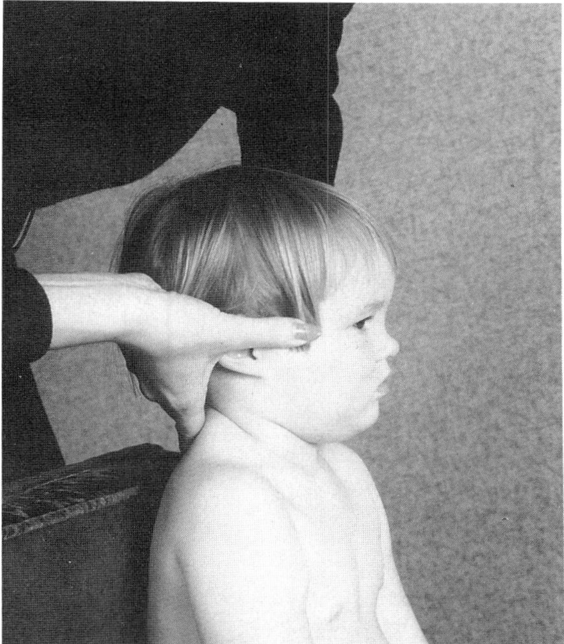

Figure 14.69. Third thoracic adjustment in the cervical chair.

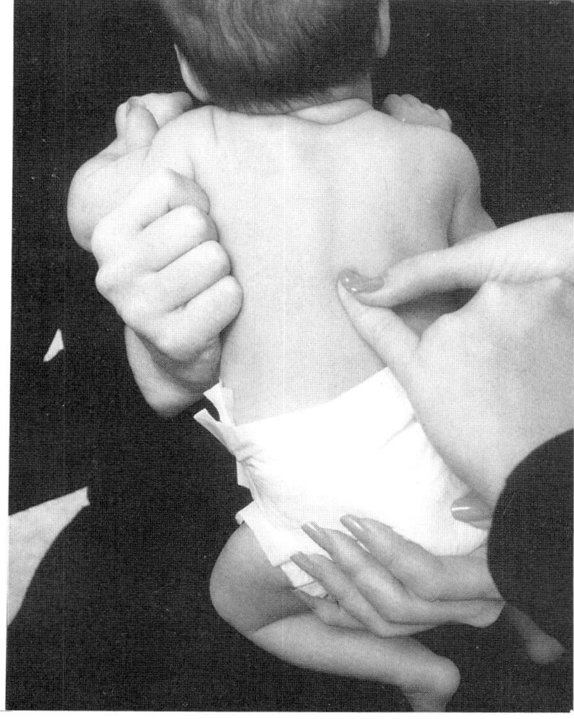

Figure 14.70. PR ninth thoracic adjustment. The parent is stabilizing this premature newborn.

corrected accordingly; however, this is usually not a primary component of the listing. The spinous process is the preferred patient contact point. A variety of patient positions and hand contacts are available to the doctor for the thoracic spine adjustment.

Three common positions are against the chest of the parent, across the lap of a parent, or across the lap of the doctor. Keeping the infant in a neutral position during the thrust and not allowing them to rotate their trunk is an important consideration. Figure 14.70 illustrates the parent holding a premature newborn for a PR ($-Z$, $+\theta Y$) ninth thoracic listing. The doctor stands on the side of spinous laterality, using the distal end of the fifth phalange on the spinous process with the distal finger of the other hand placed on top.

The infant can also be placed prone on the parent's lap. A double-thumb contact on the spinous process can be used for a posterior subluxation (Fig. 14.71). This double-thumb contact is only one of many combinations of finger contacts. The distal end of the index finger also can be used to set a posterior thoracic subluxation or a posterior and rotated segment (e.g., PL) (Fig. 14.72).

The hi-lo table can be used for patient placement of

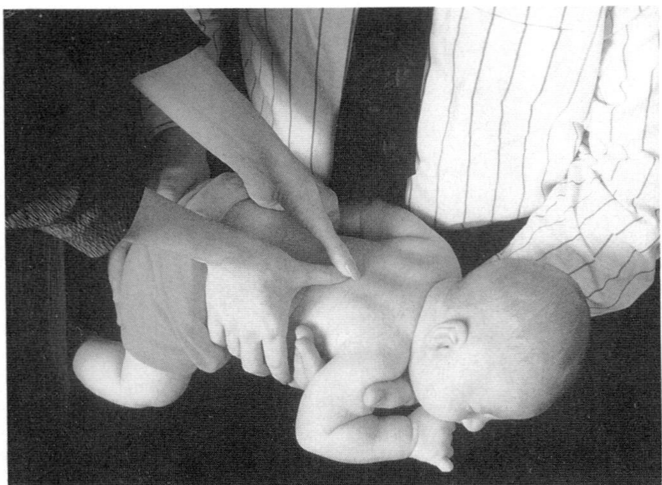

Figure 14.71. A double-thumb contact on the spinous process for a thoracic adjustment.

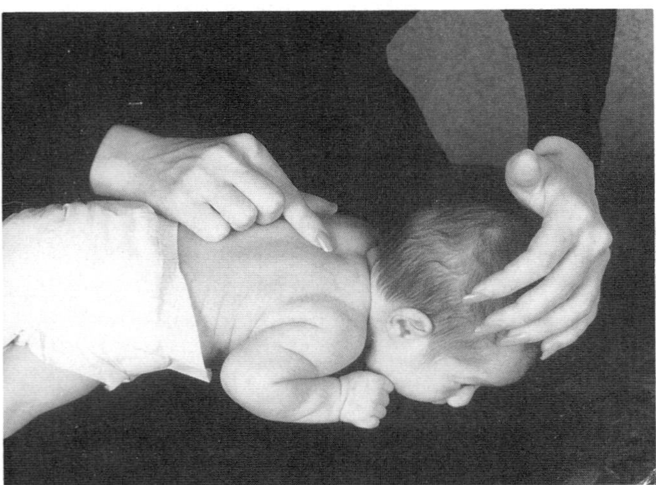

Figure 14.72. Posterior thoracic adjustment with an index finger contact. Notice the stabilization hand.

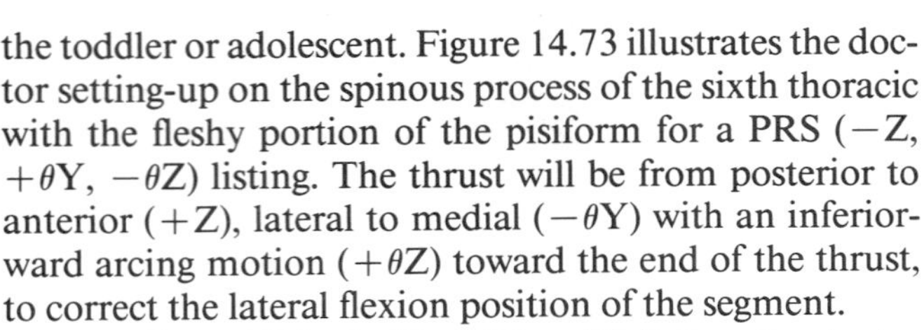

the toddler or adolescent. Figure 14.73 illustrates the doctor setting-up on the spinous process of the sixth thoracic with the fleshy portion of the pisiform for a PRS ($-Z$, $+\theta Y$, $-\theta Z$) listing. The thrust will be from posterior to anterior ($+Z$), lateral to medial ($-\theta Y$) with an inferiorward arcing motion ($+\theta Z$) toward the end of the thrust, to correct the lateral flexion position of the segment.

To adjust a PLI-t ($-Z$, $-\theta Y$, $-\theta Z$) listing, the doctor stands on the right side and the transverse process is contacted (Fig. 14.74). For a PRI-t ($-Z$, $+\theta Y$, $+\theta Z$) adjustment, the left transverse process is contacted. The hand and fingers of the contact hand should not cross the spine for a transverse process contact. The PLI-t adjustment is posterior to anterior ($+Z$), lateral to medial ($+\theta Y$), with an inferiorward arcing motion ($+\theta Z$) toward the end of the movement.

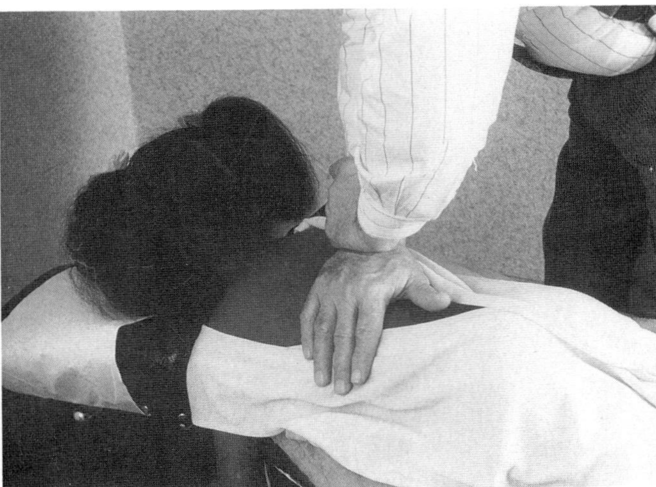

Figure 14.73. The doctor will contact with the fleshy portion of the pisiform the spinous process as shown in this adjustment for a PRS thoracic listing.

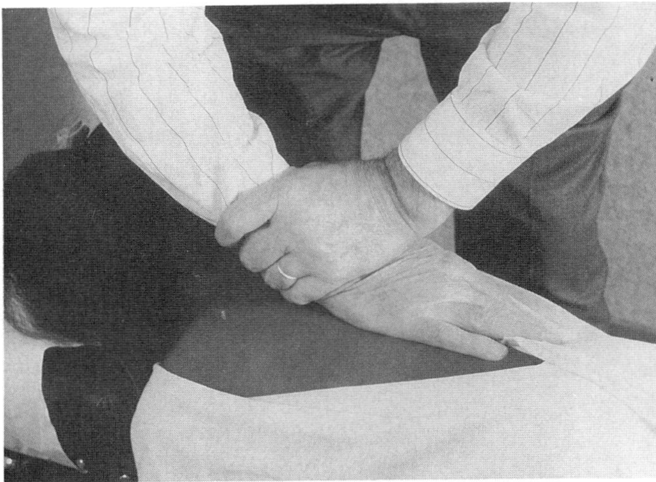

Figure 14.74. The fourth thoracic is contacted on the right transverse process for a PLI-t listing. The hands and fingers of the contact hand should not cross the spine.

An alternative set-up is a double-thumb contact placed bilaterally on the transverse processes to correct a PLI-t or PRI-t listing. For a PRI-t listing, the left thumb contacts the left transverse process. No thrust is made with the stabilization thumb (Fig. 14.75).

LUMBAR SPINE

In the newborn or infant, the major lumbar positional dyskinesia is usually posteriority ($-Z$). This will be corrected with a posterior to anterior thrust ($+Z$), using the spinous process as the short lever arm. The lap of the parent can be used to place the newborn or infant in the prone position. Figure 14.76 illustrates the distal thumb pad contact on the spinous process and the distal end of the index finger on top for stabilization. The infant also can be placed across the lap of the doctor. Figure 14.77 depicts an adjustment for a PL ($-Z$, $-\theta Y$) fifth lumbar. The doctor should place the infant's spinous laterality closest to their torso. The thrust for the PL listing is from posterior to anterior ($+Z$) and lateral to medial ($+\theta Y$). The newborn or infant also can be placed against the chest of a parent (Fig. 14.78). The doctor is shown setting-up on a midlumbar with the right thumb on the spinous process and the left thumb stabilizing the contact hand.

The side posture position also can be used for the adjustment of a variety of listings. It is recommended that a finger push contact be used instead of a pisiform, to enhance specificity (Fig. 14.79). The doctor should place an index finger on the spinous or mammillary process, depending on the listing. To support the index finger, the middle finger can be placed on top of the nailbed. The purpose of the stabilization hand is to support the upper torso in a neutral position. The parent can assist the doctor by stabilizing either the upper torso or the lower limbs to prevent the infant from rotating. There should be no axial torsion of the spine. Axial rotation would compromise the integrity of the motion segment, above and below the subluxation, especially the intervertebral disc. For a PL or PR listing, the spinous rotation is placed

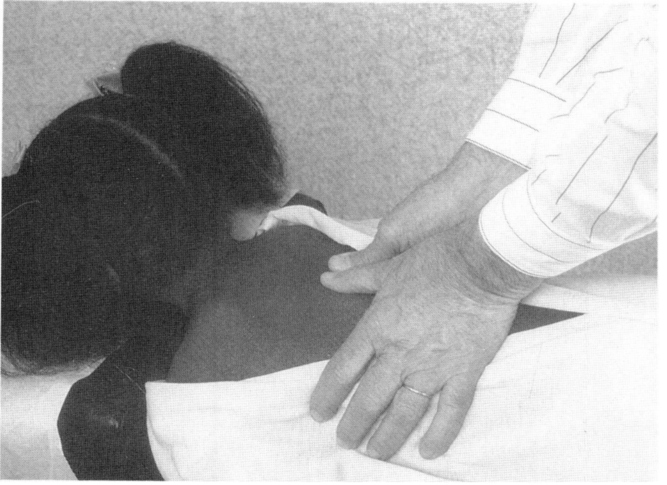

Figure 14.75. For this fourth thoracic double-thumb contact on a PRI-t listing, the thrust will be made on the left transverse process only.

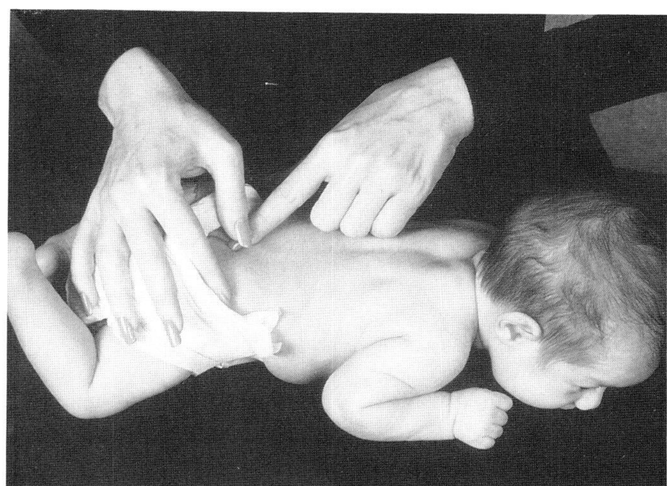

Figure 14.77. PL ($-Z$, $-\theta Y$) L5 adjustment.

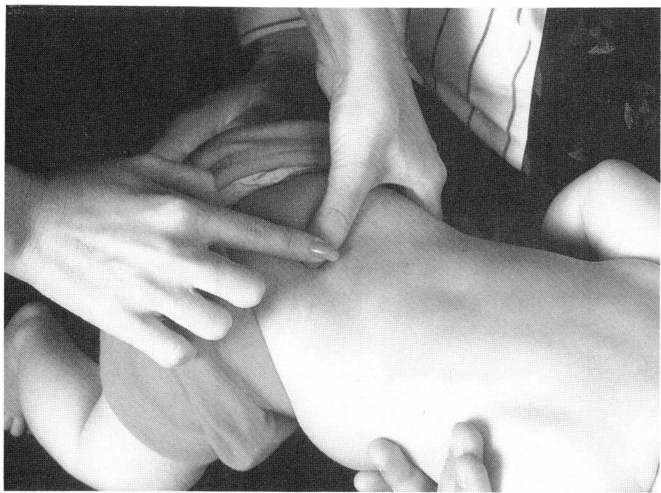

Figure 14.76. The distal end of the thumb is contacting the spinous process of the posterior fifth lumbar. The distal end of the index finger is placed on top for stabilization. The infant is further stabilized by the parent.

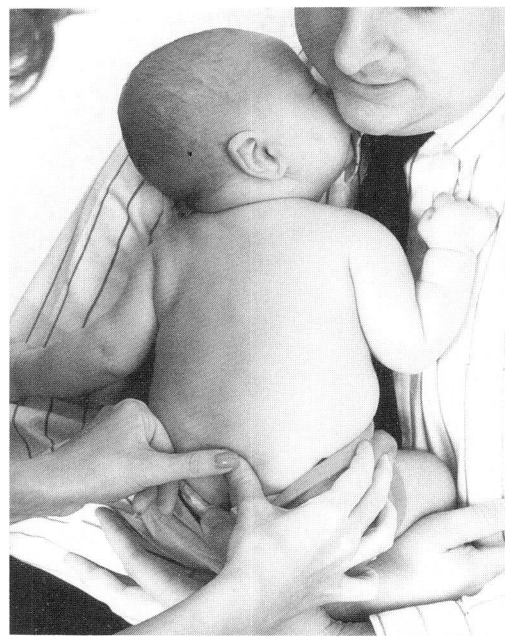

Figure 14.78. Posterior lumbar adjustment in the upright position.

toward the table. The thrust is from posterior to anterior (+Z) and lateral to medial. If a lateral flexion positional dyskinesia is present (e.g., PLS), then an inferiorward arcing motion ($-\theta Z$) should be made toward the end of the thrust. A PRI-m ($-Z, +\theta Y, +\theta Z$) listing is adjusted with the patient on their right side (spinous rotation down). The left mammillary is contacted. The thrust is from posterior to anterior (+Z) and an inferiorward arcing motion ($-\theta Z$) is applied toward the end of the thrust. Lateral flexion positional dyskinesia is rarely detected in the newborn or infant, unless a scoliosis is present. At no time should the doctor's leg be placed on the infant's or toddler's bent leg as is traditional in some long lever techniques.

The use of the parent's hand can be used to stabilize the legs if necessary. Figure 14.80 depicts a side posture fourth lumbar, PRI-m pisiform push set-up. The contact hand position is modified for a spinous process pisiform contact (e.g., PLS) (Fig. 14.81). The finger push contact can be used for a spinous or mammillary process contact. Figure 14.82 depicts a second lumbar PR listing set-up.

The forearm of the doctor should follow the disc plane line of the motion segment involved. To stabilize the pelvis of the older child, the doctor will gently bend a leg across the top bent leg of the patient. The doctor should create no force (weight or drop) into the patient during the adjustment. The stabilization hand on the older child should not press the shoulder down onto the table (Fig. 14.81).

PELVIS

Ilium

The simple or compound ilium misalignment does not commonly occur in the newborn, infant or toddler, unless it is trauma induced.

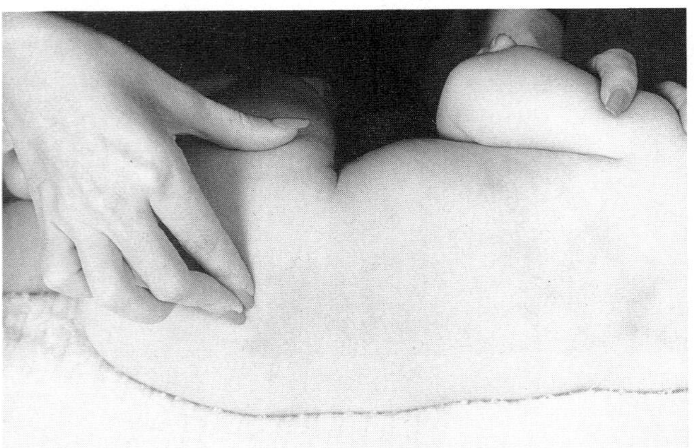

Figure 14.79. The index finger on the spinous or mammillary process will increase specificity for a push move on this lumbar vertebra. To support the index finger, the middle finger is placed over the nailbed. The purpose of the stabilization hand is to support the upper torso in a neutral position.

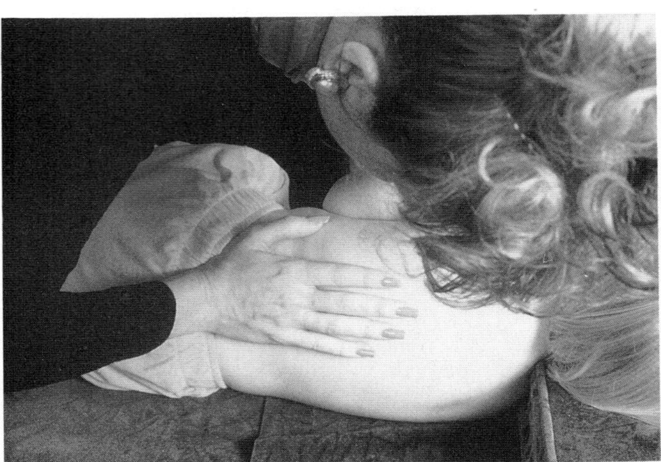

Figure 14.80. The fourth lumbar is contacted with the left mammillary up for a PRI-m adjustment.

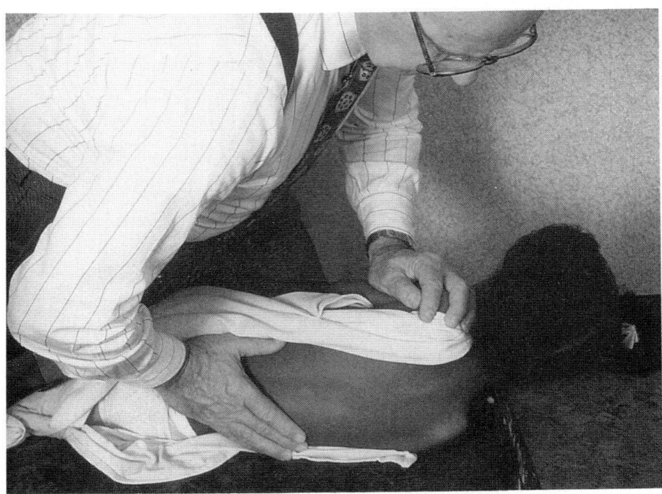

Figure 14.81. PLS L5 adjustment. The fingers of the contact hand cross the spine. To stabilize the pelvis, the doctor will gently place his or her leg across the top bent leg of the child.

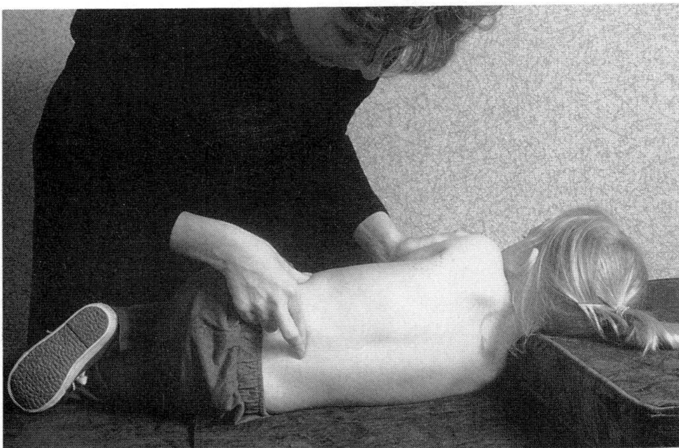

Figure 14.82. L2 PR adjustment. The spinous laterality is placed down toward the table when a finger push move is used (See Chapter 7). The stabilization hand should not pin the shoulder onto the table.

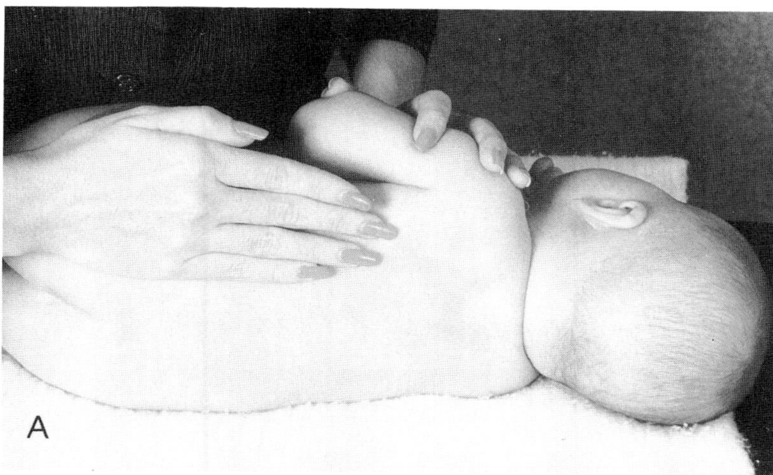

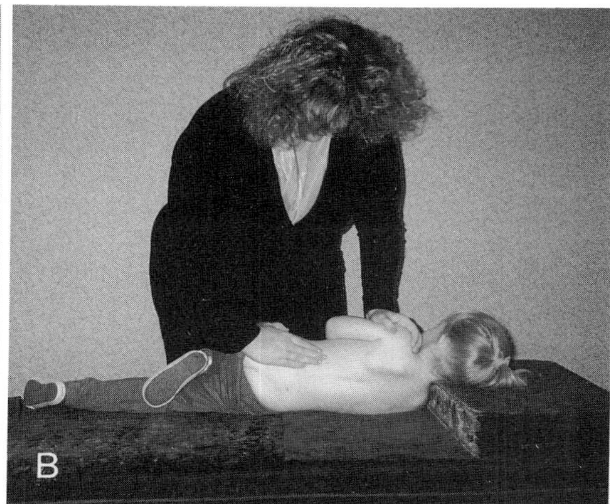

Figure 14.83. **A,** The side posture position can be used to contact the PSIS with the pisiform on the PI ilium. **B,** PI ilium adjustment for the toddler.

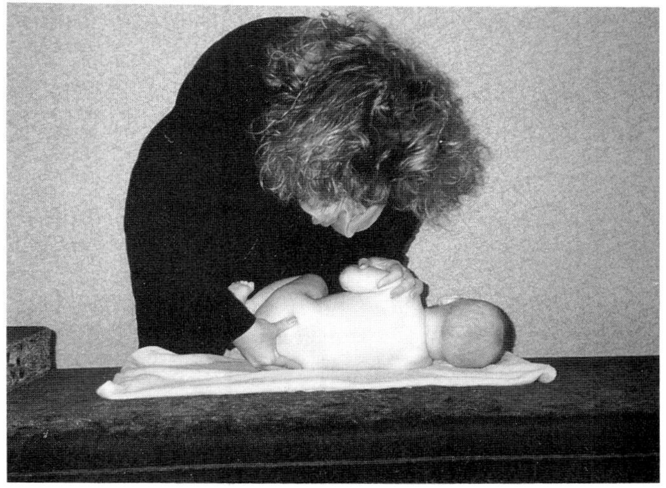

Figure 14.84. The distal end of the thumb is shown contacting the PI ilium with the involved side toward the doctor.

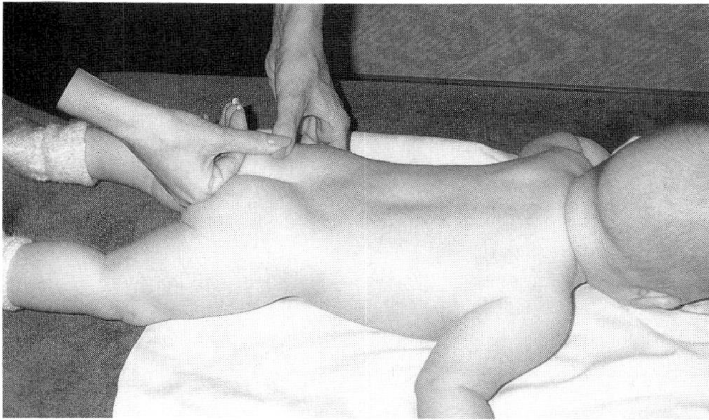

Figure 14.85. In the prone position, the PI ilium can be contacted with a distal thumb on the PSIS with the opposite thumb placed over the nailbed.

The involved side is positioned up in the side posture for a PI ($-\theta X$) ilium. Figure 14.83 illustrates a pisiform contact for a push set-up. The distal end of the thumb also can be used to contact the ilium (Fig. 14.84). A PI ilium set-up in the prone position with a finger contact is a third alternative (Fig. 14.85). The thrust is from posterior to anterior ($+Z$), with a slight inferior to superior ($+\theta X$) arc.

The forearm in all ilium listings should reflect the sacroiliac joint plane. As previously described in the lumbar section, the infant and older child should be properly stabilized.

Figure 14.86 illustrates an AS ($+\theta X$) ilium adjustment. This is performed in the side posture position with the involved side up. Contact is made on the posterior rim of the acetabulum with the pisiform. The fingers will gently rest across the buttocks of the infant. The prone position can be used for an ilium adjustment (Fig. 14.87). The thrust is from posterior to anterior ($+Z$) with a slight superior to inferior ($-\theta X$) arc.

Figure 14.88 depicts Ex ilium adjustments (involved side against the table) in the side posture position. The doctor contacts the lateral border of the PSIS of the infant/toddler with the distal ends of two or three metacarpals. The adolescent is contacted with the proximal end of the metacarpals. The prone position is depicted for a thumb contact Ex ilium (Fig. 14.89). The direction of the fingers when the doctor places the pisiform on the thumb is important as it creates a line of correction. The thrust for an Ex ilium is from lateral to medial ($+\theta Y$/lt. ilium, or $-\theta Y$/rt. ilium).

Figure 14.90 depicts adjustment for an In ilium using a pisiform contact. The involved side is placed up, and contact is made on the medial border of the PSIS. An alternative contact is to use the distal ends of two or three phalanges to finger push the In ilium (Fig. 14.91). Figure

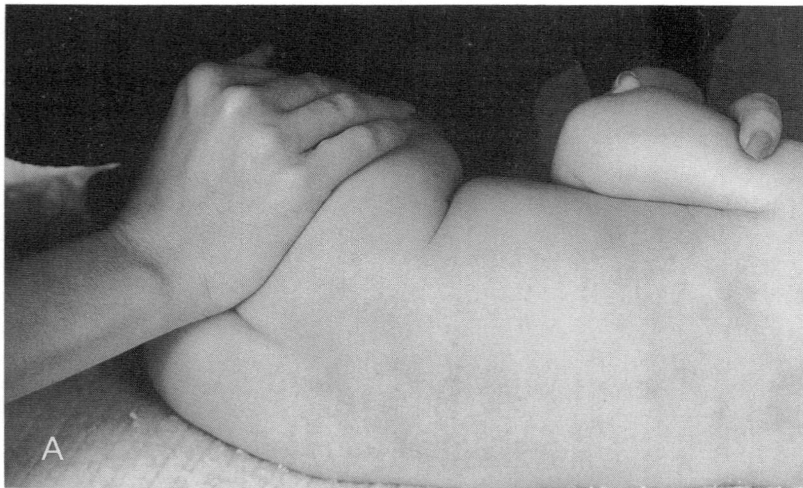

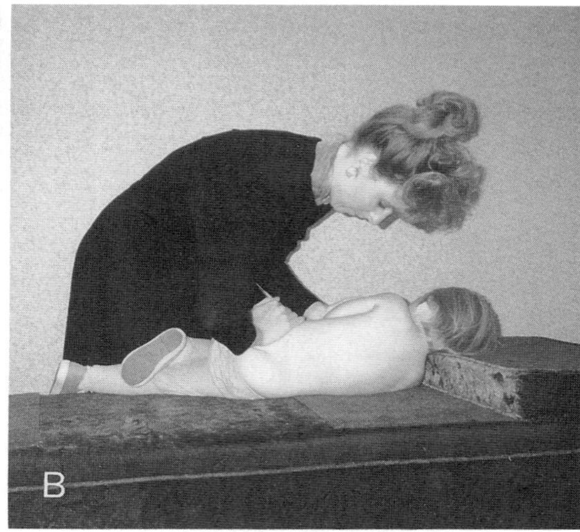

Figure 14.86. **A,** Contacting the posterior rim of the acetabulum with the pisiform on the AS ilium. With the infant, the doctor's finger will gently lie across the buttocks. **B,** AS ilium adjustment in the toddler.

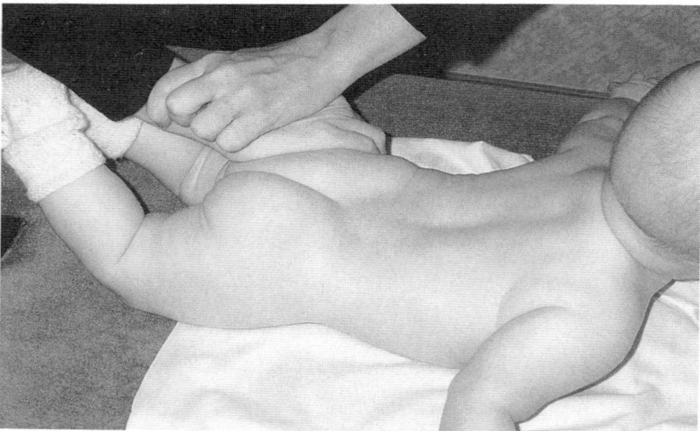

Figure 14.87. AS ilium adjustment in the prone position.

14.92 illustrates the thumb-pisiform contact for a prone In ilium adjustment of the infant. The thrust is from medial to lateral ($-\theta Y$/lt. ilium or $+\theta Y$/rt. ilium).

The side posture adjustments for a PIIn ilium using a pisiform contact are depicted in Figure 14.93. Figure 14.94 illustrates a prone position, thumb-pisiform contact for a PIIn ilium. The thrust is from posterior to anterior ($+Z$), inferior to superior ($+\theta X$), and from medial to lateral ($-\theta Y$/lt. ilium or $+\theta Y$/rt. ilium).

Figure 14.95 depicts an ASIn ilium adjustment in the side posture position. Contact is made on the posterior rim of the acetabulum with the pisiform. The doctor should always take into consideration the plane line of the sacroiliac articulation when making the adjustment. The thrust is from posterior to anterior ($+Z$), slightly superior to inferior, and medial to lateral ($-\theta Y$/lt. ilium or $+\theta Y$/ rt. ilium).

ASEx adjustments in the side posture position are illustrated in Figure 14.96. The involved side is placed toward the table. The distal portions of the metacarpals are used as the doctor's contact point for the infant. For the toddler, the proximal ends of the metacarpals will be the contact points. Contact is made on the posterior rim of the acetabulum. The thrust is from posterior to anterior ($+Z$), superior to inferior ($-Y$), and lateral to medial.

Figures 14.97 depicts the side posture position for a PIEx ilium adjustment. The contact is made by either the distal portion of the metacarpals (for newborn/infant) or the proximal portion (for a toddler/adolescent). The thrust is from posterior to anterior ($+Z$), inferior to superior ($-Y$), and from lateral to medial.

Sacrum

Posteriorly displaced sacral segments are relatively common in patients with unfused sacrums. These can be adjusted similarly to posterior subluxations of the lumbar spine. It is important that the contact be specific on the involved sacral segment.

The toddler or adolescent is usually adjusted in the side posture position similar to the adult. Careful positioning is important and the doctor should avoid unnecessary torsion by pushing with the stabilization hand. Care must be taken to avoid torquing the lower spine with the thigh stabilization. Figure 14.98 depicts a thumb contact for a posterior sacral segment in the side posture position. A distal end finger contact for a posterior sacral segment is depicted in Figure 14.99. The prone position is illustrated for a posterior sacral segment adjustment (Fig. 14.100A-B). The doctor can use a double thumb, a single thumb, or a pisiform contact on the second sacral tuber-

nal cord provide the efferent sympathetic fibers to the stomach. The anterior and posterior vagal trunks supply the parasympathetic nerve supply (37).

A study on colic by a Danish group of chiropractors (41) revealed positive results when adjustments were rendered. A second study by Klougart et al. (42) on 316 cases of infantile colic reported success within the first two weeks in 94% of the cases. Both studies warrant further controlled research in this area.

The spinal areas to note for a vertebral subluxation in these children are the thoracic region (e.g., T4 to T9) and the upper cervical region (e.g., C1-C2).

Digestive Dysfunction

A wide variety of digestive disorders can occur with the newborn, toddler, and adolescent. Common disorders that affect children range from vomiting, nausea and upset stomachs, to "picky" eating and loss of appetite leading to malnutrition.

Other than the few studies that have been performed in the area of infantile colic, little literature exists. Further research is needed in this area. The reader is referred to Chapter 13 for further discussion.

Enuresis

The condition of enuresis is the persistence beyond the age of five of involuntary discharge of urine when voluntary control should be developed. Enuresis or bedwetting normally occurs during the sleep period of the child. Boys more frequently than girls tend to manifest this disorder (39,40).

CLINICAL SIGNS AND SYMPTOMS

Nocturnal enuresis can be of two forms: persistent and regressive. Persistent enuresis is a continuous pattern of wet nights, whereas the regressive type has inconsistent recurrence after dry periods. A third manifestation of enuresis is diurnal. This is uncontrollable dribbling during the day that does not typify occasional accidents.

CHIROPRACTIC EVALUATION

The bladder receives its parasympathetic fibers from the pelvic splanchnic nerves. The nerve supply from T11, T12, L1 and L2 provide sympathetic fibers. The visceral nerve plexus also contributes both sympathetic and parasympathetic fibers (43).

A study of fourteen enuresis cases by a group of osteopaths correlated traumatic injuries with findings of interosseous lesions. Correction of the lesions produced excellent results (44). Gemmell (45) reports a case of enuresis which resolved while under chiropractic care. Future controlled studies are needed, in light of the apparently positive results of these studies.

The vertebral subluxation complex is commonly detected at the second or third sacral segments, or the fifth lumbar. A second region to evaluate is the lower thoracic and upper lumbar region (T11 to L2). The upper cervical area (e.g., C0 to C2) should also be analyzed (46).

Febrile Convulsions

The simple febrile convulsion usually occurs between the age of 6 months to approximately age 5 years. This seizure is a form of the general tonic-clonic seizure. The criteria for identification of the seizure is that the fever be greater than 38° centigrade during an attack which lasts under 15 minutes. There should be no other central nervous system infections or neurologic abnormalities. Genetic factors appear to also be related (39).

CLINICAL SIGNS OR SYMPTOMS

Before the attack, the febrile convulsion is preceded by a quick onset of increased body temperature. The nature of

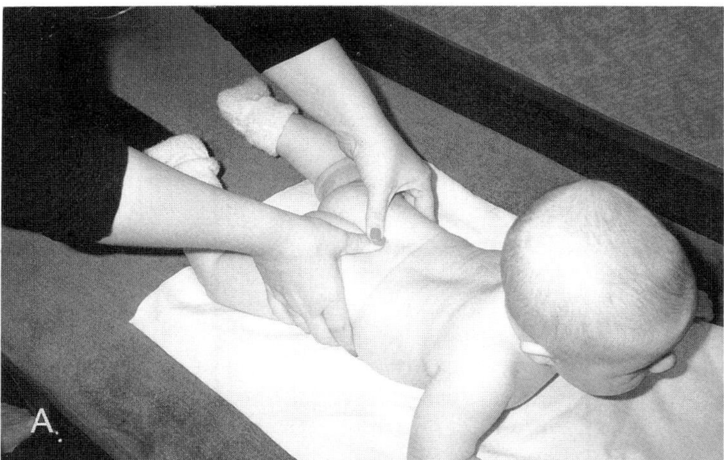

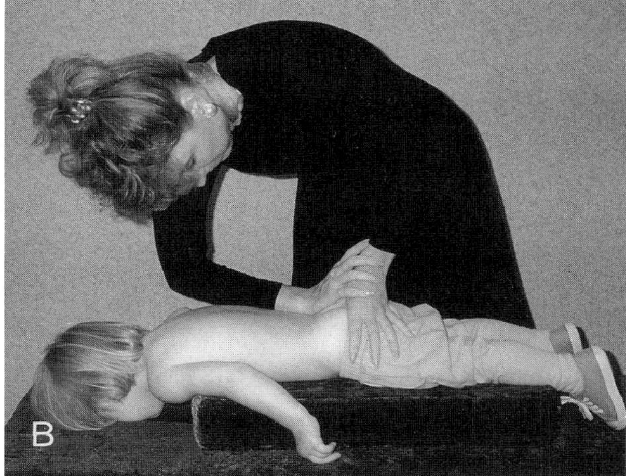

Figure 14.100. A, Double thumb contact for posterior sacral segment. **B,** Thumb-pisiform contact for a posterior sacral segment.

the seizure is tonic-clonic or atonic. Normal alertness returns soon after the brief postural stupor.

CHIROPRACTIC EVALUATION

The vertebral subluxation complex may be detected in the upper cervical region (C1 to C2) and/or the mid to lower thoracic area (T8 to T10). The author's clinical observations suggest that this disorder can be helped with chiropractic care. Please refer to Chapter 13 for additional information.

Foot Flare

Internal or external rotation of the foot can be seen unilateral or bilaterally. Foot flare is usually detected at the onset of the development of walking. In many instances by the age of 4 or 5 years, the flare will resolve by itself (27).

CHIROPRACTIC EVALUATION

The evaluation of the vertebral subluxation should be directed to the sacroiliac articulations. With a singular internal foot rotation, an Ex ilium on the same side may be involved. Bilateral internal foot rotation is commonly caused by a base posterior sacrum. External foot rotation is more commonly unilateral. On the side of foot involvement, a possible In ilium or sacral rotation (P-L or P-R) may be related.

Growing Pains

The onset of growing pains usually occurs between the ages of 3 and 6 years. The etiology is unknown.

CLINICAL SIGNS AND SYMPTOMS

Usually the child will manifest enough shin pain to interrupt sleep.

CHIROPRACTIC EVALUATION

Areas to observe for the vertebral subluxation complex are the lower lumbars (L4 and L5), the sacrum, or an ilium involvement. Gutmann (11) reported improvement with children with this disorder when an upper cervical subluxation was adjusted. Foot disorders (e.g., pronation, navicular subluxation) may also be related (See Chapter 16).

Headache

The chiropractic care for patients with headache is discussed in Chapter 13. The reader is referred for additional information. By seven years of age, approximately 37% of all children will have manifested headaches. Nearly 3% of these will be of the migraine variety. Sixty-nine percent of all adolescents will have manifested headaches by the age of 14 years. Approximately 11% are migraine in nature (39, 47).

CHIROPRACTIC EVALUATION

Regarding pediatric headaches, Lewit (15) considers the cervical spine as a frequently related site. He adjusted two groups of children suffering from migraine and nonmigraine headaches. Of the 27 migraine children in the study, 24 experienced excellent results after spinal adjustments. In the nonmigraine headache group, 28 of the 30 children obtained positive results with adjustments.

Jaundice

Jaundice is the accumulation in the skin of bilirubin. This condition is observed in 60% of term infants and 80% of preterm infants. In the extreme case scenario, the disturbance of the production, metabolism, and excretion process of bilirubin can severely impair the function of an infant (39,48).

CLINICAL SIGNS AND SYMPTOMS

The color of the skin will usually appear from shades of bright yellow to orange. Some infants will manifest poor feeding and lethargic activity levels. Lab tests can establish the amount of bilirubin accumulated.

CHIROPRACTIC EVALUATION

The liver is innervated by the sympathetic and parasympathetic (vagal) system. The celiac plexus will branch off to the hepatic plexus to the liver. This plexus will receive filaments from the right phrenic and left and right vagus nerves (43). The seventh to tenth thoracic segments originate mainly in the preganglionic sympathetic fibers and pass to the celiac plexus via the sympathetic trunk ganglia and the greater and lesser thoracic splanchnic nerves (49).

A vertebral subluxation is commonly detected at the mid to lower thoracic region (T7 to T12). The author's clinical observations suggest that the incidence of jaundice can be greatly diminished if the mother receives care during pregnancy.

This may be due to enhanced neurophysiologic function between the mother and fetus, or decreased spinal biomechanical stress on the fetus from preventing or correcting in-utero constraint, and decreased labor-delivery time. Clinical research should be conducted to evaluate the suggested hypotheses.

Otitis Media

Otitis media is an inflammation process of the middle ear. It is usually accompanied by effusion or fluid collection in the middle ear area. Several authorities suggest that by the age of three, approximately two-thirds of all children will have had at least one otitis media episode. By the age of two, one-third of all children will have experienced up to three episodes (39).

There are three classifications of otitis media: acute (< 3 weeks), subacute (3 weeks to 3 months), and chronic (>3 months). The type of the exudate will further define the different classifications (39,50).

Otitis media may be preceded by upper respiratory infection, the common cold, a sore throat, or sinusitis. The eustachian tube also may be involved and disrupted by these dysfunctional states.

CLINICAL SIGNS AND SYMPTOMS

Some children may manifest a variety of signs; however, they do not have to manifest all the clinical findings. Infants may pull on their ears or the general area. The tympanic membrane appears more inflamed in the acute stage. Concurrent signs can include fever, decreased hearing, and discharge.

CHIROPRACTIC EVALUATION

The tympanic membrane and the middle ear are supplied by several branches of nerve fibers. These nerve branches are the trigeminal (CN V), vagus (CN X), glossopharyngeal (CN IX) and facial (CN VII) (43).

At the spinal levels of C1 through C4, the cervical plexus receives motor fibers that can be traced from the tensa veli palatine (eustachian tube) to the superior cervical sympathetic ganglion (51).

Gutmann reports (11) a tendency toward ear, nose, and throat infection in children with upper cervical subluxation. Clinical observations suggest that subluxation of the mid to upper cervical region (i.e., C1 to C4), and occasionally the upper thoracic and lower cervical area is involved.

Scoliosis

The reader is encouraged to review Chapter 9 before proceeding. Chiropractic care may be most effective if a preventive approach is adopted. The writings of Smith (1) and Dunne et al. (2) suggest that in-utero constraint can cause morphogenic alterations (e.g., scoliosis) due to extrinsic forces. In a study by Dunn (3) on 6,000 breech presentations, 42% had postural scoliosis. The in-utero position of transverse lie also was considered to be another cause of scoliosis. The Webster In-Utero Constraint Turning Technique may reduce the incidence of postural scoliosis in newborns.

Farfan (30) states that asymmetric vertebrae are common in scoliosis. The vertebral body shows a decrease in vertical height on the side of curve concavity. On the side of convexity the pedicles are longer and the neural arch appears fuller.

Effective and noninvasive alternative methods for evaluating scoliosis in children (i.e., pre-school, elementary) should be a high priority for the chiropractic profession. Developing vertebrae can acquire asymmetries (4,10,13,14,17,30), which later may contribute to the development of scoliosis. Scoliosis may be greatly diminished if earlier detection and spinal adjustments are used. A preliminary study by Cooke et al. (52) used thermography to identify the presence of scoliosis in a group of adolescents. In a blinded analysis of randomly selected thermograms, the examiners correctly identified most normal and abnormal patients. The sensitivity of the thermographic examination was 98.2% and specificity was 91% (See Chapter 4). The reference test was a radiologic examination.

Thermography should be considered in the screening of adolescents for scoliosis. Its noninvasiveness should prioritize its integration into school screening programs.

All schools should have spinal education in their curriculum and adolescents should be educated regarding the spine, nervous system, vertebral subluxations (including chiropractic care as a health alternative for the individual), and scoliosis. Spinal hygiene habits should also be discussed with the objective of reducing the incidence of spinal trauma. The effect of various sporting events (See Chapter 2) on the development of spinal injuries needs to be acknowledged.

Tonsillitis

The term tonsils commonly refers to the two faucial tonsils. The adenoids refer to the pharyngeal tonsils (50). Approximately 30% of all the children in the United States have removal of their tonsils and adenoids. Only 1 to 2% of the children, however, are considered candidates who truly require the procedure (50) (See Chapter 4). Unfortunately, the hypertrophic or large tonsil in very young children is often misdiagnosed as abnormal. After the age of eight, the tonsil will usually return to its normal size, when normal atrophy begins to occur (50).

CLINICAL SIGNS AND SYMPTOMS

Acute tonsillitis is most commonly seen during the ages of four to seven but can occur throughout the childhood and into the adult years. Chronic tonsillitis is defined as recurrent or a persistent sore throat. The signs range from throat inflammation and irritation to obstruction in swallowing and breathing.

Adenoidal hypertrophy is accompanied frequently with chronic tonsillitis. Mouth breathing, snoring, and persistent rhinitis are commonly associated signs.

CHIROPRACTIC EVALUATION

The plexus that innervates the tonsillar region is formed by branches of the vagus and glossopharyngeal nerves. The pharyngeal plexus also contributes branches (43).

The mid to upper cervical region (i.e., C0-C4) should be closely examined for the presence of a vertebral subluxation complex. Gutmann (11) reports amelioration of tonsillitis in children who received upper cervical adjustments. Lewit (15) found that 92% of children with chronic tonsillitis had upper cervical subluxations. Gutmann (11) further cites the observations of Mohr who states that when the disturbance of the functional atlanto-occipital joint was corrected, no tonsillectomies were necessary.

Torticollis

This condition is sometimes referred to as "wryneck" (53). The sternocleidomastoid muscle is contracted on one side, with the head tilted toward the side of contracture and the chin rotated away. As the muscle deformity continues, a fibrotic mass can develop in the midportion of the sternocleidomastoid muscle. In chronic cases where intervention does not occur, facial asymmetry can result. There are two general forms of torticollis: congenital and acute (See Chapter 10).

CLINICAL SIGNS AND SYMPTOMS

Congenital torticollis is seen immediately or shortly after birth. The head of the supine newborn should easily rotate 90° in both directions. The decreased range of motion associated with torticollis may not be apparent until after the first week. The firm muscle mass will usually not appear unless the condition has been chronic for two to three months. Congenital torticollis has been found in 20 to 25% of breech (in-utero constraint) presentations (1,3). Birth trauma also appears to be related (8,11,53).

Acute or spastic torticollis is usually observed in the child after a mild cervical trauma (27), or after an upper respiratory or tonsillar infection (53).

If other causes are suspected, radiographic evaluation should be used to rule out Kleippel-Feil anomaly, cervical fracture, dislocation, and osseous infection (31,39,53).

CHIROPRACTIC EVALUATION

Several sources (11,27,53) have attributed upper cervical (i.e., C0 to C2) subluxation, such as atlanto-axial rotatory fixation, as a cause of torticollis.

The upper cervical region (C0 to C3) and the upper thoracic (T1 to T4) area should be evaluated for the presence of subluxation (See Chapter 10).

CHALLENGED CHILD

The handicapped child is an individual who can derive great benefits from chiropractic care. Rather than seeing the child as having physical and mental deficiencies which restrict normal achievements, the chiropractor should adopt a perspective that the child must use all resources and abilities (i.e., challenged).

Children with scoliosis, paralysis, spina bifida, cystic fibrosis, muscular dystrophy, cerebral palsy, and other disorders will have abnormal stresses placed on the spinal column and its associated components. Physical limitations from abnormal posture, inability to participate in normal physical activities, or apparatus restrictions (e.g., wheelchairs, crutches, braces) further contribute to spinal biomechanical compromise. These factors may cause a vertebral subluxation and thus nervous system dysfunction.

Optimal neurologic function is of benefit to the patient with Down syndrome, just as it is in an otherwise "normal" individual. This applies as well to mental retardation and other neurologic disorders.

Introduction of the challenged child to the chiropractic office brings its own unparalleled demands. Case histories may need to be more extensive and extra time is usually necessary. The examination (chiropractic, physical, neurologic and orthopaedic) may need to be expanded or tailored to the child's abilities and limitations.

Motion palpation and instrumentation examination can be assisted by the parent or paraprofessional. Figure 14.101 shows a 6-year-old cerebral palsy child being examined with the Nervoscope.

Radiographing these children in the office will normally require extra assistance by a parent and paraprofessional (Fig. 14.102). It may be necessary to use an outside radiologic facility in the more difficult cases.

The doctor must thoroughly evaluate the child with regard to the patient's own unique normal and abnormal spinal biomechanical functions before the adjustment. The pediatric evaluation and adjusting procedures presented earlier should be reviewed. New technical skills may be required in providing an adjustment for a challenged child. Figure 14.103 illustrates a prone double-thumb contact on a midthoracic vertebra of a cerebral palsy patient.

Attention Deficit Disorder (Hyperactive Syndrome)

The term "attention deficit disorder," or ADD, designates the central disturbances of a group of children labeled as suffering from hyperactivity, hyperkinesia, minimal brain

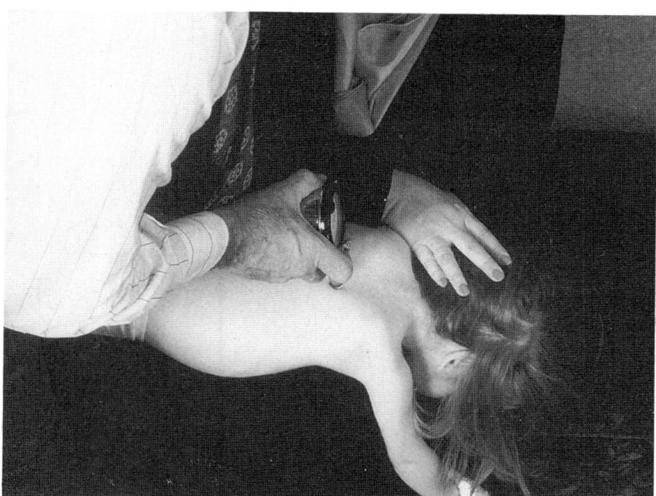

Figure 14.101. Skin temperature analysis of a cerebral palsy patient.

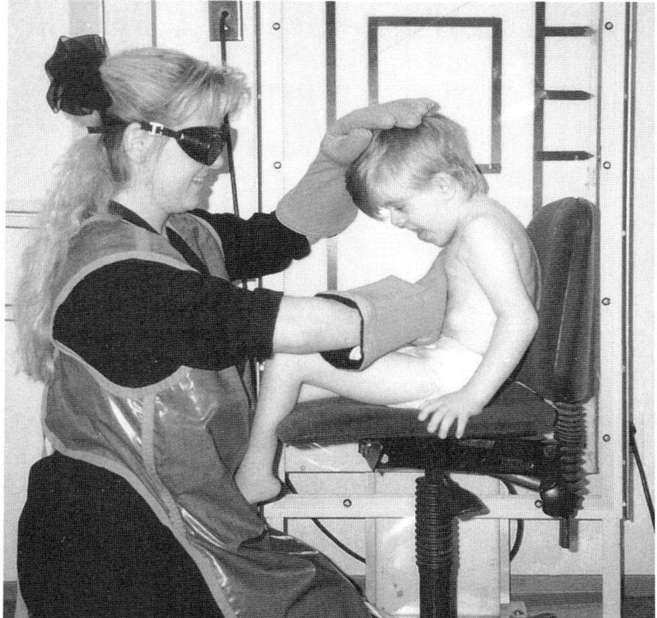

Figure 14.102. Radiographic positioning of the challenged child.

damage, and/or minimal cerebral dysfunction. Depending on the definition, an attention deficit disorder with hyperactivity is estimated to occur in 5 to 10% of school-age children (39). Hyperactivity is often overlapped with learning disabilities. The incidence of hyperactivity in boys is four to six times more frequent than found in girls (39).

CLINICAL SIGNS AND SYMPTOMS

About twice as many children with attention deficit disorder have associated motor overactivity than those who

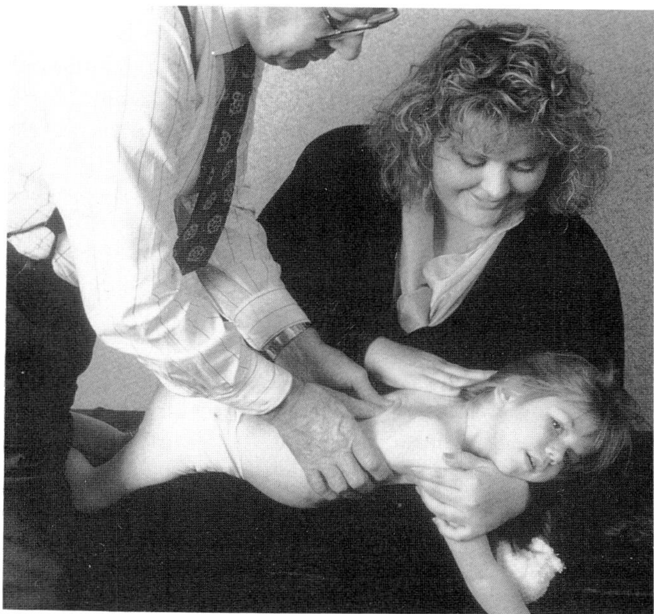

Figure 14.103. Double-thumb contact for a thoracic adjustment of a cerebral palsy patient.

do not. Evidence suggests that these two conditions have significant differences: children with ADD and hyperactive traits have been found to demonstrate aggressive behavior with little expression of guilt, more commonly poor school performance, and unpopularity with their peers (39).

Nonhyperactive children with ADD are anxious and socially withdrawn and in addition to poor academic performance, have difficulty participating in sports. In general, children with ADD have short attention spans, are distractible and impulsive, and tend to act without considering or reflecting upon the consequences of their behavior. Further, they have a low tolerance for frustration and are emotionally labile and excitable. The moods of these children tend to be neutral or oppositional.

CHIROPRACTIC EVALUATION

The upper cervical region (C0 to C3) should be analyzed for vertebral subluxation. As in the case of any patient, the entire spine should be examined, and subluxations, if present, reduced. Giesen et al. (54) demonstrated improvement in children with hyperactivity after chiropractic treatment. The authors suggest more investigation in this area, in light of the potential for nondrug intervention in children with this disorder.

Hinwood and Hinwood (25) report improvement in patients with psychic disorders (related to sympathetic fiber irritation) after cervical adjustments.

Lewit's review of the literature (15) found that patients with poor motor patterns and imbalance of muscle groups showed patterns of minimal brain dysfunction.

Cerebral Palsy

In the United States, approximately 300,000 individuals manifest this nonprogressive central motor deficit. Cerebral palsy is considered as a group of disorders with a variety of etiologies.

Several causes that have been attributed to cerebral palsy include physical trauma to the brain from birth (39), obstetric complications (47,55,56), and breech presentations and delivery (1–3).

CLINICAL SIGNS AND SYMPTOMS

There are several classifications of this disorder of impaired motor function. The clinical picture will depend on the severity of the intellectual impairment.

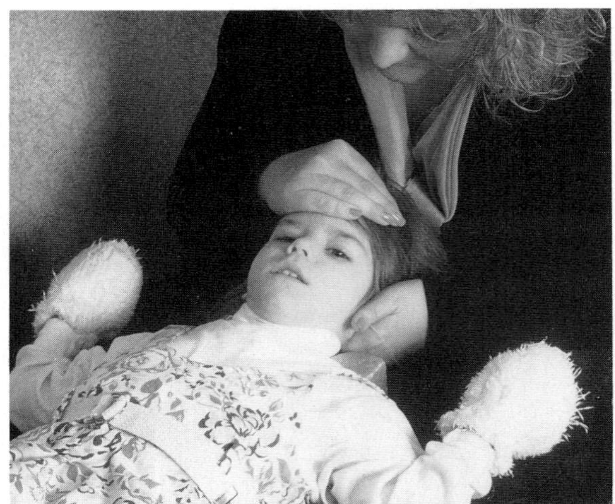

Figure 14.104. AS occiput adjustment in the supine position.

CHIROPRACTIC EVALUATION

A vertebral subluxation is often detected in the upper cervical region in these patients. An AS occiput is commonly present. The lateral cervical radiograph (both neutral and flexion view), visual inspection and palpation can assist in identifying the subluxation. In younger children, the floppy head presentation may necessitate adjusting the AS occiput in the supine position (Fig. 14.104). Because of the extensive spastic contractures, a full spinal analysis is always recommended.

Arbuckle (56) discusses the need for examining the cranium and the upper thoracic spine and providing adjustive care where indicated. Normal autonomic nervous system tone is requisite for optimal blood circulation in the brain (56).

Down Syndrome

Down syndrome is sometimes referred to as mongolism (39,57). This condition is due to an extra chromosome (21-trisomy). In the general population, one out of every 600 to 800 live births will have this chromosomal abnormality. There are two other autosomal trisomic syndromes; 18-trisomy and 13-trisomy.

CLINICAL SIGNS AND SYMPTOMS

The three more common autosomal trisomic syndromes have a wide range of clinical signs. Characteristic features are mental retardation, congenital heart disease, and abnormalities of the cranium, face, abdomen, pelvis, hands, and feet.

CHIROPRACTIC EVALUATION

Careful attention should be focused to the upper cervical region (i.e., C0-C3), because approximately 20% of these children are born without a transverse ligament of the atlas (16). Radiographic studies are mandatory to evaluate the atlanto-dental interval (ADI). The normal ADI distance is 2 to 5 mm, on a lateral cervical radiograph. Any distance greater than 5 mm is indicative of atlanto-axial ligament instability (33). A minimum of a neutral lateral cervical radiograph and flexion views are required before any cervical adjustment.

Epileptic (Seizure) Disorders

There are two classes of recurrent seizures. The first is termed "symptomatic" and occurs in response to a specific cause. This normally occurs with children under the age of two. The second class of seizure is termed "idiopathic." This seizure often persists into adulthood. Approximately 10% of all children will manifest one or more seizures during their childhood. In the adult population, only 1% will have some form of epilepsy (39,47).

CLINICAL SIGNS AND SYMPTOMS

Within the two classifications of seizures are numerous subclasses that can be differentiated with the EEG. Reviewing Chapter 13 and other sources (39,47) is suggested.

CHIROPRACTIC EVALUATION

The vertebral subluxation is commonly discovered in the upper cervical region (C0 to C2). The sacral area may also be related.

Gutmann (11) reports an adjustment of an infant suffering from cerebral spasms which were resolved when the atlas-occiput relation was corrected. The disturbance appeared only after the child had been dropped on several occasions on the head. Infantile spasms also appear to be correlated to seizure disorders (39).

CHILD-PROOFING THE CHIROPRACTIC OFFICE

Child-proofing the office is an important concern for all chiropractors who participate in a pediatric practice. When observing the office environment, one must review it with a very critical eye for younger children. Safety considerations are primary.

An area often overlooked by many is cleanliness of the office surroundings. Parents, in particular, will evaluate the office in this manner. Floor cleanliness is especially important. A few small objects to watch for are paper clips, pen tops, loose staples, and bottle caps. Younger children will not hesitate to place small objects in their mouths. These small objects are a common cause of choking accidents.

The reception room is an area of frequent use by children and this should be carefully surveyed. Sharp corners on low tables can become a road block for a running toddler. The doctor should be aware of items on table tops that could be accidentally pulled off by an adventurous little one. Lamps, art work, and plants are a few items that should be arranged differently.

Throughout the office, electrical outlets that are not in use should be covered with plastic plugs. This common electrical hazard is preventable. Other electrical concerns include frayed cords that should be replaced and the placement on floors of cords that can potentially be tripped over.

Chemical items should be put out of the reach of all children. In the bathroom and kitchen area, cleaning products should be locked-up or placed out of reach. This also should be true for any practitioner who may have physiotherapy items accessible to children.

It is advised that the office have a policy not to allow any child to go unsupervised in the adjusting or physiotherapy areas. The staff should inform parents of this policy. Electro-mechanical adjusting tables such as the hi-lo, are for use only by the doctor. This should be clearly explained to both the child and parent.

CHIROPRACTIC CARE OF PREGNANCY

From the previous discussion of in-utero constraint, it becomes obvious that pediatric care begins before the child is born. Unfortunately, little research exists regarding chiropractic care during pregnancy. The few studies that have been performed only address the issues of lumbar pain during pregnancy or labor.

One interprofessional study conducted by a chiropractor and a medical doctor (58) revealed that 75% of those women who received chiropractic adjustments during their pregnancy stated that they benefitted from care of their complaints of lumbago, dorsalgia, cervicalgia, cephalgia, and vertigo.

Diakow et al. (59) performed a retrospective study of chiropractic care and its effects on lower back pain during pregnancy and labor. The results demonstrated significant improvement in symptomatology. The majority of the women who were chiropractic patients experienced no back labor.

Low back pain and its associated complaints (e.g., leg pain) during pregnancy appears to be a common occurrence. The number of women who experience pain during pregnancy can range from 48 to 56% (60). Although a majority of these women manifest lumbar pain in their last trimester, one study (60) revealed that 28% had symptoms already by the twelfth week of gestation.

Risk factors for low back pain during pregnancy include previous back problems, a young age, and multiparity (61). There also appears to be an ethnic predisposition. Caucasians were found to be at higher risk when compared with Hispanics (60).

Many etiologies have been considered in the pathogenesis of low back pain during pregnancy. The increased biomechanical load on the spine, as well as the shape of the spine during pregnancy, may be related. Other factors include ligamentous laxity due to relaxin (which will increase ten-fold), a bulging intervertebral disc, direct fetal pressure, and vascular obstruction (60,62).

Guthrie (63) did a study on the benefits of back pressure during labor. He distributed a questionnaire to 175 women. One hundred thirty-four responded that they had experienced back labor either alone or in conjunction with front labor. During labor, 71.8% received back pressure from their husbands, and 12.6% from nurses. Those patients who received back pressure for relief of back pain, resulted in the following changes: 24% had complete relief; 41% had 80% relief; 18% had about 50% relief; and 25% had some relief. Although this was a preliminary study, Guthrie discusses the possible role of osteopathic care during labor, because of the neuroanatomic relationship of the lumbosacral region. During the first stage of labor, pain is sensed through the visceral afferent nerves that pass through Frankenhauser's ganglion in the pelvic plexus and in the middle and superior hypogastric plexus between the tenth thoracic and the first lumbar segment. The second stage of labor originates in the perineum through the second to fourth sacral segments. Uterine contractions could cause lumbar myalgia through reflex mechanisms.

Melzack and Belanger (64) found that both labor pain with back pain and low back pain during menstruation, shared common underlying mechanisms. The authors noted that low back pain was not directly caused by labor contractions, because the pain was persistent between contractions. One possible cause was reflex spasm in those skeletal muscles served by the same spinal segments as the uterus (64). If this theory is correct, then this would support the clinical observations of many chiropractors: women patients who receive adjustments before labor have a reduction in the facilitation of these spinal segments.

Burns (65,66) conducted two studies on the relationship of vertebral lesions and pregnancy in laboratory animals. The first study was the observation of vertebral lesions during pregnancy. Through clinical experience and animal experimentation, Burns justified that a relationship of the upper lumbar spinal region with the pelvic viscera existed. Further, she discovered that vertebral lesions were responsible for causing interference in the physiologic functions of the region. This study also suggested that upper cervical lesions could contribute to abnormal function of maternal physiology during the course of pregnancy. Maternal physiologic alterations reported from cervical lesions included disturbances in the circulation of the entire body due to cardiac malfunction, thyroid dysfunction, and sexual disturbances. Vertebral lesions in female laboratory animals also produced miscarriages, behavioral changes, premature births, stillbirth, "runty" offspring, and early death of the young. Burns further speculates on the clinical experiences of her colleagues with human pregnancy. Lesions of the lumbar spine, innominates and upper thoracic region, when adjusted, had some interesting effects. Females with vertebral lesions had pregnancies and labor that were more abnormal, compared with nonlesioned females. Burns also cites empirical evidence that previously sterile couples were able to conceive after osteopathic care.

The other study by Burns (65) demonstrated that maternal lumbar lesions of rabbits had effects on the development of their young. It was reported that a physiologic difference was noted between the young of lesioned mothers compared with the young of nonlesioned mothers. Physiologically, the young of lesioned mothers demonstrated stunted growth, erratic behavior, slow development and implications of anatomic deformities. Further, the study mentions various obstetrical complications occurring with mothers suffering from these lumbar lesions.

Historical work in this area demonstrates the potential neurologic effects of the vertebral subluxation complex on both the mother and unborn child. Further investigation in this or related areas is clearly warranted based on these early investigations with laboratory animals.

Fallon (67) correlates the following neurologic conditions associated with subluxation in pregnancy: meralgia paresthetica, brachial, intercostal, and sciatica neuralgia, coccydynia, carpal tunnel syndrome, Bell's palsy, and traumatic neuritis. The benefits of reduction of labor time also was reported from the case history files of Fallon. Without chiropractic care, the primigravida female labored approximately 14 hours and the multiparous female approximately 9 to 10 hours. With chiropractic care during pregnancy, she reported in primigravida cases, approximately 8 to 9 hours of labor. Multiparous females had approximately 4 to 5 hours of labor. The personal observations of this author suggests that labor time can be further reduced with appropriate chiropractic care. Visit frequency generally averages two per month up until the seventh or eight month of gestation. The frequency is then increased to approximately one visit per week until delivery. A variety of factors will contribute to the time variables of labor. It appears that chiropractic care may have an influence. The author advocates further studies in a controlled environment.

Examination

Similar chiropractic evaluation procedures that are performed on the adult can be performed on the pregnant patient. Instrumentation and static palpation rarely differs significantly for the analysis of the pregnant patient. Motion palpation and postural analysis will alter because of the hormonal influence and weight bearing changes of the musculoskeletal system. Noticeable changes expected to occur during pregnancy are an increased lumbar lordosis and sacral base angle, increased segmental mobility (particularly of the sacroiliac and pubic articulations), a shift of weight bearing to the heels, and gait alterations.

Unless previous radiographs are available for review, radiographs are usually not performed on the pregnant patient (See Chapter 5). Any female who is of child-bearing age should be required to answer on the case history form if there is a possibility of pregnancy. Whoever performs the actual task of exposing the radiographs in the office should verbally inquire if there is a possibility of pregnancy and record the answer. A sign also should be posted in the radiography room, thus informing the patient to immediately notify the staff of pregnancy. If pregnancy is confirmed, a signed waiver stating that radiographs were omitted from the examination should be placed in the patient's file before the adjustment.

In the case of cervical trauma (e.g., whiplash), one may consider limited cervical views to rule out the possibility of fracture (68). Before the radiographic procedure for the pregnant female, discussion with the patient, spouse and obstetrician may be necessary to answer any questions. The involved parties should be informed of the safety precautions provided. This should include the wearing of a full-trunk lead apron and brain, eye, and thyroid shielding.

Adjustment

During the course of pregnancy, hormonal changes will alter the function of musculature and other supporting structures. This alteration normally creates hypermobility of the spinal motion segments and innominates. It is contraindicated to introduce unnecessary rotational forces into the pregnant patient.

The proper patient placement for the adjustment is important. Referring to Chapters 6 to 11 for illustrations of the adult set-up for the cervical, thoracic, lumbar, and pelvic regions is suggested.

PELVIC BENCH

During the side posture set-up, the doctor should carefully stabilize the upper torso with a cephalic pressure, without pressing the patient's shoulder to the pelvic bench. As the abdominal region of the pregnant patient becomes larger, the doctor must occasionally compensate the stance away from the abdomen (Fig. 14.105). In the more advanced gravid female, no body-drop during the thrust phase should occur. The patient may need to be assisted in getting off the table during the last trimester (Fig. 14.106).

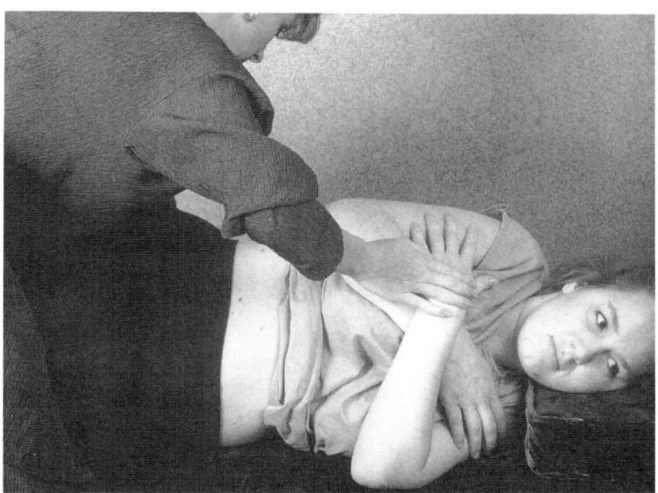

Figure 14.105. Side posture positioning of the pregnant patient.

HI-LO TABLE

The hi-lo table also can be used during the majority of the pregnancy. The hi-lo thoracic piece should be placed in a locked position to avoid rebounding during the thrust. As the stomach begins to protrude, the thoracic and lumbar pieces are separated to compensate for the baby (Fig. 14.107). As the thoracic section is raised, the face piece will eventually become out of reach for the patient. If this position is uncomfortable, the knee-chest table should be used.

KNEE-CHEST TABLE

The knee-chest table is very effective for adjusting the thoracic and lumbar spine in the pregnant patient (69) (Figs.

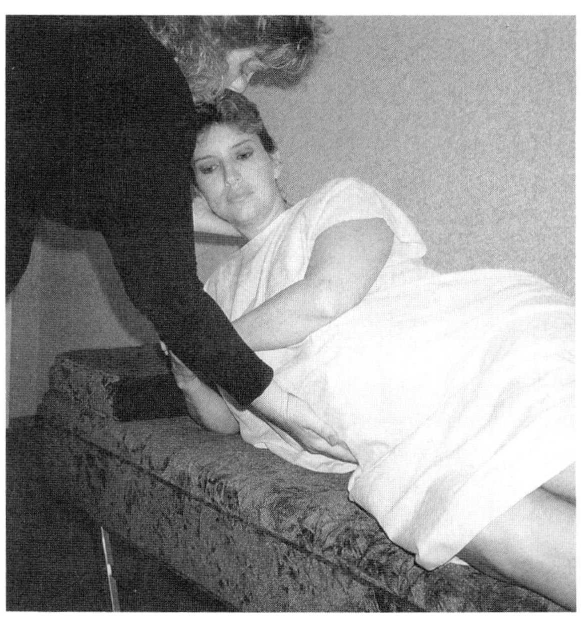

Figure 14.106. Assisting the patient.

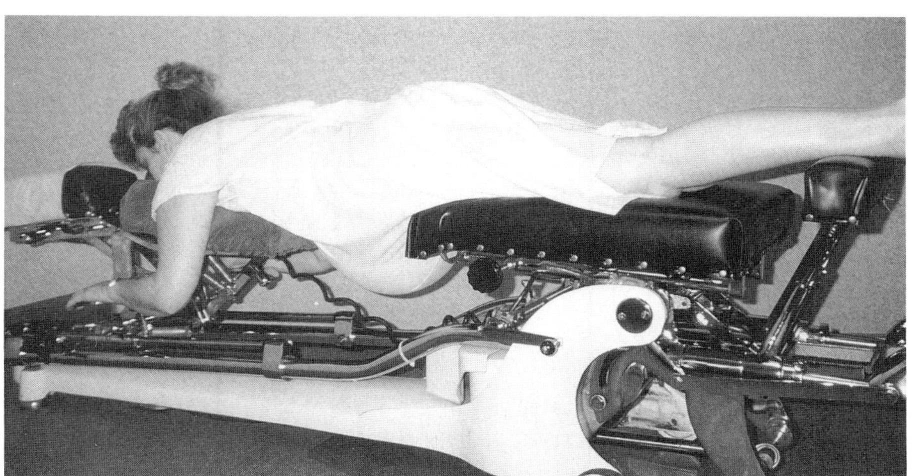

Figure 14.107. Pregnant patient positioning on the hi-lo table.

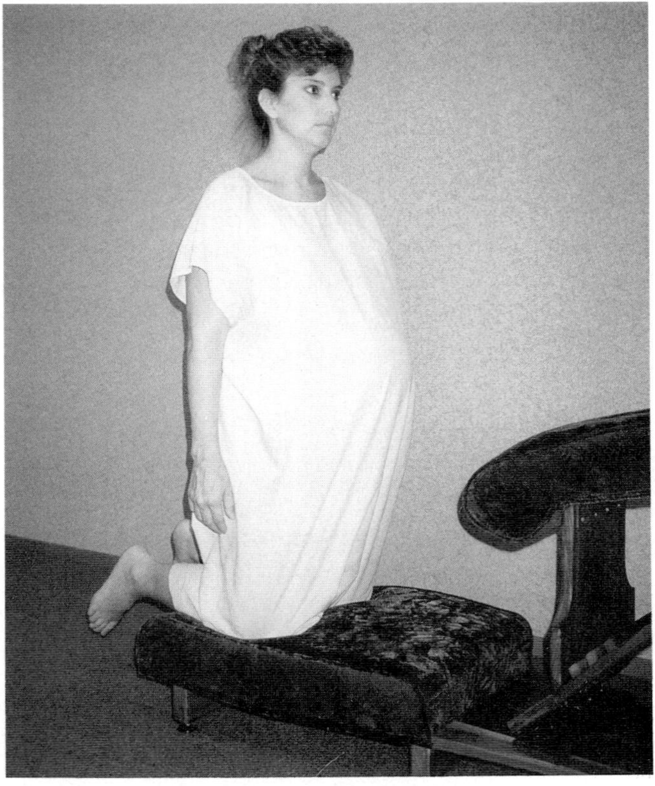

Figure 14.108. The beginning stage of patient positioning on the knee-chest table.

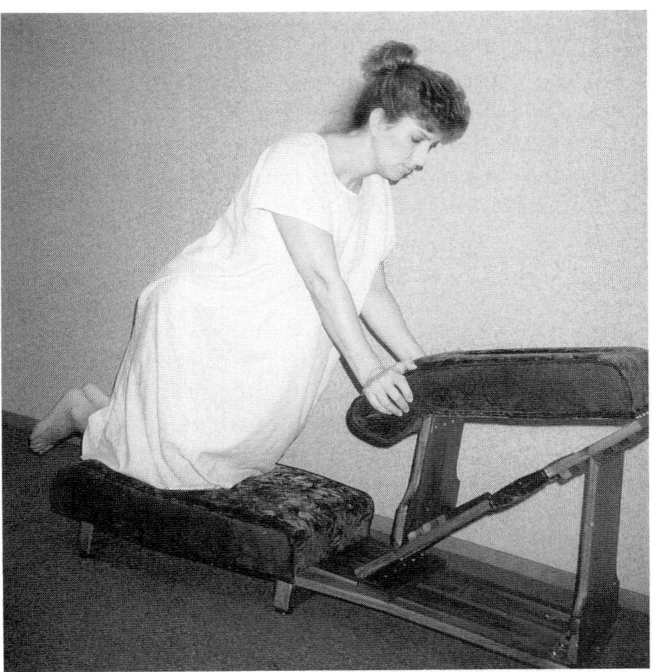

Figure 14.109. Moving into the knee-chest position.

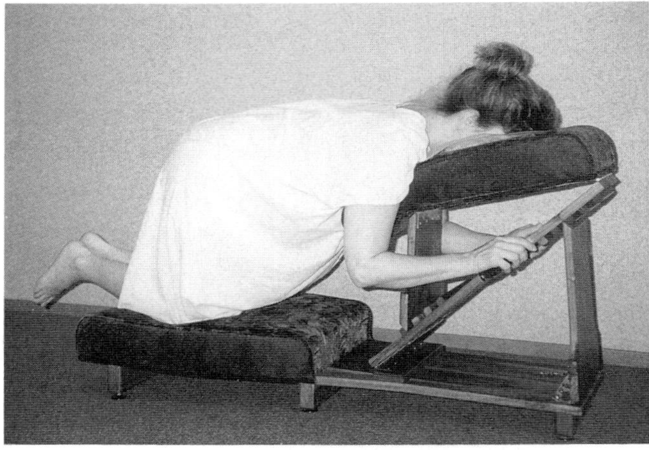

Figure 14.110. Final positioning on the knee-chest table.

14.108–14.110). The proper knee-chest procedure for patient placement, indications, contraindications and thrust, are thoroughly discussed in Chapter 7. Before the thrust, it is very important that the set-up reflect the appropriate motion segment disc and facet planes in the different regions of the spine.

Figure 14.111 illustrates the proper patient placement and doctor stance for a fifth lumbar listing. A double-thumb contact can be performed on the mammillary process in the lumbar region (Fig. 14.112). Figure 14.113 demonstrates a PLS adjustment for the eighth thoracic vertebra. At no time during the thrust stage should a toggle-recoil be performed on the knee-chest table. Rather, a set and hold (approximately 2 seconds) is recommended (See Chapter 2).

In-Utero Constraint Analysis and Reduction

At the seventh month of gestation, the previously breeched fetus turns itself down with the head engaged in the vertex (caudal) position of the pelvis. If the fetus remains in the breech (or other lie) position after the seventh month, biomechanical stress leading to in-utero constraint can cause extensive physical deformities and delivery complications.

Webster (5) has developed a technique to detect and correct the breech infant. Upon review of approximately 800 of his breech cases, Webster has stated that less than 25 cases did not respond to the care provided. After delivery of these unresponsive cases, other factors were determined to be related. With modifications by the author, the in-utero constraint analysis and correction are presented.

WEBSTER IN-UTERO CONSTRAINT TURNING TECHNIQUE

The first step involves placing the patient in a comfortable prone position, with the chin in a neutral position. The doctor lifts the patient's legs bilaterally and flexes them together toward the buttocks. The purpose of this bilateral

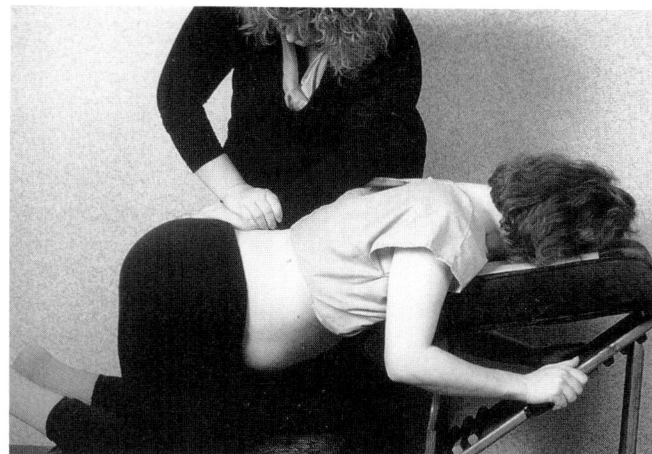

Figure 14.111. Fifth lumbar adjustment.

leg test is to determine if there is equal leg resistance. Equal leg resistance putatively indicates that the fetus is in a normal vertex position. Should the doctor discover one of the flexed legs has increased resistance (i.e., appears to push back toward the doctor), this theoretically indicates posterior sacral rotation subluxation (i.e., P-L or P-R) on the same side. Figure 14.114 illustrates increased resistance on the right leg.

The side of sacral rotation is then placed up on the pelvic bench (Fig. 14.115). The contact point of the doctor is the pisiform. This is placed between the second sacral tubercle and the posterior superior iliac spine (PSIS). The vector of thrust is from posterior to anterior (+Z) along the plane line of the articulation.

The second step involves placing the patient in a supine position. The doctor should stand on the side opposite of the sacral rotation. From this side, the doctor takes the knife edge of the inferior hand and angles it 45°

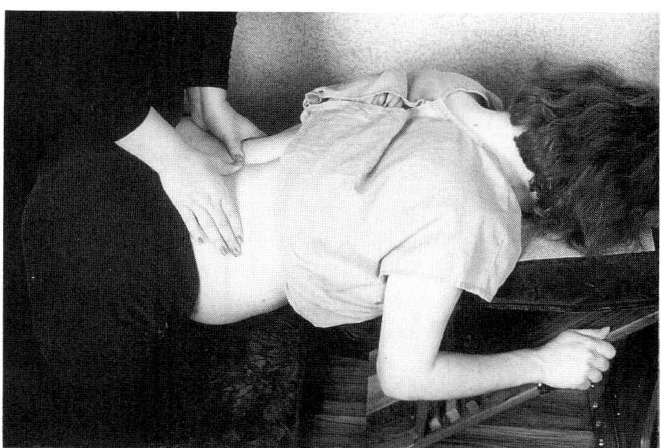

Figure 14.112. Double-thumb contact for a lumbar adjustment.

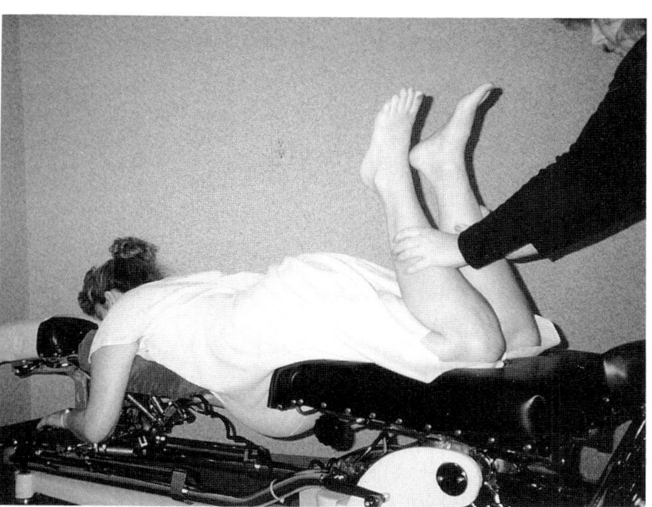

Figure 14.114. Increased resistance of the right leg.

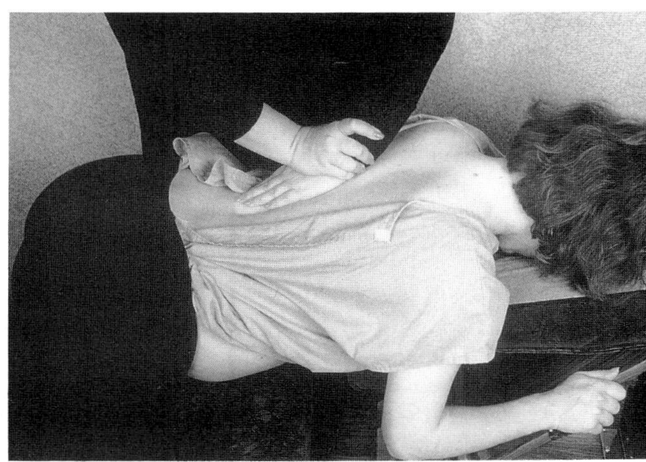

Figure 14.113. Eighth thoracic adjustment on a pregnant patient.

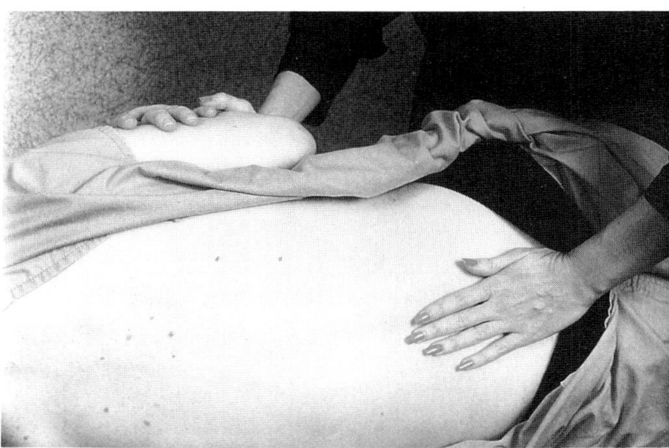

Figure 14.115. Sacral adjustment in the side posture position.

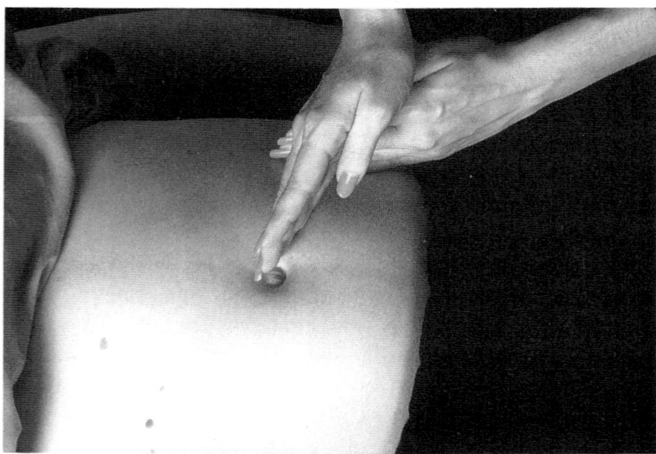

Figure 14.116. Analyzing the left side of a patient who was adjusted as a P-R sacrum.

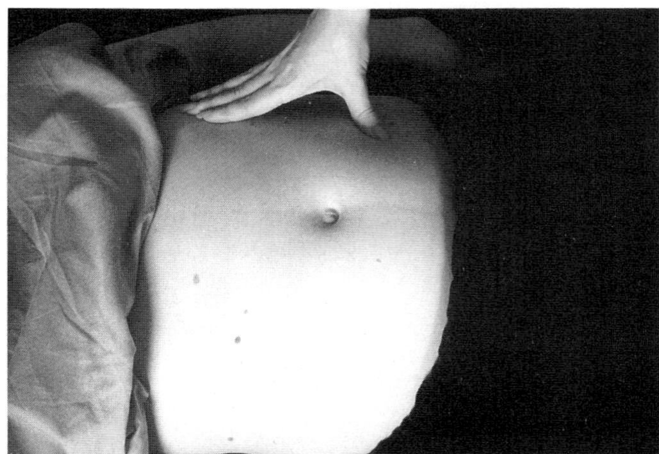

Figure 14.117. Applying pressure to the trigger point.

from the anterior-superior iliac spine (ASIS), lateral to medial and inferior to superior. With the superior hand, the knife edge is angled 45° from the umbilicus, medial to lateral and superior to inferior (Fig. 14.116). The intersection of both hands should be at a trigger point on the rectus abdominal muscle which is then contacted by the doctor's thumb. If a trigger point cannot be identified, the thumb is rotated from the bisect point in either direction, until the trigger point is discovered. The thumb should be used to apply a slight superior to inferior vector, with approximately 3 to 6 ounces of pressure (Fig. 14.117). The thumb contact point is held for approximately 1 to 2 minutes, or until the doctor feels the muscle relax under the pressure contact.

After the adjustment is made, the patient is returned to the prone position and the bilateral leg test is reevaluated. In most cases, the leg resistance will equalize. If equalization is not attained, the patient is returned to the pelvic bench and the sacrum is adjusted with more depth or amplitude. After the second adjustment, the prone position is used to analyze the leg resistance. If equalization is obtained, the doctor then moves to the third step. If equalization of the legs does not occur (a rare occurrence) after the second adjustment, the doctor is advised to halt the procedure and schedule the patient for a reevaluation the following day.

No other adjustments should be performed during any visit(s) that are specifically designed to turn the in-utero constraint infant. Clinical observations suggest that it is not unusual within three to ten visits in a 2- to 3-week time period, for positive results to occur. Equal leg resistance generally contraindicates the sacral adjustment or trigger point treatment. In rare cases, such as the complete breech and/or ventral vertex body positioning, equal resistance may be noted during the leg check. These patients should be adjusted as though a sacral base posterior is present. In addition, the trigger point contact should be made bilaterally (simultaneously).

Another rare presentation, such as the facial or brow, may require adjusting the sacral rotation as previously noted, but the trigger point contact is made on the same side of sacral rotation.

Acknowledgments

I would like to acknowledge the contributions of Drs. Susi Anrig, Daniel Anrig, Ernst Anrig, Cherie Goble, Gregory Plaugher, Larry Webster, Judy Forrester, Mark Sauter, Huldy Anrig, Dr. Richard W. Doble, Jr., and Randall Howe; the models who performed beautifully and repetitively; the children, Keane Anrig, Erin and Kirsten Medcalf, Michael Van Arsdale, Andrew Carter and Jaclynn Francis, Katie Hand, and Austin Janka; and the very expectant mothers, Dorothy Gray and Lisa Carbajal.

References

1. Graham JM. Smith's recognizable patterns of human deformation. 2nd ed. Philadelphia: WB Saunders, 1988.
2. Dunne KB, Clarren SK. The origin of prenatal and postnatal deformities. Pediatric Clin North Am 1986;33:1277–1297.
3. Dunn PM. Congenital postural deformities. Br Med Bull 1976;32:71–76.
4. Moreland MS. Morphological effects of torsion applied to growing bone. J Bone Joint Surg 1980;62B:230–237.
5. Webster LL. Chiropractic care during pregnancy. Today's Chiro 1982;Sept/Oct:20–22.
6. Paulson J. Accidental injuries. In: Behrman R, Vaughan VC, Nelson WE, eds. Nelson textbook of pediatrics, 13th ed. Philadelphia: WB Saunders, 1987:211–214.
7. Leventhal HR. Birth injuries of the spinal cord. J Pediatrics 1960;56:447–453.
8. Byers RK. Spinal-cord injuries during birth. Develop Med Child Neurol 1975;17:103–110.
9. Towbin A. Latent spinal cord and brain stem injury in newborn infants. Develop Med Child Neurol 1969;11:54–68.
10. Anderson RT. Angulation of the basiocciput in three cranial series. Current Anthropology 1983;24:226–228.

11. Gutmann G. Blocked atlantal nerve syndrome in infants and small children. ICA Int Rev Chiro 1990;July/Aug:37–42.
12. Banks BD, Beck RW, Columbus M, et al. Sudden infant death syndrome: a literature review with chiropractic implications. J Manipulative Physiol Ther 1987;10:246–252.
13. Lecture Notes. Congenital and developmental spinal biomechanics. Applied Spinal Biomechanical Engineering 1987 Postgraduate Seminar, Manchester, NH 03104.
14. Heilig D. Osteopathic pediatric care in prevention of structural abnormalities. J Am Osteopath Assoc 1949;48:478–481.
15. Lewit K. Manipulative therapy in rehabilitation of the locomotor system. London: Butterworth & Co, Ltd., 1985:23–29.
16. Menkes JH, Batzdorf U. Postnatal trauma and injuries by physical agents. In: Menkes JH, ed. Textbook of child neurology. 3rd ed. Philadelphia: Lea & Febiger, 1985:493–496.
17. Jirout J. Einfluss der einseitigen Grosshirndominanz auf das Rontgenbild der Halswirbelsaule. Radiologie 1980;20:466–469.
18. Goldberg C, Dowling FE. Handedness and scoliosis convexity: a reappraisal. Spine 1990;15:61.
19. Glasauer FE, Cares HL. Traumatic paraplegia in infancy. JAMA 1972;219:38–41.
20. Taylor AR. The mechanism of injury to the spinal cord in the neck without damage to the vertebral column. J Bone Joint Surg 1951;33B:543–547.
21. Melzak J. Paraplegia among children. Lancet 1969uly 5:45–48.
22. Fielding JW. Cervical spine injuries in children. In: Sherk HH, Dunn EJ, Eismont FJ, eds. The cervical spine. 2nd ed. Philadelphia: JB Lippincott, 1989;199:422–435.
23. Pang D, Wilberger JE. Spinal cord injury without radiographic abnormalities in children. J Neurosurg 1982;57:114–129.
24. Educational literature. Washington, DC: National Head Injury Foundation, 1991.
25. Hinwood JA, Hinwood JA. Children and chiropractic: a summary of subluxation and its ramifications. J Aust Chiro Assoc 1981;11:18–21.
26. Percy EC. Acute subluxation of the cervical spine. CMA J 1970(Oct 24).
27. Zitelli BJ, Davis HW, eds. Atlas of pediatric physical diagnosis. St. Louis: CV Mosby, 1987.
28. Plaugher G, Lopes MA, Melch PE, Cremata EE. The inter- and intraexaminer reliability of a paraspinal skin temperature differential instrument. J Manipulative Physiol Ther 1991;14:361–367.
29. Herbst RW. Gonstead chiropractic science and art. Mt. Horeb, WI: Sci-Chi Publications, 1968.
30. Farfan HF. Mechanical disorders of the low back. Philadelphia: Lea & Febiger, 1973.
31. Aker PS, Cassidy JD. Torticollis in infants and children: a report of three cases. J Can Chiro Assoc 1990;34:13–19.
32. Kent C. An overview of pediatric radiology in chiropractic. ICA Int Rev Chiro 1990;July/Aug:45–53.
33. Yochum TR, Rowe LJ. Essentials of skeletal radiology. Baltimore: Williams & Wilkins, 1987.
34. Dawson EG, Smith L. Atlanto-axial subluxation in children due to vertebral anomalies. J Bone Joint Surg 1979;61A:582–587.
35. Caffey J. The whiplash shaken infant syndrome: manual shaking by the extremities with whiplash-induced intracranial and intraocular bleedings, linked with residual permanaent brain damage and mental retardation. Pediatrics 1974;54:396–403.
36. Glasauer FE, Cares HL. Biomechanical features of traumatic paraplegia in infancy. J Trauma 1973;13:166–170.
37. Warwick R, Williams PL, eds. Gray's anatomy. 36th British ed. Philadelphia: WB Saunders, 1980.
38. Stephenson RW. Chiropractic textbook. Davenport, IA: Palmer School of Chiropractic, 1948.
39. Behrman RE, Vaughan VC. Nelson textbook of pediatrics. 13th ed. Philadelphia: WB Saunders, 1987.
40. Prugh DG, Kisley AJ. Psychosocial aspects of pediatrics and psychiatric disorders. In: Kempe HC, Silver HK, O'Brien D, Fulginiti VA, eds. Current pediatric diagnosis and treatment. 9th ed. Norwalk, CT: Appleton & Lange, 1987:730–755.
41. Nilsson N. Infantile colic and chiropractic. Euro J Chiro 1985;33:624–665.
42. Klougart N, Nilsson N, Jacobsen J. Infantile colic treated by chiropractors: a prospective study of 316 cases. J Manipulative Physiol Ther 1989;12:281–288.
43. Moore KL. Clinically oriented anatomy. 2nd ed. Baltimore: Williams & Wilkins, 1985.
44. Robuck SV. The interosseous lesion as a causative factor in enuresis and other bladder disturbances in children. J Am Osteopath Assoc 1936;36:73–74.
45. Gemmell HA, Jacobson BH. Chiropractic management of enuresis: time-series descriptive design. J Manipulative Physiol Ther 1989;12:386–389.
46. Lecture notes. Gonstead seminar of chiropractic. Mt. Horeb, WI, 1990.
47. Nellhaus G, Stumpf DA, Moe PG. Neurologic and muscular disorders. In: Kempe HC, Silver HK, O'Brien D, Fulginiti VA, eds. Current pediatric diagnosis and treatment. 9th ed. Norwalk, CT: Appleton & Lange, 1987:645–729.
48. Koops BL, Battaglia FC. The newborn infant. In: Kempe HC, Silver HK, O'Brien D, Fulginiti VA, eds. Current pediatric diagnosis and treatment. 9th ed. Norwalk, CT: Appleton & Lange, 1987: 41–97.
49. Netter FH. The CIBA collection of medical illustrations. Vol. 1 Part 1., 1983.
50. Schmitt BD, Berman S. Ear, nose and throat. In: Kempe HC, Silver HK, O'Brien D, Fulginiti VA, eds. Current pediatric diagnosis and treatment. 9th ed. Norwalk, CT: Appleton & Lange, 1987:308–340.
51. Hendricks CL, Larkin-Thier SM. Otitis media in young children. Chiropractic 1989;2:9–13.
52. Cooke ED, Carter LM, Pilcher MF. Identifying scoliosis in the adolescent with thermography: a preliminary report. Clin Orthop 1980;148:172–176.
53. Eilert RE. Orthopedics. In: Kempe HC, Silver HK, O'Brien D, Fulginiti VA, eds. Current pediatric diagnosis and treatment. 9th ed. Norwalk, CT: Appleton & Lange, 1987:622–644.
54. Giesen JM, Center DB, Leach RA. An evaluation of chiropractic manipulation as a treatment of hyperactivity in children. J Manipulative Physiol Ther 1989;12:353–363.
55. Shields JR, Schifrin BS. Perinatal antecedents of cerebral palsy. Obstet Gynecol 1988;71:899–905.
56. Arbuckle BE. The value of occupational and osteopathic manipulative therapy in the rehabilitation of the cerebral palsy victim. J Am Osteopath Assoc 1955;55:227–237.
57. Robinson A, Goodman SI, McCabe ERB. Genetic and chromosomal disorders, including inborn errors of metabolism. In: Kempe HC, Silver HK, O'Brien D, Fulginiti VA, eds. Current pediatric diagnosis and treatment. 9th ed. Norwalk, CT: Appleton & Lange, 1987:1007–1046.
58. Mantero E, Crispini L. Static alterations of the pelvic, sacral, lumbar area due to pregnancy. Chiropractic treatment. In: Mazzarelli JP, ed. Chiropractic Interprofessional Research Torino: Edizioni Minerva Medica, 1982:59–68.
59. Diakow PRP, Gadsby TA, Gadsby JB, et al. Back pain during pregnancy and labor. J Manipulative Physiol Ther 1991;14:116–118.
60. Fast A, Shapiro D, Ducommun EJ, et al. Low-back pain in pregnancy. Spine 1987;12:368–371.
61. Ostgaard HC, Andersson GBJ. Previous back pain and risk of developing back pain in a future pregnancy. Spine 1991;16:432–436.
62. Svensson HO, Andersson GBJ, Hagstad A, Jansson PO. The relationship of low-back pain to pregnancy and gynecologic factors. Spine 1990;15:371–375.

63. Guthrie RA. Lumbar inhibitory pressure for lumbar myalgia during contractions of the gravid uterus at term. J Am Osteopath Assoc 1980;80:264–266.
64. Melzack R, Belanger E. Labour pain: correlations with menstrual pain and acute low-back pain before and during pregnancy. Pain 1989;36:225–229.
65. Burns L, Vollbrecht WJ. Effects of maternal lumbar lesions upon the development of young rabbits. J Am Osteopath Assoc 1919;18:527–530.
66. Burns L. Vertebral lesions and the course of pregnancy in animals. J Am Osteopath Assoc 1923;23:155–157.
67. Fallon JM. Chiropractic and pregnancy. Int Rev Chiro 1990;46(6):39–42.
68. Heckman JD. Managing musculoskeletal problems in pregnant patients. Part 2: fractures, RA, scoliosis, and metabolic disorders. J Musculoskeletal Med 1990;7(9):17–24.
69. Plaugher G, Lopes MA. The knee-chest table: indications and contraindications. Chiropractic Technique 1990;2:163–167.

15 Extravertebral Disorders: Temporomandibular Joint, Nasal Septum, and Sinus

TRENT R. BACHMAN

In reviewing the literature on disorders of the temporomandibular joint (TMJ), two distinct characteristics are immediately apparent. First, the majority claim to be successful with their methods of correction of this malady. Second, there is little interprofessional collaboration in standardization of treatment. Therefore, in providing a contemporary approach to the diagnosis and treatment of temporomandibular disorders, it is the intent of the author to provide a concise protocol for chiropractors which also incorporates a corroboration with the various allied professionals specializing in this area. The chiropractor's unique training in detecting and correcting joint dysfunction lends a distinct advantage in providing care to patients with TMJ disorders.

Often, the most useful tool in determining the cause of temporomandibular disorders is derived from the patient history. Seldom is a singular underlying traumatic event the cause of the condition. TMJ dysfunction is considered to be a multifactorial disease (Table 15.1) (1).

When the chiropractor encounters a patient presenting with possible TMJ dysfunction, great care should be taken to avoid a tunnel vision approach that would skew the ability to derive an accurate diagnosis and provide a corrective treatment program. For TMJ disorders, as in the case of the vertebral subluxation complex, the logical and most productive course of management is to start with noninvasive reversible forms of treatment and therapy and to escalate if necessary, as the severity of the condition dictates. All too often, chiropractors are quick to refer TMJ patients to dentists and other allied health professionals when they can be managed, and often times treated, with chiropractic methods. When the severity of the condition dictates a teamwork approach, the chiropractor should refer to a dentist or other allied health professional familiar with the TMJ and with whom a working relationship can then be established. The chiropractor may also want to refer the patient to a diagnostic imaging center or a comprehensive rehabilitation facility to obtain additional information in order to get an accurate diagnosis or to incorporate adjunctive therapies that may enhance the patient's recovery. Additionally, there is a need for the chiropractor to incorporate as many objective tools available as outcome measures for manual treatment and any adjunctive therapies.

Surface Anatomy of the Temporomandibular Joint

The temporomandibular joint is situated just anterior to the external acoustic meatus and below the posterior end of the zygomatic arch. When the mouth is open, the condyles move out of the mandibular fossa into the articular tubercle, at which time a depression is noted on palpation of the joint. When palpating for the location of the TMJ, it is the posterior lateral aspect of the condyle which the clinician locates to monitor the movement through its range of motion (2).

The temporomandibular joint is a three-joint complex that consists of the head of the condyle and its articulation with the inferior border of the articular discs. The superior boundary of the joint is housed within the glenoid fossa which articulates with the superior border of the articular disc. The head of the mandibular condyle is knuckle-shaped and convex in all directions and is accepted via the articular disc into the glenoid fossa which is oval and deeply concave (Fig. 15.1).

The articular disc is described as a firm, oval, fibrous plate. When viewed in the lateral plane (Fig. 15.2), its cen-

Table 15.1.
Proposed Causes of Temporomandibular Joint Dysfunction[a]

External trauma to the joints and/or muscles
Motor vehicle accidents
Dental treatment
Orthodontia
Surgical procedures with intubation
Cervical traction
Contact sports
Occlusal disparity
Poor bite
Missing teeth
Jaw misalignment
Psychological factors
Anxiety
Tension
Nutritional factors
Nutrient deficiencies
Occlusal habits
Clenching
Bruxism
Gum chewing

[a]Modified from Thompson T, Dwyer JT, Palmer CA. Nutritional remedies for temporomandibular joint dysfunction: fact or fiction. Nutrition Today 1991; Jan/Feb:39.

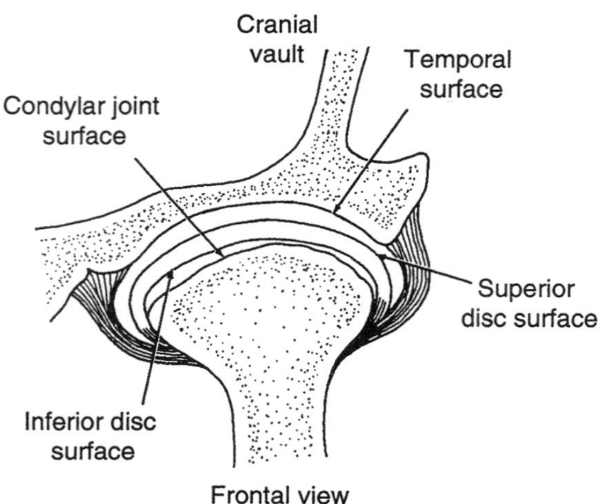

Figure 15.1. Anterior view of the temporomandibular joint illustrating the articular surfaces of the three joint complex. (Courtesy Dr. Darryl Curl.)

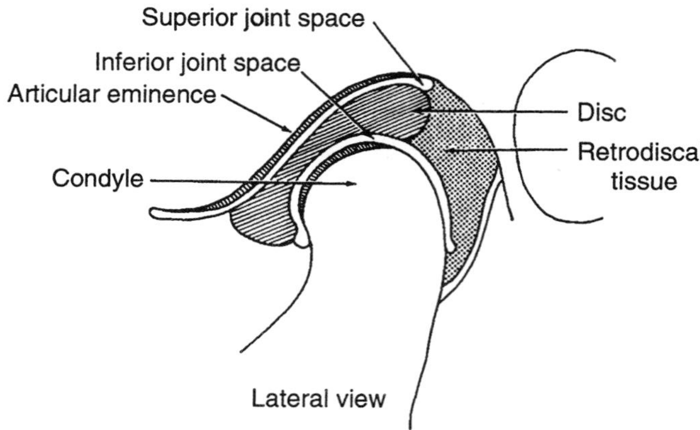

Figure 15.2. Lateral view of the temporomandibular joint compartment. The disc is non-vascularized while the retrodiscal tissue is highly vascularized. (Courtesy Dr. Darryl Curl.)

tral portion is quite thin with respect to the periphery. The posterior border is especially thick. The disc is fused to the capsule at the anterior aspect where it extends forward in front of the condyle. This allows for the attachment of the superior fibers of the lateral pterygoid muscle. The capsule is continuous posteriorly with the retrodiscal pad.

The anterior portion of the articular disc is avascular in contrast to the retrodiscal pad, which is a vascularized and innervated thick layer of connective tissue attached to the posterior wall of the capsule. The unique avascular characteristic of the articular disc is complemented by avascular fibrous layers covering the mandible and the glenoid temporal surface of the TMJ. The lack of vascularized tissue suggests the presence of considerable mechanical stresses along this portion of the joint.

The capsule and articular discs are independently attached inferiorly to the medial and lateral poles of the condyle. This unique attachment of the disc to the respective poles of the condyle assures synchronization of normal biomechanical movements by the mandible and the articular disc.

Fibrous Capsule

The fibrous capsule of the TMJ is attached to the articular tubercle of the temporal bone and along the limits of the posterior root of the zygoma. Posteriorly, the fibrous capsule arises from the posterior aspect of the articular lip. Although the capsule is strongly reinforced laterally, it tends to be loosely arranged anteriorly, posteriorly, and medially. The lateral capsular region is strongly reinforced via the temporomandibular ligament. A wide fan-shaped lateral portion and a narrow medial band comprise the two separate layers of the temporomandibular ligament. The broad fan-shaped portion of this ligament is connected along the zygomatic process of the temporal bone and its narrow portion is attached to the neck of the mandible. Its posterior fibers present a vertical arrangement between the mandible and temporal bones, whereas the anterior fibers are obliquely arranged inferiorly and posteriorly. The medial portion of the fibers travel primarily in a horizontal manner and comprise a ligamentous band which attaches to the crest of the articular tubercle and extends along the lateral pole of the mandibular condyle and attaches to the disc.

The function of the ligaments is primarily to limit movements of the mandible. The lateral fan-shaped fibers prevent the mandibular condyle from being displaced away from the articular eminence. The medial band prevents excessive retrusive movements and thus prevents the condyle from pressing against and damaging the tissues behind the articulation (3).

The sphenomandibular and the stylomandibular are considered to be the accessory ligaments of the TMJ. The stylomandibular ligament extends from the styloid process and stylohyoid ligament to the angle of the mandible. The ligament tenses when the mandible is protruded and is loose when the jaw is closed. When the jaw is at its maximal opening, this ligament is in its most relaxed state. The suggested function of the stylomandibular ligament is to limit excessive protrusive movements (3). The sphenomandibular ligament originates from the sphenoid spine and inserts onto the mandibular lingula and neck of the mandible. Shore (4) suggests that the accessory ligaments function in a restrictive manner to keep the condyle, temporal bone and articular disc firmly opposed.

Synovial Membrane

The synovial membrane consists of a highly vascularized form of connective tissue which lines the entire fibrous capsule. It also covers the superior and inferior surfaces of the retrodiscal pad and the loose connective tissues anchoring the posterior border of the disc to the capsule.

The rich vascular supply which the synovial tissue requires is located in the posterior compartment via the superficial temporal artery. Essentially, the synovial membrane lines all of the TMJ articular structures which are not subject to shearing or compressive stresses. The synovial membrane is absent in the articular surfaces subjected to compressive and shearing forces, such as the mandibular condyle, articular disc, and the temporal bone.

Masticatory Muscle Action

When examining the masticatory muscle structures for possible extracapsular involvement, the clinician must carefully evaluate the agonist as well as the antagonist muscles. The musculoskeletal system provides the mechanical power in stabilizing, positioning, and movement of the TMJ articulation. It is critical to understand that no single muscle structure acts alone in this process. In order for normal movement to be performed, a cooperative effort between the agonist muscles and the antagonist muscles is necessary. As the agonist muscles initiate joint movement, the antagonist muscles working in concert, respond in opposition by producing a graduated and controlled muscular contraction.

Muscle Tone

Muscle tonus is characterized primarily by the muscles' resistance to elongation or stretch. Clinically, muscle tonus is described as hypertonic or hypotonic. Hypertonicity relates to the muscles relative expansion in passive resistance to stretching of the muscle fibers. Hypotonicity relates to a diminished passive resistance to stretch.

Muscle Spasm

Muscle spasm is characterized by an abrupt involuntary muscle contracture, either individually or as a group. This phenomenon involves functionally related musculature and is accompanied by pain and mechanical interference to normal joint activity. When spastic muscle contraction is present, it may take the form of isometric or isotonic behavior. Isotonic muscle spasm creates a shortening of the muscle which leads to aberration in muscular movement and tone. Isometric muscle spasm produces a marked resistance to stretching and is characterized as muscular rigidity. Muscle spasm is readily observed and easily palpated on evaluation.

Muscle Splinting

Muscle splinting is characterized by an involuntary increase of tonicity of the musculature, which in turn impairs the stability and normal movement of the TMJ. It is believed that muscle splinting is a response to altered mechanical or proprioceptive sensory impulses. In contrast to muscle spasm, splinting readily returns the muscle fibers to normal tonus on cessation of the causative factor.

Clinical Implications

Often, masticatory conditions may be difficult to differentiate into exact categories, therefore hindering the administration of proper treatment. Masticatory muscle contractures are often categorized into involuntary responses and actuation of normal biomechanical movements. Muscle tonus, muscle splinting and muscle spasm are categories of involuntary responses. Muscle tonus is characterized as a varying degree of continuous contractions of a muscle at rest which furnishes mechanical stability to the craniomandibular articulation. Muscle splinting is a momentary state of hypertonicity induced by the body's protective mechanism in an attempt to stabilize a threatened articular structure. Muscle splinting in and of itself does not produce any structural muscular dysfunction and tends to present itself as a feeling of weakness and inhibition of pain. Muscle spasm is a self-perpetuating muscle protracted state of involuntary tonic contraction. It is accompanied by pain and rigidity and induces structural muscular changes.

Actuation of normal biomechanical movement consists of conscious voluntary mandibular movements such as habitual chewing, sucking, kissing, and swallowing. These types of movements are based on patterns within the central nervous system and are kept in check by sensory and proprioceptive neuroreceptors (15).

Arthrokinematics

During the full range of mandibular movement from the closed position to maximal opening, both condyles of the mandible contribute equally. Opening and closing of the mouth is achieved through coupled motion of the condyle. This coupled motion consists of rotation and translation. Opening of the mouth is first initiated by pure rotation around the horizontal axis through the two condylar heads. This rotational motion is described as a hinged movement and occurs initially between the mandibular condyle and the articular disc (Fig. 15.3). As the opening of the mouth continues, the rotational hinge motion reaches its maximum at about the first 12 to 15 mm of mandibular movement. At this point, further opening of the mouth is allowed by the translatory or gliding motion of the mandibular condyle and meniscus as it articulates along the slope of the articular eminence. Therefore, the translational component contributing to opening and closing of the mouth occurs in the superior joint compartment. Even though rotation and translation make up the coupled motion when the mouth is open, it is important to understand that each of these movements is providing the dominant activity according to the posi-

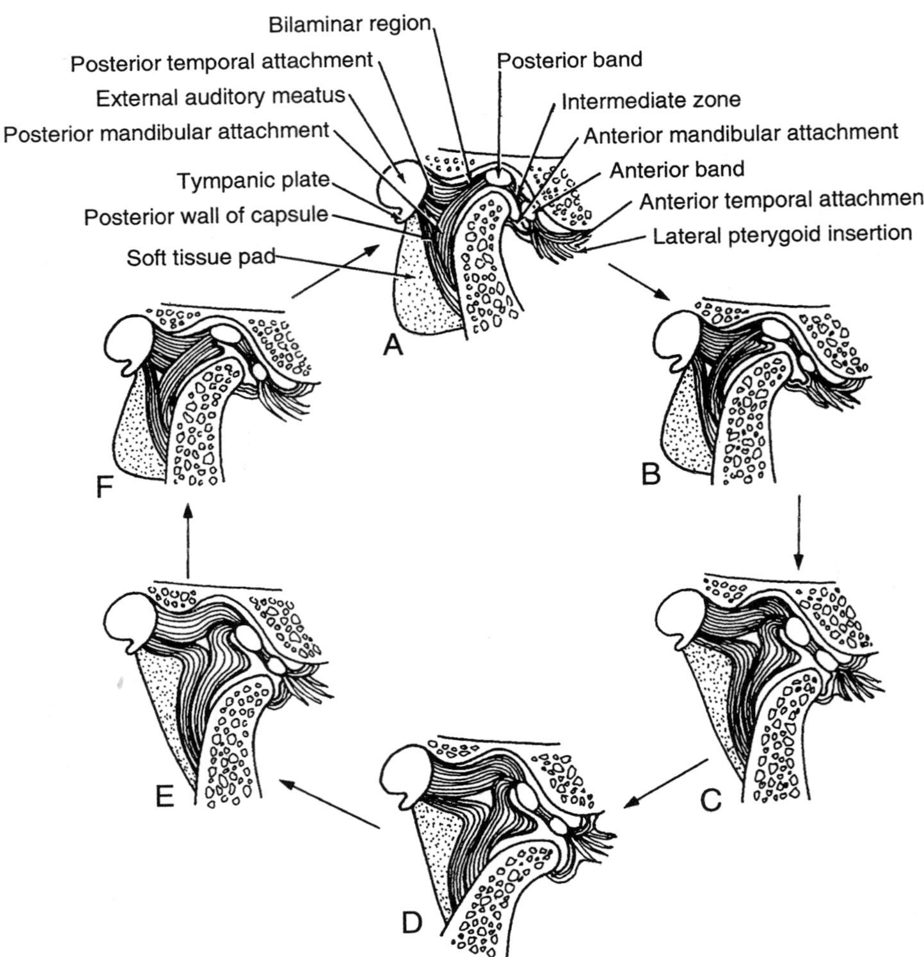

Figure 15.3. Mechanical relationships of the mandibular condyle, the articular disc, and the articular surfaces of the temporal bone during one complete opening (A-D) and closing (D-A) cycle of the jaw. Modified from Warwick R, Williams PL, eds. Gray's anatomy. 35th British ed. Philadelphia: WB Saunders, 1973:410

tion of the mandibular condyle through its range of motion.

Muscles of Mastication

The muscles of mastication are comprised of the masseter, temporalis, medial pterygoid, and the lateral pterygoid (Figs. 15.4 and 15.5). The masseter, temporalis, and the medial pterygoid exert their forces primarily in the vertical plane, such as when closing the jaw.

The lateral pterygoid is anatomically situated in the horizontal plane and it acts to stabilize the TMJ and protraction of the mandible. These muscles are innervated by the motor branches of the mandibular division of the trigeminal nerve.

The muscles of mastication, suprahyoid and infrahyoid muscles, as well as the tongue and fascia work in concert in all mandibular movements and functions of deglutition. It is therefore important that the clinician have an understanding of these individual contributors to the external temporomandibular complex. Analysis of their individual functions is integral to the assessment of the function of the temporomandibular articulation.

MASSETER

The masseter muscle is rectangular and consists of a large superficial and a smaller deep portion. It arises from the zygomatic arch to the outer surface of the mandibular ramus. It is a powerful elevator of the mandible with its superficial portion directing its force at right angles to the posteriorly ascending occlusal plane of the molars. If the mandible is in a protruded position, the fibers of the deep portion are angled downward and forward. This action of the deep portion of the muscle may act to stabilize the condyle against the articular eminence during biting and chewing actions (3).

TEMPORALIS

The fan-shaped temporalis muscle occupies the entire temporal fossa of the skull. The muscle consists of three parts: anterior, middle, and posterior. The anterior muscle fibers form the bulk of the muscle and are aligned vertically. The fibers of the middle part are aligned in an oblique manner and the posterior fibers are aligned in a horizontal fashion. The anterior and posterior muscle fibers of the temporalis act as strong elevators of the mandible as well as provide stabilization for the TMJ. The middle muscle fibers are capable of exerting strong retracting forces on the mandible.

MEDIAL PTERYGOID

The medial (internal) pterygoid muscle is a thick quadrilateral muscle which is anatomically positioned on the medial side of the mandibular ramus. This muscle is the counterpart to the masseter muscle, both functionally and anatomically. Although not as strong as the masseter muscle, the medial pterygoid assists in the movements of elevation and protrusion of the mandible. It also assists to laterally deviate the mandible to the contralateral side of contraction. The medial surface of this muscle comes into direct contact with the tensor veli palatini muscle. The tensor veli palatini muscle tenses the soft palate which results in the opening of the auditory tube during swallowing (6). The unique anatomic relationship which exists between the medial pterygoid and the tensor veli palatini muscle may contribute to eustachian tube dysfunction when the medial pterygoid muscle is influenced by aberrant forces from temporomandibular dysfunction.

LATERAL PTERYGOID

The lateral (external) pterygoid muscle is comprised of superior and inferior heads. The smaller superior head originates from the infratemporal surface of the greater sphenoid wing medial to the infratemporal crest. The larger inferior head originates from the outer surface of the lateral pterygoid plate (3). Elevation of the mandible

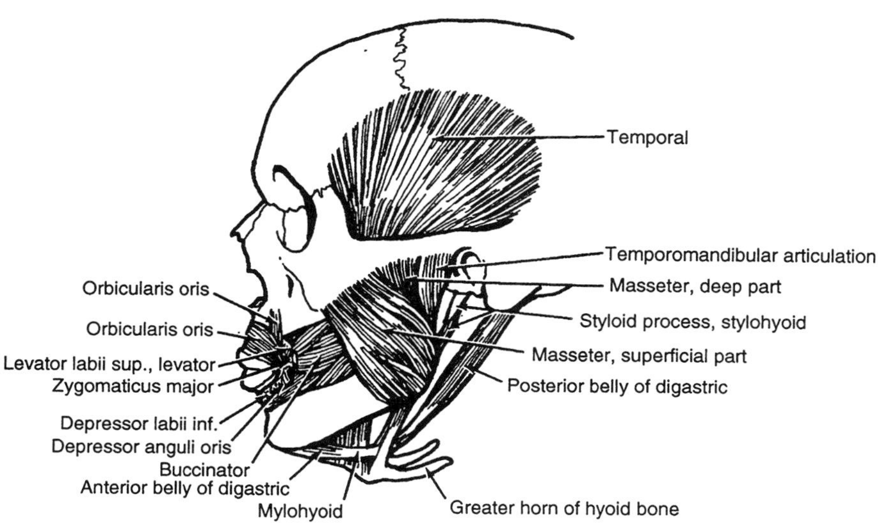

Figure 15.4. Lateral illustration of the superficial muscles of mastication which includes the musculature of the mouth and the suprahyoid muscles. Modified from Platzer W, ed. Pernkopf's Anatomy. Vol. 1. 3rd ed. Baltimore: Urban & Schwarzenberg, 1980:31.

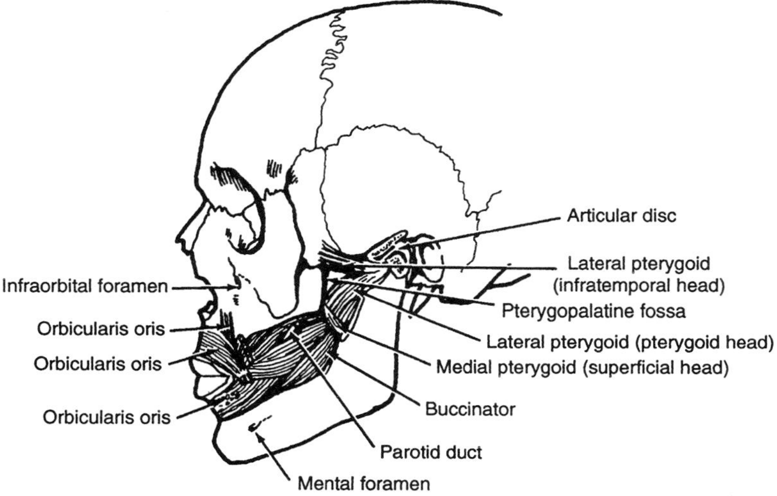

Figure 15.5. Lateral illustration of the deep muscles of mastication and the buccinator muscle. Modified from Platzer W, ed. Pernkopf's Anatomy. Vol. 1. 3rd ed. Baltimore: Urban & Schwarzenberg, 1980:31.

is achieved with contraction of the superior head, while mandibular movements of protraction and opening are achieved with contraction of the inferior head. The superior head may also function in stabilization of the mandibular condyle against the articular eminence. During biting and chewing the resultant forces are directed forward and inward, passing through the TMJ.

Resistance to opening of the jaw activates the superior head with its attachment to the articular disc and anterior portion of the meniscus. This is responsible for the forward pulling of the articular disc and meniscus, thus providing a cushion to the condyle during translational (gliding) motion. This unique action of the superior head of the lateral pterygoid muscle is vital when making a manual correction of the TMJ.

SUPRAHYOID MUSCLE GROUP

The suprahyoid muscles consist of the digastric, stylohyoid, mylohyoid, and the geniohyoid (Figs. 15.6 and 15.7). Although the suprahyoid group is technically not considered part of the muscles of mastication, they do exert an important influence in specific mandibular movements.

The digastric asserts its muscular influence in stabilizing the hyoid bone. With the hyoid in a static fixed position, the digastric assists the muscles of mastication to depress the mandible. Conversely, when the mandible is in a static fixed position, elevation of the hyoid bone will occur (7).

The digastric muscle is also thought to provide assistance during retrusive mandibular motion and functions to assist the lower head of the lateral pterygoid muscle in opening movements of the mandible (3). The stylohyoid muscle, which elongates the floor of the mouth, acts to retract and raise the hyoid bone.

The mylohyoid muscle functions in raising the floor of the mouth when deglutition is initiated with accompanied elevation of the hyoid bone. This muscle acts in mandibular movement such as depression, retrusion, and lateral deviation on the ipsilateral side of contraction.

The geniohyoid muscle is activated with mandibular movements such as depression, protrusion, and lateral deviation on the ipsilateral side. When the mandible is in the static fixed position, the geniohyoid muscle functions to elevate the hyoid bone and as an antagonist of the stylohyoid muscle will move the hyoid bone forward.

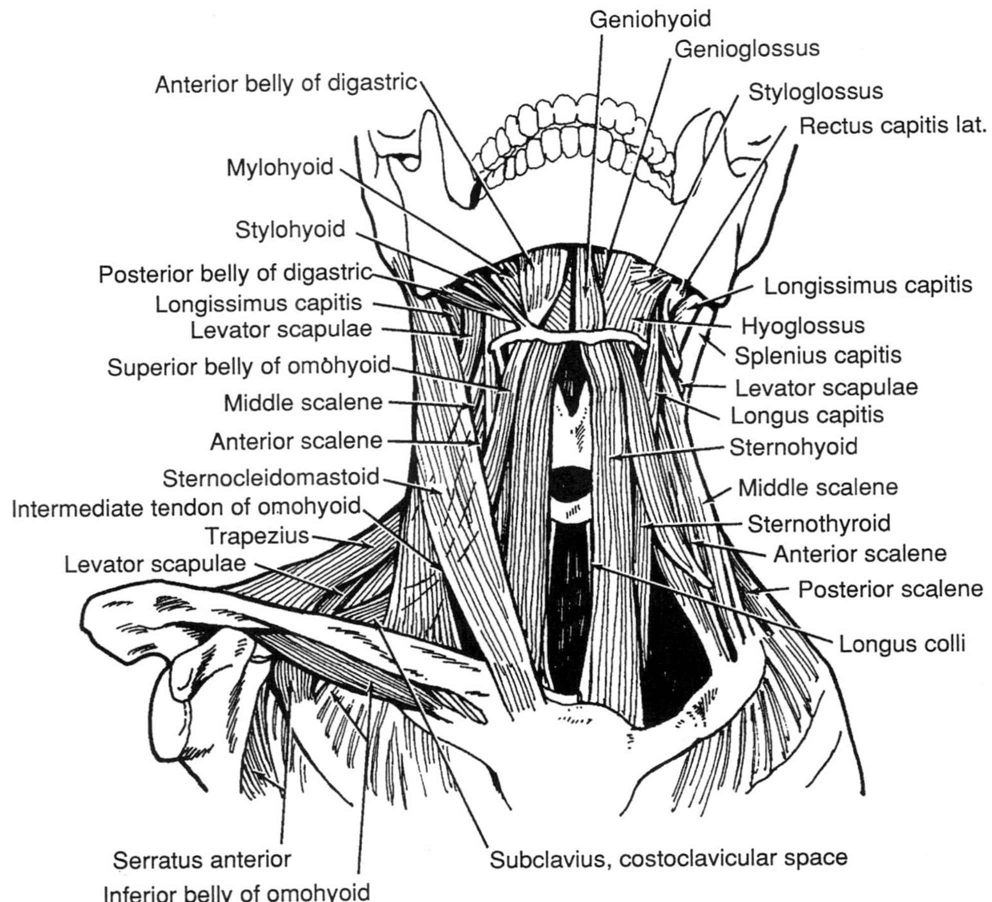

Figure 15.6. Anterior illustration of the neck musculature involved in cranium and mandibular movement. Modified from Platzer W, ed. Pernkopf's Anatomy. Vol. 1. 3rd ed. Baltimore: Urban & Schwarzenberg, 1980:263.

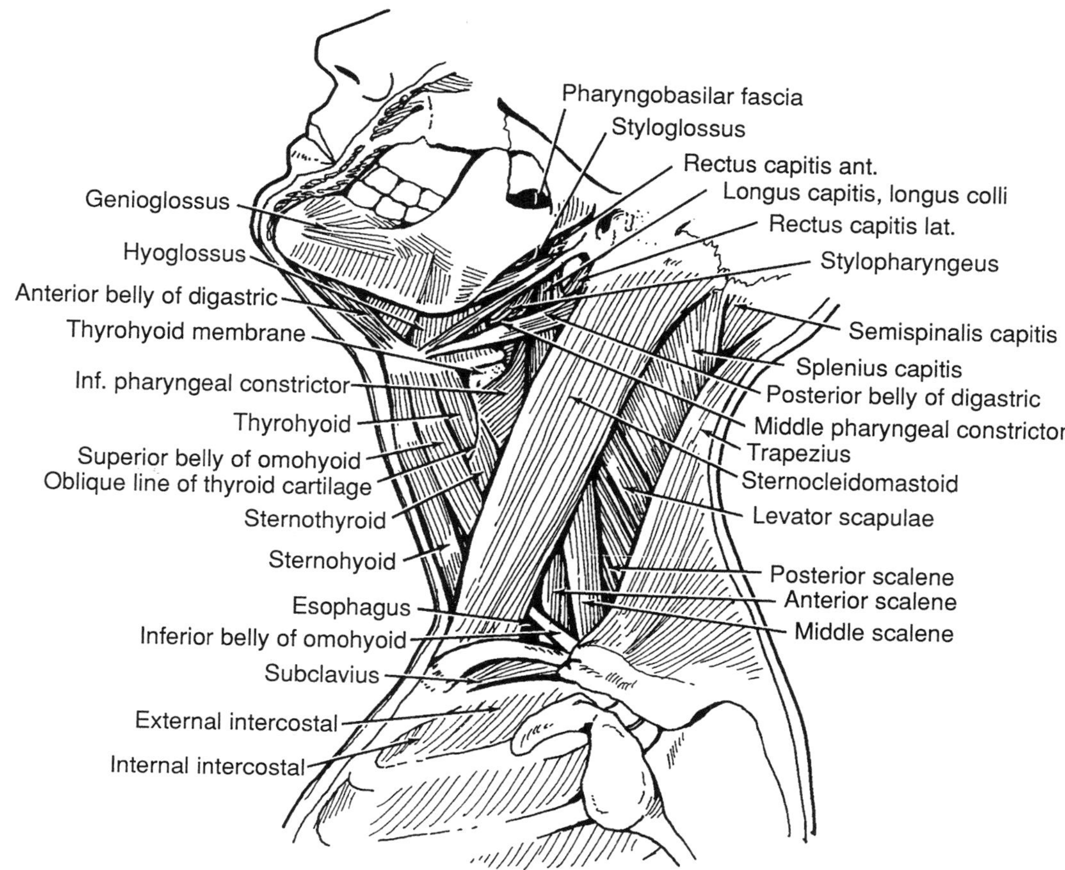

Figure 15.7. Lateral illustration of the neck musculature involved in cranium and mandibular movement. Modified from Platzer W, ed. Pernkopf's Anatomy. Vol. 1. 3rd ed. Baltimore: Urban & Schwarzenberg, 1980:264.

INFRAHYOID MUSCLE GROUP

The infrahyoid muscle group consists of the sternohyoid, sternothyroid, thyrohyoid, and the omohyoid. This muscle group provides an antagonistic force to the suprahyoid muscle group by depressing the hyoid bone and securing the hyoid during suprahyoid muscle activity (8).

Terminology

Temporomandibular dysfunction refers to a collection of symptoms associated with functional and structural disturbances of the musculature and associated soft tissue elements. Some of the most common symptoms include: clicking of the joint, limitations in the joint mechanics during mandibular motion, and head and neck pain often accompanied by tenderness in the muscles of mastication (Table 15.2). Various health care disciplines specializing in TMJ disorders acknowledge that any dysfunction, pain, or paralysis of the masticatory system that occurs independently of mandibular dysfunction is not, by definition or classification, a TMJ disorder. It must be understood that "TMJ" is a generic term, much the same as the term, "whiplash."

Table 15.3 shows the diverse clinical symptomatology of TMJ dysfunction; however, it is not intended to be an

Table 15.2.
Classification of Acute and Chronic TMJ Disorders

Acute TMJ Disorders

- I. Masticatory Muscle Disorders (External Derangements) (9)
  1. Muscle Splinting (9)
  2. Myospasms (9)
  3. Myositis (9)
  4. Myofascial Trigger Point Pain (Active) (9)
  5. Muscle Hyperactivity (10)
  6. Trismus (10)
  7. Dyskinesias (10)
- II. Disc-Interference Disorders (Internal Derangements) (9)
  1. Spontaneous Dislocation (11)
  2. Derangements of the Condyle-Disc Complex (9)
     a. Disc Displacements (11)
     b. Disc Dislocations with Reduction (11)
     c. Disc Dislocations without Reduction (11)
  3. Structural Incompatibility of the Articular Surface (9)
     a. Adhesions (Synovial Stickiness) (11)
     b. Alterations in Form (Tearing) (11)
  4. Subluxations (rarely acute) (11)
  5. Spontaneous Dislocations of the Condyle (11)
- III. Inflammatory Disorders (Capsular Derangements) (9)
  1. Synovitis (9)
  2. Capsulitis (9)
  3. Retrodiscitis (9)
- IV. Hypomobility/Hypermobility Disorders (External or Capsular Derangements) (9)
  1. Muscle Contracture (9)
  2. Ligamentous Instability (9)
- V. Postural/Proprioceptive Disorders (usually chronic) (External Derangements) (9)

Table 15.2.
Classification of Acute and Chronic TMJ Disorders—*Continued*

Chronic TMJ Disorder
- I. Masticatory Muscle Disorders (External Derangements) (9)
  1. Muscle Splinting (rare to see in chronic form) (9)
  2. Myospasms (rare to see in chronic form) (9)
  3. Myositis (9)
  4. Myofascial Trigger Point Pain (Latent) (9)
- II. Disc-Interference Disorders (Internal Derangements) (0)
  1. Derangements of the Condyle-Disc Complex (9)
     - a. Disc Displacements (9)
     - b. Disc Dislocations with Reduction (9)
     - c. Disc Dislocations without Reduction (9)
  2. Structural Incompatibility of the Articular Surface (9)
     - a. Adhesions (9)
     - b. Alterations in Form (Perforations) (9)
     - c. Osteoarthritis (10)
  3. Dislocations (rarely chronic) or Subluxations (usually chronic) of the Condyle (9)
- III. Inflammatory Disorders (Capsular Derangements) (9)
  1. Synovitis (rarely chronic) (9)
  2. Capsulitis (rarely chronic) (9)
  3. Retrodiscitis (rarely chronic) (9)
  4. Degenerative Joint Disease (11)
  5. Inflammatory Arthritis (10,11)
  6. Rheumatoid Arthritis (10)
  7. Polyarticular (10)
- IV. Hypomobility/Hypermobility Disorders (External or Capsular Derangements) (9)
  1. Muscle Contracture (9)
  2. Capsular Fibrosis (11)
  3. Coronoid Impedance (11)
  4. Ankylosis (10)
  5. Ligamentous Instability (9)
- V. Growth Disorders (External, Capsular, or Internal Derangements) (9)
  1. Hypoplasia (9)
  2. Hyperplasia (9)
  3. Neoplasia (9)
  4. Remodeling (11)
  5. Condyle Position Abnormality (11)
     - a. Retroposition (11)
     - b. Anteroposition (11)
     - c. Decreased interarticular space (11)
  6. Developmental Disturbances (10)
- VI. Postural/Proprioceptive Disorders (9) (External Derangements)

exhaustive list of the signs and symptoms of TMJ disorders. Nevertheless, it does provide the clinician an appreciation for the complexity of this syndrome.

Etiology

When the patient presents with a TMJ disorder, it is imperative that the clinician make use of all available subjective information and objective findings to derive a well-defined etiology of the condition. The diversity of the signs and symptoms of this disorder has often complicated the clinician's ability to accurately establish a diagnosis.

The nature of TMJ symptoms has made it necessary to formulate a reduction in the observable clinical symptoms to establish a more narrowed definition of the syndrome. As noted by Solberg (11), signs and symptoms of a TMJ disorder are:

Table 15.3.
Clinical Symptomatology Associated with TMJ Dysfunction

1. Asthma (12)
2. Chronic Ear Infection (12)
3. Hearing Loss (14)
4. Tinnitus (13)
5. Headaches (13)
6. Neck Pain (12)
7. Shoulder Pain (12)
8. Inflammation (14)
9. Earache (13)
10. Lingual Pain or Numbness (13,15)
11. Facial Pain (16)
12. Vertigo (dizziness) (13)
13. Sinus Congestion (12)
14. Throat Infections (12)
15. Functional Jaw Pain (14)
16. Incoordination of Mandibular Joint (13)
17. Painful Teeth and Gums (14,15)
18. Oropharyngeal Syndromes (15)
19. Speech Impairment (15)
20. Bell's Palsy (14)
21. Reflex Sympathetic Dystrophy Syndrome (16)

1. Pain and tenderness in the region of muscles of mastication and the TMJs;
2. Incoordination and sounds during condylar movement; and
3. Limitation of mandibular movement.

To rely solely on the evaluation of signs and symptoms could inadvertently cause the clinician to make an inaccurate diagnosis, with little emphasis on assessing the patient's prognosis. For example, the same TMJ pain or dysfunction may be caused by cervical nerve entrapment (vertebral subluxation complex), referred pain syndrome from a distant myofascial irritation or trigger point, intrinsic intracapsular pathology or intrinsic extracapsular pathology. The treatment for these conditions is quite different, therefore, the need for further objective evaluation is paramount. Kopp (17) states that the clinical signs and symptoms of patients with TMJ osteoarthrosis do not differ from those patients with other mandibular dysfunctions, except in crepitation of the TMJ. This lack of apparent discrimination may very well account for many of the treatment failures in the clinical management of these disorders.

In reviewing the literature on TMJ, the term "syndrome" has been used to imply that a patient may present with all the symptoms simultaneously. From a clinical perspective, this is clearly not the case.

During the consultation with the patient, the natural history of the TMJ disorder (biologic gradient) should be developed. The diagnostic process is enhanced by the clinician's ability to evaluate the soft tissue structures associated with biomechanical dysfunction and masticatory pain which are often present.

Pathomechanics

External macrotrauma and internal microtrauma should be considered in evaluating patients presenting with TMJ disorders. External macrotrauma would include acceleration/deceleration hyperextension/hyperflexion cervical spine injuries (e.g., whiplash), surgical procedures involving intubation, cervical traction, dental treatment, orthodontia treatment, contact sports, and impacts that would cause any structure of the TMJ joint to be forced beyond its elastic barrier.

Etiologies of internal microtrauma include self-imposed psychic stress causing occlusal interference (e.g., tooth clenching, grinding, and bruxism), cracked tooth syndrome, chronic periodontitis causing such conditions as excessive tooth wear, and degenerative soft tissue changes, degenerative arthritis, and inflammatory arthritis.

Derangement of the internal TMJ implies an anatomic disturbance between the temporal bone, the articular disc and the mandibular condyle. Internal derangements include restriction of translational motion of the condyle, condylar dislocation, condylar subluxation, temporal adhesions, and discondylar lesions (18).

Proprioceptor and tactile neuroreceptor activation are additional factors that must be considered probable causes of TMJ dysfunction. Traumatic forces influencing condylar malposition will produce noxious stimuli of these sensory fibers in the joint capsule, sometimes involving the periodontal membrane (18).

Malocclusion of the dentition may cause aberrances in condylar movement with resultant pain. Such irritating stimuli to the TMJ capsule is mediated by the masseteric and deep temporal nerves. A posterior condylar misalignment results in derangement of the articular disc, impingement of the retrodiscal tissue, and may cause vascular changes in the inner ear (18).

It is imperative that the clinician evaluate the entire spine, but especially the cervicothoracic area, for the presence of a VSC that could possibly cause postural abnormalities leading to acute or chronic TMJ instability. Rotational lesions of C1-C2 may also cause localized pain at the posterior margin of the joint.

Examination

The emphasis of the examination is on the neuromusculoskeletal relationships of the head, neck, and TMJ region. In obtaining a thorough history, the clinician should be particularly observant in recording the patient's subjective complaints. Often, the subjective information provides valuable clues to the location and nature of the symptoms.

Observation for the presence of asymmetry in the patient's posture, cranium, and facial architecture, dental occlusion and mandibular movement through its allowable ranges of motion may provide the clinician with valuable insight in determining if the TMJ disorder is due to extracapsular and/or intracapsular dysfunction.

Pincock and Dann (19) state that approximately 32% of the patients treated in their practice have dentofacial deformities associated with TMJ disorders. Palpation of trigger points of the involved musculature and determining the integrity of the tissue elements involved is also important.

NEUROLOGIC TESTS

Golberg (20) suggests an examination protocol consisting of a 4-minute neurologic exam. This would incorporate clinical testing and evaluation of the cranial and cervical nerves (Fig. 15.8) as well as the cerebellar and vestibular neurologic systems.

MUSCLE TESTS

Pain of the head and neck is commonly associated with TMJ disorders and masticatory dysfunction. Often, the origin of pain is myogenous in nature (21), thus necessitating a thorough orthopaedic evaluation of the TMJ and the associated masticatory muscle structures.

The primary movers involved in the opening of the mouth are the lateral pterygoid muscles. These muscles

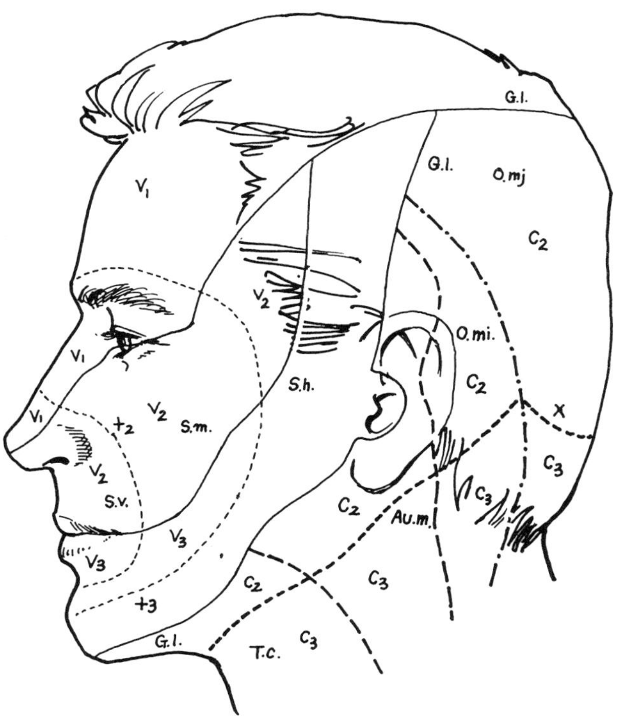

Figure 15.8. Lateral view of the head illustrating areas of innervation and nerve pressure points. The solid lines in this illustration separate the various fields which provide a guide for the clinician in examination of the head when a trauma has occurred. Trauma to the spinal nucleus of the trigeminal nerve may be easily recognized by the clinician by performing appropriate tests on the cutaneous distributions. Modified from Platzer W, ed. Pernkopf's Anatomy. Vol. 1. 3rd ed. Baltimore: Urban & Schwarzenberg, 1980:7.

clinician placing one hand just above the ...pital protuberance and the other hand under ... The patient is instructed to open the mouth ...y while the clinician applies a firm closing force to ...e chin. The muscle's strength should be noted. Care should be taken not to cause injury to potentially compromised soft tissue structures while performing the test.

The primary elevators include the masseter, temporalis, and medial pterygoid muscles. These muscles are tested by placing a separator between the patient's posterior teeth. The patient is then instructed to slowly bite down on the separator. While the patient is clenching the teeth together, the clinician should note any pain that may be elicited. As well, evaluation of the muscles' definition is essential. If the muscles are large and defined when contracting, it may indicate the patient experiences episodes of clenching or bruxism.

Lateral excursion movements of the TMJ are performed by the medial and lateral pterygoid muscles. This movement is tested by the clinician placing the contact hand on the side of the mandible and the stabilizing hand on the contralateral temporal region of the skull. The patient is instructed to resist against lateral pressure.

The medial pterygoid muscles may be evaluated bilaterally by performing a protrusive-retrusive test. To perform this procedure, the patient is instructed to protrude the jaw and resist as the clinician applies pressure to the jaw posteriorly.

Retrusive movement of the TMJ is performed by the posterior temporalis working in conjunction with the digastric muscle. This movement is tested by placing the clinician's gloved thumb intraoral on the patient's lower molars while wrapping the remaining fingers around the jaw (Fig. 15.9). The patient is instructed to resist as the clinician applies a slight pulling force to the mandible.

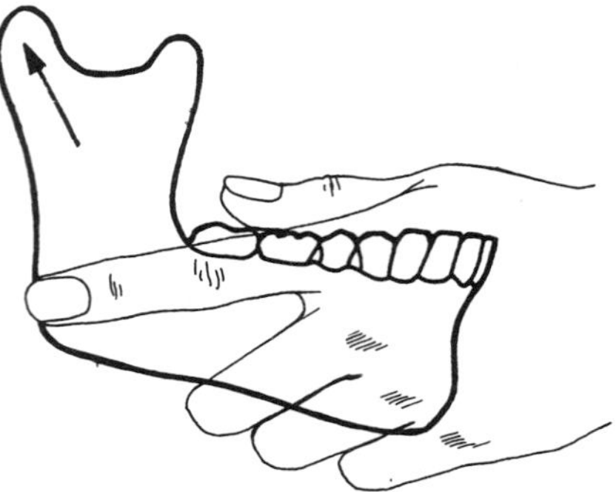

Figure 15.9. Schematic demonstrating placement of the clinician's hand while performing muscle tests and examination of TMJ articular integrity. Modified from Curl DD. Acute closed lock of the temporomandibular joint: manipulation paradigm and protocol. Chiropractic Technique 1991;3:16.

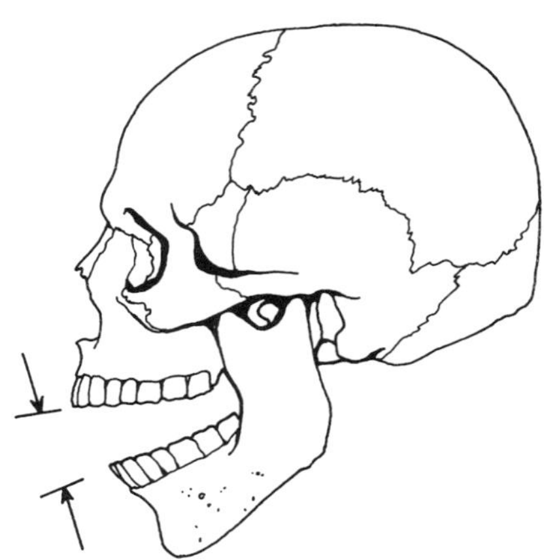

Figure 15.10. The normal range during maximal jaw opening is 40 to 60 mm.

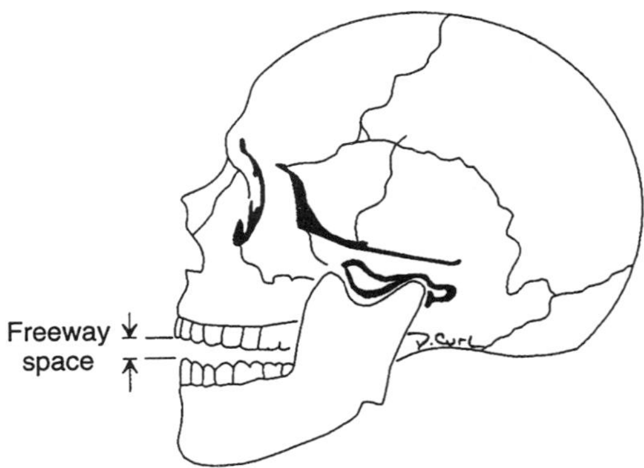

Figure 15.11. Interocclusal freeway space as demonstrated in a normal subject. (Courtesy Dr. Darryl Curl.)

INSTRUMENTATION

A vernier caliper instrument is used to measure active range of motion of normal mandibular physiologic movements. Limitations or blockages in normal mandibular motion may be due to dysfunctional musculature, capsular damage or osseous derangement (e.g., fracture, congenital defects, etc.). As previously stated, the clinician should take care not to damage already compromised tissues.

Opening. Vernier caliper instrumentation is used to evaluate the limits of mandibular movement. The upper and lower incisors are the clinician's reference point to observe movement in the vertical plane. With normal movement, the mandible stays true through the midline of the incisors. The normal range of motion is considered to be 40 to 60 mm (Fig. 15.10). The mandibular position in its neutral resting posture, which consists of nonocclusal contact, is described as the interocclusal freeway space and is approximately 3 to 5 mm (Fig. 15.11).

Instrumentation is especially useful when a lateral deviation is noted during jaw opening and is determined with bilateral measurement at the beginning and end of the deviation. This measurement is helpful in documentation of treatment effectiveness.

Protrusion. If the patient presents with a protrusive deviation, the doctor may suspect internal capsular derangements. Because protrusive movement is almost a pure translation of the TMJ bilaterally, it is reasonable to assume that any loss of synchrony of mandibular movement would be caused by dysfunction occurring in the superior joint compartment. To perform this measurement, the upper and lower incisors are brought into centric occlusion. The incisors of the mandible are then drawn forward beyond the upper incisors. Approximately 6 to 9 mm of protrusion is considered normal in the adult.

Lateral Excursion. When evaluating lateral excursion of the mandible, the chiropractor should note the presence of pain or restriction of the desired movement. Using the midline of the upper and lower incisors as the reference point, the vernier caliper instrument is used to measure the distance of lateral mandibular movement. A measurement is noted during both left and right lateral excursions to evaluate the presence of asymmetry (Figs. 15.12 and 15.13). If asymmetry exists, this finding indicates masticatory musculature dysfunction, inflammation, coronoid process impingement, or internal capsular derangement such as discal adhesions or an anteriorly dislocated disc.

Retrusion. When measuring retrusive mandibular movement, the condyles are seated on the center of the articular discs. Referred to as the close-packed position, the condyle-disc complex is bilaterally positioned in the superior and posterior portion of the TMJ fossae. Normal retrusive movement is approximately 3 to 4 mm.

Range of Motion

Assessing passive range of motion of the mandible is performed specifically to evaluate the integrity of the joint capsule and associated ligamentous structures. The range of motion evaluation is performed by testing the following temporomandibular movements: (1) open end-feel, (2) lateral glide, and (3) distractive joint play.

OPENING

Open end-feel is performed by placing a thick gauze pad over the lower incisors and applying a downward and slightly posteriorward pressure at the patient's end-range of jaw opening. For purposes of hygiene and safety, it is recommended that the doctor wear protective gloves while performing this procedure. During the procedure, the clinician should observe any aberrant joint motion or hypermobility of the supporting ligamentous structures. A normal capsular or ligamentous end-feel is described as a firm yet slightly giving sensation.

LATERAL GLIDING

Lateral glide is performed by contacting the lateral condylar poles of the TMJ with the distal tips of the first and second fingers. A slight lateral to medial pressure is applied to assess the integrity of the joint capsule and accessory ligaments. The clinician will note a short slight gliding motion with a firm end-feel if the joint is normal.

DISTRACTION

The distractive joint play procedure is performed with the patient in a seated or semirecumbent position. The clinician's gloved left thumb is pressed intraorally onto the lower molars while the remaining fingers are wrapped around the jaw. The palmar surface of the clinician's right hand cradles the skull while the tip of the index finger pal-

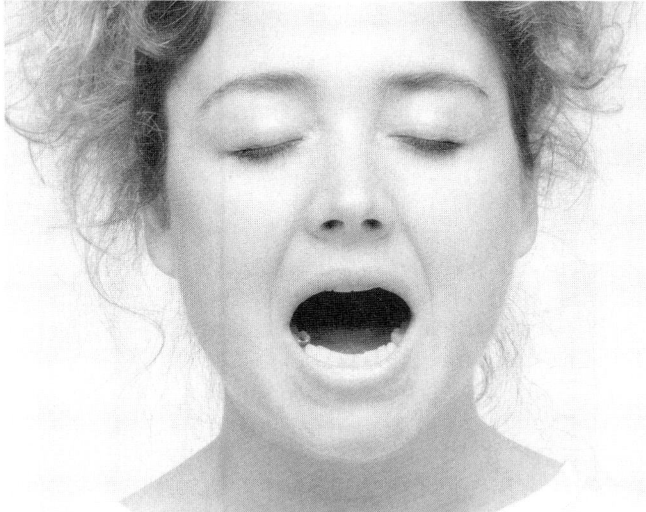

Figure 15.12. Observation of mandibular asymmetry during maximal opening.

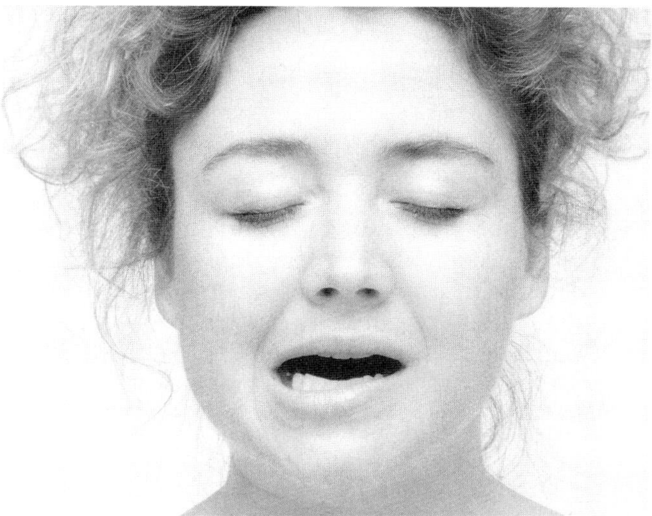

Figure 15.13. Observation of right lateral excursion on closing of the mouth. Vernier calipers are not shown. Upon closing, the middle incisors will deviate away from the side of involvement (the fixated joint).

..r motion. Again, for hygiene and safety ..ves are recommended. The clinician should .. pressure downward and slightly lateral at about ..20°. A slight gapping of the capsule with a firm end-..l is considered normal.

AUSCULTATION

The TMJ auscultation examination is performed by placing the bell end of the stethoscope over the area of the joint. The stethoscope is used to detect the presence of joint sounds during mandibular movements. Traditionally, it is considered that the occurrence of any joint sounds such as crepitus, popping, and clicking are indicative of TMJ dysfunction.

Osborne (22) describes the mechanism of reciprocal clicking on opening and closing of the jaw as it occurs during TMJ disc failure. In the resting postural position, the disc is distorted and lies on the anterior aspect of the condyle. As the mandible begins the opening movement, the disc becomes wedged ahead of the condyle. This movement becomes restrained because of the anterior attachment of the articular disc to the neck of the condyle. The involved compressive forces distorted the disc within the joint. As the potential energy increases in the distorted disc, it eventually overcomes the posterior annulus and retrodiscal restraint, and the disc pops posteriorward with an audible click. When the mandibular movement is reversed in the closing direction, the condyle tends to squeeze the disc anteriorward. The anteriorward movement of the disc is again restrained by the posterior annulus and retrodiscal tissues. As this wedging effect squeezes the disc anteriorward, the condyle snaps against the articular eminence with an articular click.

Vincent (23) and Saunders (24) suggest that the occurrence of some joint sounds on evaluation is a normal variant. When a joint noise has been ascertained by the use of auscultation, the clinician can note the type of sound and its duration, as well as when the sound occurs during mandibular gait.

JOINT PALPATION

TMJ palpation is performed to ascertain the integrity of the joint proper, as well as its related soft tissue structures. In addition, joint palpation is used to assist the auscultation examination to better differentiate the source of the joint sounds. The two methods of joint palpation are as follows:

1. The external auditory meatus is used as a point of reference in which the padded finger tip of the fifth digit is placed. This is performed with the clinician facing the patient while the patient is in a seated position. If the condyle has misaligned in an anterior to inferior direction, the clinician may feel a marked anterior position of the involved TMJ. If the condyle has misaligned in a posterior and superior direction the clinician may feel the posterior aspect of the condyle up against the pad of the finger on the involved side.
2. The external region of the joint proper will be used as a point of reference in which the finger tip of the index finger is placed. This test is performed with the clinician standing behind the seated patient. If the condyle has misaligned in an inferior position, the clinician may feel the condyle on the involved side lead the condyle of the contralateral side during opening movements of the mandible. If the condyle has misaligned in a posterior and superior direction, the clinician may feel a momentary hesitation or a lagging sensation of the involved condyle as compared to the contralateral side, during opening movements of the mandible.

While performing the palpatory joint examination, the clinician must be sensitive to the presence of pain or discomfort during opening and closing movements.

MUSCLE PALPATION

When performing a palpatory muscle examination, many of the masticatory muscles are readily accessible. The lateral pterygoid, medial pterygoid, and posterior digastric, however, are more difficult to palpate. In performing this examination the clinician should be sensitive to the presence of inflammation, edema, trigger points, and changes in muscle tonus such as splinting, guarding, or spasm. When used in conjunction with other clinical examination procedures, the information obtained from the palpatory muscle examination may be extremely useful in ascertaining a specific cause of TMJ dysfunction.

IMAGING

Although there are several imaging modalities used to objectively examine and evaluate the temporomandibular joint, only two are widely used by the chiropractic profession. They consist of magnetic resonance imaging (MRI) and plain film radiography (PFR).

MRI is used to image histologic disc alterations, remodeling of discal tissues, masticatory muscles, disc adhesions, tumors, disc perforations, osseous remodeling, and anterior and medial disc positional alterations. Tissues heavily laden with hydrogen ions produce a high signal intensity which appears as a lighter contrast on the MRI. Conversely, tissues with minimal amounts of hydrogen ions produce a low signal intensity, which appears as a darker contrast on the MRI. This characteristic makes the MRI a superior modality for evaluating the presence of capsular and disc degeneration.

Plain film radiography is perhaps the most commonly used imaging modality in evaluating the TMJ. The projections commonly used include the transorbital (anterior to posterior), lateral cephalometric (lateral skull), transcranial (lateral oblique), and submentovertex (axial). Lombardi and Preti (24,25) used PFR to measure differences in condylar position. PFR enables the clinician to observe severe osseous degenerative changes in the condyle or temporal region, as well as bone fractures or other osseous pathology. Capsular as well as extracapsular restriction of mandibular movement may also be confirmed with PFR (19).

EXAMINATION OF THE CHILD

Mechanical derangements of the TMJ and related structures from birthing injuries may be related to a variety of childhood illnesses (12,26). If these mechanical derangements are left uncorrected in the infant/child, the pathology may remain into adulthood (2). Hence, when the clinician is conducting a neuromusculoskeletal exam on an infant/child, it is imperative that the TMJ and accompanied cranial bones be incorporated as well.

It is known that restrictions in normal biomechanical movement of the craniomandibular mechanism may lead to chronic head and neck pain in infants/children (26). The infant/child may also elicit hyperactive behavior due to the physical stresses in the craniomandibular structures caused by aberrant neurologic function. These symptoms are often associated with vertebral subluxation complex of the upper cervical spine, thoracic spine or temporomandibular joint. Netter (27,28) presents two hypotheses as to the cause of asthma; vagal nerve reflex bronchospasm and intrinsic smooth muscle defect. Both of these hypotheses may be directly influenced by chiropractic manipulation and soft tissue therapy. Gillespie and Barnes (12) present a plausible explanation for the first postulate of vagal nerve reflex bronchospasm. They suggest that the mechanical motion and positional influences of the temporal bones, occiput, and the atlas as having a possible effect on the vagus nerve passing through the jugular foramen. An intrinsic smooth muscle defect of the trachea and bronchi may be mediated by patterns of myofascial soft tissue tensioning from the head, jaw and cervical spine. It is reasonable to assume that aberrant tensile forces placed on the myofascial structures would inhibit normal function of these tissues thus creating patterns of irritation.

EXAMINATION OF THE ADULT

In the adult, the clinician seeks to find the underlying cause of TMJ dysfunction, which is often a chronic biomechanical abnormality. Acute TMJ trauma does occur however (e.g., whiplash).

Royder (29) makes a case for evaluating the sacroiliac region in patients with TMJ disorders. Abnormalities in this region may create postural disturbances above, such as scoliosis, which influences the TMJ. It becomes apparent that a treatment protocol which includes the lower extremities, pelvis, and the lumbar spine is necessary as part of the regime for a TMJ disorder should dysfunction exist in related areas.

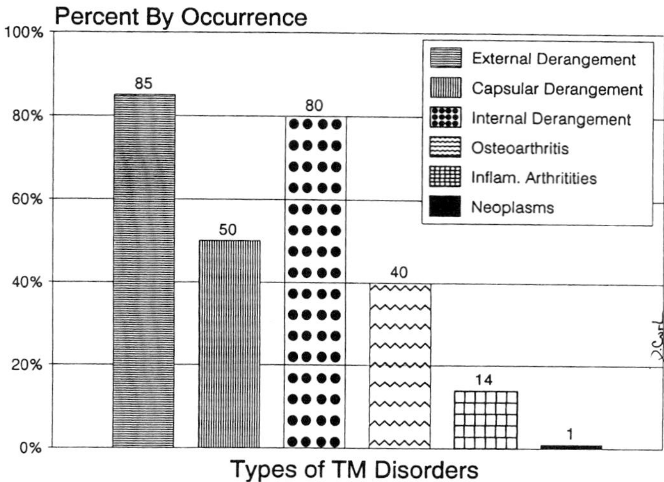

TM disorders can be categorized according to the specific nature of the underlying pathologic process

Figure 15.14. Types of TMJ disorders categorized by occurrence. In the complexity of TMJ disorders it is possible to have several of these categories present in the same patient. (Courtesy Dr. Darryl Curl.)

The cervicothoracic region should be examined and evaluated for biomechanical improprieties. Mechanical restrictions in this area may lead to dysfunction in the temporomandibular region via the scalene, spinalis capitis, splenius capitis, sternocleidomastoideus, and associated long muscles of the neck (See Figs. 15.6 and 15.7).

Somatic dysfunction of the occipitoatlantal and atlantoaxial regions can affect mandibular positioning to the extent that the suprahyoid and infrahyoid muscles would not be able to open the jaw without distortion of the TMJ on one side or the other (30).

When examining the TMJ region, the clinician must make every effort to determine if there is an intracapsular, capsular or extracapsular derangement (Fig. 15.14). It is important both diagnostically and therapeutically that the clinician's approach to evaluating TMJ dysfunction be comprehensive so that the precise location of biomechanical restraint is identified. Bell (31) describes three distinct symptomatic categories of masticatory dysfunction as follows:

1. Restriction of biomechanical mandibular movement;
2. Interference during mandibular movement; and
3. Acute malocclusion disturbances.

Intracapsular restriction is frequently caused by obstruction of the articular disc which in turn restricts mandibular movement by preventing translatory motion of the condyle. Several factors that may contribute to the obstruction of the articular disc include, fibrous adhesion formation or osseous ankylosis, altered gross tissue changes in the joint capsule due to arthritis, and trauma or functional displacement to the intracapsular tissue structures resulting in a dislocated articular disc.

...t to normal translatory movement is ...ociated with alterations in both size and ... the capsular ligament. Alterations to the cap-...gament resulting in restriction to mandibular ...ement may be the result of capsulitis (inflammatory ...dema) or capsular fibrotic adhesions due to previous episodes of capsulitis or traumatic injury. Capsular restraint has effects on condylar movement, such as protrusion opening and contralateral excursion.

Extracapsular restriction is commonly caused by contracted or immobilized mandibular elevator musculature. This may be precipitated by inflammation or neurologic dysfunction. Clinical evaluation of extracapsular restriction of mandibular movement differs from capsular restriction in that opening of the jaw is restricted, but protrusion and contralateral excursion remain fairly normal. The doctor will note a deflection of the midline incisal path with jaw opening movements. The direction in which the midline incisal path deviates depends on the location of the involved muscle(s). For example, contracture of the masseter or temporalis muscle would permit ipsilateral deflection of the midline incisal path. If the patient's deflection is induced solely by a contracted medial pterygoid muscle, the midline incisal path is deviated contralaterally.

Factors that may skew the clinician's ability to visibly note the presence of deflection with opening movement of the jaw include: contracted musculature involving the medial pterygoid muscle in conjunction with the masseter muscle, or the medial pterygoid muscle in conjunction with the temporalis muscle, and if both TMJs are involved, the presence of bilateral extracapsular restriction.

Acute malocclusion is sensed subjectively by the patient as spontaneous physical changes in the way the teeth occlude. It is common for the patient to experience pain and masticatory discomfort when the teeth are forcefully brought into maximal intercuspation. Two of the more common causes that may influence acute malocclusion are muscle spasm or changes in the TMJ, specifically the disc-condyle-eminence complex. Muscle spasm of the lateral pterygoid muscle may induce acute malocclusion by drawing the condyle forward on the ipsilateral side, thus causing occlusal disarticulation of the patient's posterior teeth and premature contact of the anterior teeth contralaterally. Spasm of the masseter muscle draws the mandible laterally, while spasm of the medial pterygoid muscle would displace the mandible medially. Trauma to the TMJ structures or osseous surface deterioration due to arthritic conditions or infection would effectively change the relationship of the disc condyle complex with the articular eminence, leading to acute malocclusion.

When examining the patient with complaints of malocclusion, it is important for the clinician to understand that such altered occlusion is often accompanied by masticatory dysfunction or pain. If pain accompanies the patient's symptoms of acute malocclusion, the doctor can expect to see an increase in the sensation of pain with maximal intercuspation, which may be relieved by biting against a separator on the ipsilateral side of involvement.

If the chiropractor suspects a cracked tooth, tooth abscess, periodontal disease, or tooth pain as being the causative factor contributing to acute malocclusion, it would be reasonable to perform a dental fremitus (percussion) test. This test is performed by simply asking the patient to sharply close the teeth together without clenching, while the clinician listens and observes for any singular striking dentition sounds and/or pain. If this test results in a positive finding, the clinician should perform a tooth-specific manual percussion test by carefully striking the individual posterior tooth with a firm, blunt sterilized metal object. To assure doctor-patient hygiene and protection, the wearing of gloves is advised. If the test elicits a positive finding for pain or tooth dysfunction, then referral to a dentist or orthodontist is appropriate.

Articular disc jamming is classically understood to be any obstruction of the disc condyle and articular eminence complex which would interfere with translatory movement of the jaw. Factors such as dysfunctional articular discal ligaments, increased passive interarticular pressure, physiologic incompatibility between articular sliding surfaces, and discal trauma are frequent causes of disc jamming. Provided that the disc condyle complex function remains undamaged, disc jamming will usually cause the patient to experience only momentary episodes of obstructed translatory movement of the jaw.

When performing a clinical assessment of a patient presenting with disc jamming, the clinician should note the following: the patient will be relatively pain-free, maximal intercuspation will not elicit symptoms of acute malocclusion, and lateral and protrusive mandibular movement will be normal and unobstructed. Disc jamming usually responds favorably to chiropractic adjustive therapy.

A functional anteriorly dislocated disc is described as an obstruction which blocks the return phase of translatory mandibular movement. A contraction of the superior lateral pterygoid muscle is often the causative factor. Because of the nonexistence of surface to surface contact of the condyle, articular disc, and articular eminence, the articular disc is trapped anterior to the mandibular condyle due to the collapsing of the articular disc spaces.

During the examination of a patient presenting with functional anterior dislocation of the articular disc, the clinician should note the following: mandibular movements within the patient's permitted range of motion will elicit noises such as grinding and grating; on maximal intercuspation the patient will sense symptoms of acute malocclusion of the posterior teeth on the ipsilateral side of involvement; and translatory mandibular movements in protrusion and lateral excursion are proportionately restricted with opening.

Functional anterior dislocation of the articular disc

appears to respond favorably to chiropractic adjustive therapy. The preferred method of manual treatment is to apply a distracting technique to stretch the superior retrodiscal lamina.

Conservative Management

The author suggests a conservative therapeutic approach be exhausted before escalating to more invasive treatment. The effectiveness of conservative management has been reported to be effective 70 to 90% of the time for patients with TMJ dysfunction and related syndromes (32). Treatment methods used include the following:

1. Application of ice, alternating every 20 minutes until the swelling has been reduced.
2. Upon the reduction of swelling, the application of moist heat packs and passive mobilization.
3. Trigger-point therapy to relax restrictive muscle tonus.
4. Superficial muscle massage utilizing spray and stretch techniques.
5. Physical therapy modalities such as ultrasound, biofeedback, and TENS unit.
6. Specific manual correction, chiropractic adjustive/manipulative therapy.

Manual Adjustive Procedures

Manual adjustive/manipulative procedures have been widely reported as being successful methods in the treatment of TMJ (10,12,33–40). The clinician has a variety of manual corrective procedures to choose from which fall into two distinct categories. The two categories include distraction and translational manual corrective methods. In this section, three of the most common TMJ misalignments will be discussed and recommendations as to the most beneficial corrective method will be made.

The types of mandibular adjustive/manipulative methods described herein are of a modified high-velocity low amplitude type. Often, the term "thrust" is used in describing a mandibular manual procedure; however, the clinician should understand that the use of a thrust is unlike adjustments of the spinal column. Loughner, Larkin and Mahan (41) demonstrated that middle ear damage can occur when tension is applied to the anterior malleolar (AML) and to a lesser degree, the discomalleolar ligaments (DML). The AML connects to the malleus with the lingula of the mandible via the sphenomandibular ligament (SML), and the DML passes from the medial retrodiscal tissue to the malleus. When the condyle is distracted inferiorly, tension was directly applied to the AML via the SML, which demonstrated the potential to cause middle ear damage. Therefore, every distractive adjustive/manipulative procedure which the clinician may choose to use, should emphasize a very low amplitude movement technique, rather than a thrust. This is to ensure that the ligamentous structures of the TMJ are not injured during the maneuver.

When using mandibular adjustive/manipulative procedures, the desired treatment outcomes are to provide alleviation of pain, reduce the presence of inflammation, reduce nerve irritation, re-establish normal motion of osseous joint structures, normalize masticatory muscle tonus, and reduce microadhesions which may exist between discal structures and the adjacent articular surfaces.

If the patient is experiencing an acute episode of TMJ dysfunction, it is suggested that the mandibular adjustive/manipulative procedures be performed on a daily basis for a two to three week period. In chronic cases, where derangement of TMJ structures has occurred, the clinician may not see a significant improvement for approximately 2 to 4 weeks. Because of the intricate structures of the TMJ and their constant bombardment of external forces, the clinician must take care to not get discouraged too quickly, if resolution of symptoms are slower than anticipated. Lawrence (32) reports the use of conservative treatment therapy for approximately 3 to 6 months before considering more invasive procedures and subsequent referral to an oral surgeon.

ACUTE CLOSED LOCK

In conditions of acute closed lock, the patient is only able to open the mouth to a distance of 13 to 20 mm. The displacement of the articular disc to an anteromedial direction is a result, in part, of the tractional forces of the superior head of the lateral pterygoid (Fig. 15.15). Acute closed lock of the TMJ is characterized by restriction of mandibular movement, absence of joint sounds during condylar motion, pain and tenderness located in the TMJ region, and acute malocclusion (42).

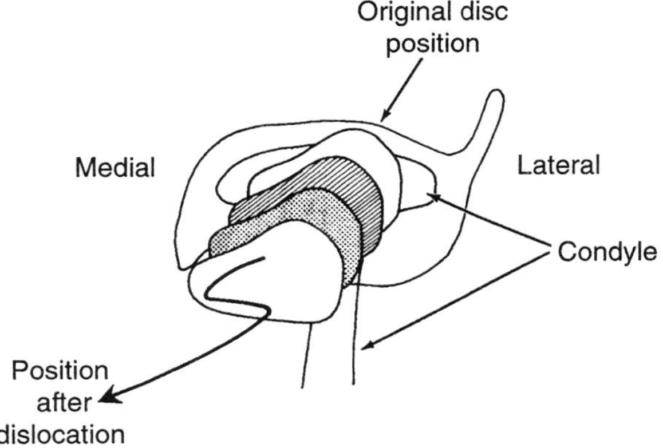

Figure 15.15. Anterior to posterior view of the left condyle demonstrating the displacement of the articular disc in an anteromedial direction. Trauma or ligamentous laxity may act to displace the disc from its normal position. The lateral pterygoid collateral ligaments and the retrodiscal tissues are additional support structures which permit displacement of the disc as a result of trauma or joint dysfunction. Modified from Curl DD. Acute closed lock of the temporomandibular joint: manipulation paradigm and protocol. Chiropractic Technique 1991;3:14

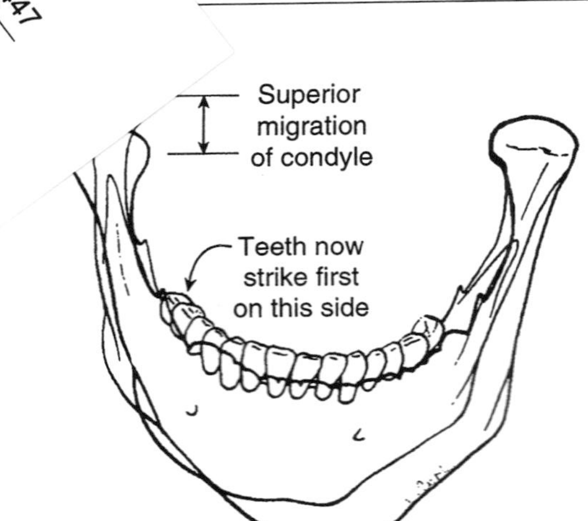

Figure 15.16. The mandibular condyle migrates into the temporal fossa when the disc is displaced. Therefore, the side of premature dental contact on closing of the mouth is the side of the disc displacement. Modified from Curl DD. Acute closed lock of the temporomandibular joint: manipulation paradigm and protocol. Chiropractic Technique 1991;3:14.

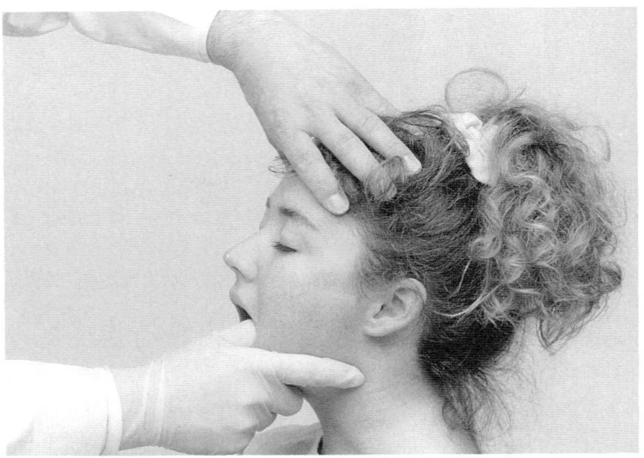

Figure 15.17. Demonstrates manual therapy in the seated position with the doctor stabilizing the patient's head. If desired, the patient's head can be stabilized with the help of an assistant.

Because of the anterior articular disc displacement, the condyle migrates into the temporal fossa posterior-lateral, thus causing premature contact of the dentition on the ipsilateral side of involvement (Fig. 15.16). This type of condylar misalignment is characterized as a posterior superior TMJ subluxation.

Name of technique procedure: Unilateral Acute Closed Lock Mandibular Distraction Maneuver (Figs. 15.17 and 15.18)

Indications: The disc is blocking translatory glide of the condyle resulting in restrictions during mandibular movement. Opening distance of the mandible is usually only 13 to 20 mm, hence, the term closed lock.

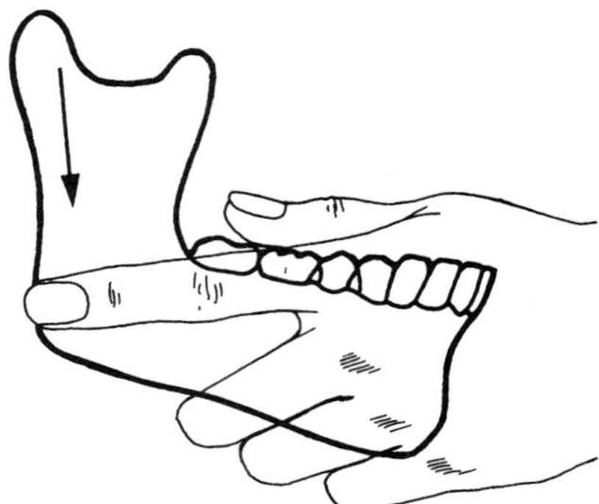

Figure 15.18. Illustration of the position of the clinician's thumb during the intraoral contact with the remaining fingers grasping the mandible firmly. As with all intraoral contacts, the clinician should wear protective gloves. Modified from Curl DD. Acute closed lock of the temporomandibular joint: manipulation paradigm and protocol. Chiropractic Technique 1991;3:16.

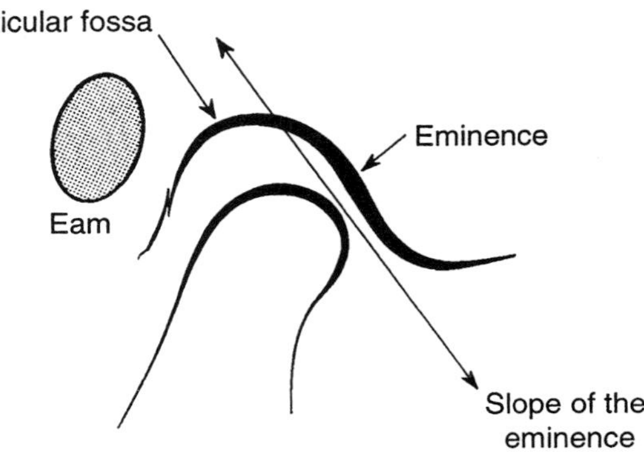

Figure 15.19. It is necessary for the clinician to first locate the slope of the eminence to evaluate the line of drive for the distractive maneuver. The slope of the eminence may be determined by first locating the articular fossa and following the eminence inferiorward and anteriorward. Modified from Curl DD. Acute closed lock of the temporomandibular joint: manipulation paradigm and protocol. Chiropractic Technique 1991;3:15.

Contraindications: All other listings, hypermobility, instability, destruction of joint capsule, fracture or infection of the TMJ complex.

Patient position: Seated or supine

Doctor's position: Standing opposite of the affected TMJ, the clinician uses an intraoral contact with the thumb placement on the last mandibular molar ipsilateral to the side of involvement.

Supporting hand: Stabilization of the patient's head.

Pattern of thrust: First, the clinician must visualize the slope of the eminence to determine the line of drive (Fig. 15.19). The distraction maneuver is produced by directing the force 90° to the slope of the articular eminence (Fig. 15.20). Once the remaining joint play has been brought to tension, the thrust is applied perpendicular and away from the slope of the eminence.

Name of technique procedure: Bilateral Acute Closed Lock Mandibular Distraction Maneuver (Figs. 15.21 and 15.22)

Indications: Bilateral disc involvement blocking translatory glide of the condyles resulting in restrictions during mandibular movement. Opening distance of the mandible is usually only 13 to 20 mm, hence, the term closed lock.

Contraindications: All other listings, hypermobility, instability, destruction of joint capsule, fracture or infection of the TMJ complex.

Patient position: Seated or supine

Doctor's position: Standing on either side of the patient using bilateral intraoral thumb contact

Supporting hand: An assistant should stabilize the patient's head.

Pattern of thrust: The bilateral distraction maneuver is produced by directing the force 90° to the slope of the articular eminence (Fig. 15.23). Once the remaining joint play has been brought to tension, the thrust is applied perpendicular and away from the slope of the eminences.

Name of technique procedure: Gonstead Unilateral Anterior-inferior condyle subluxation translational maneuver

Indications: Anteroinferior positional dyskinesia of the condyle

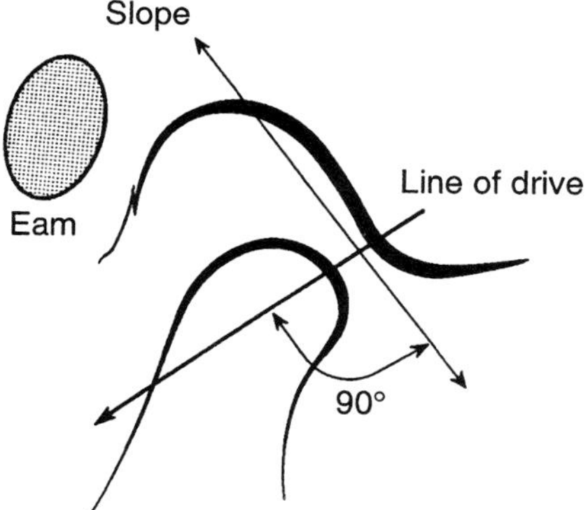

Figure 15.20. To initiate the distractive maneuver, it is necessary to gap the TMJ by acting 90° to the slope of the articular eminence at its midline. Modified from Curl DD. Acute closed lock of the temporomandibular joint: manipulation paradigm and protocol. Chiropractic Technique 1991;3:15.

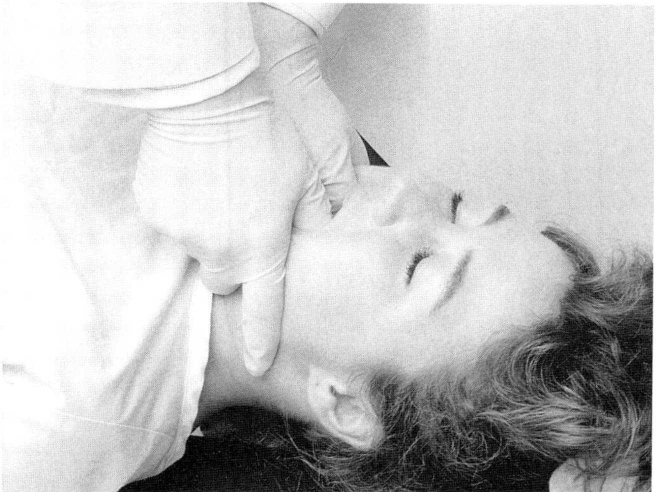

Figure 15.21. Bilateral distractive maneuver with the patient in the supine position. It may be necessary to have an assistant stabilize the patient's head into the table.

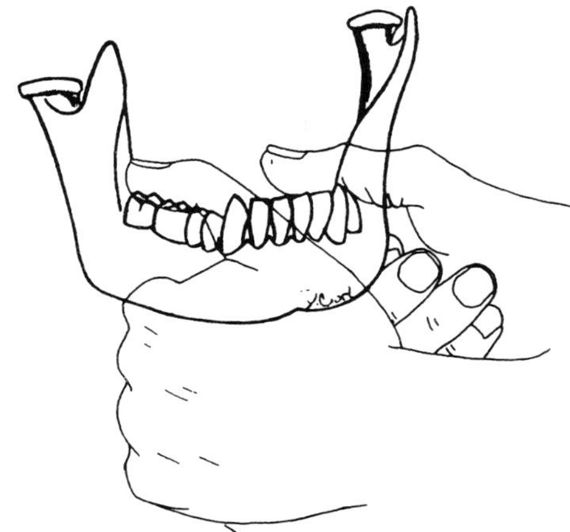

Figure 15.22. Clinician's intraoral hand placement for bilateral disc involvement using the distractive maneuver. Modified from Curl DD. Acute closed lock of the temporomandibular joint: manipulation paradigm and protocol. Chiropractic Technique 1991;3:17.

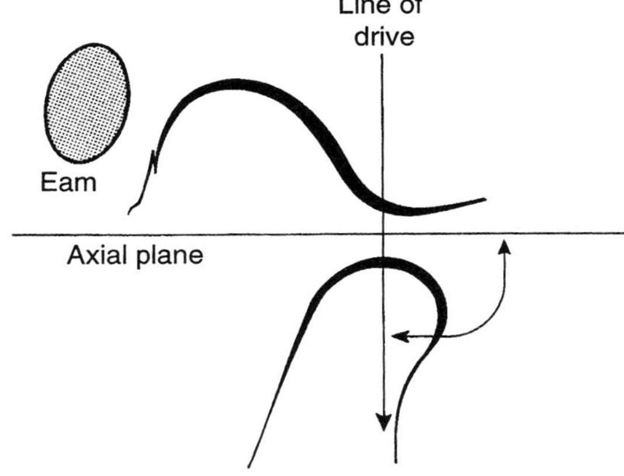

Figure 15.23. Direction in which the distractive maneuver is directed is 90° to the axial plane. The point at which recapture of the disc is inferior or anterior to the articular eminence. Modified from Curl DD. Acute closed lock of the temporomandibular joint: manipulation paradigm and protocol. Chiropractic Technique 1991;3:17.

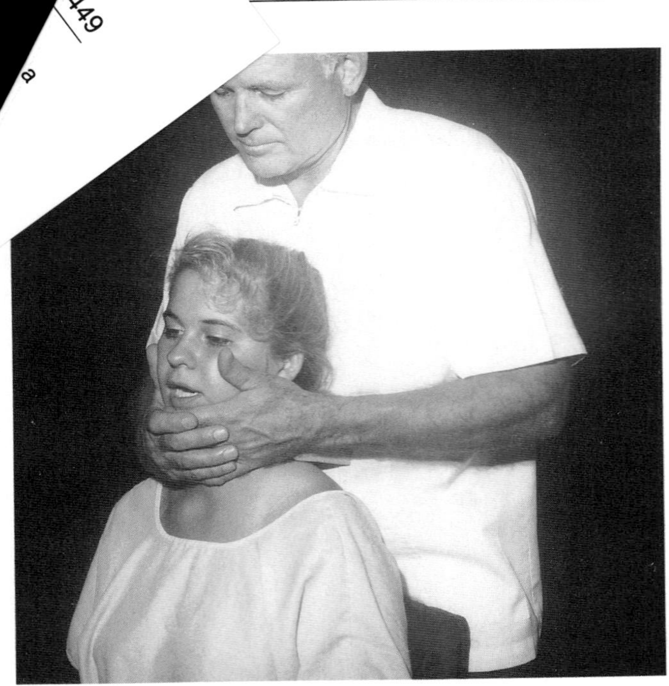

Figure 15.24. Clinician's contact hand and stabilization hand position for the seated translational adjustment.

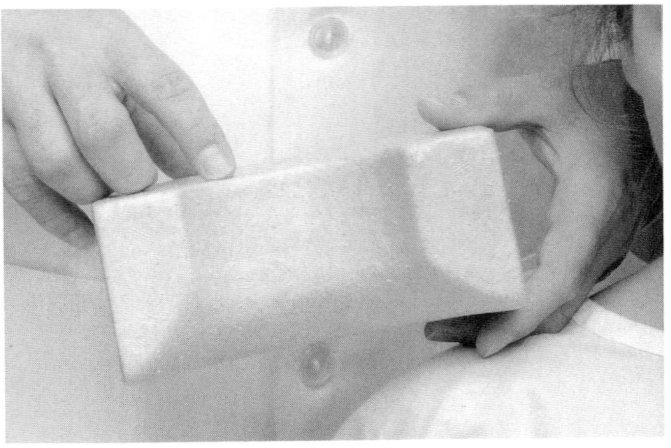

Figure 15.25. The Gonstead condyle block has a beveled and a 90° edge. The 90° edge is placed at the level of the atlas and the beveled edge rests at the base of the cervical spine.

Contraindications: All other listings, hypermobility, instability, destruction of joint capsule, fracture or infection of the TMJ complex.

Patient position: Seated

Doctor's position: Standing behind the patient, contacting the involved side first. The fingertips are placed on the chin, the pisiform on the ramus of the mandible and the thenar on the lateral pole of the condyle (Fig. 15.24).

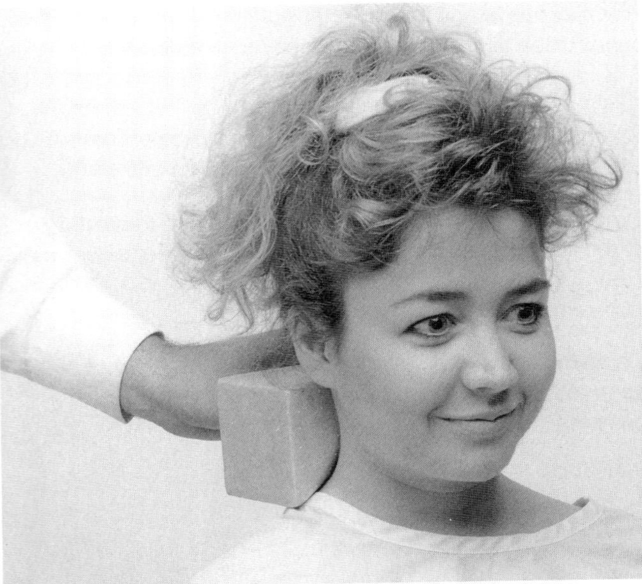

Figure 15.26. The condyle block is used to support the cervical spine so as to not traumatize the related structures during the maneuver.

Supporting hand: This hand is placed contralateral to the side of involvement with the fingertips on the chin, pisiform on the ramus of the mandible and the thenar on the lateral pole of the condyle. Also, the Gonstead condyle block is used to support the patient's neck (Figs. 15.25 and 15.26).

Pattern of thrust: The patient is first instructed to open their mouth as wide as possible (Fig. 15.27A). The patient is then instructed to slowly close their mouth as the doctor's stabilization hand pulls in a posterior direction on the contralateral side through the first ⅓ of mandibular movement. The clinician then stabilizes the jaw contralateral to the involved side by applying a medialward force with the stabilization hand (Fig. 15.27B). When this stabilizing force has been accomplished, the primary contact hand continues to follow the travel of mandibular movement with a sustained force posterior and superiorward (Fig. 15.27C). Just as the mouth is about to close, the primary contact hand will give a light and quick movement posterior, superior and medialward to re-establish the condyle into its fossa.

DEVIATED NASAL SEPTUM

The nasal septum can often be injured during sport activities such as boxing, basketball and wrestling. A blow to the nose may deviate the septal cartilage to one side.

As with any head trauma, a thorough neurologic assessment should be made to determine if emergency room referral is required. In the absence of neurologic signs or gross injury, this disorder can be managed conservatively. Contusions of the maxillary and frontal sinus areas, and the orbits, should be examined to rule out concomitant injury (e.g., fracture) to these structures.

The nose may be visibly deviated to one side. This should correlate with the mechanism of injury. There will usually be localized swelling, which can be reduced with cryotherapy. Airway occlusion may occur on the side o[illegible] deviation.

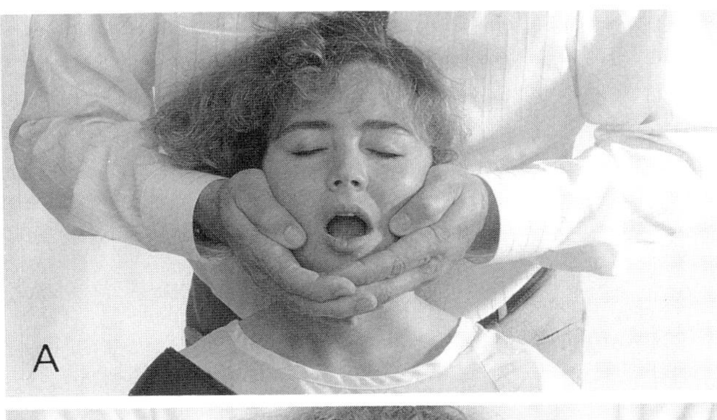

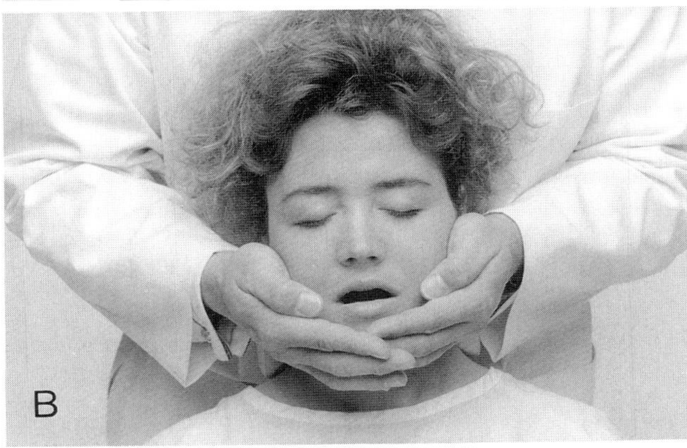

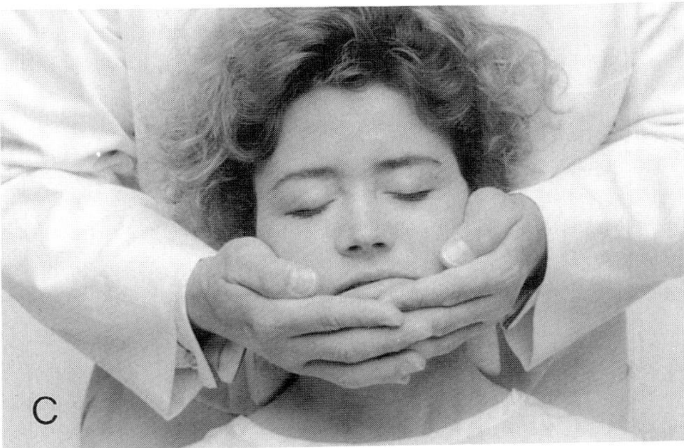

Figure 15.27. **A,** After hand position has been established and the patient's mouth is fully opened, the patient is instructed to slowly close their mouth so as to resist the manual force applied by the clinician. The resistance of the patient activates the lateral head of the pterygoid and tensions the articular disc, thereby permitting its recapture. **B,** When the patient has closed their mouth approximately one third, the supporting hand stabilizes the unaffected TMJ. **C,** The contact hand completes the translational maneuver by guiding the condyle in a posterior superior direction into the articular fossa.

Adjustment

The patient is seated for the maneuver (Fig. 15.28). The doctor should stand behind the patient, so as to visualize the deviation from an aerial view. The cartilage just inferior to the junction with the nasal bone is contacted with the thumb pad on the side of septal deviation. The stabi-

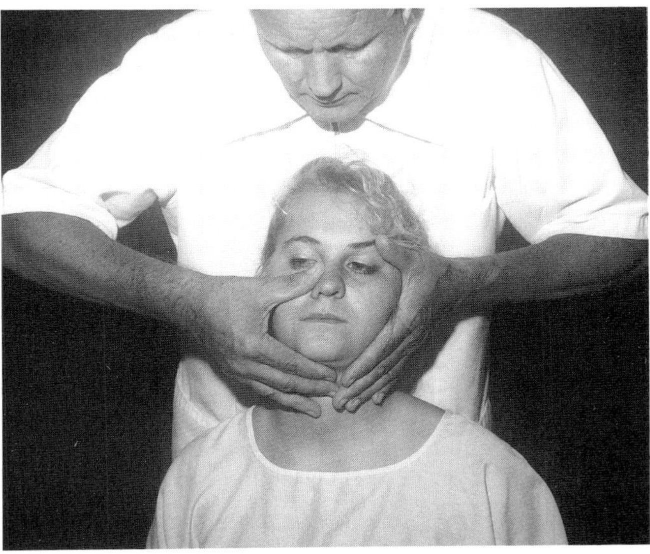

Figure 15.28. Adjustment for a deviated nasal septum (See text).

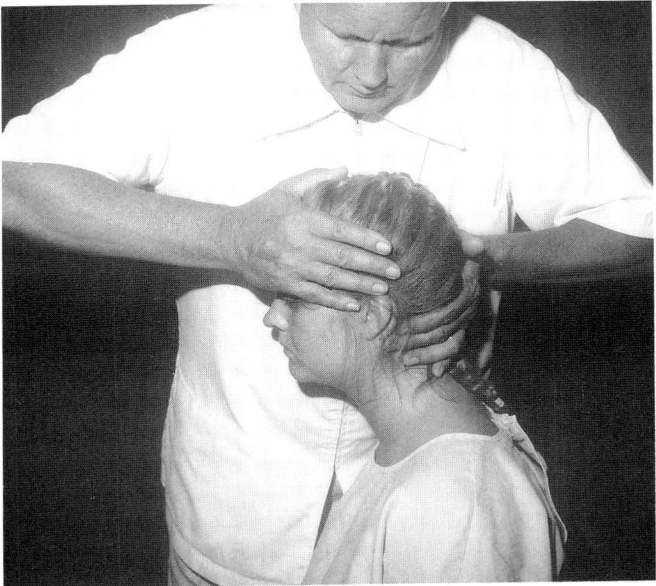

Figure 15.29. Frontal sinus adjustment. A posteriorward pressure is applied with the doctor's hand over the frontal bone. Stabilization is provided at the posterior.

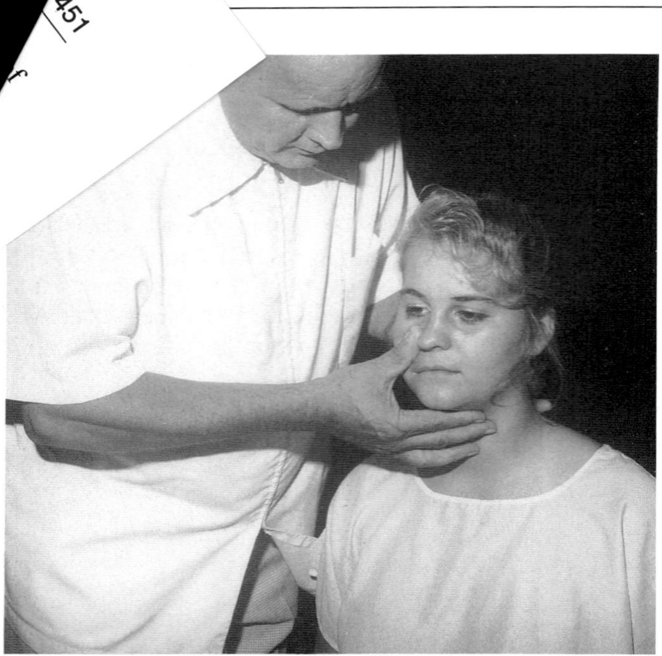

Figure 15.30. The maxillary sinus is adjusted by directing a pressure with the thumb pad in a posterior, lateral and inferiorward direction. The back of the patient's head should be supported with the stabilization hand. The fingers of the adjusting hand are used to stabilize the mandible.

lization hand should cradle the opposite side of the face. A controlled thrust is made lateral to medial and slightly superior to inferior.

SINUSES

The frontal and maxillary sinuses can be adjusted. While not a "true" articulation, a manual pressure can be applied to the areas, which may alleviate symptoms such as headache or congestion (Figs. 15.29 and 15.30).

References

1. Thompson T, Dwyer JT, Palmer CA. Nutritional remedies for temporomandibular joint dysfunction: fact or fiction? Nutrition Today 1991;26:37–42.
2. Gelb H. Clinical management of head, neck and TMJ pain and dysfunction. Philadelphia: WB Saunders, 1976.
3. Sarnat BG, Laskin DM. The temporomandibular joint. 3rd ed. Springfield, IL: Charles C Thomas, 1979: 89–90.
4. Shore NA. Temporomandibular joint dysfunction and occlusal equilibration. 2nd ed. Philadelphia: JB Lippincott, 1976.
5. Bell WE. Clinical management of temporomandibular disorders. Chicago: Year Book Medical Publishers Inc., 1982.
6. Warfel JH. The head, neck, and trunk. 4th ed. Philadelphia: Lea & Febiger, 1973:110.
7. Helland MM. Anatomy and function of the temporomandibular joint. J Orthop Sports Physical Ther 1980;1:149–151.
8. Warwick R, Williams PL. Gray's anatomy. 35th British ed. Philadelphia: WB Saunders, 1973:501–509.
9. Curl DD, Bergman TF, Taylor JAM. Head and neck pain from the temporomandibular joint and its interaction with the cervical spine. Los Angeles College of Chiropractic Relicensing Program. 1990.
10. Ash MM. Current concepts in the aetiology, diagnosis and treatment of TMJ and muscle dysfunction. J Oral Rehabil 1986;13:1–20.
11. Solberg WK. Neuromuscular problems in the orofacial region: diagnosis—classification, signs and symptoms. Int Dent J 1981;31:206–215.
12. Gillespie BR, Barnes JF. Diagnosis and treatment of TMJ, head, neck and asthmatic symptoms in children. J Craniomandibular Practice 1990;8:342–49.
13. Williamson EH. The interrelationship of internal derangements of the TMJ joint, headache, vertigo, and tinnitus: a survey of 25 patients. J Craniomandibular Practice 1990;8:301–306.
14. Gonstead Seminar of Chiropractic. Lecture Notes. Mt. Horeb, WI, 1991.
15. Isberg AM, Isacsson G, Williams WN, Loughner BA. Lingual numbness and speech articulation deviation associated with TMJ joint disc displacement. Oral Surg Oral Med Oral Pathol 1987;64:9–14.
16. Cohan BL. Reflex sympathetic dystrophy syndrome. J Craniomandibular Practice 1990;9:1:76–87.
17. Kopp S. Clinical findings in temporomandibular osteoarthrosis. J Dent Res 1977;85:434.
18. Keeling SD, Gibbs C, Hall MB, Lupkiewicz SL. Internal derangements of the TMJ: changes associated with mandibular repositioning and orthodontic therapy. Am J Orthodontics and Dentofacial Orthopedics 1989;96:363–373.
19. Pincock JL, Dann JJ. Orthognathic surgery. Calif Dent Assoc J 1991;19:31–40.
20. Golberg S. The four minute neurologic exam. Miami: Medmaster, 1987.
21. Carstensen B. Indications and contraindications of manual therapy for temporomandibular joint dysfunction. In: Grieve G, ed. Modern manual therapy. Edinburgh: Churchill Livingstone, 1986:700–705.
22. Osborne JW. The disc of the human temporomandibular joint design function and failure. J Oral Rehabil 1985;12:279–293.
23. Vincent SD, Lilly GE. Incidence and characterization of temporomandibular joint sounds in adults. J Am Dent Assoc 1988;116:203–206.
24. Saunders R, Buoncristiani R. Diagnostic and surgical arthroscopy of the temporomandibular joint. J Craniomandibular Disorders 1987;1:202–213.
25. Lombardi M, Preti G, Tomasinelli A, Debernardi C. Perceptibility of condylar displacement through transcranial radiographs and split-cast technique on dry skull. Craniomandibular Practice 1991;9:23–28.
26. Schmidt MA. Childhood ear infections. Berkeley: North Atlantic Books, 1990:77–84.
27. Netter F. The CIBA collection of medical illustrations: clinical symposia asthma. St. Caldwell, NJ, 1990;27(1&2):slide 2205.
28. Netter F. The CIBA collection of medical illustrations: clinical symposia asthma. St. Caldwell, NJ, 1990;27(1&2):slide 2203.
29. Royder JO. Structural influences in temporomandibular joint pain and dysfunction. J Am Osteopath Assoc 1981;80:460–467.
30. Hruby RJ. The total body approach to the osteopathic management of TMJ joint dysfunction. J Am Osteopath Assoc 1985;85:502–510.
31. Bell WE. Temporomandibular joint. In: Goldman HM, Forest SP, Byrd DL, et al., eds. Current therapy in dentistry. St. Louis: CV Mosby, 1968:557–584.
32. Lawrence DJ, ed. Fundamentals of chiropractic diagnosis and management. Baltimore: Williams & Wilkins, 1991:490–497.
33. Ow RK, Carlsson GE, Jemt T. Responses and evaluation of patients with temporomandibular disorders in relation to conservative treatment. Ann Acad Med Singapore 1987;16:318–321.
34. Segami N, Ken-Ichiro M, Tadahiko I, Michio F. Arthrographic evaluation of disc position following mandibular manipulation for

internal derangement with closed lock of the temporomandibular join. J Craniomandibular Disord 1990;4:99–108.
35. Herbst RW. Gonstead chiropractic science and healing art. Mt. Horeb, WI: Sci-Chi Publications, 1968.
36. Braun BL. Treatment of an acute anterior disk displacement in the temporomandibular joint: a case report. Phys Ther 1987;67:1234–1236.
37. Farrar WB. Diagnosis and treatment of anterior disc dislocation of the articular disc. NY J Dent 1971;41:348–351.
38. Hall LJ. Physical therapy treatment results for 178 patients with temporomandibular joint syndrome. Am J Otol 1984;5:183–196.
39. Christensen K. Clinical chiropractic biomechanics. 2nd e. Dubuque: Educational Division Foot Levelers, Inc., 1984:128–132.
40. Schafer R. Chiropractic management of sports and recreational injuries. 2nd ed. Baltimore: Williams & Wilkins, 1986:298–299.
41. Loughner BA, Larkin LH, Mahan PE. Discomalleolar and anterior malleolar ligaments: possible causes of middle ear damage during temporomandibular joint surgery. Oral Surg Oral Med Oral Pathol 1989;68:14–22.
42. Curl DD. Acute closed lock of the temporomandibular joint: manipulation paradigm and protocol. Chiropractic Technique 1991;3:13–18.

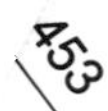

·avertebral Disorders: Upper and Lower ·emities

·EPHEN L. COLLINS, MITCHELL S. SILL, and DAVID A. GINSBERG

The spinal column has long been the primary focus of the chiropractic profession. As patients increasingly use chiropractors as their primary source of health care, the need to address other anatomic areas of dysfunction becomes increasingly important. The evaluation and treatment of disorders afflicting the extravertebral articulations have become an integral component of chiropractic practice.

As in the area of conservative spinal health care, the chiropractic approach to dysfunction of the extremities fulfills a void that has not been addressed by allopathic medicine. The area of sports medicine has expanded dramatically in recent years. The chiropractic profession has an important perspective and contribution to make with regard to athletic and recreational injuries.

This chapter is designed to assist the Doctor of Chiropractic in gaining the basic knowledge necessary to clinically address conditions of the upper and lower extremities.

The peripheral joints like those of the spine and pelvis are subject to injury which may result in articular malpositions causing abnormal biomechanical function, as well as potentially altering neural, vascular, and muscular function. It is for this reason that Gonstead (1) conceptualized a philosophical basis for including extraspinal adjusting within the purview of chiropractic care. Furthermore, normal spinal biomechanics not only contribute to, but are dependent on, the integrity of both the upper and lower extremities. To neglect these areas of the body does not provide the patient with optimal care.

The doctor should always consider that many patients presenting with chief complaints which suggest extremity pathology may actually be suffering from symptoms which are secondary to visceral pathology or lesions of the spinal column (e.g., vertebral subluxation complex).

It is the responsibility of the practitioner to arrive at a differential diagnosis through the patient history, physical examination, and special diagnostic procedures: x-ray, MRI, hematologic tests, thermography, etc. As with most diagnostic work-ups, the patient history is generally the most valuable tool.

EXAMINATION

The initial approach to the patient presenting with extremity symptoms as the chief complaint should include a comprehensive spinal evaluation to aid in the detection of the origin of the condition (Table 16.1). If and when vertebral subluxation, as well as visceral pathology, have been eliminated as possible sources of symptomatology, attention should be focused at the peripheral joint in question. Many of the conditions for which the clinician is consulted for are not the result of a macrotraumatic episode and are generally less complicated to properly diagnose. The selective extraction of historical subtleties will ultimately lead to a proper diagnosis. As it is not in the interest of this chapter to instruct on general history-taking procedures, only pertinent questions which supply data helpful in extremity care shall be discussed. Inclusion of such inquiries will be discussed within each portion of the standard health history.

I. Bibliographical Information
II. Chief Complaint
III. Present Illness
IV. Past History
V. Family History
VI. Review of Systems:
   1) Physical
   2) Sociological
   3) Psychological

Table 16.1.
Origin of Pain: Peripheral Joints vs. Vertebral Subluxation Complex (VSC)[a]

Factors	Peripheral Joint	VSC
Onset	General history of specific incident or action	Gradual or insidious
Provocative	Joint use or load	Spinal postures, stresses, aggravation
Palliative	Joint rest, support, ice, etc.	Ameliorating factors for spinal conditions
Quality of pain	Sharp, throbbing	Dull, ache
Region	Localized, specific, usually unilateral	Diffuse, difficult to isolate, possibly bilateral
Radiation	Generalized, nonspecific pattern	Dermatomal, scleratomal, myotomal
Intensity	Mild to severe	Mild to moderate
Timing	Generally correlated to joint function	Temporally related to spinal factors

[a]General information obtained during routine history procedures often leads to the specific site of the lesion.

Biographical Data

After obtaining standard data including name, address, sex, birthdate and marital status, the doctor should inquire about the patient's occupational and recreational activities. The examiner must retrieve information related to specific physical demands placed on the patient during daily life. Occupational factors include: job duties, postural demands, time commitments for work activities, and exposure to noxious agents. If the patient engages in recreational activities, be it in the form of organized activity or merely sporadic exertion, the patient is susceptible to injury. Helpful information includes all activities inherent to the patient's leisure schedule, past injuries sustained, recent changes in activity level, awareness of general conditioning techniques, and adherence to warm-up and cool-down practices.

Chief Complaint

The history of the patient's symptoms begins with the chief complaint (CC) which is a list in the patient's words of one or more symptoms (2). The duration of the various symptomatology is important as it establishes the chronicity of the condition (3).

The purpose of listing multiple symptoms as chief complaints is two-fold. They serve as meaningful leads that aid in making differential diagnoses, and they also present a prominent list to remind the doctor about what complaints prompted the patient to seek health care.

Present Illness

The present illness section is the heart of the history and frequently leads to the ultimate diagnosis of the patient. The components of the present illness include (4):

1. Onset of symptoms (O)
2. Provoking and palliative factors (P)
3. Quality of pain (Q)
4. Radiation or referral (R)
5. Severity of symptoms (S)
6. Timing and frequency of symptoms (T)

ONSET

The onset of the patient's symptoms is important diagnostically as the doctor must determine if the injury is a result of an overt macrotrauma, repetitive overuse, microtrauma or misuse (abuse). For example, the patient might state that while jogging one afternoon a sudden step into a hole resulted in a twisted ankle which caused immediate pain and swelling (macrotrauma). Another scenario would be a patient suffering from ankle pain but denying previous injury. A detailed history, in fact, reveals that the patient runs two to five miles daily on the side of a steeply crested road (microtrauma).

Table 16.2.
Generalized Pain Description and Source

Symptom	Involved Structure
Sharp pain with motion	Joint
Constant pain	Joint or Nerve
Burning/hot pain	Nerve
Sharp pain without motion	Nerve
Stabbing or shooting pain	Nerve
Tingling or numbness	Nerve
Crampy, knot or spasm	Muscle
Dull ache	Muscle or Nerve
Throbbing	Vascular

PROVOKING AND PALLIATIVE FACTORS

Provoking factors are those which the patient can perform and consistently aggravate or reproduce their symptoms. Palliative factors are just the opposite: activities or actions on the patient's behalf which decrease or alleviate symptoms. For example, a patient presenting with anterior knee pain states that symptoms increase when running down hills but decrease when resting with the knees fully extended.

QUALITY OF PAIN

The patient is asked to describe the pain (Table 16.2). This description is useful in identifying the type of tissue which serves as the source of pain (4).

RADIATION

Radiation refers to pain that has radiated and/or has been referred to another area. Although pain referred by nerve root involvement follows dermatomal patterns, pain originating from muscular pathology refers along specific myotomes. Pain of ligamentous origin will follow a scleratomal pattern. Additionally, myofascial referral patterns have also been demonstrated. The clinician should be familiar with the aforementioned referral patterns to aid in determining the origin of pain.

SEVERITY

The task of assessing a patient's level of pain can be difficult. Differing thresholds of pain and the willingness or mood of the patient are just a few of the variables to be considered. The patient should be asked to estimate the level of pain on an analog (1–10) pain scale. Grade 0 represents no symptomatology, whereas grade 10 delineates severe, debilitating pain. The grade recorded should correlate with the patient's overall presentation and behavior.

TIMING/FREQUENCY

The timing or frequency of symptoms should be noted. The doctor should inquire if the symptomatology is inter-

...orse in the morning, daytime or ...ptoms are presently getting better, are ...nchanging (5). For example, the patient ...ring occasional pain of the right shoulder ...lly follows a weekly tennis match and lasts for ...oximately 1 to 3 hours after cessation of play. This ...ould most likely indicate some type of impingement syndrome of the shoulder which is aggravated by overhead arm motions.

PAST HISTORY

Useful information includes prior injuries to the same area or to the opposite extremity. This becomes important when bilateral comparisons are made. If the doctor discovers a possible laxity of a ligament, it might be desirable to compare it with its contralateral counterpart. The doctor will need to know if there was a previous injury of the opposite joint. If a past history of injury is discovered, the doctor should ascertain if professional care was sought, and if so, what was the type, duration, and results.

FAMILY HISTORY

Historical data pertaining to the family may aid in diagnosis, either directly or indirectly. Hereditary factors can play a direct role in a patient's susceptibility to a particular injury. Indirectly, careful questioning may reveal that patients may be pressured by family members to compete in activities against their wishes, try to perform at a level higher than they are capable of, or continue to participate even when injured.

REVIEW OF SYSTEMS

The review of systems (ROS) portion of the history serves to collect data concerning past and present health and status of the bodily systems. The ROS includes information concerning physical, sociological, and psychological health, which may identify problems not previously uncovered (3). After the history, the clinician should thoroughly examine the patient to obtain additional findings which aid in the quest for an accurate diagnosis. To competently evaluate a patient, the doctor must have a comprehensive knowledge of the structures and functions of the body part or region to be examined.

Upper Extremity Examination

Examination of the upper extremity begins as the patient enters the room and exposes the bare shoulder and arm for examination. Complete exposure is essential for a comprehensive examination. Failure to fully visualize the patient greatly compromises examination efficacy.

The doctor should note the patient's willingness to use the upper extremity (5). The patient is then requested to walk to and from the doctor to demonstrate the freedom of armswing, the reciprocal movement and posture of the arms, scapular movement, and motion of the trunk. Allowing the patient to be seated once again, the examiner must consider all anatomic structures which in some way might refer symptoms to the upper extremity (Table 16.3).

It should be noted that because the upper extremity and shoulder articulate with the thorax, they form a kinetic chain. An injury or malfunction of any component of the chain may lead to compensatory pathologies elsewhere. It is for this reason that a patient with a complaint of any joint of the upper extremity receive a thorough spinal examination.

Before the initiation of the upper extremity evaluation, unless the symptomatology is directly related to an obvious localized peripheral joint or soft tissue pathology, complete general physical and spinal examination is indicated to accurately evaluate the status of the patient and arrive at the proper diagnosis. The material presented in Chapter 4 serves as a reference for the chiropractic examination of the spine.

PALPATION

Palpation is performed to 1) assess skin temperature, 2) to detect the presence of a sensory deficit, and 3) to locate and identify specific structures which are swollen or painful. A thorough knowledge of surface as well as underlying anatomy is imperative to adequately perform a palpatory examination (Fig. 16.1A-B).

NEUROLOGIC EXAMINATION

The examination of the musculoskeletal system is not adequate without a thorough assessment of the nervous system (6). It is important to keep in mind the segmental nerve supply to both the skin and muscles. Superficial sensation is assessed with a safety pin, whereas deep pain may be tested by squeezing the muscles of the limb.

Table 16.3.
Sources of Referred Pain to the Shoulder[a]

Cervical Spine
Temporomandibular Joint
Thoracic Outlet Syndrome
Sternoclavicular Joint
Acromioclavicular Joint
Scapulothoracic Joint
Costosternal Joint
Costovertebral and Costotransverse Joints
Thoracic Spine
Lumbar Spine
Carpal Tunnel Syndrome
Visceral Conditions

[a]Various sources of referral must be considered when examining the patient presenting with shoulder pain.

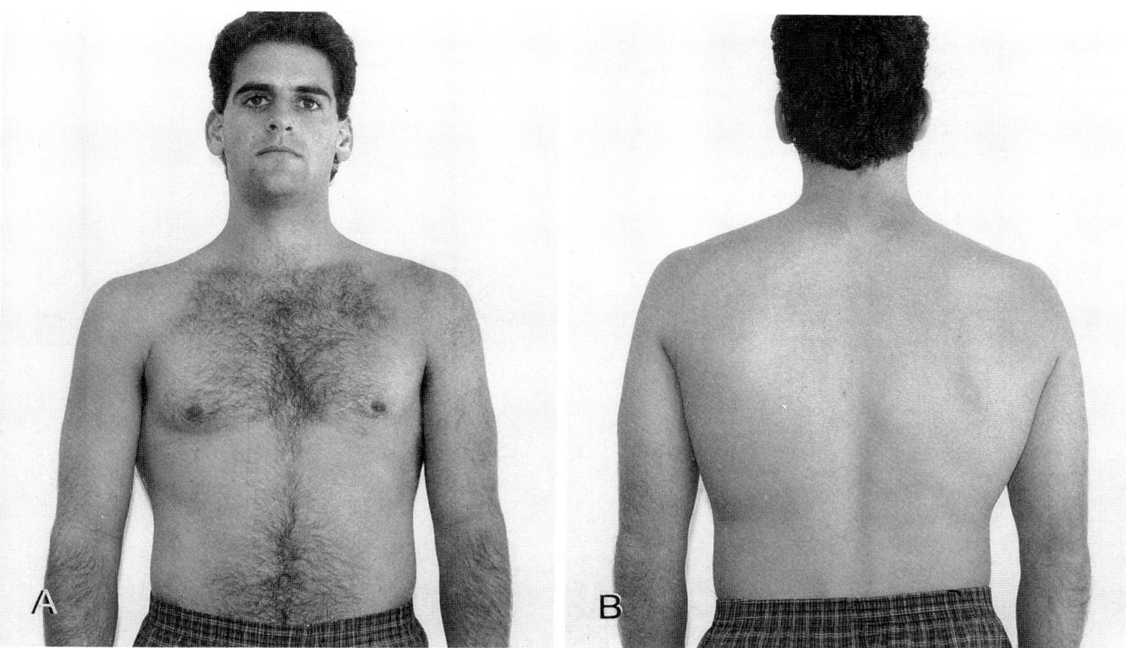

Figure 16.1. **A,** Anterior landmarks of the upper body. **B,** Posterior landmarks of the upper body.

Table 16.4.
Muscle Strength Grading[a]

Grade	Clinical Findings
0 = Zero	No contractile activity
1 = Trace	Evidence of slight muscular contractibility
2 = Poor	Complete range of motion with gravity eliminated
3 = Fair	Complete range of motion against gravity
4 = Good	Complete range of motion against gravity with some resistance
5 = Normal	Complete range of motion against gravity with full resistance

[a]Muscles are graded according to standardized examination findings.

Individual muscles should be tested for strength and graded accordingly. A numerical value of 5 represents normal muscle power, whereas a decreasing grade indicates relative loss of muscular strength (Table 16.4).

Manual muscle testing and strength loss determination are arts that the examiner must learn to master. The doctor must become proficient at isolating individual muscles and muscle groups, and grading them appropriately. Hurried or inappropriate testing methods will likely lead to missed diagnoses (7) (Table 16.5).

It should be noted that a Grade 5 is possible even in the presence of moderate muscle atrophy. If a more objective evaluation is required, an isokinetic muscle testing unit (e.g., Cybex, Merac, etc.) may be used. This evaluation allows the doctor to reliably compare right and left counterparts as well as agonist-antagonist ratios and specific muscle to body weight ratios.

Deep tendon reflexes are assessed to evaluate motor response elicited by a sensory stimulus. As in muscle testing, reflexes are graded. The grading scale most commonly used ranges from 0–4 (Table 16.6). The standard deep tendon reflexes evaluated are:

1. Biceps—C5 and C6 (musculocutaneous nerve)
2. Brachioradialis—C5 and C6 (musculocutaneous nerve)
3. Triceps—C6 to C8 (radial nerve)
4. Wrist extension—C7 and C8 (radial nerve)
5. Wrist flexion—C6 to C8 (median nerve).

RANGE OF MOTION

Active and passive ranges of motion are evaluated bilaterally with the aid of a goniometer or inclinometer. A complete range of motion assessment includes evaluation of the shoulder, elbow and wrist. Although various authors report differing ranges of motion, the more commonly accepted values are listed in Table 16.7 (8).

Active range of motion involves both contractile and noncontractile tissues; therefore, active movements alone are not specific in identifying the involved anatomic structures. It is preferred to perform the active range of motion (AROM) tests before the passive range of motion (PROM). This allows the doctor to get a general idea of the patient's range of motion while detecting any obviously restricted or painful motions.

After the AROM examination, the doctor should take the patient through the passive ranges of motion. These passive motions stress the noncontractile tissues: ligaments, joint capsule, fascia, nerves, blood vessels, and bone.

...cle Tests for Muscles Acting on the ...r Extremity

	Manual Test
...s	The patient shrugs his or her shoulders against resistance offered by the doctor.
...rratus Anterior	The patient thrusts an outstretched arm against a wall or resistance offered by the examiner.
Latissimus	The patient attempts downward and backward movement of the arm against examiner resistance.
Teres Minor	Same as latissimus dorsi. The examiner must differentiate individual muscle function by means of muscle palpation during contraction.
Rhomboids	The patient holds the hand on the hip with the arm positioned back and medial. The examiner attempts to force the arm (elbow) laterally and forward while palpating the muscle bellies.
Sternocleidomastoid	The patient rotates the head to one side and then the other against resistance provided by the doctor to the opposite temporal area.
Deltoid	The patient's arm is abducted to 90°, the examiner applies downward pressure at the elbow.
Subscapularis	With the elbow at the patient's side and flexed at 90°, the patient resists the examiner's attempt to externally rotate the arm.
Supraspinatus	The patient is instructed to abduct the shoulder 90° and bring the arm forward 30°. The forearm is pronated until the thumb points directly downward. The patient then resists downward pressure exerted by the doctor.
Infraspinatus and Teres Minor	With the elbow at the side and flexed to 90°, the patient resists the examiner's attempt to push the hand medially, thus internally rotating the humerus.
Biceps Brachii	The patient flexes a supinated forearm against resistance offered by the doctor.
Triceps Brachii	With the forearm in varying positions of flexion, the patient resists efforts of the examiner to flex the elbow.

Passive movements, such as joint play, are also performed to assess "end play" at the end of the patient's range of motion (9). Cyriax (9) describes the most commonly encountered end-play findings (Table 16.8).

Passive movements should be evaluated in the following joints and directions:

1. Sternoclavicular Joint:
   - Superior Glide
   - Inferior Glide
   - Rotation
2. Acromioclavicular Joint:
   - Anterior Glide
   - Posterior Glide
   - Rotation
3. Glenohumeral Joint:
   - Inferior Glide
   - Anterior Glide
   - Posterior Glide
   - Traction

Table 16.6.
Standard Grading of the Muscle Stretch (DTR) Reflexes

Grade	Clinical Findings
0	Areflexia
0+	Hyporeflexia
1–3	Normal
3+–4+	Hyperreflexia

Table 16.7.
Normal Range of Motion Values for the Major Joints of the Upper Extremity

Shoulder	
Flexion	180°
Extension	45°
Abduction	180°
Horizontal Adduction	135°
Internal Rotation	70°
External Rotation	90°
Elbow	
Flexion	145°
Radioulnar Joints	
Pronation	90°
Supination	90°
Wrist	
Flexion	80°
Extension	70°
Radial Deviation	20°
Ulnar Deviation	35°

4. Scapulothoracic Articulation:
   - Elevation
   - Depression
   - Protraction
   - Retraction
   - Downward Rotation
   - Upward Rotation
5. Costovertebral Joints:
   - Anterior Glide
   - Posterior Glide
6. Ulnohumeral Joint:
   - Anterior Glide
   - Posterior Glide
7. Proximal Radioulnar Joint:
   - Anterior Glide
   - Posterior Glide
8. Distal Radioulnar Joint:
   - Anterior Glide
   - Posterior Glide
9. Carpal Joints:
   - Anterior Glide
   - Posterior Glide

ORTHOPAEDIC EVALUATION

The doctor should develop a specific pattern of orthopaedic testing which will ensure a comprehensive evaluation of all structures in question while requiring the least number of postural changes on behalf of the patient.

There exist virtually hundreds of orthopaedic tests from which the doctor must select and design an evaluation program. Only some of the more commonly used tests are discussed here (5,6,10,11).

Drop Arm Test. This test evaluates the integrity of the supraspinatus tendon of the rotator cuff. The arm is passively abducted to 90°, and the patient is instructed to maintain this position. The doctor then applies downward pressure to the arm. Injury to the supraspinatus tendon will result in pain and/or weakness in the patient's inability to hold the arm up (Fig. 16.2).

Apprehension Test. The clinician passively moves the shoulder into abduction and external rotation. A history of glenohumeral dislocation or subluxation will likely bring about an apprehensive facial expression by the patient (Fig. 16.3).

Yergason's Test. The patient's elbow is flexed to 90° with the forearm pronated. The patient then supinates against resistance. Pain localized to the bicipital groove suggests bicipital tendonitis or synovitis of the tendon sheath (Fig. 16.4).

Ludington's Sign. With the patient's fingers interlocked on top of the head with the elbows back, the biceps are actively contracted. Active pathology within the bicipital groove may cause pain or crepitus (Fig. 16.5).

Table 16.8.
Common End-play Findings

Etiology	Clinical Findings
1. Capsular	Hard arrest of movements with some give
2. Spasm	Vibrant twang
3. Springy Block	A rebound is seen and felt at the extreme of the possible range
4. Tissue Approximation	Normal sensation
5. Empty	No organic resistance but the patient complains of pain
6. Bone-to-Bone	Abrupt halt when two hard surfaces meet

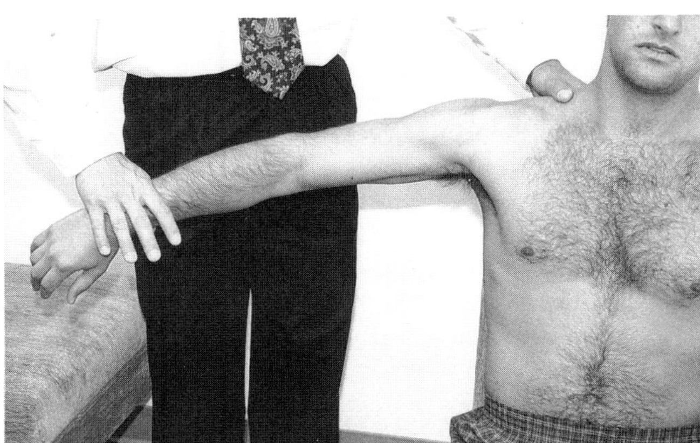

Figure 16.2. Drop arm test.

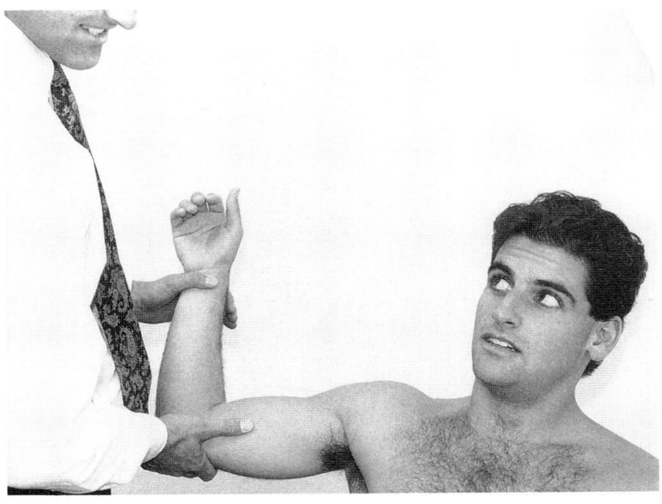

Figure 16.3. Apprehension test.

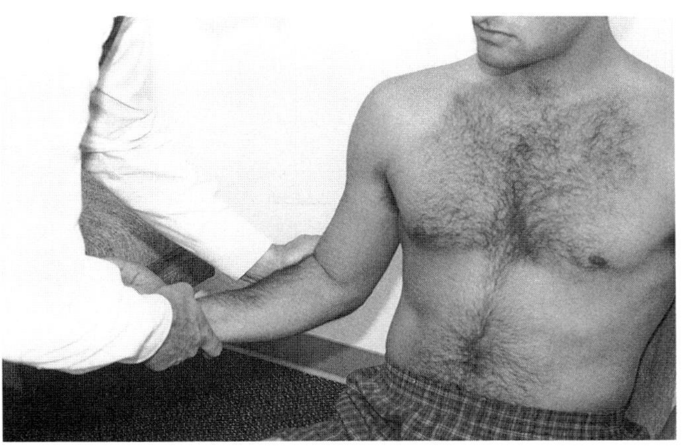

Figure 16.4. Yergason's test.

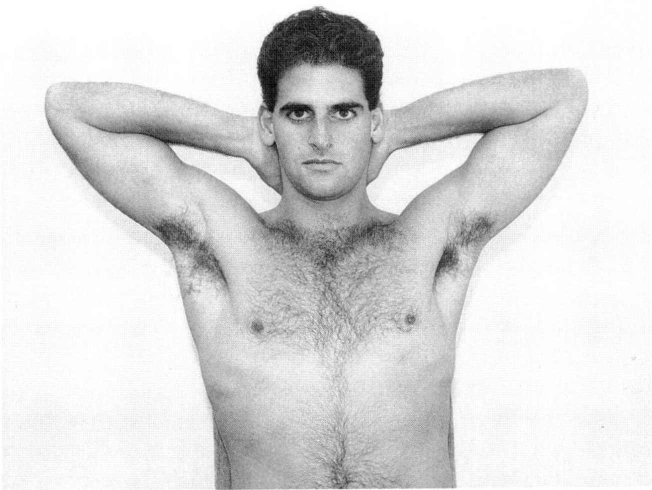

Figure 16.5. Ludington's test.

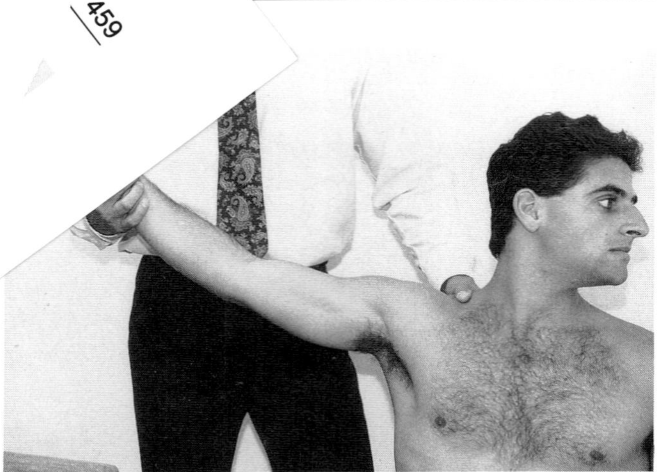

Figure 16.6. Adson's test.

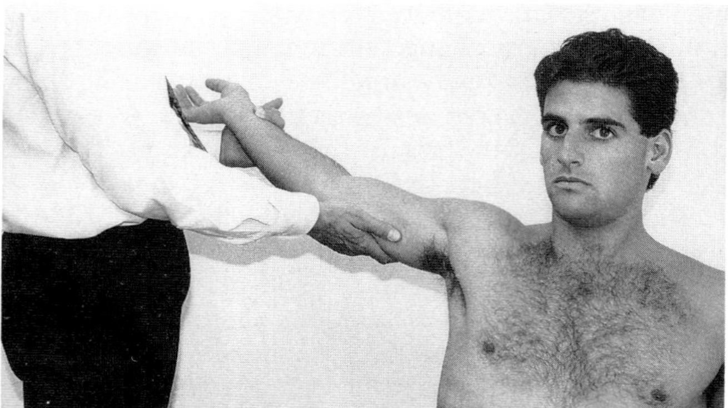

Figure 16.8. Hyperabduction test.

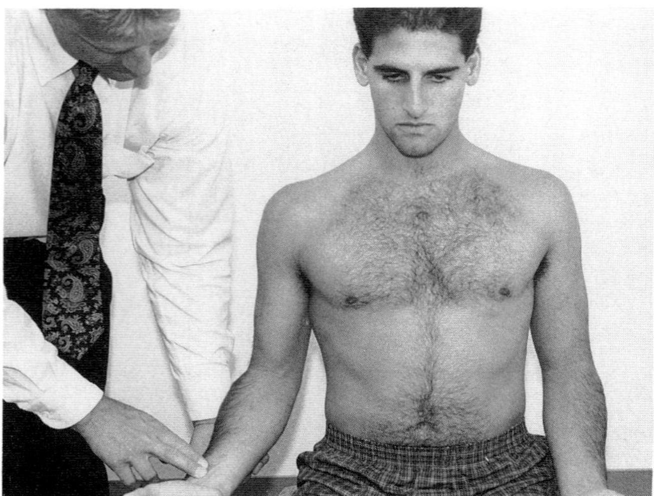

Figure 16.7. Costoclavicular test.

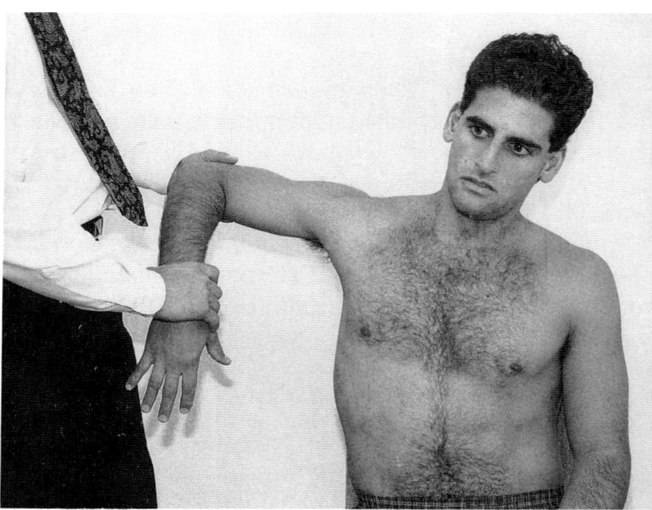

Figure 16.9. Impingement test.

Adson's Test. With the neck extended and rotated to the opposite side of the involved extremity, the patient inhales and holds the breath. The doctor simultaneously takes the patient's radial pulse. Reduction of the radial pulse and/or reproduction of upper extremity symptoms is considered a positive test. Spasm or hypertrophy of the scalene musculature is implicated (Fig. 16.6).

Costoclavicular Maneuver. There exists the possibility that the neurovascular bundle may become compressed between the clavicle and the 1st rib. The patient is instructed to draw the shoulders inferior and posterior. The doctor examines for a reduction in radial pulse, auscultates for a bruit over the mid aspect of the clavicle, and inquires about the reproduction of upper extremity symptoms (Fig. 16.7).

Hyperabduction Syndrome Test. The doctor examines the patient for a radial pulse reduction, midclavicular or axillary bruit and reproduction of upper extremity symptoms while the patient's arm is hyperabducted. Obstruction in this syndrome results from compression of the neurovascular bundle by the pectoralis minor tendon (Fig. 16.8).

Impingement Test. The arm is internally rotated and abducted while the scapula is fixed in place. Reproduction of symptoms is indicative of a shoulder impingement syndrome (Fig. 16.9).

Clunk Test. With the patient in the supine position, the examiner's hand is placed posteriorly on the humeral head, and the opposite hand holds the humeral condyles at the elbow to provide rotation motion to the arm. The patient's arm is brought into full overhead abduction, and the examiner's hand on the humeral head provides anterior force while the opposite hand rotates the humerus. A "clunk" or grinding can be felt as the humeral head hits or snaps on the labral tear (Fig. 16.10).

Spring Test. The doctor applies a slow steady inferiorward pressure to the distal clavicle and follows that action with a rapid release. The doctor observes for an upward rebound of the distal clavicle, which is indicative of a Grade II or Grade III acromioclavicular sprain (Fig. 16.11A-B).

Opposition Test. With the patient seated, the doctor applies a posterior to anterior force to the spine of the scapula and an anterior to posterior force to the distal clavicle, thus creating a shear force within the acromioclavicular joint. Production of pain or crepitus is an indication of acromioclavicular sprain or arthritis (Fig. 16.12).

Varus/Valgus Stress of the Elbow. A valgus stress applied to a slightly flexed elbow tests the integrity of the medial collateral ligament, whereas a varus stress challenges the lateral collateral ligament (Fig. 16.13A-B).

Kaplan's Test. With the patient seated, the affected upper limb is held straight out, the wrist is in slight dorsiflexion and grip strength is tested in the normal manner; this maneuver is then repeated, this time with the examiner firmly encircling the patient's forearm with both hands placed approximately 1 to 2 inches below the elbow joint line. It is a positive sign if the initial grip weakness and lateral elbow pain show a significant increase in grip strength and lessening of the pain in the elbow (6).

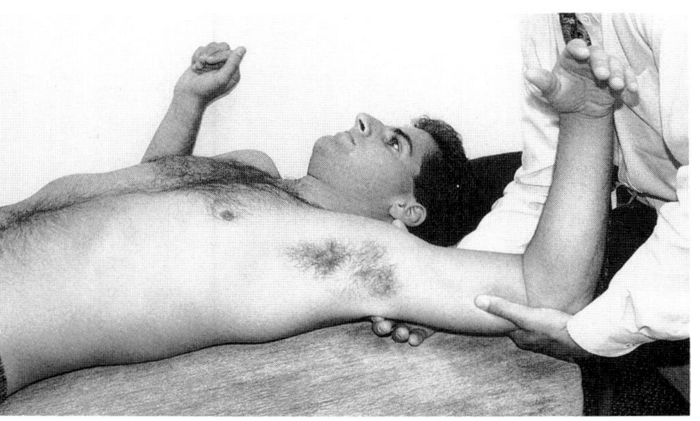

Figure 16.10. Clunk test.

Lower Extremity Examination

Much like that of the upper extremity, the examination of the lower extremity is initiated as the patient enters the room. The patient's gait should be observed on entry. The gait test should be observed during a 10-meter level walk-away, space permitting (12). Limb deformities or leg length discrepancy can often be detected. A general knowledge of gait is needed to comprehend and identify dysfunction.

Gait of the lower extremity can be divided into two phases: Stance Phase and Swing Phase. The Stance Phase encompasses the time during which the foot is in contact with the ground. The Swing Phase is the span of time when the foot leaves the ground and again returns to the ground. Both the Stance and Swing Phases can further be divided into portions of each phase (Table 16.9). Spinal biomechanics involved in gait are discussed in Chapter 2.

The gait should be scrutinized for deviations which may arise from any anatomic component of the lower extremity:

1. *Ankle and Foot:* Foot slap, toe first, flat foot, hyperpronation, supination, foot varus-valgus, toe drag, etc.
2. *Knee:* Excessive knee flexion, knee hyperextension, limited knee flexion, limited extension, genuvalgum, genuvarum, etc.
3. *Hip:* Excessive flexion, limited flexion, excessive extension, limited extension, circumduction, etc.
4. *Trunk:* Antalgic lean, posterior trunk lean, anterior trunk lean, etc.

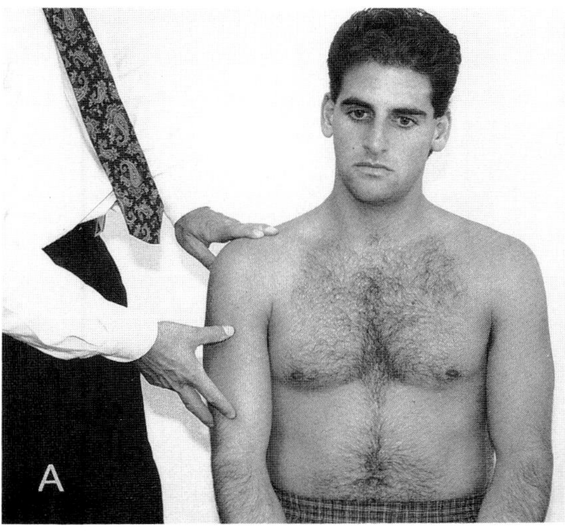

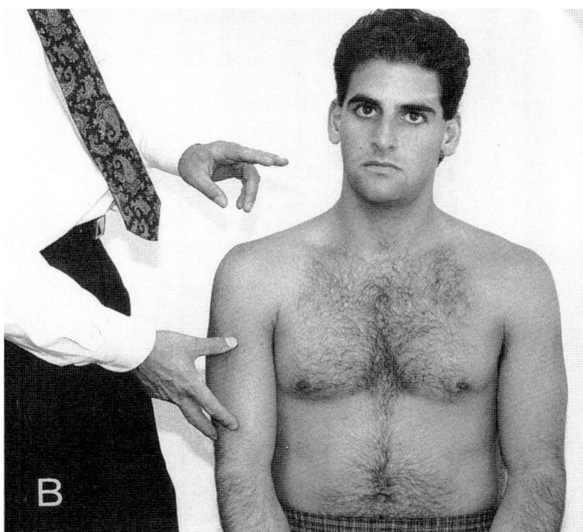

Figure 16.11A-B. Spring test.

... the lower extremity is strongly ...nesiologic performance of all of its ... All too often the doctor focuses on the ... thus limiting the span of examination and ...dering the task of proper diagnosis impossible. It ... be considered that local symptomatic treatment ...ll commonly remedy the condition in the present, only for a reaggravation later.

PALPATION

Palpation is necessary to locate and identify any painful, tender, or inflamed structure. As with all palpatory examinations, the doctor should also evaluate for skin temperature changes as well as sensory deficits. A comprehensive knowledge of all topical landmarks and underlying anatomy is required for an effective palpatory examination (Fig. 16.14A-B).

NEUROLOGIC EXAMINATION

The standard lower extremity neurologic examination begins with assessment of deep tendon reflexes (DTRs). All DTR findings should be graded and recorded using the customary 0–4 scale. The DTRs most commonly evaluated are the patellar reflex (L2-L4 innervation) and the achilles reflex (S1-S2 innervation).

The superficial nerves are evaluated by using a safety pin to compare bilateral sensation. The evaluation includes the L1 through S2 dermatomes.

STRENGTH EVALUATION

Manual muscle testing is performed bilaterally to assess general muscular strength (7) (Table 16.10).

RANGE OF MOTION

Goniometric measurements, both passive and active, of hip, knee, ankle and subtalar joint should be recorded (8,10,13). Again, authors vary on the normal values of joint ranges of motion (Table 16.11).

Passive movements or joint play should be evaluated in the following joints and directions:

1. Hip Joint:
   - Anterior Glide
   - Posterior Glide
2. Knee Joint (femorotibial):
   - Posterior Glide
   - Medial Glide
   - Lateral Glide
   - Anteromedial Rotational Glide
   - Anterolateral Rotational Glide
   - Posteromedial Rotational Glide
   - Posterolateral Rotational Glide

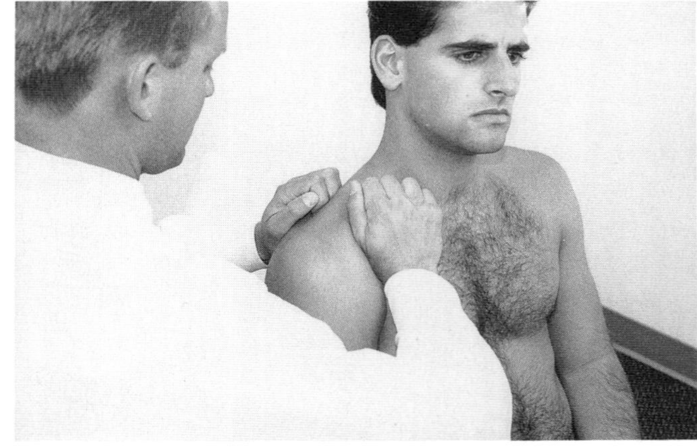

Figure 16.12. Opposition test.

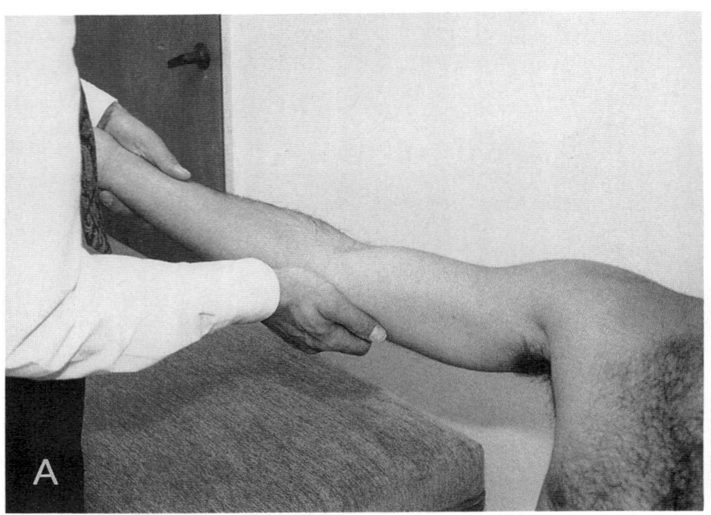

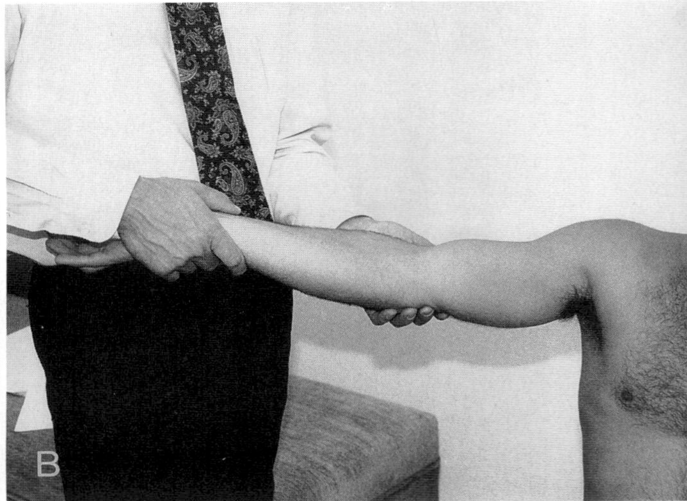

Figure 16.13. **A,** Varus test for the elbow. **B,** Valgus test for the elbow.

Table 16.9.
The Components of the Normal Gait Cycle

Stance Phase:	
1. Heel Strike:	The initiation of the stance phase when the heel first contacts the ground.
2. Foot Flat:	Following heel strike as the sole of the foot contacts the floor.
3. Midstance:	The point at which the body travels directly over the planted foot.
4. Heel-Off:	The point at which the heel of the planted foot lifts off the ground.
5. Toe-Off:	The point at which the toe of the planted foot leaves the ground.
Swing Phase:	
1. Acceleration:	The portion of the arc traveled by the swinging extremity initiated by toe-off and completed as the swinging extremity is underneath the body.
2. Midswing:	The portion of the swing when the extremity passes directly below the body.
3. Deceleration:	The portion of the swing which the extremity is decelerating in preparation for heel strike.

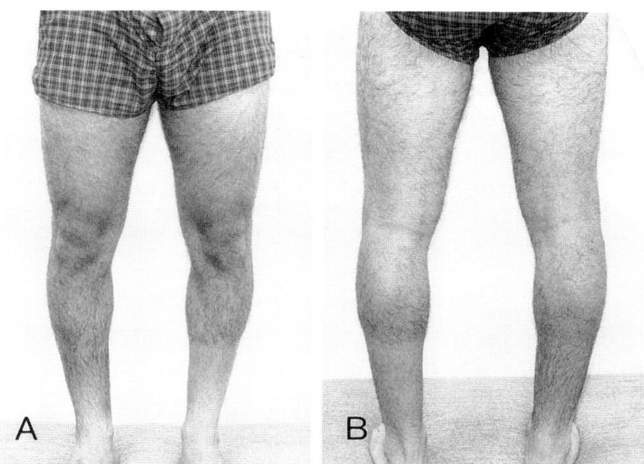

Figure 16.14. **A,** Anterior landmarks of the lower extremity. **B,** Posterior landmarks of the lower extremity.

3. Superior Tibiofibular Articulation:
   - Anterior Glide
   - Posterior Glide
   - Superior Glide (with dorsiflexion of the foot)
4. Inferior Tibiofibular Articulation:
   - Anterior Glide
   - Posterior Glide
5. Mortise Joint:
   - Anterior Glide
   - Posterior Glide
6. Subtalar Joint:
   - Medial Glide
   - Lateral Glide
   - Posterior Glide
7. Intertarsal Joints:
   - Superior Glide
   - Inferior Glide.

ORTHOPAEDIC EVALUATION

As with the evaluation of the upper extremity, there exists far too many individual orthopaedic tests to expect the clinician to perform all of them. Again, the doctor must select a variety of appropriate tests to provide a comprehensive orthopaedic evaluation of the lower extremity. The following selected orthopaedic tests are used during routine examinations:

Ober's Test. The patient is positioned in the lateral decubitus position with the lower leg slightly flexed at the hip and knee. The upper limb, the limb being tested, is abducted and extended. The knee is then flexed to 90° and the limb is allowed to drop to the table. If the limb does not drop, there might be a tight or shortened iliotibial band (10) (Fig. 16.15).

Trendelenburg Test. The patient stands on one leg. The test is positive if the hip on the non-weight-bearing side does not rise as the patient stands on one lower extremity. The indications of a positive test include hip dislocation, weakness of the hip abductors, or coxa vara (Fig. 16.16).

Abduction Test. The doctor applies a valgus stress to the knee while the ankle is stabilized in slight external rotation. The test is performed with the knee in full extension and also with the knee flexed at 20°. Excessive movement of the tibia away from the femur is indicative of damage to the medial collateral ligament (Fig. 16.17).

Adduction Test. The doctor applies a varus stress to the patient's knee while the ankle is stabilized. The test is performed with the knee in full extension and flexed to 20° to 30°. Excessive movement of the tibia away from the femur is indicative of damage to the lateral collateral ligament (Fig. 16.18).

Anterior Drawer Sign. The patient lies in the supine position with the involved knee flexed to 90°. The doctor sits atop the forefoot of the flexed limb to anchor the lower leg. With the patient's foot positioned in neutral rotation, the doctor pulls forward on the proximal portion of the posterior tibia. The test is positive if there is excessive anterior movement of the tibia with respect to the femur. A positive test is indicative of instability of the anterior cruciate ligament (Fig. 16.19).

Apley's Grinding Test. The patient is in the prone position with the knees flexed to 90°. The doctor applies a compressive force through the foot down into the knee while internally and externally rotating the tibia. A sensation of pain and/or the presence of joint crepitus is indicative of a meniscal injury (Fig. 16.20A-B). The test continues by applying a distractive force to the leg. Pain elicited by distraction implies ligamentous rather than meniscal injury.

Apprehension Test. The patient is placed in the supine position with the knees flexed to 30°. The examiner slowly displaces the patella laterally. The test is positive if the

scle Tests for the Lower Extremities

es:	Psoas Major and Iliacus (Hip Flexion)
Test:	The patient lies or is seated with legs over the edge of the table. The patient flexes the hip through the last portion of the range of motion as the doctor offers resistance at the distal femur.
Muscle:	Sartorius (Hip Flexion, Abduction and Lateral Rotation with Knee Flexion)
Test:	From a seated position, the patient flexes, abducts and laterally rotates the hip and flexes the knee. Resistance to hip flexion and abduction is provided with one hand above the joint; resistance to hip lateral rotation and knee flexion is offered by the other hand above the ankle joint.
Muscles:	Gluteus Maximus, Semitendinosus, Semimembranosus, and the Long Head of the Biceps Femoris (Hip Extension)
Test:	With the patient in the prone position, the hip is extended as the doctor offers resistance proximal to the knee joint.
Muscle:	Gluteus Medius (Hip Abduction)
Test:	The patient lies in the lateral decubitus position with the hip slightly extended beyond midline. The patient abducts the hip against resistance offered by the doctor proximal to the knee joint.
Muscles:	Adductor Magnus, Adductor Brevis, Adductor Longus, Pectineus and Gracilus (Hip Adduction)
Test:	The patient lies in the lateral decubitus position with the leg to be tested resting on the table. The doctor supports the upper leg in approximately 25° of abduction. The patient adducts the lower leg as the doctor offers resistance proximal to the knee joint.
Muscles:	Obturator Externus, Obturator Internus, Quadratus Femoris, Piriformis, Gemellus Superior and Gemellus Inferior (Hip Lateral Rotation)
Test:	The patient is seated with knee flexed to 90°. The patient laterally rotates the hip as the doctor stabilizes the lateral aspect of the knee and resists the patient's attempt to rotate the hip by applying pressure to the medial aspect of the ankle.
Muscles:	Gluteus Minimus and Tensor Fasciae Latae (Hip Medial Rotation)
Test:	Same as the lateral hip rotation test except the patient attempts to medially rotate the hip against resistance offered by the doctor to the lateral ankle.
Muscles:	Biceps Femoris, Semitendinosus, and Semimembranosus (Knee Flexion)
Test:	With the patient in the prone position, the doctor stabilizes the pelvis with one hand and offers resistance to active knee flexion with the other hand just proximal to the ankle.
Muscle:	Quadriceps Femoris (Knee Extension)
Test:	The patient sits on the table with knees flexed at 90°. The patient attempts to extend the knee while the doctor offers resistance proximal to the ankle joint.
Muscles:	Gastrocnemius and Soleus (Ankle Plantarflexion)
Test:	The patient stands on the limb to be tested and raises the heel off the floor 5 to 10 times.
Muscle:	Tibialis Anterior (Ankle Dorsiflexion and Foot Inversion)
Test:	The seated patient dorsiflexes and inverts the foot against resistance offered by the doctor. The patient should be instructed to keep the toes relaxed to avoid involvement of the extensor digitorum and hallicis longus.
Muscle:	Tibialis Posterior (Foot Inversion)
Test:	The patient lies in the lateral decubitus position with the upper ankle positioned midway between plantarflexion and dorsiflexion. The patient then inverts the ankle as the doctor stabilizes the lower leg with one hand, while providing resistance to the patient's efforts with the other.
Muscles:	Peroneus Longus and Peroneus Brevis (Foot Eversion)
Test:	The seated patient inverts the foot. The patient attempts to evert the foot as the doctor resists the motion.
Muscles:	Flexor Digitorum Longus, Flexor Digitorum Brevis, and Flexor Hallucis Longus (Flexion of Toes)
Test:	The patient flexes the proximal phalanges of the 2nd through 5th digits against resistance offered by the doctor. This test assesses the flexor digitorum brevis. Flexion of the distal phalanges with stabilization provided to the middle row of phalanges and resistance offered to the distal phalanges evaluates the strength of the flexordigitorum longus. Flexion of the 1st toe against resistance assesses the flexor hallucis longus.
Muscles:	Extensor Digitorum Longus and Extensor Digitorum Brevis
Test:	The seated patient extends the toes as the doctor stabilizes the metatarsals with one hand and offers resistance to the distal phalanges of all the toes.

patient looks apprehensive or contracts the quadriceps. A positive test is suggestive of a history of patella dislocation (Fig. 16.21).

Clarke's Sign The patient is in the supine position with the knees extended. The doctor lightly compresses the patella with the web of the hand. The patient is instructed to slowly contract the quadriceps. Inability to complete a full contraction without pain is suggestive of chondromalacia of the patella (Fig. 16.22).

Hughston Plica Test. This test is intended to identify an abnormal suprapatellar plica. The patient is in the supine position, and the doctor flexes the knee and medially rotates the tibia with one hand, while displacing the patella medialward with the opposite hand. The test is positive if a "pop" is elicited at the plica while the knee is flexed and extended by the doctor (Fig. 16.23).

Lateral Pivot Shift Test. The doctor holds the lower leg with one hand and places the other hand on the lateral proximal aspect of the leg. With the knee in full extension, a valgus stress is applied followed by internal rotation of

Table 16.11.
Commonly Accepted Joint Ranges of Motion for the Major Joints of the Lower Extremity

Hip	
Flexion	125°
Extension	10°
Abduction	45°
Adduction	10°
Internal Rotation	45°
External Rotation	45°
Knee	
Flexion	140°
Ankle	
Plantarflexion	45°
Dorsiflexion	20°
Subtalar Joint	
Inversion	35°
Eversion	20°

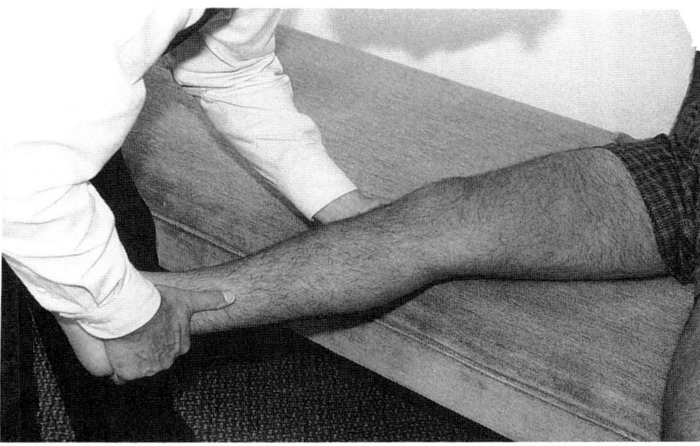

Figure 16.17. Abduction test for the knee.

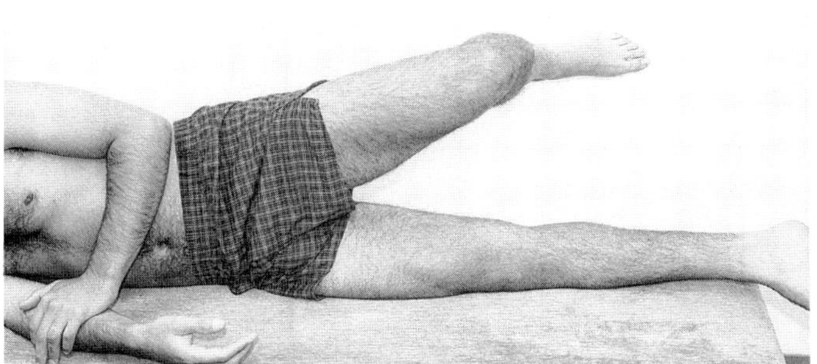

Figure 16.15. Ober's test.

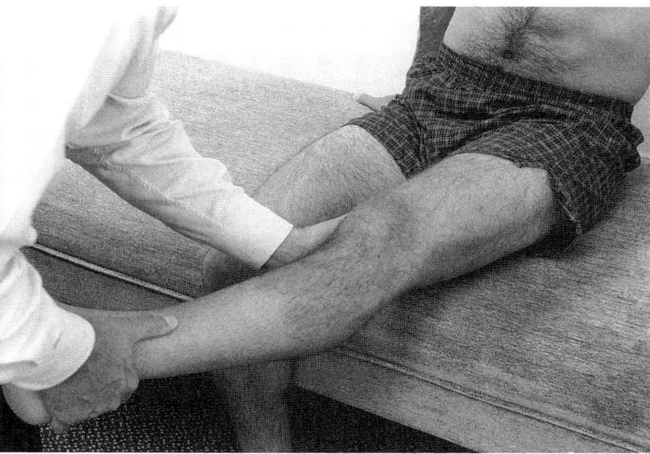

Figure 16.18. Adduction test for the knee.

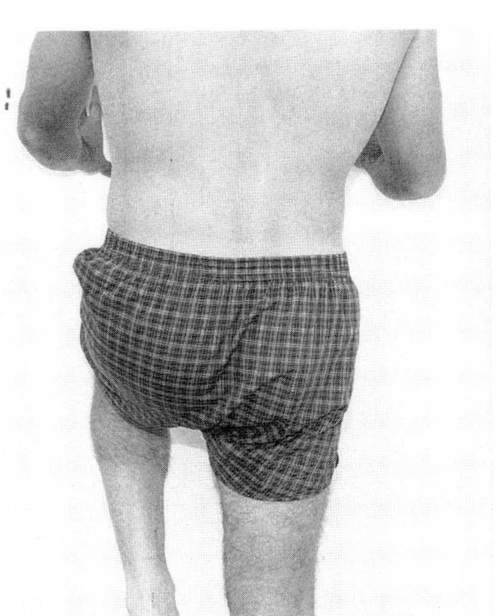

Figure 16.16. Trendelenburg's test.

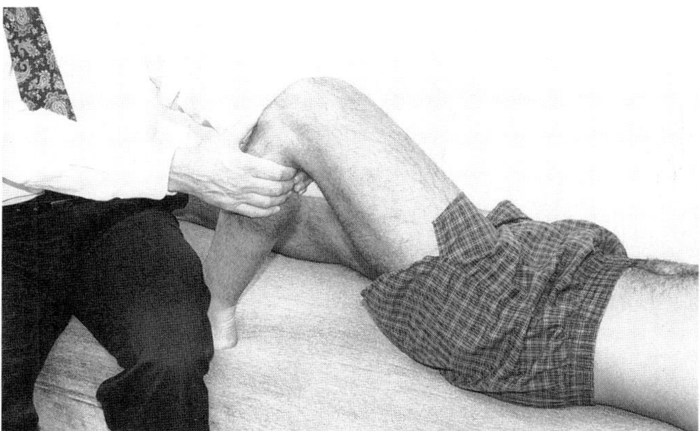

Figure 16.19. Anterior drawer test for the knee.

the leg and flexion of the knee. At approximately 30° flexion, an anterior jump of the lateral tibial plateau is suggestive of anterolateral rotatory instability (Fig. 16.24).

Reverse Pivot Shift Test. This test is intended to demonstrate posterolateral rotatory instability of the knee. With the patient in the supine position and the knee in full extension, the doctor supports the patient's knee posteriorly with one hand and the heel of the foot with the other hand. The foot is then laterally rotated. The test is positive if there is a jerk in the knee, or the tibia shifts posteriorly and the knee gives way (Fig. 16.25).

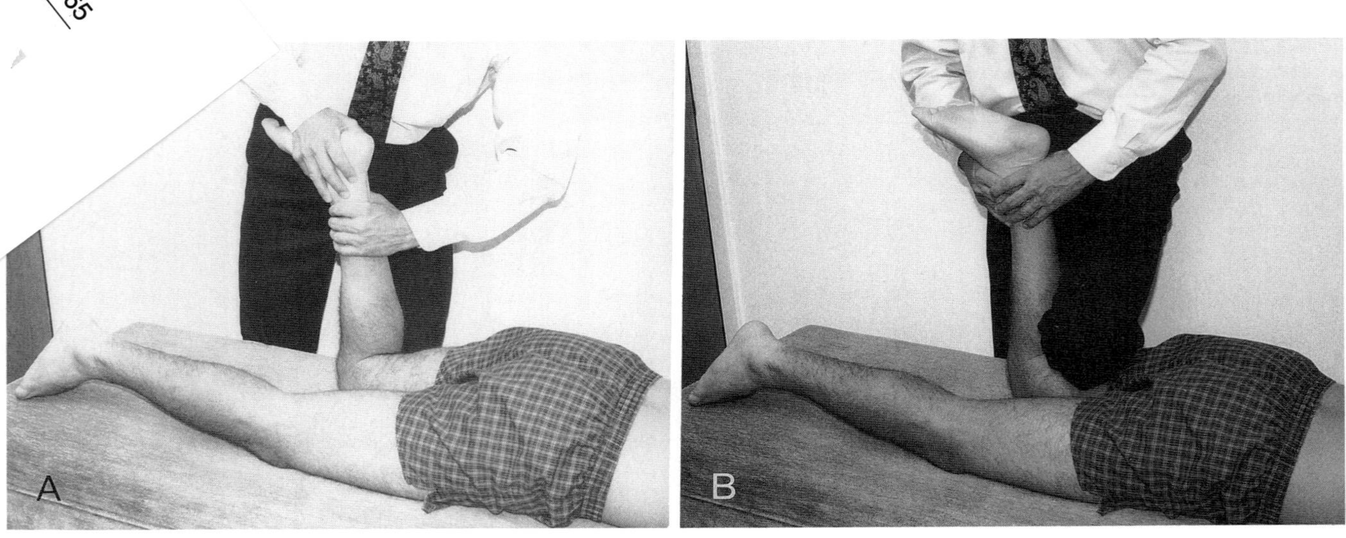

Figure 16.20. **A,** Apley's compression test. **B,** Apley's distraction test.

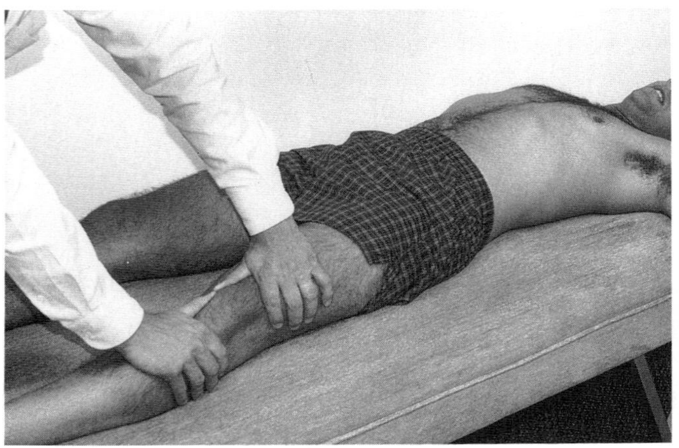

Figure 16.21. Patellar apprehension test.

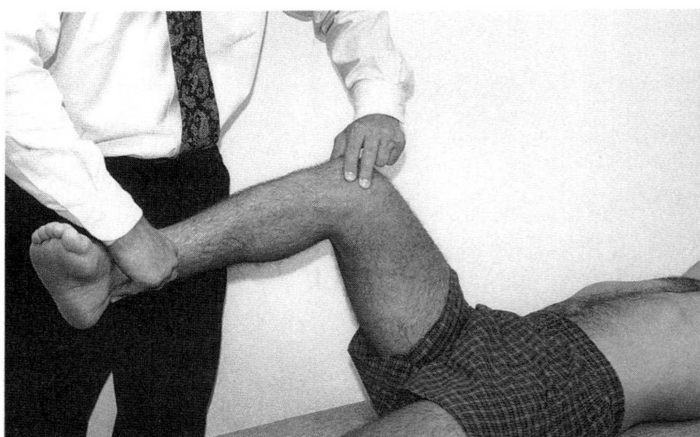

Figure 16.23. Hughston test.

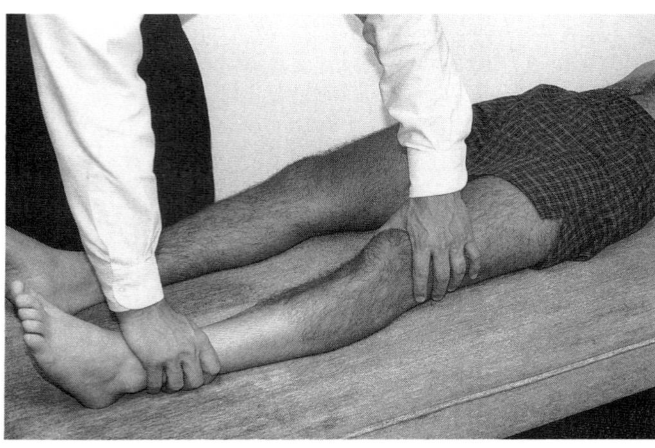

Figure 16.22. Clarke's sign.

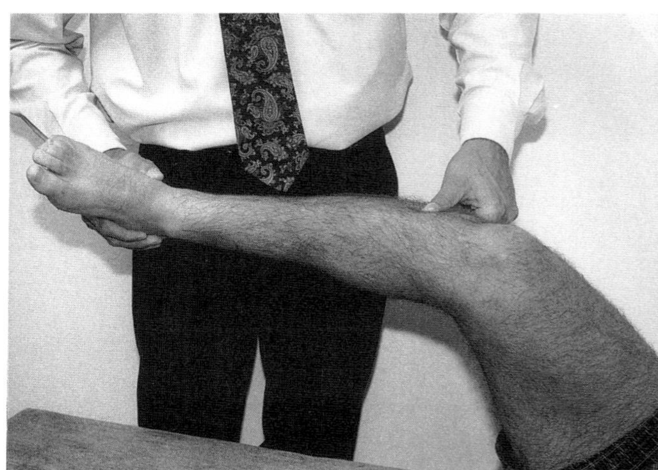

Figure 16.24. Lateral pivot shift test.

Lachman's Test. With the patient in the supine position, the doctor stabilizes the distal anterior femur with one hand and holds the proximal tibia with the other hand. The knee is held in slight flexion as the tibia is drawn forward on the femur. Excessive anterior movement of the tibia is indicative of injury to the anterior cruciate ligament (Fig. 16.26).

McMurry Test. The patient is in the supine position while the examiner holds the foot with one hand and palpates the joint line of the knee with the other. The knee is then flexed and the tibia is rotated internally and externally and then alternately positioned in internal and external rotation as the knee is fully extended. Crepitus or popping felt over the joint line may indicate a meniscal tear (Fig. 16.27).

Posterior Drawer Test. The patient is positioned as in the anterior drawer test. The doctor attempts to move the tibia posteriorly on the femur. Excessive posterior slippage is suggestive of posterior cruciate ligament damage (Fig. 16.28).

Anterior Drawer Test of the Ankle. As the anterior distal tibiofibular articulation is stabilized, the doctor holds the foot in 20° of plantarflexion and draws forward. Anterior slippage which exceeds that of the uninvolved side is indicative of anterior ankle instability (Fig. 16.29).

Homan's Sign. If, during passive dorsiflexion of the foot, deep pain is felt in the lower leg, deep vein thrombosis should be suspected.

Thompson Test. With the patient in the prone position, the doctor squeezes the middle third of the gastrocnemius. The normal result is mild plantarflexion of the foot. Absence of this is indicative of a rupture of the achilles tendon.

Quadriceps-angle (Q-angle). An indirect method of assessment of patellar tracking is the measurement of the Q-angle. The Q-angle is the measured angle formed by the line connecting the anterior superior iliac spine and the center of the patella and the line connecting the tibial tuberosity and the center of the patella (14). The measurement is made with the knees fully extended and the hips in the neutral position.

The normal values of the Q-angle are 14° for men and

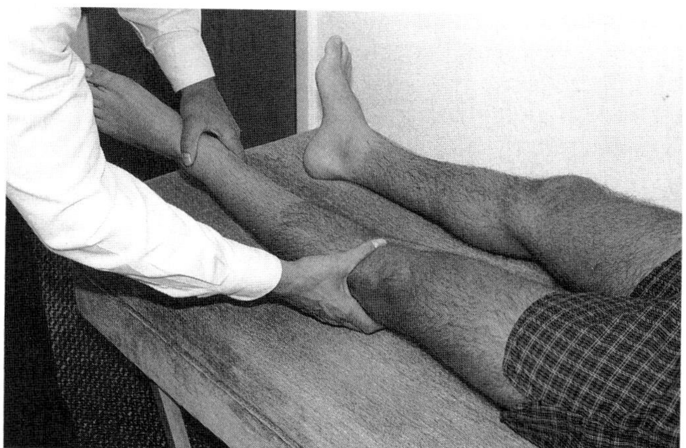

Figure 16.25. Reverse pivot shift test.

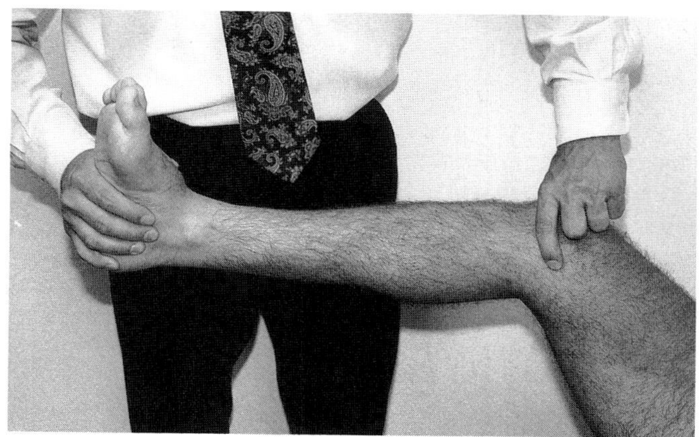

Figure 16.27. McMurry's test.

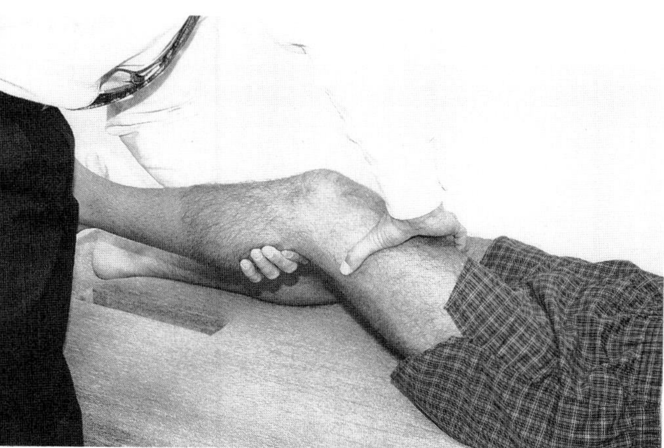

Figure 16.26. Lachman's test.

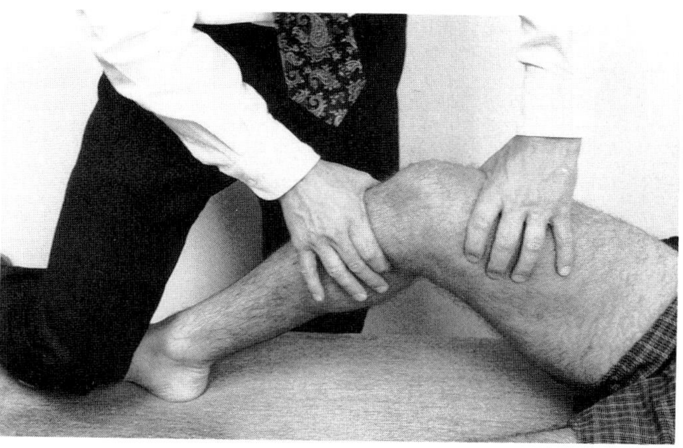

Figure 16.28. Posterior drawer test of the knee.

17° for women. Although increased Q-angles have been associated with recurrent patellar dislocation, chondromalacia, and patellar arthralgia, objective documentation of the association is limited. Fox (15) claims that the Q-angle itself is not indicative of pathology.

Also, variations in the Q-angle do not significantly alter peak torque values of knee extension when tested at 30°, 60°, and 90°/sec (15) (Fig. 16.30).

SHOULDER GIRDLE

The shoulder girdle consists of four independent linkages: the sternoclavicular joint, the acromioclavicular joint, the glenohumeral joint, and the scapulothoracic articulation.

Sternoclavicular Joint

The sternoclavicular joint is a synovial joint which allows for three planes of motion: elevation-depression, protraction-retraction, and rotation. The joint is comprised of the medial end of the clavicle, the articular surface of the manubrium, and the interposed sternoclavicular disc. Ligamentous support is provided by the costoclavicular ligament and the sternoclavicular ligament (Fig. 16.31).

KINESIOLOGY

Elevation-depression occurs around an anterior posterior axis; protraction-retraction occurs around a vertical axis; and rotation occurs around an axis running longitudinally through the clavicle. Interposed between the osseous components of the sternoclavicular joint is a fibrocartilage disc or meniscus. The disc is attached superiorly to the clavicle and inferiorly to the manubrium. It acts as a hinge during joint motion and further serves as a shock absorber when forces are transmitted along the clavicle from its lateral end. Misalignment of the sternoclavicular joint commonly results when a force is applied to the lateral aspect of the shoulder which exceeds the shock-absorbing capacities of the meniscus and the tensile strength of the supporting ligaments and joint capsule.

RADIOGRAPHIC ANALYSIS

The standard radiographic analysis of the sternoclavicular joint requires a P-A view of the involved joint. The P-A projection is often insufficient to accurately assess the status of the joint. It is occasionally necessary to obtain a tomogram of the joint.

The most common injury to the sternoclavicular joint is a sprain which occurs when the patient falls directly on the shoulder. If the force is great enough, the proximal end of the clavicle may subluxate or dislocate. With subluxation, the direction of misalignment is usually superior. Complete dislocation produces a malalignment of the proximal clavicle in a superior and medial direction.

Acromioclavicular Joint

The acromioclavicular joint is composed of the distal end of the clavicle and the acromion process of the scapula. Ligamentous support is supplied by the conoid ligament, trapezoid ligament, acromioclavicular ligament, and the coracoacromial ligament.

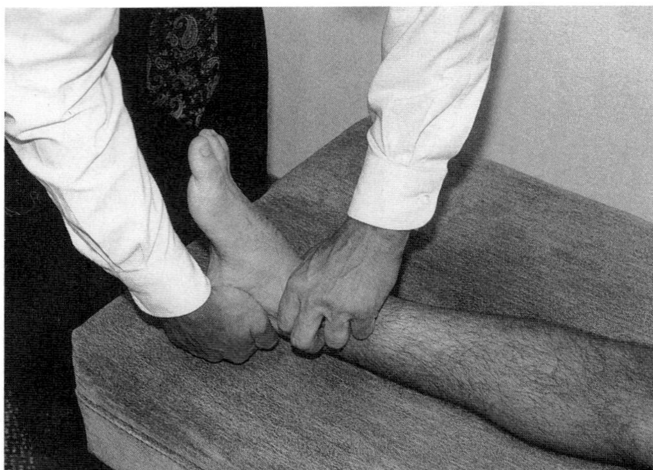

Figure 16.29. Anterior drawer test of the ankle.

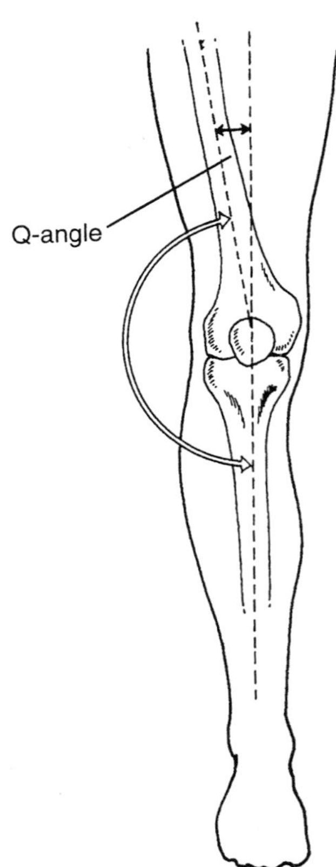

Figure 16.30. Q-angle of the knee.

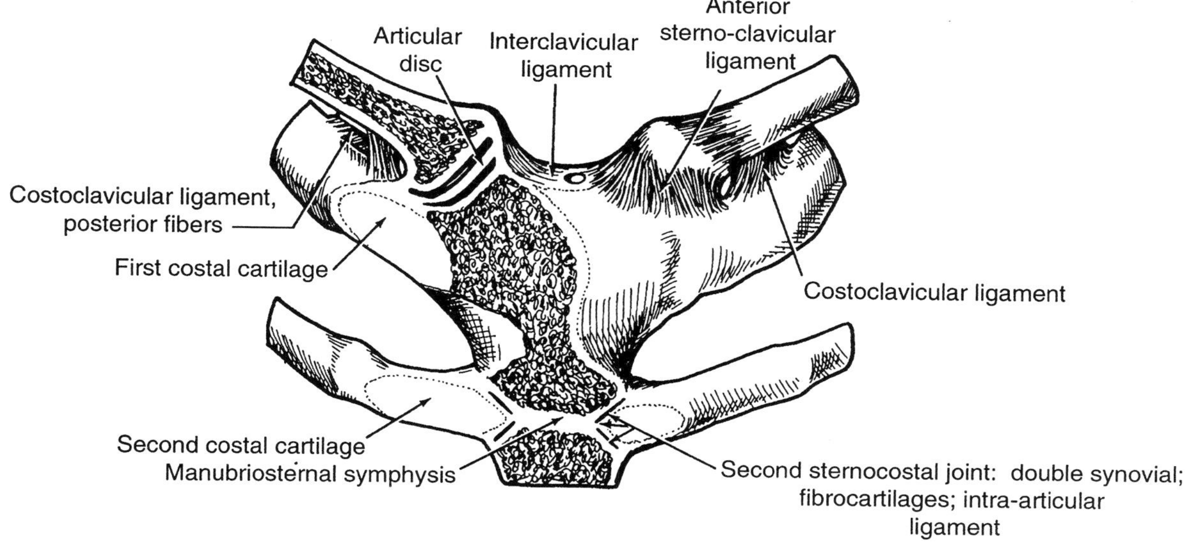

Figure 16.31. Ligamentous structures of the sternoclavicular joint. Modified from Warwick R, Williams P. Gray's anatomy. 35th British ed. Philadelphia: WB Saunders, 1980:454.

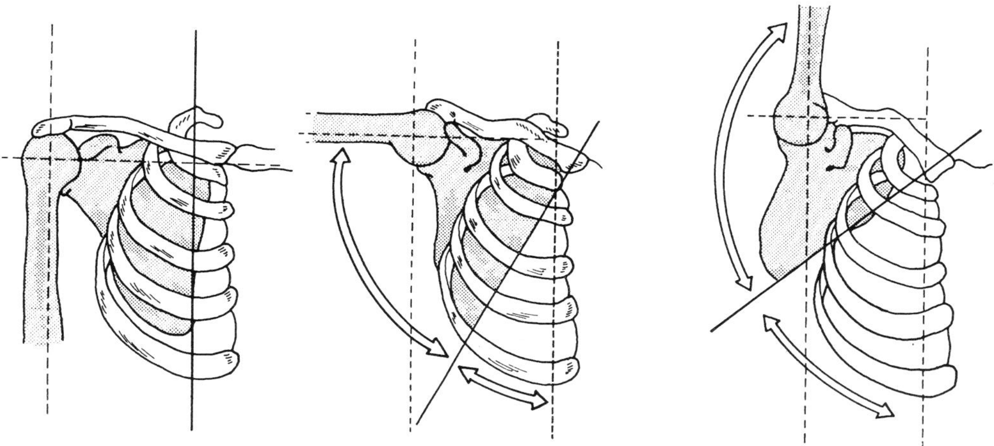

Figure 16.32. Glenohumeral abduction with scapular motion.

KINESIOLOGY

The acromioclavicular joint is a synovial, hinge-type joint which permits three definable motions to occur (8,13,16). The primary movement at the acromioclavicular joint involves rotation of the scapula around an anterior-posterior axis as noted during abduction of the shoulder. A description of shoulder abduction is required.

During abduction, the glenohumeral joint and the scapulothoracic articulation move in a 2:1 ratio, that is to say, for every 3° of abduction, 2° occur at the glenohumeral joint and one degree occurs at the scapulothoracic articulation. The scapula does not move until the shoulder has been abducted approximately 20°. From this point the glenohumeral and scapulothoracic articulation move in the 2:1 ratio. This ratio of movement continues until 120°. At this point the surgical neck of the humerus contacts the acromion and full abduction to 180° can only be completed if the humerus is externally rotated (13) (Fig. 16.32). If fixation occurs at any of the articulations of the shoulder girdle, this scapulothoracic rhythm will likely be altered, which may result in dysfunction of another joint in the region. During abduction the acromion slides on the distal clavicle in the same direction as the movement of the scapula (8,13).

There are two remaining motions allowed by the acromioclavicular joint. One movement is described as "winging," in which the scapula slides laterally around the rib cage. This motion is around the vertical axis. The final motion is referred to as "tipping" of the inferior angle of the scapula around a coronal axis. Motions at the acromioclavicular joint are very small and not clinically

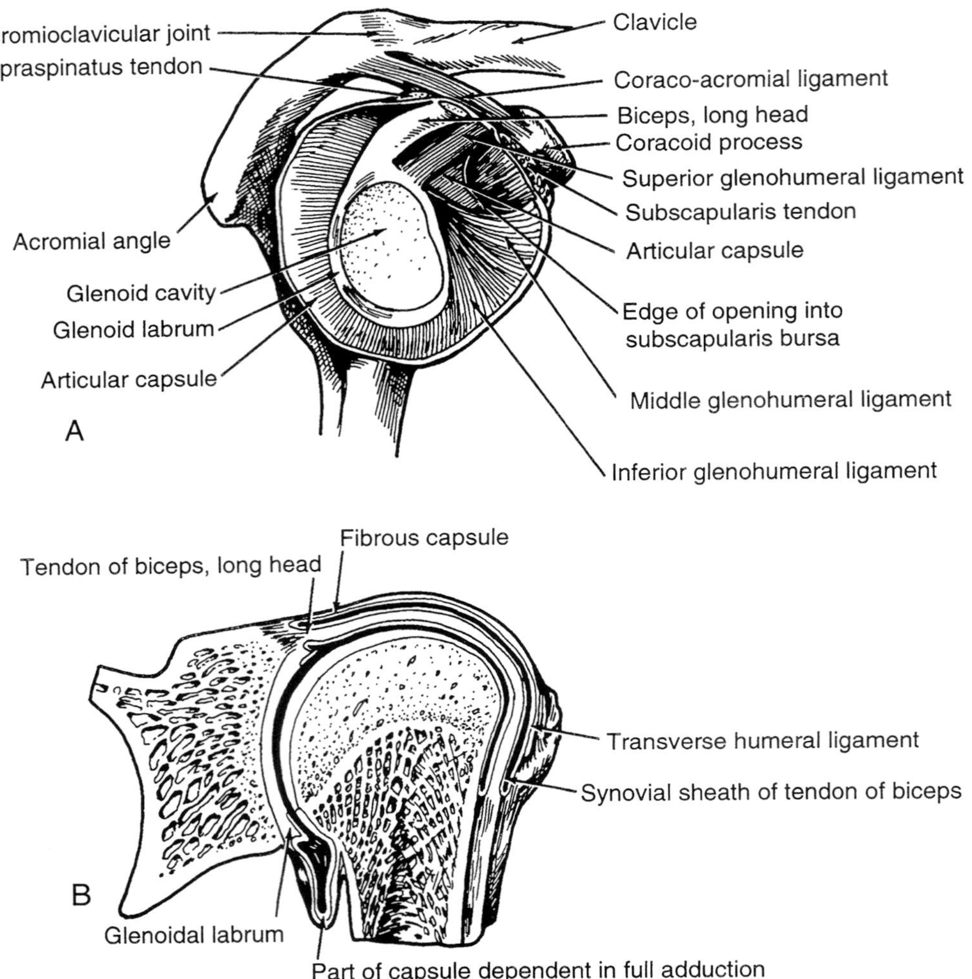

Figure 16.33. **A,** Anatomic structures of the glenohumeral joint (sagittal plane). Modified from Warwick R, Williams P. Gray's anatomy. 35th British ed. Philadelphia: WB Saunders, 1980:459. **B,** Anatomic structures of the glenohumeral joint (coronal plane). Modified from Warwick R, Williams P. Gray's anatomy. 35th British ed. Philadelphia: WB Saunders, 1980:457.

measurable, yet the few degrees of motion allowed are nonetheless fundamental for normal shoulder function.

RADIOGRAPHIC ANALYSIS

To evaluate the acromioclavicular joint, an anteroposterior radiograph of both shoulders is exposed on one film while the patient stands. Downward traction is then applied to both arms by securing 10-pound weights to the patient's wrists, and the exposure repeated. The central ray should be directed cephalically 15°. In normal studies, the acromioclavicular joint should measure 11 to 13 mm (16). A Grade II injury is noted when the acromioclavicular interval is greater than 13 mm. A Grade III separation demonstrates a large widening of the acromioclavicular interval (13mm), upward displacement of the clavicle, and widening of the coracoclavicular space.

Glenohumeral Joint

The glenohumeral joint is a synovial ball and socket, or spheroid joint which allows three degrees of motion: flexion-extension, abduction-adduction, and internal-external rotation. It is composed of the glenoid fossa of the scapula, the head of the humerus, a joint capsule, the glenoid labrum, the rotator cuff and a myriad of other structures (Fig. 16.33A-B).

KINESIOLOGY

The range of motion for each of the three axes of movement varies greatly. The range of flexion through extension varies from 190° to 240° with 120° to 180° devoted to flexion. The range of abduction varies depending on whether the humerus is internally or externally rotated. Abduction of an internally rotated humerus is measured up to 60°, whereas in full external rotation, it will abduct further to 120° to 135°. As discussed earlier, the scapulothoracic articulation is responsible for an additional 50° to 60° total shoulder abduction.

Abduction of the shoulder occurs through a combination of rolling and sliding of the humeral head on the glenoid fossa. As the humeral head rolls through abduction, it simultaneously slides inferiorly to prevent impaction of the humeral head into the acromion process (Fig. 16.34). This pattern of motion should be kept in mind as the doctor palpates the glenohumeral joint. The humerus can internally rotate 70° to 90°. External rotation ranges from 80° to 90°.

RADIOGRAPHIC ANALYSIS

To analyze the glenohumeral joint, anteroposterior radiographs are obtained with the humerus positioned first in internal rotation and then in external rotation. The glenohumeral joint normally widens during external humeral rotation. This widening should be symmetrical with that of the opposite shoulder. Excessive widening is suggestive of glenohumeral joint instability. A lateral scapular radiograph should also be performed. The lateral scapular view is beneficial in assessing the position of the humeral head. In this view, the acromion, coracoid process, and the body of the scapula form a "Y" which serves as a reference point from which the position of the humeral head can be assessed.

Normally, the humeral head lies at the junction of the three structures. If the humeral head lies either anterior, posterior, superior or inferior to this junction, then glenohumeral misalignment in that specific direction should be considered. Approximately 85% of all shoulder misalignments are anteroinferior in direction, 10 to 13% are primarily anterior in direction, and perhaps only 2% are posterior.

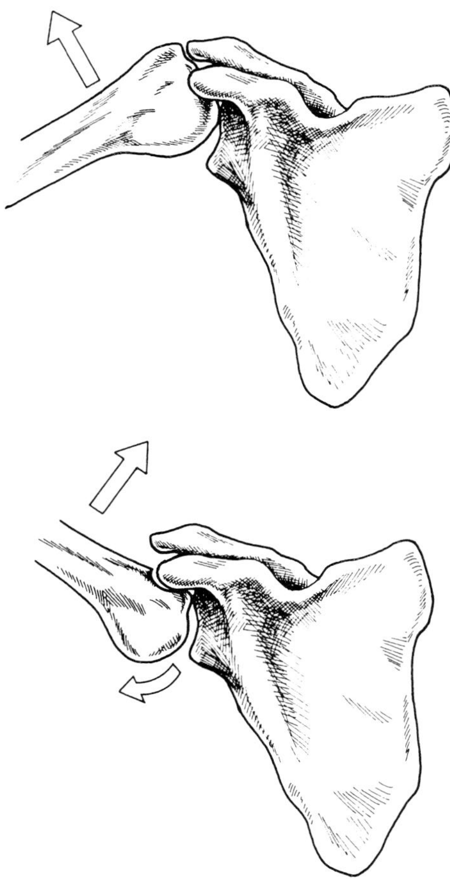

Figure 16.34. Diagram of the humeral head during abduction. Modified from Norkin CC, Levangie PK. Joint structure and function: a comprehensive analysis. Philadelphia: WB Saunders, 1983:173.

Scapulothoracic Articulation

Although the scapulothoracic articulation is not a true joint, it does consist of a relationship between the scapula and posterior thoracic wall. The scapula is normally positioned approximately two inches from midline, between the second and seventh ribs. It is from this position that the normal motions of the scapula are described. These motions consist of elevation-depression and abduction-adduction, which are translatory movements, and upward and downward rotation of the inferior tip of the scapula. It is the latter which allows for complete abduction of the shoulder. Positional stability of the scapula is provided osseously by a competent sternoclaviculo-acromion kinetic chain as well as the muscular elements (10,13) (Table 16.12).

COMMON DISORDERS OF THE SHOULDER

Shoulder Girdle

ANTERIOR DISLOCATION OF THE GLENOHUMERAL JOINT

Definition. The anterior-inferior dislocation of the glenohumeral joint is the most common type of shoulder dislocation. The injury typically occurs when the humeral head is forced anteriorly beyond the edge of the glenoid rim without spontaneous reduction.

Etiology. The displacement of the humeral head occurs when the arm is hyperabducted and externally

Table 16.12.
Muscles that Move or Stabilize the Scapula

Adduction	Abduction	Upward Rotation	Downward Rotation
Trapezius	Serratus anterior	Upper trapezius, serratus anterior	Lower trapezius, rhomboid major, rhomboid minor, levator scapulae, pectoralis minor

rotated. The acromion acts as a fulcrum at which time the head is levered out of the glenoid fossa. As this occurs, there is tearing of the inferior glenohumeral ligament, anterior capsule and possibly the glenoid labrum.

Damage to the axillary or musculocutaneous nerve may complicate this injury. If the axillary nerve is involved, the resultant disability may demonstrate slight weakness or hypesthesia over the deltoid region of the arm. If the musculocutaneous nerve is involved, it may demonstrate weakness of the biceps brachii, brachialis, and the coracobrachialis muscles. Both of these conditions usually resolve spontaneously in a matter of a few weeks to several months. Other complications may include fractures of the humerus and/or glenoid process. The most commonly associated fracture of the humerus is avulsion of the greater tuberosity.

Signs and Symptoms. The athlete-individual suffering an anterior dislocation of the shoulder usually experiences a feeling of uselessness and pain in the shoulder region with muscle tightness and tenderness about the shoulder and anterior chest region. Tingling and numbness may also be present in the arm and hand region. Further, on reduction the patient usually experiences an increase in general symptomatology.

Diagnostic Work-Up. On disrobing the patient for examination, a noticeable loss of rounding of the shoulder with a prominent acromion process will be viewed. The humeral head may be noticed inferior to the coracoid process. The patient generally presents with the affected arm held across the chest. Infrequently, the arm may hang away from the body in an externally rotated posture. Any attempt to abduct or internally rotate the arm will be resisted by the patient. Neurologic sensation can be demonstrated with a safety pin over the lateral arm (axillary nerve) and radial aspect of the forearm (musculocutaneous nerve). The remainder of the arm should be tested for other brachial plexus nerve lesions. Further testing of the brachial plexus may be aided by evaluating muscle strength in the upper extremity. Distal pulses should be evaluated for compromise of the vascular supply into the extremity. On completion of the physical examination, adequate plain film x-rays should be taken. An anterior-inferior dislocation of the shoulder will demonstrate the humeral head in the subcoracoid potential space. Complications with this type of injury may include impaction of the humeral head (Hill-Sach's defect), fracture of the greater tuberosity, and avulsion of the inferior aspect of the glenoid rim (Bankart lesion).

Depending on where the humeral head comes to rest, positional terms should be applied (e.g., subglenoid, subcoracoid and subclavicular dislocation).

Treatment. Shoulder dislocation is an acute emergency. The shoulder should be reduced to normal anatomic posture. There are a number of methods used to reduce this injury. Turek discusses the Kocher maneuver as a technique in the reduction of anterior shoulder dislocations. It basically consists of flexing the abducted arm at the elbow while maintaining slow distal inferior traction of the affected arm. While maintaining this traction, the arm should be slowly externally rotated to approximately 80°, at which time the elbow is then placed in front of the chest. The arm is then rotated internally, placing the affected hand on the opposite shoulder. Once the shoulder has been reduced, the arm should be immobilized across the chest in a sling and swathe.

An alternative method which is very effective also exists. The elbow of the affected extremity is flexed to 90° while an inferior tractional force is applied to the humerus. The shoulder is then slowly abducted and externally rotated. Reduction of the dislocation may occur during any of these steps (Fig. 16.35A,B-C,D). As with the Kocher maneuver, the arm is then placed across the body and immobilized. The period of immobilization is very controversial, ranging from 1 to 2 days (as pain subsides) up to 6 weeks. The above maneuvers required to reduce the shoulder should not be performed by the uninitiated.

The patient may be placed on electrical muscle stimulation of the pectoralis major as it inserts into the humerus within 48 hours of injury. Soft tissue manipulation including transverse frictional massage and trigger point therapy should also be applied to the muscles about the shoulder. After the immobilization phase of recovery, the shoulder should be evaluated to detect the presence of an anteroinferior humeral subluxation. If present, manual correction as discussed earlier should follow. Also, once immobilization has ceased, the glenohumeral joint should be maintained with a supportive taping procedure (Fig. 16.36).

RECURRENT TRANSIENT SUBLUXATION OF THE SHOULDER

Definition. Transient subluxation of the shoulder may cause the so called dead-arm syndrome, which is characterized by a sudden sharp or paralyzing pain when the shoulder moves forcibly into a position of maximal external rotation in elevation or is subjected to a direct blow.

Etiology. Many of the recurrent subluxations of the shoulder are subjected to forceful external rotation in positions of abduction and varying amounts of hyperextension. Other forms of recurrent subluxation occur by direct trauma (17) or repetitive inferior tractional loads. This syndrome may also occur during throwing, repetitive forceful serving in tennis, or working with the arm in a strained position above the shoulder level.

Anatomic Considerations. Most frequently, the anterior capsule is stretched or detached, allowing the humeral head to slip forward when a certain point of abduction and external rotation is reached (18).

Symptoms. It is imperative to obtain a good history of the injury. Many times the patient will complain of inter-

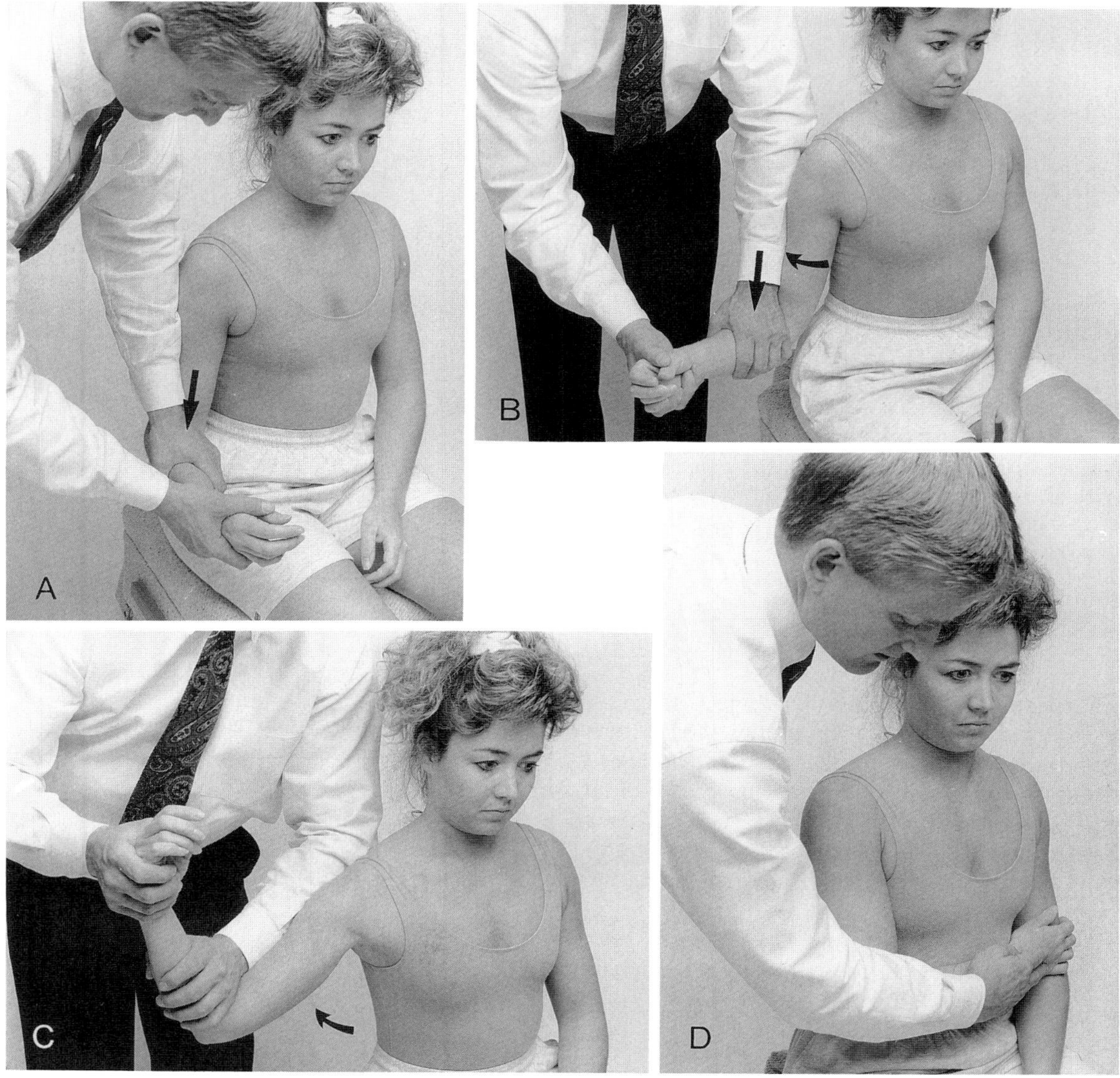

Figure 16.35A-D. Reduction technique for anteroinferior glenohumeral dislocation.

mittent shoulder pain and/or weakness, crepitus, and loss of various ranges of motion.

Diagnostic Work-Up. Passive and active ranges of motion of the shoulder demonstrate normal range without pain. Orthopaedic examination should include the apprehension test. Muscle testing should be performed for the deltoid, supraspinatus, teres minor and major, infraspinatus, subscapularis, and pectoral muscles.

Radiographically, Hill-Sach's lesions of the humeral head may be found. This deformity occurs with impaction of the humeral head on the inferior glenoid rim. A true axillary radiograph (Fig. 16.37) will show changes along the anterior rim of the glenoid.

Magnetic resonance imaging of the shoulder may aid in demonstrating anterior instability. Signs specifically related to the disruption of the anterior capsule are very commonly identified in patients with instability. One of the results of capsular stripping or detachment that occurs in these patients after the first and subsequent dislocations is a large anterior pouch, usually in association with a large subscapularis bursa. This then forms a potential space into which the humeral head can dislocate or subluxate (19).

Treatment. Initial chiropractic treatment of recurrent subluxation of the shoulder should include restoring normal position of the humeral head in the glenoid rim. Because the majority of these conditions are anterior and inferior, the humerus should be set inferior to superior and anterior to posterior. This should then be followed up with electrical muscle stimulation to the pectoralis clavicular division with a 15-second contraction time and a 45-second release time over a period of 15 minutes. This

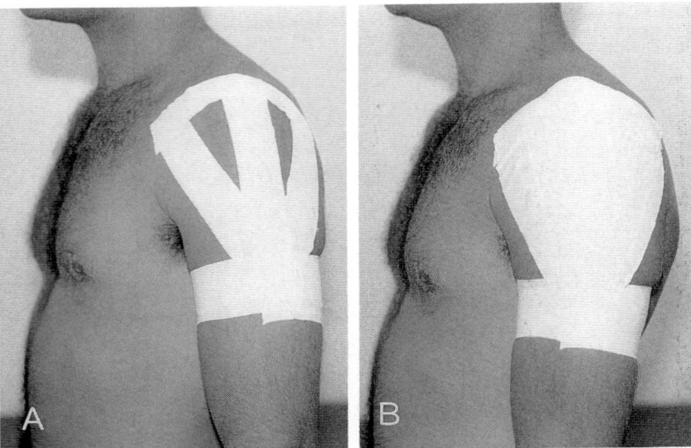

Figure 16.36. Glenohumeral supportive tape procedure. **A,** A superior anchor strip is applied proximal to the glenohumeral joint and an inferior anchor strip encompasses the mid-portion of the humerus. **B,** Closing strips are applied inferior to superior to give support to the joint.

should be performed at intervals of three times per week for 2 to 6 weeks. Supportive taping may also prove beneficial.

As with rehabilitation of any joint, full range of motion with progressive resistance is indicated within pain limits. Surgical tubing exercises may be included to improve strength and stability of the internal and external rotators of the shoulder. Soft tissue work such as transverse friction massage and trigger point therapy may also be applied to the internal and external rotators of the shoulder.

If after 4 to 8 weeks of conservative care, the shoulder remains unstable, further chiropractic or orthopaedic consultation should be obtained.

IMPINGEMENT SYNDROME

Definition. This disorder is a painful condition that most commonly results from entrapment of the supraspinatus tendon between the humeral head of the acromion, the coracoacromial ligament, or acromioclavicular clavicular joint (20–22).

Etiology. The impingement occurs between the anterior edge and undersurface of the anterior third of the acromion, the coracoacromial ligament, and at times, the acromioclavicular joint, rather than against the lateral acromion (22). When the arm is raised forward, the supraspinatus passes under the anterior edge of the acromion and the acromioclavicular joint. Further, any disorder that results in an increase volume of the rotator cuff tendons, such as hypertrophy, and arthritic degeneration, may predispose the patient to this disorder (23). Shoulder impingement syndrome has been divided into three stages:

1. *Stage 1 Edema and Hemorrhage:* This phase is characterized by edema and hemorrhage which may result from excessive overhead use in sports or work (23). Individuals usually suffering from this particular phase are 25 years of age or younger.
2. *Stage 2 Fibrosis and Tendonitis:* This phase is less common than Stage 1. It occurs with repeated episodes of overuse. The shoulder function is satisfactory for light activity but becomes symptomatic after vigorous overhead use. Commonly, individuals with this particular lesion are in the age range of 25 to 40 years (23).
3. *Stage 3 Tears of the Rotator Cuff, Biceps Ruptures and Bone Changes:* During this phase of injury, the patient is usually greater than 40 years of age. With chronic impingement and wear, tears of the rotator cuff, biceps lesions, and bone alterations may be seen at the anterior acromion and greater tuberosity (23). The earliest bone changes evidenced radiographically include a slight prominence on the greater tuberosity at the point of insertion of the supraspinatus tendon, and a traction spur at the anterior acromion which is inside the coracoacromial ligament (22).

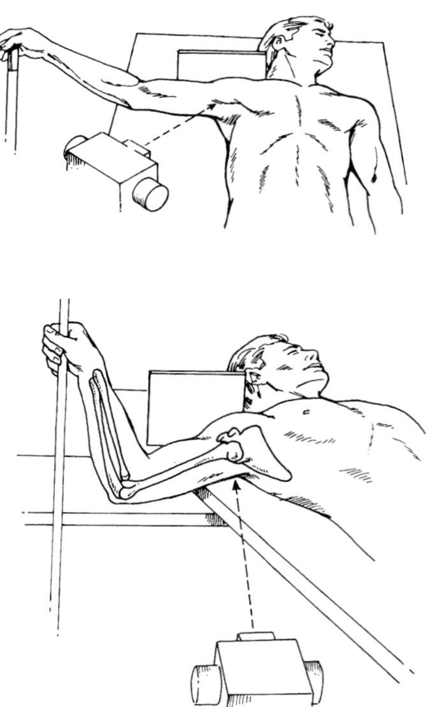

Figure 16.37. True axillary radiograph technique. Modified from Resnick D, Niwawama G. Diagnosis of bone and joint disorders. 2nd. ed. Philadelphia: WB Saunders, 1988:17.

Signs and Symptoms. Initially, the patient presents with a dull ache over the anterior, posterior, and lateral aspects of the shoulder. This is usually brought on by strenuous activity as occurs with competitive swimmers and pitchers.

The patient suffering from Stage 2 impingement syndrome will present with a persistent dull ache in the shoulder which often interferes with sleep and work. Because of the chronic inflammation in the region, there may be restrictions with shoulder movements during activities of daily living.

The Stage 3 patient demonstrates a symptomatic presentation of prolonged periods of pain, especially at night. Weakness of the shoulder may also be present.

Clinical Findings. Stage 1 impingement syndrome demonstrates: (*a*) palpable tenderness over the greater tuberosity at the supraspinatus insertion; (*b*) palpable tenderness along the anterior edge of the acromion; (*c*) a painful arc of abduction between 60° and 120° (24).

Stage 2 impingement syndrome demonstrates palpable tenderness over the greater tuberosity at the supraspinatus insertion with associated palpable tenderness along the anterior edge of the acromion. Additionally, there is: (*a*) a greater degree of soft tissue crepitus, due to scarring in the subacromial space; (*b*) a catching sensation with reversal of elevation at approximately 100°, thought to represent scar tissue entrapment beneath the acromion; and (*c*) mild limitation to both passive and active range of motion (24).

Stage 3 impingement syndrome includes all of the findings found in Stage 1 and Stage 2 as well as: (*a*) limitation to shoulder motion, active being more limited that passive; (*b*) infraspinatus atrophy; (*c*) weakness of shoulder abduction and external rotation; (*d*) biceps tendon involvement with rupture or degenerative changes, which occurs in a high percentage of patients with rotator cuff tears; and (*e*) acromioclavicular joint tenderness, especially if degenerative changes are present (24).

Diagnosis. The diagnosis of impingement syndrome can be made on the basis of a good clinical examination (25). The "impingement sign" is elicited with the patient seated and the examiner standing. Scapular rotation is prevented with one hand while the other hand raises the arm in forced forward elevation, thereby causing the greater tuberosity to impinge against the acromion (23). Another evaluation can be performed by forcibly internally rotating the forward flexed proximal humerus, which forces the greater tuberosity against the leading edge of the coracoacromial ligament, producing an impingement sign (24). Manual muscle testing may reveal weakness of the supraspinatus muscle.

Plain film radiographic alterations may include bone proliferation, eburnation, and cystic change in the greater tuberosity (26). A well-defined osseous excrescence, termed a subacromial spur, is present in some patients with this syndrome. It extends from the anterior inferior aspect of the acromion and is best visualized on an anteroposterior radiograph with 30° of caudal angulation of the x-ray beam (27). The subacromial spur appears to be a traction phenomenon created by the repetitive impingement of the greater tuberosity on the coracoacromial ligament (26).

Magnetic resonance imaging of the shoulder can play an important part in making the diagnosis of impingement syndrome. The distal supraspinatus tendon will demonstrate an increased signal intensity. This increase is probably related to a number of factors including edema and inflammatory changes, as well as mucoid degenerative changes (28). It may also be noted that the anterior acromion is at a distinctly lower positional level than the distal clavicle. Neer (22) felt that an abnormal size or position of the anterior aspect of the acromion can predispose a patient to impingement syndrome.

Treatment. Impingement syndrome should be treated conservatively in Stage 1. This should include decreased activity (limited external rotation and abduction). Applications of ice should be recommended to mitigate the acute severity. During the acute phase, stretching of the external rotators of the arm can be performed. This is a combined movement of horizontal abduction and internal rotation while blocking the scapula from movement. Further, exercises within pain-free range of motion to enhance glenohumeral range of motion, such as Codman's pendulum exercises, should be incorporated. Also, exercises to help decompress the supraspinatus should be performed. This may include strengthening the pectoralis major (sternal division), latissimus dorsi, serratus anterior, rhomboid major and minor, trapezius, and levator scapulae.

The doctor should also evaluate the painful shoulder with regard to joint fixation. This should include examination of the A-C joint, the scapulothoracic articulation, and the glenohumeral joint. If an area of fixation dysfunction is identified, the structures involved should be adjusted accordingly. Areas of fixation in the spine (cervical and thoracic) should be evaluated as well. Restoration of function in the cervical and thoracic spine will enhance neurologic function at the affected extremity.

ROTATOR CUFF LESIONS

Definition. Lesions of the rotator cuff are common in the adult. The most common site of injury is the supraspinatus tendon. In the young athlete, such lesions are probably due mainly to wear and tear of the supraspinatus tendon as it passes under the acromion process (29). The rotator cuff is made up of the following muscles: supraspinatus, infraspinatus, teres minor, and subscapularis (30).

Tears of the rotator cuff may be considered partial or complete. Partial tears are of two types: 1) the intratendonous tear and 2) deep surface tear (3). Complete tears involve the entire thickness of the tendons thus causing exposure of the humeral head. The tendon most commonly involved is the supraspinatus. Less frequently, the infraspinatus and teres minor are torn.

Etiology. The supraspinatus muscle is located between the humeral head and acromion. This "sandwich" phenomenon, with its unyielding boundaries, may result in chronic bursal inflammation and tendonitis which eventually leads to significant tendon degeneration and tearing (31). It must be noted that the coracoacromial ligament contributes to the anterior one-third of the acromial arch which also introduces compressive forces on the rotator cuff.

The supraspinatus tendon has been studied by Rathbon and McNab (32) who demonstrated a hypovascularity in the area of the supraspinatus insertion. This may help explain why tears in the rotator cuff take time to heal.

Historically, there are five mechanisms through which a rotator cuff tear can occur: an injury without fracture or dislocation of the shoulder; anterior dislocation of the shoulder; dislocation with a fracture of the greater tuberosity; chronically with or without a history of injury; and avulsion fracture of the greater tuberosity (33).

Signs and Symptoms. Patients may be of any age when they present with a cuff tear, but clearly, the majority of symptomatic rotator cuff tears occur in patients over the age of 40 (31). Commonly, the patient may present with pain in the area of the rotator cuff which is most noticeable at night. Pain may be experienced in the area of the biceps tendon which radiates cephalically towards the neck. Activities that involve raising the arm above the level of the shoulder in internal or external rotation may become awkward and painful.

Clinical Findings. Examination should include bony and soft tissue comparison of the involved shoulder with the noninjured extremity. Active and passive range of motion should be noted with particular attention to abduction and internal and external rotation. Isolated strength examination should be performed on the supraspinatus, infraspinatus, teres minor, deltoid, and the subscapularis muscles. Weakness of the supraspinatus muscle is common, as is weakness of any of the rotator cuff muscles if they are involved.

Diagnosis. Injuries to the rotator cuff have been categorized into four stages: In Stage 1, the rotator cuff becomes inflamed and contracted with concurrent muscle atrophy (34). Stage 2 lesions involve fibrous disruption without an actual tear in the muscle. Stage 3 demonstrates permanent thickening of the bursa accompanied by a 1-cm or less defect in the tissue. Stage 4 demonstrates permanent thickening of the bursa along with a tear greater than 1 cm.

Plain film examination of a shoulder with a suspected tear should aid the examiner in evaluating alignment, bony structures, and soft tissue changes. Further examination of the shoulder with a suspected tear in the rotator cuff should include magnetic resonance imaging which will help demonstrate a tear in the tissues. If a tear is identified, this examination should be followed up with arthrography to better determine the extent of the tear.

Treatment. Rotator cuff tears in Stage 1 or Stage 2 should be treated conservatively. Early management of this lesion should include passive range of motion, soft tissue mobilization, trigger point therapy as needed, and shoulder manipulation when indicated. Cryotherapy can be applied over the involved area. Stretching exercises should be performed with the arm in 90° of shoulder abduction, 90° of elbow flexion, and as much external rotation as can be achieved at the glenohumeral joint (34). A second stretching exercise will require the patient to lie diagonally on the table to allow head support while the shoulder hangs over the edge. The arm is put as far over head as possible, with the palm towards the ceiling, weight in hand, and the elbow extended (34). As pain-free range of motion increases, the patient should begin active strengthening of the damaged muscles. In terms of recovery of musculature strength and power, evidence is beginning to accumulate that isokinetic training is the most effective means of rehabilitation after injury (35–37).

If isokinetic equipment is not available, strengthening exercises can be performed using rubber tubing. In using rubber tubing, the examiner must keep in mind that early strengthening programs should be initiated during mid-range excursion of the muscle, performed rapidly and pain free. As strength increases, the arc of motion performed with the tubing increases until full pain-free motion is possible. These larger arcs are performed slowly to reduce the likelihood of "pushing" the joint through a painful range of motion.

If the shoulder arthrogram demonstrates extravasation of contrast material from the joint into the adjoining soft tissues, surgical consultation is recommended.

ADHESIVE CAPSULITIS (FROZEN SHOULDER)

Definition. Adhesive capsulitis is a condition that begins with insidious onset of pain and gradual restriction of movement in the shoulder region (38). Often, the pain associated with this condition radiates medially and cephalically into the upper back and neck. The pain is exacerbated with even minimal shoulder movement.

Etiology. The etiology of this condition remains unknown. Typically, there is an insidious onset of gradually progressive shoulder pain with marked limitation of movement. Features of this pathologic condition include microscopic evidence of chronic capsular inflammation with fibrosis and perivascular infiltration (38–40). Immunologic studies in individuals with this condition reveal that a certain percentage of patients have HLA B27 antigen (41).

Chronic cases of adhesive capsulitis are characterized by adhesions of the synovial folds, obliteration of the joint cavity, and a thickened, contracted capsule that eventually becomes fixed to the bone (39,42,43). Other factors that have been implicated include recurrent trauma to the shoulder, manual work, thyroid disease, ischemic heart disease, repeated injection of phenobarbitone and isoniazid, and diabetes.

Anatomic Considerations. Current doctrine supports Neviaser's theory that the capsule is the sight of the lesion and lends credence to the synonymous use of the terms adhesive capsulitis and frozen shoulder (44). The anteroinferior aspect of the dependent fold between the long head of the biceps and the subscapularis tendon is the region where adhesions develop within the fold itself and also at the glenoid fossa and humerus (45,46).

Signs and Symptoms. With many patients, there is a description of an onset of acute pain that progresses during the first few weeks and months. Individuals frequently complain of night pain that is manifested on awakening when rolling over on the affected side. The pain is distributed vaguely in the deltoid muscle area (44). The pain is present at rest and during activity. With time, the pain abates spontaneously; however, motion restriction persists. Some patients also complain of proximal soreness of the upper back and neck, a symptom probably attributable to the compensatory overuse of shoulder girdle muscles, such as the trapezius, rather than to referred pain from the shoulder (44). The pain associated with this condition is often described as a mild to severe ache.

Clinical Findings. Most patients are between the ages of 40 and 50 years (39). The magnitude of pain ranges from mild to severe and is characteristically described as a dull ache which is poorly localized. The pain is generally noted to be more intense at the posterior and superior aspects of the shoulder. Women frequently complain of inability to hook a bra or comb hair, whereas men experience difficulty in reaching for a wallet or the back of a shirt collar (39). Restriction of movement at first seems secondary to pain, but subsequently, measurable limitation of both active and passive range of motion in different planes is noted (38).

The syndrome usually progresses through four stages:

1. *Stage 1:* The patient usually presents with signs and symptoms of the impingement syndrome. Motion usually is restricted very little, if at all. Stage 1 is commonly misdiagnosed as rotator cuff tendonitis (47).
2. *Stage 2:* Arthroscopy demonstrates the synovium is red and thickened with adhesions visualized growing across the dependent fold of the capsule onto the humeral head. There are decreased joint spaces between the humeral head and glenoid, as well as the space between the humeral head and biceps tendon (47). Physical exam during this stage will demonstrate marked loss of motion throughout all planes with associated pain in all ranges of motion.
3. *Stage 3:* Arthroscopy demonstrates a pink synovitis that is not as marked as in Stage 2; however, the dependent fold of the capsule is noted to be half its original size. The humeral head is still positioned against the glenoid and bicipital tendon.
4. *Stage 4:* Arthroscopy demonstrates no synovitis. The dependent fold of the capsule is markedly contracted and motion is essentially lost. The humeral head continues to be pressed against the glenoid and biceps tendon.

Diagnosis. Depending on the stage, the patient will demonstrate decreased ranges of motion with associated pain. Plain film radiography in the early stages may not show any bony or soft tissue abnormalities. In long-standing cases, the most common radiographic finding is localized osteoporosis of the humeral head (48). Arthrography is the most reliable method to make the diagnosis. The arthrographic evidence of adhesive capsulitis is loss of the normally loose dependent fold of the joint and a dramatic decrease in the volume of contrast material that can be injected (47).

Clinical examination of the cervical spine should be performed. This should include, range of motion, orthopaedic, and neurologic examination. Pain sometimes radiates distally along the C5 dermatome.

Treatment. Early treatment of adhesive capsulitis should be initially conservative, with the emphasis on controlling inflammation and passive stretching of the capsular structures (47). This should be followed up with passive joint mobilization. Joint mobilization should occur in the direction of the joints accessory motion. The accessory motions are described as small spinning, gliding, rolling or distractive movements that occur between joint surfaces and are essential for normal mobility (49). As the range of motion increases in the affected shoulder, active exercises can be performed by the patient at home. Early home exercises should include pendulum and finger climbing up a wall.

Rizk et al. (38) developed a unique approach for the treatment of this condition in the acute phase. Their study reported 28 cases treated with range of motion exercises as well as pulley traction and the use of transcutaneous nerve stimulation (38). At the end of the study, the patients had 90% of full range of motion and pain-free sleep by 8 months.

Patients suffering from this condition should have the cervical spine examined. This examination should determine areas of hypomobility or fixation. Specific gentle cervical adjustments should be performed to help restore normal function.

The patient should respond to conservative treatment within 3 to 6 months. If desired clinical results are not forthcoming, an outside chiropractic or orthopaedic consultation is advised. If, however, conservative treatment continues to fail in delivering the desired results, the patient should be advised about manipulation under anesthesia. The procedure is as follows: an assistant stabilizes the scapula, the shoulder is then gently manipulated into abduction, then into flexion, and then combined with internal and external rotation (50). On completion of this maneuver, the arm is placed into 90° abduction with the use of a swathe tied to the head of the bed. Twenty-four hours postmanipulation under anesthesia, range of motion is maintained by instituting an active exercise program. This is monitored at intervals of five times a week for 2 weeks and then three times a week for the next 2 weeks (50). Manipulation under anesthesia is not without risk, because tissues are grossly torn and may develop further scarring (44). Further, manipulation also increases the possibility of fractures, dislocation, and brachial plexus injuries (40,51).

ACROMIOCLAVICULAR SEPARATION

Definition. The acromioclavicular separation is defined as partial or complete tearing of the coracoacromial ligament, acromioclavicular ligament, and coracoclavicular ligaments (trapezoid ligament, conoid ligament).

Etiology. The acromioclavicular (A-C) joint is the most commonly sprained joint in the shoulder complex. Injuries to the A-C joint occur mainly by a direct fall on the shoulder or falling on the hand of an outstretched arm. The degree of disruption of the acromioclavicular and coracoclavicular ligaments varies. The initial injury is to the acromioclavicular ligaments followed by damage to the coracoclavicular ligament.

Signs and Symptoms. Acromioclavicular joint separations have been classified into three categories: A Grade 1 (first degree) demonstrates pain and discomfort directly over the joint. The differentiation between a mild sprain and a contusion is extremely difficult, because a mild sprain does not demonstrate hypermobility, and indeed, normal motions of the shoulder girdle will elicit no pain (29). A Grade 2 (second degree) will elicit pain on forced motion of the shoulder. Pain, tenderness, and swelling will also be localized to the acromioclavicular joint. Palpatory tenderness may be noted over the coracoclavicular ligaments. Range of motion of the shoulder will be limited due to pain. A slight elevation of the acromioclavicular joint may be present. A Grade 3 (third degree) demonstrates marked swelling, and point tenderness about the joint. Point tenderness will also be noted about the coracoclavicular ligaments. There is marked elevation of the distal end of the clavicle. The patient often holds the arm, because any downward pull or motion increases the pain and discomfort from the joint.

Clinical Findings. Allman's classification of injuries to the acromioclavicular joint into Grades 1, 2, and 3 has been widely accepted (52).

Grade 1 injuries to the acromioclavicular joint demonstrate minimal tearing of the joint capsule and ligaments. The A-C articulation appears normal on visual inspection. Grade 2 A-C separation demonstrates tearing of the capsule and A-C ligament along with some tearing of the coracoclavicular ligament. The distal portion of the clavicle may demonstrate slight elevation with associated swelling and point tenderness. Point tenderness will also be noted over the coracoclavicular ligaments. Further, pain is exacerbated with abduction of the arm. Grade 3 injuries demonstrate marked elevation of the distal clavicle. This injury demonstrates complete tearing of the capsule, A-C ligaments, and coracoclavicular ligaments. There is often damage to the deltoid and trapezius muscles (53). A Grade 4 type separation has been defined although it is very rare. This is a true posterior dislocation with tearing of all ligaments and buttonhole placement of the clavicle through the fibers of the trapezius muscle.

Diagnosis. The clinical presentation and plain film radiographs assist with the diagnosis. With Grade 1 type injuries, the plain film will be essentially normal. In Grade 2 separation, the stress radiograph will demonstrate elevation of the distal clavicle. In normal studies, the acromioclavicular articulations should measure 11 to 13 mm in width (16). A Grade 2 injury will have an A-C interval greater than 13 mm. A Grade 3 acromioclavicular separation will demonstrate a marked increase in the A-C interval. There will also be an increase in the coracoclavicular space. This is due to the disruption of the conoid and trapezoid ligaments.

Treatment. With Grade 1 A-C sprains, treatment should be focused on reducing the inflammatory response to the joint. Cryotherapy should be used on and about the injured joint. Further, stabilization of the joint can be enhanced by strengthening the anterior deltoid. Soft tissue mobilization, pain-free range of motion below 90° of shoulder abduction, trigger point therapy, and transverse frictional massage should be performed around the injured joint to minimize local adhesions.

Grade 2 separations can also be treated conservatively. The distal acromioclavicular joint will demonstrate subluxation in the superior direction. Applications of ice should be placed over the affected joint. After 20 minutes of cryotherapy, the distal clavicle can be adjusted in a superior to inferior direction. Once this procedure has been completed, the arm should be placed across the body and a Kenny/Howard splint applied. This splint provides vertical control of both the acromion and clavicle in achieving and maintaining reduction. If bracing is not available or desired the distal clavicle may be secured by use of athletic tape (Fig. 16.38A-B). The splint or tape should be worn for 2 to 4 weeks. The patient can be seen on a daily basis for 5 days to ensure proper alignment of the joint. Soft tissue mobilization, trigger point therapy and transverse frictional massage can also be applied to the affected area. Applications of electrical muscle stimulation can be performed on the anterior deltoid in a strengthening mode to help assist the clavicle in maintaining its proper position. Applications of ice should be used after each treatment program. During the second through fourth week of treatment, the patient may be given home exercises to further enhance strengthening of the anterior deltoid.

Taft et al. (52) found that most patients who have a Grade 3 injury can be treated nonoperatively, using a Kenny/Howard splint. The goal is to maintain the position of the distal part of the clavicle so that its distal edge is separated from the proximal part of the acromion by only 2 to 3 mm to minimize cosmetic deformity. The

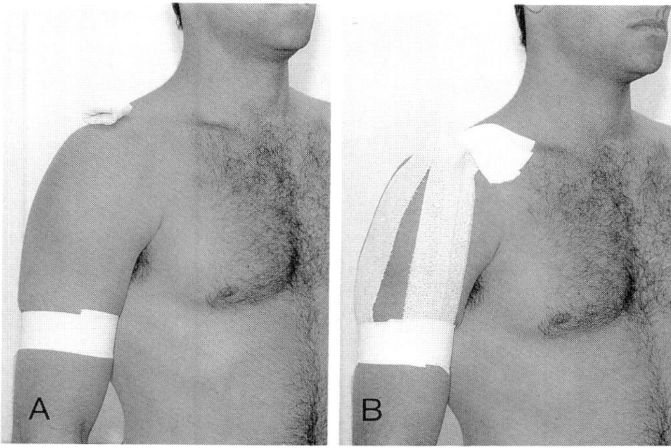

Figure 16.38. A-C sprain supportive taping procedure. **A,** A pad is placed over the distal aspect of the clavicle and an anchor strip is placed around the midportion of the humerus. **B,** Elastic tape connects the clavicular pad with the humeral anchor strip. This maintains a downward force on the clavicle allowing the soft tissue components of the joint to heal.

splint is worn for 5 to 6 weeks to allow for sufficient maturation of the collagenous scar. This will prevent a latent increase in the deformity due to the weight of the arm (52). Surgical consultation should be considered if conservative measures fail.

Elbow

The humeroulnar and humeroradial joints, which are comprised osseously of the humerus, ulna and radius, make up two functional units: a uniaxial hinge (ginglymus) joint which permits flexion and extension and a trochoid joint which allows pronation and supination of the forearm and wrist. The trochlea of the humerus articulates with the trochlear notch of the ulna, while the capitulum of the humerus opposes the head of the radius (8,13) (Fig. 16.39A-C).

The elbow is enveloped in a fibrous capsule that attaches proximally to the humerus just above the olecranon and the coranoid fossa, distally to the ulna just behind the greater sigmoid notch, and to the neck of the radius and the lesser sigmoid notch. The capsule is thin, pliable, and redundant anteriorly and posteriorly to permit freedom during flexion and extension (8). The collateral ligaments are found on the inner and outer aspects of the capsule and provide stability by checking mediolateral motion. The collateral ligaments are divided into: 1) medial collateral (internal); 2) lateral collateral (external); and 3) annular ligaments (orbicular). The medial collateral ligament extends from the lower edge of the medial epicondyle and fans out to attach to the margin of the greater sigmoid fossa. The lateral collateral ligament extends from the lower edge of the lateral epicondyle and passes distally to blend with the annular ligament. The annular ligament is composed of transversely oriented fibers that encircle the radial head and attach to the radial notch anteriorly and posteriorly (8,13,16).

KINESIOLOGY

The axis of motion around which the elbow flexes and extends is represented by a line through the centers of the capitulum and the trochlea. With the forearm held in full supination, active flexion of the elbow is approximately 135° to 145°, whereas the range for passive flexion is 150° to 160°. Extension, both passive and active, is 0° (8,13).

Because the trochlea extends further distally than does the capitulum, the axis for flexion and extension of the elbow is not fully perpendicular to the shaft of the humerus. When the elbow is positioned in full extension, the forearm deviates laterally from the humerus. This angle of deflection is known as the Carry Angle. The average angle for the male elbow is 5° and for the female, 10° to 5° (10,11) (Fig. 16.40). Significant deviations of the angle are usually the result of epiphyseal injury or fracture malunion during bone maturation. Such deviations rarely result in functional abnormalities (26).

SUPERIOR AND INFERIOR RADIOULNAR JOINTS

The superior (proximal) radioulnar joint is contained within the capsule of the elbow joint and is described as a pivot (trochoid) joint. The circular head of the radius articulates with the radial notch of the ulna. Both the inner surface of the annular ligament and the head of the radius are lined with articular cartilage. The joint allows for supination and pronation of the forearm. Pronation of the forearm is 70° to 80°. Supination of the forearm ranges from 80° to 90° (8,13). The inferior radioulnar joint is composed of the ulnar notch of the distal radius, an articular disc, and the head of the ulna (Fig. 16.41). The disc is triangular in shape with its base at the ulnar notch and its apex attached to the styloid process of the ulna. The articular surface of the radius is concave. The radius, along with the wrist and hand, rotate around the head of the ulna.

RADIOGRAPHIC ANALYSIS

The standard radiographic series for the elbow is composed of three views: anteroposterior, lateral, and a tangential (Jones) projection (54). The anteroposterior view demonstrates the distal humerus, the proximal ulna, the proximal radius, as well as the elbow joint space. This view is used to rule out osseous fracture or dislocation and joint space abnormalities. The lateral projection is useful in the detection of fractures of the olecranon process, the

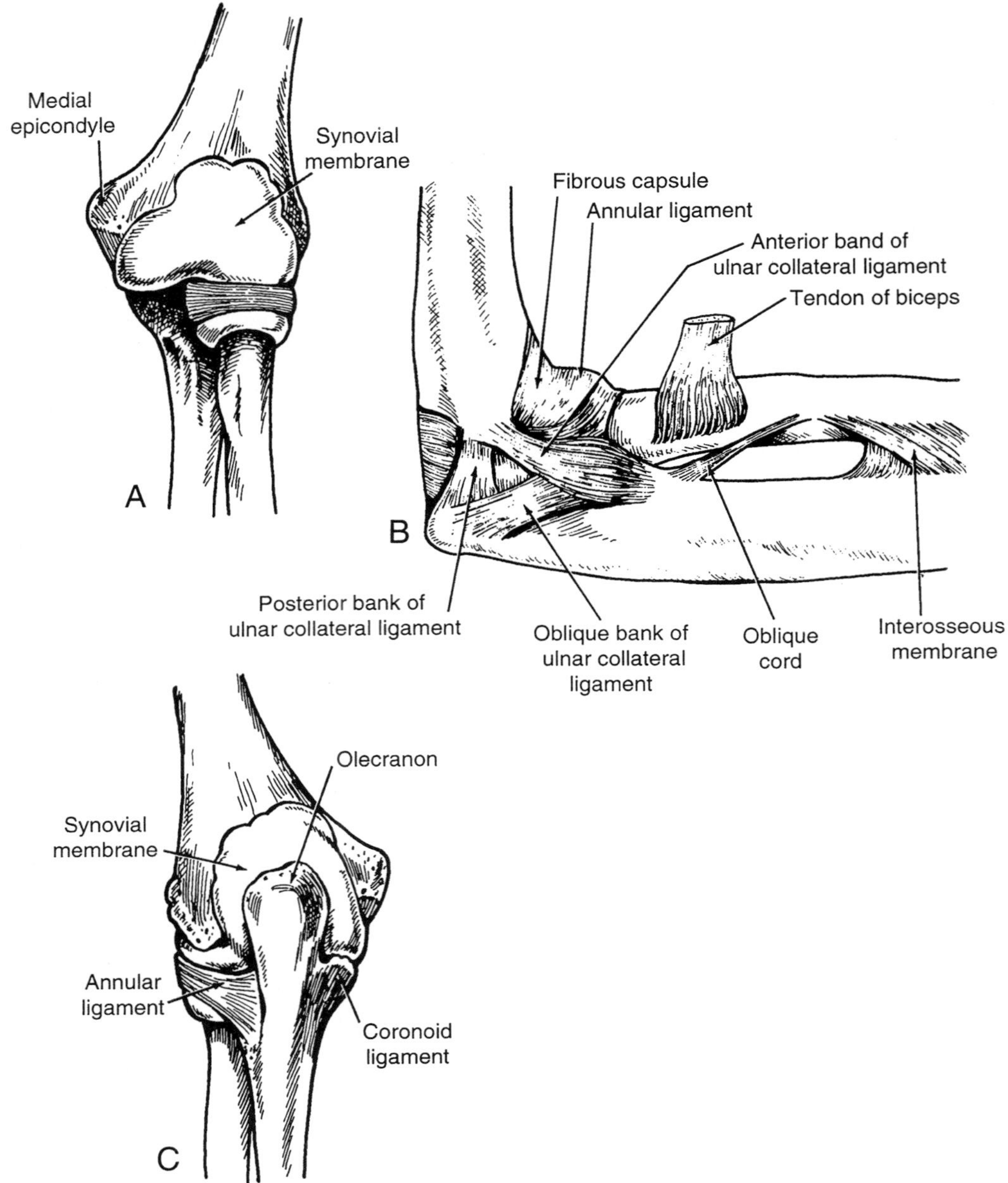

Figure 16.39. **A,** AP view of the elbow joint. Modified from Warwick R, Williams P. Gray's anatomy. 35th British ed. Philadelphia: WB Saunders, 1980:461. **B,** Medial view of the elbow. Modified from Warwick R, Williams P. Gray's anatomy. 35th British ed. Philadelphia: WB Saunders, 1980:463. **C,** PA view of the elbow joint.

radial head, and the coranoid process. The Jones view is important in the detection of intraarticular loose bodies.

Common Disorders of the Elbow

EPICONDYLITIS (MEDIAL AND LATERAL)

Definition. Epicondylitis designates a pattern of pain at the origins of either the extensors of the fingers and wrist on the lateral epicondyle of the humerus (tennis elbow), or the flexors on the medial epicondyle (little leaguer's or golfer's elbow) (55). The lateral epicondyle is said to be seven times more involved than the medial.

Etiology. Activities which require repetitive pronation and supination movements with the elbow almost fully extended are commonly present in the development of epicondylitis. Such activities include performing work with a screwdriver, hammer, lifting or ironing, or playing tennis or the violin (56).

Several pathologies have also been named with this condition: traumatic periostitis, arthritis, synovitis, sprain, adhesions of the radiohumeral joint, adhesions of the radioulnar joint, frayed or torn orbicular ligament, bursitis, tears of the extensor tendons and infection (56).

The various conditions on the lateral side which may

be labeled tennis elbow are: 1) true epicondylitis of the extensor supinator aponeurotic attachment to the lateral epicondyle; 2) radioulnar synovitis marked by development of a pannus of synovium between the radius and ulna; 3) strain in the aponeurosis itself, often directly over the radial head; and 4) radiohumeral bursitis (29). Attending injuries to the lateral aspect of the elbow may also produce avascular necrosis and osteochondral fractures. Medial lesions may develop from strains from the origin of the wrist flexors, ulnar neuritis, or ulnar nerve entrapment.

Anatomic Considerations. Lateral lesions of the elbow are commonly related to macroscopic or microscopic tears in the extensor carpi radialis brevis or the common extensor origin (55). The medial lesions primarily involve the flexor carpi radialis, pronator teres and less commonly, the palmaris longus, flexor carpi ulnaris and flexor sublimis (29). In the young athlete, problems in this region may be related to an ununited epiphysis.

Symptoms. With lateral epicondylitis, pain is noted on palpation about the radiohumeral articulation and the lateral epicondyle. A persistent ache may also be noted throughout the joint. With medial epicondylitis, pain is noted primarily at the medial epicondyle and the origin of the wrist flexors. Activities which require grasping objects with the hand and pronating and supinating movements reproduce the symptoms.

Clinical Findings. The onset of symptoms is usually gradual. A persistent dull ache appears over the lateral or medial aspect of the elbow and may be referred into the forearm. The condition is exacerbated with movements requiring grasping and twisting motions of the hand and wrist. A well-localized point of tenderness exists at one of the following sites: the epicondylar ridge, the lateral epicondyle, the lower edge of the capitulum, the lateral radiohumeral interval, or the area overlying the radial head during rotation of the forearm (16). Digital palpation may reveal articular swelling and protrusion. The shoulder complex should also be evaluated because of its possible kinetic chain effect on the elbow.

Diagnosis. Motion of the elbow should be performed for all planes. In most instances, range of motion will be complete. Point tenderness may be noted with digital palpation over the radiohumeral articulation, the lateral epicondyle or the medial epicondyle. Hypomobility may be noted with compression, distraction and medial to lateral glide of this articulation. Grip strength should be noted bilaterally. Often, the affected limb will demonstrate weakness. Orthopaedic testing includes Cozen's, Mill's, and Kaplan's tests.

The cervical spine should also be evaluated for range of motion, fixation dysfunction, muscle tightness and tenderness, and nerve root irritation.

Plain film radiography of the elbow is usually normal; however, osteochondral fragments may be found. If the condition has been long standing, a periositis may be seen. As a rule, periositis is seen only after months or years of disability (56). With acute elbow conditions, especially after trauma, the radiograph should be inspected for a Fat

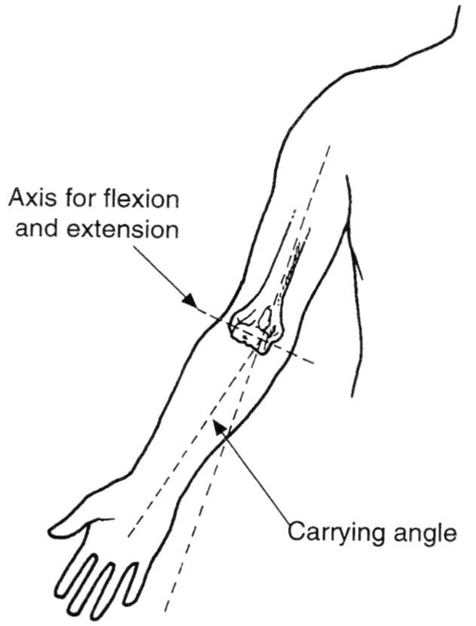

Figure 16.40. Carry angle and axis of rotation of the elbow joint. Modified from Lehmkuhl LD, Smith LK. Brunnstrom's clinical kinesiology. Philadelphia: FA Davis, 1983:149.

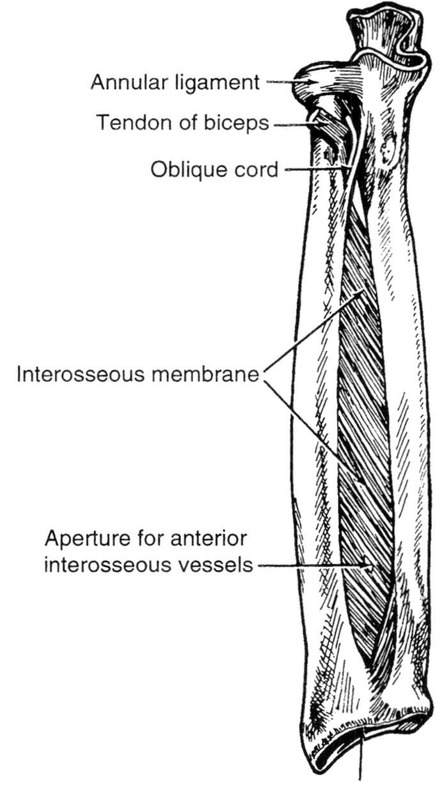

Figure 16.41. Superior and inferior radioulnar joints. Modified from Warwick R, Williams P. Gray's anatomy. 35th British ed. Philadelphia: WB Saunders, 1980:465.

Pad sign. If present, either advanced soft tissue injury or fracture is present.

Treatment. It should be emphasized that tennis elbow is a common lesion which usually responds to conservative treatment (57). Initial management should include isolation of the joint fixation followed with manipulation. Before manipulative treatment it is often necessary to mildly mobilize or "pump" the articulation to increase joint mobility. Soft tissue mobilization and trigger point therapy should be performed over the medial and lateral epicondyles, the triceps, the biceps brachii, the brachialis, the brachioradialis, the wrist flexors, and the wrist extensors. Ice massage may be performed over the involved structures.

Rehabilitative exercises for the elbow include the following:

1. Wrist flexion, extension, supination, and pronation range of motion stretches.
2. Elbow flexion, extension, supination, and pronation range of motion stretches.
3. Wrist curls and reverse curls with wrist weights.
4. Elbow curls, reverse curls, thumb up and thumb down curls with wrist weights.
5. Squeezing a rubber ball.

Supporting the elbow with a neoprene sleeve is helpful and allows for rest of the joint. The condition should resolve within 4 to 6 weeks.

Wrist and Hand

The wrist is composed of: (*a*) the distal ulna, (*b*) the proximal row of carpals consisting of the scaphoid (navicular), the lunate, the triquetrum, the pisiform, and (*c*) the distal carpal row comprised of the trapezium, the trapezoid, the capitate, and the hamate (Fig. 16.42). Discussions in this text, in regards to the wrist and hand, shall be limited to the radiocarpal joint, the midcarpal joint (the articulation between the proximal and distal rows of carpal bones), the carpometacarpal joints of digits II through V, and the carpometacarpal joint of the thumb.

RADIOCARPAL JOINT

The radiocarpal joint is classified as condyloid. The distal end of the radius is concave, and this surface articulates with a disc. Opposing the radius are the convex surfaces of the proximal scaphoid and lunate. Please note that neither the distal ulna nor the triquetrum possesses articular surfaces and is anatomically separated from the radiocarpal joint by the articular disc. Clinically, the lunate is found to be the most commonly dislocated or subluxated carpal bone while the scaphoid is the most frequently fractured carpal bone.

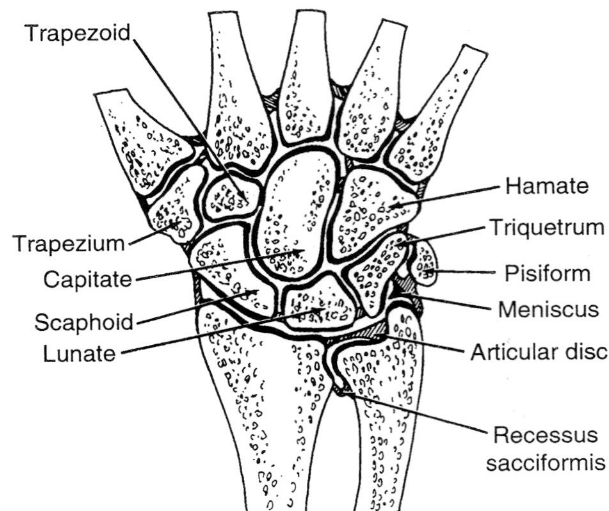

Figure 16.42. Wrist and hand. Modified from Warwick R, Williams P. Gray's anatomy. 35th British ed. Philadelphia: WB Saunders, 1980:467.

KINESIOLOGY

During flexion, the scaphoid and lunate glide posteriorly while in extension they slide anteriorly. Radial deviation primarily occurs as the distal carpals move on the proximal carpals. Ulnar deviation occurs predominantly as radiocarpal motion (8,13,58).

The normal ranges of motion for the wrist are as follows:

Flexion: 75° to 90°
Extension: 65° to 75°
Radial Deviation: 15° to 25°
Ulnar Deviation: 25° to 40°

MIDCARPAL JOINT

The midcarpal joint is the series of articulations located between the proximal and distal rows of carpal bones. It is not a true joint in terms of opposing uninterrupted articular surfaces and a joint capsule but rather a functional unit. Although small amounts of motion take place between the individual carpal bones, the majority of motion occurs at the midcarpal joint and consists primarily of flexion and extension.

CARPOMETACARPAL JOINTS OF DIGITS II AND V

The trapezoid, capitate, and hamate bones articulate with the proximal ends of the second through fifth metacarpals. Motion at these joints consists primarily of very limited amounts of flexion and extension as well as minimal amounts of rotation.

CARPOMETACARPAL JOINT OF THE FIRST DIGIT

The trapezium articulates with the proximal end of the first metacarpal. The joint is classified as saddle type. The capsule is thick and strong yet loose, which permits a great deal of motion. Flexion ranges from 40° to 90°. The joint also allows a minimal amount of abduction and adduction.

RADIOGRAPHIC ANALYSIS

The standard radiographic series for the wrist and hand includes six views: posteroanterior wrist, posteroanterior wrist with ulnar deviation, medial oblique wrist, lateral wrist, posteroanterior hand, and the oblique hand. If it is desirable to evaluate the wrist or hand independently, only the pertinent views need be obtained.

Although all of the aforementioned radiographs are useful in fracture and dislocation detection, the posteroanterior ulnar deviation projection and the lateral wrist projection are especially helpful. The posteroanterior ulnar deviation projection can be used to better visualize scaphoid fractures by distracting the fragments and widening the fracture line (59). The lateral wrist projection aids in the visualization of the carpal bones and their positional relationship to the distal radius.

Common Disorders of the Wrist

CARPAL TUNNEL SYNDROME

Definition. Carpal tunnel syndrome (CTS) is a compressive neuropathy of the median nerve. The compression occurs over the volar aspect of the wrist.

Etiology. There are many causes of carpal tunnel syndrome. The most common though is a thickening of the flexor synovalis in the carpal tunnel as a result of nonspecific inflammation of the tendons (60). Current theory cites carpal bone fixation dysfunction (subluxation) as a possible cause of local nonspecific inflammation. Numerous other causes have been linked to carpal tunnel syndrome and include gout, calcium pyrophosphate dehydrate crystal deposition disease, hydroxyapatitate crystal deposition disease, acromegaly, hypothyroidism, amyloidosis, rheumatoid arthritis, ganglion cysts, neuromas and other tumors, infection, thrombosis of the median artery, fibrosis of the tendon sheaths, muscle and bone anomalies, hemorrhage, and fractures or dislocations of the wrist (26).

Carpal tunnel syndrome occurs more often in women, in a ratio of 5 to 1. The average age of onset is between 30 to 50 years. CTS can be aggravated by activities such as sewing, peeling potatoes, using wrenches or vibratory tools, performing repetitive wrist movements, and heavy manual labor (16,61–64).

In most instances, the onset of CTS is insidious, spontaneous, and nocturnal (16).

Anatomic Considerations. The carpal groove is converted into an osseous fibrous carpal tunnel by a strong fibrous retinaculum attached to the bony margins (19). The tunnel transmits the flexor tendons and median nerve to the hand. Just proximal to the flexor retinaculum, the nerve is lateral to the tendons of the flexor digitorum superficialis but dorsal to the retinaculum. It is bound by the space in front of the retinaculum and behind the anterior surfaces of the carpal bones.

It is important to remember that the median nerve is responsible for most of the sympathetic nerve supply to the hand. This may explain the frequency of trophic disturbances associated with median nerve injury (16).

Clinical Findings. The initial onset may be a slight paresthesia which precedes the onset of the acute symptoms by several months. The paroxysms of pain, paresthesia, and numbness occur in the thumb, index, middle finger, and one-half of the ring finger (16). Atrophy and weakness may be seen in the thenar muscles.

The patient is commonly awakened after a few hours of sleep complaining of burning, aching, pricking, or pins and needles, and numbness in one or both hands (16). A deep aching sensation may be noted in the forearm, shoulder, and neck region. Difficulty may be noted with opposition of the thumb and fingers.

CTS usually develops in the dominant limb. Bilateral afflictions can occur and when this happens; it is usually first observed in the dominant limb.

Diagnosis. Physical examination will demonstrate a positive Tinel's sign (paresthesia noted over the distribution of the medial nerve after percussion over the volar aspect of the wrist) and reproduction of pain and paresthesia with the Phalen maneuver (flexion of the patient's hand at the wrist for greater than one minute) (26). The flick sign has also been noted to be beneficial in the diagnosis of this condition. The flick sign is characterized by a flicking movement of the wrist and hand, similar to that used when shaking down a thermometer. In one study, the presence of a positive flick sign accompanied electrodiagnostic abnormality in 93% of the subjects (65). A nerve conduction study should be considered to aid in obtaining the definitive diagnosis. A pneumatic-tourniquet test can be performed by inflating a tourniquet about the upper arm to exacerbate the symptoms of carpal tunnel syndrome. The cuff is placed about the upper arm and inflated above the patient's normal systolic pressure. In normal patients, a tingling sensation develops in the entire hand and fingers over the ulnar aspect of the hand approximately 2 to 3 minutes after initiation; in patient's with carpal tunnel syndrome, tingling in the thumb, index middle and ring fingers develops within 30 to 60 seconds (66). This test is based on a transient ischemia to an already compromised median nerve. Sensory and motor deficits can be determined by electromyelographic diagnostic studies.

Plain film radiographic evaluation will help rule out fractures, tumors, and arthritic changes. A carpal tunnel view will demonstrate the greater multangular, hook of the hamate, capitate and pisiform. The examiner should look for proper alignment of the tunnel as well as soft tissue or bony changes within the tunnel.

The role of MRI in the evaluation of CTS remains unclear at this time (67).

Treatment. Initially, all tasks requiring repetitive hand and wrist motion (especially extension) and equipment which causes excessive vibration to the hand and wrist should be modified or discontinued. If the offensive mechanisms are not modified, the condition could relapse or even progress into a reflex sympathetic dystrophy.

Fixation dysfunction of the radiocarpal, carpal, and carpometacarpal joints should be adjusted. Commonly present is anterior misalignment of the lunate, which approximates the tunnel, or separation of the distal radio-ulnar articulation, which subsequently stretches the transverse ligament thus compromising the carpal tunnel. The distal forearm, wrist, and hand may be supported in a cock-up splint. Rehabilitative exercises should include:

1. Active pain-free wrist range of motion stretches;
2. Grip strength increase with use of sorbathane hand exerciser performed with the hand positioned palm up, palm down, and thumb up;
3. Wrist curls, reverse curls, radial deviation, ulnar deviation, supination, and pronation with hand weights for 3 to 4 sets of 10 repetitions;

The patient should also be evaluated with regards to sleeping posture. It should be noted if the patient sleeps on the side with the arms above the head or on the stomach with the head turned sideways and the arms above the head. If either one of these sleeping postures is discovered, the patient must be instructed in proper resting posture.

Fixation dysfunction of the elbow should be adjusted. The cervical spine should also be examined for fixation-subluxations to help restore neural integrity to the upper extremity. It is commonplace to successfully treat CTS by means of conservative chiropractic cervical care.

Using an underwater technique, ultrasound may be applied to the volar surface of the wrist. Also, cryotherapy over the involved structures may be helpful.

Hip Joint

The hip joint is best described as a ball and socket joint. Unlike the glenohumeral joint, the hip offers a deep bony socket which encompasses the ball (head of the femur) constituting a very stable yet highly mobile articulation.

The bony components of the hip joint (articulatio coxae) include the spheroid-shaped head of the femur and the concave cup-like acetabulum which is formed by the union of three bones: the ilium, ischium and pubis. A horseshoe-shaped articular cartilage lines the roof of the acetabulum. The entire head of the femur is covered with articular cartilage.

The head of the femur projects from the femoral neck which angles anteriorly, superiorly, and medially, from its origin between the greater and lesser trochanters on the femoral shaft (8,13) (Fig. 16.43).

Three ligaments offer the majority of support to the hip joint: *(a)* iliofemoral ligament (Y-ligaments); *(b)* pubofemoral ligament; and *(c)* transverse ligament.

The iliofemoral ligament (IFL) is an inverted Y-shaped structure. It is the thickest and strongest part of the capsule. The IFL acts as the main stabilizer of the hip in the upright posture (Fig. 16.44). The blood vessels and nerves of the hip pass into the joint through the foramen inferior to the transverse ligament.

KINESIOLOGY

The hip joint offers three degrees of freedom: 1) flexion-extension, 2) abduction-adduction, and 3) internal-external rotation.

Flexion of the hip with the knee flexed may be continued until the thigh contacts the abdominal wall. When the knee is fully extended, tension produced by taut posterior thigh musculature limits hip flexion to approximately 75° to 90°. Extension of the hip is 0° to 10°.

Hip abduction is approximately 40° to 55° and adduction is 30° to 40°. External rotation is estimated to be 40° to 50° and internal rotation is 30° to 45° (8,13).

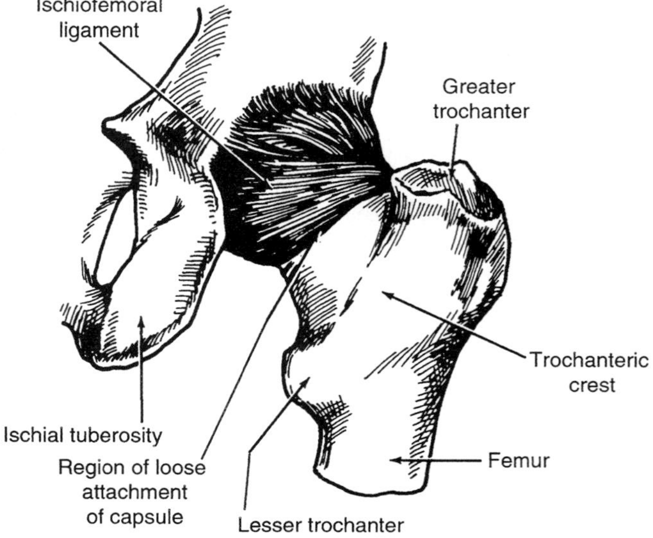

Figure 16.43. Hip joint with the joint capsule. Modified from Warwick R, Williams P. Gray's anatomy. 35th British ed. Philadelphia: WB Saunders, 1980:481.

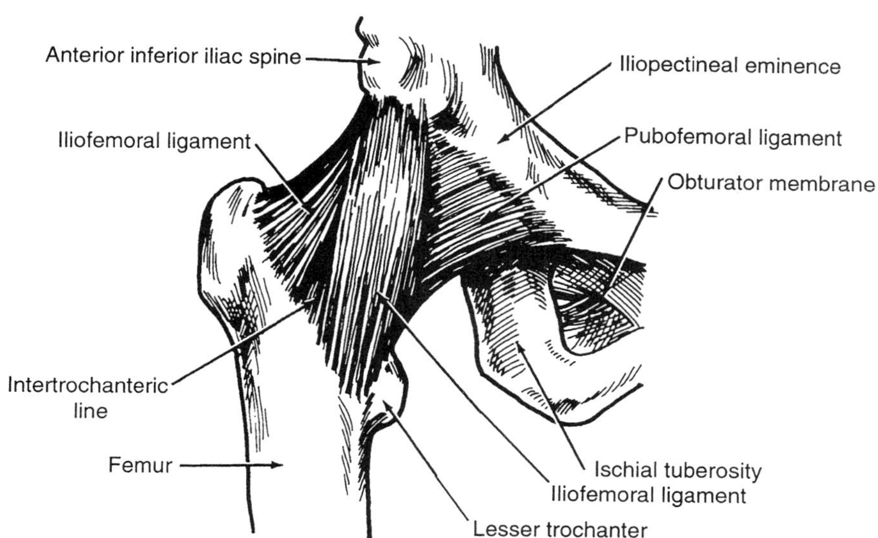

Figure 16.44. Ligaments of the hip. Modified from Warwick R, Williams P. Gray's anatomy. 35th British ed. Philadelphia: WB Saunders, 1980:481.

RADIOGRAPHIC ANALYSIS

The standard radiographic series of the hip includes three views: the anteroposterior pelvis projection, the anteroposterior acetabular projection, and the lateral pelvis projection. The radiographs should be used to rule out recent osseous fracture or dislocation, tumor, infection, and previous deformity (e.g., ischemic necrosis).

Knee

The knee complex is a modified hinge joint of two special articulations located within one joint capsule: the tibiofemoral joint and the patellofemoral joint. Also located in this region but not considered to be part of the knee joint proper is the proximal tibiofibular joint (PTF). The PTF joint does, however, play a functional role in knee motion, as well as with inferior tibiofibular joint and ankle kinematics and will be discussed in this section.

The articulating surfaces of the femur (i.e., medial and lateral condyles) are convex and symmetrical. The medial condyle is longer than the lateral. The corresponding articular surfaces of the tibia are asymmetrical and concave. The medial plateau is 50% larger than its lateral counterpart (8,10,13).

The asymmetrical nature of the articulating surfaces of the femur and tibia creates circumstances that allow movement resulting from rolling, spinning, and gliding of one bony component on the other.

The asymmetrical relationship of the femoral condyles and the tibial plateaus is compensated by the interposed cartilaginous menisci (68). These structures are curved, wedge-shaped structures that lie between the opposing articular surfaces. The menisci are attached to each other as well as the joint capsule. The medial meniscus is more oval in comparison with the more circular lateral meniscus.

The osseous components provide very little in terms of stability of the knee joint. Strength and stability depends on the integrity of local muscles and ligaments.

The anterior cruciate ligament proceeds superiorly and posteriorly from its anterior medial tibial attachment and inserts on the medial side of the lateral femoral condyle. It stabilizes the knee in extension and prevents hyperextension, as well as limiting external rotation of the tibia on the femur, and anterior displacement of the tibia relative to the femur.

The posterior cruciate ligament originates from the posterior tibia and travels anteriorly, superiorly and, medially to attach on the lateral surface of the medial femoral condyle. The posterior cruciate ligament restricts posterior displacement of the tibia on the femur as well as excessive tibial internal rotation (68).

Mediolateral stability of the knee is primarily offered by the medial (tibial) collateral ligament and the lateral (fibular) collateral ligament. The medial collateral ligament attaches to the medial aspect of the medial femoral epicondyle and inserts into the medial aspect of the proximal tibia. The lateral collateral ligament spans from the lateral epicondyle to the head of the fibula. The lateral collateral ligament has no attachment to the lateral meniscus and is separate from the joint capsule proper. Additionally, medial support is offered by the tendons of the semitendonous gracilis and sartorius. Lateral support is provided by the iliotibial band and the biceps femoris (8). The proximal tibiofibular joint is an arthrodial joint. The tendon of the biceps femoris attaches to the head of the fibula and is instrumental in providing lateral support to the knee (Fig. 16.45A-C).

KINESIOLOGY

Flexion of the knee ranges from 120° to 140°. During flexion, the femoral condyles roll and spin as well as slide

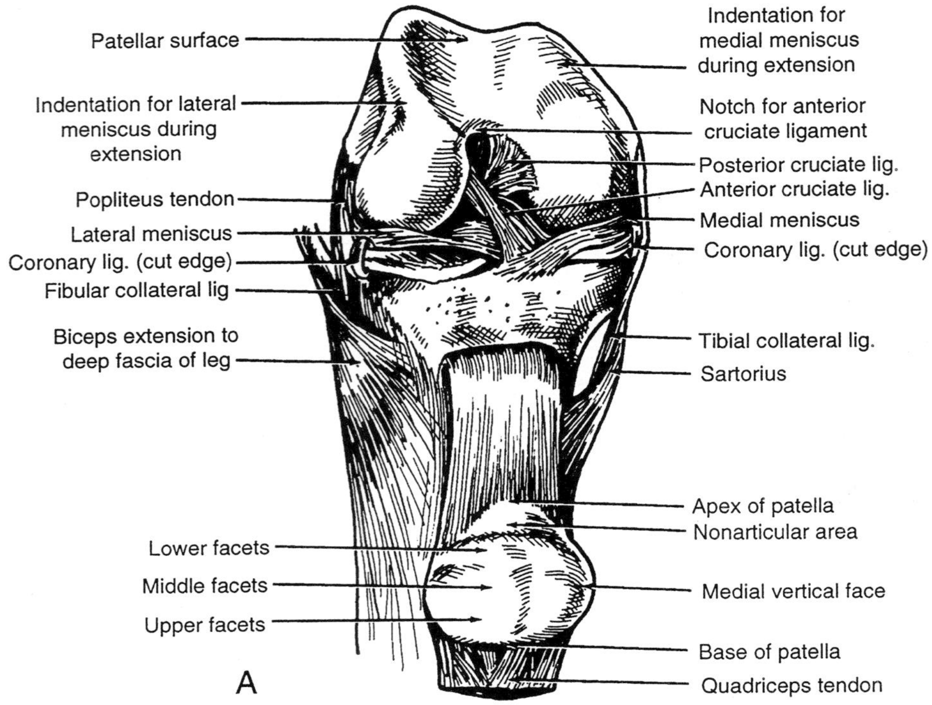

Patellar surface
Indentation for lateral meniscus during extension
Popliteus tendon
Lateral meniscus
Coronary lig. (cut edge)
Fibular collateral lig
Biceps extension to deep fascia of leg
Lower facets
Middle facets
Upper facets
Indentation for medial meniscus during extension
Notch for anterior cruciate ligament
Posterior cruciate lig.
Anterior cruciate lig.
Medial meniscus
Coronary lig. (cut edge)
Tibial collateral lig.
Sartorius
Apex of patella
Nonarticular area
Medial vertical face
Base of patella
Quadriceps tendon
A

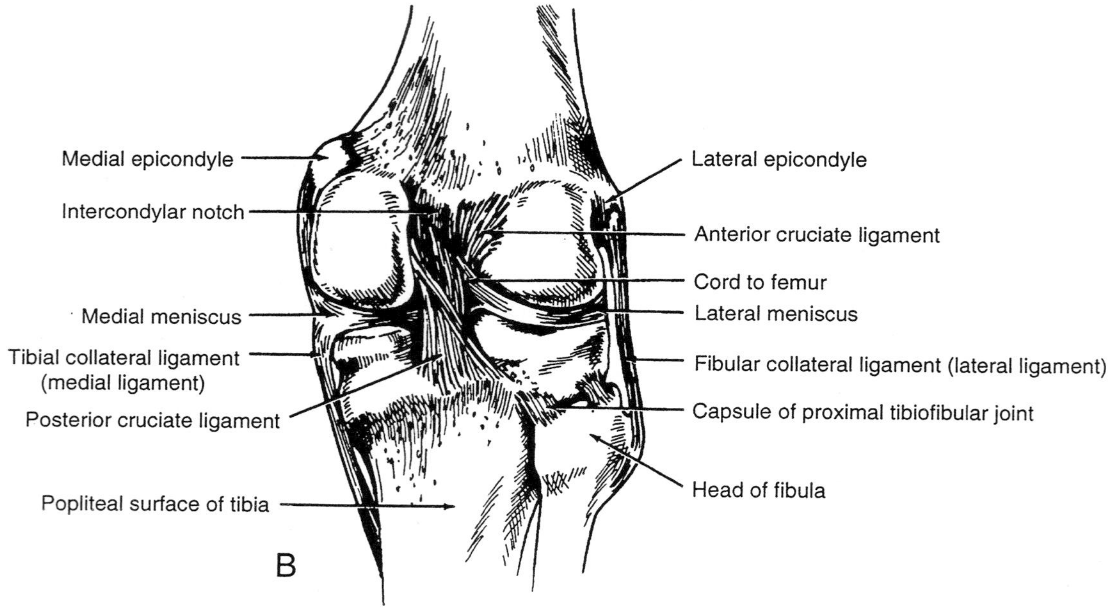

Medial epicondyle
Intercondylar notch
Medial meniscus
Tibial collateral ligament (medial ligament)
Posterior cruciate ligament
Popliteal surface of tibia
Lateral epicondyle
Anterior cruciate ligament
Cord to femur
Lateral meniscus
Fibular collateral ligament (lateral ligament)
Capsule of proximal tibiofibular joint
Head of fibula
B

Anterior cruciate ligament
Medial meniscus
Medial collateral ligament
Coronary ligament
Coronary ligament
Ilio-tibial tract
Lateral meniscus
Lateral collateral ligament
Popliteus ligament
C
Posterior cruciate ligament
Cord from lateral meniscus to medial femoral condyle

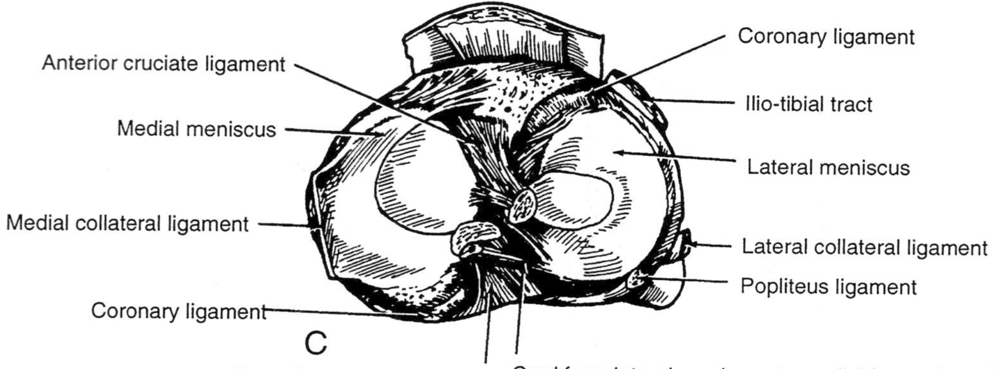

anteriorly. During extension from full flexion, the femoral condyles roll in an anterior direction while sliding posteriorly (8,13) (Fig. 16.46).

Pure rolling and spinning are impossible because the femoral articulating surfaces are much longer in the sagittal plane than are those of the tibia. Further, because the medial femoral condyle is longer than the lateral femoral condyle, the knee externally rotates approximately 5° to 10° during full extension.

With the foot planted (closed kinematic chain), the spin of the femur on the tibia during the late stages of extension causes the femur to rotate medially on the tibia. This medial rotation brings the knee into a close-packed position and is appropriately termed the "Screw Home Mechanism." To unlock the knee, the femur must rotate laterally on the tibia.

In an open kinematic chain (foot not planted), the tibia rotates laterally on the femur to produce locking (close-packed) of the knee. Unlocking of the knee is brought about by medial rotation of the tibia on the femur.

The patellofemoral joint is comprised of the triangular patella and the central groove of the femur located anteriorly between the medial and lateral condyles. During flexion and extension the central ridge of the patella slides along the central groove. Both the posterior patella and the central groove of the femur are lined with articular cartilage. The posterior surface of the patella is divided into five regions or facets: superior, inferior, medial, lateral, and odd (8,13).

During flexion, the patella slides approximately 7 to 8 mm inferiorly until it comes to rest on the inferior facet. In a closed kinematic chain, active flexion of the knee from 60° to 120° rotates the patella laterally and the lateral patellar facet is engaged. In active extension the patella glides superiorly along the central groove until it assumes a position either laterally or incongruently in contact with the lateral aspect of the central groove, or centered in the patellar groove. The patella may come to rest in either place because of the considerable variation among individuals in the configuration of the patellofemoral joint.

During active rotation at the tibiofemoral joint in the opened kinematic chain, with the knee flexed to 90°, the patella rotates in the opposite direction to the femur. For example, when lateral rotation of the femur on the tibia occurs at the tibiofemoral joint, it is accompanied by medial rotation of the patella. That is to say that the apex of the patella moves toward the medial aspect of the tibia (8,13).

The PTF joint is responsible for diminishing torsional stresses at the ankle, to decrease lateral bending of the tibia and to decrease weight-bearing torsion (69). The

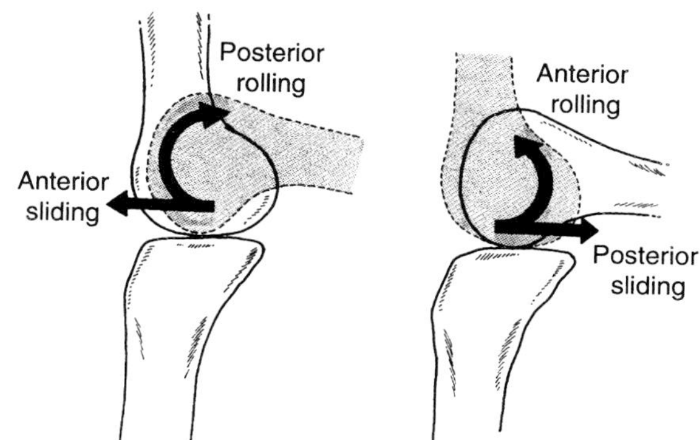

Figure 16.46. Movement of the knee during flexion and extension. Modified from Norkin CC, Levangie PK. Joint structure and function: a comprehensive analysis. Philadelphia: WB Saunders, 1983:299.

PTF joint moves superiorly and medially during ankle dorsiflexion; it moves inferiorly and laterally on ankle plantarflexion.

RADIOGRAPHIC ANALYSIS

The standard radiographic series for the knees requires two views: the weight-bearing anteroposterior bilateral knee projection and the lateral view (of the involved knee). The anteroposterior projection should be taken with the feet of the patient parallel and spaced approximately 6 to 8 inches apart.

A radiographic marking system is used to establish the relative alignment of the tibiofemoral joint. A line is drawn from a point in the center of the tibia approximately midshaft to a point in the center of the tibial plateaus. Another line is drawn from a point in the center of the femoral shaft to the center of the patella. Two additional lines are drawn on the inferior aspect of the femoral condyles (FCL) and the superior aspect of the tibial plateaus (TPL), respectively. These two lines should appear parallel. The femoral shaft line (FSL) and the tibial shaft line (TSL) should intersect one another at the joint line.

A wedging of the FCL and the TPL indicates a misalignment of the tibiofemoral joint. If the wedge is wider on the medial aspect of the joint, the medial side of the tibiofemoral joint is listed and denotes medial (M or internal-In) misalignment of the involved structure. If the wedge is wider on the lateral aspect of the tibiofemoral joint, the lateral side of the tibiofemoral joint is listed and denotes lateral (L or external-Ex) misalignment of the involved structure. The determination of whether to list the femur or the tibia is based on comparison of the involved structures and their contralateral counterparts. For example, if both tibiae appear symmetrical radio-

Figure 16.45A-C. AP, PA, and superior to inferior views of the osseous and soft tissue components of the knee. Modified from Warwick R, Williams P. Gray's anatomy. 35th British ed. Philadelphia: WB Saunders, 1980:483–4.

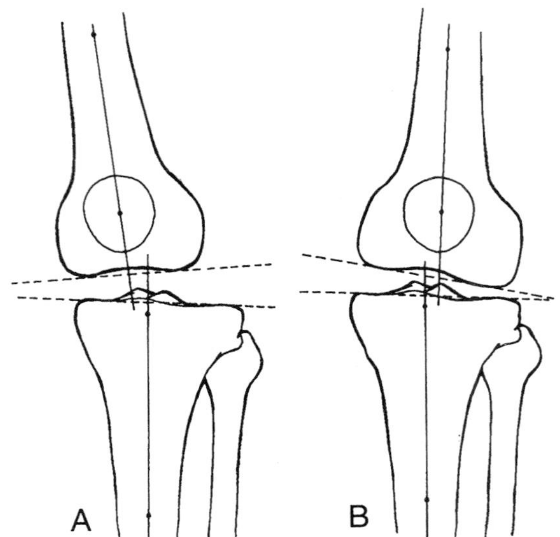

Figure 16.47. Radiographic analysis of the knee. **A,** Diagram of a PL (PEx) left tibia. **B,** Diagram of an AM (AIn) left femur.

graphically, whereas the femurs do not, the femur would be listed. If, however, the femurs are commensurable and the tibiae are not, the tibia would be listed.

The determination if rotational misalignment has occurred at the tibiofemoral joint requires comparisons of the FSL and the TSL. If when listing the femur, the FSL is positioned lateral to the TSL, the femur has rotated anteriorly on the medial aspect and the femur is listed anteromedial (AM or AIn). If the FSL is positioned medial to the TSL, the femur has rotated posteriorly on the medial aspect and is listed posteromedial (PM or PIn). If when listing the tibia, the TSL is positioned lateral to the FSL, the tibia has rotated posteriorly on the lateral aspect and is listed posterolateral (PL or PEx). Finally, if the TSL is positioned medial to the FSL, the tibia has rotated anteriorly on the lateral aspect and is listed anterolateral (AL or AEx) (Fig. 16.47A-B). The Gonstead listing protocol uses the In and Ex terminology to delineate the medial or lateral component of the misalignment. The authors have introduced the M and L terminology to more clearly depict the actual misalignment and to better correlate with recognized rotatory instability patterns of the knee.

Common Disorders of the Knee

ANTERIOR KNEE PAIN

Definition. In the past, anyone who came into the doctor's office complaining of anterior knee pain and crepitation was diagnosed with chondromalacia patella. Although this type of differential diagnosis was fairly simple, it is obvious that such generalization does not allow for successful management. Patellar tracking disorders, patellar malalignment, patellalgia, patellofemoral arthralgia, chondromalacia patella, and runner's knee are just a few of the terms used to describe a patient with anterior knee pain. More important in the diagnosis and treatment of a patient with anterior knee pain is the localization of the tissues or structures involved in the pathology. Basically, there are four general categories that encompass the many conditions that present with anterior knee pain (70). Patellar tracking and/or instability problems involve some sort of aberrant tracking or disrelationship of the patellofemoral joint. The second category is chondral and osteochondral disorders which include such conditions as osteochondritis dessicans or osteochondral fractures of the knee. The third category is soft tissue inflammatory disorders. These injuries involve pathologic soft tissue changes, specifically bursitis and tendonitis around the anterior knee. The last general category is traction apophysitis. This includes Osgood Schlatter's disease, Larsen-Johansson disease, and bipartite patella. These are inflammatory conditions of tendons or fibrocartilage at their insertions into the bone.

Etiology. Patellofemoral tracking and instability-patellofemoral malalignment is a condition caused by excessive horizontal movement of the patella during knee flexion and extension due to an increased Q angle. With a Q angle greater than 15°, the excessive patellar motion begins to wear the undersurface of the patella (70). This condition, as well as other patellar tracking problems, is more common in females because of a wider pelvis causing an increased Q angle. It is also important to consider other structural variants that may affect the Q angle, such as foot pronation, femoral anteversion, In and/or Ex ilium, and coxa vara.

Lateral patellofemoral compression syndrome is caused by a tight lateral patellar retinaculum and a weak vastus medialis muscle which creates abnormal pressure on the patellofemoral joint (70). A tight iliotibial band (ITB) or tensor fascia lata may also contribute to patellofemoral compression syndrome. Femoral anteversion and hyperpronation are other structural abnormalities that may also contribute to patellofemoral compression syndrome (71).

Some tracking disorders can be the result of patellar instability. Subluxation or dislocation of the patella occurs with an acute twisting, jumping, or deceleration injury (70). Instability of the patella, as in patellar dislocation, has been associated with patella alta (72).

Chondral and Osteochondral Disorders: Chondromalacia patella, osteochondritis dessicans, and osteochondral fractures are the result of cartilage and subchondral bone destruction due to trauma or aberrant patellar tracking. Chondromalacia patella is the result of abnormal patellar tracking and is characterized by cartilaginous destruction and bone softening.

Osteochondral fractures usually arise from a fall on or blow to the knee. They often occur in motor vehicle accidents when the knee hits the dashboard (70).

Osteochondritis dessicans of the patella is a less common osteochondral disorder. It may be initiated by trauma, has an element of avascular necrosis, and is often associated with osteochondritis dessicans in other areas.

Soft Tissue Inflammatory Disorders: The main cause of inflammatory disorders to the soft tissue of the knee is overuse injury, but acute trauma is also possible. The primary conditions are quadriceps and patellar tendonitis, prepatellar bursitis (Housemaid's knee), and pes anserine bursitis. Synovitis or an inflamed plica may also cause anterior knee pain.

Traction apophysitis disorders include Osgood Schlatter's disease, Larsen-Johansson disease, and bipartite patella. They usually occur in adolescents from overuse or direct trauma, which in an adult would ordinarily cause only tendonitis (70).

Anatomic Considerations. The clinical picture of anterior knee pain may involve chondral and osteochondral surfaces of the patellofemoral articulation, the patellar tendon, the supra/infra/and prepatellar bursa, pes anserine bursa, or the osseous and muscular structures involved in the patellar tracking mechanism. Chondral and osteochondral surfaces of the patellofemoral joint are damaged by trauma or aberrant tracking of the patellar facets over the adjacent femoral joint surfaces. The most commonly injured tendons associated with anterior knee pain are the patellar and quadriceps tendons which endure much of the stress of the quadriceps mechanism.

The pes anserine and prepatellar bursa are most commonly implicated in anterior knee pain that involves micro or macro trauma. Occasionally, the ITB bursa may cause anterior knee pain, but more commonly the ITB is involved with muscular imbalance resulting in anterior knee pain. In adolescents, the site of the proximal and distal patellar tendon insertion to the bone can be susceptible to traction apophysitis. Similarly, the fibrocartilage that connects the area of incomplete fusion in bipartite patella may become inflamed. Abnormal patellar tracking or instability may be the result of several structural abnormalities. Aberrant tracking is the result of an increased Q angle. A wide pelvis (more common in females), femoral anteversion, coxa vara, genu valgum, and hyperpronation are some of the structural abnormalities that increase the Q angle. Another major factor in abnormal patellar tracking is muscular imbalance. Most often a weak vastus medialis muscle or hypertonic quadriceps, hamstrings, or lateral structures (e.g., tensor fascia lata, ITB, extensor retinaculum) increase stress on the patellofemoral joint (71). Also, gastrocnemius muscle tightness may affect the Q angle by increasing pronation of the foot (71). It is also important to consider the effect of functional limb length differences and pelvic obliquity on the Q angle and the musculature of the lower extremity.

Symptoms. The patient may report a traumatic event but often cannot relate the onset of symptoms to a specific incident. In cases of a traumatic event, severe pain, hemarthrosis, and inability to move the knee indicate possible osteochondral fracture. In cases of subluxation, giving way with pain, and effusion of the joint are common (70). Pain may be located behind or around the patella and inferior to the patella in conditions such as infrapatellar tendonitis and Osgood Schlatter's disease. Pain may also be referred to the posterior or medial aspect of the knee.

Soft tissue inflammatory conditions are usually the result of running, jumping, or some sort of overuse activity. Kneeling tends to increase anterior knee pain. The patient may also complain of pain while ascending and descending stairs, as well as with long periods of sitting, due to the increased tension on the patella. Crepitation or clicking sounds, especially when flexing the knee are a common complaint. Intermittent swelling (associated with bursa, tendon, or synovial irritation), muscular weakness (especially vastus medialis), and burning pain in the knee may also be present. It is very important to inquire about any trauma or associated symptoms of the lumbar spine and feet.

Physical Examination. The physical examination of the patient with anterior knee pain must include complete lumbopelvic, knee, and foot evaluation. The lumbosacral area is evaluated for evidence of local joint irritation and dysfunction (especially the upper lumbars) causing referred or radicular knee pain. In addition, the low back and hip area should be inspected for anatomic or functional abnormalities (e.g., pelvic obliquity, coxa vara, and femoral anteversion) which biomechanically increase stress at the patellofemoral joint due to muscular imbalance or an increased Q angle. The foot should be examined weight-bearing and nonweight-bearing to assess for hyperpronation. This exam should include at a minimum, static weight-bearing arch analysis, gait analysis, and subtalar joint function.

The knee examination must evaluate all of the tissues represented by the four general categories associated with anterior knee pain:

1. Patellar Tracking Disorders: Visual inspection of the knee may reveal structural abnormalities such as an increased Q angle, genu valgum, patella alta or baja, femoral anteversion or external tibial rotation associated with a "squinting" or medially rotated patella (73). Varying degrees of swelling are associated with tracking disorders but more commonly with tendonitis and bursitis. Palpation may reveal tenderness around the patella or a tight lateral retinaculum and iliotibial band (ITB). Ober's test is used to identify a hypertonic ITB associated with tracking disorders. Straight leg raising test may be decreased due to hamstring tightness. Passive knee flexion to 30° and lateral pressure on the patella may cause pain or apprehension (patellar apprehension test) (73). Pain with patellar compression, or apprehension with Clarke's test is indicative of a patellar tracking disorder; however, Clarke's test has a high false positive rate in asymptomatic individuals.
2. Chondral and Osteochondral Disorders: In osteochondral fractures, the patient has difficulty moving the knee. Swell-

ing, hemarthrosis, locking or catching may be visible (70). A positive Waldron's test demonstrates palpable clicking and pain during active squatting by the patient and is an indication of chondromalacia patella. Quadriceps atrophy, especially of the vastus medialis oblique muscle, is a common finding in tracking and osteochondral disorders.

3. Soft Tissue Inflammatory Disorders: Localized tenderness and swelling over inflamed bursae or tendons may help identify involved tissues. Swelling over the anterior patella indicates prepatellar bursitis (Housemaid's knee). Effusion may be present in cases involving synovitis (74). The pes anserine bursa and infrapatellar tendon are also commonly inflamed. Active and active resisted knee extension should produce pain due to the tension placed on an inflamed patellar tendon. Passive extreme flexion will also stress an inflamed patellar tendon as well as some of the bursae in the area.
4. Traction Apophysitis: Tenderness at the superior or inferior aspect of the patellar ligament where it inserts into the patella, or pain at the tibial tuberosity is an indication of Larsen-Johansson disease or Osgood Schlatter's disease, respectively. Palpable thickening of the inferior pole of the patella or the tibial tuberosity is also a sign of traction apophysitis. In cases of a symptomatic bipartite patella, tenderness and or swelling may be present directly over the patella.

Diagnosis. The differential diagnosis of a patient with anterior knee pain involves many conditions and requires a complete history and physical examination of the knee as well as the lumbar spine and foot. Plain film knee and patellofemoral views are important in ruling out fracture, arthritides, and in diagnosing chondromalacia patella. Also of use are bone scans which show increased uptake with chondromalacia patella. Osteochondral fractures may or may not be visualized radiographically, but osteochondritis dessicans is usually visualized as a loose fragment, which may not be displaced. The traction apophysitis may be visualized as a fragmentation at the tibial tuberosity in Osgood Schlatter's disease or an elongation of the inferior pole of the patella in Larsen-Johansson disease. Radiographically, bipartite patella demonstrates a lucent line dividing the patella into two pieces. The radiographs can also be used to determine a superior or inferior patella, as well as the patellofemoral index (74). Scout views of the lumbar spine and pelvis may be indicated to aid in the discovery of pelvic obliquity or other structural abnormalities.

Treatment. The initial goal of the treatment plan is to restore normal biomechanics to both the tibiofemoral and patellofemoral joints. Rotational misalignments of the femur or tibia may underlie symptomatology. Such dysfunctional conditions must be identified and remedied. A common finding with anterior knee pain is patella alta. Patella alta is accompanied by shortening of the rectus femoris muscle. Treatment should be tailored to lengthen the muscle. The application of hydrocollator packs directly over the rectus femoris while exerting a superior to inferior pressure to the patella initiates this lengthening process. After this procedure, ice is applied to the same region. This procedure should be repeated 3 to 4 times per day for 2 to 4 weeks. This procedure effectively alters the muscular length by means of plastic deformation. A neoprene knee sleeve with an inverted horseshoe pad may be worn to stabilize the patella.

Atrophy of the vastus medialis oblique may be present. If so, restoration of normal muscular girth is indicated. If there is limitation of knee extension, the patient should be instructed to perform quadriceps sets and straight leg raises to maintain and possibly increase quadriceps strength. As normal ROM is acquired, terminal knee extensions should be incorporated. This exercise consists of knee extension exercises on a knee extension weight bench. These extensions are limited to the final 30° of extension which is effective in strengthening the vastus medialis oblique. Any rehabilitative exercise program should be immediately followed by cryotherapy for a duration of 15 to 20 minutes. The avoidance of knee flexion beyond 30° is emphasized to avoid potential aggravation of the anterior knee by placing too much tensile and compressive load on the anterior knee as seen with increased knee flexion. Along this same line of thought, the patient should be instructed not to sit with the knee flexed beyond 30° for prolonged periods of time.

With Osgood Schlatter's disease, as with other anterior knee pain conditions, the patient should lessen the load or demand they place on the knees. Activities such as bicycling, stair climbing, and hiking should be avoided. With Osgood Schlatter's disease the use of a neoprene knee sleeve with a horseshoe pad placed at the inferior pole of the patella is suggested during symptomatic periods and during challenging activities.

The pedal foundation should be evaluated for, among other things, pes planus and hyperpronation. If such conditions exist, appropriate osseous adjustive procedures should be incorporated. Occasionally the patient may require an orthotic appliance to normalize foot function.

COLLATERAL LIGAMENT INJURIES

Definition. The collateral ligaments of the knee act as prime stabilizers of the medial and lateral knee. Injury to the medial collateral ligament is the most common knee injury (75,76). Medial or lateral collateral ligament injury is usually associated with large amounts of valgus or varus force, resulting in partial or complete tearing and often involves injury to associated structures.

Etiology. Collateral ligament injuries most often occur in sports like football, hockey, or skiing, but minor sprains can occur from stepping into a hole, stumbling, or landing with the knee in a varus/valgus position.

Medial collateral ligament tears result from varus force to the knee. With the knee in slight flexion and the foot planted, isolated tears are more apt to occur.

Traumatic valgus force with the knee in full extension also results in capsular tears. If any knee rotation is present, cruciate and meniscus injury is also possible (77). Lateral collateral ligament injury is far less common and results from a varus or abduction force to the knee joint. In addition, muscular imbalance may contribute to injury.

Anatomic Considerations. The medial collateral ligament is located superficially to the middle fibers of the medial joint capsule and attaches superiorly to the adductor tubercle on the femur and inferiorly to the medial tibia deep to the pes anserine bursa. The lateral collateral ligament runs from the lateral femoral condyle to the proximal fibula and is intertwined with the arcuate ligament complex. The proximity of the collaterals to capsular ligaments and musculotendonous structures makes isolated injury uncommon.

Symptoms. Clinically, the patient reports traumatic varus or valgus injury to the knee. Inability to bear weight due to medial knee instability often indicates a Grade III tear (78). Initial ability to bear weight which later becomes impossible due to pain may indicate a Grade II tear (78). Medial or lateral knee pain and muscle spasm of varying degrees with little improvement after several weeks are the most prevalent symptoms. Mild swelling or synovial effusion is also possible. Early effusion or hemarthrosis is suggestive of cruciate or meniscal injury. Other clinical signs and symptoms often exist due to concurrent injury to the cruciates, menisci, or capsular ligaments.

Clinical Findings. Visual inspection of the knee may reveal swelling or effusion. Massive effusion or hemarthrosis indicates possible injury to associated structures. Tenderness to palpation over the medial or lateral collateral ligament helps to locate the injury. Palpation of the lateral collateral ligament is most easily performed with the knee in the Hardy position (79). In lateral collateral ligament tears, peroneal nerve dysfunction is possible (80). Therefore, foot drop and/or weak dorsiflexion or eversion may be present, indicating associated peroneal nerve damage. Active or passive knee flexion with rotation is painful. Also, the patient's ability to actively flex the knee is decreased. The most clinically relevant orthopaedic tests are varus and valgus stress testing with the knee in varying degrees of flexion.

In full extension (0° of flexion), a valgus force that produces mild laxity indicates a complete medial collateral ligament tear as well as capsular sprain. A large degree of laxity with the knee in extension indicates medial collateral, capsular, and possible cruciate ligament injury (77,78). Valgus force with the knee in 15° of flexion indicates an isolated medial collateral ligament tear, Grade I, II, or III, depending on the extent of the laxity and the end-feel. A hard end-feel is indicative of ligament integrity, while an absent or mushy end-feel indicates anatomic or functional incompetence.

Lateral collateral ligament injury is detected with the varus or adduction stress test. A positive test is characterized by laxity with the knee in zero or 30° of flexion. The degree of knee flexion and the amount of laxity determines how the sprain is graded and is similar to the grading of medial ligament injuries. Manual muscle testing of the medial (vastus medialis, gracilis, sartorius, semitend/membranous) and lateral (iliotibial band, tensor fascia lata, biceps femoris, vastus lateralis) muscles may reveal weakness or pain. Because of the large percentage of concurrent injuries associated with collateral ligament tears, a complete orthopaedic examination of the knee with careful investigation of the cruciates, menisci, and associated capsular structures should always be performed. In cases of severe pain, effusion, or muscle spasm, stress testing under anesthesia may be necessary to evaluate true ligamentous injury.

Diagnosis. A diagnosis of collateral ligament injury is made with a complete history, including mechanism of injury, positive ab/adduction stress tests and possibly other positive orthopaedic tests in the presence of concurrent ligamentous injury. Plain film radiography should be performed to rule out fracture or other bony pathology (78). Plain film ab/adduction stress radiographs or arthrography are also helpful in making the diagnosis. A stress radiograph that demonstrates a 5-mm opening is indicative of a Grade I sprain, an opening between 5 and 8 mm classifies as Grade II, and greater than 8 mm a Grade III. The most important aspect in diagnosis and subsequent treatment of collateral ligament injuries is ruling out concomitant knee injury.

Treatment. Initial treatment should consist of bracing the injured knee to provide support and avoid any potential further injury. The biomechanics of the knee should be assessed and any detected dysfunctions should be corrected. The application of ice over the involved structures helps control inflammation. The application of microcurrent may help speed the recovery rate.

The patient should be instructed on isometric contractions of the quadriceps, hamstrings, hip adductors, and abductors. Passive and active range of motion exercises should be performed to pain tolerance. As ROM normalizes, the implementation of surgical tubing and isotonic weight exercises may be included. Optimally, the patient should be evaluated isokinetically to accurately assess the level of strength loss as compared with the uninvolved extremity. An appropriate exercise regime with realistic goals can then be prescribed.

As the patient approaches a return of complete strength, balance boards may be initiated to help restore normal proprioceptive response to the knee. Further, the patient may be instructed to run in large figure-of-eight patterns. These exercises should be performed slowly initially, with increasing intensity as the patient improves.

CRUCIATE INJURIES

Definition. An estimated 50,000 anterior cruciate ligament injuries occur during the winter ski season (81).

Although cruciate ligament injuries represent one of the most common traumatic injuries to the knee, their clinical diagnosis and treatment remain extremely difficult. Injury to the cruciate ligaments are classified as partial tears, complete midsubstance tears, or avulsion of the distal end of the ligament with an osseous fragment.

In chronic anterior cruciate laxity, the ligament may be completely intact but functionally incompetent resulting in an unstable knee. Midsubstance tears appear to be more common in adults whereas avulsion injury has a higher incidence in adolescents (82).

Etiology. Cruciate ligament injuries are common in contact as well as noncontact sports. Downhill skiing and football seem to account for the most numerous occurrences of this injury.

Injuries to the anterior cruciate ligament (ACL) most commonly occur from a blow to the anterior knee causing forceful hyperextension, noncontact deceleration with internal tibial rotation, noncontact hyperextension, or a rapid change in direction (e.g., cutting). Injury to the ACL is the third most common of knee injuries.

The posterior cruciate ligament (PCL) may also be injured from a forceful hyperextension blow to the anterior knee. A fall on a flexed knee with a plantar flexed foot or blows to the tibial tubercle also damage the PCL. The speed of the incident and whether or not the foot was planted are essential in determining the degree of injury to the cruciates and supporting structures. When considering the mechanism of injury, it is important to remember that the ACL is susceptible to injury in both internal and external tibial rotation.

Anatomic Considerations. The ACL runs from the posterior medial side of the lateral femoral condyle inferiorly, anteriorly, and medially to attach to the tibia. The PCL travels from the medial femoral condyle anteriorly in an inferior, posterior and lateral direction to insert on the posterior tibia. The cruciates are surrounded by synovial tissue containing numerous blood vessels that branch off and supply the ligament. Interruption of this blood supply during injury greatly delays healing and is of importance during surgical repair (83). The cruciates prevent translation of the femur and tibia on each other, as well as controlling the amount of rolling and gliding of the femur during flexion of the knee. During knee extension, the ACL prevents meniscal trapping by the femoral condyles and anterior translation of the tibia induced by quadriceps muscle pull (84). Also of anatomic importance are the properly balanced cocontractile forces of the hamstrings and quadriceps muscle groups in reducing stress on the ACL and secondary joint restraints by drawing the tibia superior towards the femur (84).

Signs and Symptoms. The patient suffering from an ACL injury may describe hearing a pop during the traumatic blow to the anterior knee or perhaps a sudden giving way or buckling after a jump, pivot, or quick change in direction (82). If the ligament-damaging incident occurred a prolonged time before the patient reports for evaluation, they might complain of recurrent buckling, especially during athletics. Pain and swelling may or may not be present. The presence of pain with subluxation often indicates damage to the secondary restraints of the knee.

The most common complaint of a patient with PCL tear is pain with walking or ascending/descending stairs. Swelling, hemarthrosis, effusion, and muscle spasm may also be present. The patient may also describe or demonstrate with the hands a sense of buckling or giving way.

Clinical Findings. With ACL injuries, effusion or hemarthrosis of the knee joint may be visualized within 2 to 3 hours after injury. The most clinically relevant orthopaedic tests include the anterior drawer, Lachman's, and pivot shift tests. A positive Lachman's test produces anterior subluxation of the tibia on the femur with or without pain and is the most clinically useful test. The anterior drawer test may be falsely negative due to hamstring spasm or hemarthrosis, which increases the stability of the joint with the knee in 90° of flexion. The pivot shift test is said to be positive when a palpable shift in the tibia is felt when internal tibial rotation, valgus stress and flexion movements are simultaneously created by the examiner. This test may also be falsely negative due to spasm or hemarthrosis. It is important to examine the entire knee joint including the collaterals, menisci, and patellofemoral joint, as concomitant injury to these structures is not only possible but likely. Some have reported a 62% chance of meniscal damage with an ACL tear (85,86).

With the PCL patient supine and the knees flexed to 90°, the tibia on one side may appear to sag posteriorly (sag sign). In the same position, palpation of the joint line may reveal a less prominent tibial plateau medially and laterally which is analogous to the visual sag sign. The posterior drawer test may now be performed from this same position. With the foot in neutral or external rotation, a positive test is indicated by pain and laxity.

Posterior drawer testing with internal rotation of the foot is often falsely negative due to blocking by the posterior horn of the lateral meniscus and tightening of the ligament of Wrisberg (87). Isolated PCL tears are rare and are most commonly associated with posteromedial instability (associated medial collateral ligament damage) and posterolateral instability (associated arcuate ligament complex damage) (88). Anterior drawer testing may reveal a "pseudo" laxity due to posterior subluxation of the tibia with an insufficient PCL. Abduction/adduction stress tests with the knee in full extension may demonstrate laxity indicating associated collateral ligament injury. With associated arcuate ligament complex injury, the external rotation recurvatum test demonstrates relative hyperextension and varus motion of the lateral aspect of the tibia with external tibial rotation.

Diagnosis. Early detection of ACL tears is crucial because chronic laxity predisposes the menisci, collateral ligaments, articular cartilage, and patellofemoral joint to damage (89). The most accurate objective test in the diagnosis of ACL tear is MRI. Plain film radiographs of the knee are important in ruling out tibial spine and osteochondral fractures, as well as growth plate injuries in adolescents. In cases of chronic instability, signs of degenerative joint disease (e.g., joint space narrowing, osteophytes, and subchondral sclerosis) may be present. Although MRI is a good objective test, a thorough history and physical exam coupled with clinical judgment are the most important factors in diagnosing ACL tears. If confusion still exists after examination and MRI, arthroscopy can be the most definitive means of determining the extent of injury and allows for immediate surgical correction (85). Nevertheless, because of the invasiveness of the procedure and its high cost, it should be recommended cautiously.

With PCL injuries, plain film radiographs may demonstrate posterior tibial translation, avulsion of the medial adductor tubercle, or normal findings (87). Medial joint degeneration is also a possibility. As with ACL injuries, a thorough history, examination, and plain film radiographs should be performed before resorting to more expensive tests such as MRI and arthroscopy.

Treatment. In general, as with other acute injuries, cruciate injuries are managed with the application of cryotherapy and other acute-phase therapeutic modalities. Immobilization of the knee should be instituted from 3 days to 2 weeks, depending on continued pain and inflammation (90). As with other injuries of the knee, biomechanical dysfunction should be assessed and corrected. Straight leg raises and hamstring sets should be implemented the first day after injury. The patient should be instructed to avoid weight-bearing activities until pain and inflammation subside.

Range of motion exercises such as swimming and bicycling should be incorporated 2 to 4 weeks post injury. As ROM improves the patient may begin strengthening the muscles of the involved extremity. ACL patients are required to strengthen knee flexors and hip extensors, whereas PCL patients should focus on increasing the strength of the knee extensors and hip flexors.

If a conservative treatment fails to provide adequate results in terms of knee strength, stability, or level of pain, an orthopaedic consultation is indicated for the purpose of possible surgical intervention.

MENISCAL INJURIES

Definition. The menisci of the knee joint act as shock absorbers, aid in nutrition, and help to lubricate or decrease friction in the knee joint. Injury to the menisci of the knee joint occurs as a tear in the cartilage.

The medial meniscus is injured three times more often than its lateral counterpart (68). A longitudinal or bucket handle tear in the medial meniscus and a transverse tear in the lateral meniscus are the most common types. Tears toward the ends of the menisci are called horn tears.

Etiology. The menisci may be injured by noncontact compression and forceful rotation with the knee in flexion or extension (e.g., cutting on a planted foot), and/or a traumatic blow to the knee with the foot rotated. Injury of the medial meniscus is the most common knee injury.

Anatomic Considerations. The medial meniscus is a "C" shaped fibrocartilaginous structure firmly attached at the circumference to the medial tibial plateau. It is comprised of a superior meniscofemoral portion and a lower meniscotibial portion. It is attached to the semimembranosus muscle, the medial collateral ligament, and the medial joint capsule by the coronary ligament (68).

The lateral meniscus is closer to an "O" shape, and its horns are firmly attached near the tibial spines. It also has attachments to the posterior cruciate ligament, popliteus muscle, and joint capsule, but is more loosely attached laterally than its medial counterpart. The loose attachment peripherally allows for a more mobile lateral meniscus which is the reason it is injured less often than the firmly attached medial meniscus.

Functionally, the menisci move anterior during knee extension and posterior during knee flexion, avoiding pinching of the femoral condyles. Rotation with sudden flexion or extension of the knee may pinch the menisci between the femoral condyles causing a tear. Also of anatomic importance is the relative avascularity of the menisci. The horns, central zone, and outer portions are the most vascular areas (91).

Symptoms. Because of the relative avascularity of the menisci, the severity of injury cannot be graded by the degree of pain. Most of the symptoms of meniscal injury are actually caused by a synovial reaction rather than the tear itself (68). The patient may experience severe pain immediately and be forced to stop the activity. A feeling of tightness in the joint due to effusion without any pain may be the only complaint. Immediate hemarthrosis is possible and suggests injury to the surrounding capsule or the cruciates. Clicking, buckling, and intermittent joint locking may also be involved in the symptom picture. It is important not to rule out meniscal tear in the absence of locking because many knees never lock (68).

Clinical Findings. Visual inspection findings vary from mild or no swelling to massive effusion or hemarthrosis. In the latter, it is important to include capsular and cruciate ligament tests as these structures are likely to be injured with this clinical finding. The knee may demonstrate a midflexed position due to reflex inhibition of the quadriceps mechanism or to facilitate maximal capsular effusion. Depending on the chronicity of the injury, atrophy of the quadriceps will be measurable and probably visible.

It follows that active or passive extension in this individual will increase pain. Passive extension is equivalent to a bounce home test, and a springy block indicates possible meniscal tear.

Lateral meniscus injuries show lesser degrees of effusion because of their decreased peripheral attachments. Joint line tenderness is often present in meniscal injury. Important orthopaedic tests in the diagnosis of meniscal injury are McMurray's, Apley's, and Steinman's. Steinman's tenderness displacement test is positive for meniscal injury when anterior joint line tenderness with the knee extended moves posteriorly when the knee is flexed and is a good differential test for degenerative joint disease of the knee (78). Apley's test with compression and rotation will produce pain and possibly clicking with a meniscal tear, whereas pain with distraction is indicative of capsular or ligamentous injury. McMurray's test is probably the most widely used test in detecting meniscal injury; however, it is not sensitive enough to detect tears of the anterior one-third of the meniscus (68). A positive test is indicated by clicking/snapping and possibly pain when the examiner takes the knee from flexion towards extension and applies varying amounts of varus/valgus and internal/external rotation forces. O'Donoghue's test and the modified Helfet test may also be positive as well as capsular and cruciate tests with concomitant injury. In addition, supporting knee musculature may be weak, painful, or atrophied.

Diagnosis. History and physical examination are often enough to make the diagnosis of meniscal tear but may be less clear when adjacent knee structures are simultaneously injured. Differentials in a knee that clicks include osteoarthritis, chondromalacia patella, and a tight hamstring tendon. For optimal treatment, concomitant cruciate or capsular injury must also be ruled in or out.

Plain film radiography helps to rule out fractures, osteoarthritis, and chondromalacia patella. MRI and especially arthrography, aid in determining the extent and location of injury. Arthrography is also useful in detecting discoid menisci. These are normal variants that may be induced by trauma. Clinically, there may be snapping or locking, and an arthrogram may demonstrate a large joint space with a large thick meniscus (92).

Treatment of meniscal tears remains controversial. The conservative treatment of incomplete or partial tears varies. In the asymptomatic or sedentary individual, periodic monitoring and symptomatic treatment, such as cryotherapy and rest, are all that may be indicated. Even in more substantial meniscal tears, surgery may not be performed and the conservative route taken. Initially, the doctor should evaluate the knee for femoral or tibial subluxation and if present, adjustive correction should be performed. Standard acute injury therapeutics such as cryotherapy, compression, and protective bracing should be implemented. Quadriceps and hamstring sets may be performed immediately after injury. Standard lower extremity strengthening should be initiated when ROM increases and pain and inflammation subside.

Because clinical results can vary greatly from individual to individual, the patient should be advised of other potential treatment options. The age, activity level, and possible presence of rotatory instability are important considerations when pondering possible surgical referral.

PLICA SYNDROMES

Definition. Synovial plica of the knee have been reported in the literature to have an incidence of 18 to 60% in the general population (93). The broad use of nonspecific terminology and the failure to describe a distinct clinical picture are some of the reasons the diagnosis of synovial plica syndrome remains difficult.

The following use of the term plica syndrome or synovial plica refers to a clinically symptomatic knee and not merely to the presence of abnormal capsular thickening.

A synovial plica exists as an abnormal folding and thickening in a portion of the knee joint capsule due to a failure of complete involution of the embryonic septae (94–95). The fact that the symptomatic plica may mimic other knee disorders also makes diagnosis difficult.

Etiology. The synovial plica syndrome may be the result of direct trauma to the knee or an overuse type injury triggered by an increased training schedule or the high demands of competition (96). With an injury, the nonsymptomatic synovial plica becomes inflamed and edematous. Synovitis may develop, leading to fibrous tissue replacement, resulting in a thickened inelastic plica that snaps over the femoral condyles with knee movement. At this point the plica is symptomatic and the synovitis has the potential to erode the articular cartilage or the inferior surface of the patella producing chondromalacia (96).

Anatomic Considerations. There are three main types of synovial plica that vary in size, shape, and location, but all are named for the embryonic tissue from which they arose. In descending order of their frequency, they are the medial patellar, suprapatellar, and infrapatellar plica. The medial patellar plica is located in the medial knee joint capsule, parallel to the patella, and inserts into the synovium that covers the infrapatellar fat pad.

The suprapatellar plica also known as the "plica synovialis suprapatellaris," may exist as a plica that forms a compartment distinct from the rest of the joint, a septae with a small hole in it, or a fold inferior to the quadriceps tendon that inserts distally into the medial capsular wall (97–98). The asymptomatic forms of these plica appear thin, pink, and elastic, whereas the symptomatic plica are thick, white, and fibrotic (96).

The infrapatellar plica courses anterior to the anterior

cruciate ligament (ACL) and inserts over the infrapatellar fat pad distally. The infrapatellar plica is not responsible for the plica syndrome but can make diagnosis or treatment more difficult by obstructing the arthroscope or mimicking an intact ACL in the presence of complete ACL injury (98).

Symptoms. The clinical picture of a patient with plica syndrome is highly variable and mimics many conditions. Symptoms occur at any age but are most commonly found in adolescence. The patient may complain of stiffness or an achy knee that simulates an osteoarthritic condition. Many of the patient's symptoms are often worsened with activity. For example, the patient may complain of increased pain, swelling, or snapping after running, jumping or other forms of exercise. The plica syndrome is often exacerbated by ascending or descending stairs, because the large degree of flexion and extension increases capsular stress and deformation. In addition to snapping, the patient may complain of intermittent instability, another symptom mimicking meniscal injury. The patient may also describe a feeling of the patella catching during knee flexion or extension. Finally, the patient may complain of pain after long periods of sitting, mimicking the "theatre sign" associated with chondromalacia patella.

Clinical Findings. Because of the syndrome's ability to mimic many disorders of the knee, the importance of careful orthopaedic examination to detect synovial plica syndrome cannot be overemphasized. With a long-term plica syndrome, quadriceps atrophy may be present (96). On history, or during the exam, the presence of increased pain after performing resisted knee extension implicates plica syndrome. Tenderness to palpation, and sometimes thickening over the medial femoral condyle or the medial or lateral aspect of the superior pole of the patella, helps to localize the plica. In addition, the location of the pain aids in differentiating meniscal injury which is associated with joint line tenderness. This is important because Apley's and McMurray's tests are often found to be positive in synovial plica syndrome in the absence of meniscal injury. Nevertheless, careful localization of the pain will demonstrate that it is above the joint line (99). A positive plica stutter test is characterized by a palpatory jumping or stuttering of the patella between 60° and 45° when the knee is actively extended (73). In the presence of effusion, however, which is not common, this test may be falsely negative. Pain with patellar compression or passive medial movement of the patella (mediopatellar plica test) may be present in plica syndrome. The positive test is the result of the plica being pinched between the patella and the femoral condyle. Hughston's plica test is similar to the stutter test, but the leg is medially rotated and medial pressure is applied to the patella (73). A positive test is indicated with palpatory popping over the femoral condyle caused by the synovial plica.

Diagnosis. The diagnosis of synovial plica syndrome of the knee is one of exclusion and is usually made with the history, examination, and arthrography. Differential diagnoses include meniscal injury ruled out by location of the pain, osteoarthritis ruled out by history, physical exam and x-ray, inflammatory conditions such as rheumatoid arthritis which may actually cause plica syndrome ruled in with laboratory findings, chondromalacia patella demonstrated by x-ray studies, and chronic internal knee disorders such as cruciate or capsular injury detected by history, physical examination, and special tests. Plain film radiographs are usually negative in plica syndrome, but again, aid in differential diagnosis. Arthrography and fluoroscopy are the best objective tests used to visualize synovial plica; however, the finding of a synovial plica in an asymptomatic individual is not clinically significant (100).

Treatment. Treatment of a patient suffering from plica is aimed at minimizing inflammation and increasing the flexibility of the plica. Rest or abstaining from activities that require large ranges of knee flexion and extension may help prevent inflammation. Ice massage can aid in the reduction of inflammation. Underwater ultrasound, as well as transverse frictional massage are used to decrease local adhesions and increase the pliability of the plica. Stretching the hamstrings and quadriceps may also decrease symptoms. Quadriceps strengthening by means of terminal leg extensions (extension of the knees through the final 30° of extension) and quadriceps sets (isometric contractions of the quadriceps) to reduce compressive forces on the patella and anterior knee.

Further, the femorotibial joint should be analyzed for fixation dysfunction, and if present, adjustive correction should follow. If conservative treatment is unsuccessful, arthroscopic removal of the plica should be considered.

ROTATORY INSTABILITY OF THE KNEE

Definition. Rotatory instability to the knee has become one of the most complex knee problems because it is usually misdiagnosed and is therefore mistreated. It often coexists with other knee injuries but goes undiagnosed in the acute stage, thus resulting in a chronic unstable knee. Rotatory instability of the knee joint most commonly exists as anteromedial rotational instability or posterolateral rotational instability but is possible in other directions. Anteromedial rotational instability is the result of damage primarily to the medial capsular ligaments but may involve damage to the vastus medialis retinaculum, anterior cruciate ligament (ACL), or medial meniscus (101). Posterolateral rotational instability results in posterior subluxation of the lateral tibial plateau with combined external tibial spine rotation in the absence of posterior cruciate ligament (PCL) injury (102). The instability is the result of injury to the arcuate ligament complex. Concurrent distal biceps femoris tendon or iliotibial band injury may be present (102).

Etiology Anteromedial rotatory instability is created by a valgus force to the knee. The degree of knee flexion determines which portion of the medial capsular ligament will be injured. The less the amount of knee flexion, the greater the risk of extracapsular ligamentous injury (e.g., ACL, tibial collateral, medial meniscus). A varus force directed posterolaterally, contact hyperextension, and noncontact hyperextension with external tibial rotation result in posterolateral rotational instability.

Anatomic Considerations. Because rotational instability involves more than one plane of motion, several ligamentous structures must be taken into account. Posterolateral stability is provided mainly by the arcuate ligament complex, comprised of the lateral head of the gastrocnemius muscle, popliteus tendon, lateral collateral ligament, and the arcuate ligament (103,104). The biceps femoris muscle or iliotibial band may also be important, depending on the degree of knee flexion. The medial side of the knee is stabilized primarily by the various portions of the medial capsular ligament. The anterior portion of the medial joint capsule and the vastus medialis retinaculum help prevent anteromedial instability. The middle or deep portion of the medial joint capsule (meniscofemoral/tibial ligaments) and the coronary ligament also help prevent rotatory instability of the medial knee. The cruciates and menisci also provide rotational support to the knee. Functionally, the collaterals are looser, allowing for increased tibiofemoral rotation when the knee is flexed.

Symptoms. The patient with rotational instability of the knee will probably report a past history of trauma that was either surgically or nonsurgically treated but continues to give them problems. The patient most commonly reports a feeling of giving way, especially into hyperextension, rather than pain. Climbing stairs or cutting maneuvers are very difficult. Knee joint line tenderness is a common complaint. With posterolateral rotational instability, medial joint line tenderness is more common, leading the clinician to a misdiagnosis of medial meniscus tear (105). The patient with posterolateral instability may present with foot drop or sensory changes of the anterolateral lower leg and foot from peroneal nerve damage.

Clinical Findings. On physical examination of the knee, joint line palpation may reveal medial or lateral tenderness, as well as a tender arcuate ligament complex. The posterolateral tibia may be more prominent on palpation. A careful orthopaedic examination that stresses multiple structures is essential in formulating a correct diagnosis of rotational instability. A positive lateral pivot shift test (Test of MacIntosh) reproduces the giving-way sensation described by the patient and indicates anterior rotational instability (73).

The posterior medial and lateral drawer test, performed with the foot in internal and external rotation respectively, is indicative of posterior rotatory instability when laxity is present. The reverse pivot shift test (Jakob's test) is also used to detect posterior rotatory instability.

Visual inspection of the patient standing or walking may reveal a hyperextended genu varus or externally rotated tibia if posterolateral instability is present. This knee position is also reproduced by the external rotation recurvatum test. A positive abduction stress test at 0° and 30° of knee flexion also indicates posterolateral instability. Rotational instability of the knee can result in tibiofemoral misalignment with fixation. Static observation may reveal the tibiofemoral misalignment. Motion palpation of the joint line should be performed with the patient sitting and the knee flexed. The tibia is internally and externally rotated by the examiner, and tibiofemoral motion is compared bilaterally.

Motion palpation of the tibiofemoral joint is also performed by stabilizing the patient's foot between the examiner's feet and applying light ab/adduction forces with the fingers in the joint line on the medial and lateral side. Restricted motion or fixation on the medial or lateral side, compared with the opposite extremity, corresponds with anterior or posterior medial/lateral instability, respectively. For example, with posterolateral instability one might expect to find fixation in the lateral tibiofemoral joint with posterior rotation or misalignment of the tibia on the femur.

Diagnosis. The aforementioned orthopaedic tests are representative of the more common stress tests for rotational instability of the knee. Furthermore, rotational instability of the knee is rarely the result of a single ligamentous injury. Differential diagnosis includes cruciate, meniscal, iliotibial band and biceps femoris tendon injury. A thorough history and comprehensive examination that tests capsular ligaments as well as the cruciates, menisci, and musculotendonous components of the knee are imperative for proper diagnosis and treatment.

Plain film radiography, including an anterior-posterior bilateral weight-bearing knee film, is sometimes helpful in determining tibiofemoral misalignment. MRI or arthrography may be necessary to determine cruciate or meniscal injury.

Treatment. Conservative treatment of rotatory instability of the knee initially involves correction of any subluxated and dysfunctional osseous component. When correcting tibial or femoral subluxations, it is important that the doctor contacts along with the segmental contact point the joint line and underlying meniscus. Cryotherapy should be implemented to control inflammation, especially after activity. The use of a derotation brace limits possible aggravating positions. Standard strength and flexibility rehabilitation of the involved extremity should include:

1. Full ROM hip, knee, and ankle static stretching;
2. Isotonic quadriceps and hamstring exercises;
3. Forward step-ups;
4. Lateral step-ups;
5. Bicycling;
6. Rope jumping;

mediate, and lateral cuneiform; their primary functional role is allowing range of motion in plantarflexion and dorsiflexion.

The forefoot is composed of the five metatarsals and fourteen phalanges (two on the first rays and three on the second through fifth rays). Along with the three cuneiform, the primary function of the rays of the forefoot is to offer plantarflexion-dorsiflexion.

Common Disorders of the Foot

PLANTAR FASCITIS

Definition. Plantar fascitis is an inflammatory reaction of the fascial support located at the plantar aspect of the foot. A heel spur often forms at the calcaneal tuberosity where the plantar fascia inserts due to calcification resulting from traction of the plantar fascia on the periosteum.

Etiology. The condition can occur in adolescents or adults and is the result of a strain or force along the longitudinal arch of the foot that increases tension on the plantar fascia. This inflammatory condition may be the result of an acute strain to the fascia as seen with rapid acceleration or deceleration of the foot but more commonly is caused by overuse or biomechanical stresses. The condition most commonly occurs in runners who may have recently increased their mileage (112). Excessive walking can also become a problem, especially if the individual hyperpronates. Hyperpronation, pes cavus, or pes planus results in an increased tension on the plantar fascia (112).

Anatomic Considerations. The plantar fascia is a tendon-like structure that supports the arch of the foot. It is comprised of three bands that attach proximally to the calcaneal tuberosity and distally to the base of the proximal phalanges. Other anatomic considerations are the apophyseal attachment of the achilles tendon, the subtalar joint, and the calcaneocuboid joint.

Symptoms. The patient most often reports insidious onset of heel pain or pain on the medial plantar aspect of the foot but may report a sudden onset of pain and tightness after an acute trauma such as stepping off a curb or into a hole (112). The pain is most often present during or after running or long periods of walking. It may also be present with the first steps out of bed or after walking after prolonged sitting. In the latter, the pain is usually more pronounced and makes walking difficult. Pain may be reported at the insertion of the achilles tendon with an associated tendonitis. Less frequently, pain radiates up the leg or towards the toes (112).

Clinical Findings. The most clinically helpful finding is palpatory tenderness on the medial side of the heel at the insertion of the medial band or the abductor hallucis

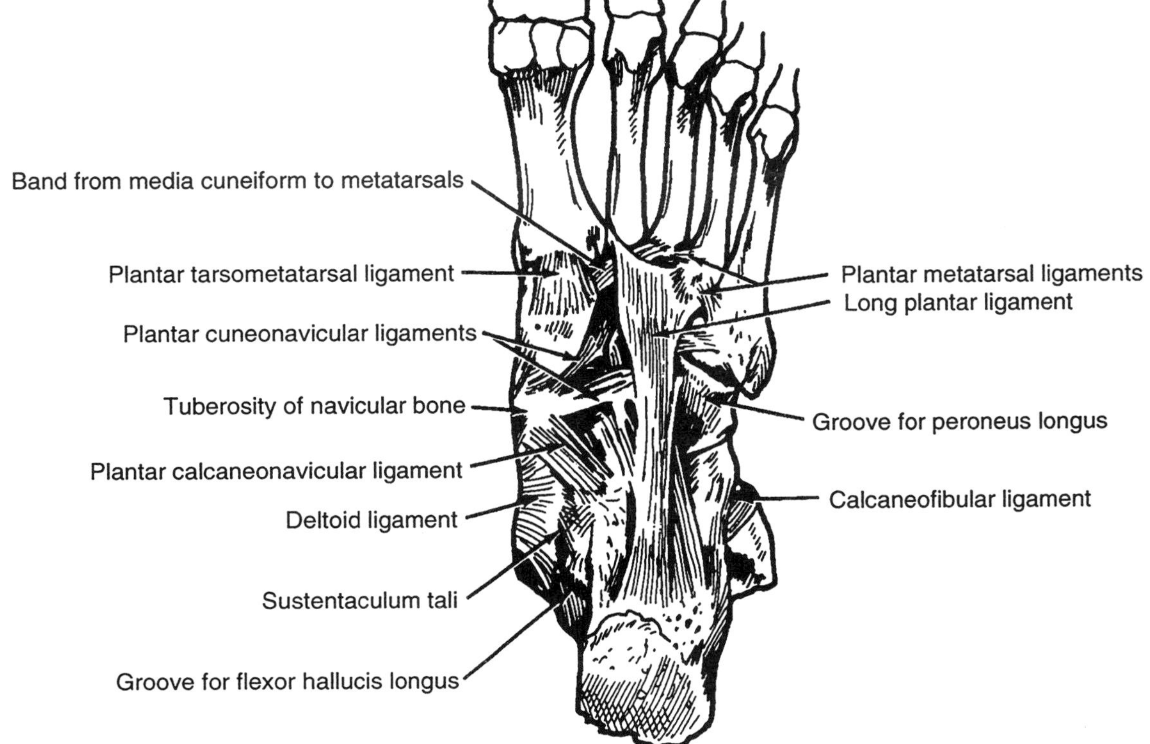

Figure 16.51. Ligaments of the foot. Modified from Warwick R, Williams P. Gray's anatomy. 35th British ed. Philadelphia: WB Saunders, 1980:498.

muscle (112). Palpatory tenderness may also be elicited over the entire plantar aspect of the calcaneus, at the insertion of the central or lateral fascial band, or at the insertion of the achilles tendon. Visual inspection of the patient weight-bearing should be performed to rule out hyperpronation, pes planus, or pes cavus deformities, which place abnormal tension on the plantar fascia. Functional leg length imbalance, a hypertonic gastrocnemius muscle or weak peroneal muscles can all cause hyperpronation resulting in plantar fascitis. The subtalar and calcaneocuboid joint should be tested for fixation and misalignment which can result in hyperpronation and abnormal foot mechanics. In the patient with radiating foot or leg pain, Tinel's test for the posterior tibial and medial calcaneal nerve is performed to rule out Tarsal Tunnel Syndrome. Examination of the lumbosacral area is indicated to rule out referred pain syndromes.

Diagnosis. The differential diagnosis of plantar fascitis includes, but is not limited to, acute strain, plantar bursitis, entrapment neuropathy, lumbosacral pathology, or rheumatic disease (112). In addition to the history and physical examination, plain film radiographs of the foot aid in the diagnosis of plantar fascitis. The most common finding is a spur at the calcaneal tuberosity (Fig. 16.52). By itself, this spur is not the cause of the pain and is also present in rheumatic diseases (112,113). If inflammatory disease (e.g., Reiter's, AS, RA, or psoriatic arthritis) is suspected, laboratory tests should be performed.

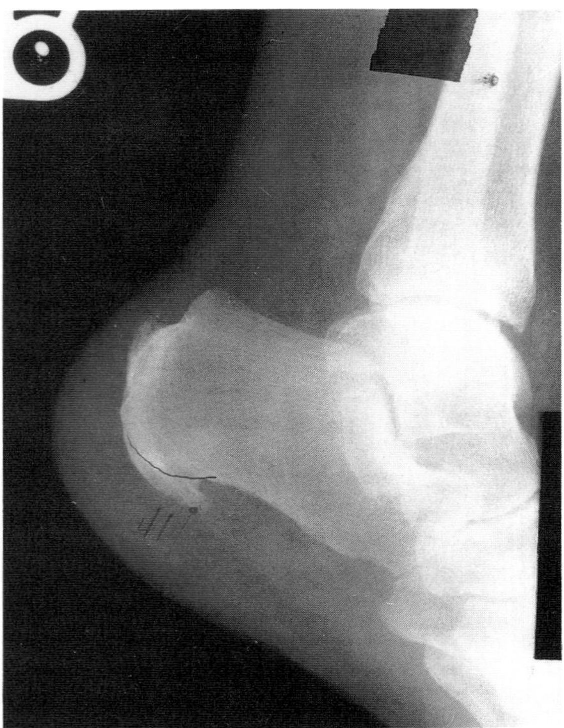

Figure 16.52. Radiograph of a calcaneal heel spur.

Treatment. Treatment of plantar fascitis initially involves the reduction and control of local inflammation by means of ice massage and ice bath submersion. The patient should be evaluated for the presence of a posterior calcaneus, inferolateral cuboid, or inferior navicular. Supportive taping or in-shoe arch supports should be used as long as symptoms persist. Toe raises and heel raises help strengthen lower leg muscles thus supporting the arch (Fig. 16.53). Towel exercises can aid in strengthening the intrinsic muscles of the foot. Rolling the arch over a wooden dowel or golf ball loosens local adhesions and provides mild symptomatic relief. In the presence of a heel spur the patient may be instructed to wear a heel cup or doughnut heel pad to reduce direct pressure on the spur. Surgical intervention is sometimes required with persistent symptomatic spurs.

HALLUX VALGUS

Definition. Hallux valgus is a subluxation of the first metatarsal phalangeal joint characterized by lateral deviation of the great toe with or without rotation, callus formation, and medial deviation of the first metatarsal head. It occurs in females more than males and may be familial or hereditary (73).

Etiology. Hallux valgus is rarely seen in societies in which shoes are not worn, and the implication of shoe wear as a primary external cause of hallux valgus is well supported by the literature (73,114). Of particular note are high heels, cowboy boots, and other narrow-toed shoes. Other causes of hallux valgus include tarsal/metatarsal fixation and misalignment, pes planus, achilles tendon contracture, and other structural abnormalities.

Anatomic Considerations. The first metatarsophalangeal joint and its supporting structures are of primary importance in hallux valgus formation. Attached by ligaments to the plantar aspect of the first metatarsal head and enveloped in the flexor hallucis brevis tendon are sesamoid bones. As the hallux valgus deformity begins to develop, the distal aspect of the great toe deviates laterally and the first metatarsal head deviates medially exposing the metatarsal head and sliding off the sesamoid complex (114). With continued external forces, a bunion is formed due to ligamentous thickening and may progress to the formation of an adventitious bursa.

Symptoms. The primary complaint is pain over the medial metatarsophalangeal joint. The patient may report varying degrees of swelling with an inability to wear certain types of shoes. The patient may experience pain at the plantar aspect of the foot in long-standing cases in which metatarsosesamoid joint degeneration has developed (114). Numbness is occasionally present in the great toe if the sensory nerves are affected.

Clinical Findings. The examination of the patient with hallux valgus should be performed weight-bearing to

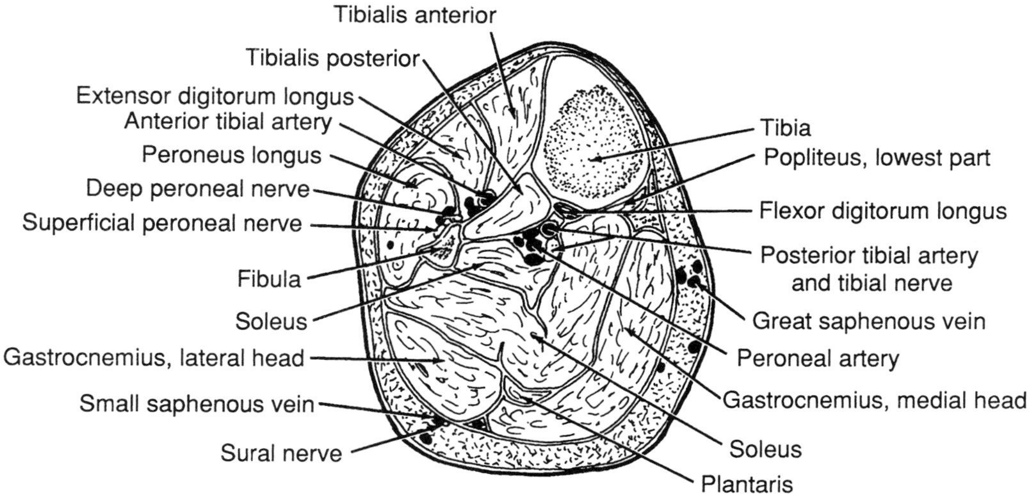

Figure 16.53. A transverse section of the lower leg.

accentuate structural and functional foot problems. The most prominent visual findings are lateral deviation of the great toe, medial deviation of the first metatarsal head, and callus formation with a large medial prominence. The first phalanx may actually overlap the second phalanx. Visual inspection may reveal hyperpronation, hammer toes, corns, or subluxation of the toes. The distance between the first and second metatarsals can appear increased. Tenderness over the bunion is present in the symptomatic patient. Neurologic and vascular examination of the foot should also be performed. The joints of the foot, particularly the subtalar, talonavicular, first tarsometatarsal, and metatarsophalangeal joints should be examined for fixation.

Diagnosis. The diagnosis of hallux valgus can be made by history and physical exam alone. The use of plain film radiography is useful in determining degenerative joint disease of the metatarsophalangeal joint. It is also helpful in detecting structural misalignment and in measuring the metatarsophalangeal and intermetatarsal angles.

Treatment. The conservative management of hallux valgus is directed toward relieving symptomatology first and possibly correcting dysfunction. The symptomatic patient should be instructed to avoid narrow-toed shoes. The primary treatment consists of correcting fixation dysfunction of the foot and ankle. Clinically, the first metatarsophalangeal joint (MPJ) is commonly subluxated. Correction of the MPJ should initially consist of passive joint mobilization and stretching followed by more vigorous corrective adjustive procedures. The patient commonly presents with overpronation of the involved foot and corrective measures, such as in-shoe arch supports or an orthotic appliance, should be considered. Strengthening exercises for the lower leg and intrinsic foot muscles can be instituted.

TARSAL TUNNEL SYNDROME

Definition. The Tarsal Tunnel Syndrome (TTS) is a peripheral nerve entrapment that may cause foot pain, sensory changes, or muscular weakness. The syndrome is the result of entrapment of the posterior tibial nerve as it passes through the tarsal tunnel on the medial side of the ankle.

Etiology. Peripheral nerve entrapments often occur at areas where the nerve is more susceptible to injury or compression. The tarsal tunnel is an opening created by bone and fascia that allows tendons, blood vessels, and nerves to pass through it. In the event of traumatic swelling and fibrous tissue deposition, however, the opening becomes narrowed and is incapable of expanding.

The syndrome may be caused by acute pronation, a varus heel with a pronated forefoot, inflammatory diseases, thrombophlebitis, benign tumors, or postcalcaneal fracture (115,116). The most common cause is after an ankle sprain. The results of the trauma are swelling and fibrous tissue infiltration which narrows the tunnel and compresses the posterior tibial nerve. The scar tissue decreases the elasticity as well as the blood supply of the nerve, thus resulting in slowed nerve conduction (117). The authors have seen posterior calcaneal or anterior talar misalignments commonly in patients suffering from TTS.

Anatomic Considerations. The tarsal tunnel is located on the medial side of the ankle and is created by the medial malleolus, calcaneus, and the tibiocalcaneal portion of the medial collateral ligament (lacinate ligament or flexor retinaculum). Contained within the TTS are the tendons of the flexor digitorum longus, flexor hallucis longus, posterior tibialis muscles, and the posterior tibial artery, vein and nerve (Fig. 16.54). The posterior tibial nerve branches off distal to the tunnel into medial and lateral plantar and calcaneal nerves that carry sensa-

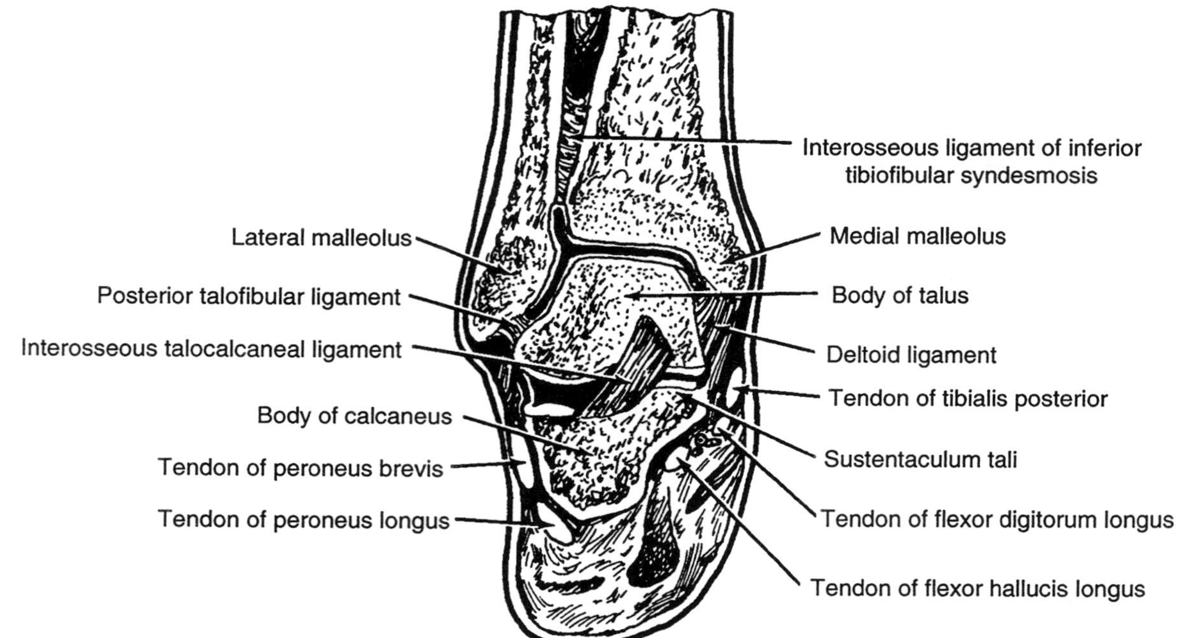

Figure 16.54. A coronal section of the ankle and rear foot. Located between the tendons of flexor hallucis longus and flexor digitorum longus is the posterior tibial nerve, artery, and vein. Modified from Warwick R, Williams P. Gray's anatomy. 35th British ed. Philadelphia: WB Saunders, 1980:496.

tion from the plantar aspect of the foot and motor impulses to the intrinsic foot muscles, respectively (118). Also of anatomic importance is the architecture of the foot. Patients with a varus heel and forefoot pronation seem to be more susceptible to developing TTS (115).

Symptoms. The onset of symptoms is usually insidious even though the cause is most often traumatic. The initial symptoms are usually intermittent and worse at the end of the day or after long periods of standing. As the condition becomes chronic, the pain becomes more intense and may even wake the patient up at night. Pain, numbness, and paresthesias are located on the plantar aspect of the foot and toes, and occasionally may radiate up the calf (115). The patient often describes a burning sensation under the ball of the foot. Activity exacerbates the symptoms, and removing the shoes or massaging the feet may relieve them. If weakness of the toe flexors is present, the patient may report difficulty in toe standing.

Clinical Findings. Examination of the lumbosacral spine must be performed to rule out referred pain. Visual inspection of the weight-bearing patient may reveal pronation or heel varus of the foot. The patient may experience tenderness to palpation where the nerve travels behind the medial malleolus. The symptoms are increased by forcing the foot into a valgus position and minimized with a varus position (117).

The most clinically useful objective tests are Tinel's and sensory testing. Tinel's test is positive when paresthesias are produced by tapping the posterior tibial nerve where it travels through the tarsal tunnel. Sensory testing to light touch, pinprick, and Wartenburg pinwheel over the plantar aspect of the foot may be positive. Weakness of the toe flexors and foot intrinsics can be discovered by resisted muscle testing. Atrophy of the foot intrinsics is also possible. Controversy exists about how common sensory and motor changes are. Applying a tourniquet above the ankle sometimes reproduces the symptoms (117). It is important to examine the skin and pulses of the foot and ankle to help differentiate vascular causes of the syndrome.

Diagnosis. Because of vague symptomatology and very few objective tests, the diagnosis of TTS is difficult. The differential diagnosis includes inflammatory disease, healing fractures, benign tumors, thrombophlebitis, and other peripheral neuropathies. Plain film radiography is useful in detecting benign tumors and posttraumatic bony changes. The most useful special test is EMG, which demonstrates slowed conduction and demyelination in Tarsal Tunnel Syndrome. Sensory nerve conduction studies are thought to be more reliable than those performed on motor nerves (119). Laboratory tests prove helpful in differentiating TTS from diabetic and heavy metal neuropathies, as well as inflammatory arthritides.

Treatment. The initial goal of treatment is to reduce local inflammation by means of local ice massage and submersion in an ice bath. Histologic examination often reveals soft tissue remodeling and scar tissue infiltration of the calcaneofibular ligament, the lateral talocalcaneal ligament, and the interosseous talocalcaneal ligament (120). Transverse frictional massage and manual mobilization of the subtalar joint also aids in the destruction of local scar tissue.

Biomechanical analysis of the subtalar joint often will reveal a posteromedially subluxated calcaneus. In this event, manual adjustment of the calcaneus is required. During the adjustive phase of care, which generally consists of two adjustments per week for 1 to 4 weeks, the use of supportive taping is advised. A figure-of-eight procedure using 2-inch self-adhering elastic tape stabilizes the subtalar joint after the adjustment. The patient should be instructed to wear the tape for 12 to 24 hours postadjustment. Supination should be controlled by use of a lateral heel wedge or an orthotic device. Supination is an aggravating factor as it stresses the interosseous talocalcaneal ligament.

Reeducation of the peroneal muscle group and soleus muscles via elastic tubing and a wobble board can help stabilize the area.

If failure to resolve this condition arises, the doctor should consider a podiatric or orthopaedic referral for further evaluation, and if appropriate, treatment.

SPECIFIC ADJUSTMENTS AND MOBILIZATIONS OF THE APPENDICULAR SKELETON

There exist virtually hundreds of various extremity adjustments that may be clinically effective. To avoid the stereotypical "jack-of-all-trades-master-of-none" label, the clinician should select maneuvers that can consistently be performed competently. This section will address a series of standard extremity adjustments which are a compilation of the authors' clinical experience.

Name of technique: Gonstead

Name of technique procedure: Costosternal Separation (Fig. 16.55).

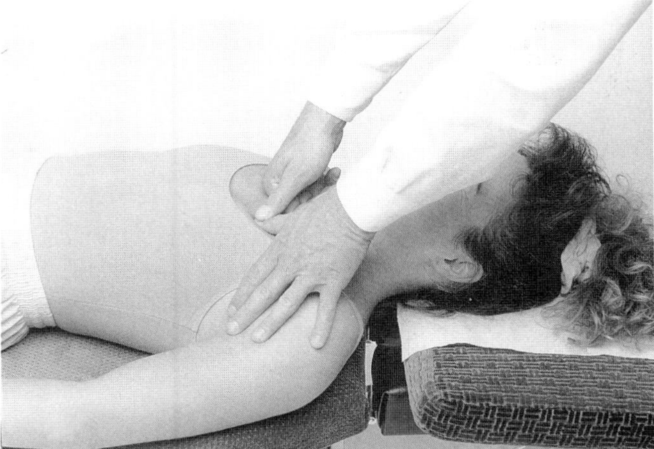

Figure 16.55. Adjustment procedure for a costosternal separation.

Indications: Localized anterior chest pain and or swelling, increased pain on deep inspiration, history of trauma to the rib cage.

Contraindications: All other listings, hypermobility, instability, rib fracture, history of pneumothorax.

Patient position: The patient is supine.

Doctor's position: The doctor stands facing the patient opposite the side of involvement.

Contact point: The doctor uses a thumb-over-thumb contact with the superior hand.

Segmental contact point: Directly over the anteriorly displaced costal cartilage.

Pattern of thrust: The maneuver is a light to moderate compression during complete expiration followed with an anterior to posterior and superior to inferior thrust.

Category by algorithm: Short lever specific contact procedure.

Name of technique: Gonstead

Name of technique procedure: Anterosuperior Proximal Clavicle Adjustment (Fig. 16.56).

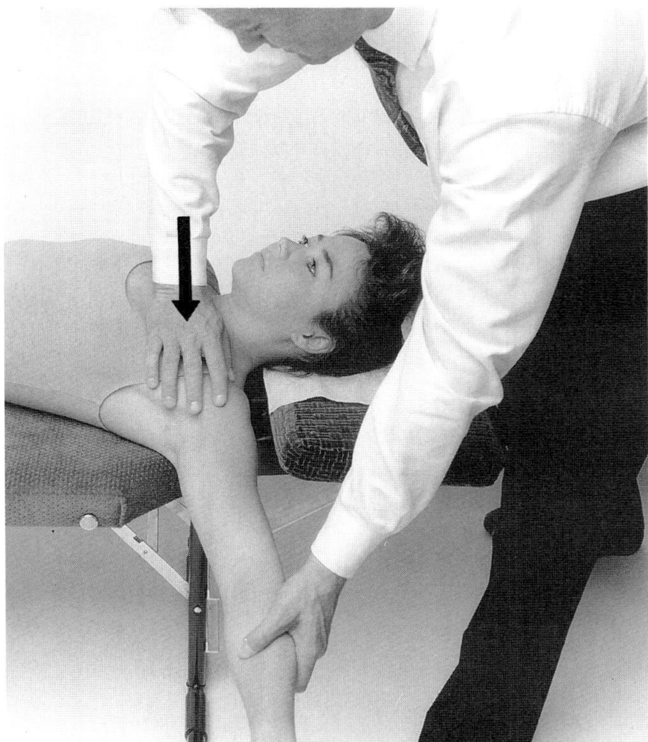

Figure 16.56. Adjustment procedure for an anterosuperior proximal clavicle.

Indications: Sternoclavicular joint pain and or swelling.

Contraindication: All other listings, hypermobility, instability, osseous fracture.

Patient position: The patient is supine, the glenohumeral joint of the involved side is positioned slightly over the edge of the bench.

Doctor's position: The doctor stands at the head of the table facing the patient while slightly favoring the involved side.

Contact point: The thenar eminence of the medial hand.

Segmental contact point: The anterosuperior aspect of the proximal end of the clavicle.

Supporting hand: The lateral hand of the doctor stabilizes the involved extremity by grasping the wrist and guiding the arm into full horizontal abduction.

Pattern of thrust: From the fully abducted position the involved extremity is slightly adducted by the supporting hand while the contact hand delivers a thrust in an anterior to posterior and superior to inferior direction.

Category by algorithm: Short lever specific contact procedure.

Name of technique: Gonstead

Name of technique procedure: Superior Distal Clavicle Adjustment (acromioclavicular joint sprain) (Fig. 16. 57A-B).

Indications: Acromioclavicular joint sprain with associated clavicular displacement.

Contraindication: All other listings, hypermobility, instability, fracture.

Patient position: The patient is seated in a cervical chair with the back in the full vertical position.

Doctor's position: The doctor stands behind the patient slightly favoring the involved side.

Contact point: The pisiform of the medial hand.

Segmental contact point: The superior aspect of the distal clavicle.

Supporting hand: The doctor's lateral hand grasps the elbow of the involved extremity which is flexed to 90° and abducts the arm to 90°.

Pattern of thrust: The lateral hand externally rotates the humerus as the medial hand initially compresses and then thrusts in a superior to inferior direction.

Category by algorithm: Short lever specific contact procedure.

Name of technique: Gonstead

Name of technique procedure: Anteroinferior Humerus Adjustment (Fig. 16.58A-C).

Indications: Anterior shoulder pain, generalized shoulder pain, bicipital tendonitis, rotator cuff tendonitis, prior shoulder dislocation, shoulder pain after lifting an object, difficulty in abduction of shoulder and arm especially above 90°.

Contraindications: All other listings, hypermobility, instability, advanced impingement syndrome, soft tissue rupture, acromioclavicular sprain, adhesive capsulitis (frozen shoulder), fracture, dislocation.

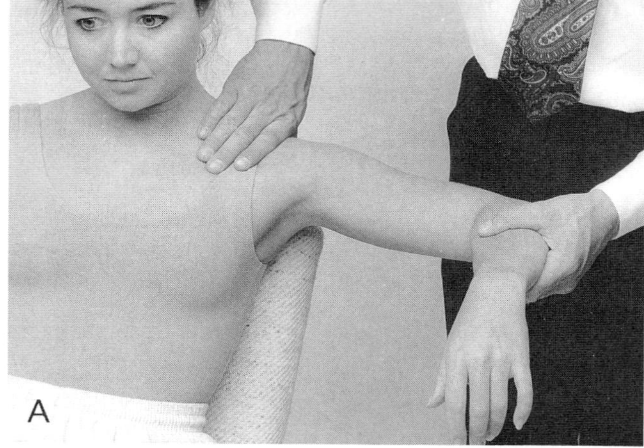

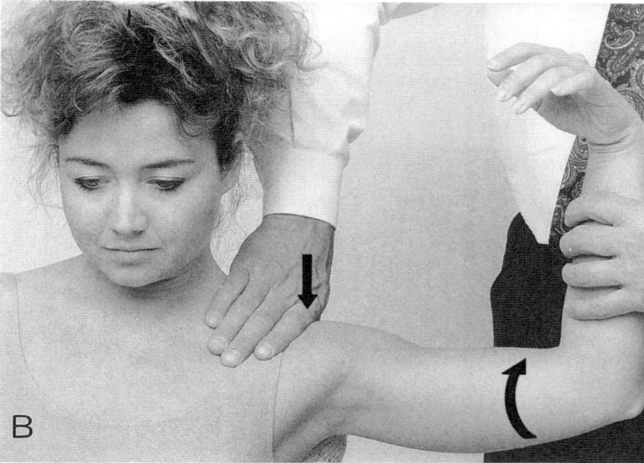

Figure 16.57A-B. Adjustment procedure for a superior distal clavicle.

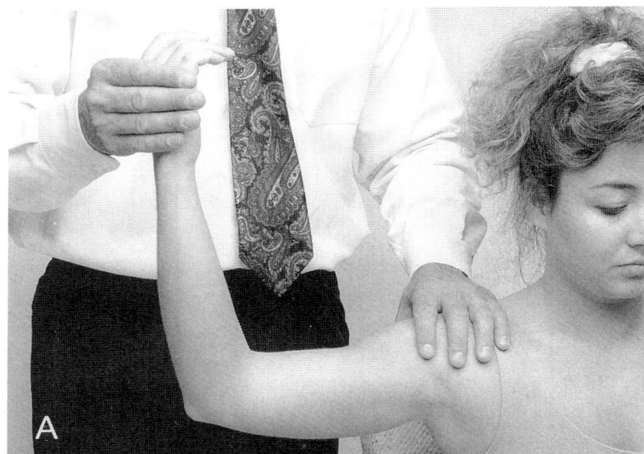

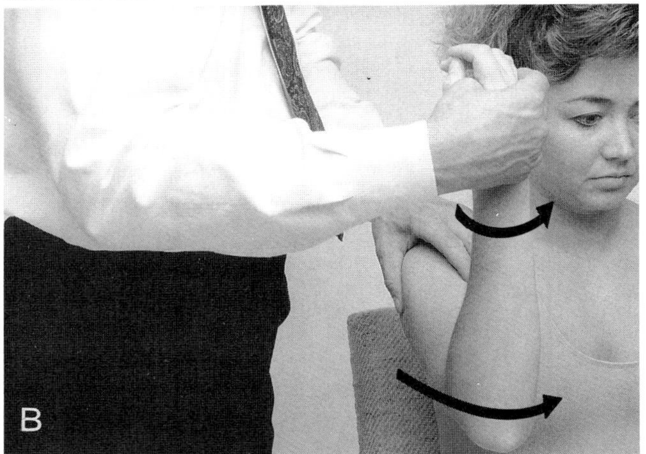

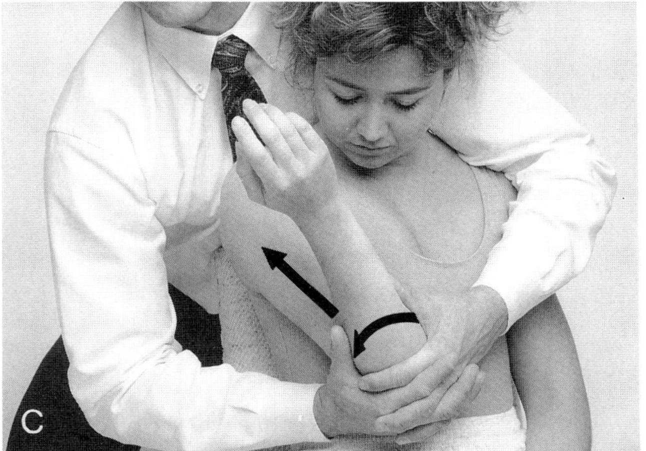

Figure 16.58A-C. Adjustment procedure for an anteroinferior humerus.

Patient position: The patient is seated in a cervical chair with the chair back positioned in the full vertical position.

Doctor's position: The doctor stands behind the patient slightly favoring the involved shoulder.

Contact point: The doctor interlocks the fingers and cups the flexed elbow of the patient on the involved side. The thumbs of both hands are placed on the medial and lateral aspects of the forearm of the involved side. The posterior aspect of the scapula on the involved side is firmly stabilized by compressing against the patient's back with the doctor's chest.

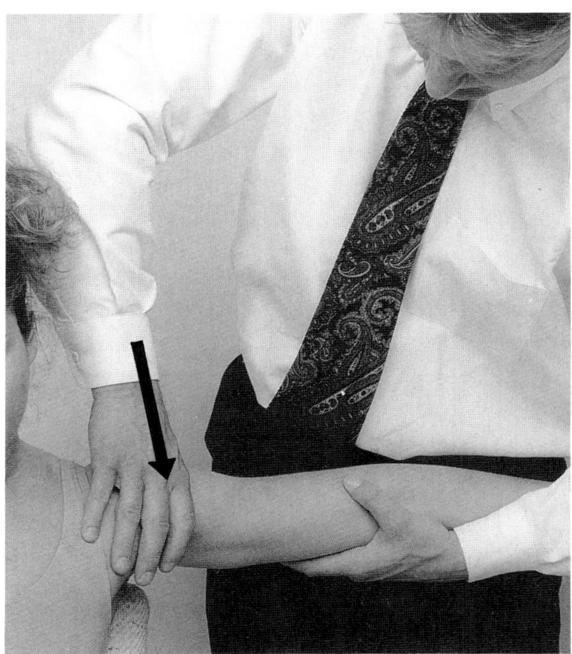

Figure 16.59. Adjustment procedure for a posterosuperior humerus.

Pattern of thrust: The doctor circumducts the involved shoulder two to five times and slightly flexes and adducts the humerus while fully flexing the elbow. The thumbs of the doctor are used to externally rotate the humerus externally. The doctor slowly lifts the arm inferior to superior to bring the glenohumeral joint to tension and then applies a light inferior to superior and anterior to posterior thrust.

Category by algorithm: Short lever specific contact procedure.

Name of technique: Gonstead

Name of technique procedure: Posterosuperior Humerus Adjustment (Fig. 16.59).

Indications: History of falling on an outstretched arm, history of posterior shoulder dislocation, impingement syndrome.

Contraindications: All other listings, hypermobility, instability, ligamentous and or tendonous rupture, fracture.

Patient position: The patient is seated.

Doctor's position: The doctor stands behind the patient favoring the involved extremity.

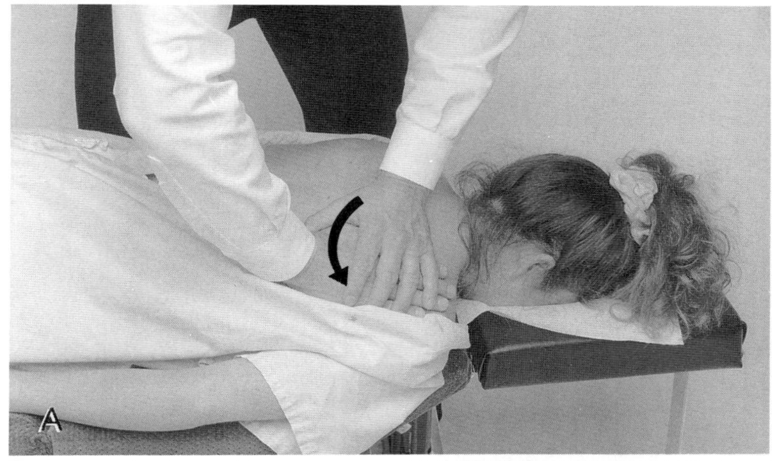

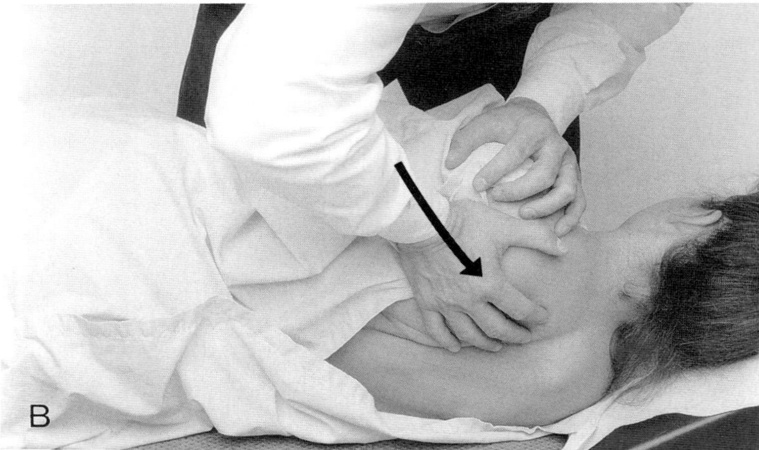

Figure 16.60. A, Adjustment procedure for a superomedial scapula. **B,** Maneuver for a superolateral scapula.

Contact point: The doctor takes a thumb web contact with the medial hand.

Segmental contact point: Posterosuperior aspect of the humeral head.

Supporting hand: The lateral hand stabilizes the involved side at the elbow. The involved limb is abducted to approximately 90° and should remain essentially parallel to the floor.

Pattern of thrust: The joint is taken to the end of joint play, directing the force of the contact hand in a posterior to anterior and superior to inferior direction. If the joint does not reduce at this point, a light thrust is delivered in the same direction.

Category by algorithm: Short lever specific contact procedure.

Name of technique: Gonstead

Name of technique procedure: Superomedial or Superolateral Scapula Adjustment (Fig. 16.60A-B).

Indications: Direct trauma, long-term spasm and/or myofascitis of the rhomboids, trapezium, and levator scapulae, abnormal scapulohumeral motion.

Contraindications: All other listings, hypermobility, instability, fracture.

Patient position: The patient is prone.

Doctor's position: The doctor stands on the opposite side of involvement reaching across the patient to the involved scapula (superomedial adjustment).

Contact point: The thenar eminence of the medial hand.

Segmental contact point: Superolateral aspect of the scapula.

Supporting hand: The lateral hand stabilizes the dorsum of the contact hand.

Pattern of thrust: A moderate thrust is delivered in a superior to inferior and medial to lateral direction while torquing superior to inferior.

Category by algorithm: Short lever specific contact procedure.

Name of technique: Gonstead

Name of technique procedure: Posterolateral Ulna Adjustment (Fig. 16.61).

Indications: Elbow trauma, inflammation of olecranon bursa, decreased elbow extension range of motion, hyperflexion injury to the elbow, history of throwing motions and sports participation.

Contraindications: All other listings, hypermobility, instability, fracture.

Patient position: The patient is seated.

Doctor's position: The doctor sits or stands slightly favoring the involved side.

Contact point: The thenar eminence of the medial hand.

Segmental contact point: The posterior aspect of the olecranon process.

Supporting hand: The lateral hand of the doctor stabilizes the involved extremity by grasping the wrist and maintaining it in full supination.

Pattern of thrust: A light thrust in a posterior to anterior and superior to inferior direction is delivered to a slightly flexed elbow.

Category by algorithm: Short lever specific contact procedure.

Name of technique: Gonstead

Name of technique procedure: Medioinferior Ulna Adjustment (Fig. 16.62).

Indications: Ulnar nerve paresthesia, wrist or elbow trauma, medial elbow pain, restricted elbow extension range of motion, history of throwing motion, sports participation.

Contraindications: All other listings, hypermobility, instability, fracture.

Patient position: The patient is seated.

Doctor's position: The doctor sits or stands facing the patient slightly favoring the involved side.

Contact point: The thenar eminence of the medial hand.

Segmental contact point: The posteromedial aspect of the olecranon process.

Supporting hand: The lateral hand of the doctor stabilizes the involved extremity by grasping the wrist and maintaining it in full supination.

Pattern of thrust: A light high velocity thrust is delivered to the slightly flexed joint in an inferior to superior and medial to lateral direction.

Category by algorithm: Short lever specific contact procedure.

Name of technique: Gonstead

Name of technique procedure: Posterolateral Radial Head Adjustment (Fig. 16.63).

Indications: Lateral epicondylitis, radial head pain and or swelling, decreased and/or painful wrist supination, history of elbow trauma, history of throwing motion, sports participation or inability to fully supinate.

Contraindications: All other listings, hypermobility, instability, fracture.

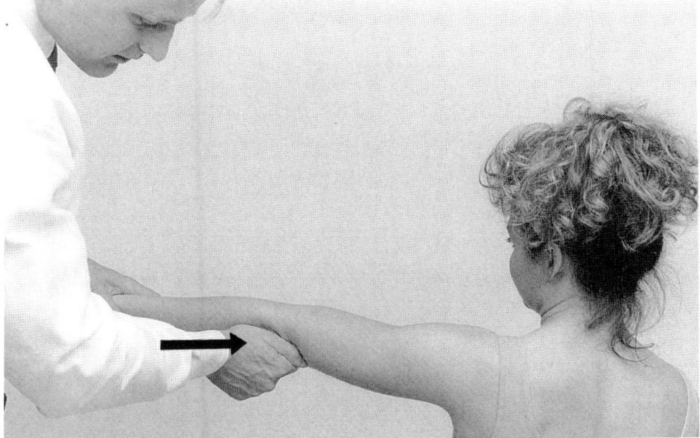

Figure 16.61. Adjustment procedure for a posterolateral ulna.

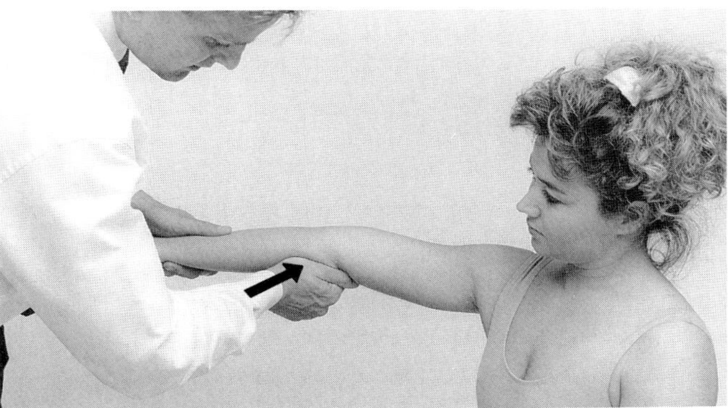

Figure 16.62. Adjustment procedure for a medioinferior ulna.

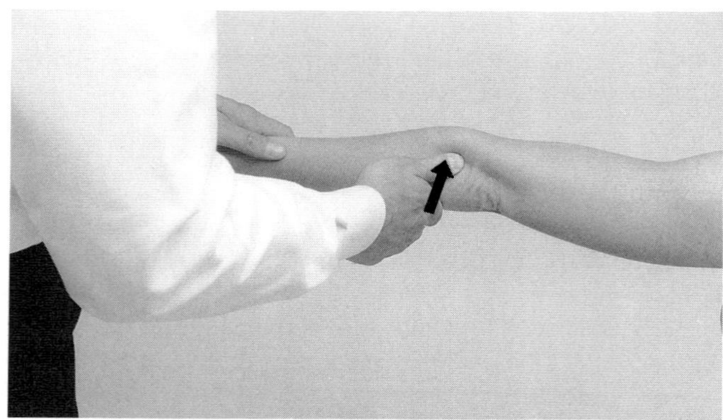

Figure 16.63. Adjustment procedure for a posterolateral radial head.

Patient position: The patient is seated.

Doctor's position: The doctor sits or stands facing the patient slightly favoring the involved extremity.

Contact point: The distal phalanx of the thumb of the lateral hand.

Segmental contact point: Posterolateral aspect of the radial head.

Supporting hand: The medial hand of the doctor stabilizes the involved extremity by grasping the wrist and maintaining it in full supination.

Pattern of thrust: A moderate thrust is delivered in a posterior to anterior and lateral to medial direction.

Category by algorithm: Short lever specific contact procedure.

Name of technique: Gonstead

Name of technique procedure: Distal Radioulnar Separation (Fig. 16.64A-B).

Indications: Wrist sprain, wrist trauma, decreased wrist range of motion, pain and/or swelling of the distal radioulnar articulation, carpal tunnel syndrome.

Contraindications: All other listings, hypermobility, instability, fracture, presence of avascular necrosis of an adjacent carpal bone.

Patient position: The patient is seated. The elbow of the involved side is flexed to 90° with the thumb pointing up.

Doctor's position: The doctor sits or stands facing the patient slightly favoring the involved side.

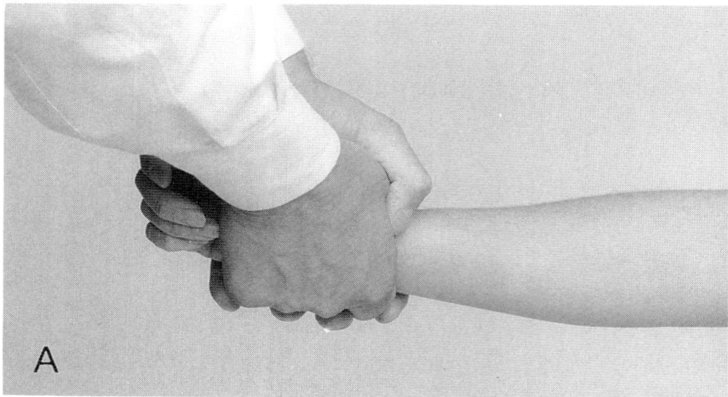

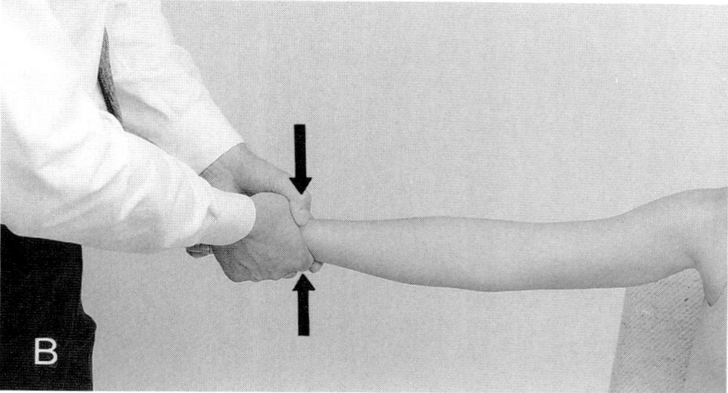

Figure 16.64. Adjustment procedure for a distal radioulnar separation. **A,** Set-up for the adjustment. **B,** Pattern of thrust.

Contact point: The doctor interlocks the fingers and wraps them and both thumbs around the distal ulna and radius. The thumbs overlie the distal radius while the intertwined fingers cradle the distal ulna.

Pattern of thrust: The distal radius and ulna are approximated by a quick "squeezing" thrust delivered by both hands of the doctor.

Category by algorithm: Short lever specific contact procedure.

Name of technique: Gonstead

Name of technique procedure: Anterior Carpal Adjustment (Fig. 16.65).

Indications: Wrist sprain, anterior wrist pain and/or swelling, ganglion cyst, loss of wrist range of motion (especially flexion), carpal tunnel syndrome.

Contraindications: All other listings, hypermobility, instability, osseous fracture, avascular necrosis of involved carpal bone, advanced osteoarthritis.

Patient position: The patient is seated.

Doctor's position: The doctor is seated or standing, facing the patient.

Contact point: The doctor takes a thumb-over-thumb contact.

Segmental contact point: The anterior aspect of the involved carpal.

Supporting hand: The fingers of both hands wrap around the hand of the involved wrist and guide the wrist from extension into flexion during the adjustment.

Pattern of thrust: The wrist is guided into slight flexion followed by a moderate thrust in an anterior to posterior direction.

Category by algorithm: Short lever specific contact procedure.

Name of technique: Gonstead

Name of technique procedure: Posterior Carpal Adjustment (Fig. 16.66).

Indications: Wrist sprain, posterior wrist pain, ganglion cyst, limitation of wrist motion (primarily extension).

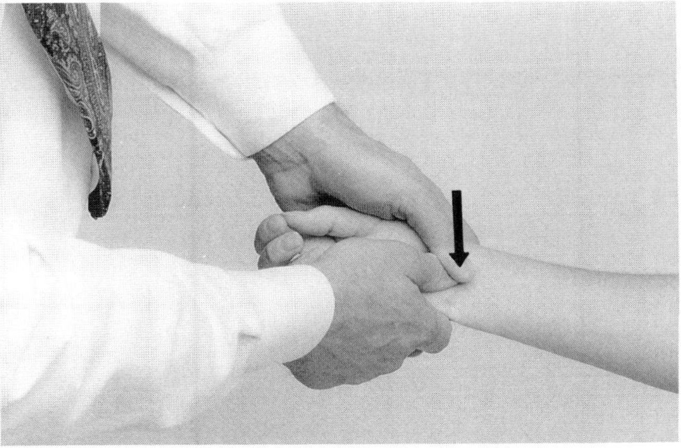

Figure 16.65. Adjustment procedure for an anterior carpal.

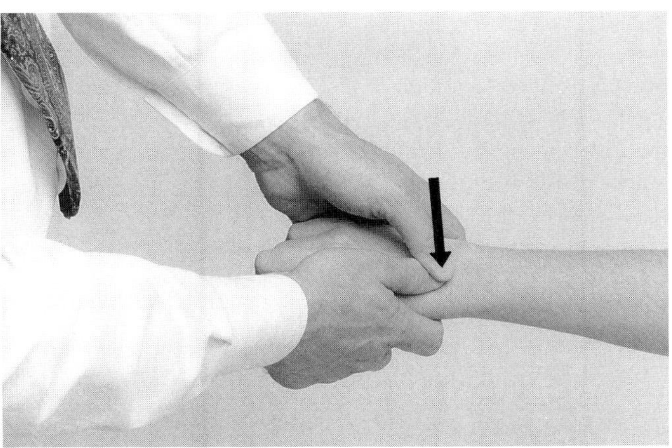

Figure 16.66. Adjustment procedure for a posterior carpal.

Contraindications: All other listings, hypermobility, instability, osseous fracture, avascular necrosis of involved carpal bone, advanced osteoarthritis.

Patient position: The patient is seated.

Doctor's position: The doctor is seated or standing, facing the patient.

Contact point: The doctor takes a thumb-over-thumb contact.

Segmental contact point: The posterior aspect of the involved carpal.

Supporting hand: The fingers of both hands wrap around the hand of the involved wrist and guide the wrist from flexion into extension during the adjustment.

Pattern of thrust: The wrist is guided into slight extension followed by a moderate thrust in a posterior to anterior direction.

Category by algorithm: Short lever specific contact procedure.

Name of technique: Gonstead

Name of technique procedure: Posterolateral Proximal First Metacarpal Adjustment (Fig. 16.67).

Indications: Pain, swelling, and/or decreased range of motion of the metacarpotrapezial articulation, deQuarvain's disease, thumb sprain.

Contraindications: All other listings, hypermobility, instability, fracture.

Patient position: The patient is seated.

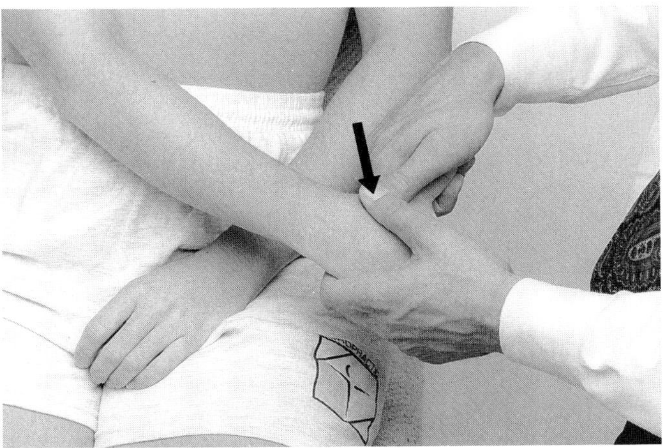

Figure 16.67. Adjustment procedure for a posterolateral proximal first metacarpal.

Doctor's position: The doctor is standing or seated facing the patient.

Contact point: The distal phalanx of the thumb of the lateral hand. The 2nd through 5th digits wrap around the involved 1st digit.

Segmental contact point: The posterolateral aspect of the proximal end of the first metacarpal.

Supporting hand: The thumb of the medial hand overlaps the contact thumb. The 2nd through 5th digits wrap around and support the hand of the involved extremity.

Pattern of thrust: Initially the involved metacarpal is distracted, followed by a thrust delivered by the thumb of the medial hand.

Category of algorithm: Short lever specific contact procedure.

Name of technique: Gonstead

Name of technique procedure: Anteromedial (AIn) Distal Femur Adjustment (Fig. 16.68A-B).

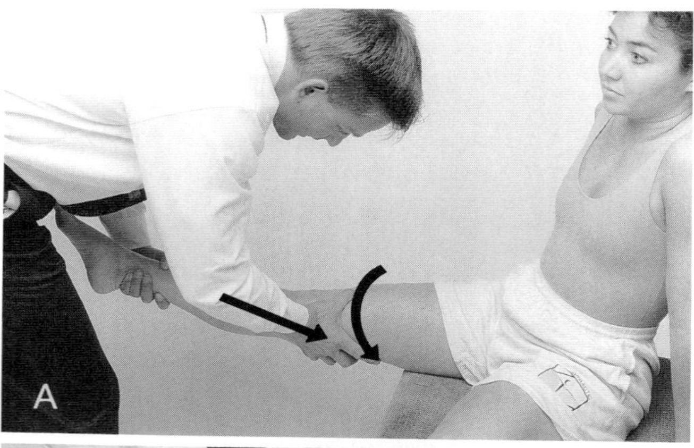

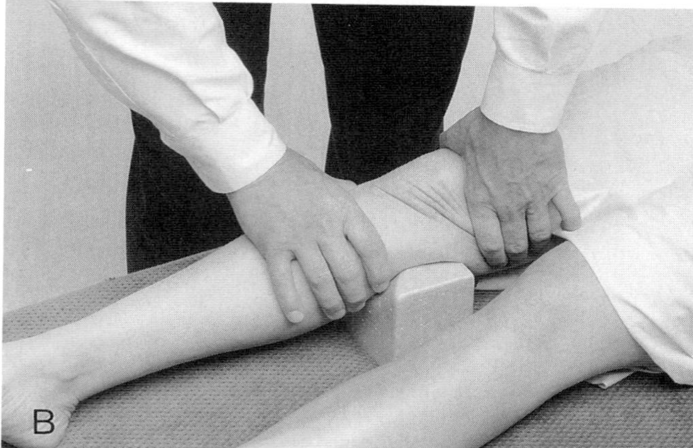

Figure 16.68. A, Adjustment procedure for an anteromedial (AIn) distal femur. **B,** Alternative maneuver for an anteromedial (AIn) distal femur.

Indications: Medial collateral ligament sprain, medial knee pain and/or swelling, joint fixation.

Contraindications: All other listings, hypermobility, instability, ligament rupture, fracture, advanced meniscal tear.

Patient position: Patient is seated.

Doctor's position: The doctor stands facing the patient favoring the subluxated knee.

Doctor's contact point: The lateral aspect of the proximal phalanx of the second digit of the medial hand or the thenar eminence.

Segmental contact point: The anteromedial aspect of the distal femur.

Supporting hand: The lateral hand stabilizes the distal tibia in external rotation.

Pattern of thrust: As the doctor slightly distracts the lower leg, the medial hand thrusts anterior to posterior and medial to lateral. Care must be taken to not thrust a semiflexed knee as to avoid hyperextending the joint.

Category by algorithm: Short lever specific contact procedure.

Name of technique: Gonstead

Name of technique procedure: Posterolateral (PEx) Proximal Tibia Adjustment (Fig. 16.69).

Indications: Lateral collateral ligament injury, posterolateral rotatory instability, lateral knee pain, joint fixation.

Contraindications: All other listings, hypermobility, instability, ligament rupture, fracture.

Patient position: Patient is prone with feet extending over the end of the pelvic bench.

Doctor's position: The doctor stands facing the patient on the opposite side of the table as the subluxated knee.

Contact point: The palmar aspect of the distal phalanx of the third digit of the superior hand.

Segmental contact point: The doctor reaches under the patient's leg from medial to lateral, contacting the posterior lateral tibia and the lateral joint line. Care should be taken not to contact the proximal fibula.

Supporting hand: The free hand supports the posterior ankle while internally rotating the lower leg.

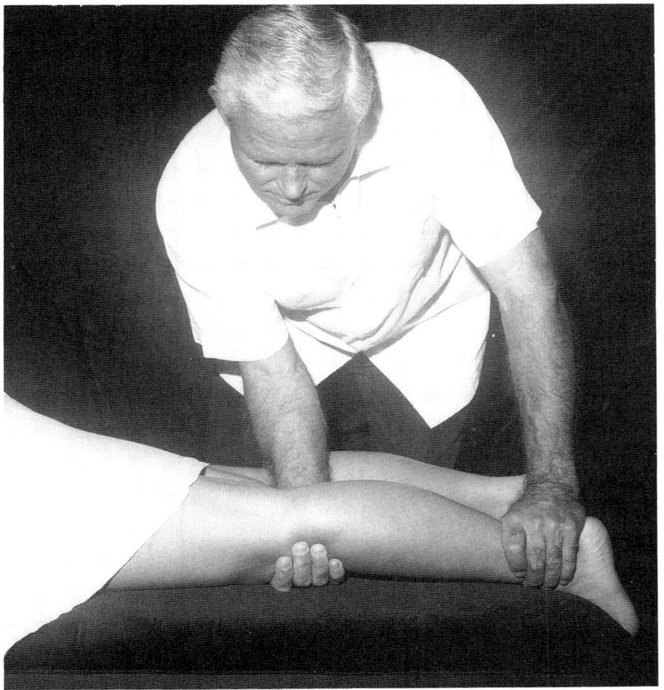

Figure 16.69. Adjustment procedure for a posterolateral (PEx) proximal tibia.

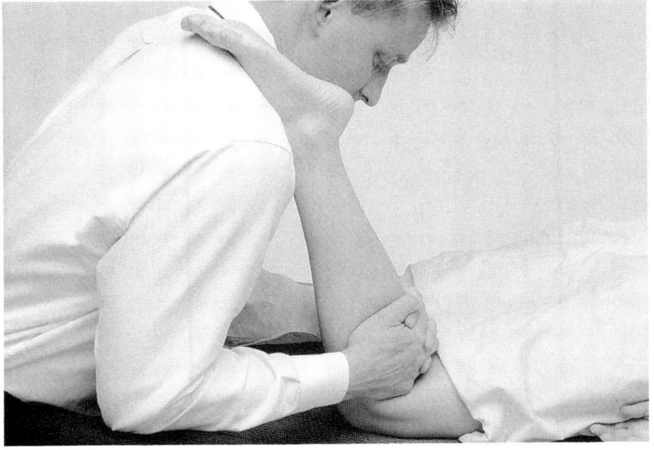

Figure 16.70. Adjustment procedure for a posterior proximal tibia.

Pattern of thrust: The thrust is posterior to anterior and lateral to medial.

Category by algorithm: Short lever specific contact procedure.

Name of technique: Gonstead

Name of technique procedure: Posterior Proximal Tibia Adjustment (Fig. 16.70).

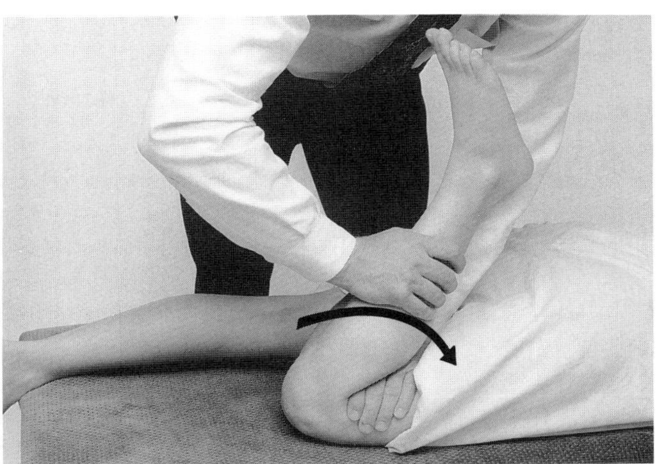

Figure 16.71. Maneuver for tibiofemoral joint traction.

Indications: History of anterior knee trauma, history of anterior cruciate ligament sprain, decreased range of motion in flexion of the knee, posterior knee pain or swelling.

Contraindications: All other listings, hypermobility, instability, posterior cruciate ligament sprain, fracture.

Patient position: Patient is placed in the prone position with the involved knee flexed to 40° to 50°.

Doctor's position: The doctor is at the feet of the patient facing cephalad.

Segmental contact point: The posterior aspect of the superior proximal tibia.

Contact point: The doctor interlocks the fingers and uses the anterolateral aspect of the right and left 5th digits to contact the patient.

Stabilization: Stabilization is provided to the lower leg by placing the dorsum of the foot of the involved side on the lateral shoulder of the doctor.

Pattern of thrust: The thrust is a medium to heavy force directed posterior to anterior.

Category by algorithm: Short lever specific contact procedure.

Name of technique: Gonstead

Name of technique procedure: Tibiofemoral Joint Traction (Fig. 16.71).

Indications: Generalized knee pain and stiffness, joint contracture, stable osteoarthritis, mild joint effusion.

Contraindications: All other listings, hypermobility, instability, fracture, patellofemoral disorders.

Patient position: The patient is prone.

Doctor's position: The doctor stands facing the patient on the side of involvement.

Contact point: The doctor uses the thumb-web of the superior hand.

Segmental contact point: The popliteal fossa of the involved knee.

Supporting hand: The inferior hand supports the involved extremity by grasping the ankle.

Pattern of thrust: The knee is slowly flexed and distracted over the contact hand by the supporting hand.

Category by algorithm: Long lever specific contact procedure.

Name of technique: Gonstead

Name of technique procedure: Anteroinferior Proximal Fibula Adjustment.

Indications: Inversion ankle sprain, lateral knee pain on walking, running, or stair climbing. Lateral knee pain on resisted knee flexion and simultaneous tibial rotation.

Contraindications: All other listings, hypermobility, instability, local fracture.

Patient position: The patient is seated.

Doctor's position: The doctor is seated, facing the patient.

Segmental contact point: The anteroinferior aspect of the fibular head.

Contact point: The thenar eminence of the lateral hand.

Supporting hand: The medial hand stabilizes the ankle.

Pattern of thrust: The thrust is directed posterior and superior.

Category by algorithm: Short lever specific contact procedure.

Name of technique: Gonstead

Name of technique procedure: Posterior Lateral Malleolus Adjustment.

Indications: Inversion ankle sprain, direct trauma to anterior distal fibula, dysfunction of the pelvis and/or lumbar spine.

Contraindications: All other listings, hypermobility, instability, fibular fracture.

Patient position: The patient is prone.

Doctor's position: The doctor stands opposite the side of segmental involvement.

Segmental contact point: The posterior border of the lateral malleolus.

Contact point: The pisiform of the inferior hand.

Supporting hand: The superior hand wraps around and supports the wrist of the contact hand.

Pattern of thrust: The thrust is directed posterior to anterior.

Category by algorithm: Short lever specific contact procedure.

Name of technique: Gonstead

Name of technique procedure: Distal Tibiofibular Separation Adjustment.

Indications: Inversion ankle sprain, eversion ankle sprain, pain on forced dorsiflexion.

Contraindications: All other listings, hypermobility, instability, medial or lateral malleolar fracture.

Patient position: The patient is supine or seated.

Doctor's position: The doctor faces the patient, at the feet.

Contact point: Both hands are used in opposition of one another. Contact is made by each thenar.

Segmental contact point: 1) internal hand contacts the medial malleoli; 2) outer hand contacts the lateral malleoli.

Pattern of thrust: The distal tibia and fibula are squeezed together by thrusting from lateral to medial on the fibula, approximating the tibia.

Category by algorithm: Short lever specific contact procedure.

Name of technique: Gonstead

Name of technique procedure: Anterior Talus Adjustment.

Indications: This misalignment is similar to anterior-inferior talus but not as common. Pain is usually localized to anterior aspect of ankle, which worsens with dorsiflexion.

Contraindications: All other listings, hypermobility, instability, talar fracture, medial or lateral malleolar fracture.

Patent position: Seated or supine on bench.

Doctor's position: Doctor is at the foot of patient, facing the patient.

Contact point: The tips of both thumbs.

Segmental contact point: The anterior aspect of the dome of the talus.

Supporting hand: The doctor wraps the 2nd to 5th digits of both hands around the plantar surface of the foot and posterior aspect of the calcaneus.

Pattern of thrust: The adjustment is initiated with the ankle in plantarflexion. The fingers around the calcaneus act as a lever to pull the talus into the mortise as the ankle is dorsiflexed, followed by delivery of a light thrust.

Category by algorithm: Short lever specific contact procedure.

Name of technique: Gonstead

Name of technique procedure: Traction Maneuver for Anteroinferior Talus (aka: lateroinferior talus).

Indications: Inversion sprain, excessive supination, anterior ankle pain, pain on dorsiflexion.

Contraindications: All other listings, hypermobility, instability.

Patient position: Patient is supine.

Doctor's position: Doctor stands at the foot of the patient, facing them.

Contact point: The 4th and 5th fingers of the doctor's medial hand.

Segmental contact point: Contact is made over the anterior-lateral aspect of talus.

Supporting hand: The area is stabilized by placing the fingers over the tops of contact hand fingers.

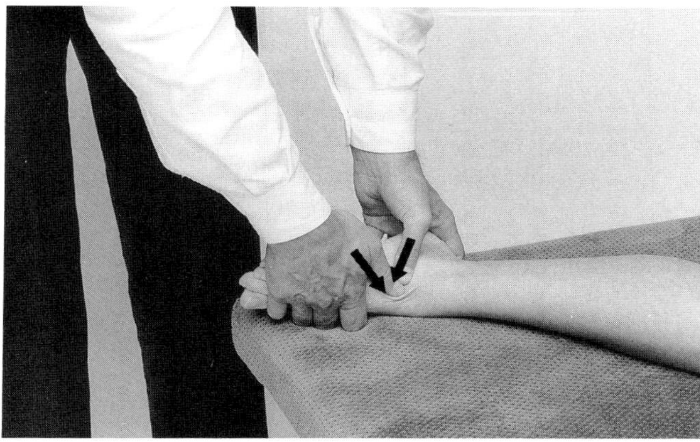

Figure 16.72. Adjustment procedure for an anteroinferior talus.

Pattern of thrust: The mortise joint is lightly distracted superior to inferior, followed by a thrusting action anterior to posterior and lateral to medial.

Category by algorithm: Short lever specific contact procedure.

Name of technique: Gonstead

Name of technique procedure: Anteroinferior Talus Adjustment (aka: lateroinferior talus) (Fig. 16.72).

Indications: Inversion sprain, excessive supination, medial ankle trauma, pain on plantar flexion.

Contraindications: All other listings, hypermobility, instability, malleolar fracture, talar dome fracture.

Patient position: The patient is seated or lying supine.

Doctor's position: The doctor stands facing the patient at the feet of the patient.

Contact point: The distal phalanx of lateral thumb.

Segmental contact point: Lateral anterior aspect of the talus.

Supporting hand: Distal phalanx of medial thumb overlaps contact point.

Pattern of thrust: The fingers are used to rock the talus and calcaneus into dorsiflexion as the thumb contact thrusts lateral to medial and anterior to posterior.

Category by algorithm: Short lever specific contact procedure.

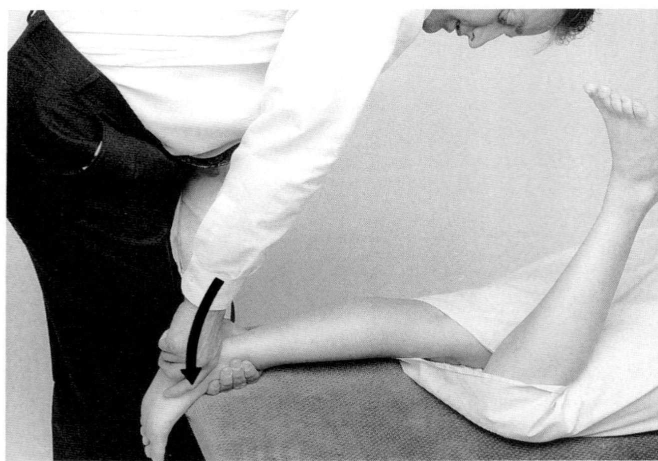

Figure 16.73. Adjustment procedure for a posterior calcaneus.

Name of technique: Gonstead

Name of technique procedure: Posterior Calcaneus Adjustment (Fig. 16.73).

Indications: Posterior calcaneal pain, pain during heel strike, heel spur, burning heel, achilles tendon injuries, tarsal tunnel syndrome.

Contraindications: All other listings, hypermobility, instability, calcaneal fractures, Sever's disease.

Patient position: The patient is prone, feet extending just over the end of the table.

Doctor's position: Doctor faces the patient at the feet of the patient.

Contact point: Thumbweb of the outer hand

Segmental contact point: Posterior aspect of the involved calcaneus.

Supporting hand: Fingers of the inner hand wrap under the anterior ankle and support the mortise joint.

Pattern of thrust: A moderate to heavy thrust is made posterior to anterior.

Category by algorithm: Short lever specific contact procedure.

Name of technique: Gonstead

Name of technique procedure: Lateral Calcaneus Adjustment.

Indications: Lateral talocalcaneal joint line pain, loss of eversion range of motion at the subtalar joint, excessive supination, increased outer heel wear on shoes.

Contraindications: All other listings, hypermobility, instability, calcaneal fracture, Sever's disease.

Patient position: The patient is prone with the feet extending over the end of the table.

Doctor's position: The doctor faces patient at the feet of the patient.

Contact point: Thumb web of the outer hand.

Segmental contact point: Posterolateral aspect of the calcaneus.

Supporting hand: Fingers of the inner hand wrap under the anterior ankle and support the mortise joint.

Patterns of thrust: A moderate to heavy thrust is made posterior to anterior and lateral to medial.

Category by algorithm: Short lever specific contact procedure.

Name of technique: Gonstead

Name of technique procedure: Medial Calcaneus Adjustment.

Indications: Medial talocalcaneal joint line pain, loss of inversion range of motion at the subtalar joint, hyperpronation, excessive medial heel wear on shoes.

Contraindications: All other listings hypermobility, instability, calcaneal fracture, Sever's disease.

Patient position: Patient is prone with feet extending over end of the table.

Doctor's position: Doctor is at the feet of the patient facing the patient.

Contact point: Thumb web of the inner hand.

Segmental contact point: Posteromedial aspect of the calcaneus.

Supporting hand: The fingers of the outer hand wrap under the anterior ankle and support the mortise joint.

Pattern of thrust: A moderate to heavy thrust is made posterior to anterior and medial to lateral.

Category by algorithm: Short lever specific contact procedure.

Name of technique: Gonstead

Name of technique procedure: Inferior Navicular Adjustment (Fig. 16.74).

Indications: Arch strain, fallen arches, hyperpronation, some varieties of shin splints.

Contraindications: All other listings, hypermobility, instability, local fracture.

Patient position: The patient is seated with the involved foot positioned in the lap of the doctor.

Doctor's position: The doctor is seated facing the patient.

Contact point: The doctor makes a double thumb or thenar contact.

Segmental contact point: Inferior-medial aspect of the navicular.

Supporting hand: The fingers of both hands wrap around and support the forefoot and midfoot.

Pattern of thrust: The foot is positioned in plantarflexion and inversion. A moderate thrust is directed inferior to superior and medial to lateral.

Category by algorithm: Short lever specific contact procedure.

Name of technique: Gonstead

Description of technique procedure: Inferior Cuneiform Adjustment (Fig. 16.75).

Indications: Loss of medial or lateral longitudinal arch, local pain and/or swelling, hyperdorsiflexion injury of the foot.

Contraindications: All other listings, hypermobility, instability, local fracture.

Patient position: The patient is prone with the knee of the involved extremity flexed to 60° to 75°.

Doctor's position: The doctor stands facing the patient at the feet of the patient.

Contact point: The doctor makes a double thumb contact.

Segmental contact point: The inferior aspect of the involved cuneiform.

Supporting hand: The fingers of both hands wrap around and support the dorsum of the foot.

Pattern of thrust: The foot is plantarflexed over the contact point followed by a light to medium inferior to superior thrust.

Category by algorithm: Short lever specific contact procedure.

Name of technique: Gonstead

Name of technique procedure: Inferior Distal Metatarsal Head Adjustment (Fig. 16.76).

Indications: Hammer toe, corn and callus formation, loss of transverse arch, turf toe.

Contraindications: All other listings, hypermobility, instability, local fracture.

Patient position: The patient is seated with the involved extremity positioned in the lap of the doctor.

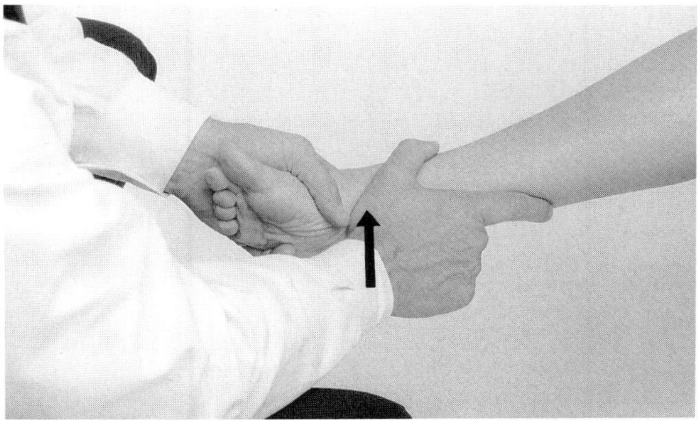

Figure 16.74. Adjustment procedure for an inferior navicular.

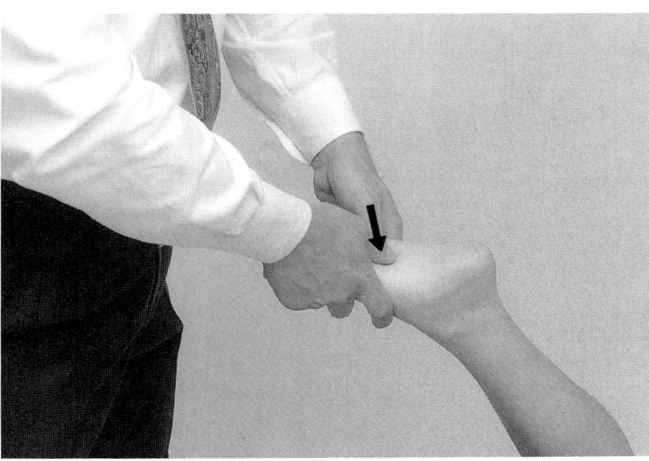

Figure 16.75. Adjustment procedure for an inferior cuneiform.

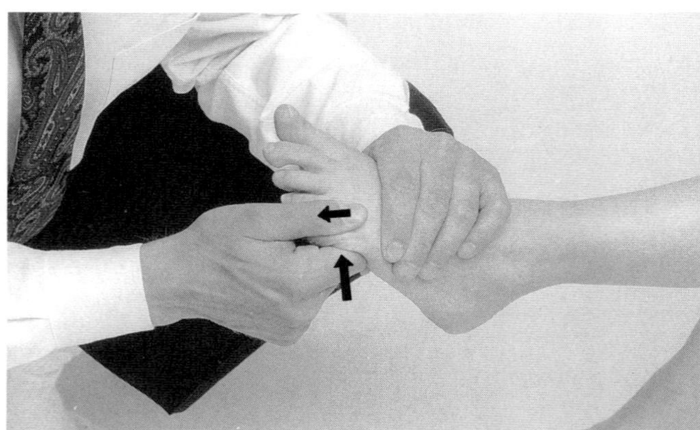

Figure 16.76. Adjustment procedure for an inferior distal metatarsal head.

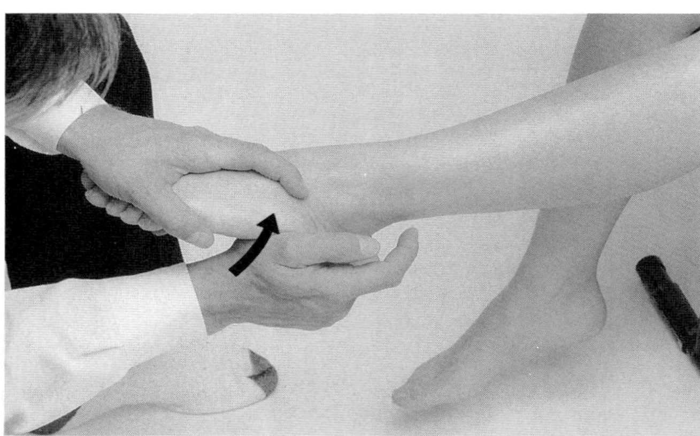

Figure 16.77. Adjustment procedure for a lateroinferior cuboid.

Doctor's position: The doctor is seated facing the patient.

Contact point: The lateral side of a flexed second proximal interphalangeal joint on the lateral hand.

Segmental contact point: The inferior aspect of the distal end of the involved metatarsal.

Supporting hand: The thumb of the contact hand wraps over the involved toe and contacts the superior aspect of the proximal end of the proximal phalanx.

Pattern of thrust: The doctor contact point is lightly thrusted inferior to superior as the supporting thumb slightly tractions the toe superior to inferior and distally.

Category by algorithm: Short lever specific contact procedure.

Name of Technique: Gonstead

Name of Technique Procedure: Lateroinferior Cuboid Adjustment (Fig. 16.77).

Indications: Lateral foot pain, loss of lateral transverse arch, arch strain, midfoot dysfunction.

Contraindications: All other listings, hypermobility, instability, local fracture.

Patient position: The patient is seated.

Doctor's position: The doctor is seated facing the patient.

Contact point: Thenar eminence of the lateral hand.

Segmental contact point: Lateroinferior aspect of the cuboid.

Supporting hand: The medial hand supports the dorsum of the foot while flexing the foot over the contact point.

Pattern of thrust: A moderate thrust is delivered in a lateral to medial and inferior to superior direction.

Category by algorithm: Short lever specific contact procedure.

References

1. Herbst RW. Gonstead chiropractic science and art. Mt Horeb, WI: Sci-Chi Publications, 1968.
2. DeGowin EL, DeGowin RL. Bedside diagnostic examination. New York: Macmillan, 1981:19–23.
3. Malasanos L, Barkauskas V, Moss M. Health assessment. St. Louis: CV Mosby, 1981:35–112.
4. Conwell TD. Documenting patient progress. Lakewood, CO: Conwell, 1990.
5. Davis G. Functional examination of the shoulder. Phys Sports Med 1981;9:82–103.
6. Post M. Physical examination of the musculoskeletal system. Chicago: Year Book Medical Publishers, Inc., 1987:9–12.
7. Daniels L, Worthington C. Muscle testing: techniques of manual examination. Philadelphia: WB Saunders, 1980:37–87.
8. Norkin CC, Levangie PK. Joint structure and function: a comprehensive analysis. Philadelphia: WB Saunders, 1983.
9. Cyriax J. Textbook of orthopaedic medicine: diagnosis of soft tissue lesions. London: Bailliere, Tindall, and Cassell, 1969:99–110.
10. Rothstein JM, Roy SH, Wolf SL. The rehabilitation specialist's handbook. Philadelphia: FA Davis, 1991:63–137.
11. Cailliet R. Shoulder pain. Philadelphia: FA Davis, 1981:82–103.
12. Mechelse K, Pompe R, Van Best JA. Kinematics and kinetic analysis. Neur Ortho 1986;2:43–53.
13. Lehmkuhl LD, Smith LK. Brunnstrom's clinical kinesiology. Philadelphia: FA Davis, 1983.
14. Lyon LK, Benz LN, Johnson KK, et al. Q-angle: a factor in peak torque occurrence in isokinetic knee extension. J Ortho Sports Phys Ther 1988:1:250–253.
15. Fox TA. Dysplasia of the quadriceps mechanism: hypoplasia of the vastus medialis muscle as related to the hypermobile patella syndrome. Surg Clin North Am 1975;55:199–226.
16. Turek S. Orthopedic principles and their application, 4th ed. Philadelphia: JB Lippincott, 1984.
17. Rowe C, Zarins B. Recurrent transient subluxation of the shoulder. J Bone Joint Surg 1981;66A:863–870.

18. Roy S, Irvin R. Sports medicine: prevention, evaluation, management, and rehabilitation. New Jersey: Prentice-Hall, 1983:182.
19. Warwick R, Williams P. Gray's anatomy. 35th British ed. Philadelphia: WB Saunders, 1973.
20. Penny JN, Welsh MB. Shoulder impingement syndromes in athletes and their surgical management. Am J Sports Med 1981;9:11–15.
21. Hawkins RJ, Kennedy JC. Impingement syndromes in athletes. Am J Sports Med 1980;8:151–157.
22. Neer CS. Anterior acromioplasty for the chronic impingement syndrome. J Bone Joint Surg 1972;54A:41–50.
23. Neer CS. Impingement lesions. Clin Orthop 1983;173:70–77.
24. Hawkins R, Abrams J. Impingement syndrome in the absence of rotator cuff tears (stage 1 and 2). Orthop Clin North Am 1987;18:373–382.
25. Kieft G, Bloen J, Rozing P, Obermann W. Rotator cuff impingement syndrome: mr imaging. Radiology 1988;166:211–214.
26. Resnick D, Niwayama G. Diagnosis of bone and joint disorders. Philadelphia: WB Saunders, 1983.
27. Cone RO, Resnick D, Danzig L. Shoulder impingement syndrome: radiographic evaluation. Radiology 1984;150:29.
28. Mink J, Deutsch A. MRI of the musculoskeletal system: a teaching file. New York: Raven Press, 1990:25.
29. O'Donohue D. Treatment of injuries to athletes. 4th ed. Philadelphia: WB Saunders, 1984.
30. Neviaser R. Treating patients with rotator cuff tears. Musculoskeletal Med 1985;3:17–23.
31. Brehms J. Rotator cuff tear: evaluation and treatment. Orthopedics 1988;11(1):69–81.
32. Rathbon JB, McNab I. The microscopic pattern of the rotator cuff. J Bone Joint Surg 1970;52B:540.
33. Neviaser R. Tears of the rotator cuff. Orthop Clin North Am 1980;2:295–306.
34. Jobe F, Moynes D. Delineation of diagnostic criteria and rehabilitation program for rotator cuff injuries. Am J Sports Med 1982;6:336–339.
35. Kenihan NA, Oakes BW. Soft tissue injury rehabilitation: isokinetics, a new concept. Aust Fam Phys 1981;10(suppl):17–20.
36. Oakes BW. Acute soft tissue injuries: nature and management. Aust Fam Phys 1982;10(suppl):3–16.
37. Steadman JR. Rehabilitation of athletic injuries. Am J Sports Med 1979;7:147
38. Rizk T, Christopher R, Pinals R, Higgins A, Frix R. Adhesive capsulitis (frozen shoulder): a new approach to its management. Arch Phys Med Rehab 1983;64:29–33.
39. Neviaser J. Adhesive capsulitis and the stiff and painful shoulder. Orthop Clin North Am 1980;11:327–331.
40. Simon WH. Soft tissue disorders of the shoulder: frozen shoulder, calcific tendinitis and bicipital tendonitis. Orthop Clin North Am 1975;6:521–539.
41. Bulgen D, Hazelman B, Voak D. HLA-B27 and frozen shoulder. Lancet 1976;1:1042.
42. Neviaser J. Painful conditions affecting the shoulder. Clin Orthop 1983;173:63–69.
43. Bateman J. The shoulder and neck. 2nd ed. Philadelphia: WB Saunders, 1978.
44. Wadsworth C. Frozen shoulder. Phys Ther 1986;66:1878–1883.
45. Fareed D, Gallivan W. Office management of frozen shoulder. treatment with hydraulic distension under local anesthesia. Clin Orthop 1989;242:177–183.
46. Quigley T. Checkrein shoulder, a type of frozen shoulder: diagnosis and treatment by manipulation and ACTH or cortisone. Clin Orthop 1982;164:4–9.
47. Neviaser J. Adhesive capsulitis. Orthop Clin North Am 1987;18(3):439–443.
48. Bland JH, Merrit JA, Boushey DR. Painful shoulder. Semin Arthritis Rheum 1977;7:21–47.
49. Nicholson G. The effects of passive joint mobilization on pain and hypomobility associated with adhesive capsulitis of the shoulder. J Sports Phys Ther 1985;6:238–246.
50. Hill J, Bogumill H. Manipulation in the treatment of frozen shoulder. Orthopedics 1988;11:1255–1260.
51. Grey RG. The natural history of "idiopathic" frozen shoulder. J Bone Joint Surg 1978;60A:564.
52. Taft T, Wilson F, Oglesby J. Dislocation of the acromioclavicular joint: an end-result study. J Bone Joint Surg 1987;69A:1045–1051.
53. Roy S, Irvin R. Sports medicine: prevention, evaluation, management, and rehabilitation. Englewood Cliffs, NJ: Prentice-Hall, 1983:174–175.
54. Mallon WJ, McNamara MJ, Urbaniak JR. Orthopedics for the house officer. Baltimore: Williams & Wilkins, 1990.
55. Conrad R, Hooper R. Tennis elbow: its course, natural history, conservative and surgical treatment. J Bone Joint Surg 1973;55A:1177–1182.
56. Cyriax JH. The pathology and treatment of tennis elbow. J Bone Joint Surg 1936;18:921–937.
57. Mazion J. Illustrated manual of neurological reflexes, signs, tests, and orthopedic signs, tests, maneuvers for office procedure. 2nd ed. Arizona City: J Mazion, 1980:253, 296, 327.
58. Wright RD. A detailed study of movement of the wrist joint. J Anat 1935;70:137.
59. Yochum TR, Rowe LJ. Essentials of skeletal radiology. Baltimore: Williams & Wilkins, 1987:76–78
60. Lawrence D. Fundamentals of chiropractic diagnosis and management. Baltimore: Williams & Wilkins, 1991:483–489.
61. Nugent G. Identifying carpal tunnel syndrome. Hosp Med 1980;16:48–49.
62. Cho D, Cho M. The electrodiagnosis of the carpal tunnel syndrome. South Dakota J Med 1989;46:5–8.
63. Physicare. The medical newsletter of the Marion Joy rehabilitation center 1988;1:4.
64. Wieslander G, Norback D, Gothe C. Carpal tunnel syndrome (CTS) and exposure to vibration, repetitive wrist movements and heavy manual work: a case study. Br J Indust Med 1989;46:43–47.
65. Pryse-Phillips W. Validation of a diagnostic sign in carpal tunnel syndrome. J Neur Neurosurg Psych 1984;47:870–872.
66. Gilliat R, Wilson G. A pneumatic-tourniquet test in the carpal tunnel syndrome. Lancet 1953;1:595–597.
67. Mink J, Deutsch A. MRI of the musculoskeletal system: a teaching file. New York: Raven Press, 1990:88–89.
68. Cailliet R. Knee pain and disability. Philadelphia: FA Davis, 1983:3–16.
69. Bressler HB, Deltoff MN. Proximal tibiofibular joint dysfunction: an overlooked diagnosis. Chiro Sports Med 1988;2:45–47.
70. Eisele SA. A precise approach to anterior knee pain. Phys Sportsmed 1991;19:127–139.
71. DeLitto A, Lehman RC. Rehabilitation of the athlete with a knee injury. Clin Sports Med 1989;8:805–857.
72. Lancourt JE, Cristine JA. Patella alta and patella infera. J Bone Joint Surg 1975;57A:1112–1115.
73. Magee DJ. Orthopedic physical assessment. Philadelphia: WB Saunders, 1987.
74. Percy EC, Strother RT. Patellalgia. Phys Sports Med 1985;13:43–58.
75. Abbott LC, Saunders J, Bost JC, Anderson CE. Injuries to the ligaments of the knee joint. J Bone Joint Surg 1944;26:503.
76. Bartel DL, Marshall JL, Schieck RA, Wang JB. Surgical repositioning of the medial collateral ligament. J Bone Joint Surg 1977;59A:107.
77. Welsh RP. Medial ligament instability of the knee. In: Welsh RP, Shephard RJ, eds. Current therapy in sports medicine. St. Louis: CV Mosby, 1985:244–246.
78. Fetto JF, Marshall JL. Medial collateral ligament injuries of the knee: a rationale for treatment. Clin Orthop 1978;132:206–217.

79. Souza T. Evaluating lateral knee pain. Chiro Sports Med 1989;3:103–110.
80. Kannus P. Nonoperative treatment of grade II and III sprains of the lateral ligament compartment of the knee. Am J Sports Med 1989;17:83–88.
81. Potera C. Knee injuries on the slopes remain a binding problem. Phys Sportsmed 1985;13:99–105.
82. Nisonson B. Anterior cruciate ligament injuries: conservative vs. surgical treatment. Phys Sportsmed 1991;19:82–89.
83. Marshall JL, Arnoczky SP, Rubin RM, Wickiewicz TL. Microvasculature of the cruciate ligaments. Phys Sportsmed 1979;7:87–91.
84. Blackburn TA. Rehabilitation of anterior cruciate ligament injuries. Orthop Clin North Am 1985;16:241–249.
85. Nisonson B. Acute hemarthrosis of the adolescent knee. Phys Sportsmed 1989;17:75–87.
86. DeHaven KE. Diagnosis of acute knee injuries with hemarthrosis. Am J Sports Med 1980;8:9–14.
87. Clancy WG, Shelbourne KD, Zoellner GB, Keene JS, Reider B, Rosenberg TD. Treatment of knee joint instability secondary to rupture of the posterior cruciate ligament. J Bone Joint Surg 1983;65A:310–322.
88. Baker CL, Norwood LA, Hughston JC. Acute combined posterior cruciate and posterolateral instability of the knee. Am J Sportsmed 1984;12:204–208.
89. Noyes FR, McGinniss GH. Controversy about treatment of the knee with anterior cruciate laxity. Clin Orthop 1985;198:61–75.
90. Middeldorf JE. Injury and treatment of the anterior cruciate ligament. Chiro Econ 1990;32:14–17.
91. Danzig L, Resnick D, Gonsalves M, Akeson WH. Blood supply to the normal and abnormal menisci of the human knee. Clin Orthop 1983;172:271–276.
92. Hermann G, Berson BL. Discoid media meniscus: two cases of tears presenting as locked knee due to athletic trauma. Am. J Sports Med 1984;12:74–76.
93. Jackson RW. The sneaky plica [Editorial]. J Rheumatol 1980;7:437.
94. Harty M, Joyce JJ. Synovial folds in the knee joint. Orthop Review 1977;7:91–92.
95. Helfet AJ. Disorders of the knee. Philadelphia: JB Lippincott, 1974.
96. Hardaker WT, Whipple TL, Basset FH. Diagnosis and treatment of the plica syndrome of the knee. J Bone Joint Surg 1980;62A:221–225.
97. Pipken G. Lesions of the suprapatellar plica. J Bone Joint Surg 1950;32A:363–369.
98. Pipken G. Knee injuries: the role of the suprapatellar plica and suprapatellar bursa in simulating internal derangements. Clin Orthop 1971;74:161–176.
99. Nottage WM, Sprague NF, Auerbach BJ, Shahriaree H. The medial patellar plica syndrome. Am J Sports Med 1983;11:211–214.
100. Deutsch AL, Resnick D, Dalinka MK, et al. Synovial plica of the knee. Diag Radiol 1981;141:627–634.
101. Slocum DB, Larson RL. Rotatory instability of the knee. J Bone Joint Surg 1968;54A:211–225.
102. Baker CL, Norwood LA, Hughston JC. Acute posterolateral rotatory instability of the knee. J Bone Joint Surg 1983;74A:614–618.
103. Hughston JC, Andrews JR, Cross MJ, Moschi A. Classification of knee ligament instabilities part I: The medial compartment and cruciate ligaments. J Bone Joint Surg 1976;58A:159–172.
104. Hughston JC, Andrews JR, Cross MJ, Moschi A. Classification of knee ligament instabilities part II: The lateral compartment. J Bone Joint Surg 1976;58A:173–179.
105. Hughston JC, Jackobsen KE. Chronic posterolateral rotatory instability of the knee. J Bone Joint Surg 1985;67A:351–359.
106. Choi J. Acute conditions incidence and associated disability. Vital Health Stat 1978;120:10.
107. Floriani LP. Ankle injury mechanism and treatment guides. Phys Sportsmed 1976;9:72–78.
108. Brostrum L. Sprained ankles: anatomic lesions in recent sprains. Acta Chiro Scand 1964;128:483–495.
109. Woodward EP. Ankle ligament surgery: experience over 18 years. Phys Sportsmed 1977;8:49–55.
110. DeCarlo MS, Talbot RW. Evaluation of ankle joint proprioception following injection of the anterior talofibular ligament. J Orthop Sports Phys Ther 1986;7:76.
111. Baumgardner GR. Technique important in ankle x-ray studies. Phys Sportsmed 1976;9:83–87.
112. Roy S. How I manage plantar fascitis. Phys Sportsmed 1983;11:127–131.
113. Seder J. How I manage heel spur syndrome. Phys Sportsmed 1987;83–85.
114. Coughlin MJ. Hallux valgus: causes, evaluation, and treatment. Postgrad Med 1984;75:174–177.
115. Radin EL. Tarsal tunnel syndrome. Clin Orthop 1983;181:167–170.
116. DeLisa JA, Saeed MA. The tarsal tunnel syndrome. Muscle and Nerve 1983;6:664–670.
117. Cailliet, R. Foot and ankle pain. Philadelphia: FA Davis, 1983.
118. Srinvasan R, Rhodes J, Seidel MR. The tarsal tunnel. Mt. Sinai J Med. 1980;47:17.
119. Oh SJ, Sarala PK, Elmor RS. Sensory nerve conduction velocity of the plantar nerves: a superior objective diagnostic test for tarsal tunnel syndrome. Trans Am Neuro Assoc 1979;103:256.
120. Hunter JL. Etiology, diagnosis, and treatment of sinus tarsi syndrome. Chiro Sports Med 1987;1:104–105.

Index

Page numbers followed by "f" denote figures; those followed by "t" denote tables.